HAMRIC & HANSON'S

ADVANCED PRACTICE NURSING

AN INTEGRATIVE APPROACH

Mary Fran Tracy, PhD, RN, APRN, CCNS, FCNS, FAAN
Associate Professor
School of Nursing, University of Minnesota
Minneapolis, Minnesota

Eileen T. O'Grady, PhD, RN, ARNP
Certified Nurse Practitioner and Wellness Coach
Founder, The School of Wellness
McLean, Virginia

Susanne J. Phillips, DNP, RN, APRN, FNP-BC, FAANP, FAAN
Associate Dean of Clinical Affairs & Clinical Professor
Sue & Bill Gross School of Nursing, University of California, Irvine
Irvine, California

edition 7

ELSEVIER

Elsevier
3251 Riverport Lane
St. Louis, Missouri 63043

HAMRIC & HANSON'S ADVANCED PRACTICE NURSING: AN INTEGRATIVE APPROACH, SEVENTH EDITION

ISBN: 978-0-323-77711-7

Previous editions copyrighted 2019, 2014, 2009, 2005, 2000, and 1996.

Library of Congress Control Number: 2022939278

Executive Content Strategist: Lee Henderson
Senior Content Development Manager: Lisa Newton
Senior Content Development Specialist: Danielle M. Frazier
Publishing Services Manager: Julie Eddy
Senior Project Manager: Abigail Bradberry
Design Direction: Amy Buxton

Printed in India

Last digit is the print number: 9 8 7 6 5 4 3 2

I would like to dedicate this book
to my advanced practice nurse colleagues,
who are inspirational as they strive every day
to provide optimal care for patients,
particularly during the pandemic crisis.
I'm extremely grateful to my family and friends, who are a constant
source of support during these challenging times.

MFT

I dedicate this book to my beloved profession,
to nurses everywhere who care deeply about the human condition.
To my advanced practice nurse colleagues,
I am filled with gratitude to be on this journey with you.
To my one and only Humayun,
who listened patiently to my editing and other woes.
Also, to our sons Liam and Conor,
who keep it real. And funny.

EO

I dedicate this book to my professional and academic mentors,
to APRN students with whom I have had the honor to share my expertise,
and to patients who have entrusted me with their health care
during the most vulnerable times.
You have all shaped the proud nurse and educator I am today.
To my husband Rob, who has provided unconditional support
throughout all my endeavors, and to Austin and
Kathryn, thank you and I love you.

SJP

CONTRIBUTORS

Cynthia Arslanian-Engoren, PhD, RN, MSN, ACNS-BC, FAHA, FNAP, FAAN
Professor
Health Behavior and Biological Sciences
University of Michigan School of Nursing
Ann Arbor, MI, United States

Melissa D. Avery, PhD, APRN, CNM, FACNM, FAAN
Editor-in-Chief
Journal of Midwifery & Women's Health
American College of Nurse-Midwives
Silver Spring, MD, United States
Emeritus Professor
School of Nursing
University of Minnesota
Minneapolis, MN, United States

Kathy Baldridge, DNP, APRN, FNP-BC, FAANP
Director of Psychometric Analysis
Advanced Practice Education Associates
Lafayette, LA, United States
Nurse Practitioner
Christus Community Clinic
Alexandria, LA, United States

Nancy P. Blumenthal, DNP, CRNP, ACNP-BC, CCTC
Lecturer and Acute Care Nurse Practitioner
Biobehavioral Health Sciences Department
University of Pennsylvania School of Nursing
Philadelphia, PA, United States

Denise Bryant-Lukosius, PhD, MScN, BScN, CON(C), HKAN
Professor
School of Nursing and Department of Oncology;
Alba DiCenso Chair in Advanced Practice Nursing
School of Nursing, Faculty of Health Sciences;
Co-Director
Canadian Centre for Advanced Practice Nursing Research
McMaster University
Hamilton, ON, Canada
Clinician Scientist and Director
Canadian Centre of Excellence in Oncology Advanced Practice Nursing
Juravinski Hospital and Cancer Centre
Hamilton, ON, Canada

Karen A. Brykczynski, PhD, RN, FNP-BC, FAANP, FAAN
Home Health Nurse
Home Health
Aspire Home Health Company, Inc,
Clearwater, FL, United States
University Distinguished Professor, Retired
School of Nursing
University of Texas Medical Branch
Galveston, TX, United States

Michelle Buck, MS, APRN, CNS
APRN Senior Policy Advisor, Retired
Nursing Regulation
National Council of State Boards of Nursing
Chicago, IL, United States

Maureen A. Cahill, MSN, APN, CNS, AOCNS
Senior Policy Advisor, Retired
Nursing Regulation
National Council of State Boards of Nursing
Chicago, IL, United States

Michael A. Carter, DNSc, DNP, FNP, GNP, FAAN
Emeritus Distinguished Professor
College of Nursing
University of Tennessee Health Science Center
Memphis, TN, United States
Adjunct Clinical Professor of Geriatrics
College of Medicine
University of Arkansas for Medical Sciences
Little Rock, AR, United States

Anne Z. Cockerham, PhD, CNM, WHNP-BC, CNE, FACNM
Professor
Midwifery and Women's Health
Frontier Nursing University
Pinehurst, NC, United States

Cindi Dabney, DNP, MSNA, BSN
Assistant Professor
Anesthesia Program
University of South Florida
Tampa, FL, United States

Margaret M. Flinter, PhD, APRN, FNP-BC, FAANP, FAAN
Senior VP and Clinical Director
Executive Leadership
Community Health Center, Inc.;
Senior Vice President and Clinical Director
Community Health Center, Inc.;
Senior Faculty
Weitzman Institute
Community Health Center, Inc.
Middletown, CT, United States

Mikel Gray, PhD, FNP, PNP, CUNP, CCCN, FAANP, FAAN
Professor
Department of Urology
University of Virginia
Charlottesville, VA, United States
Editor-in-Chief
Journal of Wound, Ostomy and Continence Nursing
United States

Lisa Hopp, PhD, RN, FAAN
Professor
College of Nursing
Purdue University Northwest
Hammond, IN, United States

Jean E. Johnson, PhD, RN, ACC, FAAN
Emerita Dean and Professor
School of Nursing
George Washington University
Washington, DC, United States

Arlene W. Keeling, PhD, RN, FAAN
Emeritus Centennial Distinguished Professor
School of Nursing
University of Virginia
Charlottesville, VA, United States

Michael J. Kremer, PhD, CRNA, CHSE, FNAP, FAAN
Professor
Adult Health & Gerontological Nursing
University Academic Affairs;
Professor
Graduate College
Rush University Medical Center
Chicago, IL, United States

Nicole Livanos, JD, MPP
Associate Director
State Advocacy & Legislative Affairs
National Council of State Boards of Nursing
Chicago, IL, United States

Patti Ludwig-Beymer, PhD, RN, CTN-A, NEA-BC, CPPS, FAAN
Associate Professor
College of Nursing
Purdue University Northwest
Hammond, IN, United States

Carole L. Mackavey, DNP, MSN, APRN, FNP-C
Assistant Professor and Masters Program Coordinator
Department of Graduate Studies
University of Texas Health Science Center at Houston
Houston, TX, United States

Eileen T. O'Grady, PhD, RN, ARNP
Certified Nurse Practitioner and Wellness Coach
Founder
The School of Wellness
McLean, VA, United States

Susanne J. Phillips, DNP, RN, APRN, FNP-BC, FAANP, FAAN
Associate Dean of Clinical Affairs and Clinical Professor
Sue & Bill Gross School of Nursing
University of California, Irvine
Irvine, CA, United States

Lynn Rapsilber, DNP, APRN, ANP-BC, FAANP
Owner
Nursing
NP Business Consultants, LLC
Torrington, CT, United States
Co-Founder
National Nurse Practitioner Entrepreneur Network
Torrington, CT, United States

Laura Reed, DNP, APRN, FNP-BC
Assistant Professor
Health Promotion and Disease Prevention
University of Tennessee Health Science Center
Memphis, TN, United States

Ellen M. Robinson, PhD, RN, HEC-C, FAAN
Nurse Ethicist
Patient Care Services, Institute for Patient Care;
Co-Chair MGH Optimum Care (Ethics) Committee
Department of Medicine;
Nurse Scientist
Yvonne L. Munn Nursing Research Center
Massachusetts General Hospital
Boston, MA, United States

Melissa A. Saftner, PhD, CNM, FACNM
Clinical Professor
School of Nursing
University of Minnesota
Minneapolis, MN, United States

Pamela Salyer, PhD, RN, BC
Adjunct Assistant Professor
School of Biomedical Informatics
University of Texas Health Science Center at Houston
Houston, TX, United States

Sue Sendelbach, PhD, APRN, CCNS
Director of Nursing Research, Retired
Abbott Northwestern Hospital
Minneapolis, MN, United States

Debora Simmons, PhD, RN, CCNS, FAAN
Assistant Professor
School of Biomedical Informatics
University of Texas Health Science Center at Houston
Houston, TX, United States

Terran W. Sims, MSN, ACNP-C, CNN-BC, COCN
GU Oncology Nurse Practitioner
Department Urology;
Course Faculty AG-ACNP
Adult Geriatrics/Critical Care
University of Virginia
Charlottesville, VA, United States

Kim Steanson, DNP, APRN, CPNP-PC/AC
Associate Professor
Vanderbilt University School of Nursing
Nashville, TN, United States

Mary Fran Tracy, PhD, RN, APRN, CCNS, FCNS, FAAN
Associate Professor
School of Nursing
University of Minnesota
Minneapolis, MN, United States

S. Brian Widmar, PhD, RN, ACNP-BC, CCRN, CNE, FAANP, FCCM
Assistant Dean for Academics and Associate Professor of Nursing
Adult-Gerontology Acute Care Nurse Practitioner Program
Vanderbilt University School of Nursing
Nashville, TN, United States

Marisa L. Wilson, DNSc, MHSc, RN-BC, CPHIMS, FAMIA, FIAHSI, FAAN
Interim Dept Chair, Associate Professor, and Specialty Track Coordinator Nursing Informatics
Family, Community, and Health Systems
The University of Alabama at Birmingham School of Nursing
Birmingham, AL, United States

Lucia D. Wocial, PhD, MS, BA, BS, HEC-C, FAAN
Senior Clinical Ethicist
John J. Lynch Center for Ethics
Medstar Washington Hospital Center
Washington, DC, United States

Frances Kam Yuet Wong, PhD, MEd, BSN, RN, FAAN, FHKAN
Chair Professor
School of Nursing
The Hong Kong Polytechnic University,
Hong Kong, China

PREFACE

Revision of this seventh edition of *Advanced Practice Nursing: An Integrative Approach* occurred during a tumultuous time. The seemingly never-ending COVID-19 pandemic, the long overdue acute acknowledgment of our perpetuation of structural racism and social injustices, and the changing political and planetary climates all impact health care and everyone's individual health in extraordinary ways. These, and other, converging events are rapidly evolving and require nimble actions for health care in general and specifically advanced practice roles and regulations. It necessitates deep (self)-reflection about the state of our health care system and the role that Advanced Practice Nurses (APRNs) play in leading and ensuring optimal health and health equity. All of this occurred during the World Health Organization's designated Year of the Nurse and Midwife—when nurses were being both revered for their courage in caring for all at great personal and mental health risk and reviled and attacked by some for their promotion of scientific evidence and practice. Revising this book during this tumultuous time has required persistence, patience, reflection, and frequent pivoting for all involved.

It has been 14 years since the Consensus Model (APRN Joint Dialogue Group, 2008) was put forth to provide uniformity in APRN role regulation to align licensure, accreditation, certification, and education. Out of 55 US nursing jurisdictions, only 18 fully meet all elements of the Consensus Model (Buck, 2021) as of this writing. Regulatory changes to respond to the pandemic have accelerated modern APRN practice that has long been promoted by the Consensus Model and might have otherwise taken years to fully achieve. It remains to be seen whether these changes will become permanent or will revert to prepandemic standards. Regardless, it is hard to imagine that APRN roles and functions won't be permanently changed. The value of nurses has never been more apparent, and APRNs are no exception.

In addition, many foundational documents to the practice of nursing were to be published or updated during the pandemic; several were unsurprisingly delayed in their publication releases. Publications such as the International Council of Nurses' (2020) *Guidelines on Advanced Practice Nursing 2020*, the National Academy of Medicine's (2021) *Future of Nursing 2020–2030 Report*, the American Association of Colleges of Nursing (2021) *The Essentials: Core Competencies for Professional Nursing Education*, and the American Nurses Association (2021) *Nursing: Scope and Standards of Practice* are all key to inform the current and future state of APRN roles and practice. We have done our best to highlight the content from these documents throughout the book while recognizing that the full impact of their meaning, interpretation, and operationalization cannot be fully understood for years.

The context of our current society and these documents only serves to underscore the ongoing importance of APRNs' skill and leadership on the basics of patient-centered care, safety, quality outcomes for all people, and increasing need for communication. These skills and leadership are essential in caring for our ever increasingly complex patient populations with multiple chronic health conditions who need and can benefit from the holistic perspective of APRNs.

The number of doctor of nursing practice (DNP) programs and DNP graduates in the nation's workforce continue to increase. The DNP-prepared APRN brings a strong set of leadership skills and the expertise to embed evidence into all kinds of practices, which is very beneficial to society. However, many people inside and outside of nursing confuse the DNP as a role within nursing rather than a degree. This book continues to provide clarity on the four specific APRN roles within the APRN umbrella term, regardless of degree type. As advanced practice education continues to evolve, we hope that the profession of nursing will work to decrease the confusion between the DNP degree and the four advanced practice nursing roles.

PURPOSE

The purpose of this book is to continue to promote the clarion call for nursing leaders, educators, and practicing clinicians to seek integrated understanding of APRNs. It explores how they are prepared and the evolving opportunities for the roles that they will create and assume given the developing health care landscape. This seventh edition continues to collate the latest trends and evidence regarding APRN competencies and roles and incorporates discussions of the new and immediate challenges in today's environment. However, there is still significant work ahead to solidify within and outside the profession the value-added benefit of APRNs as direct care providers and leaders—an imperative for patient safety and quality care around the globe. It is only through a unified voice that we can advance APRNs as a whole while we continue to support the uniqueness of each of the four APRN roles.

UNDERLYING PREMISES

We continue to advocate that advanced practice nursing be viewed in the broadest sense in this book—encompassing the entire professional understanding and enactment of APRN roles, with patients and families at the center of their purpose of existence.

It is assumed that health care policy is an ongoing process, made up of small and large revisions over decades. Policy issues surrounding APRNs are, of necessity, living, moving, and ever-changing, never more so than in today's society. The book highlights ongoing APRN policy issues in the United States, knowing that both incrementalism and the urgent pandemic-related changes can make it difficult to write with certitude around any health care policy. However, it is with certainty that we have seen new gaps in health care where APRNs can use their leadership and advocacy skills: depoliticizing the science behind our interventions, ensuring access and culturally appropriate care for all, promotion of wellbeing not only for patients but also for healthcare workers, and addressing workforce shortages.

Each APRN student comes to a graduate program with a background in nursing. Human caring and compassion for others lie at the heart of nursing. While caring is not laid out as a core APRN competency, it is assumed that each student who comes to the APRN role already embodies the Nursing Code of Ethics, Provision 1: "The nurse practices with compassion and respect for the inherent dignity, worth, and unique attributes of every person" (American Nurses Association, 2015). This has never been needed more than now, when stress on the healthcare system and workers tests our tolerance, civility, and compassion while we attempt to support our and others' resilience and efforts to reduce burnout and compassion fatigue.

ORGANIZATION

This edition continues the tradition of extensive updating and revision based on the most current evidence available. The editors and authors have incorporated content up until the final feasible moment to provide readers with the latest changes in regulatory, credentialing, and professional issues impacting APRNs. Exemplars have been updated throughout the book, and Key Summary Points at the end of each chapter emphasize the key takeaways for readers. In Part I, "Historical and Developmental Aspects of Advanced Practice Nursing," readers will note that we have removed consultation as a core APRN competency (Chapter 3). We have moved toward viewing consultation as activities that are embedded throughout APRN practice and therefore readers will find information about consultation throughout the book. In addition, the ethical decision-making competency has been reframed to the broader perspective of ethical practice. We have eliminated the chapter on evolving roles and opportunities for APRNs. While APRN roles are evolving, which may need to be addressed by revision of the Consensus Model, these natural evolutions are discussed in the role chapters. Chapter 6 has been expanded to cover additional content on the status of international APN roles and the challenges for the roles in all regions of the world. While advanced practice nursing is significantly different between the United States and other countries, there is much we can do to collaborate and learn from each other. In Part II, "Competencies of Advanced Practice Nursing," the six competencies are outlined—Direct Clinical Practice, Guidance and Coaching, Evidence-Based Practice, Leadership, Collaboration, and Ethical Practice; these competencies continue to stand the test of time as the foundational core for all APRN roles. In Part III, "Advanced Practice Roles: The Operational Definitions of Advanced Practice Nursing," each of the APRN role chapters has been updated to highlight the unique niche APRNs fill in exhibition of the core competencies through each of the specific roles. In particular, Chapter 14 has been expanded to include both the adult–gerontology acute care nurse practitioner and the pediatric acute care nurse practitioner. Of note, there are several changes in Part IV, "Critical Elements in Managing Advanced Practice Nursing Environments." Chapter 19 has been significantly revised to provide the latest information on the frequently changing world of reimbursement. Chapter 21 continues to be a rich resource for evidence demonstrating the outcomes of APRNs.

Finally, recognizing the significant impact of the complexity of technology on the health care system and the daily practice of APRNs, we have added Chapter 22, "Future Technologies Influencing APRN Practice." The chapter covers a range of important technology topics, including technology-assisted communication; diagnostic, therapeutic, and procedural devices and apps; decision support and advanced analytics; cybersecurity; and high-tech home care.

AUDIENCE

This book is intended for graduate nursing students, practicing APRNs, educators, administrators, and nursing leaders. The book will be a resource for graduate students as they learn to incorporate theory, research, policy, and practice skills into their developing roles. It provides an understanding of the common threads among APRN roles, the unique contributions of each role, and the holistic advanced skills distinct to APRNs compared with other non-nurse providers.

This book will be useful to practicing APRNs as an update for a health care environment that is constantly changing. It provides a foundation for practice and an opportunity to self-assess for areas of strength and areas for growth throughout one's APRN career. APRNs can use pertinent sections of the book with administrators to highlight role functions and documented outcomes of APRNs and how optimization of each role can be envisioned and implemented.

For educators, the book continues to serve as a comprehensive resource for use in educational APRN program curricula. Instructor resources available with this book include slides with content that corresponds to each chapter as well as each of the images in the book. In addition, an instructor resource will be a test bank of questions. These Evolve resources can be accessed at http://evolve.elsevier.com/Hamric/

APPROACH

The Editors extend a sincere and grateful thank you to the book's contributors as they have tried to maintain their work as practitioners and educators while also collaborating with us on this revision during a pandemic. It has been a challenging endeavor to complete this seventh edition revision during these chaotic and uncertain times. It has taken thoughtful consideration on the part of each author to determine how to update the chapters with meaningful detail, while still conveying the key points for the current and future practice of APRNs, notwithstanding the exact contextual changes that are yet unknown.

Quality, safety, and holistic patient care will always be the bedrock of APRN practice. APRNs are here to stay, and a united APRN approach will ensure optimal health for our patients, populations, and society.

TRANSITIONS

We are excited to welcome Dr. Susanne J. Phillips to the editor team for this seventh edition. She has been a previous contributor to the book and has been a great addition to the editor team.

In closing, it is with heavy hearts and a deep sense of responsibility that we acknowledge and mourn the passing of Ann B. Hamric on February 9, 2020. Her vision and tireless advocacy in unifying advanced practice nursing under one umbrella have helped shape our success and strengthened our power. Her clear and forceful articulation of the initial APRN model and foundational concepts has evolved to meet the needs of society, patients, and populations and has stood the test of time. She published the first edition of this book, *Advanced Nursing Practice: An Integrative Approach*, in 1996 with Judy Spross and Chuckie Hanson. We cannot adequately express the depth of our gratitude for what Dr. Hamric gave to us individually and collectively in originating this definitive book and working with us on these later editions. Her passion was palpable and we are the better for it.

Mary Fran Tracy
Eileen T. O'Grady
Susanne J. Phillips

REFERENCES

American Association of Colleges of Nursing. (2021). *The essentials: Core competencies for professional nursing education*. https://www.aacnnursing.org/Portals/42/AcademicNursing/pdf/Essentials-2021.pdf

American Nurses Association. (2015). *Code of ethics for nurses with interpretive statements*.

American Nurses Association. (2021). *Nursing: Scope and standards of practice* (4th ed.).

APRN Joint Dialogue Group. (2008). Consensus model for APRN regulation: Licensure, accreditation, certification & education. http://www.aacn.nche.edu/education-resources/APRNReport.pdf

Buck, M. (2021). An update on the Consensus Model for APRN regulation: More than a decade of progress. *Journal of Nursing Regulation*, *12*(2), 23–33.

International Council of Nurses. (2020). *Guidelines on advanced practice nursing 2020*. https://www.icn.ch/system/files/documents/2020-04/ICN_APN%20Report_EN_WEB.pdf

National Academies of Science, Engineering and Medicine. (2021). *The future of nursing 2020–2030: Charting a path to achieve health equity*. The National Academies Press. https://nam.edu/publications/the-future-of-nursing-2020-2030/

CONTENTS

PART I

Historical and Developmental Aspects of Advanced Practice Nursing

1 HISTORY AND EVOLUTION OF ADVANCED PRACTICE NURSING 2
ARLENE W. KEELING ■ ANNE Z. COCKERHAM

NURSE ANESTHETISTS 3

Early Roots 3

Documenting Outcomes 3

Resistance From Organized Medicine: Legal Challenges 4

Navigating Interprofessional Challenges at the Grassroots Level 6

Issues With Financial Reimbursement 7

Setting Educational Standards 8

NURSE-MIDWIVES 8

Early Roots: "Granny Midwives" 8

Time and Place Matter: "The Midwife Problem" 9

Place Matters: Frontier Nursing Service Midwives 9

Roots of Midwifery Education in the United States 10

Place Matters: New Mexico 11

A National Organization 11

Growth of Midwifery Practice 12

Reimbursement 12

Nurse-Midwifery Programs in the Second Half of the 20th Century 13

CLINICAL NURSE SPECIALISTS 13

Early Roots 13

Time and Place Matter: World Wars I and II 14

Legislation and Medical Specialization 14

Navigating Inter- and Intraprofessional Challenges 16

Organization and Evaluation 17

Declining Demand for Clinical Nurse Specialists 18

CNS Education and Reimbursement 19

NURSE PRACTITIONERS 19

Early Roots of Primary Care 19

The Need for Primary Care in the Mid-20th Century 21

Intraprofessional Conflict Over the NP Role 22

Support From Physicians 23

The Concept of "Advanced Practice" 23

Resistance to the NP by Organized Medicine 24

Growth, Organization, and Legislation 25

Neonatal and Acute Care Nurse Practitioners 25

Nurse Practitioner Education 26

CONCLUSION 26

KEY SUMMARY POINTS 27

REFERENCES 27

2 CONCEPTUALIZATIONS OF ADVANCED PRACTICE NURSING 31
CYNTHIA ARSLANIAN-ENGOREN

NATURE, PURPOSES, AND COMPONENTS OF CONCEPTUAL MODELS 33

CONCEPTUALIZATIONS OF ADVANCED PRACTICE NURSING: PROBLEMS AND IMPERATIVES 34

CONCEPTUALIZATIONS OF ADVANCED PRACTICE NURSING ROLES: ORGANIZATIONAL PERSPECTIVES 37

- Consensus Model for Advanced Practice Registered Nurse Regulation 37
- American Nurses Association 40
- American Association of Colleges of Nursing 41
- National Organization of Nurse Practitioner Faculties 42
- National Association of Clinical Nurse Specialists 42
- American Association of Nurse Anesthesiology 43
- American College of Nurse-Midwives 45
- International Organizations and Conceptualizations of Advanced Practice Nursing 45
- Section Summary: Implications for Advanced Practice Nursing Conceptualizations 46

CONCEPTUALIZATIONS OF THE NATURE OF ADVANCED PRACTICE NURSING 47

- Hamric's Integrative Model of Advanced Practice Nursing 48
- Conceptual Models of APRN Practice: United States Examples 49
- Conceptual Models of APRN Practice: International Examples 57
- Section Summary: Implications for Advanced Practice Nursing Conceptualizations 61

MODELS USEFUL FOR ADVANCED PRACTICE NURSES IN THEIR PRACTICE 61

- Advanced Practice Nursing Transitional Care Models 61
- Dunphy and Winland-Brown's Circle of Caring: A Transformative, Collaborative Model 62
- Donabedian Structure/Process/ Outcome Model 64

RECOMMENDATIONS AND FUTURE DIRECTIONS 65

- Conceptualizations of Advanced Practice Nursing 65
- Consensus Building Around Advanced Practice Nursing 66
- Consensus on Key Elements of Practice Doctorate Curricula 67
- Research on Advanced Practice Nurses and Their Contribution to Patients, Teams, and System Outcomes 67

CONCLUSION 68

KEY SUMMARY POINTS 68

REFERENCES 68

3 A DEFINITION OF ADVANCED PRACTICE NURSING 74

MARY FRAN TRACY

DISTINGUISHING BETWEEN SPECIALIZATION AND ADVANCED PRACTICE NURSING 76

DISTINGUISHING BETWEEN ADVANCED NURSING PRACTICE AND ADVANCED PRACTICE NURSING 77

DEFINING ADVANCED PRACTICE NURSING 78

CORE DEFINITION OF ADVANCED PRACTICE NURSING 78

- Conceptual Definition 79
- Primary Criteria 80

SIX CORE COMPETENCIES OF ADVANCED PRACTICE NURSING 84

- Direct Clinical Practice: The Central Competency 84
- Additional Advanced Practice Nurse Core Competencies 85
- Scope of Practice 86

DIFFERENTIATING ADVANCED PRACTICE ROLES: OPERATIONAL DEFINITIONS OF ADVANCED PRACTICE NURSING 87

- Workforce Data 87
- Four Established Advanced Practice Nurse Roles 87

CRITICAL ELEMENTS IN MANAGING ADVANCED PRACTICE NURSING ENVIRONMENTS 89

IMPLICATIONS OF THE DEFINITION OF ADVANCED PRACTICE NURSING 91
Implications for Advanced Practice Nursing Education 91
Implications for Regulation and Credentialing 92
Implications for Research 92
Implications for Practice Environments 93
CONCLUSION 94
KEY SUMMARY POINTS 95
REFERENCES 95

4 ROLE DEVELOPMENT OF THE ADVANCED PRACTICE NURSE 98
CAROLE L. MACKAVEY ▪ KAREN A. BRYKCZYNSKI
PERSPECTIVES ON ADVANCED PRACTICE NURSE ROLE DEVELOPMENT 99
NOVICE-TO-EXPERT SKILL ACQUISITION MODEL 99
Transition From Student to Clinician 101
ROLE CONCEPTS AND ROLE DEVELOPMENT ISSUES 101
Role Ambiguity 102
Role Incongruity 102
Role Conflict 104
ROLE TRANSITIONS 107
Advanced Practice Nurse Role Acquisition in Graduate School 107
Strategies to Facilitate Role Acquisition 110
Advanced Practice Nursing Role Implementation: Entering the Workforce .. 114
Strategies to Facilitate Role Implementation 121
Facilitators and Barriers in the Work Setting 124
Continued Advanced Practice Nurse Role Evolution 126
Evaluation of Role Development 127
CONCLUSION 129
KEY SUMMARY POINTS 130
REFERENCES 130

5 INTERNATIONAL DEVELOPMENT OF ADVANCED PRACTICE NURSING 137
DENISE BRYANT-LUKOSIUS ▪ FRANCES KAM YUET WONG
ADVANCED PRACTICE NURSING ROLES WITHIN A GLOBAL HEALTHCARE CONTEXT 137
Defining Advanced Practice Nursing 137
Global Deployment 138
Types of Advanced Practice Nursing Roles ... 138
Emerging and New Frontiers for Future Role Development 143
FACILITATING THE INTRODUCTION AND INTEGRATION OF ADVANCED PRACTICE NURSING ROLES 148
Pan-Approaches and Collaboration 148
Funding and Reimbursement Arrangements 152
Systematic Approaches to Role Planning... 153
Use and Generation of Evidence 154
NEXT STEPS IN THE GLOBAL EVOLUTION OF ADVANCED PRACTICE NURSING ROLES......... 155
CONCLUSION 155
KEY SUMMARY POINTS 156
REFERENCES 156

PART II

Competencies of Advanced Practice Nursing

6 DIRECT CLINICAL PRACTICE................168
MARY FRAN TRACY ▪ NANCY P. BLUMENTHAL
DIRECT CARE VERSUS INDIRECT CARE ACTIVITIES 169
SIX CHARACTERISTICS OF DIRECT CLINICAL CARE PROVIDED BY ADVANCED PRACTICE NURSES 172
USE OF A HOLISTIC PERSPECTIVE 173
Holism Described 173
Holism and Health Assessment 173
Nursing Model or Medical Model 175

FORMATION OF THERAPEUTIC PARTNERSHIPS WITH PATIENTS 176
Implicit Bias 179
Communication With Patients 179
Shared Decision Making 179
Cultural Influences on Partnerships 180
Therapeutic Partnerships With Noncommunicative Patients 181
EXPERT CLINICAL PERFORMANCE 182
Clinical Thinking 182
Ethical Reasoning 186
Skillful Performance 187
USE OF REFLECTIVE PRACTICE 190
USE OF EVIDENCE AS A GUIDE TO PRACTICE 191
Evidence-Based Practice 192
Theory-Based Practice 193
DIVERSE APPROACHES TO HEALTH AND ILLNESS MANAGEMENT 194
Interpersonal Interventions 194
Therapeutic Assessments and Interventions 194
Individualized Interventions 197
Complementary Therapies 197
Clinical Prevention 198
MANAGEMENT OF COMPLEX SITUATIONS 200
HELPING PATIENTS MANAGE CHRONIC ILLNESSES 202
DIRECT CARE AND INFORMATION MANAGEMENT 203
CONCLUSION 204
KEY SUMMARY POINTS 205
REFERENCES 205

7 GUIDANCE AND COACHING 212
EILEEN T. O'GRADY ■ JEAN E. JOHNSON
WHY GUIDANCE AND COACHING? 213
Patient Engagement 213
Burden of Chronic Illness 214
GUIDANCE AND COACHING DEFINITIONS 214
Guidance 215
Coaching 215
THEORIES AND RESEARCH SUPPORTING APRN GUIDANCE AND COACHING 217
Nightingale's Environmental Theory 217
Middle Range Theory of Integrative Nurse Coaching 217
Transtheoretical Model 218
Watson's Model of Caring 219
Positive Psychology 219
Growth Mindset 219
Self-Determination Theory 220
Transitions in Health and Illness 220
BUILDING RELATIONSHIPS FOR APRN GUIDANCE AND COACHING 223
Presence 223
Communication 224
Nonjudgmental (Suspending Judgment) 225
Empathy and Compassion 226
Managing Conflict 227
Partnership 227
DETERMINING PATIENT READINESS FOR CHANGE 228
Patient Readiness 228
THE "FOUR As" OF THE COACHING PROCESS 233
Agenda Setting 233
Awareness Raising 234
Actions and Goal Setting 235
Accountability 235
APRN PRACTICE PRINCIPLES FOR SUCCESSFUL GUIDANCE AND COACHING 235
Ask Questions 235
Ask Permission 236
Build on Strengths 236
Support Small Changes 237
Be Curious 237
Challenge 237
Get to the Feelings 238

BUILDING COACHING INTO PRACTICE 238
CONCLUSION 239
KEY SUMMARY POINTS 239
REFERENCES 240

8 EVIDENCE-BASED PRACTICE 243
MIKEL GRAY ■ TERRAN W. SIMS
APRNS AND THE DNP 244
EVIDENCE-BASED PRACTICE AND THE APRN 245
Identifying Evidence 245
Resources for Evidence-Based Practice 248
Quality Improvement Projects: Evaluating EBP 250
GENERATING EVIDENCE: HISTORICAL PERSPECTIVE 252
STEPS OF THE EVIDENCE-BASED PROCESS 253
Step 1: Formulate a Measurable Clinical Question 253
Step 2: Search the Literature for Relevant Studies 254
Step 3: Critically Appraise and Extract Evidence 259
Step 4: Implement Useful Findings in Clinical Decision Making 268
FROM POLICY TO PRACTICE: TIPS FOR ACHIEVING MEANINGFUL CHANGES IN PRACTICE BASED ON CURRENT BEST EVIDENCE 268
Stakeholder Engagement 271
Organizational Support 271
Clinical Leadership Support 272
Evidence-Based Practice Innovation: Feedback 273
FUTURE PERSPECTIVES 273
CONCLUSION 274
KEY SUMMARY POINTS 274
REFERENCES 274

9 LEADERSHIP 279
LAURA REED ■ MICHAEL CARTER
THE IMPORTANCE OF LEADERSHIP FOR APRNS 280
Constantly Evolving Healthcare Systems 280
Evolving Health Professional Education 281
APRN Competencies 281
LEADERSHIP: DEFINITIONS, MODELS, AND CONCEPTS 282
Leadership Models That Lead to Transformation 282
Leadership Models That Address System Change and Innovation 285
Concepts Related to Change 286
TYPES OF LEADERSHIP FOR APRNS 289
Clinical Leadership 289
Professional Leadership 290
Systems Leadership 290
Health Policy Leadership 292
CHARACTERISTICS OF APRN LEADERSHIP COMPETENCY 293
Mentoring 293
Empowering Others 295
Innovation 295
Political Activism 296
ATTRIBUTES OF EFFECTIVE APRN LEADERS 296
Timing 296
Self-Confidence and Risk-Taking 297
Communication and Relationship Building 298
Boundary Management: Balancing Professional and Personal Life 298
Self-Management/Emotional Intelligence 299
Moral Courage 300
Respect for Cultural and Gender Diversity 301
Global Awareness 302
DEVELOPING SKILLS AS APRN LEADERS 302
Factors Influencing Leadership Development 302
Personal Characteristics and Experiences 302
Strategies for Acquiring Competency as a Leader 303
DEVELOPING LEADERSHIP IN THE HEALTH POLICY ARENA 303

Using Professional Organizations to the Best Advantage 305
Internships and Fellowships 305
New Modes of Communication 305
OBSTACLES TO LEADERSHIP DEVELOPMENT AND EFFECTIVE LEADERSHIP 305
Clinical Leadership Issues 305
Professional and System Obstacles 306
Dysfunctional Leadership Styles 306
Horizontal Violence 306
STRATEGIES FOR IMPLEMENTING THE LEADERSHIP COMPETENCY 309
Developing a Leadership Portfolio 309
Promoting Collaboration Among APRN Groups 309
Networking 310
Effectively Working With Other Leaders to Advance Health Care 310
Institutional Assessment Regarding Readiness for Change 310
Followship 311
CONCLUSION 311
KEY SUMMARY POINTS 311
REFERENCES 311

10 COLLABORATION 315
CINDI DABNEY ■ MICHAEL CARTER
DEFINITION OF COLLABORATION 316
Collaboration: What It Is 316
Collaboration: What It Is Not 316
Domains of Collaboration in Advanced Practice Registered Nursing 318
Types of Collaboration 319
Interprofessional Collaboration 320
CHARACTERISTICS OF EFFECTIVE COLLABORATION 320
Clinical Competence and Accountability 321
Common Purpose 321
Interpersonal Competence and Effective Communication 321
Trust and Mutual Respect 322
Recognizing and Valuing Diverse, Complementary Culture, Knowledge, and Skills 322
Humor 322
IMPACT OF COLLABORATION ON PATIENTS AND CLINICIANS 324
Evidence That Collaboration Works 324
Research Supporting Interprofessional Collaboration 325
Effects of Failure to Collaborate 326
IMPERATIVES FOR COLLABORATION 327
Ethical Imperative to Collaborate 327
Institutional Imperative to Collaborate 328
Research Imperative to Study Collaboration 329
CONTEXT OF COLLABORATION IN CONTEMPORARY HEALTH CARE 329
Incentives and Opportunities for Collaboration 329
Challenges to Collaboration 330
PROCESSES ASSOCIATED WITH EFFECTIVE COLLABORATION 332
Recurring Interactions 332
Effective Conflict Negotiation and Resolution Skills 333
Partnering and Team Building 333
IMPLEMENTING COLLABORATION 333
Assessment of Personal, Environmental, and Global Factors 334
STRATEGIES FOR SUCCESSFUL COLLABORATION 334
Individual Strategies 334
Team Strategies 335
Organizational Strategies 335
CONCLUSION 337
KEY SUMMARY POINTS 337
REFERENCES 337

11 ETHICAL PRACTICE 341
LUCIA D. WOCIAL ■ ELLEN M. ROBINSON
FOUNDATIONS OF ETHICAL PRACTICE 342
Personal and Professional Values 344

Moral Distress 345
Clear Communication 345
Interprofessional Collaboration 346
OVERVIEW OF ETHICAL APPROACHES TO RESOLVING ETHICAL CONFLICTS 346
Principle-Based Approach 346
Casuistry Approach 347
Narrative Ethics 348
Care-Based Ethics 348
PROFESSIONAL CODES AND GUIDELINES 348
Professional Boundaries 350
GOALS OF CARE: A CLINICAL-ETHICAL FRAMEWORK TO ENHANCE APRN PRACTICE 350
Prognosis 350
Values, Beliefs, and Preferences 352
ETHICAL COMPETENCY OF APRNS 354
Knowledge Development 355
Skill Acquisition 355
Ethical Decision-Making Frameworks 356
Addressing Ethical Conflict 357
Creating Ethical Environments 357
Preventive Ethics 359
ETHICAL ISSUES AFFECTING APRN PRACTICE 361
Primary Care Issues 361
Acute and Chronic Care Issues 361
End-of-Life Complexities 362
Conscientious Objection 365
SOCIETAL ISSUES 366
Promoting Social Justice 366
Access to Resources 368
Genomics 369
COVID-19 Pandemic 369
Gun Violence 370
Participation in Research 370
LEGAL ISSUES 370
NAVIGATING BARRIERS TO ETHICAL PRACTICE AND STRATEGIES TO OVERCOME THEM 371
Barriers Internal to the APRN 371
Interprofessional Barriers 372
Patient–Provider Barriers 372
Organizational and Environmental Barriers 373
APRN WELL-BEING 373
CONCLUSION 376
KEY SUMMARY POINTS 377
REFERENCES 377

PART III

Advanced Practice Roles: The Operational Definitions of Advanced Practice Nursing

12 THE CLINICAL NURSE SPECIALIST 384
MARY FRAN TRACY ▪ SUE SENDELBACH
CLINICAL NURSE SPECIALIST PRACTICE: COMPETENCIES WITHIN THE SPHERES OF IMPACT 387
Direct Clinical Practice 391
Guidance and Coaching 394
Evidence-Based Practice 396
Leadership 398
Collaboration 401
Ethical Practice 401
CURRENT MARKETPLACE FORCES AND CONCERNS 402
Scope of Practice and Delegated Authority 405
The Future of Nursing Reports 405
Consensus Model for APRN Regulation and Implications for the Clinical Nurse Specialist 406
Reimbursement for Clinical Nurse Specialist Services 408
Availability and Standardization of Educational Curricula for Clinical Nurse Specialists 409
National Certification for Clinical Nurse Specialists 409

Variability in Individual Clinical Nurse Specialist Practices and Prescriptive Authority 410
Understanding the Similarities and Differences Between Clinical Nurse Specialists and Nurse Practitioners 410
ROLE IMPLEMENTATION 412
Evaluation of Practice 412
FUTURE DIRECTIONS 413
CONCLUSION 415
KEY SUMMARY POINTS 415
REFERENCES 415

13 THE PRIMARY CARE NURSE PRACTITIONER 420
MARGARET M. FLINTER ■ SUSANNE J. PHILLIPS
CURRENT AND HISTORICAL PERSPECTIVES ON PRIMARY CARE AND THE NURSE PRACTITIONER ROLE 422
Current Perspectives on Primary Care 422
Historical Perspective and the First Nurse Practitioners 423
Progress and Change: 1970 to the Present ... 424
THE PRIMARY CARE NURSE PRACTITIONER ... 425
Direct Clinical Practice 426
Guidance and Coaching 436
Evidence-Based Practice 437
Leadership 437
Collaboration 438
Ethical Practice 438
Going Forward With Shared Competencies for Primary Care 439
EMERGENCE OF POSTGRADUATE TRAINING IN PRIMARY CARE 439
PRIMARY CARE AND THE FEDERAL GOVERNMENT 441
Health Resources and Services Administration 441
THE PRIMARY CARE SAFETY NET 443
Community Health Centers 443
Nurse-Led Health Centers 444
School-Based Health Centers 446
Veterans Affairs 446
PRACTICE REDESIGN IN PRIMARY CARE 447
Team-Based Primary Care 447
Disruptive Innovations: From Retail Clinic to the New Primary Care Center 447
PRIMARY CARE WORKFORCE AND THE CONTEXT OF PCNP PRACTICE TODAY 448
Primary Care Nurse Practitioner Workforce 448
Where Are PCNPs Practicing Today? 448
TRENDS IN PRIMARY CARE 450
Home Care 450
Burnout: COVID-19 450
CONCLUSION 450
KEY SUMMARY POINTS 451
REFERENCES 451

14 THE ACUTE CARE NURSE PRACTITIONER 457
S. BRIAN WIDMAR ■ KIM STEANSON
EMERGENCE OF THE ACNP ROLE 458
COMPETENCIES OF THE ACNP ROLE 459
Direct Clinical Practice 461
Diagnosing and Managing Disease 461
Promoting and Protecting Health and Preventing Disease 465
Guidance and Coaching 466
Evidence-Based Practice 467
Leadership 467
Collaboration 468
Ethical Practice 468
PREPARATION OF ACNPS 469
ACNP SCOPE OF PRACTICE: LEVELS OF INFLUENCE 471
National Level (Professional Organizations) 472
State Level (Government) 473
Institutional Level 473
Service-Related Level 474
Individual Level 475
PROFILES OF THE ACNP ROLE AND PRACTICE MODELS 475

Comparison With Other Advanced Practice Nurse and Physician Assistant Roles 478

ACNPs and Physician Hospitalists 479

ACNP Practice Models 479

Outcome Studies Related to ACNP Practice 479

SPECIALIZATION OPPORTUNITIES WITHIN THE ACNP ROLE 481

Bone Marrow Transplantation Services 481

Diagnostic and Interventional Services 481

Heart Failure Services............................. 482

Orthopedic Services 482

Critical Care Teams................................ 482

Rapid Response Teams 482

Supportive and Palliative Care 482

CHALLENGES SPECIFIC TO THE ACNP ROLE.. 483

FUTURE DIRECTIONS 484

CONCLUSION... 484

KEY SUMMARY POINTS 485

REFERENCES... 485

15 THE CERTIFIED NURSE-MIDWIFE 489

MELISSA A. SAFTNER ■ MELISSA D. AVERY

MIDWIFE DEFINITIONS 490

International Definition........................... 490

US Midwife Definitions 490

HISTORICAL PERSPECTIVE 491

THE NURSE-MIDWIFERY PROFESSION IN THE UNITED STATES TODAY 491

Recognition of Nurse-Midwifery 491

Education and Accreditation 492

Certification and Certification Maintenance 493

Reentry to Practice................................. 493

Regulation, Reimbursement, and Credentialing... 493

American College of Nurse-Midwives 496

Midwifery Internationally 497

IMPLEMENTING ADVANCED PRACTICE NURSING COMPETENCIES 498

Overview of APRN and Certified Nurse-Midwife Competencies............................ 498

Direct Clinical Practice 501

Guidance and Coaching of Patients, Families, and Other Care Providers........... 502

Evidence-Based Practice 502

Leadership... 503

Collaboration 503

Ethical Practice 505

CURRENT PRACTICE OF NURSE-MIDWIFERY.. 506

Scope of Practice 506

Practice Settings 507

Certified Nurse-Midwife Practice Summary... 508

PROFESSIONAL ISSUES 508

Image.. 508

Work Life 510

Professional Liability 511

Diversity 511

Quality and Safety 514

CONCLUSION... 514

KEY SUMMARY POINTS 514

REFERENCES... 515

16 THE CERTIFIED REGISTERED NURSE ANESTHETIST 519

MICHAEL J. KREMER

BRIEF HISTORY OF CRNA EDUCATION AND PRACTICE 520

Education... 520

Certification 520

Continued Professional Competence 521

Practice.. 521

Role Differentiation Between CRNAs and Anesthesiologists............................... 522

PROFILE OF THE CRNA................................. 523

Scope and Standards of Practice 524

Education.. 524

Programs of Study 527

Nurse Anesthesia Educational Funding 529

Practice Doctorate 530
Institutional Credentialing 530
ROLE DEVELOPMENT AND MEASURES OF CLINICAL COMPETENCE 531
Direct Clinical Practice 531
Guidance and Coaching 534
Evidence-Based Practice 535
Leadership 536
Collaboration 538
Ethical Practice 541
CURRENT CRNA PRACTICE 542
Workforce Issues 543
Access to Care 543
Reimbursement 544
NURSE ANESTHESIA ORGANIZATIONS 546
American Association of Nurse Anesthesiology 546
International Federation of Nurse Anesthetists and International Practice 546
FUTURE DIRECTIONS IN CRNA PRACTICE 547
CONCLUSION 547
KEY SUMMARY POINTS 548
REFERENCES 548

PART IV

Critical Elements in Managing Advanced Practice Nursing Environments

17 MAXIMIZING APRN POWER AND INFLUENCING POLICY 554
EILEEN T. O'GRADY ▪ SUSANNE J. PHILLIPS
POLICY: HISTORIC CORE FUNCTION IN NURSING 555
POLICY: APRNS AND MODERN ROLES 555
POLICY VERSUS POLITICS 556
Health Policy 556
Politics 556
UNITED STATES FUNDAMENTALLY DIFFERS FROM THE INTERNATIONAL COMMUNITY 557
KEY POLICY CONCEPTS 559
Federalism 559
Incrementalism 559
Presidential Politics 561
APRNs, Civic Engagement, and Money 561
POLICY MODELS AND FRAMEWORKS 564
Longest Model 564
The Kingdon or Garbage Can Model 564
Knowledge Transfer Framework 565
CURRENT ADVANCED PRACTICE NURSING POLICY ISSUES 566
Framing Current Issues: Cost, Quality, Access, and the Value Agenda 566
Policy Initiatives in Health Reform 570
APRN POLITICAL COMPETENCE IN THE POLICY ARENA 571
Political Competence 572
Individual Skills 573
Moving the APRN Role Forward in Health Policy 582
EMERGING ADVANCED PRACTICE NURSING POLICY ISSUES 584
APRN Full Practice Authority 584
APRN Workforce Development 586
CONCLUSION 586
KEY SUMMARY POINTS 586
REFERENCES 587
18 MARKETING YOURSELF AS AN APRN: CONTRACTING AND NEGOTIATION 590
SUSANNE J. PHILLIPS
SELF-AWARENESS: FINDING A GOOD FIT 590
CHOOSING BETWEEN ENTREPRENEURSHIP/INTRAPRENEURSHIP 592
Characteristics for Entrepreneurship/Intrapreneurship 593
Entrepreneurial/Intrapreneurial Success 593
Challenges of Innovative Practice 593
MARKETING FOR THE NEW APRN 596
Preparing the New APRN to Market Core Competencies 596

Professional Networking 596
Communication 600
Interview Process 603
NEGOTIATION AND RENEGOTIATION 607
Business and Contractual Arrangements ... 611
Professional Issues and Practice Arrangements 612
Malpractice Insurance............................. 612
OVERCOMING INVISIBILITY........................... 614
CONCLUSION... 614
KEY SUMMARY POINTS................................ 615
REFERENCES.. 615

19 REIMBURSEMENT AND PAYMENT FOR APRN SERVICES............................617
LYNN RAPSILBER ■ KATHY BALDRIDGE
HEALTHCARE REFORM HISTORY 618
REIMBURSEMENT MODELS.......................... 621
Federally Funded Medical Coverage 621
State-Administered Medical Coverage....... 622
Third-Party Payers.................................. 624
BILLING FOR APRN SERVICES: UNDERSTANDING THE PROCESS 624
The Credentialing Process 625
Provider Panels and Contracts.................. 626
Coding Sets 627
Outpatient Billing 629
Medical Decision Making......................... 630
Inpatient Billing 633
Revenue Cycle Management 635
VALUE-BASED AND FEE-FOR-SERVICE MODELS 636
Resource-Based Relative Value Scale 636
Value-Based Payments 636
REIMBURSEMENT ISSUES AND CHALLENGES... 638
Incident-To Billing.................................. 638
Liability/Malpractice Insurance................ 640
Reimbursement Pay Parity....................... 643
BUSINESS DEVELOPMENT 643
Entrepreneurship 643
Business Ownership 644
Additional APRN Compensation Models .. 644
FUTURE TRENDS 645
CONCLUSION... 645
KEY SUMMARY POINTS.................................. 645
REFERENCES.. 645

20 UNDERSTANDING REGULATORY, LEGAL, AND CREDENTIALING REQUIREMENTS 649
MAUREEN A. CAHILL ■ MICHELLE BUCK ■ NICOLE LIVANOS
THE CONSENSUS MODEL FOR APRN REGULATION: LICENSURE, ACCREDITATION, CERTIFICATION, AND EDUCATION 650
Implementation of Consensus Model Regulation... 650
The Need for Education and Credentialing of APRNs in the US Healthcare System 652
ADVANCED PRACTICE REGISTERED NURSE MASTER'S AND DOCTORAL EDUCATION 652
BENCHMARKS OF ADVANCED PRACTICE NURSING AND EDUCATION.......................... 653
ADVANCED PRACTICE REGISTERED NURSE COMPETENCIES 653
Professional APRN Competencies............ 653
APRN Program Oversight and Accreditation... 654
APRN Role and Population Certification... 655
Postgraduate Education.......................... 655
Continued Competency Measured Through Recertification 655
Mandatory Clinical Education and Clinical Practice Requirements................. 656
ELEMENTS OF APRN REGULATION AND CREDENTIALING 656
LANGUAGE ASSOCIATED WITH THE CREDENTIALING OF APRNS 657
Titling of APRNs 657
State Licensure and Recognition 657
Institutional Credentialing....................... 658

Prescriptive Authority 659
Identifier Numbers 660
SCOPE OF PRACTICE FOR APRNS 661
STANDARDS OF PRACTICE AND STANDARDS OF CARE FOR APRNS 662
ISSUES AFFECTING APRN CREDENTIALING AND REGULATION 662
Collaborative Practice Arrangements 662
Reimbursement 663
Risk Management, Malpractice, and Negligence 664
Telehealth, Tele-practice, and Licensure Portability 666
INFLUENCING THE REGULATORY PROCESS 667
CURRENT PRACTICE CLIMATE FOR APRNS 667
Visioning for Advanced Practice Nursing 667
FUTURE REGULATORY CHALLENGES FOR APRNS 669
CONCLUSION 669
KEY SUMMARY POINTS 670
REFERENCES 670

21 APRN OUTCOMES AND PERFORMANCE IMPROVEMENT RESEARCH 673
PATTI LUDWIG-BEYMER ■ LISA HOPP
REVIEW OF TERMS 674
Why Measure Outcomes? 674
What Outcome Measures Are Important? 678
CONCEPTUAL MODELS OF CARE DELIVERY IMPACT 680
Models for Evaluating Outcomes Achieved by APRNs 680
Outcomes Evaluation Model 680
Nursing Role Effectiveness Model Adapted for Acute Care Nurse Practitioners 680
EVIDENCE TO DATE 683
Role Description Studies 683
Role Perception and Acceptance Studies 684
Care Delivery Process Studies 684
"PROCESS AS OUTCOME" STUDIES 685
PERFORMANCE (PROCESS) IMPROVEMENT ACTIVITIES 685
OUTCOMES MANAGEMENT ACTIVITIES 686
POPULATION HEALTH ACTIVITIES 686
IMPACT OF APRN PRACTICE 689
Studies Comparing APRN to Physician and Other Provider Outcomes 689
Nurse Practitioner Outcomes 695
Clinical Nurse Specialist Outcomes 695
Certified Nurse-Midwife Outcomes 696
Certified Registered Nurse Anesthetist Outcomes 696
Studies Comparing APRN and Physician Productivity 697
Relative Work Value of APRNs 697
FUTURE DIRECTIONS FOR USING OUTCOMES IN APRN PRACTICE 698
CONCLUSION 700
KEY SUMMARY POINTS 701
REFERENCES 701

22 FUTURE TECHNOLOGIES INFLUENCING APRN PRACTICE 709
DEBORA SIMMONS ■ PAMELA SALYER
ILLUSIONS OF TECHNOLOGY IN A PANDEMIC 711
MAKING SENSE OF COMPLEXITY IN HEALTH INFORMATION TECHNOLOGY 711
The Donabedian Model 711
James Reason Swiss Cheese Model 712
HUMAN-CENTERED DESIGN 713
TECHNOLOGY-ASSISTED COMMUNICATION 715
Written Communication Technologies 715
Verbal Communication Technologies 717
Nonverbal Communication Technologies 718
Visual Communication Technologies 719
Social Media as a Communication Tool 719
DIAGNOSTIC, THERAPEUTIC, AND PROCEDURAL DEVICES AND APPS 721
Diagnostic and Therapeutic Devices and Apps 721

Procedural Devices and Apps 724
SUPPORTIVE TECHNOLOGY 725
DATA, CLINICAL DECISION SUPPORT, AND ADVANCED ANALYTICS 727
Data 727
Clinical Decision Support 730
Advanced Analytics 731
CYBERSECURITY 732
Data Security and Privacy 732
States of Digital Data 732
Regulatory Compliance 733
Types of Cyberattack 734
Mobile Device Security 734
Blockchain 735
HIGH-TECH HOME CARE 735
FUTURE IMPLICATIONS OF TECHNOLOGY-ENABLED ADVANCED PRACTICE REGULATION AND GROWTH: A CALL TO PARTICIPATE 737
CONCLUSION 738
KEY SUMMARY POINTS 739
REFERENCES 739

23 USING HEALTHCARE INFORMATION TECHNOLOGY TO EVALUATE AND IMPROVE PERFORMANCE AND PATIENT OUTCOMES 744
MARISA L. WILSON
INFORMATICS AND INFORMATION TECHNOLOGY SUPPORTING IMPROVED PERFORMANCE AND OUTCOMES 746
Coding Taxonomies and Classification Systems 747
REGULATORY REPORTING INITIATIVES THAT DRIVE PERFORMANCE IMPROVEMENT 751
Current Reporting Requirements 751
New Reporting Requirements of MACRA 755
RELEVANCE OF REGULATORY REPORTING TO ADVANCED PRACTICE NURSING OUTCOMES 761
The National Provider Identifier Number ... 762
FOUNDATIONAL COMPETENCIES IN MANAGING HEALTH INFORMATION TECHNOLOGY 762
Descriptive, Predictive, and Prescriptive Data Analytics 763
FOUNDATIONAL COMPETENCIES IN QUALITY IMPROVEMENT 768
Continuous Quality Improvement Frameworks 768
Organizational Structures and Cultures That Optimize Performance Improvement 769
STRATEGIES FOR DESIGNING QUALITY IMPROVEMENT AND OUTCOME EVALUATION PLANS FOR ADVANCED PRACTICE NURSING 770
Phases of Preparing a Plan for Outcome Evaluation 770
Define the Data Elements 774
Derive Meaning From Data and Act on Results 776
Clarify Purpose of the Advanced Practice Nurse's Role 778
CONCLUSION 779
KEY SUMMARY POINTS 780
REFERENCES 780

INDEX, 783

PART I

Historical and Developmental Aspects of Advanced Practice Nursing

1

HISTORY AND EVOLUTION OF ADVANCED PRACTICE NURSING

ARLENE W. KEELING ■ ANNE Z. COCKERHAM

"No occupation can be intelligently followed or correctly understood unless it is, at least to some extent, illumined by the light of history. ..."

~ Lavinia L. Dock and Isabel M. Stewart (1938, p. 1)

CHAPTER CONTENTS

NURSE ANESTHETISTS 3
- Early Roots 3
- Documenting Outcomes 3
- Resistance From Organized Medicine: Legal Challenges 4
- Navigating Interprofessional Challenges at the Grassroots Level 6
- Issues With Financial Reimbursement 7
- Setting Educational Standards 8

NURSE-MIDWIVES 8
- Early Roots: "Granny Midwives" 8
- Time and Place Matter: "The Midwife Problem" 9
- Place Matters: Frontier Nursing Service Midwives 9
- Roots of Midwifery Education in the United States 10
- Place Matters: New Mexico 11
- A National Organization 11
- Growth of Midwifery Practice 12
- Reimbursement 12
- Nurse-Midwifery Programs in the Second Half of the 20th Century 13

CLINICAL NURSE SPECIALISTS 13
- Early Roots 13
- Time and Place Matter: World Wars I and II 14
- Legislation and Medical Specialization 14
- Navigating Inter- and Intraprofessional Challenges 16
- Organization and Evaluation 17
- Declining Demand for Clinical Nurse Specialists 18
- CNS Education and Reimbursement 19

NURSE PRACTITIONERS 19
- Early Roots of Primary Care 19
- The Need for Primary Care in the Mid-20th Century 21
- Intraprofessional Conflict Over the NP Role 22
- Support From Physicians 23
- The Concept of "Advanced Practice" 23
- Resistance to the NP by Organized Medicine 24
- Growth, Organization, and Legislation 25
- Neonatal and Acute Care Nurse Practitioners 25
- Nurse Practitioner Education 26

CONCLUSION 26

KEY SUMMARY POINTS 27

Writing in their 1938 book *A Short History of Nursing*, early nursing scholars Lavinia Lloyd Dock and Isabel M. Stewart emphasized the importance of documenting and studying the history of the nursing profession. They were correct in their observations: history offers enlightenment; it also gives new generations of nurses their cultural identity. Awareness of the history of advanced practice nursing provides essential background to our understanding of "how we got where we are today." Understanding that background can shape the profession's response to current challenges.

NURSE ANESTHETISTS

Early Roots

The roots of nurse anesthesia in the United States can be traced to the mid-19th century, shortly after the discovery of ether and chloroform as agents to induce unconsciousness during surgery. During the American Civil War (1861–1865), before the first formal US nurse training schools were opened, lay women from both the Union and the Confederacy volunteered as nurses, some assisting in surgeries by providing anesthesia. For example, according to one historical account, after the Battle of Gettysburg in 1863 Mrs. John Harris "set out from Baltimore with chloroform and stimulants" and ministered "as much as [was] in her power to the stream of wounded" (Thatcher, 1953, p. 33). In addition to lay women, Roman Catholic nuns with little or no training as nurses administered much of the anesthesia during the war (Jolly, 1927).

Following the Civil War, in 1873 three training schools for nurses opened in New York, Massachusetts, and Connecticut, providing a steady stream of graduate nurses to care for the sick. By the 1880s, some US surgeons began to employ these trained nurses to assist them in the operating room by handing them instruments or administering anesthesia. One of the most notable of these surgeons was Dr. William W. Mayo of St. Mary's Hospital in Rochester, Minnesota. In 1889 Mayo hired Edith Graham, a graduate of Women's Hospital Training School in Chicago, to be his anesthetist and office nurse.

Shortly after hiring her, Dr. Mayo taught Graham how to give anesthesia using the "open drop method" taught to him by a German physician a few years earlier. The process was quite simple. A wire frame covered with gauze was placed over the patient's mouth and nose, and the anesthetizer would slowly administer drops of chloroform or ether on the gauze until the patient lost consciousness. The key to maintaining a steady state of anesthesia was vigilant observation, something at which nurses excelled and something that was often lacking when an inexperienced medical student, more interested in the surgical procedure itself, administered the drugs (Keeling, 2014).

FACT BOX 1.1

Instructions for Administration of Chloroform (1893)

"A nurse is often called upon in private practice to administer an anesthetic, as it is not possible at every operation to have sufficient medical assistance" (p. 331). "The nurse must have at hand a hypodermic syringe (sterilized and in good order), whiskey or brandy, tincture of digitalis, a solution of strychnine, morphine, atropine, and aqua ammonia, as any of them may be called for" (p. 333).

ADAMS HAMPTON, I. (1893). THE ADMINISTRATION OF ANÆSTHETICS. IN *NURSING: ITS PRINCIPLES AND PRACTICE* (CH. 22, PP. 331–336). PHILADELPHIA: SAUNDERS.

Entrusting the delivery of anesthesia to Graham proved to be an excellent decision. From 1889 to 1893, the Mayo team performed 655 surgical operations at St. Marys Hospital. Of these, 98.3% were successful in that the patients left the hospital alive. In all cases, Edith Graham had administered the anesthesia (Pougiales, 1970).

Documenting Outcomes

Committed to continuing to employ nurses to deliver anesthesia, Dr. Mayo hired another nurse, Alice Magaw, to assist him and his son, Dr. William Mayo, when Graham left the practice in 1893 (Keeling, 2014).

Magaw delivered anesthesia to over a thousand patients from January 1, 1899, to January 1, 1900, keeping excellent records of the surgeries, the anesthesia given, and the patient outcomes. She published those results in the *St. Paul's Medical Journal*, writing (Fig. 1.1):

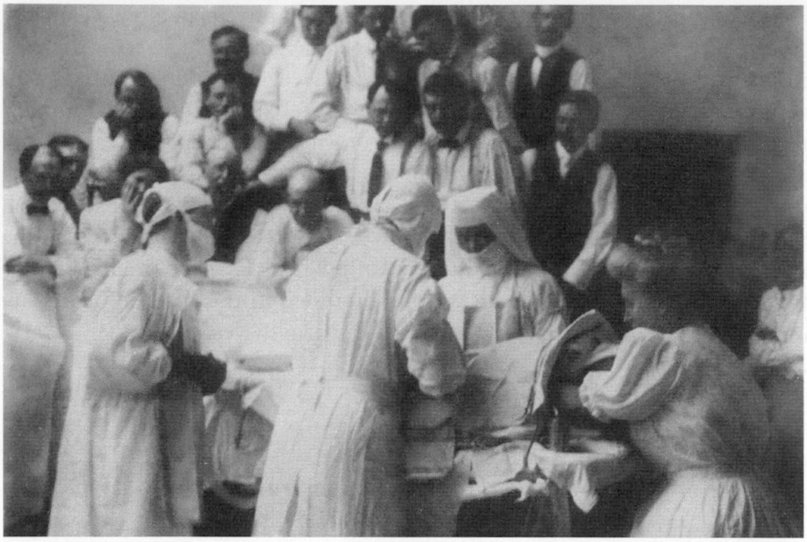

Fig. 1.1 ■ Alice McGaw in operating room at Mayo Clinic. (Courtesy Mayo Clinic Archives.)

In that time, we administered an anesthetic 1,092 times; ether alone 674 times; chloroform 245 times; ether and chloroform combined, 173 times. I can report that out of this number, 1,092 cases, we have not had an accident; we have not had occasion to use artificial respiration once; nor one case of ether pneumonia; neither have we had any serious renal results. …

(Magaw, 1900, p. 306)

Documenting and publishing the results of nurse-administered anesthesia was key to demonstrating the safety and efficacy of nurse anesthesia practice when, between 1899 and 1901, Dr. Mayo and his sons added several other nurse anesthetists to their surgical teams. Their work gained national acclaim, and both physicians and nurses from around the world visited the famous clinic to learn methods of anesthesia delivery and procedures for training nurses.

Resistance From Organized Medicine: Legal Challenges

Despite the successful outcomes in nurse anesthetists' practice, some physicians would soon challenge the legality of the nurses' practice. In the 1910s, the delivery of anesthesia was becoming increasingly based on new discoveries in medicine and science, and anesthesia was becoming a growing medical specialty. As a result, some physicians accused nurse anesthetists of practicing medicine without a license. One such challenge occurred in 1911 when the New York State Medical Society argued (unsuccessfully) that the administration of an anesthetic by a nurse violated state law (Thatcher, 1953). A year later in Ohio, the state medical board passed a resolution specifying that only physicians could administer anesthesia. Despite this resolution, nurse anesthetist Agatha Hodgins, who had been working as a nurse anesthetist with Dr. George Crile at the Cleveland Clinic since 1908, established the Lakeside Hospital School of Anesthesia in Cleveland, Ohio. Begun in 1915, the school was geared toward the preparation of nurse anesthetists. Shortly after its opening, however, a state medical society sued the Lakeside Hospital program. The lawsuit was unsuccessful and resulted in an amendment to the Ohio Medical Practice Act, legally protecting the practice of nurse anesthesia.

Despite these legal setbacks, organized medicine's opposition to the practice of nurse anesthesia continued and another lawsuit against nurse anesthetists, Frank et al. v. South et al., was filed in Kentucky in 1917. That case went to a Kentucky court of appeal, which ruled that anesthesia provided by nurse anesthetist Margaret Hatfield *did not* constitute the practice of medicine if it was given under the orders and supervision of a licensed physician (in this case,

Dr. Louis Frank). It was a landmark decision: the courts had declared nurse anesthesia legal but "subordinate" to oversight by physicians. The ruling would have lasting implications for nurse anesthetists' practice. Later in the century it would set precedent for all advanced practice registered nurse (APRN) practice. Meanwhile, throughout the United States, numerous schools for nurse anesthetists opened between 1912 and 1920, each offering 6 months of postgraduate nursing education in the specialty (Keeling, 2007).

Time and Place Matter: World War I

Organized medicine's support for nurse anesthetists increased, albeit poignantly, when the United States entered World War I in 1917. That year more than 1000 nurses were deployed to Britain and France, including nurse anesthetists. Dr. George Crile of Lakeside Hospital in Cleveland had been in charge of planning for war, and he had planned to use nurse anesthetists. When battle casualties poured into the base hospitals scattered throughout France, physicians were needed to operate; nurses would give anesthesia (Beeber, 1990).

> *During the drives, patients came in so fast. ... As soon as they were through operating on one patient, I would have to have the next patient anesthetized.*
>
> ***Nurse Anesthetist Sophie Winton, Mobile Hospital #1 (Keeling, 2007, p. 42)***

The war also created opportunities for research, and physicians and nurses began to investigate new methods for anesthesia administration. At the well-established Lakeside Hospital anesthesia program, Dr. George Crile and nurse anesthetist Agatha Hodgins experimented with combined nitrous oxide–oxygen administration. They also investigated the use of morphine and scopolamine as adjuncts to anesthesia (Keeling, 2007).

After the war, when nurse anesthetists returned to the United States, opportunities for their employment were mixed. For example, in 1922 Samuel Harvey, a Yale professor of surgery, hired Alice M. Hunt as an instructor of anesthesia at the Yale Medical School. It was a significant and prestigious appointment for a nurse. In contrast to Hunt's experience, however, many other nurse anesthetists struggled to find practice opportunities. Medicine was becoming increasingly complex and scientific and controlled by organized medical specialties intent on preserving their spheres of practice. Interprofessional conflict over disciplinary boundaries was inescapable.

Organization and Resistance From Both Nursing and Medicine

By the early 1930s, over 2000 institutions in the United States were employing nurse anesthetists, and it was soon clear that nurse anesthetists needed to organize as a specialty group to make their voices heard. In 1931 nurse anesthetist Agatha Hodgins established the National Association of Nurse Anesthetists (later renamed the American Association of Nurse Anesthesiology [AANA]) and served as the organization's first president.

Finding an affiliation for the specialty within the nursing profession itself was difficult, however. At the first meeting of the Association of Nurse Anesthetists, the group voted to affiliate with the American Nurses Association (ANA). However, the ANA denied the request; the ANA was afraid to assume legal responsibility for a group that could be charged with practicing medicine without a license. The ANA's fears were not unfounded. During the 1930s, the devastation of the national economy made jobs scarce, and because so many nurses were delivering anesthesia in so many hospitals throughout the country, nurse anesthetists were becoming an increasing threat to physicians who needed extra work giving anesthesia (Keeling, 2007).

As tensions between nurse anesthetists and their physician counterparts increased, more physicians challenged the nurses' practice. In California, the Los Angeles County Medical Association sued nurse anesthetist Dagmar Nelson in 1934 for practicing medicine without a license. Nelson won. According to the judge, "The administration of general anesthetics by the defendant Dagmar A. Nelson, pursuant to the directions and supervision of duly licensed physicians and surgeons, as shown by the evidence in this case, does not constitute the practice of medicine or surgery" (McGarrel, 1934).

In response, Dr. William Chalmers-Frances filed another suit against Nelson that again resulted in a judgment for Nelson (Chalmers-Frances v. Nelson, 1936), and once again the physicians appealed the case. In 1938 the physicians petitioned the California Supreme Court for a decision and once again the Court ruled in favor of nurse anesthetists. The case became famous. The courts had established legal precedent—the practice of nurse anesthesia was considered to be legal and within the scope of nursing practice, as long as it was done under the guidance of a supervising physician. The landmark decision soon became known as "The Captain of the Ship Doctrine" referring to the fact that the operating surgeon was "Captain of his Ship" and responsible for everything that happened in the operating room, including the nurse anesthetist's practice (Keeling, 2007).

Meanwhile, by the late 1930s the field of anesthesia was increasingly becoming a medical specialty. It was a time of increasing specialization within the field of medicine, and many subspecialties were requiring board certification to practice in a given area. The first written examination for board certification in medical anesthesiology was given in 1939. Meanwhile, demands for anesthetists, advances in the types of anesthesia available, and advances in scientific knowledge in the field of anesthesia stimulated physicians' interest in the specialty. In particular, the use of the new drug sodium pentothal required specialized knowledge of physiology and pharmacology, underscoring the emerging argument that only board-certified physicians could safely provide anesthesia. The administration of anesthesia was, in fact, becoming more complex, and anesthesiologists were developing expertise in administering drugs such as sodium pentothal and in performing endotracheal intubation and regional blocks (Waisel, 2001). Clearly, medicine was strengthening its hold on the specialty.

Time and Place Matter: World War II

World War II increased the demand for nurse anesthetists, both in civilian hospitals within the United States and in military hospitals at home and abroad (Fig. 1.2). With the attack on Pearl Harbor and America's entrance into the war in 1941, the military mobilized teams of medical and nursing personnel, sending some to Europe and others to the Pacific. Many of those would work in mobile evacuation hospitals. However, despite profound shortages of anesthetists, the US military would not grant nurse anesthetists a specific designation or a higher grade of pay. In fact, experienced nurse anesthetists worked within the status of rank-and-file general-duty nurses, even though they gave anesthesia. Later, when shortages of physicians increased the demand for nurse anesthetists at the front, military staff nurses were recruited to be trained as nurse anesthetists (Exemplar 1.1).

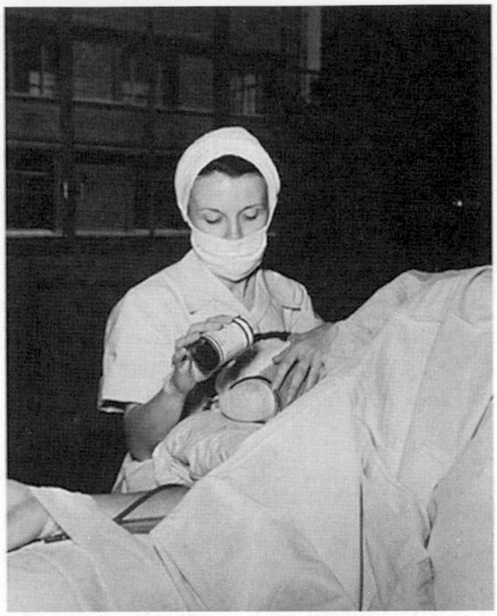

Fig. 1.2 ■ World War II nurse anesthetist giving anesthesia. (National Library of Medicine.)

Meanwhile, on the home front in the United States, while other nurses were being "refreshed" and retooled for work in general duty, nurse anesthetists continued to give anesthesia in operating rooms throughout the country. Their role was essential; thousands of physicians had left their jobs to join the military. Simply put, nurse anesthetists filled jobs vacated by physicians.

Navigating Interprofessional Challenges at the Grassroots Level

At Johns Hopkins Hospital during the 1940s, one nurse anesthetist, working with Drs. Alfred Blalock and Helen Taussig, would soon gain worldwide recognition for her work assisting in the famous "blue-baby surgeries"—named for they cyanosis the babies experienced because of a heart defect. During the first operation to repair the condition known as *tetralogy of Fallot*, nurse Olive Berger administered the anesthesia. After that, per Dr. Blalock's request, Berger administered anesthesia in the next 475 blue-baby cases. Recognized

EXEMPLAR 1.1

NURSE ANESTHETISTS IN WORLD WAR II, 1942–1945

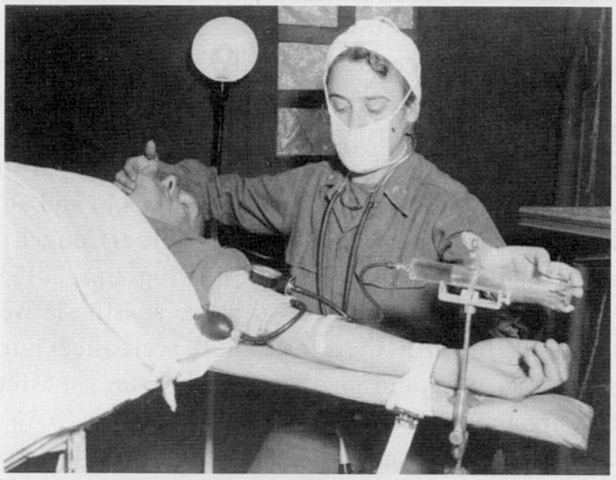

(Courtesy Bjoring Center, UVA)

During World War II, the University of Virginia sponsored the 8th Evacuation Hospital, a 750-bed mobile hospital a few miles from the front lines in Italy. There, surgical teams often operated around the clock despite air raids, heavy rains, and blackouts. Nurse anesthetists were needed for the team to keep up with the endless stream of battle casualties requiring surgery, and Dorothy Sandridge Gloor, a young surgical nurse, received "on the job training" to give anesthesia. Working alongside surgeons for 16-hour shifts, Gloor learned new skills and the specialty knowledge necessary to deliver anesthesia (Kinser, 2011).

for her expertise and skill, Berger was later appointed instructor in anesthesia at Johns Hopkins School of Medicine (Keeling, Hehman, & Kirchgessner, 2018). It was a significant achievement—one that demonstrated how a nurse anesthetist skillfully collaborated with a prestigious surgical team.

> *Lots of places had nurse anesthetists but also had a physician anesthetist in charge … but we didn't. Dr. Blalock did not want it and Dr. Blalock had great faith in us.*
>
> ***Nurse anesthetist Olive Berger (Carmel, 2015, 65)***

Time and Place Matter: Wars in Korea and Vietnam

By the 1950s, the United States was again at war, this time with Korea, and once again war provided a setting in which opportunities abounded for nurse anesthetists. By the end of the Korean War, the US Army had established several nurse anesthesia education programs, including one at Walter Reed General Hospital. That program graduated its first class in 1961—a class consisting only of men. Later, the Letterman General Hospital School of Anesthesia in San Francisco also graduated an all-male class. The significant movement of men into this nursing specialty was unprecedented and would continue when the United States entered the war in Vietnam.

As was the case in wars of other eras, the war in Vietnam (1959–1975) provided nurses with opportunities to stretch the boundaries of the discipline as they treated thousands of casualties in evacuation hospitals and aboard hospital ships. By 1968 there were more than 800 Army nurses stationed in Vietnam. Not surprising, nurse anesthetists played an active role at the front, providing vital services in the prompt surgical treatment of the wounded. Among those who served was Elwood Wilkins, a nurse anesthetist who enlisted in the US Army in 1966, the day he graduated from the nurse anesthesia program at Mayo School of Health Sciences. While on duty in Vietnam, Wilkins gave anesthesia in a busy evacuation hospital, one that was always short of supplies and one that often received 100 casualties at a time (Keeling, 2014). Opportunity was not without cost. Of the 10 nurses killed in Vietnam, 2 were nurse anesthetists (Bankert, 1989).

> *In Vietnam we practiced jungle anesthesia. You make do with what you've got. (Mayo School of Health Sciences Alumni Connection Magazine, 2009. p. 6)*
>
> ***Elwood Wilkins, Certified Registered Nurse Anesthetist***

Issues With Financial Reimbursement

Reimbursement for certified registered nurse anesthetists' practice was never clear-cut, and the financial threat certified registered nurse anesthetists (CRNAs) posed to physicians was a source of continued interprofessional conflict. Beginning in 1977, the AANA led a long and complex effort to secure third-party reimbursement under Medicare so that CRNAs could bill for their services. The organization would finally succeed in 1989. However, tensions continued to escalate, particularly in relation to malpractice policies, antitrust, and restraint of trade issues. Legal challenges ensued. In the 1980s, when anesthesiologists conspired to restrict practice privileges, the outcome of the lawsuit Oltz v. St. Peter's Community Hospital established CRNAs' right to sue for anticompetitive damages. A second case, Bhan v. NME Hospitals, Inc., et al. (1985), established CRNAs' right to be awarded damages when hospitals and physician anesthesiologists made contracts excluding nurses from practicing anesthesia. Clearly, CRNAs were winning the legal battles and overcoming practice barriers erected by hospital administrators and physicians.

Setting Educational Standards

Since it was founded in 1931, the AANA's primary focus was to improve educational standards through university affiliation and a standardized curriculum, and in 1945 the Association published its standards in the *Essentials of an Acceptable School of Anesthesiology for Graduate Registered Nurses*. At the same time the AANA instituted mandatory certification for CRNAs. This formal credentialing, specifying the requirements for the nurse anesthetist, preceded credentialing of nurses in the other specialties. Five years later the AANA's plan for accreditation of anesthesia programs was approved, and the first accreditation of programs began in 1952. Over the next decades, the AANA continued to promote university affiliation, and by 1982 the AANA board of directors set the baccalaureate degree as a requirement for nurses entering anesthesia programs (Horton, 2007a, 2007b).

The 1990s saw a significant growth in CRNA education programs, although many of the programs were very small. As the decade opened, there were 17 master's programs in nurse anesthesia; by 1999, there were 82 (Bigbee & Amidi-Nouri, 2000). Starting in 1998, *all* accredited programs in nurse anesthesia were required to be at the master's level (Horton, 2007b). However, these master's programs were not always housed in schools of nursing. They were also located in schools of medicine, allied health, and the basic sciences.

In 2007 the AANA affirmed its support that the doctor of nurse anesthesia practice (DNP) be the entry for nurse anesthesia practice by 2025 (AANA, 2007). The University of Minnesota opened the first postbaccalaureate DNP program for CRNAs in 2009 (Glass, 2009), and in 2015 the Council on Accreditation for Nurse Anesthesia Programs approved standards for a practice doctorate. According to that council, all students entering nurse anesthesia programs in and after 2022 must graduate with a doctoral degree (Council on Accreditation for Nurse Anesthesia Programs, 2015).

Soon doctoral programs in nurse anesthesia were trending. In 2017 there were 120 accredited nurse anesthesia programs in the United States, of which 62 were approved to award a doctoral degree (AANA, 2017). As of September 2020, there were 124 accredited nurse anesthetist programs in the United States and Puerto Rico, using more than 2008 clinical sites. One hundred and two of those programs awarded the doctoral degree (AANA, 2020).

NURSE-MIDWIVES

Unlike nurse anesthetists, who have only been practicing for 150 years or so, midwives have practiced since the beginning of time. Midwives entered the United States through the slave trade or during waves of European immigration. These untrained or foreign-trained women lost much of the public's esteem as childbirth became medicalized in the late 19th and early 20th centuries. As Clara Noyes, an early nurse leader, wrote "the word 'midwife,' in America, at least, is one to which considerable odium is attached, and immediately creates a mental picture of illiteracy, carelessness and general filth" (Noyes, 1912, p. 466). Women in isolated communities throughout the country, particularly in rural settings, continued to rely on lay midwives well into the 20th century.

Early Roots: "Granny Midwives"

"Granny midwives," as they were condescendingly called, were untrained or apprentice-trained women who provided the vast majority of obstetric care prior to the 1950s. Although European immigrants served in this role in northern, urban areas, the term granny midwife is most often associated with Black women in the racially segregated southern states. Typically these midwives were the only care providers for Black Southern women at a time when few hospitals admitted Black patients and there was no public funding to support physician attendance in the home. In rural southern states such as Mississippi, in which 50% of the population was Black, most women (80% of African American and 8% of White women) relied on these midwives to deliver their babies (Smith, 1994). In the 1940s in Arkansas, granny midwives attended the majority of all African American births (Bell, 1993). See Fig. 1.3.

Time and Place Matter: "The Midwife Problem"

During the Progressive Era at the turn of the 20th century, medical, nursing, and public health leaders argued that untrained midwives attending home births were the primary cause of high maternal and infant mortality rates. In 1923 physician Anna Rude lamented the "inadequacy of our laws governing midwives, which contain neither uniform provisions nor required standards" (Rude, 1923, p. 987). Soon, with the rise of obstetrics as a medical specialty, some physicians argued for the total abolition of midwives and for the legal prosecution of violators. Others, including prominent public health officials, advocated for the close regulation of midwives' practice and control over their training rather than for the elimination of midwifery practice altogether.

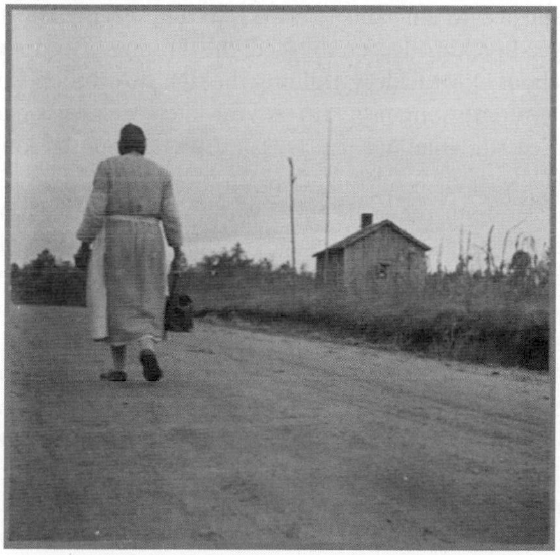

Fig. 1.3 ■ **Siloam, Greene County, Georgia, midwife.** (Library of Congress.)

Those who argued that midwives were the sole, or even the most significant, cause of poor obstetric outcomes were incorrect. From 1915 until the mid-1930s, despite an increase in physician-assisted births, maternal and infant mortality rose dramatically. In 1933 a committee of the New York Academy of Medicine reported that the maternal death rate for surgeons' practice was 9.9 per 1000 live births; for obstetricians it was 5.4 per 1000 live births. In contrast, midwives who received public health instruction and practiced in patients' homes had the lowest maternal death rate of 1.4 per 1000 live births (Litoff, 1978). In fact, the actual causes of poor obstetric outcomes in the United States were complex. They included the lack of prenatal care; inadequate education for providers of maternity care, including physicians; physician interventions during delivery, often with unproven and dangerous obstetric techniques; and high rates of puerperal infections due to patient-to-patient contamination in the growing number of women giving birth in hospitals (Cockerham, 2019).

Over time the outcome data led public health officials to conclude that something had to be done. It was apparent that increased education for obstetricians, the training and regulation of midwives, and the employment of certified nurse-midwives could improve outcomes for mothers and babies.

Place Matters: Frontier Nursing Service Midwives

To address the "midwife problem" in the economically depressed, rural mountainous area of Kentucky, Mary Breckinridge, a wealthy and politically connected nurse-midwife, founded the Frontier Nursing Service (FNS) in 1925. Having worked in post–World War I France and later having trained as a midwife in Scotland, Breckinridge was aware of the important role that trained midwives played in remote areas of the United Kingdom and was determined to bring their services to Kentucky. To do so, she recruited several British nurse-midwives and established headquarters at Wendover, a log cabin located on a mountain ridge in Leslie County. From there, the nurse-midwives provided midwifery care to mothers in the poverty-stricken community. Because there were few roads in

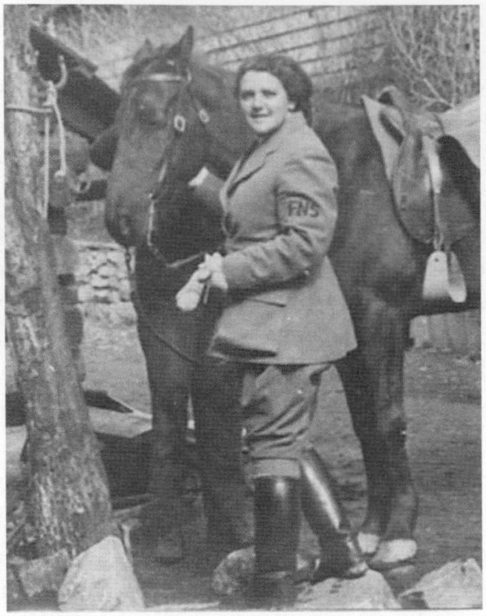

Fig. 1.4 ■ Frontier Nursing Service nurse with horse. (Courtesy of Frontier Nursing University, Versailles KY.)

the mountainous region, the nurses traveled by horseback to attend births, carrying their supplies in saddlebags. Often working by flashlight in dark, dilapidated cabins, the nurse midwives made do with what they had on hand to assist women in childbirth, lining the birthing bed with old newspapers and having the husband boil water on a woodstove (Breckinridge, 1981; Cockerham & Keeling, 2012). See Fig. 1.4.

> *The whole of the district work — is done with the aid of two pairs of saddlebags. … In these bags we have everything needed for a home delivery. …*
>
> ***(Summers, 1938, p. 1183)***

Key to measuring the effectiveness of the FNS practice was the documentation of outcomes with regard to maternal and infant morbidity and mortality. Using a comprehensive record system, the FNS nurses kept data about their practice and had the results analyzed by statisticians from the Metropolitan Life Insurance Company. These findings, reported for each series of 1000 FNS cases, provided statistical evidence of the safety and effectiveness of the FNS nurses' care in Leslie County. Indeed, the nurses' work made a difference. The maternal death rate of 12 per 10,000 live births for the first 25 years of the service's existence was dramatically lower than the national maternal mortality rates of 66.1 per 10,000 live births in 1931 and 37.6 per 10,000 live births in 1940 (Cockerham, 2019). Clearly, having trained nurse-midwives was key to that success—even if they had to be imported from the United Kingdom. What also became clear was that the United States needed its own schools for the education of nurse-midwives.

Roots of Midwifery Education in the United States

With the exception of a nurse training program at the Preston Retreat Hospital—a lying-in hospital in Philadelphia that opened in 1866—the Manhattan Midwifery School in New York City (1925–1931) was the earliest program for the education of nurse-midwives in the United States. This was followed by the School of the Association for the Promotion and Standardization of Midwifery (APSM) in New York City (Burst & Thompson, 2003). Affiliated with the Maternity Center Association, the APSM opened in 1932 and was more commonly known as the Lobenstine Midwifery School. Later, in 1934, it became known as the Maternity Center Association School of Nurse-Midwifery.

Other nurse-midwifery schools soon followed. In 1939 the entry of Britain into World War II proved to be the catalyst for Breckinridge to open a school for nurse-midwifery in Kentucky. That year, the FNS lost many of its British nurse-midwives when they returned to England to work. To address the shortage, Breckinridge established the Frontier Graduate School of Midwifery, training the first two students in a 4-month-long program. A year later, each class had three students and the program was 6 months long (Cockerham & Keeling, 2012).

At about the same time, working within the context of a racially segregated US society, two schools opened to educate Black nurse-midwives. The Tuskegee School of Nurse-Midwifery, established in September 1941, was a joint project of the Macon County Health Department, the Children's Bureau, the Julius Rosenwald Fund, Tuskegee University, and the Alabama State Department of Health (Exemplar 1.2). Its aim was to reduce high infant and maternal mortality in the Southern United States. After graduating only 31 nurse-midwives, the school closed in 1946 because of untenable working conditions leading to an inability to retain instructors (Varney & Thompson, 2016).

EXEMPLAR 1.2
NURSE-MIDWIFE MAUDE CALLEN

Nurse-midwife Maude Callen (1898–1990) was unknown outside her small South Carolina community until photojournalist W. Eugene Smith produced a 10-page photo essay about her for Life Magazine in December 1951. Callen's story was a simple one. After training at the Georgia Infirmary, Callen moved to Pineville, South Carolina, to work as a missionary nurse. "Pineville was 22 miles from the nearest hospital ... and people sent for Miss Maude when they became ill. She was available day and night." With support from the state division of maternal and child health, Callen attended a 6-month midwifery course at the Tuskegee School of Nurse-Midwifery. The first African American nurse-midwife in South Carolina, Callen held annual midwifery institutes and delivered more than 800 infants (Clark Hine, 2011, p. 133).

Another education program for Black nurse-midwives (largely overlooked in the historical record) was the Flint–Goodridge School of Nurse-Midwifery in New Orleans, Louisiana, in operation from 1942 to 1943. Relying on monies from the US Children's Bureau and the Rosenwald Fund, the Flint–Goodridge School of Nurse-Midwifery was affiliated with Dillard University and Flint–Goodridge Hospital. On June 15, 1943, 9 months after the first two students were admitted, the Flint–Goodridge School of Nurse-Midwifery graduated those two students and subsequently closed. According to the supervisor's report, it closed for economic reasons due to the national economy in World War II (Superintendent's report, 1942).

FACT BOX 1.2

Flint-Goodridge School of Nurse-Midwifery

The school is staffed by a full- time obstetrician and two graduate nurse-midwives. The course of study covers a period of 6 months. ... Pearl Harbor, with its cataclysmic portent on our nation's thinking and national economy, has had its effects on the institutions and hospitals of the nation. Flint-Goodridge has in no way escaped the effect of these events. (Superintendent's report, 1942)

Place Matters: New Mexico

Place also mattered in the use of nurse-midwives in rural Santa Fe, New Mexico, where the Catholic Maternity Institute (CMI) was founded in 1944. In the late 1930s and early 1940s, maternal and infant death rates among Spanish Americans in New Mexico were devastatingly high. Physicians were scarce, and in the rural area patients lived at long distances from any hospital. With the arrival of the trained Catholic sister nurse-midwives in Santa Fe and the opening of the CMI, many Spanish American women would receive professional maternity care for the first time in their lives. At first, the sisters attended births in patients' homes, despite the long and often difficult travel involved.

> *CMI staff nurse-midwife Sister Catherine Shean recalled: "I think one of the most beautiful [aspects] for me was when you were in the home and the baby was born and ... the mother had been cleaned up and she was ready to receive the baby. ... We would gather together the [whole] family and we would pray with them."*
> ***(cited in Cockerham & Keeling, 2010, pp. 156–157)***

A National Organization

The establishment of a formal organization of practicing nurse-midwives, the American Association of Nurse-Midwives (AANM), was key to the development of nurse-midwifery in the United States. The AANM was incorporated in 1941 under the leadership of Mary Breckinridge (News Here and There, 1942, p. 832). Three years later, in 1944, the National Organization of Public Health Nurses (NOPHN) established a section for nurse-midwives within their organization. However, there were organizational issues for the midwives when the NOPHN was absorbed by the two other major nursing organizations in the early 1950s. The American College of Nurse-Midwives (ACNM) was founded in 1955. In 1969 the AANM and the ACNM merged (Varney & Thompson, 2016).

Growth of Midwifery Practice

Public interest in natural childbirth that stemmed from the women's movement was particularly beneficial to the practice of nurse-midwifery in the 1970s; the demand for nurse-midwifery services increased dramatically during that decade. In addition, sociopolitical developments, including the increased employment of certified nurse-midwives (CNMs) in federally funded healthcare projects and the increased birth rate resulting from baby boomers reaching adulthood, converged with inadequate numbers of obstetricians to foster the rapid growth of CNM practice (Varney & Thompson, 2016).

In 1971 the ACNM, the American College of Obstetricians and Gynecologists, and the Nurses' Association of the American College of Obstetricians and Gynecologists issued a joint statement supporting the development and employment of nurse-midwives in obstetric teams directed by a physician. The joint statement, which was critical to the practice of nurse-midwifery, reflected some resolution of the interprofessional tension that had existed through much of the 20th century. However, the statement did not provide for autonomy for CNMs.

Later in the decade, the ACNM revised its definitions of CNM practice and its philosophy, emphasizing the distinct midwifery and nursing origins of the role (ACNM, 1978a, 1978b). This conceptualization of nurse-midwifery as the combination of two disciplines, nursing and midwifery, was unique among the advanced practice nursing specialties. It served to align nurse-midwives with *non-nurse* midwives (lay midwives), thereby broadening their organizational and political base. Philosophically controversial, even within nurse-midwifery, the conceptualization created some distance from other APRN specialties that saw advanced practice roles as based solely in the discipline of nursing. This distinction would continue to isolate CNMs from other APRNs for the next several decades.

Another issue that intensified in the 1980s was the escalating cost of malpractice insurance. The critical matter for insurance companies was the tension between providing coverage for a nurse-midwife's care for healthy mothers against the possibility of a complicated, high-risk delivery. Thus the cost of nurse-midwives' malpractice insurance rose from $38 a year in 1982 to about $3500 a year in 1986. This huge increase occurred during a time that midwives earned, on average, only $23,000 a year (Varney & Thompson, 2016). Because of the cost of insurance, many CNMs gave up delivering babies altogether; others sought employment in physicians' offices, public health departments, and hospitals in which they could be covered by their employers' policies. Some forfeited coverage completely (Varney & Thompson, 2016).

During the 1990s, increasing demand for CNM services resulted in a gradual expansion in the scope of nurse-midwifery practice. CNMs began to provide care to women with relatively high-risk pregnancies in collaboration with obstetricians in some of the nation's academic tertiary care centers (Rooks, 1997). During this decade, two practice models emerged: the CNM service model, in which CNMs were responsible for the care of a caseload of women determined to be eligible for midwifery care, and the CNM–physician team model. Nurse-midwives continued to make progress in establishing laws and regulations needed to support their practice. However, the struggle for prescriptive authority, given by each state, continued until 2007, when Pennsylvania's nurse-midwives, the last in the country, finally were granted prescriptive privileges (ACNM, 2007).

FACT BOX 1.3

Nurse Anesthetists as an Economic Threat in the Great Depression

Since the onset of the economic disturbance of the past few years, agitation has sprung up in certain quarters to restrict the right to administer anesthetics to ... licensed physicians thus eliminating nurse anesthetists from the field of anesthesia. We believe that the aforesaid economic disturbance and the agitation against the nurse anesthetist bear a direct relationship.

(NATIONAL ASSOCIATION OF NURSE ANESTHETISTS, BRIEF OF NANA, AMICUS CURIAE IN THE SUPREME COURT OF THE STATE OF CALIFORNIA, L.A. NO 15162, 1-2 AANA ARCHIVES CHICAGO, 1938)

Reimbursement

Conflict with the medical profession arose as obstetricians perceived a growing threat to their practices in the latter half of the 20th century. The denial of hospital privileges, attempts to deny third-party reimbursement, and state legislative battles over statutory recognition of CNMs ensued. In particular, problems concerning restraint of trade emerged. In 1980 the US Congress and the Federal Trade Commission conducted a hearing to determine the extent of the restraint of trade issues experienced by CNMs. In two cases, one in Tennessee and one in Georgia, the Federal Trade Commission obtained restraint orders against hospitals and insurance companies attempting to limit the practice of CNMs, in essence ensuring that CNMs could practice (Diers, 1991). Third-party reimbursement for CNMs was a second issue. In 1980 CNMs working under the Civilian Health and Medical Program of the Uniformed Services (CHAMPUS; now Tricare) for military dependents were the first to receive approval for reimbursement. Third party payment for CNMs was also included under Medicaid. Statutory recognition by state legislatures was a third problem that would be addressed in the 1980s. By 1984, all 50 states had recognized nurse-midwifery in their state laws or regulations (Varney & Thompson, 2016).

Nurse-Midwifery Programs in the Second Half of the 20th Century

Much like nurse anesthetist programs had done before them, the midwifery organization formed an accrediting body; the first draft of their accreditation criteria appeared in 1962. Accreditation supported the nurse-midwives' aim to control their entry criteria and their professional education. Nurse-midwifery programs in the United States provided two different credentials: certificates and, later, master's degrees as programs emerged in university settings in the late 1950s. In 1966 accreditation criteria mandated that all nurse-midwifery programs had to be affiliated with a university (Varney & Thompson, 2016). In 2017 there were 40 master's programs in nurse-midwifery and just 7 postbaccalaureate DNP nurse-midwifery programs (American Association of Colleges of Nursing [AACN], 2020). That trend is changing, however. As of 2020, 20 of 38 midwifery programs accredited by ACME offer a DNP (AACN, 2020).

In contrast with other APRN groups, midwifery leaders have not embraced the DNP as a necessary component of midwifery education. In 2012 ACNM argued that the current educational standards resulted in safe and positive outcomes for women and newborns (ACNM, 2012).

CLINICAL NURSE SPECIALISTS

Early Roots

The roots of specialization in nursing can be traced to the turn of the 20th century, when hospitals offered postgraduate courses in various specialty areas, including anesthesia, tuberculosis, operating room, laboratory, and dietetics. Private-duty nurses often "specialized," choosing to care for specific populations, like new mothers and their infants, patients with infectious diseases, babies and children, or the frail elderly. Nurse Katherine Dewitt first wrote about "specialties" in nursing in the inaugural issue of the *American Journal of Nursing*, in 1900. In it she described specialty practice and the nurse's need for continuing education (see Fig. 1.5):

> *Those who devote themselves to one branch of nursing often do so because of the keen interest they feel in it. The specialist can and should reach greater perfection in her sphere when she gives her entire time to it. Her studies should be continued in that direction, she should try constantly to keep up with the rapid advances in medical science. … The nurse who is a specialist can often supplement the doctor's work to a great extent.*
>
> ***(Dewitt, 1900, p. 16)***

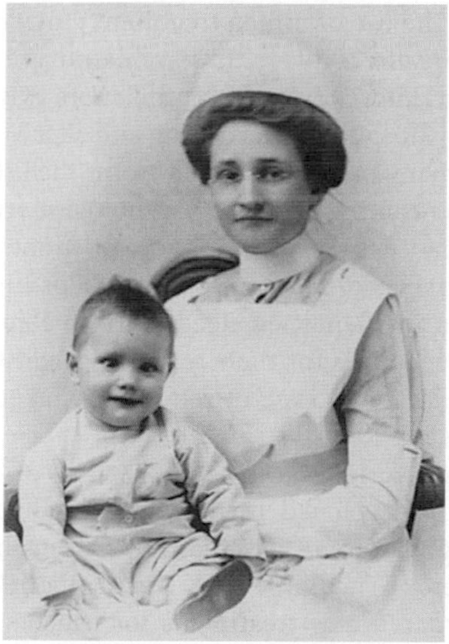

Fig. 1.5 ■ **Early specialization: Private-duty nurse with a child.** (Bjoring Center.)

Though she may have been the first to describe it, Dewitt was not the first to advocate for specialization in nursing practice. That had happened 20 years earlier, in 1880, when a training program for psychiatric nurses opened at McLean Hospital in Massachusetts (Critchley, 1985). According to nurse leader Linda Richards, the McLean Hospital maintained high standards and demonstrated "the value of trained nursing for the many persons afflicted with mental disease" (Richards, 1911, p. 109). Richards served as superintendent of nurses at the Taunton Insane Hospital for 4 years, beginning in 1899. She subsequently organized a nursing school for the preparation of psychiatric nurses at the Worcester Hospital for the Insane and finally was employed at the Michigan Insane Hospital in Kalamazoo, where she remained until 1909 (Richards, 1911). Because of her service in the field of psychiatric nursing, Richards is credited with founding the specialty.

Time and Place Matter: World Wars I and II

During the opening decades of the 20th century, Harry Stack Sullivan's classic writings and the work of Sigmund Freud dramatically changed psychiatric nursing by explaining the problems of mental illness. The emphasis on interpersonal interaction with patients as well as the use of milieu treatment provided nurses with a more direct role in the psychiatric care of hospitalized patients. Nowhere was this more evident than in military hospital wards during and after World War I, where many patients suffered from "shell shock"—a condition resulting from the psychological trauma the soldiers had experienced at the battlefront. In these wards, nurses soothed the men with soups and teas, sat with them in silence, engaged them in conversation, and gave sedatives for their recurring night terrors. It was the therapeutic use of self in a therapeutic environment (Fig. 1.6).

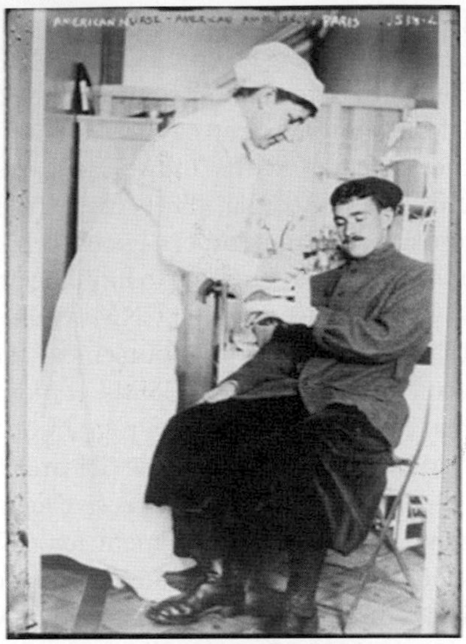

Fig. 1.6 ■ American nurse in American Ambulance Hospital, France, World War I. (Library of Congress.)

During World War II, the specialty of psychiatric nursing developed further as the public became increasingly aware of psychiatric problems in returning soldiers (Critchley, 1985). During the 1940s, physicians ordered new treatments for patients suffering mental illness. Among these were therapeutic baths and electroshock therapy, both of which required the skills of nurses who had specialized knowledge and training in their use.

> *Only the nurse skilled in her profession and with additional psychiatric background has a place in mental hospitals today.*
>
> ***(Schindler, 1942, p. 861)***

By 1943, three postgraduate programs specializing in psychiatric nursing had been established in the United States. At that time, however, the term *clinical specialist* was not used. Instead, those with advanced education in a specialty were called *nurse clinicians*. As nurse educator Frances Reiter later recalled, she first used the term nurse clinician in a speech in 1943 to describe a nurse with advanced "curative" knowledge and clinical competence committed to providing the highest quality of direct patient care (Reiter, 1966).

Legislation and Medical Specialization

Specific legislation after World War II along with a rise in medical specialization would have an effect on the profession of nursing in the mid-20th century. In 1946, after Congress passed the National Mental Health Act designating psychiatric nursing as a core discipline in mental health, federal funding for graduate and undergraduate educational programs and research in the specialty became available. As a result, psychiatric nursing was established as a graduate-level specialty, one that would lead the way for clinical nurse specialization in other areas in the next decade.

In 1954, professor of psychiatric nursing Hildegarde E. Peplau established a master's program in psychiatric nursing at Rutgers University in New Jersey. Considered a first in clinical nurse specialists (CNS) education, this program, along with the growth of specialty knowledge in psychiatric nursing that followed, provided support for psychiatric nurses to serve in new leadership roles in the care of patients with mental illness. Scholarship in psychiatric nursing flourished, including Peplau's conceptual framework for psychiatric nursing. Her book, *Interpersonal Relations in Nursing: A Conceptual Frame of Reference for Psychodynamic Nursing* (Peplau, 1952), provided theory-based practice for the specialty. Clearly, the link between academia and specialization was becoming stronger.

FACT BOX 1.4

American Nurses Association Defines Nursing Practice, 1955

The practice of professional nursing means the performance for compensation of any act in the observation, care and counsel of the ill ... or in the maintenance of health or prevention of illness ... or the administration of medications and treatments as prescribed by a licensed physician. ... The foregoing shall not be deemed to include acts of diagnosis or prescription of therapeutic or corrective measures.

(ANA, 1955)

By the mid-20th century, the rise of subspecialty medicine, particularly in the fields of cardiology, oncology, neurology, and nephrology, also had an effect on nursing. Specifically, these specialties needed nurses with an in-depth knowledge of the pathophysiology and treatment that patients with complex diagnoses required. For example, the polio epidemics of the 1940s gave rise to nursing specialization in neurogenerative diseases and their management; the inception and growth of coronary bypass surgeries in the 1950s provided impetus for nurses to learn new skills as they worked in post–cardiovascular surgical units; the discovery and use of cardiopulmonary resuscitation techniques along with new technology of cardiac monitoring gave rise to coronary care unit nursing; and changes in hospital architectural design (supported with funds from the Hill Burton Act) combined with the new concept of "progressive patient care" led to the development of numerous intensive care units, all requiring nurses with specialty knowledge to staff them.

In the 1960s clinical nurse specialization took its modern form. During this decade the Nurse Training Act of 1964 led to the creation of numerous university master's programs to prepare clinical nurse specialists. Reflecting on the impetus for the rise of these programs, Hildegarde Peplau (1965) noted that the development of areas of specialization was preceded by three social forces: (a) an increase in specialty-related information, (b) new technologic advances, and (c) a response to public need and interest. In addition to shaping most nursing specialties, these forces had a particularly strong effect on the development of the psychiatric CNS role in the 1960s. The Community Mental Health Centers Act of 1963, as well as the growing interest in child and adolescent mental health care, directly enhanced the expansion of that role in outpatient mental health care (Peplau, 1965).

FACT BOX 1.5

The Nurse Training Act, 1964

The Nurse Training Act of 1964 (H.B. 10042) authorized millions of dollars over 5 years to fund special projects and planning grants, student loans and scholarship, profession nurse traineeships, and nursing school construction. It was a "nationwide effort to alleviate critical shortages of nurses" to support "the health care of all citizens" (US Congress, 1964).

Of particular note was the development of specialization in coronary care. With the establishment of the Bethany Hospital Coronary Care Unit (CCU) in Kansas City, Kansas, in 1962 and another unit at the Presbyterian Hospital in Philadelphia, coronary care nursing soon emerged as a new area for specialization. Galvanized by space-age technology in cardiac monitoring and federal funding for regional medical programs in the mid-1960s, CCUs opened throughout the country. Working and learning together, nurses and physicians acquired specialized clinical knowledge in the area of cardiology.

Navigating Inter- and Intraprofessional Challenges

In the CCUs, nurses used their new knowledge to save patients and to acquire respect for their professional skills. Working together at the bedside, CCU nurses and cardiologists discussed clinical questions, attended joint classes in electrocardiogram ECG interpretation, and negotiated patient care responsibilities, successfully navigating interprofessional relationships at the grassroots level (Lynaugh & Fairman, 1992). In doing so, physicians and nurses together expanded nursing's scope of practice inside the CCU. As they identified cardiac arrhythmias on an ECG, administered intravenous medications, and defibrillated patients who had lethal ventricular fibrillation, CCU nurses blurred the invisible boundary separating the disciplines of nursing and medicine. CCU nurses were diagnosing and treating patients in dramatic lifesaving situations. In doing so, they challenged the very definition of nursing that had been published by the ANA only a few years earlier—a definition that would later be used to question an expanded role for nursing from within the nursing profession itself (Keeling, 2004, 2007). See Exemplar 1.3.

> *We admitted them, started an IV ... checked the blood pressure every 15 minutes for one to 2 hours, and changed the electrodes.*
>
> ***(The Hartford Unit Nurses, 1963, cited in Keeling et al., 2018, p. 312)***

As a significant number of nurses graduated from CNS master's programs in the 1970s, new CNS jobs opened in hospitals across the country. These were accompanied by an emerging sense of role ambiguity and confusion as recent graduates struggled to explain their role and their effectiveness in the clinical setting. The CNS was more than a bedside nurse; he or she had high levels of clinical expertise. The CNS role included staff and patient education, unit leadership, and/or

EXEMPLAR 1.3
"BLURRING BOUNDARIES BETWEEN MEDICINE AND NURSING"

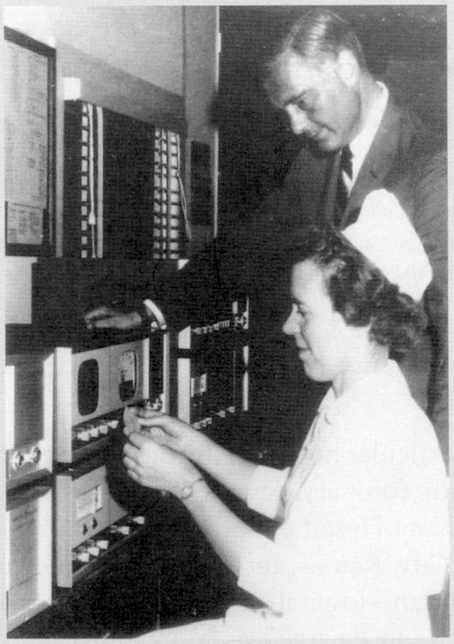

(Courtesy: Bjoring Center, UVA)

In 1962, Lawrence Meltzer, MD, of the Presbyterian Hospital in Philadelphia, proposed that the role of the nurse would be central to the new system of coronary care. Nurses would be present in the CCU round-the-clock. In July 1963, Rose Pinneo, RN, accepted the nursing leadership role in the unit. In the CCU, the nurse's clinical expertise was invaluable. As Pinneo described it:

> *Utilizing the unique combination of clinical assessment and cardiac monitoring, the nurse makes independent decisions. She determines those situations requiring her immediate intervention to save life prior to the physician's arrival or those situations that warrant calling the physician and waiting for his evaluation. It is in these precious moments that the patient's life may literally be in the hands of the nurse.*
>
> (PINNEO, 1972, p. 4)

the management of a specific population of patients (e.g., patients with diabetes who might be admitted to other hospital units for various complications) in addition to direct patient care and patient education. And, because staff nurses might envy the apparent freedom that the CNS had to come and go from a unit (to the operating room or to a clinic), they sometimes referred to the CNS as a "clipboard nurse"; that is, one who carried a clipboard of patient notes and accompanied a physician on rounds. It would take exemplary interpersonal skills as well as respect for the CNS's expertise for many of the newly minted CNSs to overcome these challenges; many simply did not (Fig. 1.7).

Organization and Evaluation

With the increase in the number of clinical nurse specialists came the need for organization at the national level. CNSs needed a voice and a means by which they could continue their education. The American Association of Critical-Care Nurses, founded in 1969 as the American Association of Cardiovascular Nurses, addressed both of these needs, as well as the nurses' desire for the opportunity to interact with their peers. Soon other specialty nurses followed their lead. Only 4 years later, a group of oncology nurses met to discuss the need for a national organization to support *their* specialty. Officially incorporated in 1975, the Oncology Nursing Society provided a forum in which nurses could discuss issues related to cancer nursing. It also provided opportunities for continuing education in the area of oncology (Lusk, 2005).

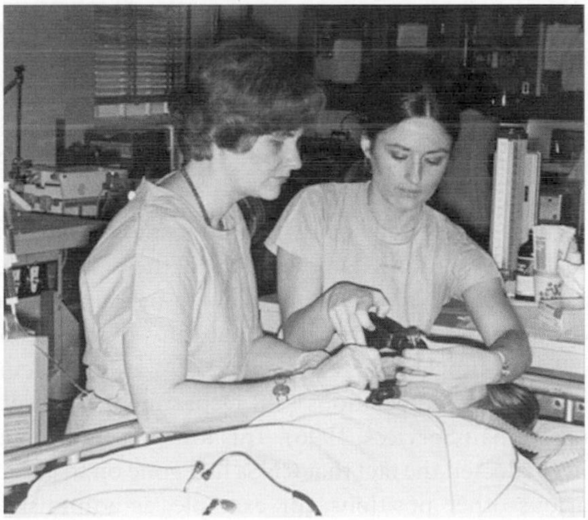

Fig. 1.7 ■ Clinical nurse specialist in cardiac unit giving oxygen. (Bjoring Center.)

The growth of these organizations was timely. In 1974 the ANA had officially recognized the CNS role, defining the CNS as an expert practitioner and change agent. The ANA also specified educational requirements for the role, identifying a master's degree as a basis for entry into CNS practice (ANA Congress of Nursing Practice, 1974). To the ANA, the CNS role was not outside the scope of nursing practice. It was a contrast to the ANA's unwillingness to include nurse anesthetists under their umbrella organization.

As with the other advanced nursing specialties of nurse anesthesia and midwifery, the development of the CNS role included early evaluation research that served to validate and promote the new role. Georgopoulos and colleagues (Georgopoulos & Christman, 1970; Georgopoulos & Sana, 1971) conducted studies evaluating the effect of CNS practice on the nursing process and outcomes in inpatient adult health-care settings. These and other studies (Ayers, 1971; Girouard, 1978) demonstrated the positive effect the CNS had on improving nursing care and patient outcomes. Moreover, with the increasing demand from society to cure illness using the latest scientific and technologic advances, hospital administrators willingly supported specialization in nursing. Many hired CNSs, particularly for their work in intensive care units.

The CNS role remained the dominant APRN role in the 1980s, with CNSs representing 42% of all APRNs (US Department of Health and Human Services, 1996). The ANA's social policy statement (ANA, 1980) clearly delineated the criteria required to assume the title of CNS and was of particular significance to the maturation of the CNS role during this decade. According to that statement:

> *The specialist in nursing practice is a nurse who, through study and supervised clinical practice at the graduate level (master's or doctorate), has become expert in a defined area of knowledge and practice in a selected clinical area of nursing. … Upon completion of a graduate program degree in*

a university graduate program with an emphasis on clinical specialization, the specialist in nursing practice should meet the criteria for specialty certification through nursing's professional society.
(ANA, 1980, p. 23)

The 1980s saw an increase in the number of CNS master's programs, research into the effectiveness of the CNS role, and concerns about the cost of employing these highly specialized nurses. By 1984, the National League for Nursing had accredited 129 programs for the preparation of CNSs. These clinically focused graduate programs were instrumental in developing and defining the CNS role, emphasizing that the role would encompass patient and staff education, direct care, and research. Concurrently, nurse researchers continued to study patient outcomes related to CNS practice. In 1987, for example, McBride and colleagues demonstrated that nursing practice, particularly in relation to documentation, improved as a result of the introduction of a CNS in an inpatient psychiatric setting. However, at about that time, healthcare cost containment raised concerns about the future of the CNS role—these highly educated nurses came with a high cost (Hamric, 1989).

Declining Demand for Clinical Nurse Specialists

By the late 1980s, many CNSs had shifted the focus of their practice away from the clinical area and instead focused on the educational and organizational aspects of the CNS role, such as orientation programs, in-service education, consultation, and administrative functions. This shift was supported by the view that CNSs were too valuable to spend their time on direct patient care (Wolff, 1984). Meanwhile, those who continued to assert that the essence of the CNS role was clinical expertise were writing on the topic (Hamric & Spross, 1983, 1989).

The increasing emphasis on cost containment during the 1980s produced legislative and economic changes that affected advanced practice nursing and the healthcare delivery system as a whole. The establishment of a prospective payment system in 1983 had a significant effect. This payment system, which used diagnosis-related groups to classify billing for hospitalized Medicare recipients, represented an effort to control rising costs by shifting reimbursement from payment for services provided to payment by case (*capitation*). As a result, hospital administrators put increasing pressure on nurses and physicians to save money by decreasing the length of time patients remained hospitalized. The emphasis on cost containment also heralded budget cuts for hospitals and the CNS role soon came under intense review. CNSs were not obviously cost-effective or overtly essential to patient care. The outcomes of the CNS role (particularly related to length of hospital stay for a patient) had not been empirically tracked. Moreover, the CNS role was poorly defined. The result was the elimination of some CNS positions by the end of the decade. The reasoning: budget cuts.

Thus the decade of the 1990s opened with decreasing employment opportunities for CNSs because of the financial problems in hospitals. Indeed, there was a need to restructure the US healthcare system to reduce costs and improve access to care. Despite the lack of job opportunities after graduation, CNS programs continued to be the most numerous of all master's nursing programs, with more than 11,000 students enrolled (National League for Nursing, 1994). The largest area of specialization was adult health–medical-surgical nursing. However, with the increasing emphasis on primary care, the rapid growth of nurse practitioner (NP) programs, the financial challenges faced by hospital administrators, and the introduction in the early 1990s of the acute care NP (ACNP) role, the number of CNS positions in hospitals continued to decline. Many nurses seeking an advanced degree entered NP programs instead.

By 1996, the National Sample Survey of Registered Nurses revealed that a significant number (7802) of CNSs had also been certified as NPs, educated to diagnose and treat health conditions. And, according to the National Sample Survey, these dual-role-prepared APRNs were more likely to be employed as NPs than as CNSs. In fact, by that time, of the 61,601 CNSs in the United States, only 23% were practicing in CNS-specific positions (US Department of Health and Human Services, 1996). This low percentage may have reflected the fact that CNSs had gone on to accept various other positions; for example, as administrators or staff educators. Others turned to academia and acquired their PhDs.

CNS Education and Reimbursement

Education for CNS practice and reimbursement for practice was complicated, in part because of the number of specialties involved and in part because of differing state laws. In many specialties, existing certification examinations were targeted to nurses who were experts by experience, not graduates of master's programs that specifically trained them for specialty practice. Thus advanced-level certification for the CNS was slow to emerge. For example, it was not until 1995 that the Oncology Nursing Society administered the first certification examination for advanced practice in oncology nursing. A further complication was that not all states recognized these examinations for APRN regulatory purposes. Organization at the national level would be key, and in 1995, the National Association of Clinical Nurse Specialists (NACNS) was formed. Soon thereafter, the Balanced Budget Act of 1997 (Balanced Budget Act, 1997) specifically identified CNSs as eligible for Medicare reimbursement. The law, providing Medicare Part B direct payment to CNSs regardless of their geographic area of practice, allowed them to be paid 85% of the fee paid to physicians for the same services. Moreover, the law's inclusion and definition of CNSs corrected the previous omission of this group from reimbursement (Safriet, 1998). The possibility of reimbursement for services was an important step in the continuing development of the CNS role; hospital administrators routinely focused on the cost of having APRNs provide patient care. By 2015 CNSs were authorized to prescribe without physician supervision in 20 states (NACNS, 2015b).

The creation of the NACNS, followed by third-party reimbursement for their services, represented two major achievements for the CNS. The NACNS developed core competencies and criteria for the evaluation of CNS graduate programs and certificates. Practice competency still varied by specialty and was overseen by 20 professional organizations, but it had to include the NACNS core competencies. In 2015 the NACNS endorsed the DNP as entry to practice for CNSs by 2030; previously they had been neutral on this question (NACNS, 2015c).

NURSE PRACTITIONERS

Early Roots of Primary Care

The early roots of what we now refer to as *primary care services* can be traced to late 19th-century urban areas of the Northeastern United States where public health nurses visited patients in their homes to assess their needs for medical care or to provide direct patient care. In Boston, the Boston Instructive District Nurses saw thousands of patients and their families; in Philadelphia, the Visiting Nurse Society met patient and family needs; and in New York, the Visiting Nurse Service of the Henry Street Settlement visited newly arrived immigrants living on the Lower East Side.

The story of the Henry Street Settlement nurses is typical. In 1893 Lillian Wald, a young graduate nurse from the New York Training School for Nurses, established the Henry Street Settlement (HSS) House on the Lower East Side of Manhattan. Its purpose was to address the needs of the poor, many of whom lived in overcrowded, rat-infested tenements. The needs of this disadvantaged immigrant community were limitless. According to one account:

> *There were nursing infants, many of them with the summer bowel complaint that sent infant mortality soaring during the hot months; there were children with measles, not quarantined; there were children with ophthalmia, a contagious eye disease; there were children scarred with vermin bites; there were adults with typhoid; … a young girl dying of tuberculosis amid the very conditions that had produced the disease.*
>
> ***(Duffus, 1938, p. 43)***

Visiting patients in their homes, the HSS nurses provided access to care to those who had none.

In addition to making home visits, the HSS nurses saw patients in the nurses' dispensary, located in the settlement house. There they treated "simple complaints and emergencies not requiring referral elsewhere." For a time, their work went unnoticed, but interprofessional conflict was inevitable. Soon, the New York Medical Society added a clause to the Nursing Registration Bill prohibiting nurses from practicing medicine. That clause would give the society an opportunity to question the HSS nurses' work and "disrupt the settlement's neighborly activities" (Buhler-Wilkerson, 2001, p. 110).

> *As the number of [HSS] ambulatory visits grew, the settlement risked attracting the unwelcome attention of the increasingly disagreeable "uptown docs."*
>
> ***(Buhler-Wilkerson, 2001, p. 110)***

To resolve the conflicts with physicians, the HSS nurses obtained standing orders from a group of Lower East Side physicians allowing the nurses to give emergency medications and treatments (Keeling, 2007). Nonetheless, conflicts with medicine surfaced again when the HHS nurses expanded their visits to areas of the city outside the Lower East Side. The situation came to a head with the collapse of the stock market in 1929, when uptown physicians saw the nurses as an economic threat. That year, the Westchester Village Medical Group accused the nurses of practicing medicine without a license. Angered by the accusation, Elizabeth MacKenzie, associate director of nurses, defended the HSS nurses in her reply:

> *My dear Dr. Black:*
> *Your letter … addressed to … the Supervisor of our Westchester Office, has been referred to me for reply. … In administering the work in that office, Miss Neary does so as a representative of the HSS Visiting Nurse Service and in accord with definite policies. … It has been the unvarying policy of the organization over the 35 years … to work in close cooperation with the medical profession doing nursing and preventive health work entirely and avoiding any semblance of the "practice of medicine" in competition with the doctors. … We will call a meeting … to which … your group will be invited for a frank discussion of our common problems.*
> *(MacKenzie, 1929)*

Although the records about this meeting are no longer available, one can assume that the meeting took place and the nurses continued to practice. Indeed, the HSS nursing service was active until the 1950s. Nonetheless, from early in the 20th century there was evidence of interprofessional conflicts whenever nurses expanded their scope of practice. There is also evidence of emerging collaboration between the professions as physicians and nurses negotiated solutions to the boundary problems. What is clear throughout is that nurses were considered "good enough" to care for the poor, whereas physicians would care for those who could pay.

Place Matters: The Frontier Nursing Service

Nurses were also deemed good enough to care for the poor in *rural* America. In addition to providing midwifery services, FNS nurses in Leslie County, Kentucky, provided care in what would later become the primary care NP role. Working out of eight clinics that covered 78 square miles in the remote mountains, the FNS nurses had considerable autonomy in providing nearly all of the primary health care for people living in that area of rural Appalachia. Nurses made diagnoses and treated patients, dispensing herbs and medicines (including morphine) with permission from their medical advisory committee. Using standing orders written by that committee, the nurses not only assisted women in childbirth but also treated a wide variety of conditions, from gunshot wounds and burns to strep throat and typhoid fever. In doing so, the nurses dispensed medicines such as aspirin, ipecac, cascara, and castor oil at their own discretion (FNS, 1948). By the late 1930s they also dispensed sulfa drugs when indicated. See Fig. 1.8.

Place Matters: Nursing in Migrant Camps and Indian Reservations

During the 1930s, when migrants from the Dust Bowl traveled to California to pick crops in the central valley, Farm Security Administration (FSA) nurses (part of President F. D. Roosevelt's New Deal program) provided most of the care the migrants received. With

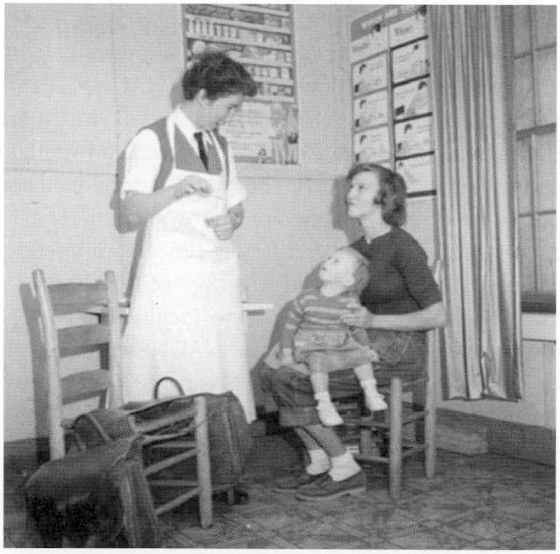

Fig. 1.8 ■ **Frontier Nursing Service well-baby check.** (Courtesy of Frontier Nursing University, Versailles KY.)

verbal approval from the camp doctor, the nurses wrote prescriptions and dispensed drugs from the clinic formulary. "They staffed well baby clinics, coordinated immunization programs … decided whether a sick migrant required referral to a physician … and provided emergency care" (Grey, 1999, p. 94).

Like the FNS nurses, FSA nurses practiced according to standing orders issued by the FSA medical offices and approved by local physicians. Essential to their practice autonomy was the tacit requirement that the patients be poor and marginalized and have little access to physician-provided medical care. Indeed, "place" mattered; when there was little access to physicians, the nurse's role expanded. See Fig. 1.9.

> *Nurses functioned pretty autonomously. They were able to do a lot of what NPs do [today] after a lot of training, but these nurses did it through experience.*
>
> ***(Grey, 1999, p. 96).***

The same requirement of little access to medical care held true for the field nurses working with the Bureau of Indian Affairs (BIA) in the first half of the 20th century. On the Navajo reservation in Arizona for example, nurses often found themselves traveling alone to see patients in their homes (hogans).

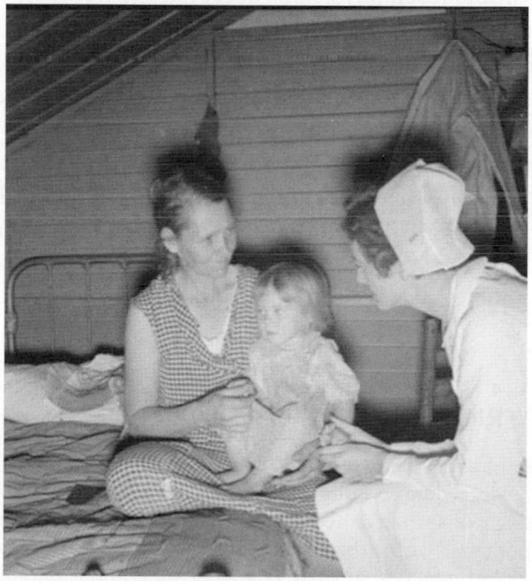

Fig. 1.9 ■ **Nurse with migrant mother.** (Courtesy Library of Congress.)

In addition to making home visits, BIA nurses were responsible for conducting well-baby "nursing conferences" under the trees as they followed nomadic tribes. The nurses' initial intent for these conferences was to teach the Navajo how to promote health and prevent disease. In actuality, these conferences became "nurse-run clinics"—Navajo mothers would arrive with sick infants and children to be seen by the nurse (Keeling, 2007).

Reporting on her work at Arizona's Teec Nos Pas in May 1931, nurse Dorothy Williams described the reality of providing much-needed care to children with ear infections, sore throats, skin infections, and other commonly occurring problems, all the while focusing in her report on the "well baby" aspects of the clinic rather than the treatments:

> *Five clinics held this week, three general and two baby clinics. Mothers bathed their babies and were given material to cut out and make gowns for baby. Preschool children were weighed, inspected, and mothers advised about diets for underweights [sic]. … Fifty treatments given.*
>
> ***(Williams, 2007, p. 139)***

Despite the minimization of treatments in her report to a supervisor in Washington, DC, it is clear that Williams was in fact providing primary care.

The Need for Primary Care in the Mid-20th Century

It was during the 1960s that the role was first described formally and implemented in outpatient pediatric clinics, originating in part as a response to a shortage of primary care physicians. As the trend toward medical specialization drew increasing numbers of physicians away from primary care, many areas of the country were designated underserved with respect to the numbers of primary care physicians. "Report after report issued by the AMA [American Medical Association] and the Association of American Medical Colleges decried the shortage of physicians in poor rural and urban areas" (Fairman, 2002, p. 163). At the same time, consumers across the nation were demanding accessible, affordable, and sensitive health care while healthcare delivery costs were increasing at an annual rate of 10% to 14% (Jonas, 1981).

The event marking the inception of the modern NP role was the establishment of the first pediatric NP (PNP) program by Loretta Ford, RN, and Henry Silver, MD, at the University of Colorado in 1965. This demonstration project, funded by the Commonwealth Foundation, was designed to prepare professional nurses to provide comprehensive well-child care and manage common childhood health problems. The 4-month program, during which certified registered nurses were educated as PNPs without requiring master's preparation, emphasized health promotion and inclusion of the family. A study evaluating the project demonstrated that PNPs were highly competent in assessing and managing 75% of well and ill children in community health settings. In addition, PNPs increased the number of patients served in private pediatric practice by 33% (Ford & Silver, 1967). Like early nurse-midwife and nurse anesthetist studies, these positive findings demonstrated support for this new nursing role. See Exemplar 1.4.

Intraprofessional Conflict Over the NP Role

The PNP role was not without significant intraprofessional controversy, particularly with regard to educational preparation. Early on, certificate programs based on the Colorado project rapidly sprang into existence. According to Ford (1991), some of these programs shifted the emphasis of PNP preparation from a nursing to a medical model. This was in contrast to the original University of Colorado demonstration project that stressed collaboration between nursing and medicine.

One of the major areas of controversy among academics was because of the fact that NPs made *medical* diagnoses and wrote prescriptions for medications, essentially stepping over the boundary between nursing and medicine outlined earlier in the century by the ANA. Because of this, some nurse educators and other nurse leaders questioned whether the NP role could be conceptualized as being within the discipline of nursing, a profession that had historically been ordered to care rather than cure (Reverby, 1987; Rogers, 1972).

Nurse theorist Martha Rogers, one of the most outspoken opponents of the NP concept, argued that the development of the NP role was a ploy to lure nurses away from nursing to medicine, thereby undermining nursing's unique role in health care (Rogers, 1972). Subsequently, nurse leaders and educators took sides for and against the establishment of educational programs for NPs in mainstream master's programs.

In 1974, a group of pro-nurse practitioner faculty, already teaching in NP programs, held their first national meeting in Chapel Hill, North Carolina. This meeting laid the foundation for the formation of the National Organization of Nurse Practitioner Faculties (NONPF). Over time, the standardization of NP educational programs at the master's level, initiated by the faculty who formed NONPF, would serve to reduce intraprofessional tension.

While nursing professors debated the discipline's responsibility to educate NPs, the NP role attracted considerable attention from health policymakers. Health policy groups such as the National Advisory Commission on Health Manpower issued statements in support of the NP concept (Moxley, 1968). At the grassroots level, physicians accepted the new role and hired NPs—they needed the help.

Early in the 1970s, the US Department of Health, Education, and Welfare Secretary Elliott Richardson established the Committee to Study Extended Roles for Nurses. This committee was charged with evaluating the feasibility of expanding nursing practice (Kalisch & Kalisch, 1986). The committee concluded that extending the scope of the nurse's role was essential to providing equal access to health care for all Americans.

EXEMPLAR 1.4

LORETTA FORD: COFOUNDER OF THE PEDIATRIC NURSE PRACTITIONER ROLE

In the 1960s in Colorado, nurse Loretta Ford and Dr. Henry Silver, a pediatrician, introduced the concept of the nurse practitioner. Both understood the potential of expanding access to health care by allowing nurses to practice to the fullest extent of advanced nursing education. The term *nurse practitioner* was coined; as Ford later explained, "We wanted to emphasize the clinical practice role" (Jacox, 2002, p. 162). According to Ford, nurse practitioners should use a nursing rather than a medical model, diagnosing and treating patients "within the context of the patient's health status, social qualities, physical characteristics, and economic realities" (Pearson, 1999, pp. 25–26).

The kind of health care Lillian Wald began preaching and practicing in 1893 is the kind the people of this country are still crying for.

(Schutt, 1971, p. 53)

The committee urged the establishment of innovative curricular designs in health science centers and increased financial support for nursing education. It also advocated standardizing nursing licensure and national certification and developing a model nurse practice law suitable for national application. In addition, the committee called for further research related to cost–benefit analyses and attitudinal surveys to assess the effect of the NP role. The report resulted in increased federal support for training programs for the preparation of several types of NPs, including family NPs, adult NPs, and emergency department NPs (Kalisch & Kalisch, 1986).

Support From Physicians

Despite the resistance to NPs within the nursing profession, physicians increasingly accepted NPs in individual healthcare practices. Working together in local practices, NPs and MDs established collegial relationships, negotiating with each other to construct work boundaries and reach agreement about their collaborative practice.

In the NP-MD dyad, negotiations centered on the NP's right to practice an essential part of traditional medicine: the process or skill set of clinical thinking … to perform a physical examination, elicit patient symptoms, … create a diagnosis, formulate treatment options, prescribe treatment and make decisions about prognosis.

(Fairman, 2002, pp. 163–164)

The proximity of a supervising physician was thought to be key to effective practice, and on-site supervision was the norm. Grassroots acceptance of the role was dependent on tight physician supervision and control of the protocols under which NPs practiced. That supervision was not without benefit to the newly certified, inexperienced NPs. According to Corene Johnson, "Initially, we had to always have a physician on site. … I didn't resent that. Actually, I needed the backup" (Fairman, 2002, p. 164). See Fig. 1.10.

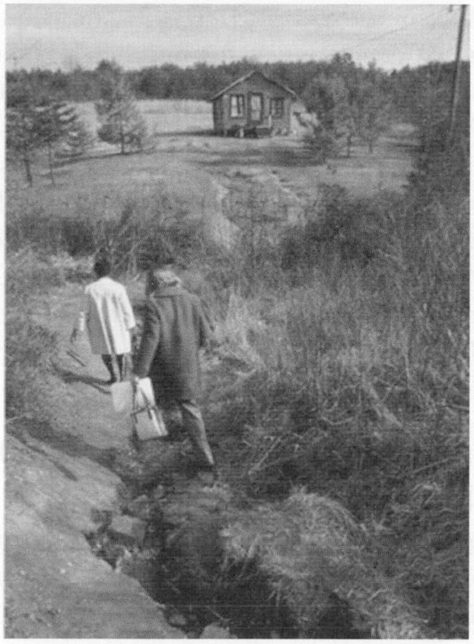

Fig. 1.10 ■ **NPs making home visit.** (Bjoring Center.)

The Concept of "Advanced Practice"

During the 1980s, the concept of advanced nursing practice began to be defined and used in the literature. In 1983 Harriet Kitzman, an associate professor at the University of Rochester, explored the interrelationships between CNSs and NPs (Kitzman, 1983). She used the term *advanced practice* throughout her discussion, applying the term not only to advanced education but also to CNS and NP practice. She noted, "Recognition for advanced practice competence is already established for both NPs and CNSs through the profession's certification programs. … advanced nursing practice cannot be setting-bound, because nursing needs are not exclusively setting-restricted" (Kitzman, 1983, pp. 284, 288). A year later, an associate professor at the University of Wisconsin–Madison, Joy Calkin, proposed a model for advanced nursing practice, specifically identifying CNSs and NPs with master's degrees as APRNs (Calkin, 1984).

During the 1980s the Council of Primary Health Care Nurse Practitioners and the Council of Clinical Nurse Specialists began to explore the commonalities of the two roles. In 1988 the councils conducted a survey of all NP and CNS graduate programs and identified considerable overlap in curricula. Subsequently, between 1988 and 1990, the two councils discussed a proposal to merge, and in 1991 the Council of Nurses in Advanced Practice was formed. Unfortunately, the merger was short-lived because of the restructuring of the ANA during the early 1990s. Nevertheless, it was an important step in the organizational coalescence of advanced practice nursing (ANA, 1991). Published in 1996, the first edition of this textbook included CRNA and CNM roles as "advanced practice nursing," reflecting an integrative vision of advanced practice. By the end of the decade, the nursing literature was increasingly using the term.

Resistance to the NP by Organized Medicine

Although physicians and NPs collaborated at the local level, organized medicine began to express its resistance to the NP role. One of the most contentious areas of interprofessional conflict involved prescriptive authority for nursing.

FACT BOX 1.6

Nurse Practitioners and Prescriptive Privileges

The fight for prescriptive authority for nurse practitioners (NPs) spanned the latter decades of the 20th century. By 1983, only Oregon and Washington granted NPs statutory, independent prescriptive authority. Other states did so with the provision that a licensed physician directly supervise the NP. How prescriptions were handled depended on the availability of the physician, negotiated boundaries of the individual physician–NP team, and the specific locality in which practice occurred. In some instances, that meant that physicians pre-signed a pad of prescriptions for the NP to use at her or his discretion; in remote area clinics, such as those in the Frontier Nursing Service, a physician might countersign NP prescriptions only once a week, and in other states the physician might write and sign a prescription at the request of the NP (Keeling, 2007). As of 2020, NPs hold prescriptive privileges in all 50 states.

As one author noted, "Nursing's efforts to obtain the legal authority to prescribe may be seen as the second chapter in the struggle over the use of the word 'diagnosing' in Nurse Practice Acts" (Hadley, 1989, p. 291). Prescriptive authority, regarded as a delegated medical act, was dependent on NPs' legal right to provide treatment. In 1971 Idaho became the first state to recognize diagnosis and treatment as part of the scope of practice of specialty nurses (Idaho Code § 54-1413, 1971). However, "As path-breaking as the statute was, it was still rather restrictive in that any acts of diagnosis and treatment had to be authorized by rules and regulations promulgated by the Idaho State Boards of Medicine and Nursing" (Safriet, 1992, p. 445). Moreover, the Drug Enforcement Act required that practitioners wishing to prescribe controlled substances obtain US Drug Enforcement Administration (DEA) registration numbers, and only those practitioners with broad prescriptive authority (e.g., physicians and dentists) could obtain these numbers (DEA, 1992).

Throughout the 1980s, NPs worked tirelessly to convince state legislatures to pass laws and establish reimbursement policies that would support their practice. Interprofessional conflicts with organized medicine, and to a lesser extent with pharmacists, centered on control issues and the degree of independence the NP was allowed. These conflicts intensified as NPs moved beyond the physician extender model to a more autonomous one. In a seminal case, Sermchief v. Gonzales (1983), the Missouri medical board charged two women's healthcare NPs with practicing medicine without a license (Doyle & Meurer, 1983). The initial ruling was against the NPs but, on appeal, the Missouri Supreme Court overturned the decision, concluding that the scope of practice of APRNs could evolve without statutory constraints (Wolff, 1984). In essence, this case provided a model for new state nurse practice acts to address issues related to APRN practice with very generalized wording, a change that allowed for expansion in the roles and functions of APRNs.

FACT BOX 1.7

Access to Cost-Effective, Quality Health Care for All Americans

In 1986, a government report titled *Nurse Practitioners, Physician Assistants and Certified Nurse-Midwives: A Policy Analysis* concluded that "within their areas of competence" NPs and CNMs provided care whose quality was "equivalent to that of care provided by physicians" (Office of Technology Assessment, 1986). Unfortunately, at the same time the report was published, the American Medical Association House of Delegates, threatened by the possibility of competition from advanced practice registered nurses, passed a resolution to "oppose any attempt at empowering nonphysicians to become unsupervised primary care providers and be directly reimbursed" (Safriet, 1992).

Growth, Organization, and Legislation

Significant growth in the numbers of NPs in practice and national organizations characterized the latter part of the 20th century. The number of NPs increased immeasurably during this time as new types of NPs developed, the most significant of which were the emergency NP, neonatal NP, family NP, and the acute care nurse practitioner. By 1984, approximately 20,000 graduates of NP programs were employed, for the most part, in settings "that the founders envisioned" (Kalisch & Kalisch, 1986, p. 715): outpatient clinics, health maintenance organizations, health departments, community health centers, rural clinics, schools, occupational health clinics, and private offices. By the late 1980s, however, based on their success in neonatal intensive care units, NPs with specialty preparation were increasingly being used in tertiary care centers (Silver & McAtee, 1988).

During this period, the multiple roles for NPs created competing interests that would affect their ability to speak with one voice on legislative issues. In an attempt to rectify this situation, the ANA established the Primary Health Care Nurse Practitioner Council. At about the same time, the American Academy of Nurse Practitioners was established in 1985 as the first organization for NPs from all specializations. In 1995 a competing NP organization was formed to serve as a "SWAT team" on policy during President Clinton's healthcare reform initiative. Named the American College of Nurse Practitioners, the new organization was seen as an umbrella organization to bring all the NP organizations together.

In the early 1990s, federal legislation regulating narcotics in the Controlled Substances Act would be of major significance to NP progress in implementing prescriptive authority. As NPs began to gain prescriptive authority for controlled substances in different states, they required a parallel authority granted by the DEA. In 1991 the DEA first responded to this situation by proposing registration for "affiliated practitioners" (DEA, 1992). This proposal called for those NPs who had prescriptive authority pursuant to a practice protocol or collaborative practice agreement to be assigned a registration number for controlled substances tied to the number of the physician with whom they worked. The proposal received much criticism specifically related to the restriction of access to health care and the legal liability of the prescribers. As a result, it was revoked in 1992. Later that year, the DEA amended its regulations by adding a category of "mid-level providers" (MLPs), who would be issued individual provider DEA numbers as long as they were granted prescriptive authority by the state in which they practiced. The MLP's number would begin with an M for mid-level provider, rather than an A or B. The MLP provision took effect in 1993, significantly expanding NPs' ability to prescribe (DEA,1993).

Neonatal and Acute Care Nurse Practitioners

One of the newer types of NPs to emerge was the neonatal NP. Originating in the late 1970s in response to a shortage of neonatologists coinciding with restrictions in the total time pediatric residents could devote to neonatal intensive care, the neonatal NP was the forerunner of the acute care NP of the 1990s. These highly skilled, experienced neonatal nurses assumed a wide range of new responsibilities formerly undertaken by pediatric residents, including interhospital transport of critically ill infants and newborn resuscitation (Clancy & Maguire, 1995).

Like the earlier neonatal NP role, the adult acute care NP (ACNP) role grew in response to residency shortages in intensive care units and new policies limiting the resident physicians to 80 hours per week. In addition, increasingly complicated tertiary care systems lacked coordination of patient care. Advanced practice nurses responded quickly to this need, building on the earlier work of Silver and McAtee (1988) to create a role that promoted quality patient care and nursing's leadership in healthcare delivery (Daly, 1997). University of Pennsylvania professors Anne Keane and Therese Richmond were among those who documented the emergence of the ACNP, referring to it at first as "The Tertiary NP" (TNP):

> *The TNP is an advanced practice nurse educated at the master's level with ... a focus on complex patients. ... The TNP can provide clinically expert specialized care in a holistic manner in a system that is often typified by fragmentation, lack of communication among medical specialists, and a loss of recognition of the patient and patient's needs as central to the care delivered .*
>
> ***(Keane & Richmond, 1993, p. 282).***

From 1992 to 1995, acute care nurse practitioner (ACNP) tracks in master's programs proliferated across the country. Soon, questions abounded concerning the content of the curriculum. To resolve these, educators met annually at ACNP consensus conferences, beginning in 1993. The ANA's Credentialing Center administered the first ACNP certification examination in December 1995. By 1997, there were 43 programs nationwide that prepared ACNPs at the master's or post-master's level (Kleinpell, 1997). In 2002 the ACNPs formally merged with the American Academy of Nurse Practitioners, with the goal of uniting primary care NPs and ACNPs under an umbrella organization. By this time, ACNPs were employed in multiple specialties, including cardiology, cardiovascular surgery, neurosurgery, emergency and trauma, internal medicine, and radiology services (Daly, 2002).

At the turn of the 21st century, the growth in the number of NP programs, an increase in prescriptive authority for NPs, and increasing practice autonomy converged to make the NP role enticing, and increasing numbers of nurses chose the NP role. The problem was that there were a number of organizations speaking for the various types of NPs. The American Academy of Nurse Practitioners continued to be active after the American College of Nurse Practitioners was founded in 1995. In addition, PNPs formed the National Association of Pediatric Nurse Associates and Practitioners (NAPNAP), and nurses interested in women's health issues formed the Association of Women's Health, Obstetric and Neonatal Nurses (AWHONN). These groups soon offered their own certification examinations, in competition with those offered by the ANA's Credentialing Center. One thing that they did agree on, however, was education for practice. In August 1993, representatives of 63 of 66 organizations attending a national nursing summit agreed to require master's education for the NP role (Cronenwett, 1995). In 2013 the American Academy of Nurse Practitioners and the American College of Nurse Practitioners merged to form the American Association of Nurse Practitioners (AANP, 2013a).

Nurse Practitioner Education

During the 1990s, the number of NPs increased dramatically in response to increasing demand, the national emphasis on primary care, and the concomitant decrease in the number of medical residencies in the subspecialties. In 1990 there were 135 master's degree and 40 certificate NP programs. Between 1992 and 1994, the number of institutions offering NP education more than doubled, from 78 to 158. In 1994 most institutions offered several tracks, which led to a total of 384 NP tracks in master's programs throughout the United States. By 1998, the number of institutions offering NP education again doubled, representing a total of 769 distinct NP specialty tracks (AACN, 1999; NONPF, 1997). Most of these programs were at the master's or post-master's level. In 2013 the number of institutions offering a master's NP degree was 368, and 92 colleges offered a postbaccalaureate DNP (AACN, 2015).

Since 2015, there has been rapid growth in the number of DNP programs for NP education nationwide. According to the DNP Directory, in 2020 there were 357 DNP programs, with more than 106 new programs in the planning stage (AACN, 2020). Clearly, the trend nationwide is toward the DNP as the requirement for NP practice.

CONCLUSION

Throughout their history APRNs have provided access to care for the underserved in both urban and rural areas. Indeed, place mattered when it came to the acceptance of their work in expanded roles. HSS visiting nurses cared for poor immigrants of the Lower East Side of New York City, FNS nurses diagnosed and treated patients in remote areas of Appalachia with the full approval of the physician committee who supervised them, and FSA nurses cared for migrants from the Dust Bowl in the Great Depression. At the battlefront in France in World War I and in Africa and Northern Italy in World War II, nurse anesthetists supported surgeons in the operating room, their role expanding as needed, in many cases to include functions that had typically been in the realm of medicine. In other cases, in newly developed intensive care units, nurses expanded their scope of practice by giving emergency treatments to patients before physicians could respond to their calls for help (Keeling, 2004).

Throughout their history, the expansion of APRN scope of practice has met both resistance and support within the nursing profession and with organized medicine. When APRNs threatened physicians' practice and income, organized medicine accused them of practicing medicine without a license. Moreover, organized nursing itself was responsible for resisting the expansion of the scope of practice of nursing, particularly when nursing leaders considered that APRN practice was a threat to nursing's traditional role. What is also clear is that APRNs have skillfully navigated intra- and interprofessional challenges, particularly at the grassroots level. In hospital settings and clinics throughout the nation, nurses and physicians worked collaboratively to provide quality patient care.

Key to APRNs' success was the creation and maintenance of education standards and certification requirements. As educational programs moved from informal, institutionally based models with a strong apprenticeship approach to more formalized graduate education programs, the credibility of APRN roles has increased. State regulations also influenced advanced nursing practice as an increasing number of states mandated a master's degree as a prerequisite for APRN licensure.

National organization has been key to progress for advanced practice nursing, and the societal effects of war have served as a catalyst to its development. Finally, economic changes, particularly in relation to healthcare financing, have had a powerful effect on the development of advanced practice nursing. The dramatic growth of managed care systems in the 1990s, in particular, presented new challenges and opportunities for APRNs related to reimbursement, scope of practice, and autonomy (Safriet, 1998). Since then, the Patient Protection and Affordable Care Act (2010) and national crisis such as the COVID-19 pandemic have led to an increased need for APRN services (ANA 2016; Lathrop & Hodnicki, 2014).

With unremitting changes in nursing and health care, it is apparent that APRN specialties will continue to evolve and diversify. What remains to be seen is whether the profession can unite on issues related to the definition of advanced practice nursing and standardized criteria for educational preparation to ensure that APRNs are permitted to practice with the autonomy experienced by other professionals. If that can be done, as the 2011 Institute of Medicine's *The Future of Nursing* report suggested, APRNs will make a significant contribution to the transformation of health care in the 21st century.

KEY SUMMARY POINTS

- APRNs have cared for underserved, impoverished patients in rural and urban areas of the nation. However, when that care competes with physicians' reimbursement for their services, organized medicine and their supporters resist, particularly in state legislative bodies, which results in interprofessional conflict.
- Documentation of the outcomes of practice helped establish the earliest nursing specialties and continues to be of critical importance to the survival of APRN practice.
- The efforts of national professional organizations, national certification, and the move toward graduate education as a requirement for advanced practice have been critical to enhancing the credibility of advanced practice nursing.
- Intraprofessional and interprofessional resistance to expanding the boundaries of the nursing discipline has occurred throughout history.
- Time and place mattered: Societal forces, including wars, the economic climate, and healthcare policy, have influenced APRN history.

REFERENCES

ACNM/ACOG/NAACOG. (1975). Joint statement on maternity care (Adopted 1/14/71). *J Nurse Midwifery, 20*, 15.

Adams Hampton, I. (1893). *Nursing. Its principles and practice for hospital and private use.* Philadelphia: Saunders.

American Association of Colleges of Nursing (AACN). (1999). *Enrollment and graduations in baccalaureate and graduate programs in nursing.* Washington, DC: Author.

American Association of Colleges of Nursing (AACN). (2015). Re-envisioning the clinical education of advanced practice registered nurses. Retrieved from https://www.aacn.nche.edu/aacn-publications/white-papers/APRN-Clinical-Education.pdf

American Association of Colleges of Nursing (AACN). (2020). DNP fact sheet. Retrieved from http://www.aacnnursing.org/News-Information/Fact-Sheets/DNP-Fact-Sheet

American Association of Nurse Anesthesiology (AANA). (2007). *AANA announces support of doctorate for entry into nurse anesthesia practice by 2025.* Park Ridge, IL: Author.

American Association of Nurse Anesthesiology (AANA). (2017). Certified Registered Nurse Anesthetists Fact Sheet. Retrieved from https://www.aana.com/membership/become-a-crna/crna-fact-sheet#:~:text=As%20of%20September%202020%2C%20there,degrees%20for%20entry%20into%20practice

American Association of Nurse Anesthesiology (AANA). (2020). Become a CRNA. See: www.aana.com/membership/become-a-crna/education

American Association of Nurse Practitioners (AANP). (2013a). About AANP. Retrieved from https://www.aanp.org/about-aanp

American Association of Nurse Practitioners (AANP). (2013b). Federal legislation. Fact sheet: Medicare reimbursement. Retrieved from https://www.aanp.org/practice/reimbursement/68-articles/325-medicare-reimbursement

American College of Nurse-Midwives (ACNM). (1978a). *Definition of a certified nurse-midwife*. Washington, DC: Author.

American College of Nurse-Midwives (ACNM). (1978b). *Philosophy*. Washington, DC: Author.

American College of Nurse-Midwives (ACNM). (2007). *News release: Pennsylvania midwives are granted prescriptive authority*. Washington, DC: Author.

American College of Nurse-Midwives (ACNM). (2012). Position statement. Midwifery education and the Doctor of Nursing Practice. Retrieved from http://www.midwife.org/Position-Statements-List

American Nurses Association (ANA). (1955). ANA board approves a definition of nursing practice. *American Journal of Nursing, 5*, 1474.

American Nurses Association (ANA). (1980). *Nursing: A social policy statement*. Kansas City, MO: Author.

American Nurses Association (ANA). (1991). *Report of the Congress on Nursing Practice to ANA Board of Directors on the merger of the Council of Clinical Nurse Specialists and the Council of Primary Health Care Nurse Practitioners into the Council of Nurses*. Washington, DC: Author.

American Nurses Association (ANA). (2016). Policy makers on the effective utilization of advanced practice registered nurses (APRNs). Retrieved from http://www.nursingworld.org/especiallyforyou/advancedpracticenurses/

American Nurses Association Congress for Nursing Practice. (1974). *Definition: Nurse practitioner, nurse clinician and clinical nurse specialist*. Kansas City, MO: American Nurses Association.

Ayers, R. (1971). Effects and development of the role of the clinical nurse specialist. In R. Ayers (Ed.), *The clinical nurse specialist: An experiment in role effectiveness and role development* (pp. 32–49). Duarte, CA: City of Hope National Medical Center.

Balanced Budget Act of 1997. Pub. L. No. 105-33 (1997).

Bankert, M. (1989). *Watchful care: A history of America's nurse anesthetists*. New York: Continuum.

Beeber, L. S. (1990). To be one of the boys: Aftershocks of the WWI nursing experience. *Advances in Nursing Science, 12*, 32–43.

Bell, P. L. (1993). "Making do" with the midwife. Arkansas's Mamie O. Hale in the 1940s. *Nursing History Review, 1*, 155–169.

Bhan v. NME Hospitals, Inc., et al. 772 F.2d 1467 (9th Cir. 1985).

Bigbee, J., & Amidi-Nouri, A. (2000). History and evolution of advanced nursing practice. In A. B. Hamric, J. A. Spross, & C. M. Hanson (Eds.), *Advanced nursing practice: An integrative approach* (2nd ed.) (pp. 3–32). Philadelphia: W. B. Saunders.

Breckinridge, M. (1981). *Wide neighborhoods: A story of the Frontier Nursing Service*. Lexington: University Press of Kentucky.

Buhler-Wilkerson, K. (2001). *No place like home: A history of nursing and home care in the United States*. Baltimore: Johns Hopkins University Press.

Burst, H. V., & Thompson, J. E. (2003). Genealogic origins of nurse-midwifery education programs in the United States. *Journal of Midwifery and Women's Health, 48*, 464–472.

Calkin, J. D. (1984). A model for advanced nursing practice. *Journal of Nursing Administration, 14*, 24–30.

Carmel, R. (2015). *Over the Drape: Olive Berger and Blue Baby Anesthesia: 1944–1954*, University of Virginia PhD dissertation.

Chalmers-Frances v. Nelson. 6 Cal.2d 402 (1936).

Clancy, G. T., & Maguire, D. (1995). Advanced practice nursing in the neonatal intensive care unit. *Critical Care Nursing Clinics of North America, 7*, 71–76.

Clark Hine, D. (2011). Taking care of bodies, babies, and business. Black women health professionals in South Carolina, 1895–1954. In E. A. Payne (Ed.), *Writing women's history* (pp. 117–141). Jackson: University Press of Mississippi.

Cockerham, A. Z. (2019). The history of midwifery in the United States. In T. King, M. Brucker, K. Osborne, & C. Jevitt (Eds.), *Varney's midwifery* (6th edition) (pp. 1–24). Burlington, MA: Jones & Bartlett.

Cockerham, A. Z., & Keeling, A. (2010). Finance and faith at the Catholic Maternity Institute, Santa Fe, New Mexico, 1944–1969. *Nursing History Review, Vol 18*, 151–166.

Cockerham, A. Z., & Keeling, A. W. (2012). *Rooted in the mountains, reaching to the world: Stories of nursing and midwifery at Kentucky's Frontier School*. Louisville, KY: Butler Books.

Council on Accreditation for Nurse Anesthesia Programs. (2015). Standards for accreditation of nurse anesthesia programs practice doctorate. Retrieved from http://home.coa.us.com/accreditation/Pages/Accreditation-Policies,-Procedures-and-Standards.aspx

Critchley, D. L (1985). Evolution of the role. In D. L. Critchley, & J. T. Maurin (Eds.), *The clinical specialist in psychiatric mental health nursing* (pp. 5–22). New York: John Wiley.

Cronenwett, L. R. (1995). Modeling the future of advanced practice nursing. *Nursing Outlook, 43*, 112–118.

Daly, B. (1997). *The acute care nurse practitioner*. New York: Springer.

Daly, B. (2002). ACNP 2002: "Where we've been and where we're going." Keynote address, April 2002. In *ACNP Consensus Conference*. Original manuscript, the Keeling Collection, Bjoring Center, University of Virginia, Charlottesville, VA.

Dewitt, K. (1900). Specialties in nursing. *American Journal of Nursing, 1*, 14–17.

Diers, D. (1991). Nurse-midwives and nurse anesthetists: The cutting edge in specialist practice. In L. H. Aiken, & C. M. Fagin (Eds.), *Charting nursing's future: Agenda for the 1990s* (pp. 159–180). New York: J. B. Lippincott.

Dock, L. L., & Stewart, I. M. (1938). *A short history of nursing* (4th edition). New York: Putnam.

Doyle, E., & Meurer, J. (1983). Missouri legislation and litigation: Practicing medicine without a license. *Nurse Practitioner, 8*, 41–44.

Drug Enforcement Administration (DEA). (1992, July 29). Rules – prior to 1998. Definition and registration of mid-Level practitioners. 21 CFR Parts 1301 and 1304. *Federal Register. (57)* 146 (p. 33465). Retrieved from: https://www.deadiversion.usdoj.gov/fed_regs/rules/prior_1998/fr0729_1992.htm

Drug Enforcement Agency (DEA). (1993, June 1). Definition and registration of mid-level practitioners. *Federal Register*. (58)103 (p. 31171). Retrieved from: https://www.deadiversion.usdoj.gov/fed_regs/rules/prior_1998/fr0601_1993.htm

Duffus, R. L. (1938). *Lillian Wald: Neighbor and crusader*. New York: Macmillan.

Fairman, J. (2002). The roots of collaborative practice: Nurse practitioner pioneers' stories. *Nursing History Review, 10*, 159–174.

Ford, L. C. (1991). Advanced nursing practice: Future of the nurse practitioner. In L. H. Aiken, & C. M. Fagin (Eds.), *Charting nursing's future: Agenda for the 1990s* (pp. 287–299). New York: J. B. Lippincott.

Ford, L. C., & Silver, H. K. (1967). The expanded role of the nurse in child care. *Nursing Outlook, 15*, 43–45.

Frank et al. v. South et al. 175 Ky. 416–428 (1917).

Frontier Nursing Service. (1948). *Medical routines*. Lexington: University of Kentucky, Frontier Nursing Service Collection.

Georgopoulos, B. S., & Christman, L. (1970). The clinical nurse specialist: A role model. *American Journal of Nursing, 70*, 1030–1039.

Georgopoulos, B. S., & Sana, M. (1971). Clinical nursing specialization and intershift report behavior. *American Journal of Nursing, 71*, 538–545.

Girouard, S. (1978). The role of the clinical nurse specialist as change agent: An experiment in preoperative teaching. *International Journal of Nursing Studies, 15*, 57–65.

Glass, L. (2009). *Leading the way, the University of Minnesota School of Nursing 1909–2009*. Minneapolis: University of Minnesota.

Grey, M. (1999). *New Deal medicine: The rural health programs of the Farm Security Administration*. Baltimore: Johns Hopkins University.

Hadley, E. (1989). Nurses and prescriptive authority: A legal and economic analysis. *American Journal of Law and Medicine, 15*(213), 245–299.

Hamric, A. B. (1989). History and overview of the CNS role. In A. B. Hamric, & J. A. Spross (Eds.), *The clinical nurse specialist in theory and practice* (2nd ed.). (pp. 3–18). Philadelphia: W. B. Saunders.

Hamric, A. B., Lindbak, S., Jaubert, S., & Worley, D. (1998). Outcomes associated with advanced nursing practice prescriptive authority. *Journal of the American Academy of Nurse Practitioners, 10*, 113–118.

Hamric, A. B., & Spross, J. (Eds.). (1983). *The clinical nurse specialist in theory and practice*. New York: Grune & Stratton.

Hamric, A. B., & Spross, J. A. (Eds.). (1989). *The clinical nurse specialist in theory and practice* (2nd ed.). Philadelphia: W. B. Saunders.

Horton, B. J. (2007a). Education news. Upgrading nurse anesthesia educational requirements (1933–2006). Part 1: Setting standards. *Journal of the American Association of Nurse Anesthetists, 75*(3), 167–170.

Horton, B. J. (2007b). Education news. Upgrading nurse anesthesia educational requirements (1933–2006). Part 2: Curriculum, faculty and students. *Journal of the American Association of Nurse Anesthetists, 75*(4), 247–251.

Idaho Code § 54-1413. (1971).

Institute of Medicine (US). Committee on the Robert Wood Johnson Foundation Initiative on the Future of Nursing. (2011). *The future of nursing: Leading change, advancing health*. Washington, DC: National Academies Press.

Jacox, A. (2002). Dr. Loretta Ford's observations on nursing's past and future. *Nursing and Health Policy Review, 1*(2), 153–164.

Jolly, E. (1927). *Nuns of the battlefield*. Providence, RI: Providence Visitor Press.

Jonas, S. (1981). *Health care delivery in the United States*. New York: Springer.

Kalisch, P. A., & Kalisch, B. J. (1986). *The advance of American nursing* (2nd ed.). Boston: Little, Brown and Company.

Keane, A., & Richmond, T. (1993). Tertiary nurse practitioners. *Image: Journal of Nursing Scholarship, 25*, 281–284.

Keeling, A. (2004). Blurring the boundaries between medicine and nursing: Coronary care nursing, circa the 1960s. *Nursing History Review, 12*, 139–164.

Keeling, A. (2007). *Nursing and the privilege of prescription*. Columbus: Ohio State University Press.

Keeling, A. (2014). *The nurses of Mayo Clinic: Caring Healers*. Rochester, MN: Mayo Clinic.

Keeling, A., Hehman, M., & Kirchgessner, J. (2018). *History of professional nursing in the United States: Toward a culture of health*. New York: Springer Publishing.

Kinser, P. (2011). "We were all in it together": Medicine and nursing in the 8th Evacuation Hospital, 1942–1945. Windows in Time (Newsletter of University of Virginia School of Nursing Center for Historical Inquiry), 7–13. Retrieved March 3, 2022 from: https://www nursing.virginia.edu/media/UVASON_CNHI_Windows_F2011_web.pdf

Kitzman, H. J. (1983). The CNS and the nurse practitioner. In A. B. Hamric, & J. A. Spross (Eds.), *The clinical nurse specialist in theory and practice* (pp. 275–290). New York: Grune & Stratton.

Kleinpell, R. M. (1997). Acute care nurse practitioners: Roles and practice profiles. *AACN Clinical Issues, 8*, 156–162.

Lathrop, B., & Hodnicki, D. R. (2014). The Affordable Care Act: Primary care and the doctor of nursing practice nurse. *Online Journal of Issues in Nursing, 19*(2).

Litoff, J. B. (1978). *American midwives: 1860 to the present*. Westport, CT: Greenwood Press.

Lusk, B. (2005). Prelude to specialization: US cancer nursing, 1920–1950. *Nursing Inquiry, 12*(4), 269–277.

Lynaugh, J. E., & Fairman, J. (1992). New nurses, new spaces: A preview of the AACN history study. *American Journal of Critical Care, 1*(1), 19–24.

MacKenzie, E. (1929). *Report of the associate director, Henry Street Visiting Nurses Service, December 15, 1928–January 15, 1929. Lillian Wald Collection*. New York: Columbia University.

Magaw, A. (1900). Observations on 1,092 cases of anesthesia from January 1, 1899 to January 1, 1900. *St. Paul's Medical Journal*, 306–311.

Mayo School of Health Sciences Alumni Connection Magazine. Fall, 2009. Pg 6. Retrieved from https://mcforms.mayo.edu/mc4100-mc4199/mc4192-1109.pdf

McBride, A. B., Austin, J. K., Chestnut, E. E., Main, C. S., Richards, B. S., & Roy, B. A. (1987). Evaluation of the impact of the clinical nurse specialist in a state psychiatric hospital. *Archives of Psychiatric Nursing, 1*, 55–61.

McGarrel, A. (1934). *Transcript on appeal, volume 1. William Chalmers-Francis and the Anesthesia Section of the LA County Medical Association v. Dagmar A. Nelson and St. Vincent's Hospital*. Chicago: AANA Executive Office, Historical Files.

Moxley, J. (1968). The predicament in health manpower. *American Journal of Nursing, 68*, 1489–1492.

National Association of Clinical Nurse Specialists. (2015a). CNS prescriptive authority by state. Retrieved from http://www.nacns.org/docs/toolkit/5-AuthorityTable.pdf

National Association of Clinical Nurse Specialists. (2015b). More clinical nurse specialists now able to practice, prescribe without physician supervision. Retrieved from http://www.nacns.org/docs/PR-PrescriptiveAuthority1512.pdf

National Association of Clinical Nurse Specialists. (2015c). NACNS position statement on the Doctor of Nursing Practice. Retrieved from http://www.nacns.org/docs/DNP-Statement1507.pdf

National League for Nursing. (1984). *Master's education in nursing: Route to opportunities in contemporary nursing, 1984–1985*. New York: Author.

National League for Nursing. (1994). *Graduate education in nursing, advanced practice nursing*. New York: Author.

National Organization of Nurse Practitioner Faculties. (1997). *Criteria for evaluation of nurse practitioner programs*. Washington, DC: National Task Force on Quality Nurse Practitioner Education.

News here and there. (1942). American Association of Nurse-Midwives. *American Journal of Nursing, 42*, 832.

Noyes, C. D. (1912). The midwifery problem. *American Journal of Nursing, 12*, 466–471.

Nurse Training Act of 1964. Pub. L. No. 88-581 (1964).

Office of Technology Assessment. (1986). *Nurse practitioners, physician assistants and certified nurse-midwives: A policy analysis*. Washington, DC: Author.

Oltz v. St. Peter's Community Hospital. CV 81-271-H-Res (D. Mont. 1986).

Pearson, L. (1999). Editor's memo. Lessons from a leader…Loretta Ford. *The Nurse Practitioner, 24*(11), 21. 25, 26.

Peplau, H. E. (1952). *Interpersonal relations in nursing: A conceptual frame of reference for psychodynamic nursing*. New York: Putnam.

Peplau, H. E. (1965). Specialization in professional nursing. *Nursing Science, 3*, 268–287.

Pinneo, R. (1972). Mastering monitoring. *Nursing, 72*(2), 22–25.

Pougiales, J. (June 1970). The first anesthetizers at the Mayo Clinic. *Journal of the American Association of Nurse Anesthetists, 38*(3), 235–241.

Reiter, F. (1966). The nurse-clinician. *American Journal of Nursing, 66*, 274–280.

Reverby, S. M. (1987). *Ordered to care: The dilemma of American nursing* (pp. 1850–1945). New York: Cambridge University Press.

Richards, L. (1911). *Reminiscences of America's first trained nurse*. Boston: Whitcomb and Barrows.

Rogers, M. E. (1972). Nursing: To be or not to be. *Nursing Outlook, 20*, 42–46.

Rooks, J. (1997). *Midwifery and childbirth in America*. Philadelphia: Temple University Press.

Rude, AE. (1923). The midwife problem in the United States. *J Amer Med Assoc, 81*, 987–992.

Safriet, B. J. (1992). Health care dollars and regulatory sense: The role of advance practice nursing. *Yale Journal on Regulation, 9*, 417–488.

Safriet, B. J. (1998). Still spending dollars, still searching for sense: Advanced practice nursing in an era of regulatory and economic turmoil. *Advanced Practice Nursing Quarterly, 4*, 24–33.

Schindler, F. (1942). Nursing in electro-shock therapy. *American Journal of Nursing, 42*, 858–861.

Schutt, B (1971). A prophet honored. Lillian D. *American Journal of Nursing, 71*, 53.

Sermchief v. Gonzales. 660 S.W.2d 683 (1983).

Silver, H. K., & McAtee, P. (1988). Speaking out: Should nurses substitute for house staff? *American Journal of Nursing, 88*, 1671–1673.

Smith, S. (1994). White nurses, Black midwives, and public health in Mississippi, 1920–1950. *Nursing History Review, 2*, 29–49.

Summers, V. (1938). Saddle bag and log cabin technic: The Frontier Nursing Service. *Inc. American Journal of Nursing, 38*, 1183–1188.

Superintendent's report, December 1942, "Flint–Goodridge Hospital of Dillard University," pp. 1–47. https://archive.org/stream/1942flin-goodridgesuperintendentsreport/1942

Thatcher, V. S. (1953). *A history of anesthesia: With emphasis on the nurse specialist*. Philadelphia: J. B. Lippincott.

US Congress. (1964). *House Committee on Interstate and Foreign Commerce, Subcommittee on Public Health and Safety, Nurse Training Act of 1964*. Washington DC: Government Printing Office.

US Department of Health and Human Services, Health Resources and Services Administration, National Center for Health Workforce Analysis. (1996). *The registered nurse population, findings from the National Sample Survey of Registered Nurses*. Rockville, MD.

Varney, H., & Thompson, J. B. (2016). *The midwife said fear not. A history of midwifery in the United States*. New York: Springer.

Waisel, D. (2001). The role of World War II and the European theater of operations in the development of anesthesiology as a physician specialty in the USA. *Anesthesiology, 94*, 907–912.

Williams, D. (2007). Field nurses' narrative report, May 1931. In A. Keeling (Ed.), *Nursing and the privilege of prescription, 1893–2000* (pp. 72–97). Columbus: Ohio State University Press.

Wolff, M. A. (1984). Court upholds expanded practice roles for nurses. *Journal of Law, Medicine and Ethics, 12*, 26–29.

2 CONCEPTUALIZATIONS OF ADVANCED PRACTICE NURSING

CYNTHIA ARSLANIAN-ENGOREN

"Every artist was first an amateur."
~ Ralph Waldo Emerson

CHAPTER CONTENTS

NATURE, PURPOSES, AND COMPONENTS OF CONCEPTUAL MODELS 33
CONCEPTUALIZATIONS OF ADVANCED PRACTICE NURSING: PROBLEMS AND IMPERATIVES 34
CONCEPTUALIZATIONS OF ADVANCED PRACTICE NURSING ROLES: ORGANIZATIONAL PERSPECTIVES 37
Consensus Model for Advanced Practice Registered Nurse Regulation 37
American Nurses Association 40
American Association of Colleges of Nursing 41
National Organization of Nurse Practitioner Faculties 42
National Association of Clinical Nurse Specialists 42
American Association of Nurse Anesthesiology 43
American College of Nurse-Midwives 45
International Organizations and Conceptualizations of Advanced Practice Nursing 45
Section Summary: Implications for Advanced Practice Nursing Conceptualizations 46
CONCEPTUALIZATIONS OF THE NATURE OF ADVANCED PRACTICE NURSING 47
Hamric's Integrative Model of Advanced Practice Nursing 48
Conceptual Models of APRN Practice: United States Examples 49
Conceptual Models of APRN Practice: International Examples 57
Section Summary: Implications for Advanced Practice Nursing Conceptualizations 61
MODELS USEFUL FOR ADVANCED PRACTICE NURSES IN THEIR PRACTICE 61
Advanced Practice Nursing Transitional Care Models 61
Dunphy and Winland-Brown's Circle of Caring: A Transformative, Collaborative Model 62
Donabedian Structure/Process/Outcome Model 64
RECOMMENDATIONS AND FUTURE DIRECTIONS 65
Conceptualizations of Advanced Practice Nursing 65
Consensus Building Around Advanced Practice Nursing 66
Consensus on Key Elements of Practice Doctorate Curricula 67
Research on Advanced Practice Nurses and Their Contribution to Patients, Teams, and System Outcomes 67
CONCLUSION 68
KEY SUMMARY POINTS 68

Concepts, models, and theories are used by advanced practice registered nurses (APRNs) to elicit histories, perform physicals, plan treatment, evaluate outcomes, and develop interpersonal relationships, as well as to help patients and families improve their health, cope with illnesses, and die with dignity. All APRNs, regardless of their years of experience and practice, rely on common processes and language to communicate with colleagues about patient care and to explain clinical situations. As such, it is important that the nursing profession and APRNs understand the language of advanced practice nursing to communicate it to each other, clients, and stakeholders.

Understanding the conceptualization of advanced practice nursing, APRN practice, similarities and differences among APRNs, and how APRNs contribute to affordable, accessible, and effective care is central to actualizing a patient-centered, interprofessional healthcare system that maximizes patient outcomes and minimizes negative consequences. Conceptualizations of advanced practice nursing include models and theories that guide the practice of APRNs. The use of theory is fundamental to the sound progress in any practice discipline. Common language and mutually understood conceptual and theoretical frameworks support communication, guide practice, and are used to evaluate practice, education, policy, and research.

Such a foundation is essential for APRNs given the proposed changes in the US healthcare system, as seen in the Patient Protection and Affordable Care Act, 2010, the *Consensus Model for APRN Regulation* (APRN Joint Dialogue Group, 2008), and *The Future of Nursing Report 2020–2030* (National Academies of Science, Engineering and Medicine [NASEM], 2021). Other forces driving a common understanding of APRNs are the increasing numbers of programs offering the doctor of nursing practice (DNP) degree, accountable care organizations, and the promulgation of interprofessional competencies (Canadian Interprofessional Health Collaborative [CIHC], 2010; Health Professions Network Nursing and Midwifery Office, 2010; Interprofessional Education Collaborative [IPEC] Expert Panel, 2016), as well as recommendations to the United States Congress to increase funding for interprofessional education and practice (National Advisory Council on Nurse Education and Practice, 2015).

In addition to efforts in the United States, nursing associations, councils, and regulatory agencies in other countries have clarified, established, and/or regulated APRN roles and practice (Canadian Nurses Association [CNA], 2013, 2016a, 2016b; International Council of Nurses [ICN] Nurse Practitioner/Advanced Practice Nursing Network, 2020; Nursing and Midwifery Board of Australia, 2014). In countries in which APRN roles exist, in addition to studies of the distinctions among roles (Carryer et al., 2018; Gardner et al., 2013, 2016), APRN educational programs are being established, for example, in Israel (Kleinpell et al., 2014), mainland China (Wong, 2018), and Singapore (Ayre & Bee, 2014; see Chapter 5). Country-specific frameworks are being developed to clarify education, scope of practice, registration and licensing, and/or credentialing (Fagerström, 2009). Although contextual factors may differ from those in the United States, global opportunities exist for clarifying and advancing APRN practice specific to a country's culture, health system, professional standards, and regulatory requirements. A sample of conceptual and theoretical models of APRN practice from various countries is presented in this chapter along with US and international conceptualizations of APRN roles.

Professional organizations with interests in licensing, accreditation, certification, and educational (LACE) issues regarding APRNs also operate from a conceptualization of advanced practice nursing, whether implicit or explicit. In this chapter, models promulgated by APRN stakeholder organizations that describe the nature of advanced practice nursing and/or differentiate between advanced and basic practice and selected models, including international, that have guided APRN practice are discussed. Problems associated with lack of a unified definition of advanced practice and imperatives for undertaking this important work exist. When practical, consensus on advanced practice nursing models should be beneficial for patients, society, and the profession. The APRN Consensus Model (APRN Joint Dialogue Group, 2008) and core competencies of APRN practice brought needed conceptual clarity to the regulation of advanced

We wish to acknowledge the previous chapter author, Judith A. Spross, PhD, RN, FAAN, for her excellent work in previous editions.

practice nursing in the United States. However, variations in scope of practice still remain between states in the United States (Phillips, 2020) and around the world (Kleinpell et al., 2014). Additionally, work is still needed to differentiate basic and advanced nursing practice and the practice of APRNs from that of other disciplines. Therefore the purposes of this chapter are as follows:

1. Lay the foundation for thinking about the concepts underlying advanced practice nursing by describing the nature, purposes, and components of conceptual models.
2. Identify conceptual challenges in defining and operationalizing advanced practice nursing.
3. Describe selected conceptualizations of advanced practice nursing.
4. Make recommendations for assessing existing models and developing, implementing, and evaluating conceptual frameworks for advanced practice.
5. Outline future directions for conceptual work on advanced practice nursing.

It is important to note that, because of the dynamic and evolving nature of health care and nursing organizations' activities in this arena, nationally and globally, readers are encouraged to consult the websites cited in this chapter for up-to-date information.

NATURE, PURPOSES, AND COMPONENTS OF CONCEPTUAL MODELS

A conceptual model is one part of the structure of nursing knowledge. Ranging from most abstract to most concrete, this structure consists of metaparadigms, philosophies, conceptual models, theories, and empirical indicators (Fawcett & Desanto-Madeya, 2013). Traditionally, key concepts in the metaparadigm of nursing are humans, the environment, health, and nursing (Fawcett & Desanto-Madeya, 2013).

Fawcett and Desanto-Madeya (2013) described a conceptual model as

> *a set of relatively abstract and general concepts that address the phenomena of central interest to a discipline, the propositions that broadly describe these concepts, and the propositions that state relatively abstract and general relations between two or more of the concepts. (p. 13)*

In addition, they noted that a conceptual model is "a distinctive frame of reference … that tells [adherents] how to observe and interpret the phenomenon of interest to the discipline" and "provide[s] alternative ways to view the subject matter of the discipline; there is no 'best' way" (Fawcett & Desanto-Madeya, 2013, p. 13). Although there is no best way to view a phenomenon, evolving a more uniform and explicit conceptual model of advanced practice nursing benefits patients, nurses, and other stakeholders (Institute of Medicine, 2011) by facilitating communication, reducing conflict, and ensuring consistency of advanced practice nursing, when relevant and appropriate, across APRN roles, and by offering a "systematic approach to nursing research, education, administration, and practice" (Fawcett & Desanto-Madeya, 2013, p. 15).

Models may help APRNs articulate professional role identity and function, serving as a framework for organizing beliefs and knowledge about their professional roles and competencies, providing a basis for further development of knowledge. In clinical practice, APRNs use conceptual models in the delivery of their holistic, comprehensive, and collaborative care (Carron & Cumbie, 2011; Dunphy, Winland-Brown, Porter, Thomas & Gallagher, 2011; Elliott & Walden, 2015; Musker, 2011). Models may also be used to differentiate among and between levels of nursing practice—for example, between staff nursing and advanced practice nursing (Gardner et al., 2013) and between clinical nurse specialists (CNSs), nurse-midwives (CNMs), and nurse practitioners (NPs; Begley et al., 2013).

Conceptual models are also used to guide research and theory development by focusing on a given concept or examining the relationships among select concepts to elucidate testable theories. For example, Gullick and West (2016) evaluated Wenger's community of practice framework to build research capacity and productivity for CNSs and NPs in Australia. Faculty, in the preparation of students for APRN roles, use conceptual models to plan curricula, to identify important concepts and their relationships, and to make choices about course content and clinical experiences (Perraud et al., 2006; Wong et al., 2010).

Fawcett and Graham (2005) and Fawcett et al. (2004) have challenged us to think about conceptual questions of advanced practice:

- What do APRNs do that makes their practice "advanced"?
- To what extent does incorporating activities traditionally done by physicians or other healthcare professionals qualify nursing practice as "advanced"?
- Are there nursing activities that are also advanced?

Because direct clinical practice is viewed as the central APRN competency, this begs the question: What does the term *clinical* mean? Does it refer only to hospitals or clinics? These questions are becoming more important given the APRN Consensus Model and given the role that APRNs are expected to play across the continua of health care as a result of ongoing changes to healthcare legislation. From a regulatory standpoint, the emphasis on a specific population as a focus of practice will lead, when appropriate, to reconceptualizing curricula to ensure that graduates are prepared to succeed in new or revised certification examinations. Hamric (2014) has noted that although some APRN competencies (e.g., collaboration) may be performed by nurses in other roles, the expression of these competencies by APRNs is different (see Chapter 3). For example, although all nurses collaborate, APRNs are expected to lead, facilitate, and role model collaboration. In addition, a unique aspect of APRN practice is that APRNs are authorized to initiate referrals and prescribe treatments that are implemented by others (e.g., physical therapy). Innovations and reforms arising from changes in healthcare legislation will ensure that APRNs are explicitly engaged in the delivery of care across care settings, including in nursing clinics and palliative care settings, and as full participants in interprofessional teams. Changes in regulations and in the delivery of health care may be the impetus that leads to new or revised conceptualizations of advanced practice nursing (e.g., defining theoretical and evidence-based differences between the care provided by APRNs and other providers and clinical staff, the role of APRNs in interprofessional teams, and specialization and subspecialization in advanced practice nursing). Working together, nursing leaders and health policymakers will be able to design a healthcare system that delivers high-quality care at reasonable cost, based on disciplinary and interdisciplinary competencies, outcomes, effectiveness, and efficacy.

In addition to a pragmatic reevaluation of advanced practice nursing concepts based on the evolution of APRN regulation and healthcare reform, important theoretical questions are being raised about the conceptualization of advanced practice nursing. Issues range from the epistemologic, philosophic, and ontologic underpinnings of advanced practice (Arslanian-Engoren et al., 2005) and the extent to which APRNs are prepared to apply nursing theory to their practices (Algase, 2010; Arslanian-Engoren et al., 2005; Karnick, 2011) to the questions about the nature of advanced practice knowledge, discerning the differences between and among the notions of specialty, advanced practice, and advancing practice (Allan, 2011; Christensen, 2009, 2011; MacDonald et al., 2006; Thoun, 2011).

In summary, questions arising from a changing health policy landscape and from theorizing about advanced practice nursing underscore the need for well-thought-out, robust conceptual models to guide APRN practice. Conceptual clarity of advanced practice nursing, what it is and is not, is important not only for patients and those in the nursing profession but also for interprofessional education (CIHC, 2010; Health Professions Network Nursing and Midwifery Office, 2010; IPEC Expert Panel, 2016) and practice (American Association of Nurse Anesthesiology [AANA], 2018). Conceptual clarity of advanced practice nursing will also inform the creation of accountable care organizations and support efforts to build teams and systems in which effective communication, collaboration, and coordination will lead to high-quality care and improved patient, institutional, and fiscal outcomes.

CONCEPTUALIZATIONS OF ADVANCED PRACTICE NURSING: PROBLEMS AND IMPERATIVES

Despite the usefulness and benefits of conceptual models, conceptual confusion and uncertainty remain regarding advanced practice nursing. One noted issue is the lack of a well-defined and consistently applied core stable vocabulary used for model building. Despite progress, this challenge remains. For example, in the United States *advanced practice nursing* is the term that is used, but the ICN and CNA use the term *advanced nursing practice*. Considerable variation is noted between the conceptual definition of advanced practice nursing and that of advanced nursing practice as used in Australia, Canada, New Zealand, the United States, Canada, and the United Kingdom (Stasa et al., 2014). Adding to this opacity is the use of the term *advanced practitioner* to describe the role of non-APRN experts in the United Kingdom and internationally (McGee, 2009). The role and functions of APRNs need to be clearly and consistently conceptualized, which is challenging when different terms are used to describe APRNs. For example, the state of Iowa in the United States uses the term *advanced registered nurse practitioner* to describe all four advanced practice nursing roles, whereas the state of Virginia uses the term *licensed nurse practitioner* to describe NPs, CNMs, and certified registered nurse anesthetists (CRNAs).

The APRN Consensus Model (APRN Joint Dialogue Group, 2008) represents a major step forward in promulgating a uniform definition of advanced practice in the United States for the purpose of regulation. However, the lack of a core vocabulary continues to make comparisons difficult because the conceptual meanings vary. Competencies are more commonly used to describe concepts of APRN practice, but reflection on and discussion of other terms such as *roles, hallmarks, functions, activities, skills*, and *abilities* continue and may contribute to the urgent need for clarification of conceptual models and a common language.

Few models of APRN practice address nursing's metaparadigm (person, health, environment, nursing) comprehensively. The problem in comparing, refining, or developing models is that concepts are often used without universal meaning or consensus and, occasionally, with no or inconsistent definitions. It is rightly anticipated that conceptual models of the field and its practice change over time. However, the evolution of advanced practice nursing and its comprehension by nurses, policymakers, and the public will be enhanced if scholars and practitioners agree on the use and definition of fundamental concepts of APRN practice.

Another challenge is the paucity of conceptual models describing the practice and outcomes of APRNs. Although the numbers of models are increasing, they remain small. Further compounding this issue is the scarcity of international and global models of APRN practice. Within the United Arab Emirates, the role of the APRN is emerging along with a road map for successful implementation (Behrens, 2018); though encouraging, no formal APRN model has been put forth to date. Models are needed that address the diverse health and cultural needs of individuals, families, and communities worldwide.

Another issue is a lack of clarity in the conceptualizations that differentiate the clinical practice of APRNs from that of registered nurses (RNs). Conceptual models can help identify key concepts and variables that distinguish the focus, levels of practice, and outcomes between and among nurses with different levels and types of academic preparation and specialty certification.

Of additional importance is clarifying and distinguishing the differences in practice of APRNs and physician colleagues. Some graduate APRN students may struggle with this issue as part of role development. The lack of conceptual clarity is apparent in advertisements that invite both NPs and physician assistants to apply for the same position. Organized medicine continues to expend resources trying to limit or discredit advanced practice nursing, even as some physician leaders work on behalf of advocating for APRNs. Barriers to APRNs' ability to practice to the full extent of their education and training as recommended by NASEM's *Future of Nursing 2020–2030* report (2021) may be the result of lack of conceptual clarity between nursing at the advanced practice level and the practice of medicine. To this end, the philosophic underpinnings of conceptual models of APRN practice need explication.

The emphasis on interprofessional education and practice is another issue in need of clarification. Interprofessional education and practice are central to accountable, collaborative, coordinated, and high-quality care. Graduate education of APRNs alongside other health professionals is beginning to take place. For example, at the University of Michigan, an interprofessional clinical decision-making course with graduate students from nursing (APRN students), pharmacy, dentistry, medicine, and social work is one of the first of its kind in the nation. Students learn together and from each other about their roles, preparation, and disciplinary foci (Sweet et al., 2017). The development of interprofessional competencies for health professionals (CIHC, 2010; Health Professions Network Nursing and Midwifery Office, 2010; IPEC Expert Panel, 2016) indicates the need for high-functioning interprofessional teams of healthcare experts to maximize patient outcomes. The existence of interprofessional competencies and emergence of promising conceptualizations of interprofessional work are critical contextual factors for elucidating and advancing conceptualizations of advanced practice nursing (Barr et al., 2005; Reeves et al., 2011). Conceptual models for APRN practice on interprofessional teams are needed to explicate the unique and critical contributions of APRNs to patient outcomes and system resources.

Among many imperatives for reaching a conceptual consensus on advanced practice nursing, most important are the interrelated areas of policymaking, licensing and credentialing, and practice, including competencies. In the policymaking arena, for example, not all APRNs are eligible to be reimbursed by insurers, and even those activities that are reimbursable are often billed "incident to" a physician's care, rendering the work of APRNs invisible (see Chapter 19). The APRN Consensus Model (APRN Joint Dialogue Group, 2008), the Patient Protection and Affordable Care Act (2010), and NASEM's *The Future of Nursing 2020–2030* (2021) call for changes to enable APRNs to work within their full scope of practice will make it easier for US policymakers to recommend and adopt changes to policies and regulations that now constrain APRN practice, eventually making the contributions of APRNs to quality care visible and reimbursable. Agreement on vocabulary and concepts such as competencies that are common to all APRN roles will maximize the ability of APRNs to work within their full scope of practice.

Although some progress has been made, there are compelling reasons for continuing dialogue and activity aimed at clarifying advanced practice nursing and the concepts and models that help stakeholders understand the nature of APRN work and the contributions of APRNs. Reaching consensus on concepts and vocabulary will serve theoretical, practical, and policymaking purposes. As the work of healthcare reform and implementing interprofessional competencies, education, and practice moves forward, there will be opportunities for the profession to conceptualize advanced practice nursing more clearly. Box 2.1 presents outcomes that come from clarification and consensus on conceptualization of the nature of advanced practice nursing.

BOX 2.1

Clarification and Consensus on Conceptualization of the Nature of Advanced Practice Nursing

1. Clear differentiation of advanced practice nursing from other levels of clinical nursing practice.
2. Clear differentiation between advanced practice nursing and the clinical practice of physicians and other non-nurse providers within a specialty.
3. Clear understanding of the roles and contributions of advanced practice registered nurses (APRNs) on interprofessional teams, enabling employers to create teams and accountable care organizations that can meet institutions' clinical and fiduciary outcomes.
4. Clear delineation of the similarities and differences among APRN roles and the ability to match APRN skills and knowledge to the needs of patients.
5. Regulation and credentialing of APRNs that protect the public and ensure equitable treatment of all APRNs.
6. Clear articulation of international, national, state, and local health policies that do the following:
   a. Recognize and make visible the substantive contributions of APRNs to quality, cost-effective health care and patient outcomes.
   b. Ensure the public's access to APRN care.
   c. Ensure explicit and appropriate mechanisms to bill and pay for APRN care.
7. A maximum social contribution by APRNs in health care, including improvement in health outcomes and health-related quality of life for the people to whom they provide care.
8. The actualization of practitioners of advanced practice nursing, enabling APRNs to reach their full potential, personally and professionally.

CONCEPTUALIZATIONS OF ADVANCED PRACTICE NURSING ROLES: ORGANIZATIONAL PERSPECTIVES

Practice with individual clients or patients is the central work of the field; it is the reason for which nursing was created. The following questions are the kinds of questions a conceptual model of advanced practice nursing should answer:

- What is the scope and purpose of advanced practice nursing?
- What are the characteristics of advanced practice nursing?
- Within what settings does this practice occur?
- How do APRNs' scopes of practice differ from those of other providers offering similar or related services?
- What knowledge and skills are required?
- How are the knowledge and skills different from those of other providers?
- What patient and institutional outcomes are realized when APRNs deliver care? How are these outcomes different from those of other providers?
- When should healthcare systems employ APRNs, and what types of patients particularly benefit from APRN care?
- For what types of pressing healthcare problems are APRNs a solution in terms of improving outcomes, quality of care, and cost-effectiveness?
- How are diversity and social determinants of health addressed in APRN conceptual models?
- What changes or revisions are needed to include?
- Are outcomes improved when APRNs deliver care guided by models that include these key concepts?

Of the conceptual models presented in this chapter, some are more narrowly focused than others, and some are more homogeneous or mixed with respect to the phenomenon studied. Still other models explain systems and the relationships between and among systems. All of these foci are important, depending on the purposes to be served. However, in the development of conceptual models, the phenomenon to be modeled must be carefully defined. For example, a model may encompass the entire field of advanced practice nursing or be confined to distinctive concepts (e.g., collaborative practice between APRNs and physicians or the difference between APRN practice and the practice of non-APRN nurses). If a phenomenon and its related concepts are not clearly defined, the model could be so inconsistent as to be confusing or so broad that its effect will be diluted.

In addition to describing concepts and how they are related, assumptions about the philosophy, values, and practices of the profession should be reflected in conceptual models. The discussion of conceptualizations of advanced practice nursing is guided by these assumptions:

1. Each model, at least implicitly, addresses the four elements of nursing's metaparadigm: persons, health and illness, nursing, and the environment.
2. The development and strengthening of the field of advanced practice nursing depend on professional agreement regarding the nature of advanced practice nursing (a conceptual model) that can inform APRN program accreditation, credentialing, and practice.
3. APRNs meet the needs of society for advanced nursing care.
4. Advanced practice nursing will reach its full potential to the extent that foundational conceptual components of any model of advanced practice nursing framework are delineated and agreed on.

Consensus Model for Advanced Practice Registered Nurse Regulation

In 2004, an APRN Consensus Conference was convened to achieve consensus regarding the credentialing of APRNs (APRN Joint Dialogue Group, 2008; Stanley et al., 2009) and the development of a regulatory model for advanced practice nursing. Independently, the APRN Advisory Committee for the National Council of State Boards of Nursing (NCSBN) was charged by the NCSBN Board of Directors with a similar task of creating a future model for APRN regulation and, in 2006, disseminated a draft of the APRN Vision Paper (NCSBN, 2006), a document that generated debate and controversy. Within a year, these groups came together to form the APRN Joint Dialogue Group, with representation from numerous stakeholder groups, and the outcome was the APRN Consensus Model (APRN Joint Dialogue Group, 2008).

The APRN Consensus Model includes important definitions of roles, titles, and population foci. Furthermore, it defines specialties and describes how to make room for the emergence of new APRN roles and population foci within the regulatory framework. A timeline for adoption and strategies for implementation were put forth, and progress has been made in these areas (see Chapter 20 for further information; only the model is discussed here). Fig. 2.1 depicts the components of the APRN Consensus Model, the four recognized APRN roles and six population foci. The term *advanced practice registered nurse* refers to all four APRN roles. An APRN is defined as a nurse who meets the following criteria (APRN Joint Dialogue Group, 2008):

- Completes an accredited graduate-level education program preparing them for one of the four recognized APRN roles and a population focus (see discussion in Chapter 3)
- Passes a national certification examination that measures APRN role and population-focused competencies and maintains continued competence by national recertification in the role and population focus
- Possesses advanced clinical knowledge and skills preparing them to provide direct care to patients; the defining factor for *all* APRNs is that a significant component of the education and practice focuses on direct care of individuals
- Builds on the competencies of RNs by demonstrating greater depth and breadth of knowledge

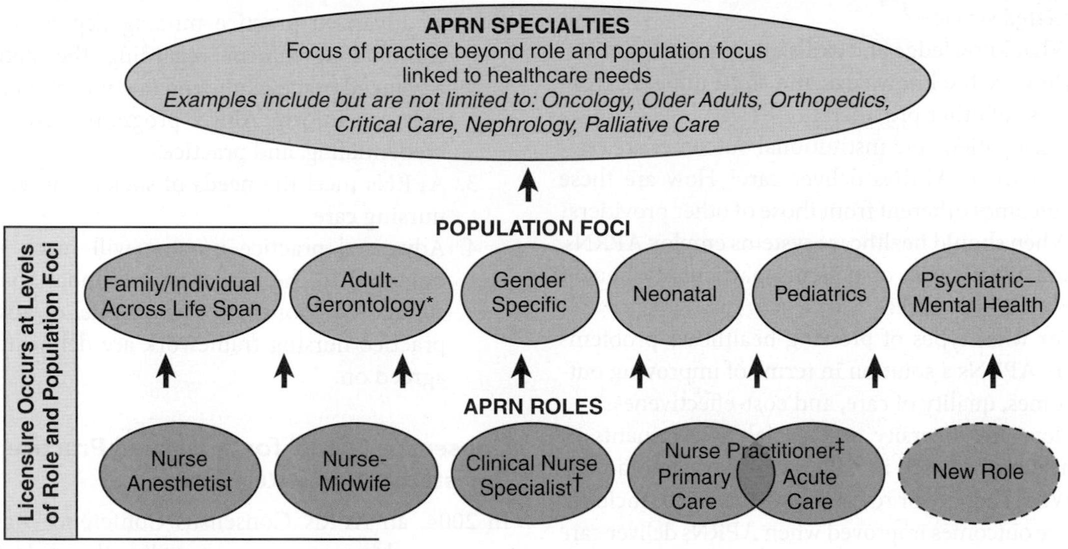

Fig. 2.1 ■ **Consensus model for APRN regulation.** This model was based on the work of the APRN Consensus Work Group and the NCSBN APRN Advisory Committee. (From *Consensus Model for APRN Regulation*, by APRN Joint Dialogue Group, 2008, http://www.aacn.nche.edu/education-resources/APRNReport.pdf., p.10). *The population focus *adult–gerontology* encompasses the young adult to the older adult, including the frail elderly. APRNs educated and certified in the adult-gerontology population are educated and certified across both areas of practice and will be titled adult-gerontology CNP or CNS. In addition, all APRNs in any of the four roles providing care to the adult population (e.g., family or gender specific) must be prepared to meet the growing needs of the older adult population. Therefore the education program should include didactic and clinical education experiences necessary to prepare APRNs with these enhanced skills and knowledge. †The clinical nurse specialist (CNS) is educated and assessed through national certification processes across the continuum from wellness through acute care. ‡The certified nurse practitioner (CNP) is prepared with the acute care CNP competencies and/or the primary care CNP competencies. At this point in time the acute care and primary care CNP delineation applies only to the pediatrics and adult-gerontology CNP population foci. Scope of practice of the primary care or acute care CNP is not setting specific but is based on patient care needs. Programs may prepare individuals across both the primary care and acute care CNP roles. If programs prepare graduates across both roles, the graduate must be prepared with the consensus-based competencies for both roles and must successfully obtain certification in both the acute and the primary care CNP roles.

and greater synthesis of data by performing more complex skills and interventions and by possessing greater role autonomy

- Is educationally prepared to assume responsibility and accountability for health promotion and/or maintenance, as well as the assessment, diagnosis, and management of patient problems, including the use and prescription of pharmacologic and nonpharmacologic interventions
- Has sufficient depth and breadth of clinical experience to reflect the intended license
- Obtains a license to practice as an APRN in one of the four APRN roles

The definition of the components of the APRN Consensus Model begins to address some of the questions about advanced practice posed earlier in this chapter. An important agreement was that providing direct care to individuals is a defining characteristic of all APRN roles. This agreement affirms a position long held by original and current editors of this text—that when there is no direct practice component in the role, one is not practicing as an APRN. It also has important implications for LACE and for career development of APRNs.

Graduate education for the four APRN roles is described in the Consensus Model document (APRN Joint Dialogue Group, 2008). It must include completion of at least three separate, comprehensive graduate courses in advanced physiology and pathophysiology, physical health assessment, and advanced pharmacology (the "three Ps"), consistent with requirements for the accreditation of APRN education programs. In addition, curricula must address three other areas—the principles of decision making for the particular APRN role, preparation in the core competencies identified for the role, and role preparation in one of the six population foci.

The Consensus Model asserts that licensure must be based on educational preparation for one of the four existing APRN roles and a population focus, that certification must be within the same area of study, and that the four separate processes of LACE are necessary for the adequate regulation of APRNs (APRN Joint Dialogue Group, 2008; see Chapter 20). The six population foci displayed in Fig. 2.1 include the individual and family across the life span as well as adult/gerontologic, neonatal, pediatric, women's health/gender-specific, and psychiatric/mental health populations. Preparation in a specialty, such as oncology or critical care, cannot be the basis for licensure. Specialization

> *indicates that an APRN has additional knowledge and expertise in a more discrete area of specialty practice. Competency in the specialty area could be acquired either by educational preparation or experience and assessed in a variety of ways through professional credentialing mechanisms (e.g., portfolios, examinations).*
>
> ***(APRN Joint Dialogue Group, 2008, p. 12)***

This was a critical decision for the group to reach, given the numbers of specialties and APRN specialty examinations in place when the document was prepared.

Even with this brief overview of the APRN Consensus Model, one sees how this model advanced the conceptualization of advanced practice nursing. It is helpful for many reasons. First, for the United States, it affirms that there are four APRN roles. Second, it is advancing a uniform approach to LACE and advanced practice nursing that has practical and policymaking effects, including better alignment between and among APRN curricula and certification examinations. Furthermore, it addresses the issue of differentiating between RNs and APRNs and has been foundational to differentiate among nursing roles. By addressing the issue of specialization, the model offers a reasoned approach for the following: (1) avoiding confusion from a proliferation of specialty certification examinations; (2) ensuring that, because of a limited and parsimonious focus (four roles and six populations), there will be sufficient numbers of APRNs for the relevant examinations to ensure psychometrically valid data on test results; and (3) allowing for the development of new APRN roles or foci to meet society's needs.

Although there are a number of noted strengths of the Consensus Model, there are also limitations. First, competencies that are common across APRN roles are not addressed beyond defining an APRN and indicating that students must be prepared "with the core competencies for one of the four APRN roles across at least one of the six population foci" (APRN Joint Dialogue Group, 2008, p. 10). The model leaves it to the different APRN roles to develop their own core competencies.

In addressing specialization, the model also leaves open the issue of the importance of educational preparation, in addition to experience, for advanced practice in a specialty, which is of particular importance to the CNS role. Additionally, Martsolf and colleagues (2020) recently raised concerns regarding the misalignment between specialty NP education, certification, and practice location and called for an evaluation of the policy and practice implications of the Consensus Model, along with an examination of the scope and scale of NP misalignment within healthcare systems.

Two years after the 2004 APRN consensus conference, the American Association of Colleges of Nursing (AACN, 2006) put forth "The Essentials of Doctoral Education for Advanced Nursing Practice." The Essentials established the DNP, the highest practice degree and the preferred preparation for specialty nursing practice. The AACN called for doctorate-level preparation of APRNs by the year 2015. DNP preparation for entry to practice has been endorsed by the Council on Accreditation of Nurse Anesthesia Educational Programs (2019), the National Association of Clinical Nurse Specialists (NACNS, 2015), and the National Organization of Nurse Practitioner Faculties (NONPF, 2015). However, the American College of Nurse-Midwives (ACNM, 2019) has not endorsed the DNP as a requirement for entry into practice for CNMs, instead supporting the completion of a graduate degree program requirement for certification and entry into clinical practice.

Although experience in an area is certainly a factor that leads to the emergence of new specialties, experience alone may be insufficient for the APRN who specializes in oncology or critical care (or another specialty) to achieve desired outcomes in timely and cost-effective ways. These are specialties in which the population's needs are many and complex and the scope of research knowledge is similarly broad and deep. These are important areas of conceptualization that need to be addressed by the American Nurses Association (ANA) and specialty professional nursing organizations, rather than by a group with a regulatory focus.

Numerous efforts are under way to implement this model in the United States. The NCSBN has an extensive toolkit to help educators, APRNs, and policymakers implement the APRN regulatory model (NCSBN, 2015). The work undertaken to produce the APRN Consensus Model (APRN Joint Dialogue Group, 2008) illustrates the power of interorganizational collaboration and is a promising example of how a model can, as Fawcett and Desanto-Madeya (2013) have suggested, reduce conflict and facilitate communication within the profession, across professions, and with the public.

American Nurses Association

As the only full-service professional organization representing the interests of the 4 million RNs in the United States through its constituent and state nurses associations and its organizational affiliates, the ANA and its constituent organizations have also been active in developing documents that address advanced practice nursing. Two of these are particularly important for the contemporary conceptualizations of advanced practice nursing. Since 1980, the ANA has periodically updated its *Social Policy Statement* (ANA, 2010). Specialization has consistently been identified as a concept that differentiates advanced practice nursing from basic nursing practice. The most recent edition of the policy notes that specialization ("focusing on nursing practice in a specific area, identified from within the whole field of professional nursing"; ANA, 2010, p. 17) can occur at basic or advanced levels and that APRNs use additional specialized knowledge and skills obtained through graduate education in their practices. According to this statement, advanced nursing practice "builds on the competencies of the registered nurse and is characterized by the integration and application of a broad range of theoretical and evidence-based knowledge that occurs as part of graduate nursing education" (ANA, 2010, p. 18). In this document, APRNs are defined as RNs who hold master's or doctoral degrees and are licensed, certified, and/or approved to practice in their roles by state boards of nursing or regulatory oversight bodies. APRNs are prepared through graduate education in nursing for one of four APRN roles (NPs, CRNAs, NMs, CNSs) and at least one of six population foci (family/individual across the life span, adult/gerontology, neonatal, pediatrics, women's health/gender-related health, psychiatric/mental health; ANA, 2010). These definitions of specialization and advanced practice are consistent with the APRN Consensus Model.

The ANA also establishes and promulgates standards of practice and competencies for RNs and APRNs. Six standards of practice and 12 standards of professional performance are described in the fourth edition of *Nursing: Scope and Standards of Practice* (ANA, 2021). Each standard is associated with competencies. Of the 18 total standards, all outline additional competencies for APRNs compared with RNs. For example, Standard 5, "Implementation," addresses the consultation and prescribing responsibilities of APRNs and Standard 12, "Leadership," addresses the competency that APRNs will model expert nursing practice to members of interprofessional teams and to consumers of health care. It is in the description of the competencies that APRN practice and the practice of nurses prepared in a specialty at the graduate level are differentiated from RN practice.

In addition to these documents, the ANA, together with the American Board of Nursing Specialties (ABNS), convened a task force on clinical nurse specialist competencies. For many reasons, including the recognition that developing psychometrically sound certifications for numerous specialties, especially for CNSs, would be difficult as the profession moved toward implementing the APRN Consensus Model, the ANA and ABNS convened a group of stakeholders in 2006 to develop and validate a set of core competencies that would be expected of CNSs entering practice, regardless of specialty (NACNS/National CNS Core Competency Task Force, 2010). This work and recent updates are discussed later in this chapter in the section on the NACNS.

American Association of Colleges of Nursing

Over the last 2 decades, the AACN has undertaken two nursing education initiatives aimed at transforming nursing education. In 2006 the AACN called for APRN preparation to be at the doctoral level in practice-based programs (DNP), with master's-level education being refocused on generalist preparation (e.g., clinical nurse leaders, staff, and clinical educators). Clinical nurse leaders are not APRNs (AACN, 2021a) and therefore are not included in this discussion of conceptualizations. Through these initiatives, and to the extent that the AACN and Commission on Collegiate Nursing Education influence accreditation, the DNP is becoming the preferred degree for most APRNs. The growth of DNP education has advanced considerably. In 2006 there were 20 DNP programs; most recently in 2019 there were 348 DNP programs (AACN, 2019). Enrollments in and graduation from DNP programs have also risen substantially (AACN, 2019).

The DNP Essentials (AACN, 2006) were composed of eight competencies for DNP graduates. For APRNs, "Essential VIII specified the foundational practice competencies that cut across specialties and are seen as requisite for DNP practice" (AACN, 2006, p. 16). Recognizing that DNP programs also prepare nurses for non-APRN roles, the AACN acknowledged that organizations representing APRNs were expected to develop Essential VIII as it related to specific advanced practice roles and to "develop competency expectations that build upon and complement DNP Essentials 1 through 8" (AACN, 2006, p. 17). These Essentials affirmed that the advanced practice nursing core includes the "three Ps" (three separate courses)—advanced health/physical assessment, advanced physiology/pathophysiology, and advanced pharmacology—and is specific to APRNs. The specialty core must include content and clinical practice experiences that help students acquire the knowledge and skills essential to a specific advanced practice role. These requirements were reconfirmed in the Consensus Model (APRN Joint Dialogue Group, 2008).

The DNP has been described as both a "disruptive innovation" (Hathaway et al., 2006) and a natural evolution for NP practice. The DNP has been endorsed as entry for APRN practice by three of the four professional association/organizations representing APRNs, with the exception of the ACNM (2019). As a result of national DNP discussions, APRN organizations have promulgated practice competencies that address doctorally prepared APRNs (e.g., ACNM, 2011b; NACNS, 2019). The NONPF (2012) now has one set of core competencies for NPs and developed population-based competencies for nurse practitioners (NONPF, 2013). Organizational positions on doctoral education are briefly explored in the discussion of APRN organizations later in this chapter.

Although not a conceptual model per se, the AACN's publication *The Essentials: Core Competencies for Professional Nursing Education* (2021b) represents a new approach to nursing education designed to provide consistency in graduate outcome. This framework conceptualizes the discipline of nursing via five key concepts: human wholeness, health, healing and well-being, environment–health relationship, and caring. It includes level 2 advanced-level nursing education subcompetencies designed to prepare nurses for advanced nursing practice specialty or advanced nursing practice roles, with specialty competencies designed to complement and build on level 2 competencies. These advanced-level nursing competencies are conceptualized to affirm a set of common competencies across APRN roles and are an important contribution to conceptual clarity about APRN practice in the United States. The Essentials provide guidance that DNP graduates attain and integrate level 2 competencies and subcompetencies for at least one APRN specialty or advanced nursing practice role and complete a scholarly project/project that the faculty will evaluate (AACN, 2021b). A discussion of APRN organizations' conceptualization of APRN practice follows, along with a discussion of the extent to which their responses to the DNP influence conceptual clarity on advanced practice nursing.

National Organization of Nurse Practitioner Faculties

The mission of the NONPF is to provide leadership in promoting quality NP education. Since 1990 the NONPF has fulfilled this mission in many ways, including the development, validation, and promulgation of NP competencies. As of 2012, there is only one set of NP core competencies (NONPF, 2012), along with recently added population-focused NP competencies (NONPF, 2013). A brief history of the development of competencies for NPs is presented here, in part because their development has influenced other APRN models.

In 1990 the NONPF published a set of domains and core competencies for primary care NPs based on Benner's (1984) domains of expert nursing practice and the results of Brykczynski's (1989) study of the use of these domains by primary care NPs (Price et al., 1992; Zimmer et al., 1990). Within each domain were a number of specific competencies that served as a framework for primary care NP education and practice.

After endorsing the DNP as entry-level preparation for the NP role, and consistent with the recommendations in the APRN Consensus Model (APRN Joint Dialogue Group, 2008), new NP core competencies were developed in 2011 and amended in 2012, with core competency content developed in 2014 (NONPF, 2011 [amended 2012], 2014) and population-focused NP competencies added in 2013. Each of the nine core competencies is accompanied by specific behaviors that all graduates of NP programs, whether master's or DNP prepared, are expected to demonstrate. Population-specific competencies for specific NP roles, together with the nine core competencies, are intended to inform curricula and ensure that graduates will meet certification and regulatory requirements.

From a conceptual perspective, these NP core and population-specific competency documents are notable for several reasons: (1) the competencies for NPs were developed collaboratively by stakeholder organizations; (2) empirical validation is used to affirm the competencies; (3) overall, the competencies are conceptually consistent with statements in the APRN Consensus Model, the DNP Essentials (AACN, 2006), and the ANA's *Nursing: Scope and Standards of Practice* 4th edition (ANA, 2021); and (4) the revised competencies are responsive to society's needs for advanced nursing care and the contextual factors that will shape NP practice for at least the next decade. In the amended 2011 NONPF competencies (NONPF, 2011, 2012), there is an emphasis on practice that is not in the APRN Consensus Model (APRN Joint Dialogue Group, 2008); patient-centered care, interprofessional care, and independent or autonomous NP practice, clearly responsive to healthcare reform initiatives, are addressed.

National Association of Clinical Nurse Specialists

The NACNS originally published the *Statement on Clinical Nurse Specialist Practice and Education* in 1998, revised it in 2004, and updated it in 2019. While acknowledging the early conceptualization of CNS practice as subroles proposed by Hamric and Spross (1983, 1989), the 2019 version differentiated CNS practice from that of other APRNs, refined the competencies of the three spheres, and renamed the

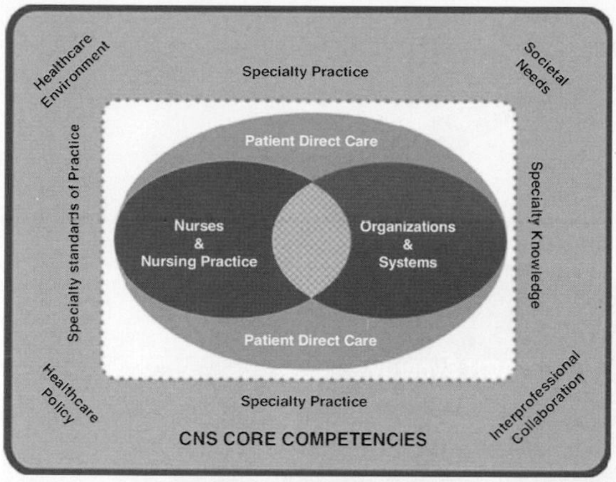

Fig. 2.2 ■ **National Association of Clinical Nurse Specialists model.** CNS practice conceptualized as core competencies in three interacting spheres is shown, as actualized in specialty practice and guided by specialty knowledge, skills/competencies, and standards of practice. (From *Statement on Clinical Nurse Specialist Practice and Education* [3rd ed.], by National Association of Clinical Nurse Specialists, 2019, Author, p. 17.)

spheres of influence to the spheres of impact. These include patient direct care, nurses and nursing practice, and organizations and systems, each of which requires a unique set of competencies (NACNS, 2019; see Fig. 2.2). The statement also outlines expected outcomes (patient, nurse, and organization) of CNS practice within each sphere of impact and competencies.

As work on the APRN Consensus Model neared completion, the NACNS and the APRN Consensus Work Group asked the ANA and the ABNS to "convene and facilitate the work of a National CNS Competency Task Force," using a standard process to develop nationally recognized education standards and competencies (NACNS/National CNS Competency Task Force, 2010, p. 3). The process of developing and validating the competencies is described in the document. Fig. 2.3 illustrates the model of CNS competencies that emerged from this work, a synthesis of the NACNS's spheres of influence (NACNS, 2004), Hamric's seven advanced practice nursing competencies (Hamric, 2009), and the Synergy Model (Curley, 1998). Subsequently, new criteria for evaluating CNS education programs were developed, based on the competencies (Validation Panel of the NACNS, 2011). The APRN Consensus Model has affected certification for CNS roles more than any other APRN role.

Several key updates were included in the most recent statement (NACNS, 2019). It combined into a single document all competencies from the original statement on CNS practice and education and updated important aspects of the 2004 Statement. Additionally, the most recent statement updated the CNS model, changed the language to spheres of impact (replacing spheres of influence), enhanced the focus on the social mandate of the CNS, enhanced the integration with and of the APRN consensus model, and expanded references.

Initially the NACNS published a white paper describing a position of neutrality regarding the DNP as an option for CNS education (NACNS, 2005). However, in 2009, the NACNS did develop core competencies for doctoral-level practice, recognizing that some CNSs would pursue advanced clinical doctorates (NACNS, 2009). Three years later, the NACNS (2012) published a *Statement on the APRN Consensus Model Implementation*, outlining the importance of grandfathering currently practicing CNSs and monitoring the implementation of the Consensus Model to ensure that its adoption would not negatively affect the ability of CNSs to practice. To this end, the competencies outlined in the NACNS 2019 *Statement on Clinical Nurse Specialist Practice and Education* apply to CNSs with graduate preparation (master's or doctorate) in nursing.

In June 2015, the NACNS issued a position statement endorsing the DNP as entry into practice for CNSs by 2030. Within this position statement, the NACNS stated support for "CNSs who pursued other graduate education to retain their ability to practice within the CNS role without having to obtain the DNP for future practice as an APRN after 2030" (NACNS, 2015, p. 2). For further information, see the NACNS website and Chapter 12.

American Association of Nurse Anesthesiology

CRNAs are recognized as APRNs within the APRN Consensus Model. Advanced practice competencies, as described in the DNP Essentials (AACN, 2006), the ANA Scope and Standards (ANA, 2021), and the APRN competencies identified in this text, are evident in the official statements of the AANA (2019, 2020). These statements include scopes of practice, standards for practice, and ethics. Chapter 16 provides a thorough discussion of CRNA practice.

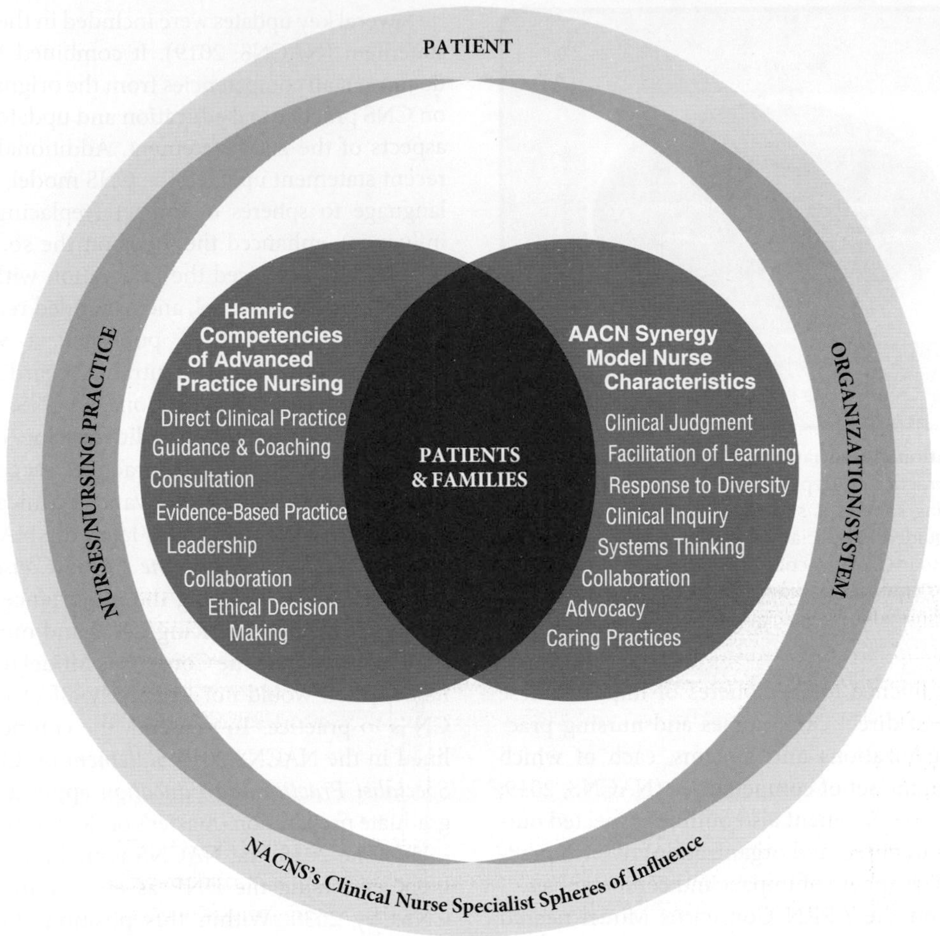

Fig. 2.3 ■ **NACNS model of CNS competencies.** (From *Clinical Nurse Specialist Core Competencies: Executive Summary 2006–2008*, by National Association of Clinical Nurse Specialists/National CNS Competency Task Force, 2010, http://www.nacns.org/docs/CNSCoreCompetenciesBroch.pdf, p. 8.)

The CRNA's scope and standards of practice are defined in two separate documents from the AANA: *Scope of Nurse Anesthesia Practice* (2020) and *Standards for Nurse Anesthesia Practice* (2019). The *Scope of Nurse Anesthesia Practice* addresses the responsibilities of CRNAs, and the *Standards for Nurse Anesthesia Practice* describe standards of professional CRNA practice. The Scope document addresses the professional role; education, licensure, certification and accountability; clinical anesthesia practice; leadership, advocacy, and policymaking; and the future of nurse anesthesia practice. The purposes of the 14 Standards are to support the delivery of patient-centered, consistent, high-quality, and safe anesthesia care and assist the public in understanding the CRNA's role in anesthesia care (AANA, 2019). The *Scope of Nurse Anesthesia Practice* and *Standards for Nurse Anesthesia Practice* provide descriptions of clinical competencies and responsibilities of CRNAs.

Initially, the AANA did not support the DNP for entry into CRNA practice and established a task force to evaluate doctoral preparation further. In 2019 the Council on Accreditation of Nurse Anesthesia Educational Programs revised its 2015 accreditation standards for nurse anesthesia education stating that students accepted into accredited entry-level programs on or after January 1, 2022, must graduate with doctoral degrees as of January 1, 2025. Further, Standard E.1 states, "The curriculum is designed to award a DNP or Doctor of Nurse Anesthesia Practice to graduate students who successfully complete graduation requirements unless a waiver for this requirement has been approved by the Council" (Council on Accreditation of Nurse Anesthesia Educational Programs, 2019). The Council on Accreditation of Nurse Anesthesia Educational Programs (2019) also includes a requirement for the "three P" courses, consistent with requirements specified in the APRN Consensus document.

American College of Nurse-Midwives

Certified nurse-midwives (CNMs) are APRNs who are recognized in the APRN Consensus Model. Advanced practice competencies, described in the DNP Essentials (AACN, 2006), the ANA Scope and Standards (ANA, 2021), and the APRN competencies are apparent in the official statements of the ACNM (2011a, 2011c). These statements include scopes of practice, standards for practice, and ethics. Chapter 15 presents a thorough discussion of CNM practice.

The scope of practice for CNMs (and certified midwives who are not nurses) has been defined in four ACNM documents: *Definition of Midwifery and Scope of Practice of Certified Nurse-Midwives and Certified Midwives* (ACNM, 2011a), the *Core Competencies for Basic Midwifery Practice* (ACNM, 2012a), *Standards for the Practice of Midwifery* (ACNM, 2011c), and the *Code of Ethics with Explanatory Statements* (ACNM, 2015a). The core competencies are organized into 16 hallmarks describing the art and science of midwifery and the components of midwifery care. The components of midwifery care include professional responsibilities, midwifery management processes, fundamentals, and care of women and of the newborn, within which are prescribed competencies. According to the definition, "CNMs are educated in two disciplines: nursing and midwifery" (ACNM, 2011a, p. 1). Competencies "describe the fundamental knowledge, skills and behaviors of a new practitioner" (ACNM, 2012a, p. 1). The hallmarks, components, and associated core competencies are the foundation on which midwifery curricula and practice guidelines are based.

In addition to the competencies, there are eight ACNM standards that midwives are expected to meet (ACNM, 2011c) and a code of ethics (ACNM, 2015a). The standards address issues such as qualifications, safety, patient rights, culturally competent care, assessment, documentation, and expansion of midwifery practice. Three ethical mandates related to the ACNM mission of midwifery to promote the health and well-being of women and newborns within their families and communities are identified in the ethics code.

As of 2010, CNMs entering practice must earn a graduate degree, complete an accredited midwifery program, and pass a national certification examination (see Chapter 15 for detailed requirements; ACNM, 2011a); the type of graduate degree is not specified. The ACNM does recognize the value of doctoral education as a valid and valuable path for CNMs, as evidenced by a statement on the practice doctorate in midwifery, including competencies (ACNM, 2011b). Although not cited, these competencies align with those in the DNP Essentials (AACN, 2006); the ACNM recognizes that there are other paths for a practice doctorate in midwifery. At the present time, the ACNM (2019) does not support the DNP as a requirement for entry into nurse-midwifery practice. Reasons cited are (1) midwifery practice is safe, based on the rigor of their curriculum standards and outcome data; (2) there is inadequate evidence to justify the DNP as a mandatory educational requirement for CNMs; and (3) the costs of attaining such a degree could limit the applicant pool and access to midwifery care (ACNM, 2012b, 2015b). Midwifery organizations have recently addressed the aspects of the 2008 Consensus Model that they support and identified those aspects that are of concern (ACNM et al., 2011).

International Organizations and Conceptualizations of Advanced Practice Nursing

In this section, issues of a common language and conceptual framework for advanced practice nursing are addressed. International perspectives on advanced practice nursing are covered more extensively in Chapter 5.

The ICN Nurse Practitioner/Advanced Practice Nursing Network (2020) defines a nurse practitioner/advanced practice nurse as "a registered nurse who has acquired the expert knowledge base, complex decision-making skills and clinical competencies for expanded practice, the characteristics of which are shaped by the context and/or country in which s/he is credentialed to practice." A master's degree is recommended for entry level (ICN Nurse Practitioner/Advanced Practice Nursing Network, 2020). Key concepts include educational preparation, the nature of practice, and regulatory mechanisms. The statement is necessarily broad, given the variations in health systems, regulatory mechanisms, and nursing education programs in individual countries.

In 2008 the CNA published *Advanced Nursing Practice: A National Framework*, which defined advanced nursing practice, described educational preparation and regulation, identified the two APRN roles (CNS and NP), and specified competencies in clinical practice, research, and leadership. In addition, they have issued position statements on advanced nursing practice (CNA, 2007) that affirm the key points in the national framework document and define and describe the roles and contributions to health care of NPs (CNA, 2009b) and CNSs (CNA, 2009a). In 2010 the CNA published a Core Competency Framework for NPs, which included the incorporation of theories of advanced practice nursing. The CNA (2019) published the Pan-Canadian framework for advanced practice nursing, which not only distinguishes the role of the CNS from that of the NP but also strengthens it and aligns it with ICN competencies.

Furthermore, leaders have undertaken an evidence-based, patient-centered, coordinated effort (called a decision support synthesis) to develop, implement, and evaluate the advanced practice nursing roles of the CNS and NP in Canada (DiCenso et al., 2010), a process different from the one used to advance these roles in the United States. This process included a review of 468 published and unpublished articles and interviews conducted with 62 key informants and four focus groups that included a variety of stakeholders. The purpose of this work was to "describe the distinguishing characteristics of CNSs and NPs relevant to Canadian contexts"; identify barriers and facilitators to effective development and use of advanced practice nursing roles; and inform the development of evidence-based recommendations that individuals, organizations, and systems can use to improve the integration of advanced practice nurses into Canadian health care (DiCenso et al., 2010, p. 21). The European Specialist Nurses Organisations (2015) defined 10 core (generic) competencies of CNS practice in Europe. The competencies address clinical role, patient relationship, patient teaching/coaching, mentoring, research, organization and management, communication and teamwork, ethics and decision making, leadership/policymaking, and public health. The competencies were developed to clarify the role of the CNS and include advanced knowledge in anatomy, physiology, pathophysiology, and pharmacology, similar to the APRN Consensus Model. It is expected that CNSs will collaborate with other health professionals to deliver high-quality patient care to ensure safety, quality of care, and equity of access to promote health and prevent disease.

Section Summary: Implications for Advanced Practice Nursing Conceptualizations

From this overview of organizational statements that clarify and advance APRN practice, it is clear that, nationally and internationally, stakeholders are actively defining advanced practice nursing. Progress in this area includes global agreement that this level of clinical nursing practice is advanced and builds on basic nursing education. As such, it requires additional education and is characterized by additional competencies and responsibilities. In the United States the consensus on an approach to APRN regulation was critical for the following reasons: (1) clarifying what an APRN is and the role of graduate education and certification in licensing APRNs, (2) ensuring that APRNs are fully recognized and integrated in the delivery of health care, (3) reducing barriers to mobility of APRNs across state lines, (4) fostering and facilitating ongoing dialogue among APRN stakeholders, and (5) offering common language regarding regulation.

Although there may not be unanimous agreement on the DNP as the requirement for entry into advanced practice nursing, the promulgation of the document fostered dialogue nationally and within APRN organizations on the clinical doctorate (whether or not it is the DNP) as a valid and likely path for APRNs to pursue. As a result, each APRN organization has taken a stand on the role of the clinical doctorate for those in the role and has developed or is developing doctoral-level clinical competencies. In doing so, it appears that the needs of their patients, members, other constituencies, and contexts have been considered. Until the time when a clinical doctorate becomes a requirement for entry into practice for all APRN roles, the development of doctoral-level competencies for APRN roles will help stakeholders distinguish between master's- and clinical doctorate–prepared APRNs with regard to competencies.

Although important differences exist between roles and across countries, a common identity for APRNs resulting from policy and regulatory initiatives would facilitate communication within and outside the profession, consistent with assertions by Styles (1998) and Fawcett and Desanto-Madeya (2013) on the purposes of models. There are important differences among APRN organizations regarding such issues as doctoral preparation, which is also consistent with Fawcett and Desanto-Madeya's assertion that there is not one best model.

The level of consensus regarding regulation in the United States reflects considerable and laudable progress, paving the way for policies and healthcare system transformations that will enable APRNs to be able to more fully ensure access to health care and improve its quality. The processes that have led to this juncture in the United States have required openness, civility, a willingness to disagree, and wisdom. Finally, there are at least two different approaches (collaborative policymaking in the United States and an evidence-based approach in Canada) to determine how best to assess contributions of APRNs and develop ways to integrate APRNs more fully into healthcare infrastructures in order to maximize their benefits to patients and populations. The global APRN community can examine these processes for insights on how to adapt them to suit their particular context.

The organizational models described address professional roles, licensing, accreditation, certification, education, competencies, and clinical practice. The descriptive statements about APRN roles and competencies demonstrate the common elements that exist across all APRN roles. These include a central focus on and accountability for patient care, knowledge and skills specific to each APRN role, and a concern for patient rights. The published definitions, standards, and competencies offer models against which similarities and differences among APRN roles and practices can be distinguished, educational programs can be developed and evaluated, and knowledge and behaviors can be measured for certification purposes. These will also assist practitioners to understand, examine, and improve their own practice and develop job descriptions. As advanced practice nursing moves forward in the United States and globally, the profession will continue to define situations in which a conceptual consensus, as well as alternative conceptualizations, will serve the public and the nursing profession.

CONCEPTUALIZATIONS OF THE NATURE OF ADVANCED PRACTICE NURSING

The APRN role-specific models promulgated by professional organizations raise several questions, such as:

- What is common across APRN roles?
- Can an overarching conceptualization of advanced practice nursing be articulated?
- How can one distinguish among basic, expert, and advanced levels of nursing practice?

Several authors have attempted to discern the nature of advanced practice nursing and address these questions. The extent to which all APRN roles are considered is not always clear; some only focus on CNS and NP roles.

Select frameworks are presented here that address the nature of advanced practice nursing. From the present review of a number of frameworks, the concepts of roles, domain, and competency are among those most commonly used to explain advanced practice nursing. However, meanings are not consistent. Hamric's model (2014), which uses the terms *roles* and *competencies*, is the only one that is integrative—that is, it explicitly considers all four APRN roles. Because it is integrative, has remained relatively stable since 1996, has informed the development of the DNP Essentials (AACN, 2006) and CNS competencies, and is widely cited, it is discussed first, enabling the reader to consider the extent to which important concepts are addressed by other models. Otherwise, the models are discussed in chronologic order and include examples from both US and international conceptual models of APRN practice.

Hamric's Integrative Model of Advanced Practice Nursing

One of the earliest efforts to synthesize a model of advanced practice that would apply to all APRN roles was developed by Hamric (1996). Hamric, whose early conceptual work was done on the CNS role (Hamric & Spross, 1983, 1989), proposed an integrative understanding of the core of advanced practice nursing, based on literature from all APRN specialties (Hamric, 1996, 2000, 2005, 2009, 2014; see Chapter 3). Hamric proposed a conceptual definition of advanced practice nursing and defining characteristics that included primary criteria (graduate education, certification in the specialty, and a focus on clinical practice with patients) and a set of core competencies (direct clinical practice, collaboration, guidance and coaching, evidence-based practice, ethical decision making, consultation, and leadership). This early model was further refined, together with Hanson and Spross in 2000 and 2005 (Hamric, 2000, 2005), based on dialogue among the editors. Key components of the original model (Fig. 2.4) include the primary criteria for advanced

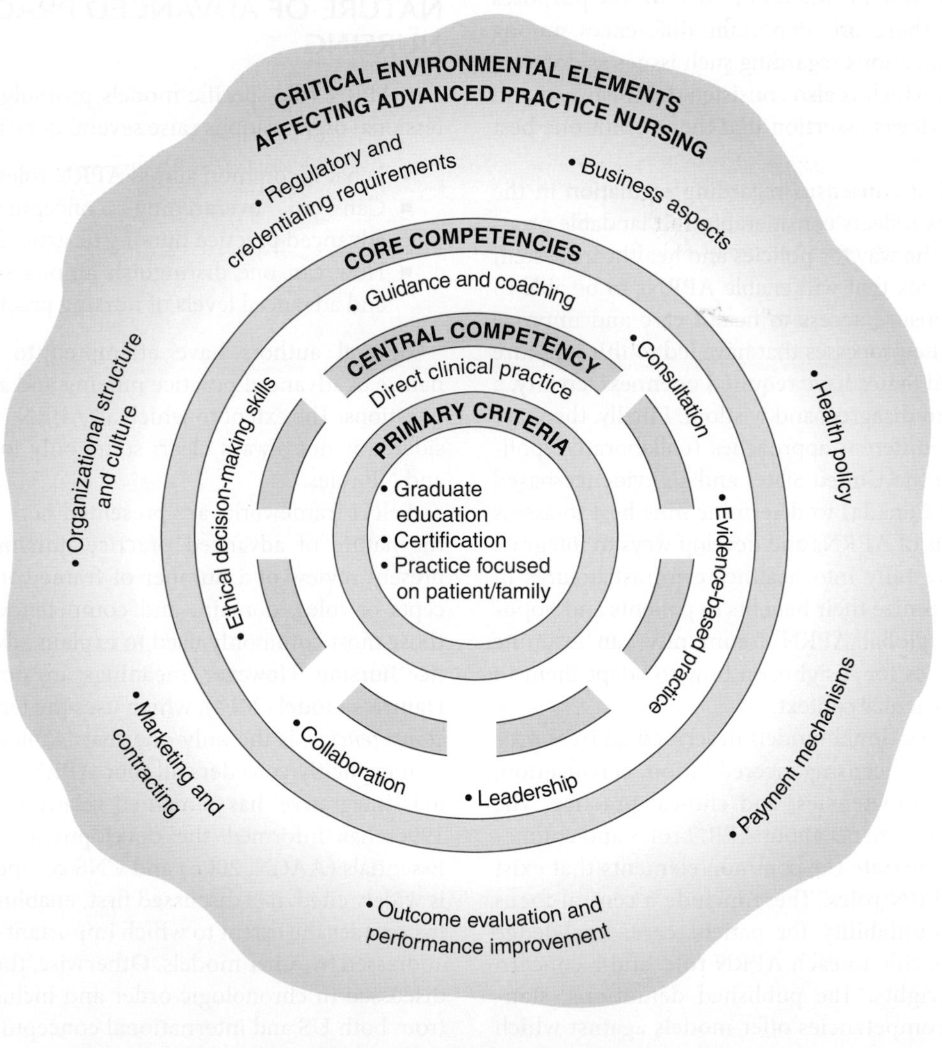

Fig. 2.4 ■ **Hamric's model of advanced practice nursing.** (5th edition, Chapter 3)

nursing practice, seven advanced practice competencies with direct care as the core competency on which the other competencies depend, and environmental and contextual factors that must be managed for advanced practice nursing to flourish.

The revisions to Hamric's original model highlight the dynamic nature of a conceptual model, and that essential features remain the same (Chapter 3, Fig. 3.4). Models are refined over time according to changes in practice, research, and theoretical understanding. The inherent stability and robustness of Hamric's model are noteworthy, particularly in light of the many potentially transformative advanced practice nursing initiatives being developed. This model forms the understanding of advanced practice nursing used throughout this text and has provided the structure for each edition of the book. Hamric's model has been used by contributors to this text to further elaborate specific competencies such as guidance and coaching (see Chapter 7) and ethical practice (see Chapter 11). It has also informed the development of the DNP Essentials (AACN, 2006) and the revised CNS competencies and is widely cited in the advanced practice literature, which provides further evidence of its contribution to conceptualizing advanced practice nursing.

In addition, integrative literature reviews provide further support for Hamric's integrative conceptualization of advanced practice nursing. Mantzoukas and Watkinson's (2007) literature review sought to identify "generic features" of advanced nursing practice; seven generic features were identified (see Box 2.2).

BOX 2.2

Seven Generic Features

1. Use of knowledge in practice.
2. Critical thinking and analytic skills.
3. Clinical judgment and decision making.
4. Professional leadership and clinical inquiry.
5. Coaching and mentoring.
6. Research skills.
7. Changing practice.

From "Review of Advanced Nursing Practice: The International Literature and Developing the Generic Features," by S. Mantzoukas and S. Watkinson, 2007, *Journal of Clinical Nursing, 16*, 28–37 (https://doi.org/10.1111/j.1365-2702.2006.01669.x).

The first three generic features are consistent with the direct care competency in Hamric's model; these three characteristics seem directly related to clinical practice, which supports direct care as a central competency. The remaining four features are consistent with the three competencies of leadership, guidance and coaching, and evidence-based practice in Hamric's model.

Similarly, an integrative literature review of CNS practice by Lewandowski and Adamle (2009) affirmed the direct care, collaboration, consultation, systems leadership, and coaching (patient and staff education) competencies in Hamric's model. Ten countries were represented in their review, and their findings were organized using the NACNS's three spheres of influence (since reconceptualized/relabeled as spheres of impact). Within the first sphere, management of complex or vulnerable populations, they found three essential characteristics—expert direct care, coordination of care, and collaboration. In the sphere of educating and supporting interdisciplinary staff, substantive areas of CNS practice were education, consultation, and collaboration. Within the system sphere, CNSs facilitate innovation and change. These findings lend support for the integration of Hamric's model with the NACNS model of CNS core competencies (NACNS, 2019; NACNS/National CNS Competency Task Force, 2010).

Conceptual Models of APRN Practice: United States Examples

Fenton's and Brykczynski's Expert Practice Domains of the CNS and NP

Some of the early work describing the practice domains of APRNs (CNSs and NPs) was conducted by Fenton (1985) and Brykczynski (1989), using Benner's model of expert nursing practice (Benner, 1984). To fully appreciate their contributions to the understanding of advanced practice, it is important to highlight some of Benner's key findings about nurses who are experts by experience. Although Benner's seminal work, *From Novice to Expert* (1984), has been used in the conceptualization of advanced practice nursing, it is important to note that Benner has not studied advanced practice nurses; her model was based on the expert practice of clinical nurses. Fenton's and Brykczynski's studies represent an extension of Benner's findings and theories to advanced practice nursing.

The early work of Benner and associates informed the development of the first NONPF competencies, graduate curricula in schools of nursing, models of practice, and the standards for clinical promotion. A noted contribution of this early work was that it "put into words what they had always known about their clinical nursing expertise but had difficulty articulating" (Benner et al., 2009, p. xix). It is perhaps this impact that led to the sustained integration of Benner's studies of experts by experience into the APRN literature, including descriptions and development of competencies.

Through the analysis of clinical exemplars discussed in interviews, Benner (1984) derived a range of competencies that resulted in the identification of seven domains of expert nursing practice. Within this lexicon, these domains are a combination of roles, functions, and competencies, although the three were not precisely differentiated. The seven domains are the helping role, administering and monitoring therapeutic interventions and regimens, effective management of rapidly changing situations, diagnostic and monitoring function, teaching and coaching function, monitoring and ensuring the quality of healthcare practices, and organizational and work role competencies.

Fenton (1985) and Brykczynski (1989) each independently applied Benner's model of expert practice to APRNs, examining the practice of CNSs and NPs, respectively. Fenton and Brykczynski (1993) jointly compared their earlier research findings to identify similarities and differences between CNSs and NPs. They verified that nurses in advanced practice were indeed experts, as defined by Benner, showing they were experts by more than experience alone. They identified additional domains and competencies of APRNs (Fig. 2.5). Across the top of Fig. 2.5 are the seven domains identified by Benner and the additional domain found in CNS practice (Fenton, 1985), that of consultation provided by CNSs to other nurses *(rectangular dotted box, top right)*. Under this box are two new CNS competencies *(hexagonal boxes)*. The third *(rounded)* box is a new NP competency identified by Brykczynski in 1989. In this study of NPs, Brykczynski identified an eighth domain (the management of health and illness in ambulatory care settings) and recognized it as a qualitatively different expression from the first two domains identified by Benner. For NPs, the new competencies were a result of the integration of the diagnostic–monitoring and administering–monitoring domains.

The figure also reveals new CNS and NP competencies identified by Fenton and Brykczynski's work. New CNS competencies were identified under the organization and work role domain (e.g., providing support for nursing staff) and the helping role, in addition to the consulting domain and competencies. New NP competencies were noted in seven of the eight domains (e.g., detecting acute or chronic disease while attending to illness under the diagnostic–administering domains). By examining the extent to which APRNs demonstrate the seven domains found in experts by experience and uncovering differences, the findings offer insight into the differences between expert and advanced practice. In addition, Fenton and Brykczynski's work described ways in which the CNS and NP roles may differ with regard to practice domains and competencies.

These early findings suggest that a deeper understanding of advanced practice could be beneficial to understanding and conceptualizing advanced nursing practice. Benner's methods could be applied to studies of advanced practice nursing, with the following aims: (1) to confirm Fenton and Brykczynski's findings in CNS and NP roles and identify new domains and competencies across all four APRN roles, (2) to understand how APRN competencies develop in direct-entry graduate and RN graduate students, and (3) to compare the non-master's-prepared clinician's competencies with the APRN's competencies to distinguish components of expert versus advanced practice nursing. Studies focused on how APRNs acquire expertise in APRN and interprofessional competencies could inform future conceptualizations of advanced practice nursing.

Calkin's Model of Advanced Nursing Practice

Calkin's model (1984) was the first to explicitly distinguish the practice of experts by experience from advanced practice nursing of CNSs and NPs. Calkin developed the model to help nurse administrators differentiate advanced practice nursing from other levels of clinical practice in personnel policies. The model proposed that this could be accomplished by matching patient responses to health problems with the skill and knowledge levels of nursing personnel. In Calkin's

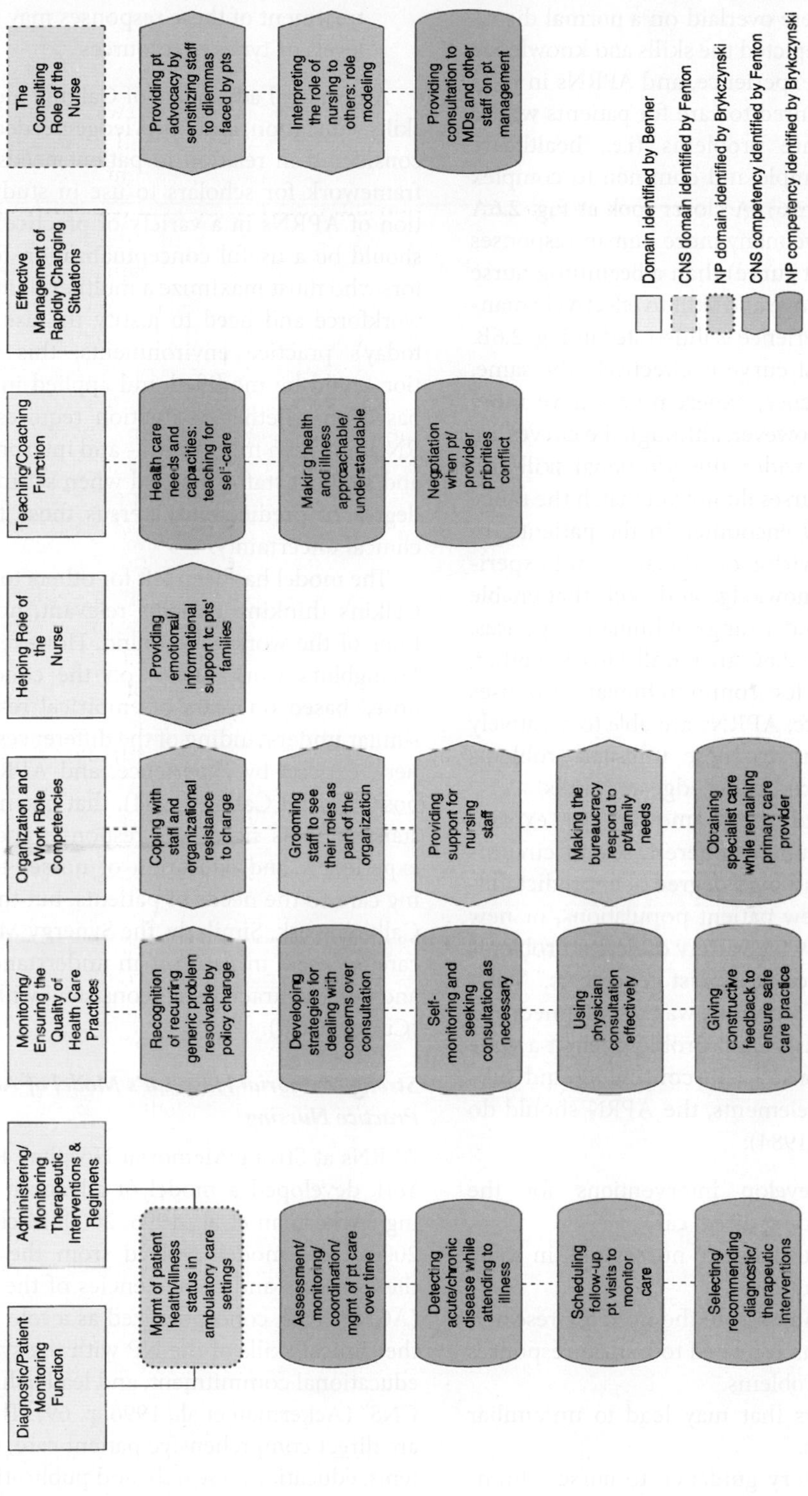

Fig. 2.5 ■ **Fenton's (1985) and Brykczynski's (1989) expert practice domains of the CNS and NP.** *Mgmt,* Management; *pt,* patient. (From "Qualitative Distinctions and Similarities in the Practice of Clinical Nurse Specialists and Nurse Practitioners," by M. V. Fenton and K. A. Brykczynski, 1993, *Journal of Professional Nursing, 9*[6], p. 317.)

model, three curves were overlaid on a normal distribution chart. Calkin depicted the skills and knowledge of novices, experts by experience, and APRNs in relation to knowledge required to care for patients whose responses to healthcare problems (i.e., healthcare needs) ranged from simple and common to complex and complicated (Fig. 2.6). A closer look at Fig. 2.6A shows that patients have many more human responses (the highest and widest curve) than a beginning nurse would have the knowledge and skill to effectively manage. The impact of experience is illustrated in Fig. 2.6B. The highest and widest curve is effectively the same, but because of experience, expert nurses have more knowledge and skill. However, although the curves are higher and somewhat wider, the additional skill and knowledge of expert nurses do not yet match the range of responses they may encounter in the patients. In Fig. 2.6C, APRNs, by virtue of education and experience, do possess the knowledge and skills that enable them to respond to a wider range of human responses. The three curves in Fig. 2.6C are parallel to each other, suggesting that even as less common human responses arise in clinical practice, APRNs are able to creatively and effectively respond to these unusual problems because of their advanced knowledge and skills.

Calkin (1984) used the framework to explain how APRNs perform under different sets of circumstances—when there is a high degree of unpredictability, new conditions, new patient populations, or new sets of problems and a wide variety of health problems requiring the services of "specialist generalists." What APRNs do in terms of functions was also defined. For example, when patients' health problems elicit a wide range of human responses with continuing and substantial unpredictable elements, the APRN should do the following (Calkin, 1984):

- Identify and develop interventions for the unusual by providing direct care.
- Transmit this knowledge to nurses and, in some settings, to students.
- Identify and communicate the need for research or carry out research related to human responses to these health problems.
- Anticipate factors that may lead to unfamiliar human responses.
- Provide anticipatory guidance to nurse administrators when the changes in the diagnosis and treatment of these responses may require altered levels or types of resources.

A principal advantage of Calkin's model is that the skills, education, and knowledge needed by nurses are considered in relation to patient needs. It provides a framework for scholars to use in studying the function of APRNs in a variety of practice situations and should be a useful conceptualization for administrators who must maximize a multilevel interprofessional workforce and need to justify the use of APRNs. In today's practice environments, this conceptualization could be modified and applied in other settings based on whether a situation requires an APRN or RN and which mix of intra- and interprofessional staff and support staff is needed when settings have a high degree of predictability versus those that have high clinical uncertainty.

The model has been left for others to test. Although Calkin's thinking remains relevant, no new applications of the work were found. However, Brooten and Youngblut's work (2006) on the concept of "nurse dose," based on years of empirical research, offers a similar understanding of the differences among beginners, experts by experience, and APRNs. They proposed, as did Calkin (1984), that one needs to understand patients' needs and responses and the expertise, experience, and education of nurses to match nursing care to the needs of patients, but they did not cite Calkin's work. Similarly, the Synergy Model in critical care is based, in part, on an understanding of patient and nurse characteristics consistent with Calkin's ideas (Curley, 1998).

Strong Memorial Hospital's Model of Advanced Practice Nursing

APRNs at Strong Memorial Hospital, Rochester, New York developed a model of advanced practice nursing (Ackerman et al., 1996, 2000; Mick & Ackerman, 2000). The model evolved from the delineation of the domains and competencies of the acute care NP (ACNP) role, conceptualized as a role that "combines the clinical skills of the NP with the systems acumen, educational commitment, and leadership ability of the CNS" (Ackerman et al., 1996, p. 69). The five domains are direct comprehensive patient care, support of systems, education, research, and publication and professional leadership. All domains have direct and indirect

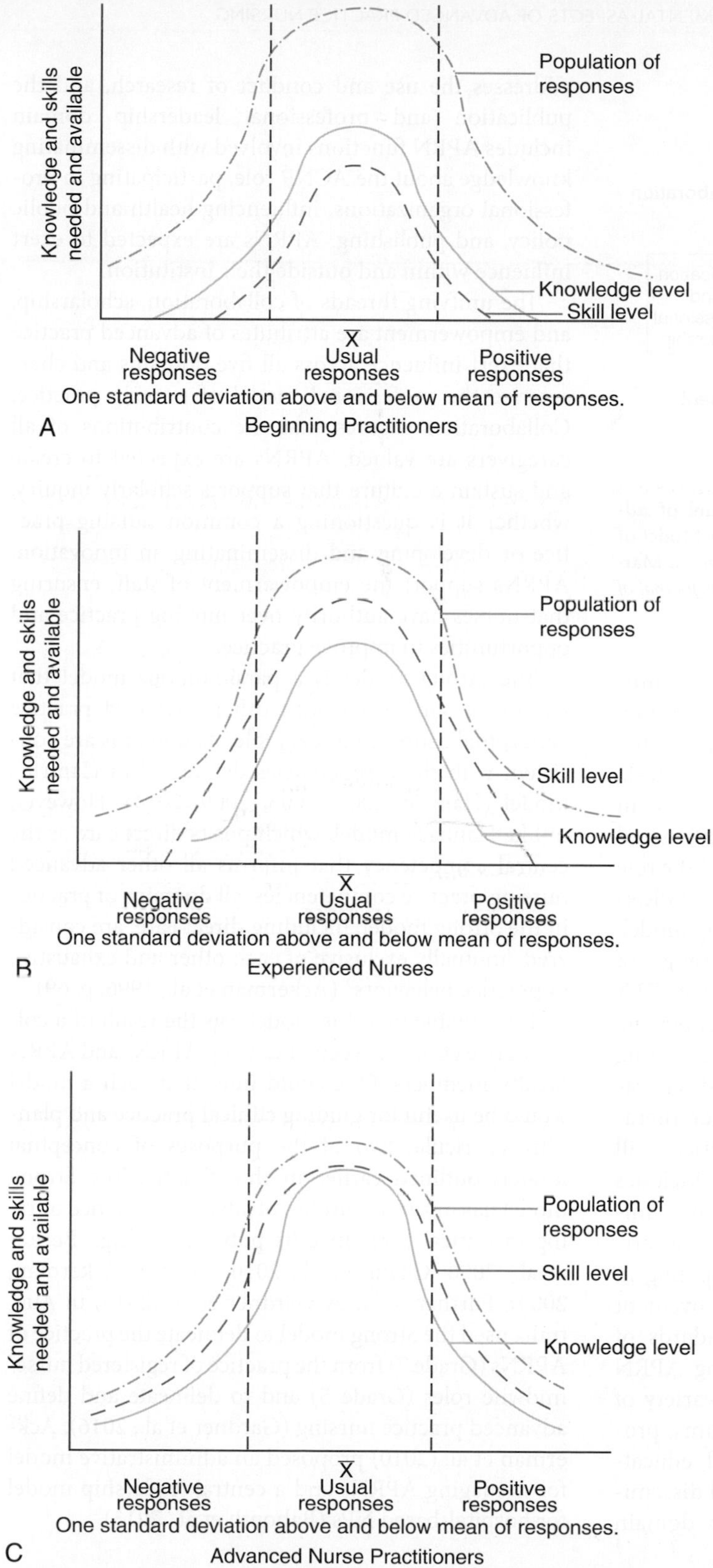

Fig. 2.6 ■ Calkin's model of advanced nursing practice. Patient responses correlated with the knowledge and skill of (A) beginning practitioners, (B) experienced nurses, and (C) advanced practice nurses (APNs). (From "A Model for Advanced Nursing Practice," by J. D. Calkin, 1984, *Journal of Professional Nursing, 14*, p. 25-26.)

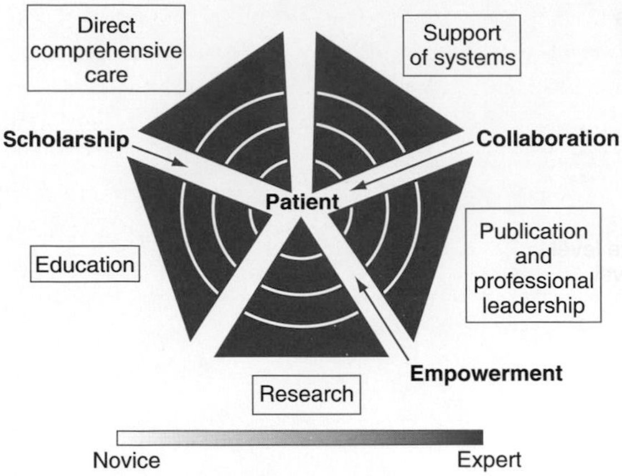

Fig. 2.7 ■ **The Strong Memorial Hospital's model of advanced practice nursing.** (From "Development of a Model of Advanced Practice," by M. H. Ackerman, L. Norsen, B. Martin, J. Wiedrich, and H. J. Kitzman, 1996, *American Journal of Critical Care, 5*, p. 69.)

activities associated with them. In addition, three unifying threads influence each domain: collaboration, scholarship, and empowerment, which are illustrated as circular and continuous threads (Ackerman et al., 1996; Fig. 2.7). These threads are operationalized in each practice domain. Ackerman et al. (2000) noted that the model is based on an understanding of the role development of APRNs; the concept of novice (APRN) to expert (APRN) is foundational to the Strong model.

Direct comprehensive care includes a range of assessments and interventions performed by APRNs (e.g., history taking, physical assessment, requesting and/or performing diagnostic studies, performing invasive procedures, interpreting clinical and laboratory data, prescribing medications and other therapies, and case management of complex, critically ill patients). The support of systems domain includes indirect patient care activities that support the clinical enterprise and serve to improve the quality of care. These activities include consultation, participating in or leading strategic planning, quality improvement initiatives, establishing and evaluating standards of practice, precepting students, and promoting APRN practice. The education domain includes a variety of activities (e.g., evaluating educational programs, providing formal and informal education to staff, educating patients and families, and identifying and disseminating educational resources). The research domain addresses the use and conduct of research, and the publication and professional leadership domain includes APRN functions involved with disseminating knowledge about the ACNP role, participating in professional organizations, influencing health and public policy, and publishing. APRNs are expected to exert influence within and outside their institution.

The unifying threads of collaboration, scholarship, and empowerment are attributes of advanced practice that exert influence across all five domains and characterize the professional model of nursing practice. Collaboration ensures that the contributions of all caregivers are valued. APRNs are expected to create and sustain a culture that supports scholarly inquiry, whether it is questioning a common nursing practice or developing and disseminating an innovation. APRNs support the empowerment of staff, ensuring that nurses have authority over nursing practice and opportunities to improve practice.

The Strong model is a parsimonious model that has many similarities with other advanced practice conceptualizations. For example, its domains are consistent with the competencies delineated in Hamric's model (Hamric, 2000, 2005, 2009, 2014). However, unlike Hamric's model, which posits direct care as the central competency that informs all other advanced nursing practice competencies, all domains of practice in the Strong model, including direct care, are considered "mutually exclusive of each other and exhaustive of practice behaviors" (Ackerman et al., 1996, p. 69).

It is notable that this model was the result of a collaborative effort between practicing APRNs and APRN faculty members. One could infer that such a model would be useful for guiding clinical practice and planning curricula, two of the purposes of conceptual models outlined earlier in this chapter. The Strong model has informed studies of advanced practice nursing in critical care since its publication (e.g., Becker et al., 2006; Chang et al., 2010; Mick & Ackerman, 2000). Further work by Gardner et al. (2013) in Australia used the Strong model to delineate the practice of APRNs (Grade 7) from the practice of registered nurse/midwife roles (Grade 5) and to delineate and define advanced practice nursing (Gardner et al., 2016). Ackerman et al. (2010) proposed an administrative model for managing APRNs and a central leadership model for hospital-based NPs (Bahouth et al., 2013).

Texas Children's Hospital Transformational Advanced Professional Practice APRN Model

The Strong Memorial Hospital model has also influenced the development of the Texas Children's Hospital transformational advanced professional practice (TAPP) APRN model (Elliott & Walden, 2015; Fig. 2.8). To better reflect the current conceptualization of the APRN role, two additional domains of professional practice were added to the Strong model: quality and safety and credentialing and regulatory practice. Professional ethics was also added as a unifying conceptual strand.

The essence of the APRN role within this model is direct, comprehensive, family-centered care. The TAPP

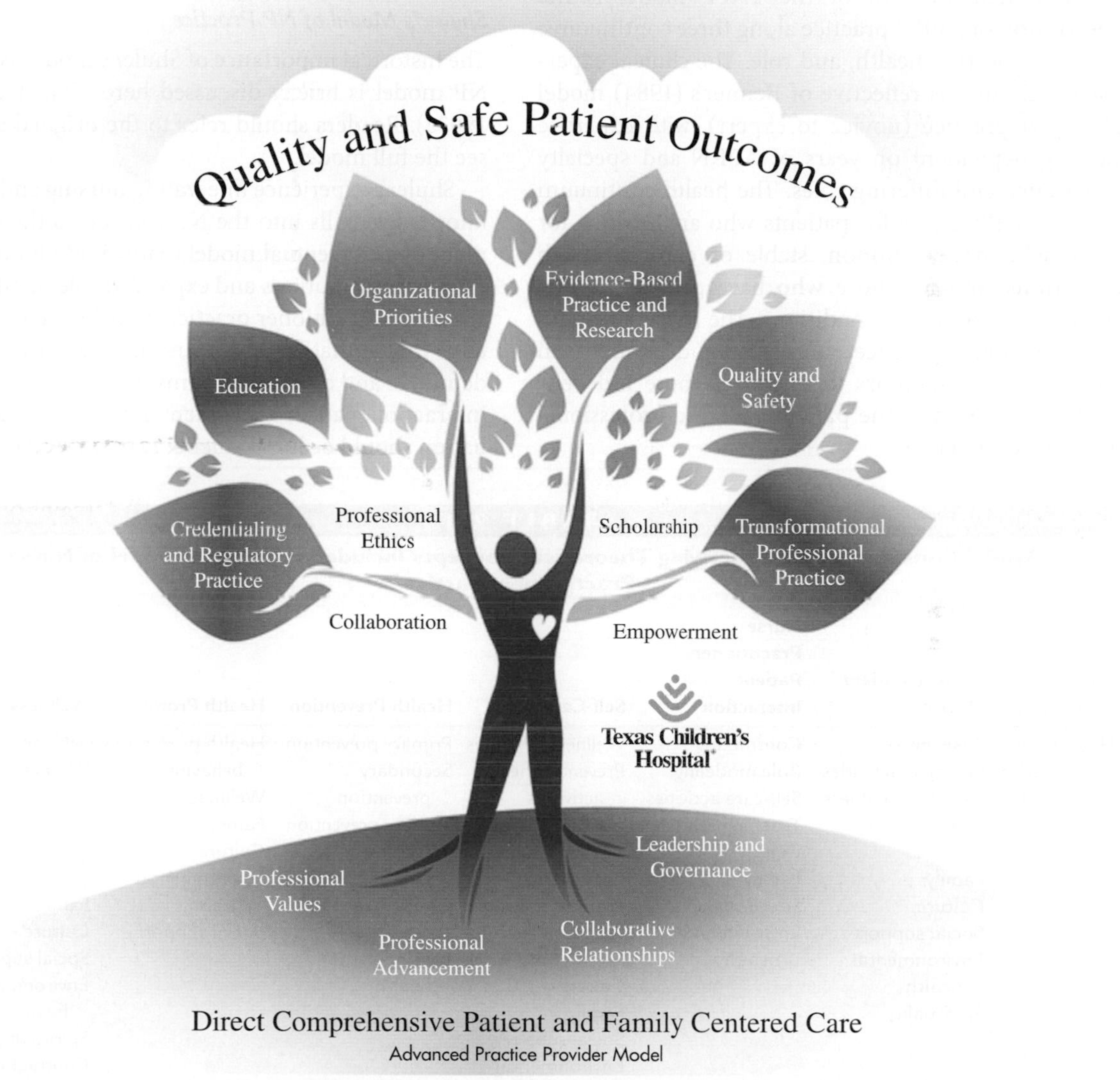

Fig. 2.8 ■ **Elliott and Walden's transformational advanced professional practice model.** (From "Development of the Transformational Advanced Professional Practice Model," by E. D. Elliott and M. Walden, 2015, *Journal of the American Association of Nurse Practitioners, 27*[9], p. 481.)

model includes this single patient care domain along with six professional development domains: organizational priorities, quality and safety, evidence-based practice and research, education, transformational professional practice, and credentialing and regulatory practice. The model recognizes that the amount of time and effort APRNs devote to the execution of the six professional development domains may vary dependent on needs of the system, patient population, and strengths and interest of individual APRNs.

An added strength of the TAPP model is the description of APRN practice along three continuums: clinical expertise, health, and role. The clinical expertise continuum is reflective of Benner's (1984) model of expert practice (novice to expert), with expertise varying dependent on years of APRN and specialty experience and differing roles. The health continuum includes APRN care for patients who are healthy; for those who have common, stable or chronic health conditions; and for those who have complex, acute, critical, or rare health conditions. The role continuum of professional practice ranges from dependent on colleagues and mentors to assume a more independent role in each of the patient care and professional domains of practice.

Although the authors indicated the model can be easily adapted to all four APRN roles, they also included physician assistants, thereby diluting the emphasis on models that conceptualize the unique practice of APRNs. In addition, because the NONPF core competencies (2011 [amended 2012]) were used along with the APRN Consensus Model (APRN Joint Dialogue Group, 2008) to develop the TAPP model, future work should test the appropriateness of this model for APRNs in roles other than the NP role.

Shuler's Model of NP Practice

The historical importance of Shuler's model as an early NP model is briefly discussed here (Shuler & Davis, 1993a). Readers should refer to the original article to see the full model.

Shuler's experience integrating nursing and medical knowledge skills into the NP role led to the development of a conceptual model that would illuminate the unique contributions and expanded role of NPs. Shuler's nurse practitioner practice model is a complex systems model that is holistic and wellness oriented. It is definitive and detailed in terms of how the NP–patient interaction, patient assessment, intervention, and evaluation should occur (Shuler & Davis, 1993a). Table 2.1

TABLE 2.1

Model Constructs and Underlying Theoretical Concepts Included in Shuler's Model of Nurse Practitioner Practice

Model Constructs	Holistic Patient Needs	Nurse Practitioner–Patient Interaction	Self-Care	Health Prevention	Health Promotion	Wellness
Underlying theoretical concepts	Basic needs Wellness activities Health and illness Psychological health Family Culture Social support Environmental health Spirituality	Contracting Role modeling Self-care activities Teaching/learning Culture Family Social support Environmental health	Wellness activities Preventive health activities Health promotion activities Compliance Problem solving Teaching/learning Contracting Culture Family Social support Environmental health	Primary prevention Secondary prevention Tertiary prevention Preventive health behavior Family Culture Environmental health	Health promotion behavior Wellness Family Culture Environmental health Social support	Self-care activities Wellness activities Disease prevention activities Health promotion activities Family Culture Social support Environmental health Spirituality Contracting Teaching/learning

From "The Shuler Nurse Practitioner Practice Model: A Theoretical Framework for Nurse Practitioner Clinicians, Educators, and Researchers, Part 1," by P. A. Shuler and J. E. Davis, 1993a, *Journal of the American Academy of Nurse Practitioners, 5,* 11–18.

outlines key model constructs and related theories. Knowing that these familiar concepts are embedded in this comprehensive model may help readers appreciate its potential usefulness.

Shuler's model is intended "to impact the NP domain at four levels: theoretical, clinical, educational, and research" (Shuler & Davis, 1993a, p. 17). The model addresses important components of advanced practice nursing: (1) nursing's metaparadigm (person, health, nursing, and environment), (2) the nursing process, (3) assumptions about patients and NPs, and (4) theoretical concepts relevant to practice. The model could be characterized as a network or system of frameworks.

Clinical application of Shuler's model is intended to describe the NP's expanded nursing knowledge and skills "into medicine," the benefits for NP and patient, and a framework whereby NP services can be evaluated (Shuler & Davis, 1993b). Shuler and Davis (1993b) published a lengthy template for conducting a visit. Although it is difficult to imagine ready implementation into today's busy NP practices, Shuler and colleagues' clinical applications of the model have been published by Shuler (2000), Shuler and Davis (1993b), and Shuler et al. (2001). In the current healthcare environment, the circle of caring model (Dunphy, Winland-Brown, Porter, Thomas & Gallagher, 2011) may be more useful for addressing some of the issues that led Shuler to create her model—integrating nursing and skills traditionally associated with medicine while learning the NP role and retaining a nursing focus while providing complex diagnostic and therapeutic interventions.

Conceptual Models of APRN Practice: International Examples

SickKids APRN Framework

A conceptual model of APRN (CNS and NP) practice was developed in Canada for the care of children and adolescents (LeGrow et al., 2010). The model was informed by four other models: the Strong Memorial Hospital model (King & Ackerman, 1995; Mick & Ackerman, 2000), the illness beliefs model (Wright et al., 1996), the five practices of exemplary leadership (Kouzes & Posner, 2002), and the CNA's (2000) advanced nursing practice national framework, which includes APRN competencies. SickKids is a family-centered model that was designed to capture the essence of the pediatric APRN role in five domains: pediatric clinical practice, research and scholarly activities, interprofessional collaboration, education and mentorship, and organization and system management. It is applicable to various pediatric practice settings across the continuum of care from the community to the hospital.

The model has been implemented throughout the organization. It has provided a common language for the conceptualization of the APRN role, to establish common expectations and competencies, establish professional development opportunities, and develop a competency-based performance evaluation. This is a promising model to conceptualize the APRN role. However, research is needed to assess the ability of the model to evaluate the effect and outcomes of pediatric APRN practice.

Model of Exemplary Midwifery Practice

In 2000, Kennedy introduced a model of exemplary midwifery practice to identify essential characteristics, specific outcomes, processes of care provided, and their relationship to specific health outcomes of women and/or infants (Fig. 2.9). The development of the model was informed by critical and feminist theories and a Delphi study using input from recipients of midwifery care and exemplary midwives, not all of whom were master's- or doctorally prepared APRNs.

The model is schematically presented as three concentric spheres. The inner sphere describes three dimensions of exemplary midwifery practice: therapeutics, caring, and the profession. *Therapeutics* illustrates how and why midwives choose and use specific therapies. *Caring* depicts how the midwife demonstrates care for and about the client, and the dimension of the *profession* examines how exemplary practice might be enhanced and accepted. The middle sphere of the model depicts five processes of exemplary midwifery practice: support for the normalcy of birth, vigilance and attention to detail, creation of a setting that is respectful and reflects the woman's needs, respect for the uniqueness of the woman and family, and updates on knowledge, personal and peer review, and balance of professional and personal life. Lastly, the outer sphere depicts five qualities of exemplary midwifery practice: (1) exceptional clinical skills and judgment, knowledge of self and limits, clinical objectivity, confidence, intelligence, and intellectual curiosity;

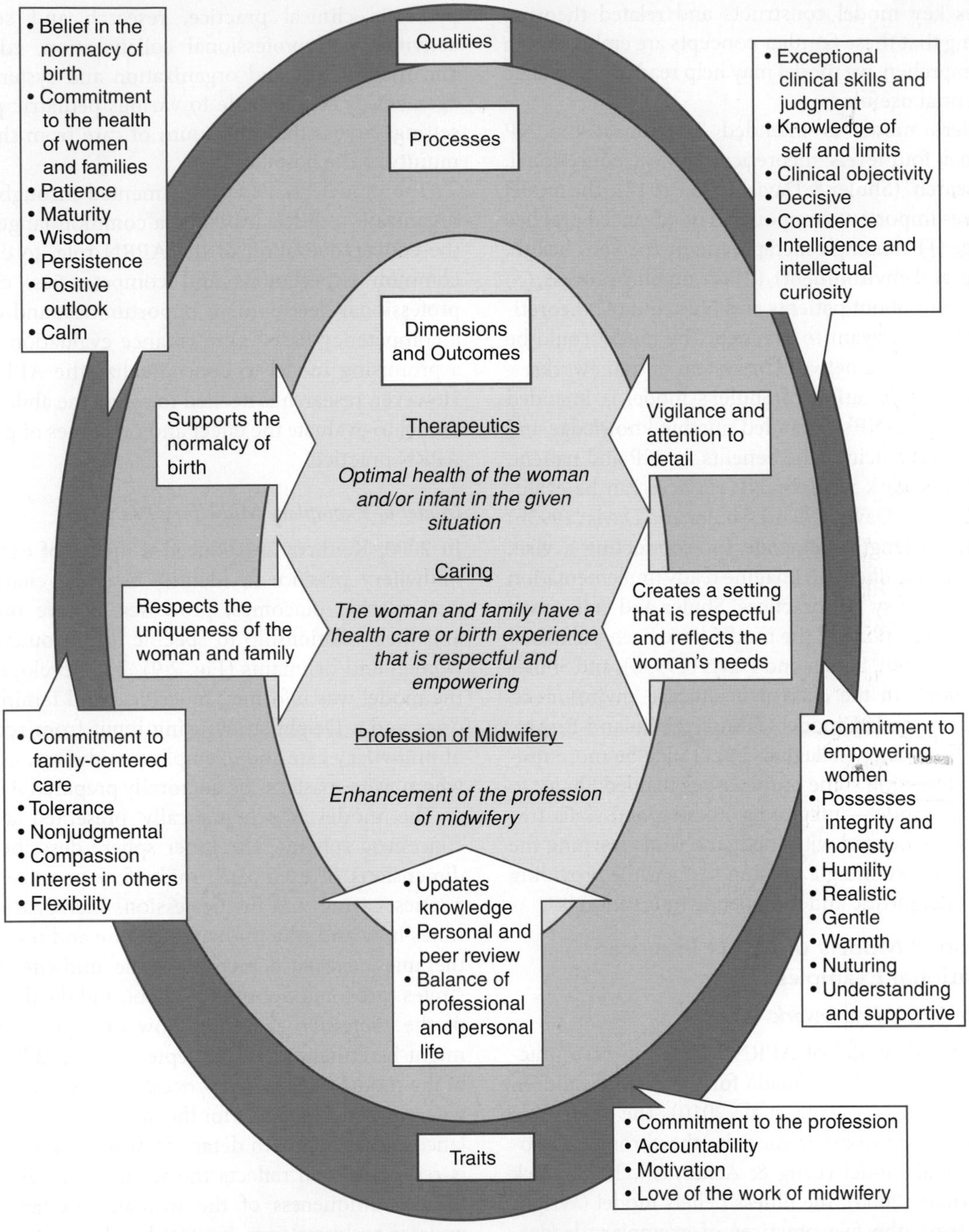

Fig. 2.9 ■ **Kennedy's abstract model of the dimensions of exemplary midwifery practice.** (From "A Model of Exemplary Midwifery Practice: Results of a Delphi Study," by H. P. Kennedy, 2000, *Journal of Midwifery & Women's Health, 45*[1], p. 8.)

(2) commitment to empowering women, integrity and honesty, humility, realistic, gentle, warmth, nurturing, and understanding and supportive; (3) commitment to the profession, accountability, motivation, love of the work of midwifery; (4) commitment to family-centered care, tolerance, nonjudgmental, compassion, interest in others, flexibility; and (5) belief in the normalcy of birth, commitment to the health of women and families, and the characteristics of patience, maturity, wisdom, persistence, positive outlook, and calm.

Although laudable efforts have been made to develop a conceptual model of exemplary midwifery practice, additional work is needed. For example, conceptual and operational definitions of the multiple concepts and the relationships among and between them need further clarification. In addition, because not all CNM participants in this study were educated and trained as APRNs, the model needs to be examined and tested in APRN-prepared CNMs to evaluate its utility and its ability to guide APRN CNM practice and improve outcomes for women and their families.

Conceptual Framework of ACNP Role and Perceptions of Team Effectiveness

A conceptual framework from Canada by Kilpatrick et al. (2013) was developed using cross-case analysis to describe key concepts that affect ACNP role enactment, boundary work, and perceptions of team effectiveness (Fig. 2.10). The development of the conceptual framework was influenced by the conceptual

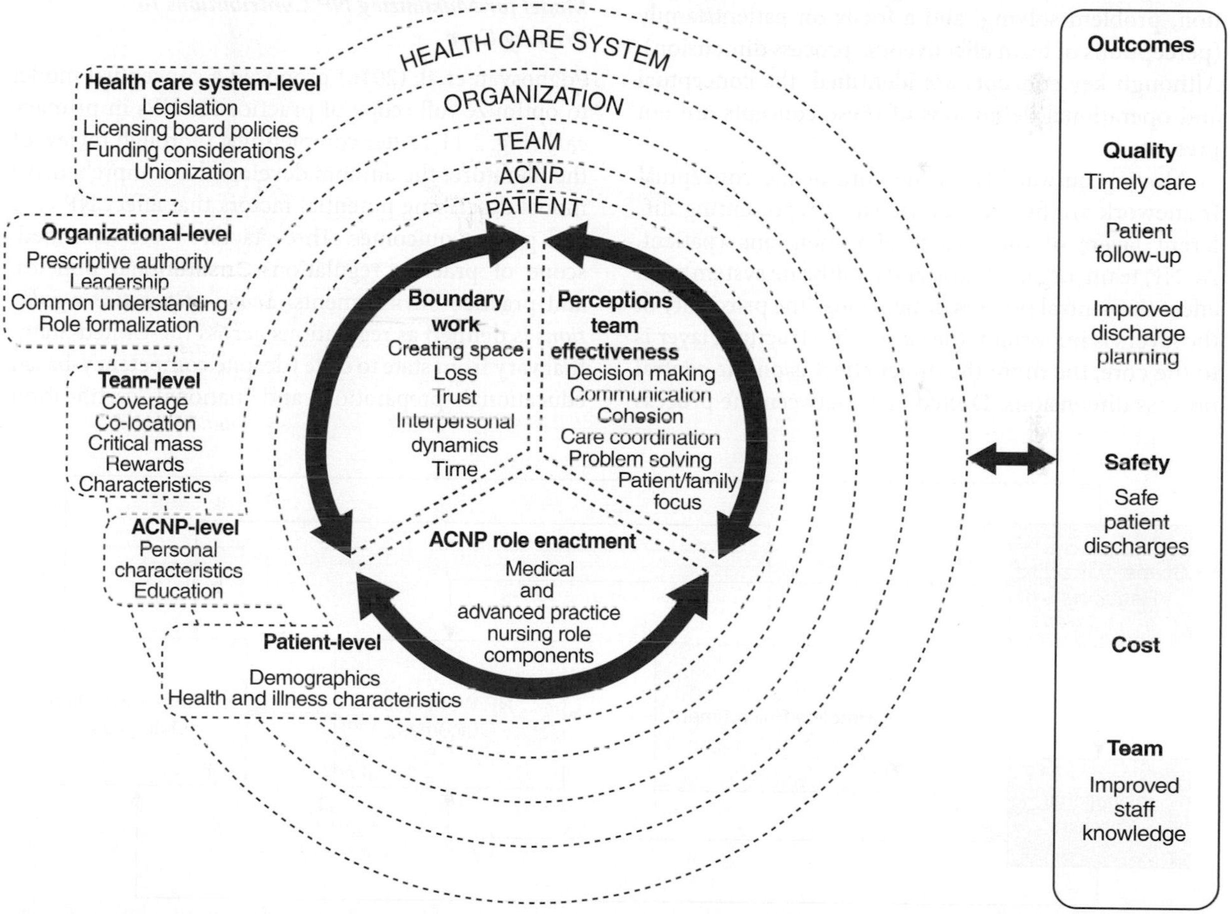

Fig. 2.10 ■ Kilpatrick et al.'s conceptual framework of ACNP role enactment, boundary work, and perceptions of team effectiveness. (From "Conceptual Framework of Acute Care Nurse Practitioner Role Enactment, Boundary Work, and Perceptions of Team Effectiveness," by K. Kilpatrick, M. Lavoie-Tremblay, L. Lamothe, J. A. Ritchie, and D. Doran, 2013, *Journal of Advanced Nursing, 69*[1], p. 211.)

framework of Sidani and Irvine (1999) for evaluating the NP role in the acute care setting and the Donabedian (1966, 2005) model of quality care that incorporates structures, processes, and outcomes.

Presented as multiple concentric circles, this conceptual framework has three central process dimensions at its core: ACNP role enactment, boundary work, and perceptions of team effectiveness. There is a bidirectional relationship proposed between the central process dimensions. Key concepts are identified within each central process dimension and include medical and advanced practice nursing and role (ACNP role enactment process dimension); creating space, loss, trust, interpersonal dynamics, and time (boundary work process dimension); and decision making, communication, cohesion, care coordination, problem solving, and a focus on patient/family (perceptions of team effectiveness process dimension). Although key concepts are identified, the conceptual and operational definitions of these concepts are not presented.

Moving outward from the core of the conceptual framework are five concentric rings representing different layers of the structural dimensions (patient, ACNP, team, organization, and healthcare system) that affect the central process dimensions. The proximity of the layers is important: the closer the structural layer is to the core, the more the direct effect is on the central process dimensions. Dotted lines between the process and structural dimensions represent the bidirectional relationship between the dimensions. Outcomes indicators include quality (timely care, patient follow-up, improved discharge planning), safety (safe patient discharges), cost, and team (improved staff knowledge).

Given the recent emphasis on teamwork and the enactment of highly functioning interprofessional teams to achieve improved patient outcomes, this framework is timely and novel because it focuses on the impact of ACNPs on teamwork. Future work should focus on the measurement of outcomes specific to and reflective of APRN care in light of the current scope of practice legislation, organizational support for the role, and patient and family perceptions of team effectiveness.

Model for Maximizing NP Contributions to Primary Care

Poghosyan et al. (2016) proposed a conceptual model to optimize full scope of practice for NPs in primary care (Fig. 2.11). After completing a thorough review of the literature, the authors developed a comprehensive model describing potential factors that affect NP care and patient outcomes. Three factors were identified: scope of practice regulations, institutional policies, and practice environments. *Scope of practice regulations* is defined as regulations across the United States that vary from state to state (despite competency-based educational preparation and national certification

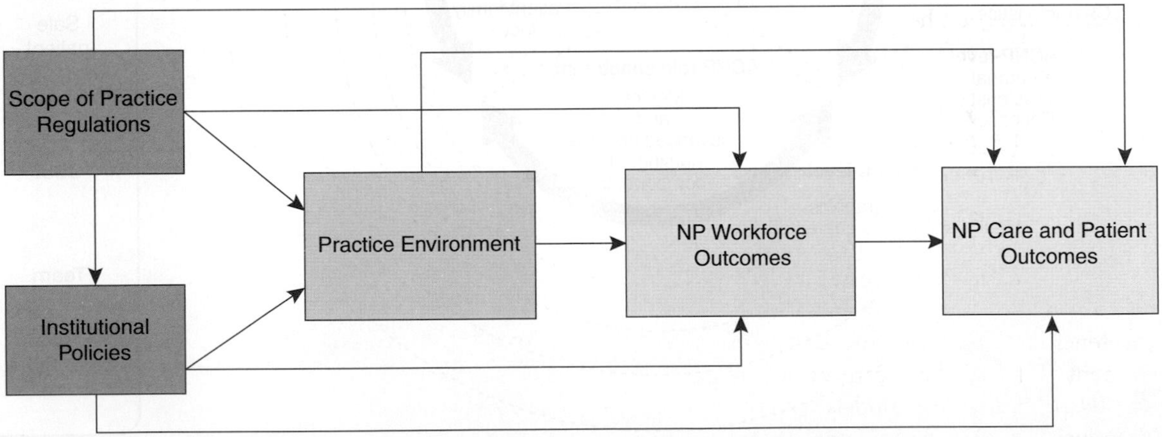

Fig. 2.11 ■ **Poghasyan et al.'s proposed model for maximizing contributions to primary care.** (From "Optimizing Full Scope of Practice for Nurse Practitioners in Primary Care: A Proposed Conceptual Model," by L. Poghosyan, D. R. Boyd, and S. P. Clarke, 2016, *Nursing Outlook, 64*[2], p. 148.)

examinations) that create barriers to NPs' abilities to practice to their full education and training, thereby creating barriers to optimal NP practice (e.g., hospital admitting privileges, recognition of primary care provider status, prescribing autonomy). *Institutional policies* are described as idiosyncratic differences between organizations even within the same state or jurisdiction that negatively affect an NP's ability to deliver patient care. These include restriction in NP practice beyond state legislation or regulation. *Practice environments* that support NP practice are defined as those that promote high-quality patient care and maximize the effectiveness and utility of primary care NPs. Positive practice environments promote favorable relationships between NPs and physicians and NPs and administration that support independent NP practice. Additionally, effective communication, similar vision and prioritization of care, and teamwork support a favorable practice environment for primary care NPs. Lastly, negative issues that affect NP workforce outcomes include high workloads, complex patients, rapidly changing administrations, and organization structures. These negative issues can lead to job stress, job dissatisfaction, burnout, and turnover.

The authors are commended on their work to develop a conceptual model to optimize full scope of practice for primary care NPs. As the authors noted, additional research is needed to fully understand the impact of restricted scope of practice and institutional policies on NP care and patient outcomes. Although the relationships between and among the variables will need to be tested, the model holds the potential to inform policy, practice, and patient outcomes.

Section Summary: Implications for Advanced Practice Nursing Conceptualizations

When one considers conceptualizations of advanced practice nursing described by professional organizations and individual authors, similarities and differences emerge. Many conceptual models address competencies that APRNs must possess. All are in agreement that the direct care of patients is central to APRN practice. Most models affirm two or more competencies identified by Hamric, and some models emphasize some competencies more than others. Some models (e.g., the Calkin and Strong models) address the issue of skill mix as it relates to APRNs, an issue of concern to administrators who hire APRNs. A notable difference across models is the extent to which the concept of environment as it relates to APRN practice is addressed. Another noted difference in the models is that only the Hamric model addresses all four APRN roles (CNS, CRNA, CNM, and NP). In the next section, selected models that APRNs may find useful as they develop and evaluate their own practices are described.

MODELS USEFUL FOR ADVANCED PRACTICE NURSES IN THEIR PRACTICE

Advanced Practice Nursing Transitional Care Models

There are several models of transitional care in which care is provided by APRNs. Early work by Brooten et al. (1988) continues to inform these models of APRN care (e.g., Partiprajak et al., 2011) and illustrates how a theory of clinical care can be studied to obtain a better understanding of the work of APRNs. It is a model that has evolved but has resulted in steady contributions to understanding and improving APRN practice. This theoretical and empirical steadfastness has had a significant influence on the new policies evolving as the United States undergoes healthcare reform.

Using a conceptual model proposed by Doessel and Marshall (1985), Brooten et al. integrated this framework into their evaluation of outcomes of APRN transitional care with different clinical populations. APRN transitional care was defined as "comprehensive discharge planning designed for each patient group plus APN home follow-up through a period of normally expected recovery or stabilization" (Brooten et al., 2002, p. 370). Brooten's model was intended to address outlier patient populations (e.g., those whose care, for clinical reasons, was likely to cost more). Across all studies, care was provided by NPs and/or CNSs whose clinical expertise was matched to the needs of the patient population. In these studies, APRN care was associated with improved patient outcomes and reduced costs.

Research by Brooten, Naylor, and others (Bradway et al., 2012) who have studied transitional care by

APRNs has provided empirical support for several elements important to a conceptualization of advanced practice nursing. In a summary of the studies conducted, the investigators identified several factors that contribute to the effectiveness of APRNs: content expertise, interpersonal skills, knowledge of systems, ability to implement change, and ability to access resources (Brooten et al., 2003). This finding provides empirical support for the importance of the APRN competencies of direct care, collaboration, coaching, and systems leadership.

Two other important findings were the existence of patterns of morbidity within patient populations and an apparent dose effect (i.e., outcomes seemed to be related to how much time was spent with patients, number of APRN interactions with patients, and numbers and types of APRN interventions; Brooten et al., 2003). Subsequently, based on this finding of a dose effect, Brooten and Youngblut (2006) proposed a conceptual explanation of "nurse dose." Their explanation suggests that nurse dose depends on patient and nurse characteristics. For the nurse, differences in education and experience can influence the dose of nursing needed.

The concept of nurse dose, which has empirical support, may enable the profession to differentiate more clearly among novice, expert, and advanced levels of nursing practice. Taken together, findings from this program of research suggest that characteristics of patients and characteristics and dose of APRN interventions are important to the conceptualization of advanced practice nursing. Finally, the fact that this program of research has used NPs and CNSs to intervene with patients provides support for a broad conceptual model of APRN practice that encompasses APRN characteristics, competencies, patient factors, environment, and other concepts that can inform role-specific models.

Although there have been other studies of APRNs providing transitional care, Brooten's work is highlighted because of the additional analyses that were done and the ultimate influence on health policy of this program of research (e.g., Naylor, 2012). The findings help understand the APRN characteristics and interventions that contributed to the success of the interventions and a model of care that evolved from the skilled care provided by APRNs.

The effect of the research conducted by Naylor et al. (2013) using the translational care model, in which APRNs are the primary coordinators of care, provide home visits, and collaborate with the patient, family caregivers, and healthcare colleagues (physicians, nurses, social workers, and other health team members), is evident in many of the provisions of the ACA and its implementation (Naylor et al., 2011). The Community-Based Care Transitions Program was created by Section 3026 of the ACA and is being implemented by the Centers for Medicare & Medicaid Services Partnership for Patients (2017).

Dunphy and Winland-Brown's Circle of Caring: A Transformative, Collaborative Model

A central premise of Dunphy and Winland-Brown's model (1998) is that the healthcare needs of individuals, families, and communities are not being met in a healthcare system dominated by medicine in which medical language (i.e., the *International Classification of Diseases*, 10th Revision, Clinical Modification codes) is the basis for reimbursement. They proposed the circle of caring to foster a more active and visible nursing presence in the healthcare system and to explain and promote medical-nursing collaboration. Dunphy and Winland-Brown's transformative model (Dunphy, Winland-Brown, Porter, Thomas, & Gallagher, 2011; Fig. 2.12) is a synthesized problem-solving approach to advanced practice nursing that builds on nursing and medical models (Dunphy & Winland-Brown, 1998).

The authors argued that a model such as theirs is needed because nursing and medicine have two different traditions, with the medical model being viewed as reductionistic and the nursing model being regarded as humanistic. Neither model, by itself, provided a structure that allowed APRNs to be recognized for their daily practice and the positive patient health outcomes that can be attributed to APRN care. The model's authors viewed the development of nursing diagnoses as an attempt to differentiate nursing care from medical care, but because few nursing diagnoses are recognized by current reimbursement systems, the nursing in APRN care was rendered invisible.

The circle of caring model was proposed to incorporate the strengths of medicine and nursing in a transforming way. The conceptual elements are the

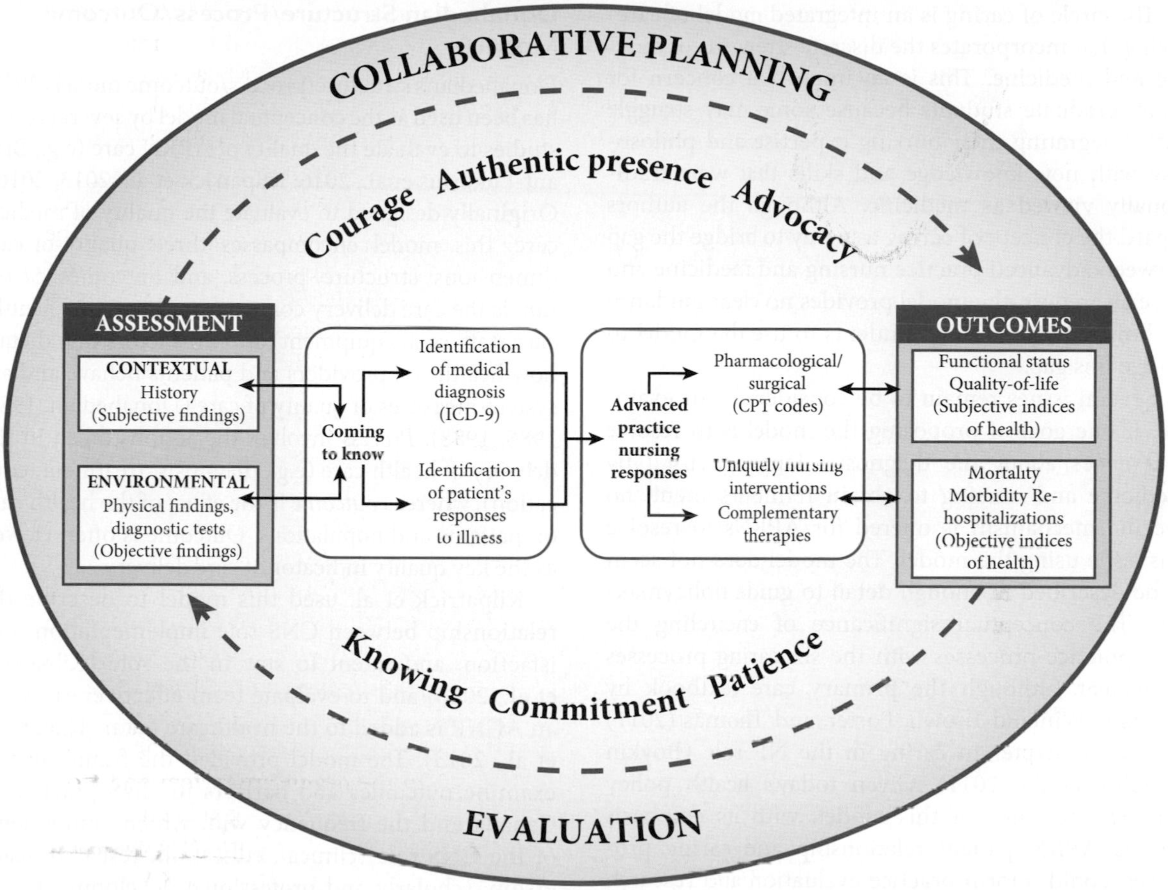

Fig. 2.12 ■ **Dunphy and Winland-Brown's circle of caring model. NP, Nurse practitioner.** (From "Primary Care in the Twenty-First Century: A Circle of Caring," by L. M. Dunphy, J. E. Winland-Brown, B. O. Porter, D. J. Thomas, and L.M. Gallagher, in L. M. Dunphy, J. E. Winland-Brown, B. O. Porter, and D. J. Thomas [Eds.], *Primary Care: The Art and Science of Advanced Practice Nursing* [3rd ed., p. 16], 2011, FA Davis.)

processes of assessment, planning, intervention, and evaluation, with a feedback loop. Integrating a nursing model with a traditional medical model permits the following to occur:

- The assessment and evaluation are contextualized, incorporating subjective and environmental elements into traditional history taking and physical examination.
- The approach to therapeutics is broadened to include holistic approaches to healing and makes nursing care more visible.
- Measured outcomes include patients' perceptions of health and care, not just physiologic outcomes and resource use.

The assessment–planning–intervention–evaluation processes in linear configuration are encircled by caring. Caring is actualized through interpersonal interactions with patients and caregivers to which NPs bring patience, courage, advocacy, authentic presence, commitment, and knowing (Dunphy & Winland-Brown, 1998; Dunphy, Winland-Brown, Porter, Thomas, & Gallagher, 2011). Conceptual definitions of these terms would add to the understanding of how these processes interact with and affect the care provided by APRNs. The authors suggested that the model promotes the incorporation of the lived experience of the patient into the provider–patient interaction and that the process of caring is a prerequisite to APRNs providing effective and meaningful care to patients.

The circle of caring is an integrated model of caregiving that incorporates the discrete strengths of nursing and medicine. This is an important concern for many graduate students because some may struggle with integrating their nursing expertise and philosophy with new knowledge and skills that were traditionally viewed as medicine. Although the authors regard the concept of caring as a way to bridge the gap between advanced practice nursing and medicine and raise awareness, the model provides no clear guidance on how faculty can help students to use the model to bridge this gap.

Several issues remain to be considered. For example, if one goal of proposing the model is to resolve differences about the diagnostic language used by medicine and nursing to obtain reimbursement, no specific mechanism is offered for APRNs to resolve this issue using the model. The model does not seem to be described in enough detail to guide policymaking. The conceptual significance of encircling the four practice processes with the six caring processes is unclear, although the primary care textbook by Dunphy, Winland-Brown, Porter, and Thomas (2011) devotes a chapter to caring in the NP role (Boykin & Schoenhofer, 2011). Given today's health policy context, the value of this model, with its emphasis on the APRN–patient relationship and caring processes, could inform practice evaluation and research on APRN practices. For example, the circle of caring model has been used for the development of an online risk assessment of mental health (McKnight, 2011), evaluation of medication adherence (Palardy & March, 2011), and neonatal transport (J. Thomas, 2011). In addition, the primary care textbook (Dunphy et al., 2011) is informed by their circle of caring model.

Given the emphasis on interprofessional education and efforts to distinguish advanced practice nursing from medical practice, empirical testing of this model is warranted. This testing would help determine whether the model has the following features: (1) is applicable to all APRN roles, (2) has the potential to be used to distinguish expert by experience practice from advanced practice, (3) is viewed by other disciplines as having an interprofessional focus that would promote collaboration, and (4) will result in more visibility for NPs and other APRNs in the healthcare system.

Donabedian Structure/Process/Outcome Model

Donabedian's structure/process/outcome model (2005) has been used as the conceptual model by several recent studies to evaluate the quality of APRN care (e.g., Bryant-Lukosius et al., 2016; Kilpatrick et al., 2013, 2016). Originally designed to evaluate the quality of medical care, this model encompasses three quality-of-care dimensions: structure, process, and outcomes. *Structure* is the care delivery context (e.g., hospitals, healthcare staff, cost, equipment) and the factors that dictate how healthcare providers and patients behave and are system measures of quality of care (Donabedian, 1980, 1986, 1988). *Process* involves the actions taken in the delivery of health care (e.g., diagnosis, treatment, education), whereas *outcome* is the effect of the health care on patients and populations. Outcome is often viewed as the key quality indicator of care delivery.

Kilpatrick et al. used this model to describe the relationship between CNS role implementation, satisfaction, and intent to stay in the role (Kilpatrick et al., 2016) and to evaluate team effectiveness when an ACNP is added to the healthcare team (Kilpatrick et al., 2013). The model provided the framework to examine outcomes and barriers to CNS practice in Canada and the frequency with which components of the CNS role (clinical, education, research, leadership, scholarly and professional development, and consultation) were enacted. Findings indicated that CNS role components of clinical and research, along with balanced scholarly and professional development and consultation activities, were associated with role satisfaction. Additional research is needed to determine whether implementation of the CNS role influences intention to remain in or actual departure from the role.

Guided by the Donabedian model, Bryant-Lukosius et al. (2016) developed an evaluation framework to inform decisions about the effective utilization of APRNs in Switzerland (Fig. 2.13). An international group of stakeholders (e.g., APRNs, APRN educators, administrators, researchers) from Canada, Germany, Switzerland, and the United States convened to develop and refine the framework. The developed framework is deliberately broad and flexible to respond to the evolving APRN roles in Switzerland. Key concepts of

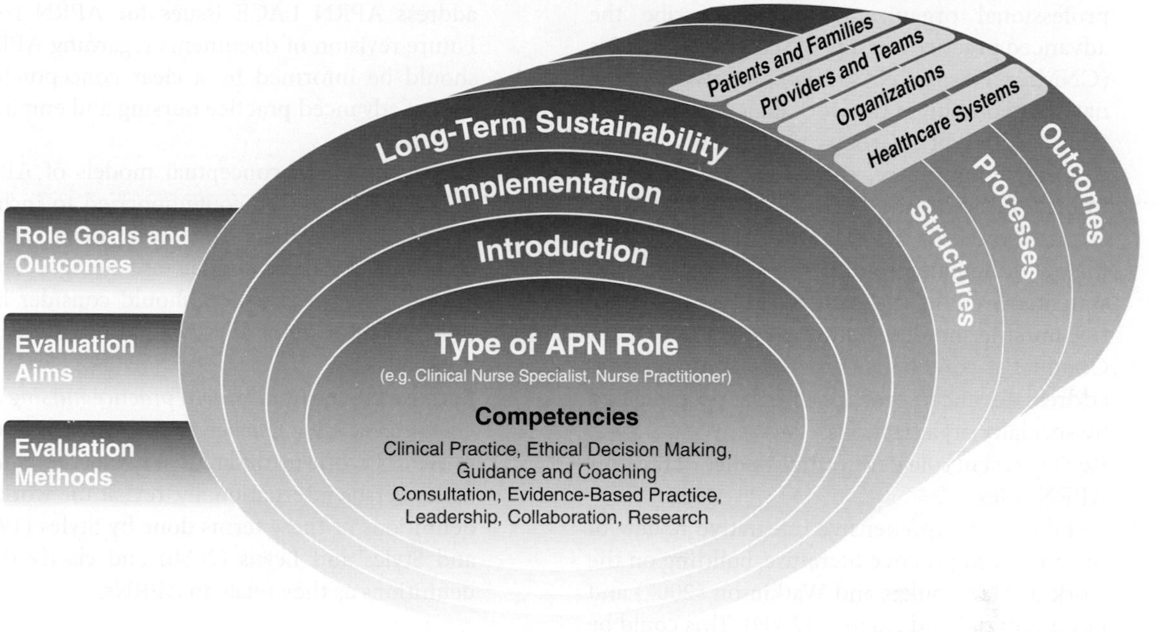

Fig. 2.13 ■ **Bryant-Lukosius education framework matrix—key concepts for evaluating advanced practice nursing roles.** (From "Framework for Evaluating the Impact of Advanced Practice Nursing Roles," by D. Bryant-Lukosius, E. Spichiger, J. Martin, H. Stoll, S. D. Kellerhals, M. Fliedner, Grossman, F., Henry, M., Hermann, L., Koller, A., & Schwendimann, R., 2016, *Journal of Nursing Scholarship, 48*[2], p. 204.)

the model are introduction stage, implementation, and long-term sustainability. The introduction stage includes the type of APRN and corresponding competencies. The implementation stage focuses on the resources (e.g., policies, education, funding) to support the different APRN roles and promote the optimal utilization and implementation of the role. Long-term sustainability focuses on long-term benefits and impact of APRN roles (e.g., consumers, system, providers) in Switzerland. Because the role of the APRN is in its early stage, the authors have indicated their plan to engage in concerted efforts with policymakers and other stakeholders to actively involve them in its use and application. Several resources have been developed to actualize this (e.g., toolkit, evaluation plan template).

RECOMMENDATIONS AND FUTURE DIRECTIONS

Given the variety of conceptualizations and inconsistency in terminology, it is not surprising that APRN students and practicing APRNs would find the conceptualization of advanced practice nursing confusing. The challenge for APRNs (students and practicing nurses) is to find a model that works for them and that enables them to understand and evaluate their practices and attend to the profession's efforts to create a coherent, stable, and robust conceptualization of advanced practice nursing.

Conceptualizations of Advanced Practice Nursing

This overview of extant models of advanced practice nursing is necessarily cursory, primarily focused on Western literature (Canada, Europe, United States). Although there is some agreement on selected elements of advanced practice, differences remain regarding the conceptualization of the ARPN. To promote a unified conceptualization of advanced practice nursing, the following recommendations are put forth:

1. Conduct a rigorous content analysis of the statements published by national and international

professional organizations that describe the advanced practice nursing of recognized APRNs (CNMs, CNSs, CRNAs, NPs). This would be a natural evolution of the work done by the APRN Consensus Work Group, the NCSBN APRN Advisory Committee, the CNA, and others to inform future work. As part of this analysis, an assessment of the extent to which nursing's metaparadigmatic concepts are integrated into statements about the nature of advanced practice nursing should be undertaken.

2. Conduct a content analysis of statements that address advanced practice nursing promulgated by specialty organizations.
3. Review recent role delineation studies of the four APRN roles.
4. Conduct a comprehensive integrative review of the advanced practice literature, building on the work of Mantzoukas and Watkinson (2007) and Lewandowski and Adamle (2009). This could be modeled on the work of Reeves et al. (2011) and their conceptualization of interprofessional education, identifying concepts and relationships that need further development.
5. Synthesize results to collaboratively propose a definition of advanced practice nursing to be used nationally and globally.
6. Create a common structure for organizational statements about APRNs that ensures nursing concepts are included:
   a. Definition of nursing and advanced practice nursing
   b. Specification of assumptions
   c. Incorporation of the metaparadigmatic elements (persons, health and illness, nursing, environment) into scopes and introductions to key documents
   d. Referencing documents such as the ANA's social policy statement and the ICN's statements on nursing
7. Implement a structure for organizations and associations developing statements regarding advanced practice nursing to explicate the foundational and philosophic underpinnings of each statement. Use the results from recommendations 1 through 5 above to inform revisions to standards and other documents that address APRN LACE issues for APRN roles. Future revision of documents regarding APRNs should be informed by a clear conceptualization of advanced practice nursing and empirical evidence.
8. The evolution of conceptual models of APRN practice needs to be contemporized to include concepts of diversity and social determinants of health. As these models are being adapted and modified, evaluation should consider how they impact care for all as well as for all diverse APRNs.
9. Because the terms *advanced practice nursing* and *advanced nursing practice* are being used to refer to APRN work in different ways in the United States versus internationally, revisit the work on definitions of these terms done by Styles (1998) and Styles and Lewis (2000) and clarify these definitions as they relate to APRNs.

Consensus Building Around Advanced Practice Nursing

A priority for the profession is a collaboratively developed conceptualization of advanced practice nursing and what is common across the various APRN roles. Achieving this is a prerequisite for building consensus among APRNs, stakeholder organizations, and policymakers and ensuring that all patients will benefit from advanced practice nursing. The APRN Consensus Model, at the time it was released, represented substantial progress in this area with regard to regulation. However, it is now dated and in need of revision. Studies are under way worldwide (see Chapter 5) that could inform efforts to refine conceptualizations of advanced nursing practice. Ongoing development of consensus on advanced practice nursing should involve:

- Periodic updates on the progress of nationwide implementation of the regulatory model—successes and challenges (note that the NCSBN periodically updates state-by-state maps on its website [https://www.ncsbn.org/5397.htm]).
- Communication between national and global APRN accrediting and certification bodies. Because US nurse anesthetists and nurse-midwives operate under different accrediting and certification bodies and mechanisms than CNSs

and NPs, their experience may be helpful in countries in which nurses and midwives are regulated separately or where nurse anesthesia is not a practice role.

- Consensus of common terms used in documents describing APRN practice.

It is evident from this review that there is still a need for common language to describe advanced practice nursing. Clear articulation and consensus of the conceptual differences among terms such as *essentials*, *competencies*, *hallmarks*, and *standard of care* are needed among the various users within the profession and among other stakeholders. The responses of the AANA, ACNM, NACNS, and NONPF to the DNP initiative and concerns about selective implementation of the APRN Consensus Model are likely to influence the evolution of advanced practice nursing in the next decade. The extent to which we reach agreement within the profession will affect policy related to advanced practice and whether the public recognizes and requests the services of APRNs. Disagreement on the nature and credentialing of advanced practice nursing should be resolved by continued efforts to foster true consensus by:

- Addressing the legitimate concerns of these organizations (e.g., impact on access to care, concerns about certification or grandfathering existing APRNs)
- Establishing priorities for negotiation and resolution by stakeholder groups and initiating a process to find common ground and address disagreements
- In the face of disagreements, working toward agreement on a common identity to facilitate public understanding of APRN roles

These consensus-building efforts are needed if our profession is to remain attractive to new nurses and new APRNs and to make room for evolving APRN roles.

Consensus on Key Elements of Practice Doctorate Curricula

The recently released Essentials (AACN, 2021b) addresses previous concerns regarding variability in DNP curricula content (Ketefian & Redman, 2015) and a reduced emphasis of DNP programs on theory (Whall, 2005) by providing consensus regarding the standard competencies for professional practice at the doctorate of practice level. Included in these competencies is expectation DNP graduates will be prepared to think theoretically, ethically, and conceptually as socially responsible and competent clinicians. Although the ACNM does not currently support the practice doctorate for entry into practice and the AANA has delayed endorsing doctoral preparation for entry into practice until 2025 and the NACNS until 2030, APRN organizations have prepared doctoral-level competencies that are consistent with those proposed in the DNP.

Research on Advanced Practice Nurses and Their Contribution to Patients, Teams, and System Outcomes

Theory-based research on APRNs' contributions to improved patient outcomes and cost-effectiveness is needed to inform and validate the conceptualizations of advanced practice nursing. Increased knowledge about advanced practice nursing is critical (see Chapter 21). The worth of any service depends on the extent to which practice meets the needs and priorities of healthcare systems, the public policy arena, and society in general. In addition to research that links advanced practice nursing with outcomes, the following recommendations are put forth:

1. Promising conceptual models of advanced practice nursing should be refined based on research that validates key concepts and tests theoretical propositions associated with these models.
2. Studies are needed to examine advanced practice nursing across APRN roles and between physician and APRN practices and APRN and PA practices with regard to processes and outcomes. Studies conducted across APRN roles can determine whether the assumption that a core set of competencies is used by all APRNs is valid and that the activities of APRNs can differentiate one APRN role from another. The studies of APRN and physician practice can identify the factors that distinguish APRN practice from physician practice as a basis for understanding differences in outcomes and developing proposals to optimally use each provider to achieve high-quality, patient-centered, cost-effective care.

3. As conceptualizations of interprofessional teams evolve, the roles and contributions of APRNs and their interdisciplinary colleagues to outcomes need examination.

When there is a better empirical understanding of the similarities and differences across APRN roles and between physicians and APRNs, this knowledge must be packaged and presented to colleagues in other disciplines, policymakers, and the public. These data will be key to educating physician colleagues, healthcare consumers, and policymakers about the meaning and relevance of advanced practice nursing to the health of our society.

CONCLUSION

Consensus regarding a conceptual model of advanced practice nursing is needed to guide practice, research, and public policy. The future of advanced practice nursing depends on the extent to which practice meets the needs and priorities of society, healthcare systems, and the public policy arena. A stable, robust model of advanced practice nursing will serve to guide the development of advanced practice nursing and ensure that patients will have access to APRN care.

Issues, limitations, and imperatives related to conceptualizing advanced practice nursing have been identified in this review of conceptual models of APRN practice. The nursing profession, nationally and internationally, remains at a critical juncture with regard to advanced practice nursing. In each country in which APRNs practice, the need to move forward with a unified voice on this issue is urgent if APRNs and the nursing profession as a whole are to fulfill their social contract with individuals, institutions, and communities. A unified conceptualization of advanced practice nursing focuses the efforts of the profession on preparing APRNs, promulgating policies, and fostering research to enable the realization of the outcomes, including maximizing the social contribution of APRNs to the health needs of society and promoting the actualization of APRNs.

KEY SUMMARY POINTS

- Conceptualizations of advanced practice nursing include models and theories that guide the practice of APRNs.
- Conceptual models can and do differentiate practice among and between levels of nursing practice and between APRNs and other healthcare providers. Conceptual and practical clarity is needed to differentiate advanced nursing practice from advanced practice nursing.
- Conceptual consensus is needed to clarify concepts and models that help stakeholders understand the nature of APRNs' work and their contributions to patient, nurse, and system outcomes. APRN practice statements need to explicate the philosophic and foundational underpinnings.
- Collaborative development of the conceptualization of advanced practice nursing and community across the various roles is a priority. A common identity will facilitate stakeholder understanding of APRN roles. Consensus-building efforts are needed to attract new nurses and new APRNs to our profession and to make room for evolving APRN roles.
- National and international efforts are under way to develop a unified consensus on the conceptualization of advanced practice nursing. However, despite these efforts, differences continue regarding the conceptualization of the APRN.
- A lack of unanimous agreement continues to exist regarding the educational preparation of APRNs and whether or not a DNP or other doctoral education is required for entry into practice.
- Research is needed on how APRNs acquire expertise in APRN and interprofessional competencies to inform future conceptualizations of advanced practice nursing.

REFERENCES

Ackerman, M. M., Clark, J., Reed, T., Van Horn, L., & Francati, M. (2000). A nurse practitioner–managed cardiovascular intensive care unit. In J. Hickey, R. Ouimette, & S. Venegoni (Eds.), *Advanced practice nursing: Changing roles and clinical applications* (pp. 470–480). Lippincott.

Ackerman, M. H., Mick, D., & Witzel, P. (2010). Creating an organizational model to support advanced practice. *The Journal of Nursing Administration, 40*, 63–68.

Ackerman, M. H., Norsen, L., Martin, B., Wiedrich, J., & Kitzman, H. J. (1996). Development of a model of advanced practice. *American Journal of Critical Care, 5*, 68–73.

Algase, D. L. (2010). Essentials of scholarship for the DNP: Are we clear yet? *Research and Theory for Nursing Practice, 24*, 91–93.

Allan, H. (2011). Advancing nursing practice: Redefining the theoretical and practical integration of knowledge. *Journal of Clinical Nursing, 20*, 873–881. *Journal of Clinical Nursing, 20*, 2687–2688.

American Association of Colleges of Nursing. (2006). The essentials of doctorate education for advanced nursing practice. Retrieved from https://www.aacnnursing.org/Portals/42/Publications/DNPEssentials.pdf

American Association of Colleges of Nursing. (2019). DNP fact sheet. Retrieved from https://www.aacnnursing.org/Portals/42/News/Factsheets/DNP-Factsheet.pdf

American Association of Colleges of Nursing. (2021a). Clinical nurse leader (CNL): Frequently asked questions. Retrieved from http://www.aacn.nche.edu/cnl/CNLFAQ.pdf

American Association of Colleges of Nursing (2021b). The Essentials: Core competencies for professional nursing education. Retrieved from https://www.aacnnursing.org/Education-Resources/AACN-Essentials

American Association of Nurse Anesthesiology. (2018). Patient-driven interdisciplinary practice: Position statement. Retrieved from https://www.aana.com/docs/default-source/practice-aana-com-web-documents-(all)/patient-drive-interdisciplinary-practice.pdf

American Association of Nurse Anesthesiology. (2019). Standards for nurse anesthesia practice. Retrieved from https://www.aana.com/docs/default-source/practice-aana-com-web-documents-(all)/standards-for-nurse-anesthesia-practice.pdf?sfvrsn=e00049b1_18

American Association of Nurse Anesthesiology. (2020). Scope of nurse anesthesia practice. Retrieved from https://www.aana.com/docs/default-source/practice-aana-com-web-documents-(all)/scope-of-nurse-anesthesia-practice.pdf?sfvrsn=250049b1_6

American College of Nurse-Midwives. (2011a). Definition of midwifery and scope of practice of certified nurse-midwives and certified midwives. Retrieved from http://www.midwife.org/ACNM/files/ACNMLibraryData/UPLOADFILENAME/000000000266/Definition%20of%20Midwifery%20and%20Scope%20of%20Practice%20of%20CNMs%20and%20CMs%20Feb%202012.pdf

American College of Nurse-Midwives. (2011b). The practice doctorate in midwifery. Retrieved from http://www.midwife.org/ACNM/files/ACNMLibraryData/UPLOADFILENAME/000000000260/Practice%20Doctorate%20in%20Midwifery%20Sept%202011.pdf

American College of Nurse-Midwives. (2011c). Standards for the practice of midwifery. Retrieved from http://www.midwife.org/ACNM/files/ACNMLibraryData/UPLOADFILENAME/000000000051/Standards_for_Practice_of_Midwifery_Sept_2011.pdf

American College of Nurse-Midwives. (2012a). Core competencies for basic midwifery practice. Retrieved from http://www.midwife.org/ACNM/files/ACNMLibraryData/UPLOADFILENAME/000000000050/Core%20Competencies%20June%202012.pdf

American College of Nurse-Midwives. (2012b). Position statement: Midwifery education and the Doctor of Nursing Practice (DNP). Retrieved from http://www.midwife.org/ACNM/files/ACNMLibraryData/UPLOADFILENAME/000000000079/Midwifery%20Ed%20and%20DNP%20Position%20Statement%20June%202012

American College of Nurse-Midwives. (2015a). Code of ethics with explanatory statements. Retrieved from https://www.midwife.org/ACNM/files/ACNMLibraryData/UPLOADFILENAME/000000000293/Code-of-Ethics-w-Explanatory-Statements-June-2015.pdf

American College of Nurse-Midwives. (2015b). Position statement: Mandatory degree requirements for entry into midwifery practice. Retrieved from http://www.midwife.org/ACNM/files/ACNMLibraryData/UPLOADFILENAME/000000000076/Mandatory-Degree-Requirements-June-2015.pdf

American College of Nurse-Midwives. (2019). Midwifery education and doctoral preparation. https://www.midwife.org/acnm/files/acnmlibrarydata/uploadfilename/000000000079/PS%20Midwifery%20Education%20and%20Doctoral%20Preparation%20190927.pdf

American College of Nurse-Midwives, Accreditation Commission for Midwifery Education, & American Midwifery Certification Board. (2011). Midwifery in the United States and the Consensus Model for APRN regulation. Retrieved from http://www.midwife.org/ACNM/files/ccLibraryFiles/Filename/000000001458/LACE_White_Paper_2011.pdf

American Nurses Association. (2010). *Nursing's social policy statement* (3rd ed.). Author.

American Nurses Association. (2021). *Nursing: Scope and standards of practice* (4th ed.). Author.

APRN Joint Dialogue Group. (2008). Consensus Model for APRN regulation: Licensure, accreditation, certification & education. Retrieved from http://www.aacn.nche.edu/education-resources/APRNReport.pdf

Arslanian-Engoren, C., Hicks, F. D., Whall, A. L., & Algase, D. L. (2005). An ontological view of advanced practice nursing. *Research and Theory for Nursing Practice, 19*, 315–322.

Ayre, T. C., & Bee, T. S. (2014). Advanced practice nursing in Singapore. *Proceedings of Singapore Healthcare, 23*(14), 269–270.

Bahouth, M. N., Ackerman, M., Ellis, E. E., Fuchs, J., McComiskey, C., Stewart, E. S., & Thomson-Smith, C. (2013). Centralized resources for nurse practitioners: Common early experiences among leaders of six large health systems. *Journal of the American Association of Nurse Practitioners, 25*(4), 203–212.

Barr, H., Freeth, D., Hammick, M., Koppel, I., & Reeves, S. (2005). The evidence base and recommendations for interprofessional education in health and social care. In H. Barr, I. Koppell, S. Reeves, M. Hammick, & D. Freeth (Eds.), *Effective interprofessional education: Argument, assumption and evidence* (pp. 2–4). Blackwell.

Becker, D., Kaplow, R., Muenzen, P., & Hartigan, C. (2006). Activities performed by acute and critical care advanced practice nurses: American Association of Critical-Care Nurses study of practice. *American Journal of Critical Care, 15*, 130–148.

Begley, C., Elliott, N., Lalor, J., Coyne, I., Higgins, A., & Comiskey, C. M. (2013). Differences between clinical specialist and advanced practitioner clinical practice, leadership, and research roles, responsibilities, and perceived outcomes (the SCAPE study). *Journal of Advanced Nursing, 69*(3), 1323–1337.

Behren, S. A. (2018). International nursing: Constructing an advanced practice registered nurse practice in the UAE: Using innovation to address cultural implications and challenges in an international enterprise. *Nursing Administration Quarterly, 42*(1), 83–90.

Benner, P. (1984). *From novice to expert*. Menlo Park, CA: Addison-Wesley.

Benner, P., Tanner, C., & Tesla, C. (2009). *Expertise in nursing practice: Caring, clinical judgment and ethics*. Springer Publishing Company.

Boykin, A., & Schoenhofer, S. O. (2011). Caring and the advanced practice nurse. In L. M. Dunphy, J. E. Winland-Brown, B. O. Porter, & D. J. Thomas (Eds.), *Primary care: The art and science of advanced practice nursing* (3rd ed.) (pp. 19–23). F. A. Davis.

Bradway, C., Trotta, R., Bixby, M., McPartland, E., Wollman, M., Kapustka, H., McCauley, K., & Naylor, M. D. (2012). A qualitative analysis of an advanced practice nurse–directed transitional care model intervention. *The Gerontologist, 52*, 394–407.

Brooten, D., Brown, L., Munro, B., York, R., Cohen, S., Roncoli, M., & Hollingsworth, A. (1988). Early discharge and specialist transitional care. *Image–the Journal of Nursing Scholarship, 20*, 64–68.

Brooten, D., Naylor, M., York, R., Brown, L., Munro, B. H., Hollingsworth, A. O., Cohen, S. M., Finkler, S., Deatrick, J., & Youngblut, J. M. (2002). Lessons learned from testing the quality cost model of advanced practice nursing (APN) transitional care. *Journal of Nursing Scholarship, 34*, 359–375.

Brooten, D., & Youngblut, J. (2006). Nurse dose as a concept. *Journal of Nursing Scholarship, 38*, 94–99.

Brooten, D., Youngblut, J., Deatrick, J., Naylor, M., & York, R. (2003). Patient problems, advanced practice nurse (APN) interventions, time and contacts among five patient groups. *Journal of Nursing Scholarship, 35*, 73–79.

Bryant-Lukosius, D., Spichiger, E., Martin, J., Stoll, H., Kellerhals, S. D., Fliedner, M., Grossman, F., Henry, M., Hermann, L., Koller, A., & Schwendimann, R. (2016). Framework for evaluating the impact of advanced practice nursing roles. *Journal of Nursing Scholarship, 48*(2), 201–209.

Brykczynski, K. A. (1989). An interpretive study describing the clinical judgment of nurse practitioners. *Scholarly Inquiry for Nursing Practice, 3*, 75–104.

Calkin, J. D. (1984). A model for advanced nursing practice. *The Journal of Nursing Administration, 14*, 24–30.

Canadian Interprofessional Health Collaborative. (2010). A national interprofessional competency framework. Retrieved from http://www.cihc.ca/files/CIHC_IPCompetencies_Feb1210.pdf

Canadian Nurses Association (CNA). (2000). *Advanced nursing practice: A national framework*. Author.

Canadian Nurses Association (CNA). (2007). Position statement: Advanced nursing practice. Retrieved from http://www2.cna-aiic.ca/CNA/documents/pdf/publications/PS60_Advanced_Nursing_Practice_2007_e.pdf

Canadian Nurses Association (CNA). (2008). Advanced nursing practice: A national framework. Retrieved from http://www2.cna-aiic.ca/CNA/documents/pdf/publications/ANP_National_Framework_e.pdf

Canadian Nurses Association (CNA). (2009a). CNA position on clinical nurse specialist. Retrieved from http://www2.cna-aiic.ca/CNA/documents/pdf/publications/PS104_Clinical_Nurse_Specialist_e.pdf

Canadian Nurses Association (CNA). (2009b). Position statement: The nurse practitioner. Retrieved from http://www2.cna-aiic.ca/CNA/documents/pdf/publications/PS_Nurse_Practitioner_e.pdf

Canadian Nurses Association (CNA). (2010). Canadian nurse practitioner core competency framework. Retrieved from https://www.cna-aiic.ca/~/media/cna/files/en/competency_framework_2010_e.pdf?la=en

Canadian Nurses Association (CNA). (2013). Strengthening the role of the clinical nurse specialist in Canada: Pan-Canadian roundtable discussion summary report. Retrieved from https://www.cna-aiic.ca/~/media/cna/page-content/pdf-fr/clinical_nurse_specialist_role_roundtable_summary_e.pdf?la=en

Canadian Nurses Association (CNA). (2016a). The nurse practitioner position statement. Retrieved from https://hl-prod-ca-oc-download.s3-ca-central-1.amazonaws.com/CNA/2f975e7e-4a40-45ca-863c-5ebf0a138d5e/UploadedImages/documents/The_Nurse_Practitioner_Position_Statement_2016.pdf

Canadian Nurses Association (CNA). (2016b). Clinical nurse specialist position statement. Retrieved from https://hl-prod-ca-oc-download.s3-ca-central-1.amazonaws.com/CNA/2f975e7e-4a40-45ca-863c-5ebf0a138d5e/UploadedImages/documents/Clinical_Nurse_Specialist_Position_Statement_2016.pdf

Canadian Nurses Association (CNA). (2019). Advanced practice nursing: A Pan-Canadian framework. Retrieved from https://www.cna-aiic.ca/-/media/cna/page-content/pdf-en/advanced-practice-nursing-framework-en.pdf?la=en&hash=76A98ADEE62E655E158026DEB45326C8C9528B1B

Carron, R., & Cumbie, S. A. (2011). Development of a conceptual nursing model for the implementation of spiritual care in adult primary healthcare settings by nurse practitioners. *Journal of the American Academy of Nurse Practitioners, 23*, 552–560.

Carryer, J., Wilkinson, J., Towers, A., & Gardner, G. (2018). Delineating advanced practice nursing in New Zealand: A national survey. *International Nursing Review, 65*(1), 24–32.

Centers for Medicare & Medicaid Services Partnership for Patients. (2017). About the partnership. Retrieved from https://partnershipforpatients.cms.gov/about-the-partnership/community-based-care-transitions-program/community-basedcaretransitionsprogram.html

Chang, A. M., Gardner, G. E., Duffield, C., & Ramis, M. (2010). A Delphi study to validate an advanced practice nursing tool. *Journal of Advanced Nursing, 66*, 2320–2330.

Christensen, M. (2009). Advancing practice in critical care: A model of knowledge integration. *Nursing in Critical Care, 14*, 86–94.

Christensen, M. (2011). Advancing nursing practice: Redefining the theoretical and practical integration of knowledge. *Journal of Clinical Nursing, 20*, 873–881.

Council on Accreditation of Nurse Anesthesia Education Programs. (2019). Standards for accreditation of nurse anesthesia programs: Practice doctorate. Retrieved from http://home.coa.us.com/accreditation/Documents/Standards%20for%20Accreditation%20of%20Nurse%20Anesthesia%20Programs%20-%20Practice%20Doctorate,%20revised%20October%202015.pdf

Curley, M. A. Q. (1998). Patient–nurse synergy: Optimizing patients' outcomes. *American Journal of Critical Care, 7*, 64–72.

DiCenso, A., Martin-Misener, R., Bryant-Lukosius, D., Bourgeault, I., Kilpatrick, K., Donald, F., Kaasalainen, S., Harbman, P., Carter, N., Kioke, S., & Abelson, J. (2010). Advanced practice nursing in Canada: Overview of a decision support synthesis. *Nursing Leadership, 23*, 15–34. Special issue.

Doessel, D., & Marshall, J. (1985). A rehabilitation of health outcomes in quality assessment. *Social Science and Medicine, 21*, 1319–1328.

Donabedian, A. (1966). Evaluating the quality of medical care. Part 2: Health services research 1. A series of papers commissioned by the Health Services Research Study Section of the United States Public Health Service, October 15–16, 1965. *The Milbank Memorial Fund Quarterly, 44*(3), 166–206. Supplement.

Donabedian, A. (1980). Methods for deriving criteria for assessing the quality of medical care. *Medical Care Review, 37*(7), 653–698.

Donabedian, A. (1986). Quality assurance in our health care system. *Quality Assurance and Utilization Review, 1*(1), 6–12.

Donabedian, A. (1988). The quality of care: How can it be assessed?. *JAMA: The Journal of the American Medical Association, 260*(12), 1743–1748.

Donabedian, A. (2005). Evaluating the quality of medical care. *The Milbank Quarterly, 83*(5), 691–729.

Dunphy, L. M., & Winland-Brown, J. E. (1998). The circle of caring. A transformative model of advanced practice nursing. *Clinical Excellence for Nurse Practitioners, 2*(4), 241–247.

Dunphy, L. M., Winland-Brown, J. E., Porter, B. O., & Thomas, D. J. (Eds.) (2011). *Primary care: The art and science of advanced practice nursing* (3rd ed.). F. A. Davis.

Dunphy, L. M., Winland-Brown, J. E., Porter, B. O., Thomas, D. J., & Gallagher, L. M. (2011). Primary care in the twenty-first century: A circle of caring. In L. M. Dunphy, J. E. Winland-Brown, B. O. Porter, & D. J. Thomas (Eds.), *Primary care: The art and science of advanced practice nursing* (3rd ed.) (pp. 3–18). F. A. Davis.

Elliott, E. D., & Walden, M. (2015). Development of the transformational advanced professional practice model. *Journal of the American Association of Nurse Practitioners, 27*(9), 479–487.

European Specialist Nurses Organisations. (2015). Competencies of the Clinical Nurse Specialist (CNS): Common plinth of competencies for the common training framework of each specialty. Retrieved from https://www2.rcn.org.uk/__data/assets/pdf_file/0006/651129/ESNO_Competences_of_CNS-19_10_2015_Final.pdf

Fagerström, L. (2009). Developing the scope of practice and education for advanced practice nurses in Finland. *International Nursing Review, 56*, 269–272.

Fawcett, J., & Desanto-Madeya, S. (2013). *Contemporary nursing knowledge: Analysis and evaluation of nursing models and theories* (3rd ed.). F. A. Davis.

Fawcett, J., & Graham, I. (2005). Advanced practice nursing: Continuation of the dialogue. *Nursing Science Quarterly, 18*, 37–41.

Fawcett, J., Newman, D., & McAllister, M. (2004). Advanced practice nursing and conceptual models of nursing. *Nursing Science Quarterly, 17*, 135–138.

Fenton, M. V. (1985). Identifying competencies of clinical nurse specialists. *The Journal of Nursing Administration, 15*, 31–37.

Fenton, M. V., & Brykczynski, K. A. (1993). Qualitative distinctions and similarities in the practice of clinical nurse specialists and nurse practitioners. *Journal of Professional Nursing, 9*(6), 313–326.

Gardner, G., Chang, A. M., Duffield, C., & Doubrovsky, A. (2013). Delineating the practice profile of advanced practice nursing: A cross-sectional survey using the modified Strong Model of Advanced Practice. *Journal of Advanced Nursing, 69*(9), 1931–1942.

Gardner, G., Duffield, C., Doubrovsky, A., & Adams, M. (2016). Identifying advanced practice: A national survey of a nursing workforce. *International Journal of Nursing Studies, 55*, 60–70.

Gullick, J. G., & West, S. H. (2016). Building research capacity and productivity among advanced practice nurses: An evaluation of the Community of Practice model. *Journal of Advanced Nursing, 72*(3), 605–619.

Hamric, A. B. (1996). A definition of advanced practice nursing. In A. B. Hamric, J. A. Spross, & C. M. Hanson (Eds.), *Advanced nursing practice: An integrative approach* (pp. 25–41). WB Saunders.

Hamric, A. B. (2000). A definition of advanced practice nursing. In A. B. Hamric, J. A. Spross, & C. M. Hanson (Eds.), *Advanced practice nursing: An integrative approach* (2nd ed.) (pp. 53–73). Saunders Elsevier.

Hamric, A. B. (2005). A definition of advanced practice nursing. In A. B. Hamric, J. A. Spross, & C. M. Hanson (Eds.), *Advanced practice nursing: An integrative approach* (3rd ed.) (pp. 85–108). Saunders Elsevier.

Hamric, A. B. (2009). A definition of advanced practice nursing. In A. B. Hamric, J. A. Spross, & C. M. Hanson (Eds.), *Advanced practice nursing: An integrative approach* (4th ed.) (pp. 75–94). Saunders Elsevier.

Hamric, A. B. (2014). A definition of advanced practice nursing. In A. B. Hamric, J. A. Spross, M. F. Tracy, & E. T. O'Grady (Eds.), *Advanced practice nursing: An integrative approach* (5th ed.) (pp. 67–85). Saunders Elsevier.

Hamric, A. B., & Spross, J. A. (1983). A model for future clinical specialist practice. In A. B. Hamric, & J. A. Spross (Eds.), *The clinical nurse specialist in theory and practice* (pp. 291–306). Grune & Stratton.

Hamric, A. B., & Spross, J. A. (1989). *The clinical nurse specialist in theory and practice* (2nd ed.). WB Saunders.

Hathaway, D., Jacob, S., Stegbauer, C., Thompson, C., & Graff, C. (2006). The practice doctorate: Perspectives of early adopters. *The Journal of Nursing Education, 45*, 487–496.

Health Professions Network Nursing and Midwifery Office, Department of Human Resources for Health, World Health Organization. (2010). Framework for action on interprofessional education and collaborative practice. Retrieved from http://whqlibdoc.who.int/hq/2010/WHO_HRH_HPN_10.3_eng.pdf

International Council of Nurses Nurse Practitioner/Advanced Practice Nursing Network. (2020). Definition and characteristics of the role. Retrieved from https://international.aanp.org/Practice/APNRoles

Institute of Medicine (US), Committee on the Robert Wood Johnson Foundation Initiative on the Future of Nursing. (2011). *The future of nursing: Leading change, advancing health*. National Academies Press.

Interprofessional Education Collaborative Expert Panel. (2016). *Core competencies for interprofessional collaborative practice: 2016 update*. Interprofessional Education Collaborative.

Karnick, P. M. (2011). Theory and advanced practice nursing. *Nursing Science Quarterly, 24*, 118–119.

Kennedy, H. P. (2000). A model of exemplary midwifery practice: Results of a Delphi study. *Journal of Midwifery & Women's Health, 45*(1), 4–19.

Ketefian, S., & Redman, R. W. (2015). A critical examination of development in nursing doctoral education in the United States. *Revista Latino-Americana de Enfermagem, 23*(3), 363–371.

Kilpatrick, K., Lavoie-Tremblay, M., Lamothe, L., Ritchie, J. A., & Doran, D. (2013). Conceptual framework of acute care nurse practitioner role enactment, boundary work, and perceptions of team effectiveness. *Journal of Advanced Nursing, 69*(1), 205–217.

Kilpatrick, K., Tchouaket, E., Carter, N., Bryant-Lukosius, D., & DiCenso, A. (2016). Relationship between clinical nurse specialist role implementation, satisfaction, and intent to stay. *Clinical Nurse Specialist, 30*(3), 159–166.

King, K. B., & Ackerman, M. H. (1995). An educational model for the acute care nurse practitioner. *Critical Care Nursing Clinics of North America, 7*(1), 1–7.

Kleinpell, R., Scanlon, A., Hibbert, D., Ganz, F., East, L., Fraser, D., Wong, F., & Beauchesne, M. (2014). Addressing issues impacting advanced nursing practice worldwide. *Online Journal of Issues in Nursing, 19*(2), 4.

Kouzes, J. M., & Posner, B. Z. (2002). *The leadership challenge* (3rd ed.). John Wiley and Sons.

LeGrow, K., Hubley, P., & McAllister, M. (2010). A conceptual framework for advanced nursing practice in a pediatric tertiary care setting: The SickKids' experience. *Nursing Leadership, 23*(2), 32–46.

Lewandowski, W., & Adamle, K. (2009). Substantive areas of clinical nurse specialist practice: A comprehensive review of the literature. *Clinical Nurse Specialist, 23*, 73–92.

MacDonald, J., Herbert, R., & Thibeault, C. (2006). Advanced practice nursing: Unification through a common identity. *Journal of Professional Nursing, 3*, 172–179.

Mantzoukas, S., & Watkinson, S. (2007). Review of advanced nursing practice: The international literature and developing the generic features. *Journal of Clinical Nursing, 16*, 28–37.

Martsolf, G. R., Gigli, K. H., Reynolds, B. R., & McCorkle, M. (2020). Misalignment of specialty nurse practitioner and the Consensus Model. *Nursing Outlook, 68*(4), 385–387.

McGee, P. (2009). *Advanced practice in nursing and the allied health professions* (3rd ed.). Wiley-Blackwell.

McKnight, S. (2011). Risk assessment in the electronic age: Application of the Circle of Caring Model. *Online Journal of Nursing Informatics, 15*(3). Retrieved from http://ojni.org/issues/?p=911

Mick, D., & Ackerman, M. (2000). Advanced practice nursing role delineation in acute and critical care: Application of the Strong Model of advanced practice. *Heart and Lung: The Journal of Critical Care, 29*, 210–221.

Musker, K. P. (2011). Nursing theory–based independent nursing practice: A personal experience of closing the theory–practice gap. *Advances in Nursing Science, 34*, 67–77.

National Advisory Council on Nurse Education and Practice. (2015). *Incorporating interprofessional education and practice into nursing: Thirteenth Report to the Secretary of the Department of Health and Human Services and the United States Congress*. U.S. Health Resources & Services Administration.

National Academies of Sciences, Engineering, and Medicine (NASEM). (2021). *The future of nursing report 2020-2030: Charting a path to achieve health equity*. The National Academies Press. https://doi.org/10.17226/25982

National Association of Clinical Nurse Specialists. (1998). *Statement on clinical nurse specialist practice and education*. Author.

National Association of Clinical Nurse Specialists. (2004). *Statement on clinical nurse specialist practice and education* (2nd ed.). Author.

National Association of Clinical Nurse Specialists. (2005). White paper on the nursing practice doctorate. Retrieved from http://www.nacns.org/docs/PaperOnNPDoctorate.pdf

National Association of Clinical Nurse Specialists. (2012). National Association of Clinical Nurse Specialists' statement on the APRN Consensus Model implementation. Retrieved from http://www.nacns.org/docs/NACNSConsensusModel.pdf

National Association of Clinical Nurse Specialists. (2015). NACNS position statement on the Doctor of Nursing Practice. Retrieved from https://nacns.org/advocacy-policy/position-statements/position-statement-on-the-doctor-of-nursing-practice/

National Association of Clinical Nurse Specialists. (2019). *Statement on clinical nurse specialist practice and education* (3rd ed.). Author.

National Association of Clinical Nurse Specialists/Doctoral Competency Task Force for Clinical Nurse Specialist Competencies. (2009). Core practice doctorate clinical nurse specialist competencies. http://nacns.org/wp-content/uploads/2016/11/CorePracticeDoctorate.pdf

National Association of Clinical Nurse Specialists/National CNS Competency Task Force. (2010). Clinical nurse specialist core competencies: Executive summary 2006–2008. Retrieved from http://www.nacns.org/docs/CNSCoreCompetenciesBroch.pdf

National Council of State Boards of Nursing. (2006). Evidence-Based Nursing Education for Regulation (EBNER). Retrieved from https://www.ncsbn.org/Final_06_EBNER_Report.pdf

National Council of State Boards of Nursing. (2015). APRN Consensus Model toolkit. Retrieved from https://www.ncsbn.org/739.htm

National Organization of Nurse Practitioner Faculties (NONPF). (2011). Nurse practitioner entry level competencies. Retrieved from http://www.nonpf.com/associations/10789/files/IntegratedNPCoreCompsFINALApril2011.pdf

National Organization of Nurse Practitioner Faculties (NONPF). (2012). Nurse practitioner entry level competencies. Retrieved from http://www.nonpf.com/associations/10789/files/NPCoreCompetenciesFinal2012.pdf

National Organization of Nurse Practitioner Faculties (NONPF). (2013). Population-focused nurse practitioner competencies. Retrieved from https://cdn.ymaws.com/www.nonpf.org/resource/resmgr/Competencies/CompilationPopFocusComps2013.pdf

National Organization of Nurse Practitioner Faculties (NONPF). (2014). Nurse practitioner core competencies content. Retrieved from http://c.ymcdn.com/sites/nonpf.site-ym.com/resource/resmgr/Competencies/NPCoreCompsContentFinalNov20.pdf

National Organization of Nurse Practitioner Faculties (NONPF). (2015). The Doctorate of Nursing Practice NP preparation: NONPF perspective 2015. Retrieved from https://cdn.ymaws.com/www.nonpf.org/resource/resmgr/DNP/NONPFDNPStatementSept2015.pdf

Naylor, M. D. (2012). Advancing high value transitional care: The central role of nursing and its leadership. *Nursing Administration Quarterly, 36*(2), 115–126.

Naylor, M. D., Aiken, L. H., Kurtzman, E. T., Olds, D. M., & Hirschman, K. B. (2011). The care span: The importance of transitional care in achieving health reform. *Health Affairs, 30*, 746–754.

Naylor, M. D., Bowles, K. H., McCauley, K. M., Maccoy, M. C., Mailin, G., Pauly, M. V., & Krakauer, R. (2013). High-value transitional care: Translation of research into practice. *Journal of Evaluation in Clinical Practice, 19*, 727–733.

Nursing and Midwifery Board of Australia. (2014). Nurse practitioner standards for practice. Retrieved from http://www.nursingmidwiferyboard.gov.au/Codes-Guidelines-Statements/Professional-standards/nurse-practitioner-standards-of-practice.aspx

Palardy, L. G., & March, A. L. (2011). The Circle of Caring Model: Medication adherence in cardiac transplant patients. *Nursing Science Quarterly, 24*, 120–125.

Partiprajak, S., Hanucharurnkul, S., Piaseu, N., Brooten, D., & Nityasuddhi, D. (2011). Outcomes of an advanced practice nurse–led type 2 diabetes support group. *Pacific Rim International Journal of Nursing Research, 15*(4), 288–304.

Patient Protection and Affordable Care Act, 42 U.S.C. § 18001 (2010).

Perraud, S., Delaney, K. R., Carlson, S. L., Johnson, M. E., Shephard, R., & Paun, O. (2006). Advanced practice psychiatric mental health nursing, finding our core: The therapeutic relationship in 21st century. *Perspectives in Psychiatric Care, 42*, 215–226.

Phillips, S. J. (2020). 32nd annual APRN legislative update: Improving access to high-quality, safe, and effective healthcare. *The Nurse Practitioner, 45*(1), 28–55.

Poghosyan, L., Boyd, D. R., & Clarke, S. P. (2016). Optimizing full scope of practice for nurse practitioners in primary care: A proposed conceptual model. *Nursing Outlook, 64*(2), 146–155.

Price, M. J., Martin, A. C., Newberry, Y. G., Zimmer, P. A., Brykczynski, K. A., & Warren, B. (1992). Developing national guidelines for nurse practitioner education: An overview of the product and the process. *The Journal of Nursing Education, 31*, 10–15.

Reeves, S., Goldman, J., Gilbert, J., Tepper, J., Silver, I., Suter, E., & Zwarenstein, M. A. (2011). A scoping review to improve conceptual clarity of interprofessional interventions. *Journal of Interprofessional Care, 25*, 167–174.

Shuler, P. A. (2000). Evaluating student services provided by school-based health centers: Applying the Shuler nurse practitioner practice model. *The Journal of School Health, 70*, 348–352.

Shuler, P. A., & Davis, J. E. (1993a). The Shuler nurse practitioner practice model: A theoretical framework for nurse practitioner clinicians, educators, and researchers, Part 1. *Journal of the American Academy of Nurse Practitioners, 5*, 11–18.

Shuler, P. A., & Davis, J. E. (1993b). The Shuler nurse practitioner practice model: Clinical application, Part 2. *Journal of the American Academy of Nurse Practitioners, 5*, 73–88.

Shuler, P. A., Huebscher, R., & Hallock, J. (2001). Providing wholistic health care for the elderly: Utilization of the Shuler nurse practitioner practice model. *Journal of the American Academy of Nurse Practitioners, 13*, 297–303.

Sidani, S., & Irvine, D. (1999). A conceptual framework for evaluating the nurse practitioner role in acute care settings. *Journal of Advanced Nursing, 30*(1), 58–66.

Spross, J. A., Hamric, A. B., Hall, G., Minarik, P., Sparacino, P. S. A., & Stanley, J. M. (2004). *Working statement comparing the clinical nurse leader and clinical nurse specialist roles: Similarities, differences, and complementarities*. American Association of Colleges of Nursing.

Stanley, J. M., Werner, K. E., & Apple, K. (2009). Positioning advanced practice registered nurses for health care reform: Consensus on APRN regulation. *Journal of Professional Nursing, 25*, 340–348.

Stasa, H., Cashin, A., Buckley, T., & Donoghue, J. (2014). Advancing advanced practice—clarifying the conceptual definition. *Nurse Education Today, 34*(3), 356–361.

Styles, M. M. (1998). An international perspective: APN credentialing. *Advanced Practice Nursing Quarterly, 4*(3), 1–5.

Styles, M. M., & Lewis, C. (2000). Conceptualizations of advanced nursing practice. In A. B. Hamric, J. A. Spross, & C. M. Hanson (Eds.), *Advanced nursing practice: An integrative approach* (2nd ed.) (pp. 25–41). WB Saunders.

Sweet, B. V., Madeo, A., Fitzgerald, M., House, J., Pardee, M., Zebrack, B., Sweier, D., Hornyak, J., Arslanian-Engoren, C., Mattison, D., & Dubin, L. (2017). Moving from individual roles to functional teams: A semester-long course in case-based decision making. *Journal of Interprofessional Care, 7*, 11–16.

Thomas, J. (2011). The Circle of Caring Model for neonatal transport. *Neonatal Network, 30*(1), 14–20.

Thoun, D. S. (2011). Specialty and advanced practice nursing: Discerning the differences. *Nursing Science Quarterly, 24*, 216–222.

Validation Panel of the National Association of Clinical Nurse Specialists. (2011). Criteria for the evaluation of clinical nurse specialist, master's, practice doctorate, and post-graduate certificate educational programs. Retrieved from http://www.nacns.org/docs/CNSEducationCriteria.pdf

Whall, A. L. (2005). "Lest we forget": An issue concerning the Doctorate in Nursing Practice (DNP). *Nursing Outlook, 53*(1), 1.

Wong, F. K. Y. (2018). Development of advanced nursing practice in China: Act local and think global. *International Journal of Nursing Sciences, 5*(2), 101–104.

Wong, F. K. Y., Peng, G., Kan, E. C., Li, Y., Lau, A., Zhang, L., Leung, A. F., Liu, X., Leung, V. O., Chen, W., & Li, M. (2010). Description and evaluation of an initiative to develop advanced practice nurses in mainland China. *Nurse Education Today, 30*(4), 344–349.

Wright, L. M., Watson, W. L., & Bell, J. M. (1996). *Beliefs: The heart of healing in families and illness*. New York: Basic Books.

Zimmer, P., Brykczynski, K., Martin, A., Newberry, Y., Price, M., & Warren, B. (1990). *National guidelines for nurse practitioner education*. National Organization of Nurse Practitioner Faculties.

3 A DEFINITION OF ADVANCED PRACTICE NURSING

MARY FRAN TRACY

"Not being heard is no reason for silence."
~ Victor Hugo

CHAPTER CONTENTS

DISTINGUISHING BETWEEN SPECIALIZATION AND ADVANCED PRACTICE NURSING 76
DISTINGUISHING BETWEEN ADVANCED NURSING PRACTICE AND ADVANCED PRACTICE NURSING 77
DEFINING ADVANCED PRACTICE NURSING 78
CORE DEFINITION OF ADVANCED PRACTICE NURSING 78
Conceptual Definition 79
Primary Criteria 80
SIX CORE COMPETENCIES OF ADVANCED PRACTICE NURSING 84
Direct Clinical Practice: The Central Competency 84
Additional Advanced Practice Nurse Core Competencies 85
Scope of Practice 86
DIFFERENTIATING ADVANCED PRACTICE ROLES: OPERATIONAL DEFINITIONS OF ADVANCED PRACTICE NURSING 87
Workforce Data 87
Four Established Advanced Practice Nurse Roles 87
CRITICAL ELEMENTS IN MANAGING ADVANCED PRACTICE NURSING ENVIRONMENTS 89
IMPLICATIONS OF THE DEFINITION OF ADVANCED PRACTICE NURSING 91
Implications for Advanced Practice Nursing Education 91
Implications for Regulation and Credentialing 92
Implications for Research 92
Implications for Practice Environments 93
CONCLUSION 94
KEY SUMMARY POINTS 95

This chapter considers two central questions that provide the foundation for this book:

- Why is it important to define carefully and clearly what is meant by the term *advanced practice nursing*?
- What distinguishes the practices of advanced practice registered nurses (APRNs) from those of other nurses and other healthcare providers?

Advanced practice nursing is considered here as a concept, not a role, a set of skills, or a substitution for physicians. Rather, it is a powerful idea, the origins of which date back more than a century. Such a conceptual definition provides a stable core understanding for all

The author wishes to acknowledge Ann B. Hamric for her visionary and thoughtful work in the inception and ongoing evolution of this foundational chapter.

APRN roles (see Chapter 2), it promotes consistency in practice that can aid others in understanding what this level of nursing entails, and it promotes the achievement of value-added patient outcomes and improvement in healthcare delivery processes. Advanced practice nursing is a relatively new concept in nursing's evolution (see Chapter 1). Although debates and dissension are necessary and even healthy in forging consensus, ultimately the profession must agree on the key issues of definition, education, credentialing, and practice. Such agreement is critically important to the survival, as well as the growth, of advanced practice nursing. In the international context, although these issues may be defined differently by different countries, in country standardization is likewise essential. In this chapter, advanced practice nursing is defined and the scope of practice of APRNs is discussed. Various APRN roles are differentiated and key factors influencing advanced practice in healthcare environments are identified. The importance of a common and unified understanding of the distinguishing characteristics of advanced practice nursing is emphasized.

The advanced practice of nursing builds on the foundation and core values of the nursing discipline. APRN roles do not stand apart from nursing; they do not represent a separate profession, although references to "the nurse practitioner (NP) profession," for example, are seen in the literature. It is the nursing core that contributes to the distinctiveness seen in APRN practices as compared to non-nursing providers such as physician assistants. According to the American Nurses Association (ANA, 2010), nursing practice has seven essential features:

> *... provision of a caring relationship that facilitates health and healing; attention to the range of human experiences and responses to health and illness within the physical and social environments; integration of assessment data with knowledge gained from an appreciation of the patient or the group; application of scientific knowledge to the processes of diagnosis and treatment through the use of judgment and critical thinking; advancement of professional nursing knowledge through scholarly inquiry; influence on social and public policy to promote social justice; and, assurance of safe, quality, and evidence-based practice. (p. 9)*

These characteristics are equally essential for advanced practice nursing. Core values that guide nurses in practice include advocating for patients; respecting patient and family values and informed choices; viewing individuals holistically within their environments, communities, and cultural traditions; and maintaining a focus on disease prevention, health restoration, and health promotion (ANA, 2015a; Friberg & Creasia, 2011; Hood, 2014). These core professional values also inform the central perspective of advanced practice nursing.

Efforts to standardize the definition of advanced practice nursing have been ongoing since the 1990s (American Association of Colleges of Nursing [AACN], 1995, 2006, 2021; ANA, 1995, 2003, 2010; APRN Joint Dialogue Group, 2008; Hamric, 1996, 2000, 2005, 2009, 2014; Hamric & Tracy, 2019; National Council of State Boards of Nursing [NCSBN], 1993, 2002). However, full clarity regarding advanced practice nursing has not yet been achieved, even as this level of nursing practice spreads around the globe. The growing international use of APRNs with differing understandings in various countries has only complicated the picture (see Chapter 5). The International Council of Nurses (ICN) continues to build upon their initial work in standardizing the definition and description of advanced practice nursing, recognizing it will continue to evolve. Advanced practice nursing roles are developing at different rates across the globe, scopes of practice and educational preparation vary, and there are debates about who is, and who is not, an APRN, among other challenging issues (ICN, 2020; Schober & Stewart, 2019).

Despite this lack of clarity (Burns-Bolton & Mason, 2012; Dowling et al., 2013; Pearson, 2011), emerging consensus on key features of the concept is increasingly evident. The definition developed by Hamric has been relatively stable throughout the seven editions of this book. The primary criteria used in this definition are now standard elements used in the United States and, increasingly, elsewhere to regulate APRNs. Similarly, consensus is growing in understanding advanced practice nursing in terms of core competencies. Even authors who deny a clear understanding of the advanced practice nursing concept propose competencies—variously called *attributes*, *components*, or *domains*—that are generally consistent with, although not always as complete as, the competencies proposed here.

It is important to distinguish the conceptual definition of advanced practice nursing from regulatory requirements for any APRN role (NCSBN, 2021a). Of necessity, regulatory understandings focus on the more basic and measurable primary criteria of graduate educational preparation, advanced certification in a particular population focus, and practice in one of the four common APRN roles: nurse practitioner (NP), clinical nurse specialist (CNS), certified registered nurse anesthetist (CRNA), and certified nurse-midwife (CNM). This approach is clearly seen in the APRN definition outlined in the *Consensus Model for APRN Regulation* (APRN Joint Dialogue Group, 2008) and has been very helpful and influential in standardizing state requirements for APRN licensure across the United States. Although necessary for regulation, this approach does not constitute an adequate understanding of advanced practice nursing. Limiting the profession's understanding of advanced practice nursing to regulatory definitions can lead to a reductionist approach that results in a focus on a set of concrete skills and activities, such as diagnostic acumen or prescriptive authority. Understanding the advanced practice of the nursing discipline requires a definition that encompasses broad areas of skilled performance (the competency approach). As Chapter 2 notes, conceptual models and definitions are also useful for providing a robust framework for graduate APRN curricula and for building an APRN professional role identity.

DISTINGUISHING BETWEEN SPECIALIZATION AND ADVANCED PRACTICE NURSING

Before the definition of advanced practice nursing can be explored, it is important to distinguish between specialization in nursing and advanced practice nursing. Specialization involves the development of expanded knowledge and skills in a selected area within the discipline of nursing. All nurses with extensive experience in a particular area of practice (e.g., pediatric nursing, trauma nursing) are specialized in this sense. As the profession has advanced and responded to changes in health care, specialization and the need for specialty knowledge have increased. The AACN's (2021) revised *Essentials: Core Competencies for Professional Nursing Education* also delineates specialization at an advanced education level that includes areas such as informatics and education. Thus few nurses are generalists in the true sense of the word. Although family NPs traditionally represented themselves as generalists, they are specialists in the sense discussed here because they have specialized in one of the many facets of health care—namely, primary care. As noted in Chapter 1, early specialization involved primarily on-the-job training or hospital-based training courses, and many nurses continue to develop specialty skills through practice experience and continuing education. Examples of currently evolving specialties include genetics nursing, forensic nursing, and clinical transplant coordination. As specialties mature, they may develop graduate-level clinical preparation and incorporate the competencies of advanced practice nursing for their most advanced practitioners (Hanson & Hamric, 2003); examples include critical care, oncology nursing, and palliative care nursing.

The nursing profession has responded in various ways to the increasing need for specialization in nursing practice. The creation of specialty organizations, such as the American Association of Critical-Care Nurses and the Oncology Nursing Society, has been one response. The creation of APRN roles—the CRNA and CNM roles early in nursing's evolution and the CNS and NP roles more recently—has been another response. A third response has been the development of specialized faculty, nursing researchers, and nursing administrators. Nurses in all of these roles can be considered specialists in an area of nursing (e.g., education, research, administration); some of these roles may involve advanced education in a clinical specialty as well. However, they are not necessarily advanced practice nursing roles.

Advanced practice nursing includes specialization but also involves expansion and educational advancement (ANA, 2015b; Cronenwett, 1995). As compared with basic nursing practice, APRN practice is further characterized by the following: (1) acquisition of new practice knowledge and skills, particularly theoretical and evidence-based knowledge, some of which overlaps the traditional boundaries of medicine; (2) significant role autonomy; (3) responsibility for health promotion in addition to the diagnosis and management of patient problems, including prescribing pharmacologic and nonpharmacologic interventions; (4) the greater complexity of clinical decision making and leadership in organizations and environments; and (5) specialization at the level of a particular APRN role and population focus (ANA, 2015b; APRN Joint Dialogue Group, 2008).

It is necessary to distinguish between specialization as understood in this chapter and the term *population focus*. The framers of the Consensus Model for APRN regulation were interested in licensing and regulating advanced practice nursing in two broad categories. The first was regulation at the level of role—CNS, NP, CRNA, or CNM. The second category was termed *population focus* and, although not explicitly defined, six population foci were identified: family and individual across the life span, adult–gerontology, pediatrics, neonatal, women's health and gender-related, and psychiatric/mental health. These foci are at different levels of specialization; for example, family and individual across the life span is broad, whereas neonatal is a subspecialty designation under the specialty of pediatrics. Therefore population focus is not synonymous with specialization and should not be understood in the same light. As the Consensus Model states:

> *Education, certification, and licensure of an individual must be congruent in terms of role and population foci. APRNs may specialize but they cannot be licensed solely within a specialty area. In addition, specialties can provide depth in one's practice within the established population foci. … Competence at the specialty level will not be assessed or regulated by boards of nursing but rather by the professional organizations.*
>
> ***(APRN Joint Dialogue Group, 2008, p. 6)***

DISTINGUISHING BETWEEN ADVANCED NURSING PRACTICE AND ADVANCED PRACTICE NURSING

The terms *advanced practice nursing* and *advanced nursing practice* have distinct definitions and cannot be seen as interchangeable. In particular, recent definitions of advanced nursing practice do not clarify the clinically focused nature of advanced practice nursing. For example, the third edition of *Nursing's Social Policy Statement* defines the term advanced nursing practice as "characterized by the integration and application of a broad range of theoretical and evidence-based knowledge that occurs as part of graduate nursing education" (ANA, 2010, p. 9). This broad definition has evolved from the AACN's *Position Statement on the Practice Doctorate in Nursing* (AACN, 2004), which recommended doctoral-level educational preparation for individuals at the most advanced level of nursing practice. The doctor of nursing practice (DNP) position statement (AACN, 2004) advanced a broad definition of advanced nursing practice as the following:

> *… any form of nursing intervention that influences health care outcomes for individuals or populations, including the direct care of individual patients, management of care for individuals and populations, administration of nursing and health care organizations, and the development and implementation of health policy. (p. 3)*

A definition this broad goes beyond advanced practice nursing to include other advanced specialties not involved in providing direct clinical care to patients, such as administration, policy, informatics, and public health (AACN, 2021). One reason for such a broad definition was the desire to have the DNP degree be available to nurses practicing at the highest level in many varied specialties, not only those in APRN roles. A decision was reached by the original task force (AACN, 2004) that the DNP degree was not to be a clinical doctorate, as was advocated in early discussions (Mundinger et al., 2000), but, rather, a practice doctorate in an expansive understanding of the term *practice*. It is important to understand that the DNP is a *degree*, much as is the master's of science in nursing, and not a *role*; DNP graduates can assume varied roles, depending on the specialty focus of their program. Some of these roles are not APRN roles as advanced practice nursing is defined here.

In the revised *Essentials*, AACN uses the term *advanced nursing practice specialty* versus *advanced nursing practice role* (i.e., APRN). However, even in this revised document, AACN interchanges the terms *advanced nursing practice role* and *advanced practice nursing role* (AACN, 2021). The nuances in the differences between these terms have not been clear to nurses in education and practice, professionals outside of nursing, and, at times, even DNP graduates themselves. As a result, the specific distinctions between the advanced specialties (such as administration) and APRN roles continue to require clarification. The current confusion in the United States also has global implications, though the international community more recently is using the term advanced nursing practice when referring to direct care roles that are comparable to US APRN roles (ICN, 2020; see Chapter 5).

Advanced practice nursing is a concept that applies to nurses who provide direct patient care to individual patients and families. As a consequence, APRN roles involve expanded clinical skills and abilities and require a different level of regulation than non-APRN roles. These skills afford APRNs unique perspectives in making broader practice decisions for individuals and populations specifically in their specialty areas. This text focuses on advanced practice nursing and the varied roles of APRNs. The revised *Essentials*' discussion on both the advanced level of education of APRNs and those in specialty areas includes requirements for clinical practicums of direct and indirect care; the specific meaning of this is unclear at this time.

DEFINING ADVANCED PRACTICE NURSING

As noted, the concept of advanced practice nursing continues to be defined in various ways in the nursing literature. The Ovid Medline database defines the Medical Subject Heading of advanced practice nursing as:

> *evidence-based nursing, midwifery and healthcare grounded in research and scholarship. Practitioners include nurse practitioners, clinical nurse specialists, nurse anesthetists and nurse midwives.*
>
> ***(US National Library of Medicine, 2021)***

This description is vague and relies primarily on a delineation of roles.

Advanced practice nursing is often defined as a constellation of four roles: the NP, CNS, CNM, and CRNA (APRN Joint Dialogue Group, 2008; Stanley, 2011). For example, the fourth edition of ANA's *Nursing: Scope and Standards of Practice* does not provide a definition of advanced practice nursing but uses a regulatory and role-based definition of APRNs:

> *a subset of graduate-level prepared registered nurses who have completed an accredited graduate-level education program preparing the nurse for special licensure recognition and practice for one of the four recognized APRN roles: certified registered nurse anesthetist (CRNA), certified nurse-midwife (CNM), clinical nurse specialist (CNS), or certified nurse practitioner (CNP). APRNs assume responsibility and accountability for health promotion and/or maintenance, as well as the assessment, diagnosis, and management of healthcare consumer problems, which includes the use and prescription of pharmacologic and non-pharmacologic interventions (APRN Joint Dialogue Group, 2008). Some clinicians in this classification began APRN practice prior to the current educational preparation requirement and have been grandfathered to hold this designation.*
>
> ***(ANA, 2021, pp. 2–3)***

In the past, some authors discussed advanced practice nursing only in terms of selected roles such as the NP and CNS roles (Lindeke et al., 1997; Rasch & Frauman, 1996) or the NP role exclusively (Hickey et al., 2000; Mundinger, 1994). Defining advanced practice nursing in terms of particular roles limits the concept and denies the unfortunate reality that some nurses in the four APRN roles are not using the core competencies of advanced practice nursing in their practice. These definitions are also limiting because they do not incorporate evolving and emergent APRN roles. Thus although such role-based definitions are useful for regulatory purposes, it is preferable to define and clarify advanced practice nursing as a concept without reference to particular roles.

CORE DEFINITION OF ADVANCED PRACTICE NURSING

The definition proposed in this chapter builds on and extends the understanding of advanced practice nursing proposed in the first six editions of this text. Important assertions of this discussion are as follows:

- Advanced practice nursing is a function of educational and practice preparation and a constellation of primary criteria and core competencies.

- Direct clinical practice is the central competency of any APRN role and informs all the other competencies.
- All APRNs share the same core criteria and competencies, although the actual clinical skill set varies depending on the needs of the APRN's specialty patient population.

A definition should also clarify the critical point that advanced practice nursing involves advanced nursing knowledge and skills; it is not a medical practice, although APRNs perform expanded medical therapeutics in many roles. Throughout nursing's history, nurses have assumed medical roles. For example, common nursing tasks such as blood pressure measurement and administration of chemotherapeutic agents were once performed exclusively by physicians. When APRNs begin to transfer new skills or interventions into their repertoire, these become nursing skills, informed by the clinical practice values of the profession.

Actual practices differ significantly based on the particular role adopted, the specialty practiced, and the organizational framework within which the role is performed. Despite the need to keep job descriptions and job titles distinct in practice settings, it is critical that the public's acceptance of advanced practice nursing be enhanced and confusion decreased. As Safriet (1993, 1998) noted, nursing's future depends on reaching consensus on titles and consistent preparation for title holders. It is imperative for the nursing profession to be clear, concrete, and consistent about APRN titles and their functions in discussions with nursing's larger constituencies: consumers, other healthcare professionals, healthcare administrators, and healthcare policymakers.

Conceptual Definition

Advanced practice nursing is the patient-focused application of an expanded range of competencies to improve health outcomes for patients and populations in a specialized clinical area of the larger discipline of nursing.[a]

In this definition, the term *competencies* refers to a broad area of skillful performance; six core competencies combine to distinguish nursing practice at this level. Competencies include activities undertaken as part of delivering advanced nursing care directly to patients. Some competencies are processes that APRNs use in all dimensions of their practice, such as collaboration and leadership. At this stage of the development of the nursing discipline, competencies may be based in theory, practice, or research. Although the discipline is expanding its research-based evidence to guide practice, an expanded ability to use theory also is a key distinguishing feature of advanced practice nursing. In addition, a strong experiential component is necessary to develop the competencies and clinical practice expertise that characterize APRN practice. Graduate education and in-depth clinical practice experiences work together to develop the APRN.

The definition also emphasizes the patient-focused and specialized nature of advanced practice nursing. APRNs expand their capability to provide and direct care, with the ultimate goal of improving patient and specialty population outcomes; this focus on outcome attainment is a central feature of advanced practice nursing and the main justification for differentiating this level of practice. Finally, the critical importance of ensuring that any type of advanced practice is grounded within the larger discipline of nursing is made explicit.

Certain activities of APRN practice overlap with those performed by physicians and other healthcare professionals. However, the experiential, theoretical, and philosophic perspectives of nursing make these activities advanced nursing when they are carried out by an APRN. Advanced practice nursing further involves highly developed nursing skill in areas such as guidance and coaching, as well as the performance of select medical interventions. Particularly with regard to physician practice, the nursing profession needs to be clear that advanced practice nursing is embedded in the nursing discipline—*the advanced practice of nursing is not the junior practice of medicine.*

Advanced practice nursing is further defined by a conceptual model integrating three primary criteria and six core competencies, one of them central to the others. This discussion and the chapters in Part II of this text isolate each of these core competencies to clarify them. The reader should recognize that this is

[a]The term *patient* is intended to be used interchangeably with *individual* and *client.*

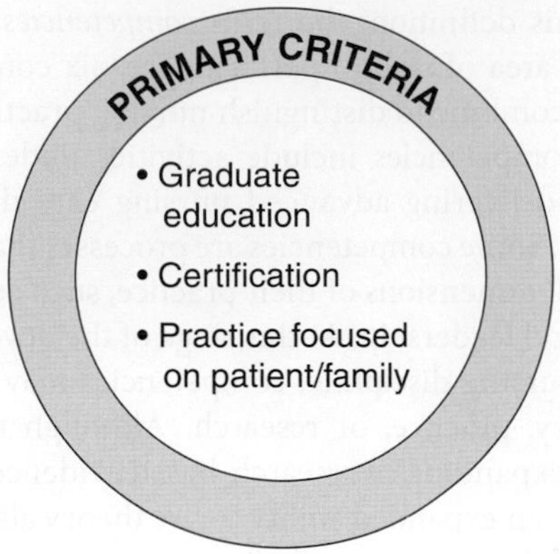

Fig. 3.1 ■ Primary criteria of advanced practice nursing.

only a heuristic device for clarifying this conceptualization of advanced practice nursing. In reality, these elements are integrated into an APRN's practice; they are not separate and distinct features. The concentric circles in Figs. 3.1 through 3.3 represent the seamless nature of this interweaving of elements. In addition, an APRN's skills function synergistically to produce a whole that is greater than the sum of its parts. The essence of advanced practice nursing is found not only in the primary criteria and competencies demonstrated but also in the synthesis of these elements into a unified composite practice that conforms to the conceptual definition just presented.

Primary Criteria

Certain criteria (or qualifications) must be met before a nurse can be considered an APRN. Although these baseline criteria are not sufficient in and of themselves, they are necessary core elements of advanced practice nursing. The three primary criteria for advanced practice nursing are shown in Fig. 3.1 and include an earned graduate degree with a concentration in an advanced practice nursing role and population focus, national certification at an advanced level, and a practice focused on patients and their families. As noted, these criteria are most often the ones used by states to regulate APRN practice because they are objective and easily measured (see Chapter 20).

Graduate Education

First, the APRN must possess an *earned graduate degree with a concentration in an APRN role.* This graduate degree may be a master's or a DNP. Advanced practice students acquire specialized knowledge and skills through study and supervised practice at the graduate level. Curricular content includes theories and research findings relevant to the core of a particular advanced nursing role, population focus, and relevant specialty. For example, a CNS interested in palliative care will need coursework in CNS role competencies, the adult population focus, and the palliative care specialty. Because APRNs assess, manage, and evaluate patients at the most independent level of clinical nursing practice, all APRN curricula contain specific courses in advanced health and physical assessment, advanced pathophysiology, and advanced pharmacology (the "three Ps"; AACN, 2021; APRN Joint Dialogue Group, 2008). Expansion of practice skills is acquired through faculty-supervised clinical experience, with master's programs requiring a minimum of 500 clinical hours and DNP programs requiring 1000 hours. As noted earlier in the ANA definition, there is current consensus that a master's education in nursing is a baseline requirement for advanced practice nursing; nurse-midwifery was the latest APRN specialty to agree to this requirement in 2009 (American College of Nurse-Midwives [ACNM], 2015).

Why is graduate educational preparation necessary for advanced practice nursing? Graduate education is a more efficient and standardized way to inculcate the complex competencies of APRN-level practice than nursing's traditional on-the-job or apprentice training programs. As the knowledge base within specialties has grown, so, too, has the need for formal education at the graduate level. In particular, the skills necessary for evidence-based practice and the theory base required for advanced practice nursing mandate education at the graduate level.

Some of the differences between basic and advanced practice in nursing are apparent in the following: the range and depth of APRNs' clinical knowledge; APRNs' ability to anticipate patient responses to health, illness, and nursing interventions; their ability to analyze clinical situations and explain why a phenomenon has occurred or why a particular intervention has been chosen; the reflective nature of their practice; their skill in assessing and addressing nonclinical variables that influence patient care; and their attention to the consequences of care and improving patient outcomes. Because of the interaction and integration of graduate education in nursing and extensive clinical experience, APRNs are able to exercise a level of discernment in clinical judgment that is unavailable to other experienced nurses (Spross & Baggerly, 1989).

Professionally, requiring at least master's-level preparation is important to create parity among APRN roles so that all can move forward together in addressing policymaking and regulatory issues. This parity advances the profession's standards and ensures more uniform credentialing mechanisms. Moving toward a doctoral-level educational expectation may also enhance nursing's image and credibility with other disciplines. Decisions by other healthcare providers, such as pharmacists, physical therapists, and occupational therapists, to require doctoral preparation for entry into their professions provided compelling support for nursing to establish the practice doctorate for APRNs to achieve parity with these disciplines (AACN, 2006). Nursing has a particular need to achieve greater credibility with medicine. Organized medicine has historically been eager to point to nursing's internal differences in APRN education as evidence that APRNs are inferior providers.

The clinical nurse leader (CNL) role represents a different understanding of the master's credential. Historically, master's education in nursing was, by definition, specialized education (see Chapter 1). However, the master's-prepared CNL is described as an "advanced generalist"; "a masters-educated nurse prepared for practice across the continuum of care within any healthcare setting in today's changing healthcare environment" (AACN, 2013, p. 4). The revised *Essentials* (AACN, 2021) document is intended to address advanced-level nursing education and does not distinguish between master's and DNP preparation. Even though CNLs have expanded leadership skills and graduate-level education, they are clearly not APRNs. APRN graduate education is highly specialized and involves preparation for an expanded scope of practice, neither of which characterizes CNL education. With the revised *Essentials*, it is even more important that the preparation of CNLs is clearly differentiated from that of the CNS for example. The existence of generalist and APRN specialty master's programs has the potential to confuse consumers, institutions, and nurses alike; it is incumbent on educational programs to clearly differentiate the curricula for generalist CNL versus specialist APRN roles to avoid role confusion for these graduates. It is likewise important that CNL graduates understand that they are not APRNs.

The AACN's proposed 2015 deadline for APRNs to be prepared at the DNP level was heavily debated (Cronenwett et al., 2011) and was not realized, even though the number of DNP programs increased dramatically (from 20 programs in 2006 to 357 in 2020 with an additional 106 new DNP programs in the planning stages; AACN, 2020). Master's-level programs that prepare APRNs are continuing at this point in time.

Certification

The second primary criterion that must be met to be considered an APRN is professional certification for practice at an advanced level within a clinical population focus. The continuing growth of specialization has dramatically increased the amount of knowledge and experience required to practice safely in modern healthcare settings. National certification examinations have been developed by specialty organizations at two levels. The first level that was developed tested the specialty knowledge of experienced nurses and not knowledge at the advanced level of practice. More recently, organizations have developed APRN-specific certification examinations in a specialty. CNM and CRNA organizations were farsighted in developing certifying examinations for these roles early in their history (see Chapter 1). As regulatory groups, particularly state boards of nursing, increasingly use the certification credential as a component of APRN licensure, the certification landscape continues to change. As noted, the Consensus Model has mandated regulation of APRNs at a role and population focus level (APRN Joint Dialogue Group, 2008), accelerating the development of more broad-based APRN certification examinations.

National certification at an advanced practice level is an important primary criterion for advanced practice nursing. Continuing variability in graduate curricula makes sole reliance on the criterion of graduate education insufficient to protect the public. Although standardization in educational requirements for each APRN role has improved over the last decade, it is difficult to argue that graduate education alone can provide sufficient evidence of competence for regulatory purposes. National certification examinations provide a consistent standard that must be met by each APRN to demonstrate beginning competency for an advanced level of practice in their role. Certification also enhances title recognition in the regulatory arena, which promotes the visibility of advanced practice nursing and enhances the public's access to APRN services.

It is critically important that certifying organizations work to clarify the certification credential as appropriate only for currently practicing APRNs. Given the centrality of the direct clinical practice component to the definition of advanced practice nursing, certification examinations must establish a significant number of hours of clinical practice as a requirement for maintaining APRN certification. Some faculty and nursing leaders who do not maintain a direct clinical practice component in their positions have been allowed to sit for certification examinations and represent themselves as APRNs. Statements such as "Once a CNS, always a CNS," which are heard with NPs and CNMs as well, perpetuate the mistaken notion that an APRN title is a professional attribute rather than a practice role. Such a misunderstanding is confusing inside and outside of nursing; by definition, these individuals are no longer APRNs. This requires collaboration between academic institutions and healthcare organizations to support faculty to maintain a clinical practice as it is increasingly difficult to practice clinically above and beyond the faculty role.

As noted, the Consensus Model focuses regulatory efforts on these broad role and population foci rather than on particular specialties, although some specialties are represented (e.g., neonatal NPs). This decision not to recognize established APRN certification examinations in specialties such as oncology or critical care for state licensure purposes has challenged the CNS role more than other APRN specialties. The American Nurses Credentialing Center has become the dominant certifying organization for State Board of Nursing–supported CNS examinations. The number of examination options for CNSs has significantly decreased with Consensus Model implementation; the American Nurses Credentialing Center website (https://www.nursingworld.org/our-certifications/, March 10, 2022) maintains a listing of currently available CNS examinations. It is likely that the types of APRN certification examinations offered may continue to evolve as the Consensus Model evolves. Even though APRN regulation is becoming more standardized, a need exists for the continued development of specialty examinations at the advanced practice nursing level, particularly for CNS specialties; as it stands now, many CNSs have to take the broad-based certification examination recognized by their state in addition to an APRN-level specialty certification examination necessary for their practice. Another unintended consequence of the limitations set by recognizing only six population foci is that educational programs have closed CNS concentrations given the lack of a sanctioned certification examination in the specialty. Although other factors also influenced these decisions, not recognizing specialty examinations for regulatory purposes is a key factor in these closures. This issue is starting to impact NPs as well, as some are becoming increasingly specialized in areas such as diabetes care, pain management, and emergency care (Schumann & Tyler, 2018).

The limited population foci sanctioned at present can be seen as a first step in standardizing regulation; the Consensus Model report noted the expectation that additional population foci would evolve. Even with these transitional issues, the Consensus Model represents an important standardization of APRN regulation and has helped cement the primary criterion of certification as a core regulatory requirement for APRN licensure.

Practice Focused on Patient and Family

The third primary criterion necessary for one to be considered an APRN is a practice focused on patients and their families. As noted in describing DNP graduates, the AACN DNP Essentials Task Force differentiated APRNs from other roles using this primary criterion. They noted two general role categories (AACN, 2006):

> *roles which specialize as an advanced practice nurse (APN) with a focus on care of individuals; and roles that specialize in practice at an aggregate, systems, or organizational level. This distinction is important as APRNs face different licensure, regulatory, credentialing, liability, and reimbursement issues*

than those who practice at an aggregate, systems, or organizational level. (p. 17)

While not clearly delineated, the revised *Essentials* recognizes a difference between advanced-level graduates in an advanced nursing practice specialty and those in an advanced nursing practice role (i.e., APRNs; AACN, 2021). This criterion does not imply that direct practice is the only activity that APRNs undertake, however. APRNs also educate others, participate in leadership activities, and serve as consultants (Bryant-Lukosius et al., 2016); they understand and are involved in practice contexts to identify and effect needed system changes; they also work to improve the health of their specialty populations (AACN, 2021). However, to be considered an APRN role, the patient/family direct practice focus must be primary.

Historically, APRN roles have been associated with direct clinical care. Recent work is solidifying this understanding. The Consensus Model (APRN Joint Dialogue Group, 2008) has made clear that the provision of direct care to individuals as a significant component of their practice is *the* defining factor for all APRNs. The centrality of direct clinical practice is further reflected in the core competencies presented in the next section.

Why limit the definition of advanced practice nursing to roles that focus on clinical practice to patients and families? There are many reasons. Nursing is a practice profession. The nurse–patient interface is at the core of nursing practice; in the final analysis, the reason that the profession exists is to render nursing services to individuals in need of them. Clinical practice expertise in a given specialty develops from these nurse–patient encounters and lies at the heart of advanced practice nursing. Ongoing direct clinical practice is necessary to maintain and develop an APRN's expertise. Without regular immersion in practice, the cutting-edge clinical acumen and expertise found in APRN practices cannot be sustained. For example, CNSs who are required to function at a healthcare organization system level may be relegated to expertise in only one or two spheres of impact (i.e., nurses and nursing personnel sphere, organizations and systems sphere). Without interaction in the patient direct care sphere, they must rely on the perspective of others (e.g., nurses, administrators) in planning and carrying out improvement activities and policies rather than using their advanced assessment and evaluation skills to fully understand problems and develop potential solutions.

If every specialized role in nursing were considered advanced practice nursing, the term would become so broad as to lack meaning and explanatory value. Distinguishing between APRN roles and other specialized roles in nursing can help clarify the concept of advanced practice nursing to consumers, other healthcare providers, and even other nurses. In addition, the monitoring and regulation of advanced practice nursing are increasingly important issues as APRNs work toward more authority for their practices (see Chapter 20). If the definition of advanced practice nursing included nonclinical roles, development of sound regulatory mechanisms would be impossible.

It is critical to understand that this definition of advanced practice nursing is not a value statement but, rather, a differentiation of one group of nurses from other groups for the sake of clarity within and outside the profession. Some nurses with specialized skills in administration, research, and community health have viewed the direct practice requirement as a devaluing of their contributions. Some faculty who teach clinical nursing but do not themselves maintain an advanced clinical practice have also thought themselves to be disenfranchised because they are not considered APRNs by virtue of this primary criterion. Perhaps this problem has been exacerbated with use of the term *advanced*, because this term can inadvertently imply that nurses who do not fit into the APRN definition are not advanced (i.e., are not as well prepared or highly skilled as APRNs).

No value difference exists between nurses in broad specialties and APRNs; both groups are equally important to the overall growth and strengthening of the profession. The profession must be able to differentiate its various roles without such differentiation being viewed as a disparagement of any one group. We must be able to say what advanced practice nursing is not, as well as what it is, if we are to ensure clarity of the concept within and outside the profession. As the AACN (2021) has noted, all nurses—whether their focus is clinical practice, educating students, conducting research, planning community programs, or leading nursing service organizations—are valuable and necessary to the integrity and growth of the discipline. However, all nurses, particularly those with advanced degrees, are not the same, nor are they necessarily APRNs. Historically, the profession has had difficulty differentiating itself and has struggled with the prevailing lay notion that "a nurse is a nurse is a nurse." This antiquated view does not match the reality and increasing complexity of the healthcare arena, nor does it celebrate the diverse contributions of all the various nursing roles and specialties.

SIX CORE COMPETENCIES OF ADVANCED PRACTICE NURSING

Direct Clinical Practice: The Central Competency

As noted earlier, the primary criteria are necessary but insufficient elements of the definition of advanced practice nursing. Advanced practice nursing is further defined by a set of six core competencies that are enacted in each APRN role. The first core competency of direct clinical practice is central to and informs all of the others (see Fig. 3.2). In one sense, it is "first among equals" of the six core competencies that define advanced practice nursing. Although APRNs do many things, excellence in direct clinical practice provides the foundation necessary for APRNs to execute the other competencies, such as collaboration, guidance and coaching, and leadership within organizations.

However, clinical expertise alone should not be equated with advanced practice nursing. The work of Patricia Benner and colleagues (Benner, 1984; Benner et al., 1996, 1999, 2008) is a major contribution to an understanding of clinically expert nursing practice. These researchers extensively studied expert nurses in acute care clinical settings and described the engaged clinical reasoning and domains of practice seen in clinically expert nurses. Although some of the participants in this research were APRNs (in the most recent report [Benner et al., 1999], 16% of the nurse participants were APRNs), most were nurses with extensive clinical experience who did not have APRN preparation. Calkin (1984) has characterized these latter nurses as "experts by experience." (See Chapter 2 for a discussion of Calkin's conceptual differentiation between levels of nursing practice.) Benner and colleagues did not discuss differences in the practices of APRNs as compared with other nurses that they have studied. They stated that "'Expert' is not used to refer to a specific role such as an advanced practice nurse. Expertise is found in the practice of experienced clinicians and advanced practice nurses" (Benner et al., 1999, p. 9).

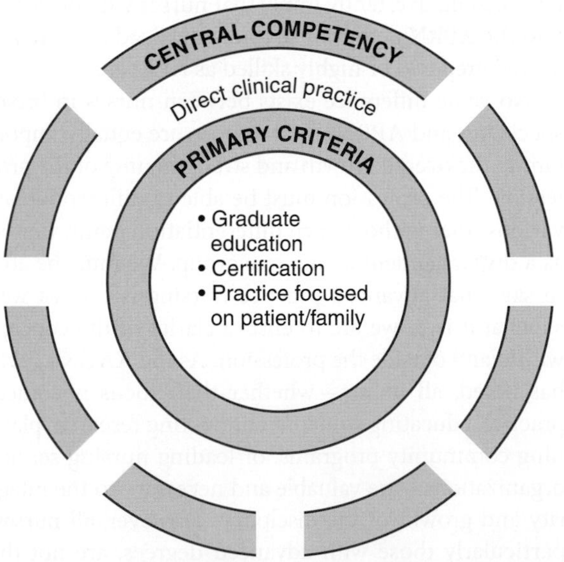

Fig. 3.2 ■ Central competency of advanced practice nursing.

Although clinical expertise is a central ingredient of an APRN's practice, the direct care practice of APRNs is distinguished by six characteristics: (1) use of a holistic perspective, (2) formation of therapeutic partnerships with patients, (3) expert clinical performance, (4) use of reflective practice, (5) use of evidence as a guide to practice, and (6) use of diverse approaches to health and illness management (see Chapter 6). These characteristics help distinguish the practice of the expert by experience from that of the APRN. APRN clinical practice is also informed by a population focus (AACN, 2021), because APRNs work to improve the care for their specialty patient population, even as they care for individuals within the population. As noted, experiential knowledge and graduate education combine to develop these characteristics in an APRN's clinical practice. It is important to note that the "three Ps" that form core courses in all APRN programs (pathophysiology, pharmacology, and physical assessment) are not separate competencies in this understanding but provide baseline knowledge and skills to support the direct clinical practice competency.

The specific content of the direct practice competency differs significantly by specialty. For example, the clinical practice of a CNS dealing with critically ill children differs from the expertise of an NP managing the health maintenance needs of older adults or a

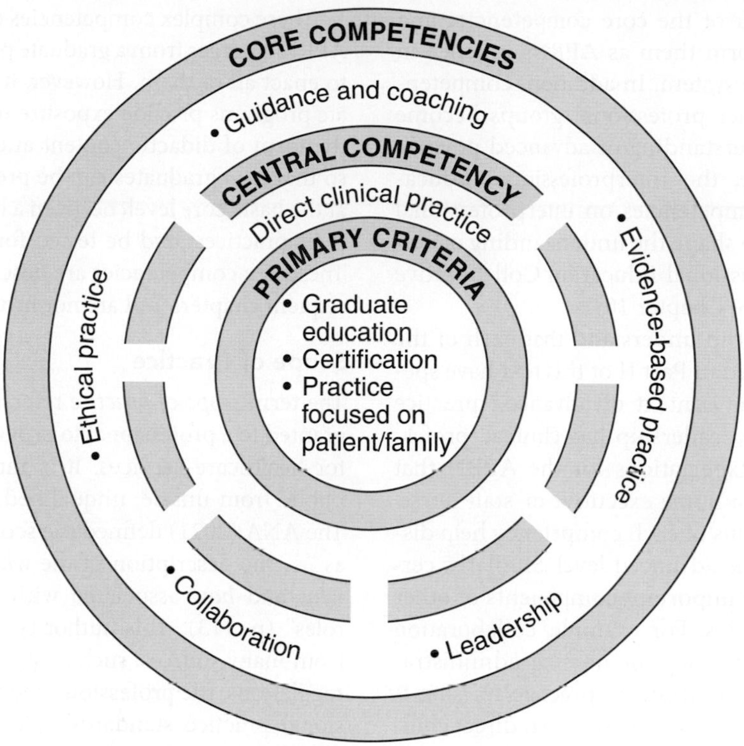

Fig. 3.3 ■ Core competencies of advanced practice nursing.

CRNA administering anesthesia in an outpatient surgical clinic. In addition, the amount of time spent in direct practice differs by APRN specialty. CNSs in particular may spend most of their time in activities other than direct clinical practice (see Chapter 12). Thus it is important to understand this competency as a central defining characteristic of advanced practice nursing rather than as a particular skill set or expectation that APRNs only engage in direct clinical practice.

Additional Advanced Practice Nurse Core Competencies

In addition to the central competency of direct clinical practice, five other competencies further define advanced practice nursing regardless of role function or setting. As shown in Fig. 3.3, these additional core competencies are as follows:

- Guidance and coaching
- Evidence-based practice
- Leadership
- Collaboration
- Ethical practice

These competencies have repeatedly been identified as essential features of advanced practice nursing. In addition, each role is differentiated by some unique competencies (see the specific role chapters in Part III of this text). The nature of the patient population receiving APRN care, organizational expectations, emphasis given to specific competencies, and practice characteristics unique to each role distinguish the practice of one APRN group from others. Each APRN role organization publishes role-specific competencies on their websites: the National Association of Clinical Nurse Specialists (NACNS) for CNSs (www.nacns.org), the National Organization of Nurse Practitioner Faculties for NPs (www.nonpf.org), the ACNM for CNMs (www.acnm.org), and the American Association of Nurse Anesthesiology for CRNAs (www.aana.com). There is a dynamic interplay between the core APRN competencies and each role; role-specific expectations grow out of the core competencies and similarly serve to inform them as APRNs practice in a changing healthcare system. In addition, competencies promoted by other professional groups become important to the understanding of advanced practice nursing; for example, the Interprofessional Education Collaborative competencies on interprofessional practice are helping to shape the understanding of collaboration (Interprofessional Education Collaborative Expert Panel, 2016; see Chapter 10).

It is also important to understand that each of the competencies described in Part II of this text have specific definitions in the context of advanced practice nursing. For example, leadership has clinical, professional, and systems expectations for the APRN that differ from those for a nurse executive or staff nurse. These unique definitions of each competency help distinguish practice at the advanced level. Similarly, certain competencies are important components of other specialized nursing roles. For example, collaboration is an important competency for nursing administrators. The uniqueness of advanced practice nursing is seen in the synergistic interaction between direct clinical practice and this constellation of competencies. In Fig. 3.3, the openings between the central practice competency and these additional competencies represent the fact that the APRN's direct practice skill interacts with and informs all the other competencies. For example, APRNs collaborate with other providers who seek their practice expertise to plan care for specialty patients. They are able to provide expert guidance and coaching for patients going through health and illness transitions because of their direct practice experience and insight.

The core competencies are not unique to APRN practices. Physicians and other healthcare providers may have developed competency in some of them. Experienced staff nurses may master several of these competencies with years of practice experience. These nurses are seen as exemplary performers and are often encouraged to enter graduate school to become APRNs. What distinguishes APRN practice is the *expectation* that every APRN's practice encompasses all of these competencies and seamlessly blends them into daily practice encounters. This expectation makes APRN practice unique among that of other providers.

These complex competencies develop over time. No APRN emerges from a graduate program fully prepared to enact all of them. However, it is critical that graduate programs provide exposure to each competency in the form of didactic content and practical experience so that new graduates can be prepared to utilize them at the basic core level, be given a base on which to build their practices, and be tested for initial credentialing. These key competencies are described in detail in subsequent chapters and are not further elaborated here.

Scope of Practice

The term *scope of practice* refers to the legal authority granted to a professional to provide and be reimbursed for healthcare services. It is intended to protect the public from unsafe, unqualified healthcare providers. The ANA (2021) defined the scope of nursing practice as "… the description of the *who, what, where, when, why,* and *how* associated with nursing practice and roles" (p. 113). This authority for practice emanates from many sources, such as state and federal laws and regulations, the profession's code of ethics, and professional practice standards. For all healthcare professionals, scope of practice is most closely tied to state statutes; for nursing in the United States, these statutes are the nurse practice acts of the various states. As previously discussed, APRN scope of practice is characterized by specialization; expansion of services provided, including diagnosing and prescribing; and autonomy to practice (APRN Joint Dialogue Group, 2008). The scopes of practice also differ among the various APRN roles; various APRN organizations have provided detailed and specific descriptions for their particular role. Carving out an adequate scope of APRN practice authority has been a historic struggle for most of the advanced practice groups (see Chapter 1), and this continues to be a hotly debated issue among and within the health professions. Significant variability in state practice acts continues, such that APRNs can perform certain activities in some states, notably prescribing certain medications and practicing without physician supervision, but may be constrained from performing these same activities in other states (NCSBN, 2021a). The Consensus Model's proposed regulatory language can be used by states to achieve consistent scope of practice language and standardized APRN regulation (APRN Joint Dialogue Group, 2008).

Although more than 2 decades old, a report by the Pew Health Professions Commission (Finocchio et al. & Taskforce on Health Care Workforce Regulation, 1998) remains relevant today. The Taskforce noted that the tension and turf battles between professions and the increased legislative activities in this area "clog legislative agendas across the country (p. ii)." These battles are costly and time-consuming, and lawmakers' decisions related to scope of practice are frequently distorted by campaign contributions, lobbying efforts, and political power struggles rather than being based on empirical evidence. More recently, while the National Academy of Medicine reported that progress continues on a state-by-state basis in achieving full practice authority for APRNs, there are still many states where APRNs have reduced or restricted practice authority (National Academies of Sciences, Engineering, & Medicine [NASEM], 2016; Phillips, 2021; see Chapter 20 for further discussion). In addition, the National Academy of Medicine highlighted the fact that medical staff member and hospital privileging criteria are inconsistent due to state laws as well as business preferences. Opposition by some physician associations and physicians is ongoing and has been a significant barrier. Much work remains to be done. The National Academy of Medicine recommended that the coalition of stakeholders to remove these barriers needs to be expanded and diversified to increase collaboration in improving health care for patients (NASEM, 2021).

DIFFERENTIATING ADVANCED PRACTICE ROLES: OPERATIONAL DEFINITIONS OF ADVANCED PRACTICE NURSING

As noted earlier, it is critical to the public's understanding of advanced practice nursing that APRN roles and resulting job titles reflect actual practices. Because actual practices differ, job titles should differ. The following corollary is also true—if the actual practices do not differ, the job titles should not differ. For example, some institutions have retitled their CNSs *clinical coordinators* or *clinical educators*, even though these APRNs are practicing consistently with the practices of a CNS. This change in job title renders the CNS practice less clearly visible in the clinical setting and thereby obscures CNS role clarity. An example is in Virginia, where state regulators label advanced practice nurses as licensed nurse practitioners for all four APRN roles, further sowing confusion in health care and the public. As noted, differences among roles must be clarified in ways that promote understanding of advanced practice nursing, and the Consensus Model (APRN Joint Dialogue Group, 2008) clarifies appropriate titling for APRNs.

Workforce Data

It is difficult to obtain accurate numbers for APRNs by role, particularly for those prepared as CNSs. The US Bureau of Labor Statistics has separate classifications for NPs, CRNAs, and CNMs in their Standard Occupational Classification listing, so some data are collected when the Bureau does routine surveys. However, CNSs are not listed as a separate role in the classification system; rather the role is subsumed under the general registered nurse (RN) classification (US Bureau of Labor Statistics, 2021a, 2021b). The Bureau of Labor Statistics has refused to add a CNS classification despite repeated attempts to convince them otherwise. Therefore the latest APRN role numbers are based on the respective organizational data for consistency (Table 3.1).

It is essential to have accurate tracking of APRN numbers by distinct role as well as by geographic distribution and basic demographic statistics. Gathering data only on select APRN roles or as subcategories of the RN role diminishes the profession's ability to actively and appropriately advocate for patients on a national level for needed care that can best be provided by APRNs.

Four Established Advanced Practice Nurse Roles

Advanced practice nursing is applied in the four established roles and in emerging roles. These APRN roles can be considered to be the operational definitions of the concept of advanced practice nursing. Although each APRN role has the common definition, primary criteria, and competencies of advanced practice nursing at its center, each has its own distinct form. Some of the distinctive features of the various roles are listed here. Differences and similarities among roles are further explored in Part III of this text.

TABLE 3.1

Number of APRNs by Category in the United States

APRN Role	Numbers	Source	Website
Nurse practitioner	>234,000	American Association of Nurse Practitioners National Nurse Practitioner Database	www.aanp.org/all-about-nps/np-fact-sheet
Clinical nurse specialist	>89,000	National Association of Clinical Nurse Specialists	www.nacns.org/docs/APRN-Factsheet.pdf https://nacns.org/2020/09/clinical-nurse-specialists-associations-sign-agreement-uniting-92000-north-american-cnss/
Certified registered nurse anesthetist	>66,000	American Association of Nurse Anesthesiology	www.aana.com/ceandeducation/becomeacrna/Pages/Nurse-Anesthetists-at-a-Glance.aspx https://www.aana.com/membership/become-a-crna/crna-fact-sheet
Certified nurse-midwife	>12,800	American College of Nurse-Midwives	www.midwife.org/Essential-Facts-about-Midwives

The NACNS (2019) has distinguished CNS practice by characterizing three "spheres of impact" in which the CNS operates. These include the patient direct care sphere, the nurses and nursing practice sphere, and the organizations and systems sphere (see Chapter 12). A CNS is first and foremost a clinical expert who provides direct care to patients with complex health problems. CNSs not only learn collaboration processes, as do other APRNs, but also function as formal consultants to nursing staff and other care providers within their organizations. Developing, supporting, and educating nursing staff and other interprofessional staff to improve the quality of patient care comprise a core part of the nurses and nursing practice sphere. Managing system change in complex organizations to build teams and improve nursing practices and effecting system change to enable better advocacy for patients are additional role expectations of the CNS. Expectations regarding sophisticated evidence-based practice activities have been central to this role since its inception.

NPs, whether in primary care or acute care, possess advanced health assessment, diagnostic, and clinical management skills that include pharmacology management. Their focus is expert direct care, managing the health needs of individuals and their families. Incumbents in the classic NP role provide primary health care focused on wellness and prevention; NP practice also includes caring for patients with minor, common acute conditions and stable chronic conditions (see Chapter 13). The acute care NP (ACNP) brings practitioner skills to a specialized patient population within the acute care setting. The ACNP's focus is the diagnosis and clinical management of acutely or critically ill patient populations in a particular specialized setting. Acquisition of additional medical diagnostic and management skills, such as interpreting computed tomography and magnetic resonance imaging scans, inserting chest tubes, and performing lumbar punctures, also characterizes this role (see Chapter 14).

The CNM (see Chapter 15) has advanced health assessment and intervention skills focused on women's health and childbearing. CNM practice involves independent management of women's health care. CNMs focus particularly on pregnancy, childbirth, the postpartum period, and neonatal care, but their practices also include family planning, gynecologic care, primary health care for women through menopause, and treatment of male partners for sexually transmitted infections (ACNM, 2020). The CNM's focus is on providing direct care to a select patient population.

CRNA practice (see Chapter 16) is distinguished by advanced procedural and pharmacologic management of patients undergoing anesthesia. CRNAs practice independently, in collaboration with physicians, or as employees of a healthcare institution. Like CNMs, their primary focus is providing direct care to a select patient population. Both CNM and CRNA practices are also distinguished by well-established national standards and certification examinations in their specialties.

These differing roles and their similarities and distinctions are explored in detail in subsequent chapters. It is expected that other roles may emerge as health care continues to change and new opportunities become apparent. This brief discussion underscores the rich and varied nature of advanced practice nursing and the necessity for retaining and supporting different APRN roles and titles in the healthcare marketplace. At the same time, the consistent definition of advanced practice nursing described here undergirds each of these roles, as will be seen in Part III of this text.

CRITICAL ELEMENTS IN MANAGING ADVANCED PRACTICE NURSING ENVIRONMENTS

The healthcare arena is increasingly fluid and changeable; some would even say it is chaotic. Advanced practice nursing does not exist in a vacuum or a singular environment. Rather, this level of practice occurs in a wide variety of healthcare delivery environments. These diverse environments are complex admixtures of interdependent elements, as noted in Fig. 3.4. The term *environment* refers to any milieu in which an APRN practices, ranging from a community-based rural healthcare practice for a primary care NP to a complex tertiary healthcare organization for an ACNP. Certain core features of these environments dramatically shape advanced practice and must be managed by APRNs in order for their practices to survive and thrive (Fig. 3.4). Although not technically part of the core definition of advanced practice nursing, these environmental features are included here to frame the understanding that APRNs must be aware of these key elements in any practice setting. Furthermore, APRNs must be prepared to contend with and shape these aspects of their practice environment to be able to enact advanced practice nursing fully.

The environmental elements that affect APRN practice include the following:

- Managing reimbursement and payment mechanisms
- Dealing with marketing and contracting considerations
- Understanding legal, regulatory, and credentialing requirements
- Understanding and shaping health policy considerations
- Strengthening organizational structures and cultures to support advanced practice nursing
- Using technology to optimize patient care
- Enabling outcome evaluation and performance improvement

With the exception of organizational structures and cultures, Part IV of this text explores these elements in depth. Discussion of organizational considerations is presented in Chapter 4 and woven throughout the chapters in Part III.

Common to all of these environmental elements is the increasing use of technology and the need for APRNs to master various new technologies to improve patient care and healthcare systems. The ability to use information systems and technology and patient care technology is an essential element of graduate-level curricula (AACN, 2021). Electronic technology in the form of electronic health records, coding schemas, communications, Internet use, and provision of care across state lines through telehealth practices is changing healthcare practice. These changes, in turn, are reshaping all six APRN core competencies. Proficiency in the use of new technologies is increasingly necessary to support clinical practice, implement quality improvement initiatives, and provide leadership to evaluate outcomes of care and care systems (see Chapters 22 and 23).

Managing the business and legal aspects of practice is increasingly critical to APRN survival in the competitive healthcare marketplace. All APRNs must understand current reimbursement issues, even as changes related to the Patient Protection and Affordable Care Act (2010) and the Medicare Access and CHIP Reauthorization Act (2015) are being debated, re-debated, and advanced. Payment mechanisms and legal constraints must be managed, regardless of setting. Given the increasing competition among physicians, APRNs, and nonphysician providers, APRNs must be prepared to market their services assertively and knowledgeably. Marketing oneself as a new NP in a small community may look different from marketing oneself as a CNS in a large health system, but the principles are the same (Chapter 18). Marketing considerations often include the need to advocate for and actively create positions

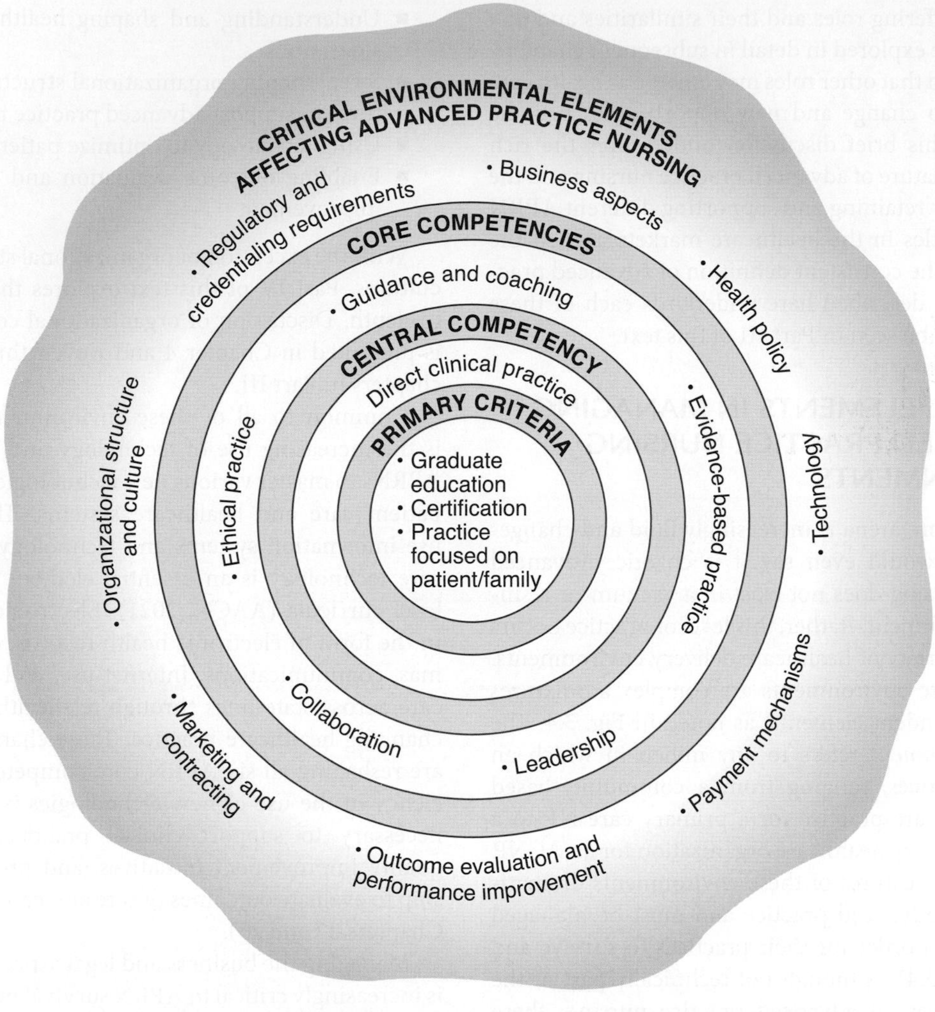

Fig. 3.4 ■ Critical elements in advanced nursing practice environments.

that do not currently exist. Contract considerations are much more complex at the APRN level, and all APRNs, whether newly graduated or experienced, must be prepared to enter into contract negotiations.

Health policy at the state and federal levels is an increasingly potent force shaping advanced practice nursing; regulations and policies that flow from legislative actions can enable or constrain APRN practices. Variations in the strength and number of APRNs in various states attest to the power of this environmental factor. Organizational structures and cultures, whether those of a community-based practice or a hospital unit, are also important facilitators of or barriers to advanced practice nursing; APRN students must learn to assess and intervene to build organizations and cultures that strengthen APRN practice. Finally, APRNs are accountable for the use of evidence-based practice to ensure positive patient and system outcomes. Measuring the favorable impact of advanced practice nursing on these outcomes and effecting performance improvements are essential activities that all APRNs must be prepared to undertake because continuing to demonstrate the value of APRN practice is a necessity in chaotic practice environments (Chapter 21).

Special mention must be made of healthcare quality. Reimbursement is being increasingly tied to quality metrics, with higher expectations for transparency of quality outcomes by providers. As quality concerns have escalated, more attention is being focused on quality metrics for all settings (see Chapter 23). As noted in the *Future of Nursing 2020–2030* report, it is imperative that issues such as structural racism, social determinants of health, and diversity in the healthcare workforce be acknowledged and addressed (NASEM, 2021). Achieving quality health care for all is dependent on resolving these issues in order to ensure even the basic first step of equitable access to the healthcare system and appropriate care and treatment. APRNs are an important part of the solution to ensuring quality outcomes for their specialty populations. Quality is not itself a competency or an environmental element, but it is an important feature that should be evident in the processes that APRNs use and the outcomes that they achieve. For example, coaching for wellness should demonstrate the quality processes of a therapeutic nurse–patient relationship and the patient being a partner with the APRN in achieving wellness outcomes. The importance of APRN involvement in quality initiatives can be seen in the work of the Nursing Alliance for Quality Care, a national partnership of organizations, consumers, and other stakeholders in the safety and quality arena (http://www.naqc.org).

IMPLICATIONS OF THE DEFINITION OF ADVANCED PRACTICE NURSING

A number of implications for education, regulation and credentialing, practice, and research flow from this understanding of advanced practice nursing. The Consensus Model (APRN Joint Dialogue Group, 2008) makes the important point that effective communication among legal and regulatory groups, accreditors, certifying organizations, and educators (licensing, accreditation, certification, and education [LACE]) is necessary to advance the goals of advanced practice nursing. Decisions made by each of these groups affect and are affected by all the others. Historically, advanced practice nursing has been hampered by the lack of consensus in APRN definition, terminology, educational and certification requirements, and regulatory approaches. The Consensus Model process, by combining stakeholders from each of the LACE areas, took a giant step forward toward the profession's achieving needed consensus on APRN practice, education, certification, and regulation.

Implications for Advanced Practice Nursing Education

Graduate programs should provide anticipatory socialization experiences to prepare students for their chosen APRN role. Graduate experiences should include practice in all of the competencies of advanced practice nursing, not just direct clinical practice. For example, students who have no theoretical base or guided practice experiences in collaboration skills or clinical, professional, and systems leadership will be ill-equipped to demonstrate these competencies on assuming a new APRN role. In addition, APRN students need to understand the critical elements in healthcare environments, such as the business aspects of practice and healthcare policy that must be managed if their practices are to survive and grow.

All APRN roles require at least a specialty master's education; master's programs are continuing for the foreseeable future even as the DNP degree is being developed in many institutions. The profession has embraced a wide variety of graduate educational models for preparing APRNs, including direct-entry programs for non-nurse college graduates and RN-to-master's of science in nursing programs. However, three of the four APRN professional organizations have endorsed doctoral preparation as entry into APRN practice (the AANA by the year 2025 [AANA, 2007], the NACNS by the year 2030 [NACNS, 2015], and the National Organization of Nurse Practitioner Faculties by 2025 [2018]). Ensuring quality and standardization of APRN education in the various specialties is imperative if the profession is to guarantee a highly skilled, uniformly educated APRN workforce to the public. The definition of advanced practice nursing used here can serve as a guide for developing quality courses and clinical practice experiences that prepare APRN students to practice at an advanced level.

It is imperative that nursing leaders and DNP faculty continue to provide increased clarity for the terms advanced nursing practice and advanced practice nursing. The differences between the two, despite being significant in the practice setting, are easily lost on the majority of RNs and even DNP graduates not prepared in an APRN role. Lack of clarity about this distinction has created ongoing problems as DNP graduates prepared in areas other than as an APRN confuse their combined graduate preparation and their RN clinical experience with being an APRN. This type of confusion about roles within nursing only perpetuates the ongoing lack of clarity when communicating with physicians and policymakers (Carter et al., 2013, 2014) and compromises the progress that APRNs have made in the practice arena.

Implications for Regulation and Credentialing

Significant progress has been made toward an integrative view of APRN regulation over the past decade, culminating in the LACE regulatory framework detailed in the Consensus Model. In particular, the primary criteria of graduate education, advanced certification, and focus on direct clinical practice for all APRN roles proposed in Hamric's definition have been affirmed as the key elements in regulating and credentialing APRNs (APRN Joint Dialogue Group, 2008). Such internal cohesion can go a long way toward removing barriers to the public's access to APRN care.

The Consensus Model has been an important unifying force within the APRN community. The regulatory clarity in this document has increasingly been seen in other national statements, and the work was highlighted in the Institute of Medicine's (IOM) report, *The Future of Nursing* (IOM, 2011). The NCSBN has embarked on the "APRN Campaign for Consensus," a nationwide effort to have this model enacted in all states. However, as of August 2021, only 16 states and two territories have fully implemented the Consensus Model into legislation (NCSBN, 2021b).

The IOM report also has given rise to action coalitions, funded by the AARP Foundation and the Robert Wood Johnson Foundation, in numerous states (Campaign for Action, n.d.). The Campaign for Action has a dual focus, implementing solutions to the challenges facing the nursing profession and strengthening nurse-based approaches to transform how Americans receive quality health care. Although the Campaign for Action is broader in scope than just advanced practice nursing, many of the solutions for transforming health care involve APRNs being able to practice to the full extent of their education. It is critically important for all APRNs to be aware of and involved in these efforts.

One implication for credentialing flows from the diverse specialty and role base of advanced practice nursing. APRNs must practice and be certified in the specific population focus and role for which they have been educated. APRNs who wish to change their specialty, population focus, or APRN role need to return to school for education targeted to that area. The days are past when a primary care NP could take a job in a specialized acute care practice without further education to prepare for that specialty. This issue of aligning APRN job expectations with education and certification is not always well understood by practice environments, educators, or even APRNs themselves. However, the need to ensure congruence between an APRN's specialty, education, certification, role, and subsequent practice has been identified by regulators; more stringent regulations regarding this issue have been promulgated (NCSBN, 2021a).

Implications for Research

As noted in Chapter 8, one of the core competencies of advanced practice nursing is the use of an evidence base in an APRN's practice and in changing the practice environment to incorporate the use of evidence. The practice doctorate initiative identified the increased need for leadership in evidence-based practice and for application of knowledge to solve practice problems and improve health outcomes as reasons for moving to the DNP degree for APRN practice (AACN, 2006); the emphasis has continued in the revised *Essentials* document (AACN, 2021). If research is to be relevant to healthcare delivery and to nursing practice at all levels, APRNs must be involved. APRNs need to recognize the importance of advancing the profession's and healthcare system's knowledge about effective patient care practices and to realize that they are a vital link in building and translating this knowledge into clinical practice.

Related to this research involvement is the necessity for more research differentiating basic and advanced practice nursing and identifying the patient populations that benefit most from APRN intervention. For example, there is compelling empirical evidence that APRNs can effectively manage chronic disease—preventing or mitigating complications, reducing rehospitalizations, and increasing patients' quality of life. This evidence is presented in the chapters in Part III of this text and in Chapter 21. Linking advanced practice nursing to specific patient outcomes remains a major research imperative for this century. It is interesting to note the increasing research being conducted in international settings as more countries implement advanced practice nursing and study the effectiveness of these new practitioners.

Similarly, research is needed on the outcomes of the different APRN educational pathways in terms of APRN graduate experiences and patient outcomes. Such data would be invaluable in continuing to refine advanced practice education. Outcomes achieved by graduates from DNP programs need similar study in comparison to master's-level APRN graduates; in critiquing the need for the DNP degree, Fulton and Lyon (2005) noted the absence of research data on whether there are weaknesses in current master's-level graduates.

Finally, it is incumbent upon DNP faculty to ensure that APRNs understand their role in evidence-based practice vis-à-vis research. In fact, faculty themselves continue to struggle with knowledge and understanding of evidence-based practice and its use in the completion of the scholarly DNP project (AACN, 2015; Dols et al., 2017). Translational, evidence-based practice change, and quality improvement projects are the proper foci for DNP projects; such projects require a complex skill set that is the focus of DNP evidence-based practice courses. DNP students are not sufficiently educated in the particulars of the formal research process to be prepared to conduct independent research successfully, and faculty have an important responsibility to assist the student to identify an appropriate topic. Unfortunately, it is not uncommon to encounter APRN DNP projects that are not an implementation of evidence-based practice or a clinical change project to bring research evidence to influence practice, but rather involve the conduct of a research study. The DNP-prepared APRN is an evidence-based practice expert who evaluates and generates internal evidence, translates research into sustainable practice changes, and uses research to make practice decisions that improve the quality of patient care (AACN, 2021; Melnyk, 2016). Without this important understanding, nursing runs the risk of implying that advancing the science of nursing through research no longer requires PhD preparation. Such a misunderstanding could lead practice institutions to hire DNP graduates with the intention that they conduct rigorous independent research. It could also substantially delay the translation of research findings into clinical practice.

Implications for Practice Environments

Because of the centrality of direct clinical practice, APRNs must hold on to and make explicit their direct patient care activities. They must also articulate the importance of this level of care for patients. In addition, it is important to identify those patients who most need APRN services and ensure that they receive this care.

APRN roles require considerable autonomy and authority to be fully enacted. Practice settings have not always structured APRN roles to allow sufficient autonomy or accountability for achievement of the patient and system outcomes that are expected of advanced practitioners. It is equally important to emphasize that APRNs have expanded responsibilities—expanded authority for practice requires expanded responsibility for practice. APRNs must demonstrate a higher level of responsibility and accountability if they are to be seen as legitimate providers of care and full partners on provider teams responsible for patient populations. This willingness to be accountable for practice will also promote consumers' and policymakers' perceptions of APRNs as credible providers in line with physicians.

The APRN leadership competency mandates that APRNs serve as visible role models and mentors for other nurses (see Chapter 9). Leadership is not optional in APRN practice; it is a requirement. APRNs must be a visible part of the solution to the healthcare system's problems. For this goal to be realized, each APRN must practice leadership in their daily activities. In practice environments, APRNs need structured time and opportunities for this leadership, including mentoring activities with new nurses.

New APRNs require a considerable period of role development before they can master all of the components and competencies of their chosen role, which has important implications for employers of new APRNs. Employers should provide experienced preceptors, some structure for the new APRN, and ongoing support for role development (see Chapter 4 for further recommendations).

As a result of government titling, it is becoming common in the practice setting to label APRNs (as well as physician assistants) as "mid-level providers." The very use of this term for an APRN implies a hierarchical (and therefore a "less than") structure for all of nursing. If the APRN is "mid-level," then the implication is that the physician is at the top and the RN is thus positioned at the bottom of the care provider structure (Boyle, 2011). This is contrary to the reality that all healthcare providers bring unique and valued expertise to the care of patients; the professional leading the care at any given point in a patient's health encounter is dependent on the needs of the patient and the provider with the corresponding expertise. This concern extends to the use of the term *Advanced Practice Provider*, which also combines APRNs with roles such as physician assistants. It is important that APRNs distinguish their roles when they are lumped into categories with other providers.

Finally, APRN roles must be structured in practice environments to allow APRNs to enact advanced nursing skills rather than simply substitute for physicians. It is certainly necessary for APRNs to gain additional skills in medical diagnosis and therapeutic interventions, including the knowledge needed for prescriptive authority. However, *advanced practice nursing is a value-added complement to medical practice, not a substitute for it*. This is true in both the primary care and acute care arenas; it may well be that substituting APRNs for physicians in classic, medically driven care configurations is not the best use of APRN skills. Because APRN competencies include those of partnering with patients, use of evidence, and coaching skills, APRNs may be more effectively used in wellness programs, working with chronically ill patients to strengthen their self-management and adherence, designing and implementing educational programs for patients with complex needs and facilitators of a coordinated approach in patients with complex acute care needs. New sustainable business models are needed that are more collaborative and configure teams in innovative ways to minimize fragmentation of care and make the best use of the APRN as a value-added complement to the traditional medical team.

As physician shortages increase, particularly the number of physicians prepared in family practice and hospitalist practices, this distinction between advanced practice nursing and medical practice must be clear in the minds of employers, insurers, and APRNs themselves. As advanced practice nursing evolves, it is becoming clear that APRNs represent an evident choice for patients seeking care. Consequently, understanding what APRNs bring to health care must be articulated to multiple stakeholders to enable informed patient choice. A competency-based definition of advanced practice nursing aids in this articulation, so that APRNs are not just seen as physician substitutes.

CONCLUSION

Since the first edition of this text in 1996, substantial progress has been made toward clarifying the definition of advanced practice nursing. This progress is enabling APRNs, educators, administrators, and other nursing leaders to be clear and consistent about the definition of advanced practice nursing so that the profession speaks with one voice.

This is a critical juncture in the evolution of advanced practice nursing as national attention on nursing and recommendations for nursing's central role in redesigning the healthcare system are increasing. The revised *Essentials* will require a thoughtful, comprehensive evaluation and approach to competency-based graduate-level education that distinguishes between DNP-prepared APRNs and other DNP-prepared nurses in order to decrease confusion. APRNs must continue to clarify that the advanced practice of nursing is not the junior practice of medicine but represents an important alternative practice that complements rather than competes with medical practice. In some cases, patients need advanced nursing and not medicine; identifying these situations and matching APRN resources to patients' needs are important priorities for transforming the current healthcare system. APRNs must be able to articulate their defining characteristics clearly and forcefully so that their practices will survive and thrive amid continued cost cutting in the healthcare sector.

For a profession to succeed, it must have internal cohesion and external legitimacy, and it must have them at the same time (Safriet, 1993). Clarity about the core definition of advanced practice nursing and recognition of the primary criteria and competencies necessary for all APRNs enhance nursing's internal cohesion. At the same time, clarifying the differences among APRNs and showcasing their important roles in the healthcare system enhance nursing's external legitimacy.

KEY SUMMARY POINTS

- The advanced practice of nursing is not the junior practice of medicine; advanced practice nursing is a complement to, not a substitute for, medical practice.
- There is a clear and distinct difference between the terms *advanced practice nursing* and *advanced nursing practice*, and this difference needs to be clearly elucidated, especially as the terms are used on a global basis.
- The three primary criteria of an earned graduate degree with a concentration in an advanced practice nursing role and population focus, national certification at an advanced level, and a practice focused on patients and their families are necessary but not sufficient to define advanced practice nursing.
- The DNP is an academic *degree*, not a *role*.
- All APRNs share the same core criteria and competencies, although the actual clinical skill set varies, depending on the needs of the APRN's specialty patient population.

REFERENCES

American Association of Colleges of Nursing. (1995). *The essentials of master's education for advanced practice nursing.* Washington, DC: Author.

American Association of Colleges of Nursing. (2004). *Position statement on the practice doctorate in nursing.* Washington, DC: Author.

American Association of Colleges of Nursing. (2006). *The essentials of doctoral education for advanced nursing practice.* Washington, DC: Author.

American Association of Colleges of Nursing. (2013). Competencies and curricular expectations for clinical nurse leader education and practice. https://www.aacnnursing.org/Portals/42/AcademicNursing/CurriculumGuidelines/CNL-Competencies-October-2013.pdf

American Association of Colleges of Nursing. (2015). The Doctor of Nursing Practice: Current issues and clarifying recommendations. Report from the Task Force on the implementation of the DNP. www.aacn.nche.edu/aacn-publications/white-papers/DNP-Implementation-TF-Report-8-15.pdf

American Association of Colleges of Nursing. (2020). DNP fact sheet. https://www.aacnnursing.org/News-Information/Fact-Sheets/DNP-Fact-Sheet

American Association of Colleges of Nursing. (2021). The Essentials: Core competencies for professional nursing education. https://www.aacnnursing.org/Portals/42/AcademicNursing/pdf/Essentials-2021.pdf

American Association of Nurse Anesthesiology. (2007). AANA announces support of doctorate for entry into nurse anesthesia practice by 2025. http://www.aana.com/newsandjournal/News/Pages/092007-AANA-Announces-Support-of-Doctorate-for-Entry-into-Nurse-Anesthesia-Practice-by-2025.aspx

American College of Nurse-Midwives. (2015). Position statement: Mandatory degree requirements for entry into midwifery practice. https://www.midwife.org/acnm/files/ACNMLibraryData/UPLOADFILENAME/000000000076/Mandatory-Degree-Requirements-June-2015.pdf

American College of Nurse-Midwives. (2020). Core competencies for basic midwifery practice. https://www.midwife.org/acnm/files/acnmlibrarydata/uploadfilename/000000000050/ACNMCoreCompetenciesMar2020_final.pdf

American Nurses Association. (1995). *Nursing's social policy statement.* Washington, DC: Author.

American Nurses Association. (2003). *Nursing's social policy statement* (2nd ed.). Washington, DC: Author.

American Nurses Association. (2010). *Nursing's social policy statement* (3rd ed.). Silver Spring, MD: Author.

American Nurses Association. (2015a). *Code of ethics for nurses with interpretive statements.* Silver Spring, MD: Author.

American Nurses Association. (2015b). *Nursing: Scope and standards of practice* (3rd ed.). Silver Spring, MD: Author.

American Nurses Association. (2021). *Nursing: Scope and standards of practice* (4th ed.). Silver Spring, MD: Author.

American Nurses Credentialing Center. (n.d.). Our certifications. https://www.nursingworld.org/our-certifications. March 10, 2022.

APRN Joint Dialogue Group. (2008). Consensus Model for APRN regulation: Licensure, accreditation, certification & education. http://www.aacn.nche.edu/education-resources/APRNReport.pdf

Benner, P. (1984). *From novice to expert.* Addison-Wesley.

Benner, P., Hooper-Kyriakidis, P., & Stannard, D. (1999). *Clinical wisdom and interventions in critical care.* Saunders.

Benner, P., Hughes, R. G., Sutphen, M. (2008). Clinical reasoning, decisionmaking, and action: Thinking critically and clinically. In Patient Safety and Quality: An evidence-based handbook for nurses. Agency for Healthcare Research and Quality. Agency for Healthcare Research and Quality. Chapter 6. http://ovidsp.ovid.com/ovidweb.cgi?T=JS&PAGE=reference&D=medp&NEWS=N&AN=21328745

Benner, P., Tanner, C. A., & Chesla, C. A. (1996). *Expertise in nursing practice: Caring, clinical judgment, and ethics.* Springer.

Boyle, D. A. (2011). Are you a mid-level provider, a physician extender, or a nurse? *Oncology Nursing Forum, 38*(5), 497.

Bryant-Lukosius, D., Spichiger, E., Martin, J., Stoll, H., Kellerhals, S. D., Fliedner, M., Grossman, F., Henry, M., Herrmann, L., Koller, A., Schwendimann, R., Ulrich, A., Weibel, L., Callens, B., & De Geest, S. (2016). Framework for evaluating the impact of advanced practice nursing roles. *Journal of Nursing Scholarship, 48*(2), 201–209.

Burns-Bolton, L., & Mason, D. J. (2012). Commentary on: Molding the future of advanced practice nursing. *Nursing Outlook, 60,* 241–249.

Calkin, J. D. (1984). A model for advanced nursing practice. *Journal of Nursing Administration, 14*, 24–30.

Campaign for Action. (n.d.). State action coalitions. Retrieved September 27, 2021 from http://campaignforaction.org/our-network/state-action-coalitions/

Carter, N., Dobbins, M., Hoxby, H., Ireland, S., Peachy, G., & DiCenso, A. (2013). Knowledge gaps regarding APN roles: What hospital decision makers tell us. *Nursing Leadership (Toronto, Ont), 26*(4), 60–75.

Carter, N., Lavis, J. N., & MacDonald-Rencz, S. (2014). Use of modified Delphi to plan knowledge translation for decision makers: An application in the field of advanced practice nursing. *Policy, Politics, & Nursing Practice, 15*(3–4), 93–101.

Cronenwett, L. R. (1995). Molding the future of advanced practice nursing. *Nursing Outlook, 43*, 112–118.

Cronenwett, L. R., Dracup, K., Grey, M., McCauley, L., Meleis, A., & Salmon, M. (2011). The Doctor of Nursing Practice: A national workforce perspective. *Nursing Outlook, 59*, 9–17.

Dols, J. D., Hernandez, C., & Miles, H. (2017). The DNP project: Quandries for nursing scholars. *Nursing Outlook, 65*(1), 84–93.

Dowling, M., Beauchesne, M., Farrelly, F., & Murphy, K. (2013). Advanced practice nursing: A concept analysis. *International Journal of Nursing Practice, 19*(2), 131–140.

Finocchio, L. J., Dower, C. M., Blick, N. T., & Gragnola, C. M., the Taskforce on Health Care Workforce Regulation. (1998). *Strengthening consumer protection: Priorities for health care workforce regulation*. Pew Health Professions Commission.

Friberg, E. E., & Creasia, J. L. (2011). *Conceptual foundations: The bridge to professional nursing practice* (5th ed.). Mosby.

Fulton, J., & Lyon, B. (2005).The need for some sense making: Doctor of Nursing Practice. *OJIN: The Online Journal of Issues in Nursing,10(3)*, Manuscript 3.

Hamric, A. B. (1996). A definition of advanced nursing practice. In A. B. Hamric, J. A. Spross, & C. M. Hanson (Eds.), *Advanced nursing practice: An integrative approach* (pp. 42–56). WB Saunders.

Hamric, A. B. (2000). A definition of advanced nursing practice. In A. B. Hamric, J. A. Spross, & C. M. Hanson (Eds.), *Advanced nursing practice: An integrative approach* (2nd ed.) (pp. 53–73). Saunders.

Hamric, A. B. (2005). A definition of advanced practice nursing. In A. B. Hamric, J. A. Spross, & C. M. Hanson (Eds.), *Advanced practice nursing: An integrative approach* (3rd ed.) (pp. 85–108). Saunders.

Hamric, A. B. (2009). A definition of advanced practice nursing. In A. B. Hamric, J. A. Spross, & C. M. Hanson (Eds.), *Advanced practice nursing: An integrative approach* (4th ed.) (pp. 75–94). Saunders.

Hamric, A. B. (2014). A definition of advanced practice nursing. In A. B. Hamric, J. A. Spross, & C. M. Hanson (Eds.), *Advanced practice nursing: An integrative approach* (5th ed.) (pp. 67–85). Elsevier.

Hamric, A. B., & Tracy, M. F. (2019). A definition of advanced practice nursing. In M. F. Tracy, & E. T. O'Grady (Eds.), *Advanced practice nursing: An integrative approach* (pp. 61–79). Elsevier.

Hanson, C. M., & Hamric, A. B. (2003). Reflections on the continuing evolution of advanced practice nursing. *Nursing Outlook, 51*, 203–211.

Hickey, J. V., Ouimette, R. V., & Venegoni, S. L. (2000). *Advanced practice nursing: Changing roles and clinical applications* (2nd ed.). Lippincott.

Hood, L. J. (2014). *Leddy and Pepper's conceptual bases of professional nursing* (8th ed.). Lippincott Williams & Wilkins.

Institute of Medicine (US), Committee on the Robert Wood Johnson Foundation Initiative on the Future of Nursing. (2011). *The future of nursing: Leading change, advancing health*. The National Academies Press.

International Council of Nurses. (2020). Guidelines on advanced practice nursing 2020. https://www.icn.ch/system/files/documents/2020-04/ICN_APN%20Report_EN_WEB.pdf

Interprofessional Education Collaborative Expert Panel (2016). Core competencies for interprofessional collaborative practice: 2016 Update. https://ipec.memberclicks.net/assets/2016-Update.pdf

Lindeke, L. L., Canedy, B. H., & Kay, M. M. (1997). A comparison of practice domains of clinical nurse specialists and nurse practitioners. *Journal of Professional Nursing, 13*, 281–287.

Medicare and CHIP Reauthorization Act (MACRA). (2015). Public Law 114-10, 114th Congress. https://www.congress.gov/114/plaws/publ10/PLAW-114publ10.pdf

Melnyk, B. M. (2016). The doctor of nursing practice degree = evidence-based practice expert. *Worldviews on Evidence-based Nursing, 13*(3), 183–184.

Mundinger, M. O. (1994). Advanced practice nursing: Good medicine for physicians? *New England Journal of Medicine, 330*, 211–214.

Mundinger, M. O., Cook, S., Lenz, E., Piacentini, K., Auerhahn, C., & Smith, J. (2000). Assuring quality and access in advanced practice nursing: A challenge to nurse educators. *Journal of Professional Nursing, 16*, 322–329.

National Academies of Sciences, Engineering, & Medicine (NASEM). (2016). *Assessing the progress on the Institute of Medicine report The Future of Nursing*. The National Academies Press.

National Academies of Sciences, Engineering, & Medicine (NASEM). (2021). *The future of nursing 2020–2030: Charting a path to health equity*. The National Academies Press.

National Association of Clinical Nurse Specialists. (2015). NACNS position statement on the Doctor of Nursing Practice. http://www.nacns.org/docs/DNP-Statement1507.pdf

National Association of Clinical Nurse Specialists. (2019). *Statement on clinical nurse specialist practice and education* (3rd ed.). Reston, VA: Author.

National Council of State Boards of Nursing. (1993). *Position paper on the regulation of advanced nursing practice*. Chicago: Author.

National Council of State Boards of Nursing. (2002). *Position paper on the regulation of advanced practice nursing*. Chicago: Author.

National Council of State Boards of Nursing. (2021a). APRN campaign for consensus: Moving toward uniformity in state laws. https://www.ncsbn.org/campaign-for-consensus.htm

National Council of State Boards of Nursing. (2021b). APRN Consensus implementation status. https://www.ncsbn.org/5397.htm

National Organization of Nurse Practitioner Faculties. (2018). NONPF DNP Statement May 2018. https://www.nonpf.org/news/400012/NONPF-DNP-Statement-May-2018.htm

Patient Protection and Affordable Care Act, 42 U.S.C. § 18001 (2010).

Pearson, H. (2011). Concepts of advanced practice: What does it mean? *British Journal of Nursing, 20*, 184–185.

Phillips, S. J. (2021). 33rd Annual APRN legislative update: Unprecedented changes to APRN practice authority in unprecedented times. *Nurse Practitioner, 46*(1), 27–55.

Rasch, R. F. R., & Frauman, A. C. (1996). Advanced practice in nursing: Conceptual issues. *Journal of Professional Nursing, 12*, 141–146.

Safriet, B. J. (1993). *Keynote address: One strong voice. Presented at the National Nurse Practitioner Leadership*. Summit: Washington DC, February 1993.

Safriet, B. J. (1998). Still spending dollars, still searching for sense: Advanced practice nursing in an era of regulatory and economic turmoil. *Advanced Practice Nursing Quarterly, 4*, 24–33.

Schober, M., & Stewart, D. (2019). Developing a consistent approach to advanced practice nursing worldwide. *International Nursing Review, 66*(2), 151–153.

Schumann, L., & Tyler, D. O. (2018). Challenges and successes in specialty practice: Focus on emergency nurse practitioners. *JAANP, 30*(10), 353–355.

Spross, J. A., & Baggerly, J (1989). Models of advanced practice. In A. B. Hamric, & J. A. Spross (Eds.), *The clinical nurse specialist in theory and practice* (2nd ed.) (pp. 19–40). Saunders.

Stanley, J. M. (2011). *Advanced practice nursing: Emphasizing common roles* (3rd ed.). F. A. Davis.

US Bureau of Labor Statistics. (2021). *Occupational employment statistics*: Occupational Employment and Wages. May, 2021 29–1141 Registered Nurses. https://www.bls.gov/oes/current/oes291141.htm

US Bureau of Labor Statistics. (2021). *Occupational employment statistics. May 2020*: Occupational Profiles. https://www.bls.gov/oes/current/oes_stru.htm#29-0000

US National Library of Medicine. (2021). Advanced practice nursing. MeSH descriptor data 2022. https://meshb-prev.nlm.nih.gov/record/ui?name=Advanced%20Practice%20Nursing

4 ROLE DEVELOPMENT OF THE ADVANCED PRACTICE NURSE

CAROLE L. MACKAVEY ■ KAREN A. BRYKCZYNSKI

"Predictions for APRNs in the twenty-first century are for a bright future in all settings."

~ Loretta C. Ford

CHAPTER CONTENTS

PERSPECTIVES ON ADVANCED PRACTICE NURSE ROLE DEVELOPMENT 99
NOVICE-TO-EXPERT SKILL ACQUISITION MODEL 99
Transition From Student to Clinician 101
ROLE CONCEPTS AND ROLE DEVELOPMENT ISSUES 101
Role Ambiguity 102
Role Incongruity 102
Role Conflict 104
ROLE TRANSITIONS 107
Advanced Practice Nurse Role Acquisition in Graduate School 107
Strategies to Facilitate Role Acquisition 110
Advanced Practice Nursing Role Implementation: Entering the Workforce 114
Strategies to Facilitate Role Implementation 121
Facilitators and Barriers in the Work Setting 124
Continued Advanced Practice Nurse Role Evolution 126
Evaluation of Role Development 127
CONCLUSION 129
KEY SUMMARY POINTS 130

This chapter explores the complex processes of advanced practice registered nurse (APRN) role development, with the objectives of providing the following: (1) an understanding of related concepts and research; (2) anticipatory guidance for APRN students; (3) role facilitation strategies for new APRNs, APRN preceptors, faculty, administrators, and interested colleagues; and (4) guidelines for continued role evolution. This chapter consolidates literature from all of the APRN specialties—including clinical nurse specialists (CNSs), nurse practitioners (NPs), certified nurse-midwives (CNMs), and certified registered nurse anesthetists (CRNAs)—to present a generic process relevant to all APRN roles. Some of this literature is foundational to understanding issues of role development for all APRN roles and, although dated, remains relevant. This chapter has been expanded to include international APRN role development experiences. To reflect the literature indicating that APRN role transition occurs as two distinct processes, the discussion is separated into (1) the educational component of APRN role acquisition and (2) the occupational or work component of role implementation. This division in the process of role development is intended to clarify and distinguish the changes occurring during the role transitions experienced during the educational period (role acquisition) and the changes occurring during the actual performance of the role after program completion (role implementation). Strategies for enhancing APRN role development are described. The chapter concludes with summary comments and suggestions to facilitate future APRN role development and evolution.

Role development in advanced practice nursing is described here as a process that evolves over time. The process is more than socializing and taking on a new role. It involves transforming one's professional identity (Benner, 2011; Jarvis-Selinger et al., 2012) and the progressive development of the core advanced practice competencies (see Chapter 3). The scope of nursing practice has expanded and contracted in response to societal needs, political forces, and economic realities (see Chapter 1). Historical evidence suggests that the expanded role of the 1970s was common nursing practice during the early 1900s among public health nurses (DeMaio, 1979; see Chapter 1). However, the core of nursing is not defined by the tasks nurses perform. This task-oriented perspective is inadequate and disregards the complex nature of nursing.

PERSPECTIVES ON ADVANCED PRACTICE NURSE ROLE DEVELOPMENT

Professional role development is a dynamic ongoing process that, once begun, spans a lifetime. The concept of graduation as commencement, whereby one's career begins on completion of a degree, is central to understanding the evolving nature of professional roles in response to personal, professional, and societal demands (Gunn, 1998). Professional role development literature in nursing is abundant and complex, involving multiple component processes, including the following: (1) aspects of adult development, (2) development of clinical expertise, (3) modification of self-identity through initial socialization in school, (4) embodiment of ethical comportment (Benner et al., 2010), (5) development and integration of professional role components, (6) subsequent resocialization in the work setting, (7) evolving technology, and (8) advances in healthcare knowledge and practice. Similar to socialization for other professional roles, such as those of attorney, physician, teacher, and social worker, the process of becoming an APRN involves aspects of adult development and professional socialization. The professional socialization process in advanced practice nursing involves identification with and acquisition of the behaviors and attitudes of the advanced practice group to which one aspires (Waugaman & Lu, 1999). This includes learning the specialized language, skills, and knowledge of the particular APRN group; internalizing its values and norms; and incorporating these into one's professional nursing identity and other life roles (Cohen, 1981).

NOVICE-TO-EXPERT SKILL ACQUISITION MODEL

Acquisition of knowledge and skill occurs in a progressive movement through the stages of performance from novice to expert, as described by Dreyfus and Dreyfus (1986, 2009), who studied diverse groups, including pilots, chess players, and adult learners of second languages. The skill acquisition model has broad applicability and can be used to understand many different skills, ranging from playing a musical instrument to writing a research grant. The most widely known application of this model is Benner's (1984) observational and interview study of clinical nursing practice situations from the perspective of new nurses and their preceptors in hospital nursing services. Although this study included several APRNs, it did not specify a particular education level as a criterion for expertise. As noted in Chapter 3, there has been some confusion about this criterion. The skill acquisition model is a situation-based model, not a trait model. Therefore the level of expertise is not an individual characteristic of a particular nurse but is a function of the nurse's familiarity with a particular situation in combination with their educational background. This model could be used to study the level of expertise required for other aspects of advanced practice nursing, including guidance and coaching, evidence-based practice, leadership, collaboration, and ethical practice.

Fig. 4.1 shows a typical APRN role development pattern in terms of this skill acquisition model. A major implication of the novice-to-expert model for advanced practice nursing is the claim that even

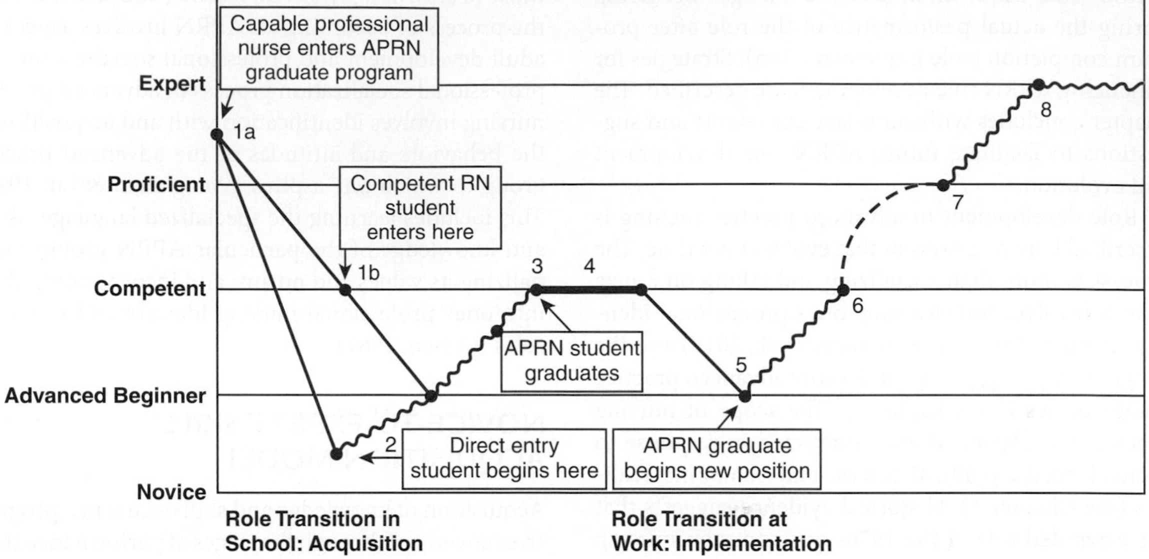

Fig. 4.1 ■ **Typical APRN role development pattern.** *1a,* APRN students may begin graduate school as proficient or expert nurses. *1b,* Some enter as competent RNs, with limited practice experience. Depending on previous background, the new APRN student will revert to novice level or advanced beginner level on assuming the student role. *2,* A direct-entry APRN student or non-nurse college graduate student with no experience would begin the role transition process at the novice level. *3,* The graduate from an APRN program is competent as an APRN student but has no experience as a practicing APRN. *4,* A limbo period is experienced while the APRN graduate searches for a position and becomes certified. *5,* The newly employed APRN reverts to the advanced beginner level in the new APRN position as the role trajectory begins again. *6,* Some individuals remain at the competent level. There is a discontinuous leap from the competent to the proficient level. *7,* Proficiency develops only if there is sufficient commitment and involvement in practice along with embodiment of skills and knowledge. *8,* Expertise is intuitive and situation specific, meaning that not all situations will be managed expertly. (See text for details.) Note: Readers may refer to the Dreyfus skill acquisition model for further details (Benner, 1984; Benner et al., 2009; Dreyfus & Dreyfus, 1986, 2009). For the purpose of illustration, this figure is more linear than the individualized role development trajectories that actually occur.

experts can be expected to perform at lower skill levels when they enter new situations or positions. Hamric and Taylor's (1989) report that an experienced CNS starting a new position experiences the same role development phases as a new CNS graduate, only over a shorter period, supports this claim. The same pattern can be expected with new doctor of nursing practice (DNP) graduates; they experience similar role development phases upon assuming a new position, but they go through phases more quickly because they are informed by broader education and experience (Glasgow & Zoucha, 2011).

The overall trajectory expected during APRN role development is shown in Fig. 4.1; however, each APRN experiences a unique pattern of role transitions and life transitions concurrently. For example, a professional nurse who functions as a mentor for new graduates may decide to pursue an advanced degree as an APRN. As an APRN graduate student, they will experience the challenges of acquiring a new role, the anxiety associated with learning new skills and practices, and the dependency of being a novice. At the same time, if this nurse continues to work as a registered nurse, their functioning in this work role will be at the competent, proficient, or expert level, depending on experience and the situation. On graduation, the new APRN may experience a limbo period during which they are no longer a student and not yet an APRN, while searching for a position and meeting certification requirements (see Chapter 20). Once in a new APRN position, this nurse may experience a return to the advanced beginner stage as they proceed through the phases of role implementation.

Transition From Student to Clinician

The new graduate APRN has demonstrated competence as an APRN student but has no experience as a practicing APRN. Abundant nursing literature reports that the first year of clinical practice constitutes a major transitional period (Urbanowicz, 2019). No matter which profession or skill the neophyte is trying to master, there is a distinction between "doing" and "being" that is crucial to understanding this work transition (Jarvis-Selinger et al., 2012). Competency and identity merge in taking on new skilled practices. Perhaps the most significant implication of the skill acquisition model is the need to accrue experience in actual situations over time, so that practical and theoretical knowledge are refined, clarified, personalized, and embodied, forming an individualized repertoire of experience that guides practice. New graduates often report that they were not adequately prepared for actual practice and lack confidence. These feelings of inadequacy arise not only from gaining experience in managing the pervasive uncertainties in clinical practice (Brykczynski, 1991) but also from their fledgling status wherein they have not been involved in actually "doing" the new practices often enough or long enough to "become" comfortable with them. There is a complex, holistic process whereby a new clinician provides care and interacts with significant others such as patients, other providers, family members, peers, and administrators and responds to them as their confidence and competence gradually build over time. Orientation programs have existed for some time to support new clinical employees. More recently, postgraduate clinical fellowships or residencies are being developed in response to the increased complexities and demands of current clinical practice to support new APRNs and facilitate their transition during the crucial first year of practice (Bryant & Parker, 2020).

Even after making the transition to an APRN role, progression in role implementation is not a linear process. As Fig. 4.1 indicates, there are discontinuities, with movement back and forth as the trajectory begins again. Years later, the APRN may decide to pursue another APRN or leadership role. The processes of role acquisition, role implementation, and novice-to-expert skill development will again be experienced—although altered and informed by previous experiences—as the postgraduate student acquires additional skills and knowledge. Role development involves multiple, dynamic, and situational processes, with each new undertaking being characterized by passage through earlier transitional phases and with some movement back and forth, horizontally or vertically, as different career options are pursued.

Direct-entry students who are non-nurse college graduates and APRN students with little or no experience as nurses before entry into an APRN graduate program would be expected to begin their APRN role development at the novice level (see Fig. 4.1). Some evidence indicates that these inexperienced nurse students in APRN programs avoid the role confusion associated with letting go of the traditional registered nurse (RN) role that is commonly reported with experienced nurse students (Heitz et al., 2004). This finding has implications for APRN education as the profession moves toward competency-based education and the DNP as the preferred educational pathway for APRN preparation (American Association of Colleges of Nursing [AACN], 2021).

Another significant implication of the Dreyfus model (Dreyfus & Dreyfus, 1986, 2009) for APRNs is the observation that the quality of performance may deteriorate when performers are subjected to intense scrutiny, whether their own or that of someone else (Roberts et al., 1997). The increased anxiety experienced by APRN students during faculty on-site clinical evaluation visits or during videotaped testing of clinical performance in simulated situations is an example of responding to such intense scrutiny. As the profession encourages new nurses to move more rapidly into APRN education, students, faculty, and educational programs must search for creative ways to incorporate the practical and theoretical knowledge necessary for advanced practice nursing. Discussing unfolding cases is a useful approach for teaching the clinical reasoning in transition that is so essential for clinical practice (Benner et al., 2010; Day et al., 2012).

ROLE CONCEPTS AND ROLE DEVELOPMENT ISSUES

This discussion of professional role issues incorporates role concepts described by Hardy and Hardy (1988) and Schumacher and Meleis (1994), along with the concept that different APRN roles represent different subcultural groups within the broader nursing culture (Leininger, 1994). Building on Johnson's (1993) conclusion that NPs have three voices, Brykczynski (1999b) described APRNs as tricultural and trilingual. They share background knowledge, practices, and skills of three cultures—biomedicine, mainstream nursing, and everyday life. They are fluent in the languages of biomedical science, nursing knowledge and skill, and everyday parlance. Some APRNs (e.g., CNMs) are socialized into a fourth culture as well, that of midwifery. Others are also fluent in more than one everyday language.

The concepts of role stress and strain discussed by Hardy and Hardy (1988) are useful for understanding the dynamics of role transitions (see Table 4.1). Hardy and Hardy described *role stress* as a social structural condition in which role obligations are ambiguous, conflicting, incongruous, excessive, or unpredictable. *Role strain* is defined as the subjective feeling of frustration, tension, or anxiety experienced in response to role stress. The highly stressful nature of the nursing profession needs to be recognized as the background within which individuals seek advanced education to become APRNs (Waddill-Goad, 2019). Role strain can be minimized by the identification of potential role stressors, development of coping strategies, and rehearsal of situations designed for application of those strategies. However, the difficulties experienced by neophytes in new positions cannot be eliminated. As noted, expertise is holistic, involving embodied perceptual skills (e.g., detecting qualitative distinctions in pulses or types of anxiety); formation of character, identity, and ethical judgment; shared background knowledge; and cognitive ability. A school–work, theory–practice, ideal–real gap will remain because of the nature of human skill acquisition, which occurs over time, and the undetermined nature of actual clinical practice. Bridging this gap requires engaged clinical reasoning in transitions and consideration of patient preferences, practice standards, costs, clinical outcomes, and numerous other aspects that vary with each situation.

Bandura's (1977) social cognitive theory of self-efficacy may be of interest to APRNs in terms of understanding what motivates individuals to acquire skills and what builds confidence as skills are developed. Self-efficacy theory—a person's belief in their ability to succeed—has been used widely to further understanding of skill acquisition with patients (Jiang et al., 2019; Mata et al., 2019). Self-efficacy theory has also been applied to mentoring APRN students (Hayes, 2001) and training healthcare professionals in skill acquisition (Parle et al., 1997). Attention to varied learning styles, different neurocognitive processes involved in learning, and APRN students as adult learners is important for teaching (Burns et al., 2006; Kumar et al., 2013).

Role Ambiguity

Role ambiguity (see Table 4.1) develops when there is a lack of clarity about expectations, a blurring of responsibilities, uncertainty regarding role implementation, and the inherent uncertainty of existent knowledge. According to Hardy and Hardy (1988), role ambiguity characterizes all professional positions and might be positive in that it offers opportunities for creative possibilities. It can be expected to be more prominent in professions undergoing change, such as those in the healthcare field. To minimize uncertainty about roles in interprofessional educational experiences and promote successful interprofessional practice, a focus on the following key components is important: awareness of one's own professional role, understanding the professional roles of others, leadership skills, principles of teamwork, and conflict negotiation skills and knowledge (MacDonald et al., 2010). Role ambiguity has been widely discussed in relation to the CNS role (Bryant-Lukosius et al., 2010; Hamric, 2003; see also Chapter 12), but it is also a relevant issue for other APRN roles (Faraz, 2017; Kelly & Mathews, 2001), particularly as APRN roles evolve (Stahl & Myers, 2002).

Role Incongruity

Role incongruity is intrarole conflict, which Hardy and Hardy (1988) described as developing from two sources. Incompatibility between skills, abilities, and role obligations is one source of role incongruity. An example of this is an adult APRN hired to work in an emergency department with a large percentage of pediatric patients. Such an APRN will find it necessary to enroll in a family NP or pediatric NP program to gain the knowledge necessary to eliminate this role incongruity. This is a growing issue as NP roles become

TABLE 4.1
Selected Role Concepts

Concept	Definition	Examples
Role stress	A situation of increased role performance demand	Returning to school while maintaining work and family responsibilities The expectation of increased workload (number of patients seen) Keeping up with rapidly changing technology Technology intruding on patient relationships Coping with restrictions related to payment system limitations
Role strain	Subjective feeling of frustration, tension, or anxiety in response to role stress	Feeling of decreased self-esteem when performance is below expectations of self or significant others
Role stressors	Factors that produce role stress	Financial, personal, or academic demands and role expectations that are ambiguous, conflicting, excessive, or unpredictable Pandemic created fear about personal safety and the stress of the overwhelming volume of patients, high acuity, and increased mortality rate
Role ambiguity	Unclear expectations, diffuse responsibilities, uncertainty about subroles	Recent graduates' uncertainty about role expectations Some degree of ambiguity exists in all professional positions because of the evolving nature of roles and expansion of skills and knowledge
Role incongruity	A role with incompatibility between skills and abilities and role obligations or between personal values and self-concept and role obligations	An adult nurse practitioner in a role requiring pediatric skills and knowledge Difficulty of incorporating holistic nursing aspects of care into medical model
Role conflict	Occurs when role expectations are perceived to be mutually exclusive or contradictory	Role conflict between advanced practice registered nurses (APRNs) and other nurses and between APRNs and physicians
Role transition	A dynamic process of change over time as new roles are acquired	Changing from a staff nurse to an APRN role Advancing from a master's-prepared APRN to a doctor of nursing practice–prepared APRN
Role insufficiency	Feeling inadequate to meet role demands	New APRN graduates experiencing feelings of inadequacy due to increased workload expectations and documentation requirements of electronic health records Change from solo practice or clinic to hospital requirements through mergers and acquisitions
Role supplementation	Anticipatory socialization	Role-specific educational components in a graduate program (e.g., clinical preceptorship experience with an APRN or interviewing a practicing APRN)

Adapted from "Role Stress and Role Strain," by M. E. Hardy and W. L. Hardy, in M. E. Hardy and M. E. Conway (Eds.), *Role Theory: Perspectives for Health Professionals* (2nd ed., pp. 159–239), 1988, Appleton & Lange; and "Transitions: A Central Concept in Nursing," by K. L. Schumacher and A. I. Meleis, 1994, *Image: The Journal of Nursing Scholarship, 26,* 119–127.

more specialized. Another source of role incongruity is incompatibility among personal values, self-concept, and expected role behaviors. An APRN interested primarily in clinical practice may experience this incongruity if the position that they obtain requires performing administrative functions. An example comes from Banda's (1985) study of psychiatric liaison CNSs in acute care hospitals and community health agencies. She reported that they viewed consultation and teaching as their major functions, whereas research and administrative activities produced role incongruity.

Role Conflict

Role conflict develops when role expectations are perceived to be contradictory or mutually exclusive. APRNs may experience conflict with varying demands of their role as well as intraprofessional and interprofessional role conflict

Intraprofessional Role Conflict

APRNs experience intraprofessional role conflict for a variety of reasons. The historical development of APRN roles has been fraught with conflict and controversy in nursing education and nursing organizations, particularly for CNMs (Varney, 1987), NPs (Ford, 1982), and CRNAs (Gunn, 1991; see also Chapter 1). Relationships among these APRN groups and nursing as a discipline have improved markedly in recent years, but difficulties remain (Fawcett et al., 2004). The degree to which APRN roles demonstrate a holistic nursing orientation as opposed to a more disease-specific medical orientation remains problematic (Judge-Ellis & Wilson, 2017).

Communication difficulties that underlie intraprofessional role conflict occur in four major areas: (1) at an organizational level, (2) in educational programs, (3) in the literature, and (4) in direct clinical practice. Kimbro (1978) initially described these communication difficulties in reference to CNMs, but they are relevant for all APRN roles. The fact that CNSs, NPs, CNMs, and CRNAs each have specific organizations with different certification requirements, competencies, and curricula creates boundaries and sets up the need for formal lines of communication. Communication gaps occur in education when courses and textbooks are not shared among APRN programs, even when more than one specialty is offered in the same school. Specialty-specific journals are another formal communication barrier because APRNs may read primarily within their own specialty and not keep abreast of larger APRN issues. In clinical settings, some APRNs may be more concerned with providing direct clinical care to individual patients, whereas staff nurses and other APRNs may be more concerned with 24-hour coverage and smooth functioning of the unit or institution. These differences may set the stage for intraprofessional role conflict.

During the 1980s and 1990s, when there was more confusion about the delineation of roles and responsibilities between RNs and NPs, RNs would sometimes demonstrate resistance to NPs by refusing to take vital signs, obtain blood samples, or perform other support functions for patients of NPs (Brykczynski, 1999a), and these negative behaviors were not addressed by their supervisors. These behaviors are suggestive of horizontal violence (a form of hostility), which may be more common during nursing shortages (Thomas, 2003). Roberts (1983) first described horizontal violence among nurses as oppressed group behavior wherein nurses who were doubly oppressed as women and as nurses demonstrated hostility toward their own less powerful group, instead of toward the more powerful oppressors. Recognizing that intraprofessional conflict among nurses is similar to oppressed group behavior can be useful in the development of strategies to overcome these difficulties (Bartholomew, 2006; G. A. Farrell, 2001). According to Rounds (1997), horizontal violence is less common among NPs as a group than among RNs generally. Over the years, as the NP role has become more accepted by nurses, there appear to be fewer cases of these hostile passive-aggressive behaviors, often currently referred to as *bullying*, toward NPs. However, they have been reported in APRN transition literature (Heitz et al., 2004; Kelly & Mathews, 2001). Heath (2014) identified courage as a key factor to address bullying, including "courage to stand up to a bully in a nonthreatening manner and courage to speak up if bullying is witnessed or experienced" (p. 441). Commitment to a zero-tolerance policy is the most effective strategy to confront bullying (Edmonson & Zelonka, 2019; Sherman, 2021).

One way to address these issues would be to include APRN position descriptions in staff nurse orientation programs. Curry (1994) claimed that thorough orientation of staff nurses to the APRN role, including clear guidelines and policies regarding responsibility issues, is an important component of successful integration of NP practice in an emergency department setting; this is also applicable to other roles and settings. Another significant strategy for minimizing intraprofessional role conflict is for the new APRN, and APRN students, to spend time getting to know the nursing staff to establish rapport and learn as much as possible about the new setting from those who really know what is going on—the nurses. This action affirms the value and significance of nurses and nursing and sets up a positive atmosphere for collegiality and intraprofessional role cooperation and collaboration. In Kelly and Mathews's (2001) study of new NP graduates, such a strategy was exactly what new NPs regretted not having incorporated into their first positions.

Interprofessional Role Conflict

Conflicts between physicians and APRNs constitute the most common situations of interprofessional conflict. Major sources of conflict for physicians and APRNs are the perceived economic threat of competition, limited resources in clinical training sites, lack of experience working together, and the historical hierarchy. Clarifying professional roles can mitigate power struggles, facilitate the integration of new roles, and foster interprofessional collaboration (Brault et al., 2014). In their study, Blackwell & Faraci (2021) found both NPs and physicians use similar integrating styles to address conflict. The integrating conflict resolution approach highlights mutual respect and collaboration. Providing physicians and nurse practitioners with education and training related to conflict resolution would be beneficial and enhance collaboration (Blackwell & Faraci, 2021). The relationship between anesthesiologists and CRNAs is an exemplar of ongoing conflict and clearly depicts interprofessional role conflict between physicians and APRNs (Exemplar 4.1).

One way to promote positive interprofessional relationships is to provide education and practice experiences that include APRN students, medical students, and both physician and APRN faculty to enhance mutual understanding of both professional roles (Trotter et al., 2019). Developing such interprofessional educational experiences is difficult because of different professional standards, academic calendars, and clinical schedules. However, these obstacles can be overcome if these interdisciplinary activities are considered essential for improved healthcare delivery and if they have sufficient administrative support (Wynia et al., 2012). Recent examples of successful interprofessional education (IPE) include CRNA and physical therapy students' anatomy review course (Williams et al., 2018); nursing, pharmacy, and medical students' simulation-based IPE scenario using a telehealth robot (Scott et al., 2020); and perinatal IPE simulation with varied APRN students, physician assistant students, obstetrics–gynecology residents, and accelerated BSN students (Trotter et al., 2019).

The issues of professional territoriality and physician concern about being replaced by advanced practice nurses were reported by Lindblad et al. (2010) from an ethnographic study of the first four graduates in 2005 from the first CNS program in Sweden. The CNSs and general practitioners agreed that the usefulness of the CNSs would have been greater if they had been able to prescribe medications and order treatments. After working with the CNSs, the general practitioners saw them more as an additional resource and complement rather than a threat. By 2009, there were 16 CNSs working in the new role in primary health care. The numbers of advanced practice nurses have increased gradually in Sweden. A study by Altersved et al. (2011) indicated that the CNS is recognized as a resource to increase accessibility to more holistic primary care; however, the barriers of limited autonomy and lack of prescriptive authority need to be addressed to further role development.

The complementary nature of advanced practice nursing to medical care is a foreign concept for some physicians, who view all health care as an extension of medical care and see APRNs simply as physician extenders. This misunderstanding of advanced practice nursing underlies physicians' opposition to independent roles for nurses because they believe that APRNs want to practice medicine without a license (see Chapters 1 and 3). In fact, numerous earlier studies of APRN practice have demonstrated that advanced practice roles incorporate a holistic approach that blends elements of nursing and medicine (S. J. Brown, 1992; Brykczynski, 1999a, 1999b; Fiandt, 2002; Grando, 1998; Johnson, 1993). However, when APRNs are viewed by physicians as direct competitors, it is understandable that some physicians would be reluctant to be involved in assisting with APRN education (National Commission on Nurse Anesthesia Education, 1990). In addition, some nurse educators have believed that physicians should not be involved in teaching or acting as preceptors for APRNs. Improved relationships between APRNs and physicians will require redefinition of the situation by both groups.

EXEMPLAR 4.1

INTERPROFESSIONAL ROLE CONFLICT: THE CASE OF CERTIFIED REGISTERED NURSE ANESTHETISTS AND ANESTHESIOLOGISTS

Certified registered nurse anesthetists (CRNAs) are advanced practice registered nurses who administer more than 45 million anesthetics to patients each year (American Association of Nurse Anesthesiology [AANA], 2020). For many years, nurse anesthetists have provided high-quality anesthesia care in a variety of settings. They are the primary anesthesia providers in rural US hospitals, as noted on the AANA website (www.aana.com). According to the AANA (2019), more than 49,000 CRNAs provide quality anesthesia care to more than 65% of all patients undergoing surgical or other medical interventions that necessitate the services of an anesthetist (see Chapter 16). The fact that nurse anesthetists predated the first physician anesthesiologists by many years (see Chapter 1) may partly explain why the relationship between anesthesiologists and CRNAs has historically been interpreted by anesthesiologists as one of direct competition, thus creating an adversarial stance. Over the years, this relationship might be characterized as a cold war with overt offensives mounted periodically by anesthesiologists.

In 1970, CRNAs outnumbered anesthesiologists by a ratio of 1.5:1. By 2000, anesthesiologists outnumbered CRNAs (Blumenreich, 2000). Currently there are an equal number of practicing CRNAs and anesthesiologists and approximately 1300 anesthesia assistants actively practicing in the United States (AANA, 2019). Twenty-seven states currently allow CRNAs to practice independently. The thrust toward independent practice continues to gain momentum. CRNAs will soon outnumber anesthesiologists in the next few years as current students graduate and enter the workforce. This is one of the factors underlying conflicts over CRNA autonomy (see the AANA website, www.aana.com, for updates on this issue). Another factor is the decision made by the Centers for Medicare and Medicaid Services, after study of the available evidence in 1997, to reimburse nurse anesthetists directly under Medicare (Kleinpell, 2001).

In response, The American Society of Anesthesiologists and the American Medical Association launched a major campaign against CRNA autonomy in the operating room, claiming that supervision of CRNAs by physicians is essential for public safety (Kleinpell, 2001; Stein, 2000). Despite the very active political action committee of the American Nurses Association, the struggle with physicians over limiting the scope of practice of CRNAs is ongoing and reflects the experiences of other advanced practice nurse groups as well. An example of this continuing struggle is the Scope of Practice Partnership (SOPP), a coalition formed by the American Medical Association with other physician organizations to mount initiatives to limit the scope of practice of nonphysician clinicians (Waters, 2007). SOPP funds investigations into the educational preparation and licensure requirements of healthcare providers with the goal of opposing autonomous practice. SOPP targets all nonphysician providers (Lindeke & Thomas, 2010).

A current issue of role delineation and conflict is anesthesiologists' efforts to categorize CRNAs and anesthesiologist assistants (AAs) on the same level as mid-level clinicians. Both are "nonphysician anesthetists"; however, the fundamental difference is that an AA works under the direct supervision of the physician and is trained using the medical model of education. The relationship between nonphysician anesthesia providers mimics the adversarial relationship that previously existed between physician assistants and nurse practitioners. Collegial relationships among the nonphysician providers may be more beneficial for both groups. The American Academy of Anesthesiologist Assistants (2019) website identifies 10 accredited programs for AAs in the United States and 1800 practicing AAs. There are 121 accredited CRNA programs in the United States and 92 nurse anesthesia programs approved for the entry-level degree of doctorate in nursing practice (AANA, 2019). CRNAs are currently educated at the master of science in nursing level; however, by 2025, all CRNAs will be required to have a doctorate for entry into practice (AANA, 2007). Thus the CRNA is achieving what nursing has been struggling with for the past few decades. The quality of care and patient safety provided by the CRNA has been well documented in peer-reviewed journals (AANA, 2019). Yet physicians continue to verbalize the need for supervision, citing patient safety and ignoring the evidence. Role acceptance is an ongoing issue for all APRNs. Progress is being made, but active participation and a strong voice are still needed to facilitate the much-needed change.

The advocacy of the Interprofessional Education Collaborative Expert Panel (2016) for an interprofessional vision for all health professionals and the recommendation by the Institute of Medicine (2003) that the health professional workforce be prepared to work in interdisciplinary teams underscore the imperative of interprofessional collaboration (see Chapter 10). Competency in interprofessional collaboration is critical for APRNs because it is central to APRN practice (K. Farrell et al., 2015). This content is incorporated into the leadership and interprofessional partnership components of the AACN (2021), *The Essentials: Core Competencies for Professional Nursing Education*.

Some interesting research has emerged on this issue in Canada and Europe. A participatory action research study conducted in British Columbia, Canada, indicated that NPs viewed collaboration as both a philosophy and a practice: "They cultivated collaborative relations with clients, colleagues, and healthcare leaders to address concerns of role autonomy and role clarity, extend holistic client-centered care and team capacity, and create strategic alliances to promote innovation and system change" (Burgess & Purkis, 2010, p. 300). Of particular importance is the fact that the NP participants described themselves as being nurses first and practitioners second. This is significant because when role emphasis is on physician replacement and support rather than on the patient-centered, health-focused, holistic nursing orientation to practice, the nursing components of the role become less valued and invisible (Bryant-Lukosius et al., 2004). Medically driven and illness-oriented health systems tend to devalue these value-added components of APRN roles, and reimbursement mechanisms for including these aspects of care are lacking.

Fleming and Carberry (2011) reported on a grounded theory study of expert critical care nurses transitioning to advanced practice in an intensive care unit setting in Scotland. Initial perceptions were that the advanced practice nursing role was closely aligned with medical practice, but later perceptions supported earlier studies that the advanced practice nursing role was characterized by an integrated, holistic, patient-centered approach to care, which was close to the medical model but different because it was carried out within an expert nursing knowledge base. The authors determined that further research is needed to explore the outcomes of this integrated practice. This is the research imperative for advanced practice nursing—to demonstrate the impact of the holistic nursing approach to care on patient outcomes.

Nurse-midwives have been in the forefront of developing collaborative relationships with physicians for many years. All APRN groups would benefit from attention to the progress that CNMs have made in collaboration with physicians. The joint practice statement of the American College of Obstetricians and Gynecologists (ACOG) and the American College of Nurse-Midwives (ACNM, 2011) has served as a model for other APRN groups. It highlights key principles for improving communication, working relationships, and seamlessness in the provision of women's health services. ACNM and ACOG released an updated joint practice statement that builds on the previous document by clarifying the meaning of team-based care, improving the definition of collaboration, stating a shared commitment to ensuring access to appropriate levels of care for all women, and expanding the workforces of both groups (ACNM, 2018).

ROLE TRANSITIONS

Role transitions are defined here as dynamic processes of change that occur over time as new roles are acquired (see Table 4.1). The middle-range transitions theory of Meleis et al. (2000) has been widely used in both undergraduate and graduate education. It can be helpful for understanding and addressing the situational transitions associated with APRN role development and has been the framework for APRN research (Barnes, 2015; Dillon et al., 2016; Tracy, 2017). Five essential factors influence role transitions (Schumacher & Meleis, 1994): (1) personal meaning of the transition, which relates to the degree of identity crisis experienced; (2) degree of planning, which involves the time and energy devoted to anticipating the change; (3) environmental barriers and supports, which refer to family, peer, school, and other components; (4) level of knowledge and skill, which relates to prior experience and school experiences; and (5) expectations, which are related to such factors as role models, literature, and media. The role strain experienced by individuals in response to role insufficiency (see Table 4.1 for definitions) that accompanies the transition to APRN roles can be minimized, although certainly not completely prevented, by individualized assessment of these five essential factors, development of strategies to cope with them, and rehearsal of situations designed for application of these strategies. Entering graduate school may be associated with a ripple effect of concurrent role transitions in family, work, and other social arenas (Klaich, 1990).

Advanced Practice Nurse Role Acquisition in Graduate School

The personal meaning of role transitions has been a major focus of APRN role development literature over the years, with alterations in self-identity and self-concept emerging as a consistent theme and role acquisition experiences sometimes described as identity crises (Roberts et al., 1997). Studies of APRN role acquisition in school are outlined in Table 4.2.

In their study of NP students, Roberts et al. (1997) reported findings similar to those observed decades earlier by E. M. Anderson et al. (1974). The description by E. M. Anderson et al. of NP students' progression from dependence to interdependence being accompanied by regression, anxiety, and conflict was found to be similar to observations made by Roberts et al. (1997) in graduate NP students over a period of 6 years (see Table 4.2). For many years, we (the authors) and our NP faculty colleagues have observed similar role transition processes in teaching role and clinical courses for graduate NP students. In a discussion of role transition experiences for neonatal NPs (NNPs), Cusson and Viggiano (2002) made the important point that even positive transitions are stressful.

Roberts et al. (1997) identified three major areas of transition as students progressed from dependence to interdependence: (1) development of professional competence, (2) change in role identity, and (3) evolving relationships with preceptors and faculty. The lowest level of competence coincided with the highest level of role confusion. This occurred at the end of the first semester and the beginning of the second semester in the three-semester program examined. Roberts et al. observed that the most intense transition period typically occurred at the end of the students' first clinical immersion experience.

Developing Competence

Roberts et al. (1997) described the first transition as involving an initial feeling of loss of confidence and competence accompanied by anxiety. Initial clinical experiences were associated with the desire to observe rather than provide care, the inability to recall simple facts, the omission of essential data from history taking, feelings of awkwardness with patients, and difficulty prioritizing data. The students' focus at this time was almost exclusively on acquiring and refining assessment skills and continued development of physical examination techniques. By the end of the first semester, students reported returning feelings of confidence and the regaining of their former competence in interpersonal skills. Although they were still tentative about diagnostic and treatment decisions, students reported feeling more comfortable with patients as some of their basic nursing abilities began to return.

Role Identity Transitions

Transitions in nursing role identity occurring during the first two stages were associated with feelings of role confusion. Students were dismayed at how slowly and inefficiently they were performing in clinical situations and reported feelings of self-doubt and lack of confidence in their abilities to function in the real world of health care. They sought shortcuts in attempts to increase their efficiency. They reported profound feelings of responsibility regarding diagnostic and treatment decisions and, at the same time, increasingly realized the limitations of clinical practice when they were confronted with the real-life situations of their patients. They recalled finding it easy to second-guess physicians' decisions in their previous nursing roles, but now they found those decisions more problematic when they were responsible for making them. This is the point that Cusson and Viggiano (2002) were making when they commented, in reference to NNPs, that the infant really does look different when viewed from the head of the bed rather than the side of the bed. They explained that

> *rather than taking orders, as they did as staff nurses, neonatal NPs must synthesize incredibly complex information and decide on a plan of action. Experienced neonatal nurses often guide house staff regarding care decisions and writing orders to match the care that is being given. However, the shift in responsibility to actually writing the orders can be very intimidating.*
>
> ***(Cusson & Viggiano, 2002, p. 24)***

Roberts et al. (1997) observed that a blending of the APRN student and the former nurse developed during stage II of the transition process as students renewed their appreciation for their previous interpersonal skills as teachers, supporters, and collaborators and again perceived their patients as unique individuals in the context of their life situations. Students developed increased awareness of the uncertainty involved in the process of making definitive diagnostic and treatment decisions. Despite current attempts to reduce diagnostic and

TABLE 4.2

APRN Student Role Transition Studies in School: Role Acquisition[a]

Researchers	Method	Participants	Noteworthy Findings
E. M. Anderson et al. (1974)	Descriptive observational study	NP students in a graduate program, a postbaccalaureate certificate program, and a continuing education program University of Minnesota	Four-stage process of NP role development: Complete dependence Developing competence Independence Interdependence
Roberts et al. (1997)	Descriptive study of observations of students and written clinical journals	100 NP students over 6 years University of Massachusetts	Four-stage transition process identified by E. M. Anderson et al. (1974) was validated in this study
Steiner et al. (2008)	Descriptive correlational questionnaire	208 FNP graduates Wyoming and Idaho	Follow-up to Heitz et al.'s (2004) study to validate educational phase findings Preceptor guidance was found to be a greater positive force than faculty guidance
Spoelstra and Robbins (2010)	Descriptive qualitative thematic analysis	24 MSN students in first semester role course Michigan	Overarching theme: the essence of nursing Three subthemes: Importance of building a framework for advanced nursing practice Importance of direct care Importance of professional leadership supported by ethical values
Fleming and Carberry (2011)	Grounded theory	Two cohorts: five critical care nurse advanced practice trainees in first cohort, four in second cohort Intensive care units Scotland	Transition occurred in four areas: Finding a niche Coping with pressures Feeling competent Internalizing the role
Ares (2014)	Online survey descriptive correlational design Nurse Self-Description form (NSDF) Nurses Professional Values Scale-Revised (NPVS-R)	225 CNS students near graduation and new graduates prior to employment from 73 CNS programs	Students found to have strong CNS self-concept and reported feeling prepared to practice in CNS role Faculty, preceptors, and mentors facilitated role socialization
Tracy (2015)	Qualitative pilot study; three focus groups	17 CRNA students: 12 in second year of didactic course work, 5 in fifth month of full-time residency training	Factors found to positively influence student CRNA role transition were the following: Preceptor guidance and support Mentoring by faculty and peers Both self- and group reflection Variety of training experiences Working with CRNAs in various practice settings

[a]Studies are listed in chronologic order.

CNS, Clinical nurse specialist; *CRNA,* certified registered nurse anesthetist; *FNP,* family nurse practitioner; *MSN,* master of science in nursing; *NP,* nurse practitioner.

treatment uncertainty through evidence-based practice, a basic degree of uncertainty is still inherent in clinical practice. Although these insights served to demystify the clinical diagnostic process, the students' anxiety about providing care increased. Learning about strategies to cope with clinical decision making in situations of uncertainty, such as ruling out the worst-case scenario, seeking consultation, and monitoring patients closely with phone calls and follow-up visits, can decrease anxiety and promote increased confidence (Brykczynski, 1991).

Evolving Relationships

The transition in the relationships between students and preceptors and students and faculty in the study by Roberts et al. (1997) involved students feeling anxious that they were not learning enough and would never know enough to practice competently. Students felt frustrated and perceived that faculty and preceptors were not providing them with all the information they needed. During the third stage, as they felt more confident and competent, students began to question the clinical judgments of their preceptors and faculty. This process is thought to help students advance from independence to interdependence—the last stage of the transition process. Much of the conflict at this juncture appeared to derive from students' feelings of "ambivalence about giving up dependence on external authorities" (Roberts et al., 1997, p. 71) such as preceptors and faculty and assuming responsibility for making independent judgments based on their own assessments from their clinical and educational experiences and the literature.

Fleming and Carberry's (2011) qualitative study of critical care nurse advanced practice trainees in Scotland provides confirmation of the experiences described here. They noted the trainees' feelings of inadequacy associated with moving from expert to novice and their anxiety and frustration over dealing with the role ambiguity of moving into a hybrid nursing and medical role. After a 12-month period, the trainees found their role "characterized by an integrated holistic patient-centered approach to care" (Fleming & Carberry, 2011, p. 74).

Influence of Prior Nursing Experience

Until recently, the literature on APRN role acquisition in school has focused exclusively on individuals who were already nurses. A commonly held assumption among nurses is "the more clinical experience, the better" for acquiring the necessary knowledge and skill to take on complex APRN roles. At least 1 year of nursing practice is typically preferred for admission to APRN programs. The process of role acquisition for students in direct-entry APRN master's programs that admit non-nurse college graduates may differ because these individuals were not functioning as nurses before they entered the program. For additional information regarding this topic, the reader is referred to the qualitative study reported by Rich and Rodriguez (2002). In their qualitative study of family nurse practitioner (FNP) role transition, Heitz et al. (2004) found differences in role acquisition experiences between FNP students who were inexperienced nurses and FNP students who were experienced nurses. Feelings of insecurity, inadequacy, vulnerability, and being overwhelmed were typical, but role confusion was reported primarily by the more experienced RN students as they went through the process of letting go of the RN role and taking on the FNP role. It will be interesting to observe whether this finding holds true for students transitioning directly from the bachelor of science in nursing to the DNP.

Strategies to Facilitate Role Acquisition

The anticipatory socialization to APRN roles that occurs in graduate education is analogous to a process that Kramer (1974) described for undergraduate RNs called *immunization*. This same process is referred to as *role supplementation in transitions theory* (Schumacher & Meleis, 1994). The overall objective is to expose students to as many real-life experiences as possible during the educational program to minimize reality shock and role insufficiency on graduation and initial role implementation. Role content can be incorporated into APRN curricula in a variety of ways, including (1) in the overall framework for designing an APRN curriculum, (2) in a specific role course (see, e.g., Spoelstra & Robbins, 2010), (3) as part of specific assignments, and (4) in role seminars that span an entire curriculum. Hamric and Hanson (2003) asserted that it is an ethical mandate for all APRN educators, regardless of specialty, to provide graduates with up-to-date knowledge of professional role and regulatory issues in addition to concentration on clinical competence. The importance of explicit role preparation for the complex and challenging roles of graduates of DNP programs is recognized in the curriculum proposed by the AACN (2006). The reenvisioned *Essentials: Core Competencies for Professional Nursing Education* addresses eight concepts central to professional nursing practice that will serve to bridge the gap between education and practice (AACN, 2021). If there is not a separate APRN role course, careful attention must be paid to this curriculum component so that it does not become integrated out of existence.

Specific strategies for facilitating role acquisition can be categorized according to three major purposes: (1) role rehearsal; (2) development of clinical knowledge and skills, including strategies for dealing with uncertainty; and (3) creation of a supportive network (see Table 4.3). Rites of passage can be useful for signifying advancement to a new level of practice and set the stage for role rehearsal. The Willow Ceremony is a rite of passage developed at the University of Wyoming to commemorate beginning an APRN program (Burman et al., 2007). The willow is a metaphor for APRNs being strong and well grounded in nursing with many roots, yet flexible. In 2012 when University of Texas Medical Branch School of Nursing in Galveston, Texas, inaugurated its DNP program, the faculty adapted the Willow Ceremony to distinguish the DNP program from the master's-level NP programs. Goal statements from students' admission essays were used in the formal ceremony and students found it very meaningful. The ceremony has been conducted annually except for the years impacted by a major hurricane and the pandemic.

Role Rehearsal

For adequate role rehearsal, APRN students should experience all aspects of the core competencies (Ares, 2014; see also Chapter 3) directly while faculty and fellow students are available to help them process or debrief these experiences. Faculty can help students by identifying periods of high role acquisition stress in their particular program so that support can be built in during those periods. APRN students should be cautioned that other nurses, physicians, other providers, and administrators in the work setting may value only clinical expertise and not the other core competencies. Strategies for enhancing understanding of how the core competencies are embedded in each APRN role include preparation of short-term and long-term goals to use as guides in the development of professional portfolios, analysis of existing position descriptions, and development of the ideal position description. These are also helpful for guiding students in their search for an initial APRN position.

Clinical Knowledge Development

The development of clinical knowledge and skills for APRN role acquisition can be promoted by planning for realistic clinical experiences with the support of faculty and preceptors nearby. Steiner et al. (2008) pointed out the importance of teaching students how to learn and how to use resources to find out what they need to know. Emphasis on realism and a holistic situational perspective are important in clinical experiences for helping students understand that the complex clinical judgments involved in APRN assessment and management of patient situations over time are not simply technical medical knowledge but a hybrid of nursing and medical knowledge and experience. Teaching and learning experiences for all of the APRN role components should integrate elements of research and theory and be incorporated into specialty APRN courses to build on the knowledge gained in the traditional graduate core and clinical support courses in the curriculum. APRN students and new graduates can benefit from familiarity with role transition processes by not expecting to be able to demonstrate all APRN role components fully and expertly immediately on graduation.

Clinical mentoring by preceptors is an important component of ensuring realistic clinical learning experiences and socialization into advanced practice nursing roles (AACN, 2015b; Burns et al., 2006; Donley et al., 2014; Tracy, 2015). APRN student enrollment has increased markedly in the face of APRN faculty shortages, and APRN students enter clinical training experiences across the curriculum with varied skill levels (AACN, 2015b). Identifying qualified and available preceptors is challenging and time consuming for faculty and support staff (Multidiscipline Clerkship/Clinical Training Site Survey, 2014). Students are matched with qualified APRN and non-nurse preceptors to provide learning opportunities, ensure development of required clinical skills, and foster the team concept. Course objectives, the advanced practice essentials (whether master's or doctoral), core competencies

TABLE 4.3

Strategies to Promote APRN Role Acquisition in School

Purpose	Strategies	Implementation
Role rehearsal	Rite of passage	Ceremony to signify moving into development of a new role
	Role course	Provide overall framework for APRN role development and begin anticipatory guidance role development thread for entire program
	Directly experience all core skills	Faculty and students monitor experience in all core competencies
	Create professional marketing portfolio	Prepare an electronic portfolio containing, for example: philosophy of care, résumé, clinical experiences, ideal position description, salary data, certification details, and APRN brochures
	Lifelike role negotiation seminar	Invite interprofessional guests
	Identify with a role model or mentor	Develop mentee relationship with an APRN and maintain contact throughout the APRN program
	Burning question interviews	Develop a list of important questions to ask APRNs relevant to future role satisfaction
	Panel discussions	Faculty and students can plan discussion with various panels to increase understanding of issues such as potential positions available, practice settings, and other health team members
	Critical incident presentations	Prepare an in-depth self-evaluation of a role conflict situation experienced in learning the APRN role and share this with peers and faculty
	Interprofessional educational experiences	Shared courses in, for example, assessment, pharmacology, ethical and legal issues, and service learning experiences
Develop clinical knowledge and skills	Realistic clinical immersion experiences	Clinical experiences need to reflect the real world of practice as much as possible
	Clinical conferences	Discussion of clinical experiences with faculty and peers promotes clinical understanding
	Clinical situation narrative seminars	Share full contextual details of situations to promote understanding of aspects of embedded clinical practice knowledge
	Case study analysis	Clinical examples make classroom learning more concrete and memorable
	Clinical logs	Maintain an electronic log of all patients seen, with pertinent details such as age, diagnosis, interventions, and outcomes
	Final clinical preceptorships	A final semester of clinical practice helps put it all together
	Faculty practice	Maintenance of faculty clinical competence enhances the credibility of APRN faculty
Create a support network	Establish a peer support system	Join local, state, and national APRN groups
	Share self- and peer evaluations	Learn to be comfortable with giving and receiving feedback for improvement
	Faculty-student-preceptor social functions	Foster an APRN-supportive environment among faculty, clinicians, students, staff, and administrators
	Establish a pattern for continuing education	Subscribe to selected APRN journals, participate in APRN conferences, and keep a record of continuing education hours
	Create a virtual community	Establish electronic mail, social media, and Internet connections
	Establish a self-monitoring system	Select a framework for self-evaluating role performance to keep track of progress in role transition over time
	Form a self-care program	Develop healthcare practices to maintain and improve health, such as stress management and getting adequate sleep, rest, exercise, and a nutritious diet

Adapted from "Chart 1-6: Strategies to Promote NP Role Acquisition in School," by K. A. Brykczynski (2000). Chart 1.6 p 61. In P. Meredith & N. M. Horan (Eds.), *Adult Primary Care* (p. 16)., Philadelphia: WB Saunders.

for the specific APRN role, and a preceptor learning agreement provide the basic structure and overall direction for faculty, preceptors, and students. Clinical faculty are responsible for conducting site visits and convening clinical conferences to evaluate learning. APRN course faculty are responsible for student, clinical faculty, preceptor, and clinical site evaluation and overall maintenance of high-quality educational standards. APRN students are linked with preceptors for one-on-one guidance in developing clinical skills and judgment. This apprenticeship model of education is time intensive and costly (AACN, 2015b).

All of these challenges require APRN educational programs to explore new and alternative models for providing clinical training, including increased use of low- and high-fidelity simulation to support clinical experiences and to evaluate students, and increased attention to interprofessional practice (AACN, 2015b). In 2012 the Centers for Medicare and Medicaid Services (CMS) launched the Graduate Nurse Education (GNE) Demonstration project, a 5-year project designed to increase training opportunities for APRN students as a way to increase primary care providers. The CMS provided reimbursement for eligible hospitals to participate in the demonstration project in five major cities (Hospital of the University of Pennsylvania, Philadelphia, PA; Duke University Hospital, Durham, NC; Scottsdale Healthcare Medical Center, Scottsdale, AZ; Rush University Medical Center, Chicago, IL; and Memorial Hermann-Texas Medical Center Hospital, Houston, TX). The hospitals partnered with accredited advanced practice nursing programs and reimbursed preceptors for training NP students (American Association of Nurse Practitioners [AANP], 2012). Incentivizing community preceptors with educational opportunities, documentation of preceptor hours for recertification, and library access may motivate participation in the student-preceptor collaborative relationships (AACN, 2015b; Donley et al., 2014). The GNE project was a success as APRN enrollment grew in the demonstration project schools (University of Pennsylvania, 2017). Collaboration between schools of nursing and healthcare agencies in developing more formal systems of rewards and benefits that facilitate professional development and career mobility for preceptors is imperative for enhancing their recruitment and retention (AACN, 2015a; Donley et al., 2014).

In 2020, with the onset of COVID 19, social distancing, and masking, telehealth, and telemedicine rapidly expanded to allow providers to maintain consistent contact with their patients. NP students are introduced to telehealth and take advantage of the extended reach provided using a virtual technological platform. Telehealth offers an opportunity to reduce health disparity in areas with limited provider coverage. Not only does telehealth aid in communication with patients and reduce travel expense but it can also reduce referrals. Providers can more readily consult specialists to discuss treatment options. Telehealth visits offer real time face-to-face communication, data collection, and review of diagnostic testing all through a virtual platform (Mechanic et al., 2020).

Finally, and perhaps most important, an overall strategy for enhancing APRN clinical knowledge and skill is for faculty to maintain competency in clinical practice. Clinical competency enhances the faculty's ability to evaluate students clinically, discuss clinically relevant examples in classes, serve as preceptors for students, and evaluate the care provided in clinical preceptorship sites. The clinical competence of faculty is important to prevent a wide gap between education and practice, enhance faculty credibility, and foster realistic expectations for new APRN graduates.

Developing a Supportive Network

Establishing a peer support system, planning social functions with faculty and preceptors, and creating a virtual community can facilitate the development of a support network. The importance of forming a support network was emphasized by study findings (Kelly & Mathews, 2001; Kleinpell-Nowell, 2001). Computer literacy is critical for networking and access to the high-quality materials available on websites, in literature searches, and on smartphones. Students need expanded informatics skills and understanding of emerging technologies, including genetics and genomics, less-invasive diagnostic tools and treatments, three dimensional printing, robotics, biometrics, electronic health records, computerized provider order entry, and clinical decision support, to enhance their ability to practice (Huston, 2013). Neurocognitive theory provides evidence-based approaches to improving learning incorporating a wide variety of multimedia tools. Instructional design has added visual comprehension through videos, simulation, and interactive programs (O. R. Anderson et al., 2014).

The establishment of a system for self-directed learning activities during the first few years after program completion forms the basis for maintaining competence throughout one's career (Gunn, 1998). The formation of a process for lifelong learning should be initiated during the APRN educational program as students create a computer-based self-monitoring system that includes clinical and role transition experiences over time to serve as a reality check or timetable. On graduation, continuing education program attendance could be incorporated into this monitoring system to facilitate compilation of necessary documentation for certification, along with ongoing self-evaluation and role development. This information can be incorporated into students' online portfolios to centralize all career materials in one place (Green et al., 2014).

Students need to be encouraged to develop and maintain self-care practices during their stressful educational experiences that they can continue when they move into the challenges of the practice arena. Faculty can serve as role models for healthy lifestyles and incorporate analysis of self-care practices into assignments to aid students in developing improved well-being. Students invariably develop renewed appreciation from these self-care assignments for how difficult it is to change health habits, and they can share knowledge they gain from these learning experiences with peers and patients.

Advanced Practice Nursing Role Implementation: Entering the Workforce

After successfully emerging from the APRN educational process, new APRN graduates face yet another transition, from the student role to the professional APRN role, referred to as *role implementation* in this text (see Fig. 4.1). APRN graduates can experience attitudinal, behavioral, and value conflicts as they move from the academic world, in which holistic care is highly valued, to the work world, in which organizational efficiency is paramount. The process of APRN role implementation is another situational transition (Schumacher & Meleis, 1994) that is described here as a progressive movement through three or four phases or stages. In the APRN role development literature the term *phase* is used by some and the term *stage* is used by others (Poronsky, 2013). One term is often favored over another in different fields; for example, in pharmacology, drug trials are referred to in different *phases*, whereas in human development the term *stage* is preferred. For the discussion here, the terms *phase* and *stage* are used as cited in the different studies (see Table 4.4).

TABLE 4.4

APRN Role Transition Studies in Practice: Role Implementation[a]

Researchers	Method	Participants	Noteworthy Findings
Baker (1979)	Retrospective interviews	4 CNSs California	Four-phase role development: Orientation Frustration Implementation Reassessment
Hamric and Taylor (1989)	Questionnaire	100 CNSs US national	Seven-phase role development: Orientation Frustration Implementation Integration Frozen Reorganization Complacent

TABLE 4.4

APRN Role Transition Studies in Practice: Role Implementation—cont'd

Researchers	Method	Participants	Noteworthy Findings
M. A. Brown and Olshansky (1997)	One-year longitudinal grounded theory	35 FNPs first year in practice Washington	Four-stage transition: Laying the foundation Launching Meeting the challenge Broadening the perspective
Kelly and Mathews (2001)	Focus group	21 recent NP graduates Illinois	Lack of control over workload Lack of support from nurses and physicians Loss of previous relationships Role ambiguity Difficulty incorporating holistic care and health promotion Personal satisfaction, increased confidence and autonomy Network of supportive peers helpful for coping with demands
Heitz et al. (2004)	Grounded theory Telephone interviews	9 recent FNP graduates Western United States	Role transition occurs in two phases Phase 1 occurs in graduate school Faculty guidance was found to be a dominant force Greater role confusion was experienced by students with more RN experience prior to entering the program Phase 2 occurs in practice over a 6-month to 2-year period following graduation
Chang et al. (2006)	Qualitative inquiry	10 acute care NPs during first year of practice Taiwan	Findings similar to M. A. Brown and Olshansky's (1997) study However, only three phases were described as follows: Role ambiguity—similar to laying the foundation Role acquisition—similar to launching Role implementation—covers both meeting the challenge and broadening the perspective
Gardner et al. (2007)	Secondary analysis of qualitative interview data Capability was theoretical framework	15 NPs practicing in Australia and New Zealand Duration of NP practice ranged from 3 months to 3 years	Findings indicating attributes of capability evident in NP practice include the following: Knowing how to learn Works well with others Creative High level of self-efficacy
Gould and Wasylkiw (2007)	Qualitative interviews	7 NPs rural New Brunswick, Canada Most 2 years in practice, one 7 years in practice, and one 25 years in practice	Main themes: Holistic nursing philosophy differs from traditional medicine Barriers to new role Need to describe role to patients Varying support from physicians System issue—salary position preferable to fee for service for NP to have more time Pioneering outlook optimistic about new dimension of health care for future

Continued

TABLE 4.4

APRN Role Transition Studies in Practice: Role Implementation—cont'd

Researchers	Method	Participants	Noteworthy Findings
Cusson and Strange (2008)	Descriptive qualitative survey questionnaire	70 NNPs from 1–28 years in NNP practice; mean 13.9 years 21 US states	Major themes described as follows: Ambivalence re: adequacy of preparation for role Transition to NNP role described as difficult, uncomfortable, and stressful Making it as a real NNP—1 year was a consistent benchmark Helpers—support of neonatologists, staff nurses, and unit managers Hinderers—poor professional behavior of some staff nurses and other NNPs
Sullivan-Bentz et al. (2010)	Descriptive qualitative focused ethnography Narrative analysis	23 recent NP graduates during first year of practice 21 coparticipants (physicians and NPs) Ontario, Canada	M. A. Brown & Olshansky's (1997) four-stage transition model formed the conceptual framework for the study Findings from this study reflected many of the findings from the earlier study. By the end of the first year, NPs transitioned from feeling overwhelmed to feeling confident in their new role
Glasgow and Zoucha (2011)	Descriptive and interpretive phenomenology	9 DNP graduates: 3 faculty, 4 practice, 1 dual faculty and practice, 1 executive position Pennsylvania and New Jersey	Shared themes: Changing context of DNP practice: uncertainty, misunderstanding, tension Feelings of confidence and empowerment in making decisions more autonomously Finding one's way and responding to opportunity
Llahana and Hamric (2011)	Questionnaire based on Hamric and Taylor's (1989) questionnaire	334 DSNs nationwide in UK	Validated experience of all 7 role development phases from Hamric and Taylor's (1989) study by at least one DSN An eighth phase, transition, was identified for experienced DSNs who moved from one practice setting to another after having moved through the implementation and integration phases
Desborough (2012)	Grounded theory	7 NPs in interviews; 5 of these in focus group Australia	Five major themes: Developing clinical practice guidelines Collaborating with the multidisciplinary team Developing legitimacy and clinical credibility Communicating Transitioning to practice
Jones et al. (2015)	Qualitative 2 focus groups and 13 individual interviews	23 NP graduates from ANP, GNP, FNP, and WHCNP programs in Western United States Majority in practice more than 1 year	Four domains of NP graduate experiences and concerns: Getting boots on Older people are more complex Very different as a provider NP has scope of practice; PA a job description

TABLE 4.4

APRN Role Transition Studies in Practice: Role Implementation—cont'd

Researchers	Method	Participants	Noteworthy Findings
Barnes (2015)	Descriptive cross-sectional survey questionnaire NP Role Transition Scale (NPRTS)	352 NPs at National NP conference in United States 6 months to 23 years in practice, mean 7.7 years	Formal orientation was significantly associated with successful NP role transition Prior RN experience neither promoted nor inhibited NP role transition Factor analysis showed three dimensions explaining NP role transition: Developing comfort and building confidence Understanding of NP role by others Collegial support
Dillon et al. (2016)	Descriptive correlational comparative design pilot study Casey Fink Graduate NP Experience Survey	34 acute care NPs with 6 months to 3 years in practice 75% had >5 years prior ICU/ED experience Most had orientation 8 weeks or less 25% no orientation	No significant differences were found in successful role transition and retention of NPs with 0–4 years' prior ICU/ED nursing experience versus more than 4 years Organizational support, communication, and leadership were most important elements influencing successful transition into ACNP role High turnover: 52% left their first NP position in <2 years
Faraz (2017)	Descriptive cross-sectional study using an online survey Instruments: Social Support Questionnaire, Role Ambiguity Scale, Confidence Scale, Misener NP Job Satisfaction Scale, Anticipated Turnover Scale	177 NPs national US practicing in primary care setting from 3 to 12 months	Professional autonomy and role ambiguity were the variables most predictive of turnover intention Ways to provide support for sufficient autonomy among NPs with minimal experience need to be developed to promote job satisfaction and retention
Tracy (2017)	Qualitative descriptive phenomenographic design using online recruitment and interviewing Transition theory was theoretical framework	15 CRNAs began practice during last 4 years Midwestern United States	Factors promoting CRNA role transition were identified as follows: Mastery of self-efficacy and confidence Expert mentoring and guidance Supportive work environment Peer support Previous experience in work setting as a student CRNA Factors impeding CRNA role transition were identified as follows: Practice limitations Lack of orientation and preceptor Hostile work environment Need for diverse case complexity and sufficient workload

Continued

TABLE 4.4

APRN Role Transition Studies in Practice: Role Implementation—cont'd

Researchers	Method	Participants	Noteworthy Findings
Ares (2018)	Quantitative survey Career Commitment subscale Imposter Phenomenon Scale	68 nurses 2.5–4 years following graduation from CNS program 2 comparison groups were formed based on employment as a CNS or not being employed as a CNS. Nearly half of the sample were employed as CNSs	Many of the participants reported that they were practicing the CNS role but their titles and position descriptions did not reflect the CNS title Significant experiences of the imposter phenomenon were reported Findings from the Career Commitment subscale were not conclusive
Bowie et al. (2019)	Qualitative cross-sectional study Content analysis of interviews	10 DNP graduates from 7 different schools in United States; 9 were postmasters DNP graduates and 1 was a BSN to DNP graduate 9 supervisors	Overall theme was: Being a change agent Subthemes were as follows: Belonging at the table Engaged sense of agency Leading with and through others
Thompson (2019)	Quantitative nonrandomized pretest–posttest single-group study design Revised NPRTS survey Intervention: role transition webinar	30 NPs Midwestern United States Target was NP graduates in first 3 months of practice but >20% graduated 16 months before and almost half graduated 9 months before as a result of study timing	The webinar was shown to have statistically significant positive influence on NPs' reported perceptions of NP role transition

[a]Studies are listed in chronologic order.

ACNP, Acute care nurse practitioner; *ANP,* adult NP; *CNS,* clinical nurse specialist; *CRNA,* certified registered nurse anesthetist; *DSN,* diabetes specialist nurse; *ED,* emergency department; *FNP,* family NP; *GNP,* geriatric NP; *ICU,* intensive care unit; *MSN,* masters of science in nursing; *NNP,* neonatal nurse practitioner; *NP*, nurse practitioner; *PA,* physician assistant; *WHCNP,* women's healthcare NP.

CNS Role Implementation Studies

Three early studies (Baker, 1979; M. A. Brown & Olshansky, 1997; Hamric & Taylor, 1989) describing the experiences of APRN graduates provide a foundation for understanding the ongoing process of transition into practice. The first study of APRN graduate role development by Baker (1979) was a retrospective interview study conducted with four CNS graduates that described a four-phase process of role development. Next, Hamric and Taylor's (1989) national questionnaire study of 100 CNSs in practice delineated seven phases of CNS role development (see Table 4.4). They found that 40 of the 42 CNSs in practice for 3 years or less experienced progression through the first three phases, which were identical to the first three phases identified by Baker. Most of the CNS respondents went through these three phases within 2 years. Integration, the fourth phase they identified, was typically reached after 3 to 5 years of practice in the CNS role. Three additional phases—frozen, reorganization, and complacent—were described that shared a negative, nonproductive character that were identified with 27% of the CNSs studied. In a later study conducted by Llahana and Hamric (2011), similar negative phases were identified with 58% of the British diabetes specialist nurses studied.

Nurse Practitioner Role Transition Study

In 1997, M. A. Brown and Olshansky described a four-stage transition process in their qualitative longitudinal study of FNPs during their first year of practice. Their characterization of this role transition process as moving from limbo to legitimacy is supported by Cusson and Strange's (2008) findings that 1 year in practice constituted a consistent benchmark for NNPs moving from ambivalence to making it as a real NNP and by Sullivan-Bentz et al.'s (2010) observation that NPs transition from feeling overwhelmed to feeling confident by the end of the first year of practice. The four-stage process identified by M. A. Brown and Olshansky is outlined in Table 4.4. The first stage, laying the foundation, was not described in previous literature. During this stage, new graduates take certification examinations, obtain necessary recognition or licensure from state boards of nursing, and look for positions. This stage has been shortened because of the availability of online certification examinations.

The second stage, launching, was defined as beginning with the first NP position and lasting at least 3 months. During this stage, the new graduate NP experiences the anxiety associated with the crisis of confidence and competence that accompanies taking on a new position and the return to the advanced beginner skill level. As the advanced beginner becomes increasingly aware of the number of elements relevant to actual performance in the role, they may become overwhelmed with the complexity of the skills required for the role and exhausted by the effort required for mastery. New NPs in Kelly and Mathews's (2001) study described similar experiences of exhaustion and frustration with lack of control over time. This is the at-work version of the crisis of confidence and competence experienced during stage 1 of the in-school role acquisition process (Roberts et al., 1997).

Imposter Phenomenon

The feeling of being "an imposter" or "a fake," described by Ares (2018) and Huffstutler and Varnell (2006), was first reported in the psychology literature in reference to high-achieving women (Clance & Imes, 1978). The imposter phenomenon (IP) has been identified as a factor affecting both male and female dental, medical, nursing, and pharmacy students and is thought to impede the career advancement of women in medicine (Armstrong & Shulman, 2019). There has been an explosion of interest in this topic over the last decade both in academic research and in popular media (Feenstra et al., 2020). While most commonly associated with women, this phenomenon occurs in both genders (Bravata et al., 2020; Haney et al., 2018). Those experiencing the imposter phenomenon tend to discount their accomplishments as the result of luck, hard work, or an error instead of their own abilities. They shy away from seeking promotions or career advancement, secretly harboring fear of being exposed as a fraud.

Personal feelings associated with this phenomenon generalized anxiety, lack of self-confidence, depression, and frustration—are commonly reported by APRNs experiencing the frustration phase or launching stage. It is related to feeling unable to meet one's own expectations and those of others (Clance & Imes, 1978) and feelings of inadequacy and constantly being tested (Arena & Page, 1992). This phenomenon is typically a temporary experience associated with taking on a new role or beginning a new job. The Heitz et al. (2004) study related similar role transition experiences of self-doubt, disillusionment, and turbulence and also reported that engaging in positive self-talk was helpful. They suggested that issues of gender and age may underlie differing perceptions of personal commitments and sacrifices as obstacles to surmount in role transition. Ares (2018) reported that the imposter phenomenon can be ameliorated by quality mentorship, peer support, and realistic expectations to ease the transition to practice. Haney et al. (2018) developed a workshop for interprofessional students to address this issue.

Clance and Imes (1978) coined the term *imposter phenomenon*, yet it is often referred to as the imposter syndrome in lay and sometimes research literature suggesting individual dysfunction requiring diagnosis and treatment. Feenstra et al. (2020) advocated reframing this phenomenon in the larger context of society rather than focusing on it as a problem of individuals and consistently using the original term *phenomenon* instead of *syndrome*. By viewing it as a systemic issue rather than an individual clinical syndrome, it can be addressed more broadly at institutional and organizational levels.

Commonalities Between CNS and NP Transition Studies

Although M. A. Brown and Olshansky (1997) did not relate their findings about NP role transition to Hamric and Taylor's (1989) findings about CNS role development, there are many similarities in the results of the two studies. The characteristics of M. A. Brown and Olshansky's launching stage are similar to those described by Hamric and Taylor for the frustration phase. M. A. Brown and Olshansky's third stage, meeting the challenge, is associated with feelings of regaining confidence and increasing competence. This stage has much in common with Hamric and Taylor's implementation phase, which is noted for returning optimism and enthusiasm as expectations are realigned. M. A. Brown and Olshansky's last stage, broadening the perspective, is characterized by feelings of legitimacy and competency as NPs. This last stage is similar to Hamric and Taylor's fourth phase of integration, during which the role is expanded and refined.

Does RN Experience Help With Role Integration?

The majority of NP role transition studies have been conducted with recent graduates; therefore there are scant data to indicate whether or not NPs move on to the fourth phase of integration or develop any of the negative phases identified by Hamric and Taylor (1989) with CNSs or Llahana and Hamric (2011) with diabetes specialist nurses. Rich (2005) investigated the relationship between duration of experience as an RN and NP clinical skills in practice among 150 NPs who graduated within 4 years from three universities in the Northeast United States. Findings from the NP self-report data indicated that duration of practice experience as an RN was not correlated with level of competency in NP practice skills. "An unexpected finding was that there was a significant negative correlation between years of experience as an RN and NP clinical practice skills as assessed by the collaborating physicians" (Rich, 2005, p. 55). The finding that collaborating physicians rated the NPs as more clinically competent than the NPs rated themselves (Rich, 2005) would be expected for NPs in the frustration phase or launching stage (see Table 4.4). Inclusion of assessments of role development and clinical competency in APRN follow-up studies would be helpful for building on the existing knowledge base.

Expect the First Year to Be Challenging

A consistent finding in APRN role development studies in the first year of APRN practice is commonly associated with a significantly difficult process of transition (Twine, 2018). APRN programs are designed to prepare graduates for *beginning*, entry-level clinical competency. The questionnaire study conducted by Hart and Macnee (2007) at two national NP conferences found that 51% of NPs perceived that they were only somewhat or minimally prepared for actual practice. NPs in the Jones et al. (2015) study reported that rather than feeling inadequately prepared for the NP role, their concern was more about not being prepared for their first job as an NP. They desired to transition into practice more swiftly and fully. They used technology for decision support, valued mentor relationships as vital to successful role integration and progression, and felt that a postgraduate residency program would be helpful. The demands of the current healthcare system can be overwhelming for new APRNs coping with the transition to practice.

Clinical residency programs were developed to address role transition issues of new APRN graduates (Bush & Lowry, 2016; Flinter, 2011; Sargent & Olmedo, 2013; Thabault et al., 2015). They are typically a year in length and are designed to enhance new graduate transition into practice, promote quality patient care, and increase NP retention and satisfaction. Flinter (2011) pointed out the need to advocate for federal funding to support graduate APRN residency training. The fact that graduate NP residents are licensed and certified and their services are billable can help offset some of the costs of such programs (Exemplar 4.2).

EXEMPLAR 4.2

POSTGRADUATE TRAINING

"Nursing is the only discipline that does not require a doctoral degree and/or have a systematic approach to residency training for advanced practice roles" (Harper et al., 2017, p. 50). The term residency has been controversial in nursing due to its traditional association with medical training. Meissen (2019) clarified that residency refers to postgraduate programs in a major field, such as primary care, while fellowship signifies postgraduate programs in a subspecialty, such as gastroenterology.

Flinter (2005) noted that clinical practice residencies are becoming more accepted and are increasing in hospital settings to support postbaccalaureate nurse entry into practice. Recognizing the difficult transition of new advanced practice registered nurses (APRNs) into initial clinical practice in community health centers, the Weitzman Center piloted the first formal postgraduate residency training program for new family nurse practitioners led by Flinter (2011). At least half of the residency program is devoted to direct clinical practice, and residents also learn about shared decision making and collaborative practice (Painter et al., 2019; Rugen et al., 2014).

In 2011 the Institute of Medicine (IOM) recommended the completion of residency programs for all new graduate nurses, including APRNs (IOM, 2011). Nurse practitioner (NP) postlicensure clinical training programs have expanded rapidly with now more than 100 postgraduate training programs for NPs/physician assistants (PAs), spanning from primary care to cardiothoracic surgery (Association of Post Graduate APRN Programs, 2019a, 2019b).

Zapakta et al. (2014) reported that four major themes emerged from the NP fellowship experience studied, including (1) the importance of bridging into professional practice (student to autonomous clinician), (2) expanded appreciation of health professionals' roles (trained in silos), (3) commitment to interprofessional teamwork, and (4) benefit of mentorship (lack of mentorship). Many reports indicate that residency programs do ease the role transition experienced by new graduate NPs. However, there is little data to support improved patient outcomes as a result of the residency experience (Meissen, 2019; Rugen et al., 2014). Currently, NP postgraduate clinical training lacks federal funding, unlike physician residencies. Salaries for NP postgraduate clinical training vary considerably depending on specialty.

The author asked NP participants from the residency program at the Michael E. DeBakey VA Medical Center, Center for Excellence in Primary Care, what was learned during their residency. One NP reported: "During the 1-year residency, I learned what I knew and what I was confident in, and more importantly, I learned my weaknesses. I was able to get practical clinical experience initially with supervision that then progressed to independence." Another NP stated:

> *There was a professional role identity aspect that is learned, which affects the team dynamics and time management. You are now giving the order versus following it out; it's a new role. It took some getting used to having the nursing team take care of simple jobs like wound care.*

Another NP commented:

> *It was a mindset necessary to break. "Oh, I'll just do it since the patient is with me now." It is important to ensure the entire team works to the full extent of his or her license for clinic efficiency and patient care. Of course, we do help out in times of need for the same reason clinical efficiency.*

NPs in the VA residency program worked in an interdisciplinary environment and learned to function as part of a team. The program combined formal and informal learning, improving critical thinking skills as well as providing clinical support for new graduates. The NP participants very clearly identified the positive impact of the residency program on their role transition. Many of the NP residents became VA employees. Residency programs for NP graduates promote increased confidence, improved retention, and better decision making with the experience obtained.

Strategies to Facilitate Role Implementation

The phases described by Hamric and Taylor (1989) are used here to structure discussion of strategies to facilitate transitions during APRN role implementation (see Table 4.5). The postgraduate clinical training programs for new graduates noted earlier constitute an overall approach for enhancing transition through the first three phases of postgraduate role implementation typically experienced during the first year of practice. A national collaboration of NP organizations has recommended that these postgraduate programs be referred to as "fellowships" rather than "residencies" to minimize confusion because they are not required for

TABLE 4.5

Strategies to Promote APRN Role Implementation in Practice

Transition Phase	Strategy
Orientation	Follow a structured orientation plan, residency, or fellowship program
	Circulate literature on APRN roles
	Network with peers
	Identify role model or mentor
	Join local, state, and national APRN groups
	Identify your expectations
Frustration	Schedule debriefing sessions with experienced APRN
	Discuss your expectations and how they fit in real-world application
	Plan for longer patient appointments initially
	Schedule administrative time
	Collaborate with other providers
	Learn time-saving tips
	Engage in positive self-talk
	Practice well-being habits of self-care
Implementation	Reassess demands, priorities, goals—modify expectations
	Schedule a 6-month evaluation
	Collaborate with other specialties—seek opportunities to co-treat with other specialties
	Learn from repetitive practice
	Learn ways to manage uncertainty
	Assemble mobile clinical resource applications
Integration	Schedule a 12-month evaluation
	Plan for role refinement and expansion
	Continue intraprofessional and interprofessional collaboration
	Continue debriefing sessions
	Continue seeking verification and feedback from colleagues

APRN, Advanced practice registered nurse.
Adapted from "Role Development of the Advanced Practice Nurse," by K. A. Brykczynski. (2014). In A. B. Hamric, C. M. Hanson, M. F. Tracy, & E. T. O'Grady (Eds.), *Advanced Practice Nursing: An Integrative Approach* (5th ed., pp. 98–100), 2014, Elsevier Saunders.

entry into practice, as are clinical residencies for physicians (American Association of Nurse Practitioners NP Roundtable, 2014).

Orientation Phase

The importance of being patient and recognizing that it takes time to develop fully in a new APRN role was stressed by NPs in Kleinpell-Nowell's surveys (1999, 2001). A strategy to facilitate role implementation for all APRNs during the orientation phase is development of a structured orientation plan (Barnes, 2015; Goldschmidt et al., 2011). Sharrock et al. (2013) described the contribution of clinical supervision to support nurses transitioning into new advanced practice roles. Ares (2018) and M. A. Brown and Olshansky (1997) noted the importance of clarification of values, needs, and expectations and of recognition that transitional experiences are time-limited. They also noted the importance of anticipatory guidance and realizing that these transition experiences follow a common pattern in new graduates. An APRN in a new position, whether experienced in the role or not, needs to be aware of the importance of being informed about the organizational structure, philosophy, goals, policies, and procedures of the agency.

Networking was emphasized by NPs in Kleinpell-Nowell's surveys (1999, 2001; see also Kleinpell, 2005). Peer support within and outside of the work setting is important, as noted by CNSs (Hamric & Taylor, 1989), NPs (Kelly & Mathews, 2001), and CRNAs (Tracy, 2017). New NPs stressed the importance of getting to know other nurses in the work setting, gaining their respect, and forming key alliances with them to enhance optimal functioning in their new position (Kelly & Mathews, 2001). Designating a more experienced APRN in the work setting as a mentor can be helpful and provide support for any APRNs new to a position (Sullivan-Bentz et al., 2010). APRNs who serve as preceptors for students can be particularly effective mentors for new graduates (Hayes, 2005). The importance of careful selection of a mentor was reported by NPs in the study by Kelly and Mathews (2001). Additional strategies suggested for networking within the system include developing peer support groups, being accessible to colleagues by phone or email, and getting involved in interdisciplinary groups (Sullivan-Bentz et al., 2010). APRNs should be encouraged to join local APRN groups for peer support, legislative and political updates, and networking opportunities. Numerous Internet sites are also available for networking, as noted earlier.

Page and Arena (1991) recommended that CNSs schedule and devote the major portion of their time during the orientation phase to direct patient care to solidify the clinical expert role. They also suggested making appointments with nursing leaders, physicians, and other healthcare professionals during this phase to garner administrative support. They recommended distributing business cards and making the job description available for discussion. They also counseled new CNSs to withhold suggestions for change until they have had the opportunity to assess the system more fully. When a new APRN joins the staff of an organization, the administrator should send a letter describing the APRN's background experiences and new position to key people in the organization.

Bridging Initial Transition Gaps

Gardner et al.'s (2007) study of NPs in Australia and New Zealand identified attributes of capability including self-efficacy, knowing how to learn, and creativity as essential complements to competency for successful NP practice. Tracy (2017) found factors similar to Gardner et al.'s of the importance of self-efficacy, mentoring, and peer support for promoting transition to practice for CRNAs. In a study of NPs in rural Canada, Gould and Wasylkiw (2007) reported that a holistic nursing philosophy of care, a pioneering outlook, and preference for a salaried position were helpful for NP practice transition. Organizational support, communication, and leadership were identified as most important for promoting transition to the ACNP role in the Dillon et al. (2016) study. They reported that turnover was greater than 50% for ACNPs during the first year of practice. In Faraz (2017), national NP study professional autonomy and ambiguity were the variables most predictive of turnover intention (see Table 4.4). Ares (2018) found that CNS graduates working in positions without CNS titles contributed to role confusion and ambiguity. APRNs can keep track of their role transition process by setting specific time-limited goals, forming peer networks, and seeking out mentors.

Frustration Phase

Hamric and Taylor (1989) observed that the frustration phase might come and go and may overlap other phases. They noted that painful affective responses are typical of this difficult phase. They suggested that monthly sessions for sharing concerns with a group of peers and an administrator might facilitate movement through this phase. Strategies identified as helpful for energizing movement from the frustration phase to the implementation phase include the following: obtaining assistance with time management (Allen, 2001), participating in support groups to ameliorate feelings of inadequacy, engaging in discussions for conflict resolution and role clarification (Desborough, 2012), reassessing priorities and setting realistic expectations (Jones et al., 2015), and focusing on short-term, visible goals.

Page and Arena (1991) suggested keeping a work portfolio to document activities so that APRN progress is more readily visible and accessible. This can be an expansion of the online portfolio and self-monitoring system initiated during the APRN program. M. A. Brown and Olshansky (1997) noted that organized sources of support such as phone calls, seminars, planned meetings with mentors, and scheduled time for consultation can significantly decrease feelings of anxiety. They noted that recognition of the discomfort arising from moving from expert back to novice and the realization that previous expertise can be valuable in the new role may help reduce feelings of inadequacy. They suggested that new APRNs request reasonable time frames for initial patient visits because novices take longer than experienced practitioners, and this may be key to successful adjustment to a new position.

Implementation Phase

During this phase, it is important for the APRN to reassess demands and expectations to prevent feeling overwhelmed. Priorities may need to be readjusted and short-term goals may need to be reformulated. M. A. Brown and Olshansky (1997, 1998) observed that competence and confidence are fostered through repetition. They also recommend scheduling a formal evaluation after approximately 6 months in which feedback about areas of strength and those needing improvement can be ascertained. Strategies mentioned as important during this time include seeking administrative support through involvement in meetings, maintaining visibility in clinical areas, and developing in-service programs with input from staff (Page & Arena, 1991). After some time in the implementation phase, APRNs may plan and execute small-scale projects to demonstrate their effectiveness in their new role.

Integration Phase

Hamric and Taylor's (1989) survey data indicated that CNSs maximize their role potential during the integration phase, which typically occurs after 3 years in practice. Satisfactory completion of the earlier phases appears to be essential for passage into this phase. One strategy for enhancing and maintaining optimal role implementation during this phase is having a trusted colleague who can act as a safe sounding board for "feedback, constructive criticism, and advice" (Hamric & Taylor, 1989, p. 79). During this phase, it is important to have a plan to guide continued role expansion and refinement, such as the portfolio mentioned earlier. Seeking appointment to key committees is important to increase recognition of APRNs in the organization. Administrative support and constructive feedback from a trusted mentor continue to be important. Development of a promotional system that offers professional advancement in the APRN practice role through additional benefits or financial incentives remains a challenge for practitioners and administrators.

Facilitators and Barriers in the Work Setting

Facilitators

Aspects of the work setting exert a major influence on APRN role definitions and expectations, thereby affecting role ambiguity, role incongruity, and role conflict. The need for ongoing peer and administrative support is a theme throughout the literature on role development, beginning with the student experience and extending into practice. Administrative factors that should be considered include whether APRNs are placed in line or staff positions; whether they are unit-based, population-based, or in some other arrangement; who evaluates them; and whether they report to administrative or clinical supervisors. The placements of various APRN positions may differ, even within one setting, depending on size, complexity, and distribution of the patient population (Andrews et al., 1999). Issues of professional versus administrative authority underlie the importance of the structural placement of the APRN within the organization. Effectiveness of the APRN role is enhanced when there is a mutual fit between the goals and expectations of the individual and the organization. Clarification of goals and expectations before employment and periodic reassessments can minimize conflict and enhance role development and effectiveness. Baird and Prouty (1989) maintained that the organizational design should have enough flexibility to change as the situation changes. Weiner (2009) described a theory of organizational readiness for change that can promote more flexible and promising approaches to improving healthcare delivery.

Practical strategies identified by Bonnel et al. (2000) for initiating NP practice in nursing facilities included proactive communication, developing a consistent system for visits, setting up the physical environment, and building a team approach to care. Credibility and advanced clinical nursing practice were recognized as facilitators by Ball and Cox (2004). Keating and colleagues (2010) noted that some organizations successfully increased their numbers of NPs by using measures such as reallocation of resources and creating a common nursing and medical budget. They encouraged continued exploration of role implementation issues and development of methods to address them to realize the potential benefits of NP practice to the healthcare delivery system. DiCenso, Martin-Misener et al. (2010), Bryant-Lukosius et al. (2010) delineated standardization of requirements, adequate resources, interprofessional education, legislation and regulation, needs assessment and understanding of role, stakeholder involvement, and a pan-Canadian approach as factors enabling role integration of advanced practice nurses in Canada. Doerksen (2010) reported on a study of professional development and mentorship needs of advanced practice nurses in Canada that identified needs for both formal and informal mentorship and administrative support as important for full role implementation. Sargent and Olmedo (2013) described a funded postgraduate residency program that facilitated role transition for APRNs, improved their retention and satisfaction, and also enhanced quality of patient care. In their review of the process of reframing professional boundaries that occurs when new professional roles are introduced, Niezen and Mathijessen (2014) identified individual knowledge, skill and confidence, legislation, socioeconomic influences, and policy as factors that could be barriers or potential facilitators.

The ability to incorporate teaching and counseling into the patient encounter may be a function of skill development gained with experience in the APRN role. This observation may be used as a rationale for structuring more time for visits and fewer total patients for new APRNs, with gradual increases in caseloads as experience is accrued. Older research has indicated that NPs incorporate counseling and teaching into the flow of patient visits—capturing the teachable moment (Brykczynski, 1999a; Johnson, 1993). Demands to see more patients in less time can impinge on the possibility of incorporating more holistic aspects into patient encounters. Current and emerging delivery models that redesign primary care payment systems, moving from volume to value, and include incentives for patient-centered care performance and optimal outcomes are promising for APRNs because these payment systems highlight and support the additional dimensions of care that APRNs can provide (Calsyn & Lee, 2012). Judge-Ellis and Wilson (2017) advocated for the implementation of models of care based on patient satisfaction and outcomes that illuminate the unique nursing dimensions of NP practice. Kleinpell et al. (2019) reported a systematic review that identified multiple positive outcomes for APRNs in the acute care setting, including decreased length of stay, improved nursing and physician satisfaction, decrease in cost of care, and decreased readmission rates. Kurtzman and Barnow (2017) reported that no statistically significant differences were detected in NP or PA care compared with MD care. Patients were more likely to receive health education and counseling such as smoking cessation counseling when seen by NPs (Kurtzman & Barnow, 2017). Autonomy and positive relationships with physicians were identified as facilitators in a recent review by Schirle et al. (2018).

Barriers

Factors found to impede NP role development include pressure to manage care for large numbers of patients, resistance from staff nurses, and lack of understanding of the NP role (Andrews et al., 1999; Kelly & Mathews, 2001). Ball and Cox (2004) identified conflict, resistance, gender bias, political awareness, and established values as barriers to APRN role implementation. Keating et al. (2010) reported on a study of perceived barriers to progression and sustainability of NP roles in emergency departments 10 years after they were introduced in Victoria, Australia. The main barriers identified were lack of organizational support, legislative constraints, and lack of ongoing funding for advanced practice nursing education. Lack of structured orientation programs was considered a barrier to APRN role transition by Goldschmidt and colleagues (2011). Sargent and Olmedo (2013) recognized limited time for physicians and experienced APRNs to mentor new APRNs as an impediment to APRN role development. Role confusion, lack of specific practice guidelines, and remuneration issues were barriers noted by Doetzel et al. (2016) with APRNs in the emergency department. Other constraints operating in today's healthcare settings that affect not only APRNs but also other providers and office staff include new billing and coding guidelines, Health Insurance Portability and Accountability Act regulations, major healthcare reform with a focus on outcomes, monitoring for fraud and abuse, sexual harassment, and demands to integrate technology into practice. Organizational-level policy restrictions, lack of professional recognition, and lack of role clarity were identified as barriers by Schirle et al. (2018).

Continued Advanced Practice Nurse Role Evolution

CNMs, CRNAs, NPs, and CNSs have attained positive recognition and support in clinical positions in many settings in the United States. However, despite the increasing familiarity and popularity of these APRN roles, some healthcare settings have used few, if any, APRNs and some staff members have had minimal experience working with APRNs. In some areas of the United States, physicians or physician assistants are preferred over APRNs. Even experienced APRNs can expect to encounter resistance to full implementation of their roles if they seek positions in institutions with no history of employing APRNs. Andrews and colleagues (1999) described their experiences introducing the NP role into a large academic teaching hospital. They delineated helpful strategies for marketing a new NP role to staff, patients, and the surrounding community, as well as ways to set up the necessary infrastructure to support the new role in the institution. They referred to this process as evolutionary.

The meaning of the evolution of established APRN roles varies according to the type of APRN role. The emphasis on cost containment in the healthcare delivery system led to the trend of having acute care NPs staff intensive care units to compensate for the shortage of house staff physicians (Rosenfeld, 2001). Then ACNP practice broadened from an intensive care unit focus to diverse settings including specialty clinics and private practice groups (Kleinpell, 2005; Kleinpell-Nowell, 2001). New roles for APRNs will develop as telehealth continues to expand (Rincon et al., 2020). Evolution of APRN roles is also reflected in the expansion of practice to multiple areas or sites. Although responsibility for multiple areas in the same facility has been typical of many CNS roles for years, it is an evolutionary process for most other APRN roles. Multisite roles might signify practice responsibilities at different sites or multiple areas of responsibility in the same site, and they may combine inpatient and outpatient responsibilities (Stahl & Myers, 2002). Stahl and Myers's clinical practices (see Exemplar 4.3) are models for APRN practice evolving to multiple sites, which constitutes a strategy for extending APRN resources and trying to use them more efficiently.

As individual APRNs mature into their respective roles and become more competent and confident in all role components, greater acceptance of the unique nature of APRN practice can be expected. In their study of CNSs, Hamric and Taylor (1989) found that freedom to develop their unique APRN role, availability of feedback from a mentor, support to broaden their influence and take on new projects, and recognition of their contributions enabled experienced CNSs to stay energized in their clinical practice roles. As Peplau (1997) advocated, nurse leaders must emphasize what nurses do for patients. The claim that APRN practice incorporates active patient participation, patient education, family assessment, involvement and support, and community awareness and connections (Neale, 1999) needs to be documented. For example, Kelly and Mathews (2001) found that graduates with 1 to 7 years of experience as NPs found it difficult to adhere to ideals of holistic care and health promotion, given the pressures of the clinical situation.

Continued research that demonstrates positive outcomes of APRN care is essential for APRN practice to make an impact on healthcare policy (Kapu & Kleinpell, 2012; see also Chapter 17). Rashotte (2005) advocated for dialogic forms of research (dialogic approaches employ conversation to explore meanings) to evoke the more holistic and humanistic aspects of what it means to be an APRN to complement the predominant instrumental and economic perspectives underlying most APRN research. Brykczynski's (2012) interpretive phenomenologic study of how NP faculty incorporate holistic aspects of care into teaching NP students is an example of such dialogic research. More research activity and increasing involvement in the larger arena of health policy may also represent continuing role evolution for APRNs. Getting involved in research activities as a coinvestigator or collaborator is a way for APRNs to remain engaged and challenged and to avoid moving into negative phases (Lambert & Housden, 2017). It also offers opportunities for interprofessional collaboration.

DNP preparation is another example of APRN role evolution. The DNP-prepared APRN brings an advanced skill set to health care with deeper understanding of research and technology. DNP-prepared APRNs are educated to translate evidence into practice, promote collaboration and interprofessional teamwork,

EXEMPLAR 4.3

EVOLVING APRN ROLES IN MULTISITE PRACTICES

Expansion of practice to multiple sites is one way in which advanced practice registered nurse (APRN) practice is evolving. Stahl is a clinical nurse specialist whose practice has evolved from the full range of clinical nurse specialist practice for four medical cardiac units at a tertiary care center to also include support primarily in education, consultation, and program development at two additional hospitals. Myers is an adult nurse practitioner who directs a hepatitis C program for a specialty physician group with 11 physicians at nine practice locations, and she also provides direct care for patients at four of the sites. Stahl and Myers (2002) relied on Quinn's (1996) wisdom for developing the leader within by expecting to "build the bridge as you walk on it" (p. 83) and learning "how to get lost with confidence" (p. 86). Their commitment to being continuous learners is a useful model for APRNs to follow as they experience the situational transitions that are inevitable as clinical practices evolve.

Self-mastery and commitment are the keys to meeting the needs of a multisite practice. Setting realistic expectations, maintaining healthy personal and professional boundaries, and establishing attainable goals can contribute to success in multisite practice. Practice challenges such as supervision and role requirements may differ from institution to institution. Inconsistency in electronic health records creates challenges for documentation. Various healthcare systems require users to attend training sessions for healthcare policies and electronic medical records, while others are not fully integrated. Hospital mergers and/or acquisitions of solo practices and community clinics impose regulatory requirements on the APRN that may not have previously existed. APRNs are required to apply for privileges to practice in hospitals. This mandated credentialing process can take up to 12 weeks and limit practice until completed. Additionally, the onboarding processes in different institutions present APRNs with multiple challenges in policy and procedures not usually present in solo practice.

Barriers still exist preventing APRNs from practicing to the full extent of their education and training (Hain & Fleck, 2014). Twenty-eight states have granted full practice authority; however, 14 states still require physician oversight for a specific number of hours or years of practice. In May of 2016 the US Department of Veterans Affairs (VA) announced a proposal for APRN full practice authority. On December 14, 2016, the VA granted full practice authority to three APRN roles to practice to the full extent of their education, training, and certification, regardless of state restrictions that limit such full practice authority, except for applicable state restrictions on the authority to prescribe and administer controlled substances, when such APRNs are acting within the scope of their VA employment. Unfortunately, certified registered nurse anesthetists were not included in the VA's full practice authority under the final rule (US Department of Veteran's Affairs, 2016). There are over 5769 APRNs working within the VA system (US Department of Veteran's Affairs, 2016).

---

and advocate and lead change in healthcare policy to improve patient outcomes (see Exemplar 4.4).

Evaluation of Role Development

Evaluation is fundamental to enhancing role implementation (see Chapter 21). Development of a professional portfolio to document APRN accomplishments can be useful for performance and impact (process and outcome) evaluation. Performance evaluation for APRNs should include self-evaluation, peer review, and administrative evaluation (Cooper & Sparacino, 1990; Hamric & Taylor, 1989). Use of a competency profile can be helpful for organizing evaluation in a dynamic way that allows for changes in role implementation over time as expertise, situations, and priorities change (Callahan & Bruton-Maree, 1994). APRNs can review the competency models available and select one to use for their ongoing competency profile (Sastre-Fullana et al., 2014). The competency profile can be used to assess performance in each of the core APRN competencies. APRN programs need to include content and skill development regarding self-evaluation and peer evaluation of role implementation so that individuals can learn to monitor their practice and identify difficulties early to avoid moving into negative developmental phases, noted earlier: frozen, reorganization, and complacent (Hamric & Taylor, 1979).

Outcome evaluation is important to demonstrate the effectiveness of each APRN role, to document the impact of APRN practice on quality of care, and to overcome APRN invisibility (O'Grady, 2008). Ongoing development of appropriate outcome evaluation measures, particularly for patient outcomes, is important (Bryant-Lukosius et al., 2016; Ingersoll et al., 2000; see Chapter 21). The existence of a reward system to provide for career advancement through a clinical ladder

EXEMPLAR 4.4
DNP: THE CHANGING FACE OF HEALTH CARE

The dual purpose of the doctorate of nursing practice (DNP) proposed by the American Association of Colleges of Nursing (AACN, 2004) was for nurses to provide advanced clinical care and leadership in clinical settings and to increase the numbers of clinical nursing faculty in academic settings (Beeber et al., 2019). AACN published the Essentials for DNP programs in 2006. Three institutions, Columbia University, The University of Tennessee Health Science Center, and the University of Texas Health Science Center, pioneered a clinical practice doctorate for APRNs prior to AACN's recognition of the DNP as the preferred model for APRNs (Mundinger & Carter, 2019). The earlier clinical practice doctorate focused on increased depth and breadth of clinical practice knowledge and skills.

The decision by AACN (2004) to allow nonclinical practice programs along with clinical practice programs to offer the same DNP degree had several consequences. Lack of clarity regarding the role of the graduates of these distinctly different programs led to ambiguity and confusion particularly in nonacademic settings. Academic institutions that had insufficient faculty prepared to provide advanced clinical practice programs were able to offer DNP programs in leadership and administration, and these programs proliferated at a much higher rate than clinical programs so that by 2018 only 15% of DNP programs focused on advanced clinical training (Martsolf & Sochalski, 2019).

The primary impetus for development of clinical DNP programs originated from an explosion of chronic illness coupled with aging of the population, which resulted in an influx of patients presenting with complex clinical problems in both acute and primary care settings. Shortages of both primary and acute care providers have increased with population growth, and reduction in clinical hours allowed for physician residents in hospitals increased the demand for APRNs in acute care settings (Kleinpell et al., 2015). The new face of health care supports the need for advanced clinical skills and leadership. Strong interprofessional collaboration is critical to successfully managing the current patient population. The clinical DNP responds to the need for advanced clinical skills and knowledge and increased collaboration with other disciplines at the systems level. The DNP is prepared with increased clinical and advocacy skills on which he or she can capitalize to effect policy change and quality improvement in health care.

DNP programs have grown in number and diversity with nonclinical programs greatly outnumbering clinical programs. Clinical DNP program graduates are filling clinical faculty roles. The roles of DNP graduates in nonacademic settings continue to evolve as new DNP graduates enter the healthcare system. Nurse entrepreneur, nurse executive, clinical educator, and nurse informaticist are some of the nonclinical positions being filled by DNP graduates. The evolution of the DNP role has contributed to the expansion of DNP programs and the adaptation of existing DNP programs to meet the changing needs of the healthcare system. Many DNP programs have implemented specialization paths (psych-mental health, executive, informatics, and education) to prepare students for the diverse opportunities available. The specialization pathway is in its infancy and is not consistent across the country. All accredited programs will be guided by the 10 domains in the updated essentials established by the AACN (2021).

DNP preparation is empowering. Educated for professional leadership, the DNP-prepared APRN exemplifies the Institute for Healthcare Improvement's Triple Aim principles of improving the patient experience of care (including quality and satisfaction), improving the health of populations, and reducing the per capita cost of health care (O'Dell, 2016; Stiefel & Nolan, 2012). Bodenhiemer and Sinsky (2015) identified a concern with widespread healthcare provider burnout and dissatisfaction and have recommended revision of the Triple Aim to a Quadruple Aim. The Quadruple Aim adds improving the work life of healthcare providers as another essential principle for enhancing patient care.

As a result of the diversity in DNP programs, new DNP-prepared APRNs encounter a degree of uncertainty and anxiety while looking for the best career opportunity to demonstrate their advanced skills and knowledge (Glasgow & Zoucha, 2011). While acceptance of the DNP role is growing, new DNPs face challenges including physician resistance and role ambiguity (or lack of role clarity), resulting in role strain. One might speculate that DNP-prepared APRNs move through the transitions in school and after graduation more quickly because of their advanced repertoire of both clinical and general life experience; however, further investigation is needed.

Along with increased awareness of the DNP, DNP-prepared APRN graduates report that advanced preparation has put them on equal ground with other healthcare professionals. There is a sense of interprofessional equality (Bowie at al., 2019). Research shows us the new DNP graduate is prepared to work in a multidisciplinary team and lead change in their organizations to improve the patient outcomes in populations (Bowie et al., 2019). The DNP role is evolving and the need for role clarity is paramount. DNP education is critical to advancing knowledge and clinical skills for advanced practice nurses (Hendricks-Ferguson et al., 2015). The complexities of health care and advances in technology and research increase the need for the doctorally prepared APRN.

program and accrual of additional benefits is particularly important for retaining APRNs in clinical roles. In less-structured situations, APRNs can negotiate for periodic reassessments and salary increases through options such as profit sharing.

The evaluation process broadens to incorporate interprofessional review when APRN practice includes hospital privileges, prescriptive privileges, and third-party reimbursement (Holley, 2016). This expansion of the evaluation process has positive and negative aspects. Advantages to the review process associated with securing and maintaining hospital privileges include the many factors considered in the evaluation, the variety of perspectives, and the visibility afforded APRNs. APRNs should seek key positions on hospital review committees to promote APRN roles within the organization. A major difficulty in implementing interdisciplinary peer review is lack of interaction between and among the students of the various health professional groups during their formative educational programs. The resurgence of interest in developing and implementing interprofessional educational experiences between nursing students and medical students is encouraging (Berger-Estilita et al. 2020; Interprofessional Education Collaborative Expert Panel, 2016).

CONCLUSION

Role development experiences for APRNs are described as consisting of two distinct transition processes. the first is referred to here as *role acquisition*, which occurs in school, and the second as *role implementation*, which occurs in practice after graduation. The limits of the educational process in preparing graduates for the realities of the work world are acknowledged. Students, faculty, preceptors, and administrators need to be informed about the human skill acquisition process and its stages, processes of adult and professional socialization, identity transformation, role acquisition, role implementation, and overall career development. Knowing (theoretical knowledge) and actually experiencing (practical knowledge) are different phenomena, but at least students and new graduates can be forewarned about the transition experiences in school and the turbulence that can be expected during the first year of practice. Anticipatory guidance for students can be provided through role rehearsal experiences, such as clinical preceptorships and role seminars. Students need to be encouraged to begin networking with practicing APRNs through local, state, and national APRN groups. This networking is especially important for APRNs who will not be practicing in proximity to other APRNs. Experienced APRNs and new APRN graduates can form mutually beneficial relationships.

Although anticipatory socialization experiences in school can facilitate role acquisition, they cannot prevent the transition that occurs with movement into a new position and actual role implementation. APRN programs should have a firm foundation in the real world. However, a certain degree of incongruence or conflict between academic ideals and work world reality will continue to exist (Ormond & Kish, 2001). APRNs must take a leadership role in guiding and directing planned change and guard against the mere maintenance of the status quo. Establishing mentor programs, structured orientation programs, and postgraduate fellowship or residency programs for new APRNs in the work setting are ways to develop and maintain support for the positive developmental phases of role implementation and minimize role strain.

APRN role development has been described as dynamic, complex, and situational. It is influenced by many factors, such as experience; level of expertise; personal and professional values; setting; specialty; relationships with coworkers; aspects of role transition; life transitions; organizational, system, and political realities; evolving technology; and advances in clinical practice. Frameworks for understanding APRN role development processes have been discussed, along with strategies for facilitating the dual transitions of role acquisition in school and role implementation upon graduation. Ongoing evolution of APRN roles in response to organizational and healthcare system changes and demands will continue. Future research studies to assess the applicability of this information to all APRN specialty groups are needed to further the understanding of APRN role development, guide educational and work setting innovations, and support health policy recommendations.

KEY SUMMARY POINTS

- Application of the Dreyfus situational model of skill acquisition to APRN role development depicts the acquisition of skills and knowledge as developing over time in stages from novice to expert, with the whole process evolving over time in cycles of progression and regression occurring as new skills and knowledge are acquired and new situations are encountered and mastered.
- APRN role development consists of two distinct processes: (1) role acquisition is the process of APRN role transition that takes place during the APRN educational program and (2) role implementation is the process of APRN role transition that occurs in the work setting following program completion.
- Conceptual understanding of role concepts and role development issues and familiarity with APRN research describing APRN role transition and implementation processes can enhance role acquisition and implementation experiences for individual APRNs, minimize the strain of role transitions, promote continued role evolution, and lead to educational innovations, improved health policy and regulations, and increased quality of health care.

REFERENCES

Allen, D. (2001). *Getting things done: The art of stress-free productivity*. Penguin Books.

Altersved, E., Zetterlund, L., Lindblad, U., & Fagerström, L. (2011). Advanced practice nurses: A new resource for Swedish primary healthcare teams. *International Journal of Nursing Practice, 17*, 174–180.

American Academy of Anesthesiologist Assistants. (2020). Certified registered nurse anesthetists' fact sheet. https://www.aana.com/about-us

American Association of Colleges of Nursing. (2004). Position statement on the practice doctorate in nursing. https://www.aacnnursing.org/Portals/42/News/Position-Statements/DNP.pdf

American Association of Colleges of Nursing. (2006). The essentials of doctoral education for advanced nursing practice. http://www.aacn.nche.edu/DNP/pdf/Essentials.pdf

American Association of Colleges of Nursing. (2015a). DNP fact sheet. http://www.aacn.nche.edu/media-relations/fact-sheets/dnp

American Association of Colleges of Nursing. (2015b). Re-envisioning the clinical education of advanced practice registered nurses, March 2015. http://www.aacn.nche.edu/aacn-publications/white-papers/APRN-Clinical-Education.pdf

American Association of Colleges of Nursing. (2021). The Essentials: Core Competencies for Professional Nursing Education. https://www.aacnnursing.org/Education-Resources/AACN-Essentials

American Association of Nurse Anesthesiology. (2007). AANA announces support of doctorate for entry into nurse anesthesia practice by 2025. http://www.aana.com/newsandjournal/News/Pages/092007-AANA-Announces-Support-of-Doctorate-for-Entry-into-Nurse-Anesthesia-Practice-by-2025.aspx

American Association of Nurse Anesthesiology. (2019). Qualifications and capabilities of the certified registered nurse anesthetist. https://www.aana.com/search?keyword=qualifications

American Association of Nurse Practitioners. (2012). CMS releases graduate nursing education demonstration FAQs. https://www.aanp.org/legislation-regulation/news/federal-news/111-articles/federal-news/599-cms-releases-graduate-nursing-education-demonstration-faqs-and-extends-deadline

American Association of Nurse Practitioners NP Roundtable. (2014). Nurse practitioner perspective on education and post-graduate training. https://www.aanp.org/images/documents/policy-toolbox/nproundtablestatementmay6th.pdf

American College of Nurse Midwives (ACNM). (2018). American College of Nurse Midwives and American College of Obstetricians and Gynecologists Announce new joint statement of practice relations. https://www.midwife.org

American College of Obstetricians and Gynecologists/American College of Nurse-Midwives. (2011). Joint statement of practice relations between obstetrician-gynecologists and certified nurse-midwives/certified midwives. http://www.acog.org/~/media/News%20Releases/nr2011-03-31.pdf

Anderson, E. M., Leonard, B. J., & Yates, J. A. (1974). Epigenesis of the nurse practitioner role. *American Journal of Nursing, 74*, 1812–1816.

Anderson, O. R., Love, B. C., & Tsai, M. J. (2014). Editorial. Neuroscience perspectives for science and mathematics learning in technology-enhanced learning environment. *International Journal of Science and Mathematics Education, 12*(3), 467–474.

Andrews, J., Hanson, C., Maule, S., & Snelling, M. (1999). Attaining role confirmation in nurse practitioner practice. *Clinical Excellence for Nurse Practitioners, 3*, 302–310.

Arena, D. M., & Page, N. E. (1992). The imposter phenomenon in the clinical nurse specialist role. *Image–the Journal of Nursing Scholarship, 24*, 121–125.

Ares, T. (2014). Professional socialization of students in clinical nurse specialist programs. *Journal of Nursing Education, 53*(11), 631. 2014.

Ares, T. (2018). Role Transition after clinical nurse specialist education. *Clinical Nurse Specialist, 32*(2), 71–80. doi:10.1097/NUR.0000000000000357

Armstrong, M. J., & Shulman, L. M. (2019). Tackling the imposter phenomenon to advance women in neurology. *Neurology. Clinical practice, 9*(2), 155–159. doi:10.1212/CPJ.0000000000000607

Association of Post Graduate APRN Programs. (2019a). Program Master List https://apgap.enpnetwork.com/page/24301-program-master-list

Association of Post Graduate PA Programs. (2019b). Post Graduate PA Program Listing. https://appap.org/programs/postgraduate-pa-np-programs-listings/

Baird, S. B., & Prouty, M. P. (1989). Administratively enhancing CNS contributions. In A. B. Hamric, & J. A. Spross (Eds.), *The clinical nurse specialist in theory and practice* (2nd ed.) (pp. 261–283). WB Saunders.

Baker, V. (1979). Retrospective explorations in role development. In G. V. Padilla (Ed.), *The clinical nurse specialist and improvement of nursing practice* (pp. 56–63). Nursing Resource. Wakefield.

Ball, C., & Cox, C. L. (2004). Part 2: Core components of legitimate influence and the conditions that constrain or facilitate advanced nursing practice in adult critical care. *International Journal of Nursing Practice, 10*, 10–20.

Banda, E. E. (1985). *Role problems, role strain: Perception and experience of clinical nurse specialist. Unpublished master's thesis*, Boston University School of Nursing.

Bandura, A. (1977). Self-efficacy: Toward a unifying theory of behavioral change. *Psychological Review, 84*, 191–215.

Barnes, H. (2015). Exploring the factors that influence nurse practitioner role transition. *The Journal of Nurse Practitioner, 11*(2), 178–183.

Bartholomew, K. (2006). *Ending nurse-to-nurse hostility: Why nurses eat their young and each other*. Opus Communications.

Beeber, A. S., Palmer, C., Waldrop, J., Lynn, M. R., & Jones, C. B. (2019). The role of Doctor of Nursing Practice-Prepared nurses in practice settings. *Nursing Outlook, 67*, 354–364.

Benner, P. (1984). *From novice to expert: Excellence and power in clinical nursing practice*. Addison-Wesley.

Benner, P. (2011). Formation in professional education: An examination of the relationship between theories of meaning and theories of the self. *Journal of Medicine and Philosophy, 36*, 342–353.

Benner, P., Sutphen, M., Leonard, V., & Day, L. (2010). Educating nurses. A call for radical transformation. Carnegie Foundation for the Advancement of Teaching.

Benner, P., Tanner, C. A., & Chesla, C. A. (2009). *Expertise in nursing practice: Caring, clinical judgment and ethics* (2nd ed.). Springer.

Berger-Estilita, J., Fuchs, A., Hahn, M., Chiang, H., & Greif, R. (2020). Attitudes towards Interprofessional education in the medical curriculum: A systematic review of the literature. *BMC Medical Education, 20*(1) 254-254. doi:10.1186/s12909-020-02176-4

Blackwell, C. W., & Faraci, N. (2021). Conflict resolution between physicians and nurse practitioners. *Journal of the American Association of Nurse Practitioners, 33*(11), 931–937. doi:10.1097/JXX.0000000000000491

Blumenreich, G. A. (2000). Legal briefs: Supervision. *AANA Journal, 68*, 404–409.

Bodenhiemer, T., & Sinsky, C. (2015). From triple to quadruple aim: Care of the patient requires care of the provider. *Annals of Family Medicine, 12*(6), 573–576.

Bonnel, W., Belt, J., Hill, D., Wiggins, S., & Ohm, R. (2000). Challenges and strategies for initiating a nursing facility practice. *Journal of American Academy of Nurse Practitioners, 12*, 353–359.

Bowie, B. H., DeSocio, J., & Swanson, K. M. (2019). The DNP degree: Are we producing the graduates we intended? *The Journal of Nursing Administration, 49*(5), 280–285.

Brault, I., Kilpatrick, K., D'Amour, D., Contandriopoulos, D., Chouinard, V., Dubois, C. A., Perroux, M., & Beaulieu., M. D. (2014). Role clarification processes for better integration of nurse practitioners into primary healthcare teams: A multiple-case study. *Nursing Research and Practice, 2014*(2014), 170514–170519. doi:10.1155/2014/170514

Bravata, D. M., Watts, S. A., Keefer, A. L., Madhusudhan, D. K., Taylor, K. T., Clark, D. M., Nelson, R. S., Cokley, K. O., & Hagg, H. K. (2020). Prevalence, predictors, and treatment of imposter syndrome: A systematic review. *Journal of General Internal Medicine, 35*(4), 1252–1275. doi:10.1007/s11606-019-05364-1

Brown, M. A., & Olshansky, E. F. (1997). From limbo to legitimacy: A theoretical model of the transition to the primary care nurse practitioner role. *Nursing Research, 46*, 46–51.

Brown, M. A., & Olshansky, E. F. (1998). Becoming a primary care nurse practitioner: Challenges of the initial year of practice. *The Nurse Practitioner, 23*(46), 52–66.

Brown, S. J. (1992). Tailoring nursing care to the individual client: Empirical challenge of a theoretical concept. *Research in Nursing and Health, 15*, 39–46.

Bryant, S., & Parker, K. (2020). Participation in a nurse practitioner fellowship to instill greater confidence, job satisfaction, and increased job retention. *Journal of the American Association of Nurse Practitioners, 32*(10), 645–651. doi:10.1097/JXX.0000000000000313

Bryant-Lukosius, D., Carter, N., Kilpatrick, K., Martin-Misener, R., Donald, F., Kaasalaninen, S., et al. (2010). The clinical nurse specialist role in Canada. *Nursing Leadership, 23*, 140–166.

Bryant-Lukosius, D., Spichiger, E., Martin, J., Stoll, H., Kellerhals, S. D., Fliedner, M., et al. (2016). Framework for evaluating the impact of advanced practice nursing roles. *Journal of Nursing Scholarship, 48*(2), 201–209.

Brykczynski, K. A. (1991). Judgment strategies for coping with ambiguous clinical situations encountered in family primary care. *Journal of the Academy of Nurse Practitioners, 3*, 79–84.

Brykczynski, K. A. (1999a). An interpretive study describing the clinical judgment of nurse practitioners. *Scholarly Inquiry for Nursing Practice: An International Journal, 13*, 141–166.

Brykczynski, K. A. (1999b). Reflections on clinical judgment of nurse practitioners. *Scholarly Inquiry for Nursing Practice: An International Journal, 13*, 175–184.

Brykczynski, K. A. (2012). Clarifying, affirming, and preserving the nurse in NP education and practice. *Journal of the Academy of Nurse Practitioners, 24*, 554–564.

Brykczynski, K. A. (2014). Role development of the advanced practice nurse. Table 4-4: Phases of Advanced Practice Nurse Role Development and Table 4-5: Transition Stages in First Year of Primary Care Practice. In A. B. Hamric, C. M. Hanson, M. F. Tracy, & E. T. O'Grady (Eds.), *Advanced practice nursing: An integrative approach* (5th ed.) (pp. 98–100). Elsevier Saunders.

Brykczynski, K. A. (2000). Strategies to promote NP role acquisition in school. Chart 1.6, p 61. In P. Meredith, & N. M. Horan (Eds.), *Adult primary care* (pp. 16). WB Saunders.

Burgess, J., & Purkis, M. E. (2010). The power and politics of collaboration in nurse practitioner role development. *Nursing Inquiry, 17*, 297–308.

Burman, M. E., Hart, A. M., Conley, V., Caldwell, P., & Johnson, L. (2007). The Willow ceremony: Professional socialization for nurse practitioner students. *Journal of Nursing Education, 46*(1), 48. doi:10.3928/01484834-20070101-10

Burns, C., Beauchesne, M., Ryan-Krause, P., & Sawin, K. (2006). Mastering the preceptor role: Challenges of clinical teaching. *Journal of Pediatric Health Care, 20*(3), 172–183.

Bush, C. T., & Lowry, B. (2016). Postgraduate nurse practitioner education: Impact on job satisfaction. *The Journal for Nurse Practitioners, 12*(4), 226–234.

Callahan, L., & Bruton-Maree, N. (1994). Establishing measures of competence. In S. D. Foster, & L. M. Jordan (Eds.), *Professional aspects of nurse anesthesia practice* (pp. 275–290). FA Davis.

Calsyn, M., & Lee, E. O. (2012). Alternatives to fee-for-service payments in health care. https://www.americanprogress.org/issues/healthcare/reports/2012/09/18/38320/alternatives-to-fee-for-service-payments-in-health-care/

Centers for Medicare and Medicaid Services. (2012). Graduate nurse education demonstration. https://innovation.cms.gov/Files/fact-sheet/GNE-Fact-Sheet.pdf

Chang, W., Mu, P., & Tsay, S. (2006). The experience of role transition in acute care nurse practitioners in Taiwan under the collaborative practice model. *Journal of Nursing Research, 14*(2), 83–91.

Clance, P., & Imes, S. (1978). The imposter phenomenon in high achieving women: Dynamics and therapeutic intervention. *Psychotherapy: Theory Research and Practice, 15*, 241–247.

Cohen, H. A. (1981). *The nurse's quest for a professional identity*. Addison-Wesley.

Cooper, D. M., & Sparacino, P. S. A. (1990). Acquiring, implementing, and evaluating the clinical nurse specialist role. In P. S. A. Sparacino, D. M. Cooper, & P. A. Minarik (Eds.), *The clinical nurse specialist: Implementation and impact* (pp. 41–75). Appleton & Lange.

Curry, J. L. (1994). Nurse practitioners in the emergency department: Current issues. *Journal of Emergency Nursing, 20*, 207–215.

Cusson, R. M., & Strange, S. (2008). Neonatal nurse practitioner role transition: The process of reattaining expert status. *Journal of Perinatal and Neonatal Nursing, 22*, 329–337.

Cusson, R. M., & Viggiano, N. M. (2002). Transition to the neonatal nurse practitioner role: Making the change from the side to the head of the bed. *Neonatal Network, 21*(2), 21–28.

Day, L., Cooper, P. L., & Scott, W. M. (2012). Using unfolding cases in primary care coursework for nurse practitioner students: Prepared to certify or prepared to practice? In *Presentation abstract, National Organization of Nurse Practitioner Faculties (NONPF) 38th Annual Meeting*, Charleston, SC. Conference April 13-16, /2012.

DeMaio, D. (1979). The born-again nurse. *Nursing Outlook, 27*, 272–273.

Desborough, J. L. (2012). How nurse practitioners implement their roles. *Australian Health Review, 36*, 22–26.

DiCenso, A., Bryant-Lukosius, D., Martin-Misener, R., Donald, F., Abelson, J., Bourgealt, I., et al. (2010). Factors enabling advanced practice role integration in Canada. *Canadian Journal of Nursing Leadership*, special issue, *23*, 211–238.

Dillon, D., Dolansky, M. A., Casey, K., & Kelley, C. (2016). Factors related to successful transition to practice for acute care nurse practitioners. *AACN Advanced Critical Care, 27*(2), 173–182.

Doerksen, K. (2010). What are the professional development and mentorship needs of advanced practice nurses? *Journal of Professional Nursing, 26*(3), 141–151.

Doetzel, C. M., Rankin, J. A., & Then, K. L. (2016). Nurse practitioners in the emergency department. Barriers and facilitators for role implementation. *Advanced Emergency Nursing Journal, 38*(1), 43–55.

Donley, R., Sr., Flaherty, M. J., Sr., Sarsfield, E., Burkhard, A., O'Brien, S., & Anderson, K. M. (2014). Graduate clinical nurse preceptors: Implications for improved intra-professional collaboration. *The Online Journal of Issues in Nursing, 19*(3), 9.

Dreyfus, H. L., & Dreyfus, S. E. (1986). *Mind over machine: The power of human intuition and expertise in the era of the computer*. Free Press.

Dreyfus, H. L., & Dreyfus, S. E. (2009). The relationship of theory and practice in the acquisition of skill. In P. Benner, C. A. Tanner, & C. A. Chesla (Eds.), *Expertise in nursing practice: Caring, clinical judgment and ethics* (2nd ed.) (pp. 1–23). Springer.

Edmonson, C., & Zelonka, C. (2019). Our own worst enemies: The nurse bullying epidemic. *Nursing Administration Quarterly, 43*(3), 274–279. doi:10.1097/NAQ.0000000000000353

Education, National Commission on Nurse Anesthesia (1990). Summary of commission findings: Issues and review of supporting documents. *Journal of the American Association of Nurse Anesthesiology, 58*, 394–398.

Faraz, A. (2017). Novice nurse practitioner workforce transition and turnover intention in primary care. *The Journal of American Nurse Practitioners, 29*, 26–34.

Farrell, G. A. (2001). From tall poppies to squashed weeds: Why don't nurses pull together more? *Journal of Advanced Nursing, 35*, 26–33.

Farrell, K., Payne, C., & Heye, M. (2015). Integrating interprofessional collaboration skills into the advanced practice registered nurse socialization process. *Journal of Professional Nursing, 31*(1), 5–10.

Fawcett, J., Newman, D. M. L., & McAllister, M. (2004). Advanced practice nursing and conceptual models of nursing. *Nursing Science Quarterly, 17*, 135–138.

Feenstra, S., Begeny, C. T., Ryan, M. K., Rink, F. A., Stoker, J. I., & Jordan, J. (2020). Contextualizing the impostor "syndrome." *Frontiers in Psychology, 11*, Article 575024. doi:10.3389/fpsyg.2020.575024

Fiandt, K. (2002). Finding the nurse in nurse practitioner practice: A pilot study of rural family nurse practitioner practice. *Clinical Excellence for Nurse Practitioners, 5*, 13–21.

Fleming, E., & Carberry, M. (2011). Steering a course towards advanced nurse practitioner: A critical care perspective. *Nursing in Critical Care, 16*, 67–76.

Flinter, M. (2005). Residency programs for primary care nurse practitioners in federally qualified health centers: A service perspective. *Online Journal of Issues in Nursing, 10*(3). doi:10.3912/OJIN.Vol10No03Man05

Flinter, M. (2011). From new nurse practitioner to primary care provider: Bridging the transition through FQHC-Based residency training. *Online Journal of Issues in Nursing, 17*(1) PMID: 22320872.

Ford, L. C. (1982). Nurse practitioners: History of a new idea and predictions for the future. In L. H. Aiken (Ed.), *Nursing in the 1980s: Crises, opportunities, challenges* (pp. 231–247). JB Lippincott.

Gardner, A., Hase, S., Gardner, G., Dunn, S. V., & Carryr, J. (2007). From competence to capability: A study of nurse practitioners in clinical practice. *Journal of Clinical Nursing, 17*, 250–258.

Glasgow, M. E. S., & Zoucha, R. (2011). Role strain in the doctorally prepared advanced practice nurse. In H. M. Dreher, & M. E. S. Glasgow (Eds.), *Role development for doctoral advanced nursing practice* (pp. 213–226). Springer Publishing.

Goldschmidt, K., Rust, D., Torowicz, D., & Kolb, S. (2011). Onboarding advanced practice nurses: Development of an orientation program in a cardiac center. *Journal of Nursing Administration, 41*(1), 36–40.

Gould, O. N., & Wasylkiw, L. (2007). Nurse practitioners in Canada: Beginnings, benefits, and barriers. *American Academy of Nurse Practitioners, 19*, 165–171.

Grando, V. T. (1998). Articulating nursing for advanced practice nursing. In T. J. Sullivan (Ed.), *Collaboration: A health care imperative* (pp. 499–514). McGraw-Hill.

Green, J., Wyllie, A., & Jackson, D. (2014). Electronic portfolios in nursing education: A review of the literature. *Nurse Education in Practice, 14*(1), 4–8.

Gunn, I. P. (1991). The history of nurse anesthesia education: Highlights and influences. Report of the National Commission on Nurse Anesthesia Education. *Journal of the American Association of Nurse Anesthesiology, 59*, 53–61.

Gunn, I. P. (1998). Setting the record straight on nurse anesthesia and medical anesthesiology education. *CRNA: The Clinical Forum for Nurse Anesthetists, 9*, 163–171.

Hain, D., & Fleck, L. (2014). Barriers to nurse practitioner practice that impact healthcare redesign. *The Online Journal of Issues in Nursing, 19*(2), 2. doi:10.3912/OJIN.Vol19No02Man02

Hamric, A. B. (2003). Defining our practice: A personal perspective [letter to the editor]. *Clinical Nurse Specialist, 17*, 75–76.

Hamric, A. B., & Hanson, C. M. (2003). Educating advanced practice nurses for practice reality. *Journal of Professional Nursing, 19*, 262–268.

Hamric, A. B., & Taylor, J. W. (1989). Role development of the CNS. In A. B. Hamric, & J. Spross (Eds.), *The clinical nurse specialist in theory and practice* (2nd ed.) (pp. 41–82). WB Saunders.

Haney, T. S., Birkholz, L., & Rutledge, C. (2018). A workshop for addressing the impact of the imposter syndrome on clinical nurse specialists. *Clinical Nurse Specialist, 32*(4), 189–194. doi:10.1097/NUR.0000000000000386

Hardy, M. E., & Hardy, W. L. (1988). Role stress and role strain. In M. E. Hardy, & M. E. Conway (Eds.), *Role theory: Perspectives for health professionals* (2nd ed.) (pp. 159–239). Appleton & Lange.

Harper, D., McGuinnes, T., & Johnson, J. (2017). Clinical residency training: Is it essential to the Doctor of Nursing Practice for nurse practitioner preparation. *Nursing Outlook, 65*(1), 50–57.

Hart, A. M., & Macnee, C. L. (2007). How well are nurse practitioners prepared for practice: Results of 2004 questionnaire study? *Journal American Academy of Nurse Practitioners, 19*(1), 35–46.

Hayes, E. F. (2001). Factors that facilitate or hinder mentoring in the nurse practitioner preceptor/student relationship. *Clinical Excellence for Nurse Practitioners, 5*, 111–118.

Hayes, E. (2005). Mentoring research in the NP preceptor/student relationship. *Journal American Academy of Nurse Practitioners, 19*(1), 35–46.

Heath, L. A. (2014). An analysis of horizontal violence and bullying within the workplace. *Midwifery Digest, 24*(4), 436–443.

Heitz, L. J., Steiner, S. H., & Burman, M. E. (2004). RN to FNP: A qualitative study of role transition. *Journal of Nursing Education, 43*, 416–420.

Hendricks-Ferguson, V. L., Akard, T. F., Madden, J. R., Peters-Herron, A., & Levy, R. (2015). Contributions of advanced practice nurses with a DNP degree during palliative and end-of-life care of children with cancer. *Journal of Pediatric Oncology Nursing, 32*(1), 32–39.

Holley, S. L. (2016). Ongoing professional performance evaluation: Advanced practice registered nurse practice competency assessment. *The Journal for Nurse Practitioner, 12*(2), 67–74.

Huffstutler, S. Y., & Varnell, G. (2006). The imposter phenomenon in new nurse practitioner graduates. Retrieved from http://www.medscape.com/viewarticle/533648

Huston, C. (2013). The impact of emerging technology on nursing care: Warp speed ahead. *The Online Journal of Issues in Nursing, 18*(2), 1. doi:10.3912/OJIN.Vol18No02Man01

Ingersoll, G. L., McIntosh, E., & Williams, M. (2000). Nurse-sensitive outcomes of advanced practice. *Journal of Advanced Practice, 32*, 1272–1281.

Institute of Medicine. (2003). *Health professions education: A bridge to quality*. National Academies Press.

Institute of Medicine. (2011). *The Future of Nursing: Leading Change, Advancing Health*: National Academies Press. doi:10.17226/12956.

Interprofessional Education Collaborative Expert Panel. (2016). *Core competencies for interprofessional collaborative practice: Report of an expert panel*. Interprofessional Education Collaborative.

Jarvis-Selinger, S., Pratt, D. D., & Regehr, G. (2012). Competency is not enough: Integrating identity formation into the medical education discourse. *Academic Medicine: Journal of the Association of American Medical Colleges, 87*(9), 1185–1190.

Jiang, X., Wang, J., Lu., Y., Jiang, H., & Li, M. (2019). Self-efficacy-focused education in persons with diabetes: A systematic review and meta analysis. *Psychology Research and Behavior Management, 12*, 67–79.

Johnson, R. (1993). Nurse practitioner-patient discourse: Uncovering the voice of nursing in primary care practice. *Scholarly Inquiry for Nursing Practice: An International Journal, 7*, 143–157.

Jones, J., Kotthoff-Burrell, E., Kass-Wolff, J., & Brownrigg, V. (2015). Nurse practitioner graduates "speak out" about the adequacy of their educational preparation to care for older adults: A qualitative study. *The Journal of the American Association of Nurse Practitioner, 27*, 698–706.

Judge-Ellis, T., & Wilson, T. (2017). Continuing education: Time and NP practice: Naming, claiming, and explaining the role of nurse practitioners. *The Journal for Nurse Practitioners, 13*, 583–589. doi:10.1016/j.nurpra.2017.06.024

Kapu, A. N., & Kleinpell, R. (2012). Developing nurse practitioner associated metrics for outcomes assessment. *Journal of the American Association of Nurse Practitioners, 25*(6), 289–296.

Keating, S. F. J., Thompson, J. P., & Lee, G. A. (2010). Perceived barriers to the sustainability and progression of nurse practitioners. *International Emergency Nursing, 18*, 147–153.

Kelly, N. R., & Mathews, M. (2001). The transition to first position as nurse practitioner. *Journal of Nursing Education, 40*, 156–162.

Kimbro, C. D. (1978). The relationship between nurses and nurse-midwives. *Journal of Nurse-Midwifery, 22*, 28–31.

Klaich, K. (1990). Transitions in professional identity of nurses enrolled in graduate educational programs. *Holistic Nursing Practice, 4*, 17–24.

Kleinpell, R. (2001). Nurse anesthetists hold fast under physicians' blast of supervision ruling. *The Nursing Spectrum, 11*, 26–27.

Kleinpell, R. (2005). Acute care nurse practitioner practice: Results of a 5-year longitudinal study. *American Journal of Critical Care, 14*, 211–221.

Kleinpell, R, Grabenkort, W. R., Kapu, A. N., Constantine, R., & Sicoutris, C. (2019). Nurse practitioners and physician assistants in acute and critical care: A concise review of the literature and data 2008–2018. *Critical Care Medicine, 47*(10), 1442–1449. doi:10.1097/CCM.0000000000003925

Kleinpell, R., Ward, N. S., Kelso, L. A., Mollenkopf F. P., Jr., & Houghton, D. (2015). Provider to patient ratios for nurse practitioners and physician assistants in critical care units. *American Journal of Critical Care, 24*, e16–e21.

Kleinpell-Nowell, R. (1999). Longitudinal survey of acute care nurse practitioner practice: Year 1. *AACN Clinical Issues, 10*, 515–520.

Kleinpell-Nowell, R. (2001). Longitudinal survey of acute care nurse practitioner practice: Year 2. *AACN Clinical Issues, 12*, 447–452.

Kramer, M. (1974). *Reality shock*. Mosby.

Kumar, S., Fathima, M. P., & Mohan, S. (2013). Impact of neurocognition on teaching competency. *Innovare Journal of Education, 1*(1), 7–9. Retrieved from https://www.academia.edu/12652954/IMPACT_OF_NEUROCOGNITION_ON_TEACHING_COMPETENCY

Kurtzman, E. T., & Barnow, B. S. (2017). A comparison of nurse practitioners, physician assistants, and primary care physicians' patterns of practice and quality of care in health centers. *Medical Care, 55*(6), 615–622. doi:10.1097/MLR.0000000000000689

Lambert, L. K., & Housden, L. M. (2017). NP engagement in research. *Canadian Oncology Nursing Journal, 27*(1), 107–110.

Leininger, M. M. (1994). The tribes of nursing in the United States. *Journal of Transcultural Nursing, 6*, 18–22.

Lindblad, E., Hallman, E., Gillsjö, C., Lindblad, U., & Fagerström, L. (2010). Experiences of the new role of advanced practice nurse in Swedish primary health care—A qualitative study. *International Journal of Nursing Practice, 16*, 69–74.

Lindeke, L. L., & Thomas, K. K. (2010). The SOPP and the Coalition for Patients' Rights: Implications of continuing interprofessional tension for PNPs. *Journal of Pediatric Health Care, 24*, 62–65.

Llahana, S. V., & Hamric, A. B. (2011). Developmental phases and factors influencing role development in diabetes specialist nurses: A UK study. *European Diabetes Nursing, 8*, 18–23a.

MacDonald, M. B., Bally, J. M., Ferguson, L. M., Lee Murray, B., Fowler-Kerry, S. E., & Anonson, J. M. S. (2010). Knowledge of the professional role of others. A key inter-professional competency. *Nurse Education in Practice, 10*, 238–242.

Martsolf, G. R., & Sochalski, J. (2019). The need for advanced clinical education for nurse practitioners continues despite expansion of Doctor of Nursing Practice Programs. *Policy, Politics and Nursing Practice, 20*(4), 183–185.

Mata, Á., Azevedo, K., Braga, L., Medeiros, G., Oliveira Segundo, V., Bezerra, I., Pimenta, I.D.S.F., Nicolas, I. M. & Piuvezam, G. (2019). Training programs in communication skills to improve self-efficacy for health personnel: Protocol for a systematic review and meta-analysis. *Medicine, 98*(33). doi:10.1097/MD.0000000000016697 p.e16697-e16697.

Mechanic, O. J., Persaud, Y., & Kimball, A. B. (2020). *Telehealth systems*. StatPearls Publishing. https://www.ncbi.nlm.nih.gov/books/NBK459384/

Meissen, H. (2019). Nurse practitioner residency and fellowship programs: The controversy still exists. *Journal of the American Association of Nurse Practitioners, 31*, 381–383. doi:10.1097/JXX.0000000000000255

Meleis, A. I., Sawyer, L. M., Im, E. O., Hilfinger-Messias, D. K., & Schumacher, K. (2000). Experiencing transitions: An emerging middle range theory. *Advances in Nursing Science, 23*(1), 12–28.

Multi-discipline Clerkship/Clinical Training Site Survey. (2014). Recruiting and maintaining US clinical training sites: Joint report of the 2013, Multi-discipline Clerkship/Clinical Training Site Survey. https://members.aamc.org/eweb/upload/13-225%20WC%20Report%20FINAL.pdf

Mundinger, M. O., & Carter, M. A. (2019). Potential crisis in NP preparation in the US. *Policy, Politics, and Nursing Practice, 20*(2), 57–63.

Neale, J. (1999). Nurse practitioners and physicians: A collaborative practice. *Clinical Nurse Specialist, 13*, 252–258.

Niezen, M. G. H., & Mathijssen, J. J. P. (2014). Reframing professional boundaries in healthcare: A systematic review of facilitators and barriers to task reallocation from the domain of medicine to the nursing domain. *Health Policy, 117*, 151–169.

O'Dell, D. G. (2016). How do DNPs fit into the Triple Aim? The DNP-prepared professional is emerging as a catalyst of change. Advance for NPs and PAs. http://nurse-practitioners-and-physician-assistants.advanceweb.com/DNP-Center/Columns/DNP-Report/How-Do-DNPs-Fit-Into-the-Triple-Aim.aspx

O'Grady, E. T. (2008). Advanced practice registered nurses: The impact on patient safety and quality. Chapter 43. In R. G. Hughes (Ed.), *Patient safety and quality: An evidence-based handbook for nurses* (pp. 1–20). Agency for Health Care Research and Quality.

Ormond, C., & Kish, C. P. (2001). Role acquisition. In D. Robinson, & C. P. Kish (Eds.), *Core concepts in advanced practice nursing* (pp. 269–285). Mosby.

Page, N. E., & Arena, D. M. (1991). Practical strategies for CNS role implementation. *Clinical Nurse Specialist, 5*, 43–48.

Painter, J., Sebach, A. M., & Maxwell, L. (2019). Nurse practitioner transition to practice: Development of a residency program. *The Journal for Nurse Practitioners, 15*, 688–691.

Parle, M., Maguire, P., & Heaven, C. (1997). The development of a training model to improve health professionals skills, self-efficacy, and outcome expectancies when communicating with cancer patients. *Social Science & Medicine, 44*, 231–240.

Peplau, H. (1997). Keynote address *Presented at the International Congress of Nurses*.

Poronsky, C. B. (2013). Exploring the transition from registered nurse to family nurse practitioner. *Journal of Professional Nursing, 29*, 350–358.

Quinn, R. E. (1996). *Deep change: Discovering the leader within*. Jossey-Bass.

Rashotte, J. (2005). Knowing the nurse practitioner: Dominant discourses shaping our horizons. *Nursing Philosophy, 6*, 51–62.

Rich, E. R. (2005). Does RN experience relate to NP clinical skills? *The Nurse Practitioner, 30*, 53–56.

Rich, E. R., & Rodriguez, L. (2002). A qualitative study of perceptions regarding the non-nurse college graduate nurse practitioner. *Journal of the New York State Nurses' Association, 33*(2), 31–35.

Rincon, T. A., Bakshi, V., Beninati, W., Carpenter, D., Cucchi, E., Davis, T. M., Dreher, J., Hiddleson, C., Johansson, M. K., Katz, A. W., & Olff, C. (2020). Describing advanced practice provider roles within critical care teams with Tele-ICUs: Exemplars from seven US health systems. *Nursing Outlook, 68*, 5–13.

Roberts, S. J. (1983). Oppressed group behavior: Implications for nursing. *Advances in Nursing Science, 5*, 21–30.

Roberts, S. J., Tabloski, P., & Bova, C. (1997). Epigenesis of the nurse practitioner role revisited. *Journal of Nursing Education, 36*, 67–73.

Rosenfeld, P. (2001). Acute care nurse practitioners: Standard in ambulatory care, they're also useful in hospitals. *American Journal of Nursing, 101*, 61–62.

Rounds, L. R. (1997). The nurse practitioner: A healing role for the nurse. In P. B. Kritek (Ed.), *Reflections on healing: A central nursing construct* (pp. 209–223). National League for Nursing.

Rugen, K. W., Watts, S. A., Janson, S. L., Angelo, L. A., Nash, M., Zapapta, S. A., Brienza, R., Gillman, S. C., Bowen, J. L., & Saxe, J. M. (2014). Veterans Affairs Centers for Excellence in Primary Care Education: Transforming nurse practitioner education. *Nursing Outlook, 62*(2), 78–88.

Sargent, L., & Olmedo, M. (2013). Meeting the needs of new-graduate nurse practitioners: A model to support transition. *The Journal of Nursing Administration, 43*(11), 603–610.

Sastre-Fullana, P., De Pedro-Gomez, J. E., Bennasar-Veny, M., Serrano-Gallardo, P., & Morales-Asencio, J. M. (2014). Competency frameworks for advanced practice nursing: A literature review. *International Nursing Review, 61*, 534–542.

Schirle, L., Norful, A., Rudner, N., & Poghosyan, L. (2018). Organizational facilitators and barriers to optimal APRN practice environments: An integrative review. *Health Care Management Review, 45*(4), 311–320. doi:10.1097/HMR.0000000000000229

Schumacher, K. L., & Meleis, A. I. (1994). Transitions: A central concept in nursing. *Image–the Journal of Nursing Scholarship, 26*, 119–127.

Scott, A., Dawson, R. M., Mitchell, S., & Catledge, C. (2020). Simulation-based interprofessional education in a rural setting: The development and evaluation of a "remote-in" telehealth scenario. *Nursing Education Perspectives, 41*(3), 187–189. doi:10.1097/01.NEP.0000000000000461

Sharrock, J., Javen, L., & McDonald, S. (2013). Clinical supervision for transition to advanced practice. *Perspectives in Psychiatric Care, 49*, 118–125.

Sherman, R. O. (2021). Bullying during time of turbulence. *Emerging Nurse Leader*. https://www.emergingrnleader.com/bullyingduringatimeofturbulance/

Spoelstra, S. L., & Robbins, L. B. (2010). A qualitative study of role transition from RN to APN. *International Journal of Nursing Education Scholarship, 7*(1), 1–14.

Stahl, M. A., & Myers, J. (2002). The advanced practice nursing role with multisite responsibilities. *Critical Care Nursing Clinics of North America, 14*, 299–305.

Stein, T. (2000). Struggling for autonomy: Dispute between CRNAs and anesthesiologists continues. *Nurseweek (California Statewide Edition), 13*, 31.

Steiner, S. H., McLaughlin, D. G., Hyde, R. S., Brown, R. H., & Burman, M. E. (2008). Role transition during RN to FNP education. *Journal of Nursing Education, 47*(10), 441–447.

Stiefel, M., & Nolan, K. (2012). A guide to measuring the Triple Aim: Population health, experience of care, and per capita cost. IHI Innovation Series white paper. Institute for Healthcare Improvement. http://www.ihi.org/resources/pages/ihiwhitepapers/aguidetomeasuringtripleaim.aspx

Sullivan-Bentz, M., Humbert, J., Cragg, B., Legault, F., Laflamme, C., Bailey, P. H., & Doucette, S. (2010). Supporting primary health care nurse practitioners' transition to practice. *Canadian Family Physician, 56*, 1176–1182.

Thabault, P., Mylott, L., & Patterson, A. (2015). Describing a residency program developed for newly graduated nurse practitioners employed in retail health settings. *Journal of Professional Nursing, 31*(3), 226–232.

Thomas, S. P. (2003). Horizontal hostility: Nurses against themselves: How to resolve this threat to retention. *American Journal of Nursing, 103*(10), 87–91.

Thompson, A. (2019). An educational intervention to enhance nurse practitioner role transition in the first year of practice. *The Journal of American Association of Nurse Practitioners, 31*(1), 24–32.

Tracy, A. (2015). A pilot study on student nurse anesthetists' views on CRNA role transition. *Anesthesia E- Journal, 3*(1). https://anesthesiaejournal.com/index.php/aej/article/view/26

Tracy, A. (2017). Perceptions of certified registered nurse anesthetists on factors affecting their transition from student. *AANA Journal, 85*(6), 438–444.

Trotter, K., Blazar, M., Muckler, V., Kuszajewski, M., & Molloy, M. (2019). Perinatal IPE simulation can improve collaborative competencies. *Journal of Interprofessional Education & Practice, 15*, 30–33. doi:10.1016/j.xjep.2019.01.011

Twine, N. (2018). The first year as a nurse practitioner: An integrative literature review of the transition experience. *Journal of Nursing Education and Practice, 8*(5), 54–62.

University of Pennsylvania. (2017). *Medicare graduate nursing education demonstration increases primary care workforce*. https://www.nursing.upenn.edu/live/news/940-medicare-graduate-nurse-education-demonstration

Urbanowicz, J. (2019). APRN transition to practice: Program development tips. *The Nurse Practitioner, 44*(12), 50-55. https://doi.org/10.1097/01.NPR.0000605520.88939.d1

US Department of Veterans Affairs. (2016). *VA grants full practice authority to advance practice registered nurses*. Press Release. https://www.va.gov/opa/pressrel/pressrelease.cfm?id=2847

Varney, H. (1987). *Nurse-midwifery* (2nd ed.). Blackwell Scientific.

Waddill-Goad, S. M. (2019). Stress, fatigue, and burnout in nursing. *Journal of Radiology Nursing, 38*(1), 44–46. hhttps://doi10.1016/j.jradnu.2018.10.005

Waters, R. (2007). Scope of practice legislative fights expected to return in 2007. *The Journal for Nurse Practitioners, 3*, 194–196.

Waugaman, W. R., & Lu, J. (1999). From nurse to nurse anesthetist: The relationship of culture, race, and ethnicity to professional socialization and career commitment of advanced practice nurses. *Journal of Transcultural Nursing, 10*, 237–247.

Weiner, B. J. (2009). A theory of organizational readiness for change. *Implementation Science. 4*(67), 1–9. https://doi.org/10.1186/1748-5908-4-67

Williams, C., Gensheimer, C., Halle, J., & Moss, P. (2018). Student perspectives of an interprofessional education experience for nurse anesthetist students and physical therapy students in a cadaver-based anatomy review course. *Open Access Library Journal,* 5, 1–15. doi:10.4236/oalib.1104782

Wynia, M. K., Von Kohorn, I., & Mitchell, P. H. (2012). Challenges at the intersection of team-based and patient-centered health care. Insights from an IOM working group. *The Journal of the American Medical Association, 308*(13), 1327–1328. https://doi.org/10.1001/jama.2012.12601

Zapakta, S. A., Conelius, J., Edwards, J., Meyer, E., & Brienza, R. (2014). Pioneering a primary care adult nurse practitioner interprofessional fellowship. *Journal of Nurse Practitioners, 10*(6), 378–386.

5

INTERNATIONAL DEVELOPMENT OF ADVANCED PRACTICE NURSING

DENISE BRYANT-LUKOSIUS ■ FRANCES KAM YUET WONG

"Learn to think continentally."
~ Alexander Hamilton

CHAPTER CONTENTS

ADVANCED PRACTICE NURSING ROLES WITHIN A GLOBAL HEALTHCARE CONTEXT 137
Defining Advanced Practice Nursing 137
Global Deployment 138
Types of Advanced Practice Nursing Roles 138
Emerging and New Frontiers for Future Role Expansion 143
FACILITATING THE INTRODUCTION AND INTEGRATION OF ADVANCED PRACTICE NURSING ROLES 148
Pan-Approaches and Collaboration 148
Funding and Reimbursement Arrangements 152
Systematic Approaches to Role Planning 153
Use and Generation of Evidence 154
NEXT STEPS IN THE GLOBAL EVOLUTION OF ADVANCED PRACTICE NURSING ROLES 155
CONCLUSION 155
KEY SUMMARY POINTS 156

In the midst of a global pandemic, the landmark year of 2020 as the International Year of the Nurse and the Midwife has heightened understanding of the central role nurses play to improve global health and strengthened awareness of advanced practice nurses as an integral component of the dynamic and contemporary nursing workforce countries require to meet challenging population health and health service needs. Thus the position to expand the international development of advanced practice nursing (APN) roles has never been stronger. Internationally, APN roles are on the threshold of new development and expansion that will include the first-time introduction of the roles in some countries and improved health systems integration in countries where roles are established. Within the global healthcare context, this chapter examines the current state of defining, deploying, and utilizing five types of APN roles, emerging frontiers where there is progress in introducing APN roles, and new frontiers for APN role development. Evidence-informed strategies for facilitating the introduction of APN roles are explored and the next steps for supporting the global development of the roles are also identified.

ADVANCED PRACTICE NURSING ROLES WITHIN A GLOBAL HEALTHCARE CONTEXT

Defining Advanced Practice Nursing

There is international agreement that clinical practice involving the direct care of patients and families, groups, communities, or populations is a defining feature of APN roles and that these roles require an expanded range of competencies in addition to those for the basic practice of a registered nurse (International Council of Nurses [ICN], 2020). The integration of clinical practice with competencies related to education, professional and organizational leadership, evidence-informed practice, and research is what makes the roles advanced. However, just as the nursing profession is at different stages of development in countries around the world, so, too, is the development of APN roles. Reflecting the evolving nature of APN roles globally, the ICN (2020) broadly defines the advanced practice nurse[1] as a

> *generalist or specialized nurse who has acquired through additional graduate education (minimum of a master's degree) the expert knowledge base, complex decision-making skills and clinical competencies for expanded practice, the characteristics of which are shaped by the context and/or country in which s/he is credentialed to practice. (p. 6)*

Common features of APN roles include a master's degree from an accredited APN education program; formal mechanisms for credentialing (i.e., licensure, registration, certification); integration of research, education, and leadership with advanced clinical competencies; and regulatory mechanisms for autonomous and expanded scope of practice (ICN, 2020). These features are consistent with the regulatory framework for the advanced practice registered nurse (APRN) in the United States related to licensure, accreditation, certification, and education (LACE; APRN Joint Dialogue Group, 2008). However, LACE features have more detailed role requirements rather than recommendations, as suggested by the ICN (2020).

Global Deployment

Strong global demand for APN roles has been evident since 2001 and the launch of the ICN's International Nurse Practitioner/Advanced Practice Nurse Network (INP/APNN; Bryant-Lukosius & Martin-Misener, 2016). Internationally, the absolute number of advanced practice nurses is unknown, as few health human resource systems are in place to monitor global APN role deployment, and at country levels there are absent or inconsistent methods for identifying nurses in these roles. However, 53% (78/147) of the countries who contributed to the recent World Health Organization (WHO, 2020) report on the state of the world's nursing identified as having APN roles. APN roles are found mainly in high-income countries, of which Canada, the United Kingdom, and the United States have the most established roles with decades of experience (see Chapter 1). In the last decade, APN roles have spread to high-income countries such as Chile and Singapore (Aguirre-Boza et al., 2019; Woo et al., 2019) and upper-middle-income countries like Jordan and South Africa (Christmals & Armstrong, 2019; Zahran et al., 2012). To date, there has been limited reporting on APN roles in low- or lower-middle-income countries. Recent publications suggest that the concept of APN is being considered in several of these countries and that APN roles requiring master's education are emerging in countries such as India, Angola, and Mongolia (Christmals & Armstrong, 2019; Scanlon, Murphy et al., 2019).

In the last decade, interest in APN roles has intensified as a result of WHO (2010) directives to meet the 2015 Millennium Development Goals for improving global health. It was recognized that national healthcare systems could be improved by enhancing nursing roles to address provider shortages, overcome inequities through universal health coverage, and improve care quality. Priorities included establishing postbasic nursing education programs to support advanced clinical practice (WHO, 2010); introducing specialized and APN roles to meet population health and health service needs, especially for primary health care (WHO, 2012); and developing career pathways for APN roles (WHO, 2015b).

Types of Advanced Practice Nursing Roles

In the United States the regulatory framework for the APRN is specific to four certified roles: the nurse anesthetist (NA), nurse-midwife (NM), nurse practitioner (NP), and clinical nurse specialist (CNS; APRN Joint Dialogue Group, 2008). The introduction of these longstanding roles varies in other countries, but internationally the CNS and NP roles are the most common types of APN roles (Heale & Rieck-Buckley, 2015). In the last 20 years, the nurse consultant (NC) has emerged as a new type of APN role (Baldwin et al., 2013).

[1]In the United States there is a clear regulatory framework and role title of advanced practice registered nurse (APRN) for nurses working in nurse practitioner, clinical nurse specialist, nurse-midwife, or nurse anesthetist roles. In this chapter the term advanced practice nurse is used to reflect the international variability in APN role titling and regulation.

Nurse-Midwife

Midwifery is one of the oldest health professions, dating back to the Stone Age (Barnawi et al., 2013). As the profession evolved, a variety of sociocultural factors influenced the development of nursing and non-nursing midwifery roles, including NMs (have nursing and midwifery education), midwives (have midwifery but no nursing education), nurses, traditional birthing attendants, and generalist and specialist physicians. The International Confederation of Midwives (ICM, 2019) has developed competencies for basic midwifery practice that apply, but are not specific to, advanced roles. The education of NMs is variable, ranging from 2 to 6 years, with about half completing at least 4 years of training (United Nations Population Fund [UNFPA], 2014). This suggests that not all NMs have a master's degree as recommended by the ICN (2020) for APN roles. NMs who meet ICM (2019) competencies have a scope of practice that includes prevention, health promotion, detecting complications, accessing medical care, and providing emergency measures within a primary healthcare framework. They work in varied settings, including the home, community, hospital, clinics, birthing centers, or health units.

Improving maternal–child health by expanding midwifery services and, in particular, increasing the number of NMs and midwives is a global priority (UNFPA, 2011). Major drivers are high maternal and infant morbidity and mortality rates, especially in low- and middle-income countries, as well as the increasing costs of medicalized care and growing use of unnecessary and expensive interventions such as cesarean sections (Renfrew et al., 2014). The importance of NMs and midwives for improving maternal–child care cannot be overstated. A report has shown that NMs and midwives with the appropriate education and who are regulated to meet ICM competencies for practice can deliver 87% of reproductive and postpartum care (UNFPA, 2014). Since 2010, collaboration among the United Nations, the ICM, and the WHO led to a series of consensus meetings with agreement on strategic priorities and reporting on key indicators as the basis for strengthening the global midwifery workforce through ongoing data assessment and monitoring (Day-Stirk et al., 2014). These data show that NMs make up a very small proportion or about 5% of the midwifery workforce (UNFPA, 2014). Despite smaller numbers, NMs spend more time delivering sexual and reproductive health and maternal–newborn care compared with nurses and generalist physicians, accounting for 14% of full-time equivalents (UNFPA, 2014).

There is limited data on the deployment of NMs in advanced roles where graduate education is required. Publications are predominately from the United States, where there are 12,000 NMs who are autonomous providers with prescriptive authority in all 50 states (American College of Nurse-Midwives [ACNM], 2019; Chapter 15). NMs are one of the largest groups of midwifery providers in the United States (ACNM, 2019) but are most prominent in rural communities with fewer obstetric providers (Kozhimannil et al., 2016).

Nurse Anesthetist

Globally, the current state of the NA workforce is not well described. In the results of international surveys published over 20 years ago, 107 countries were found to have nurses providing anesthesia care (McAuliffe & Henry, 1996, 1998). Survey results demonstrated the significant magnitude of anesthesia nursing in developed and developing countries. Nurses were involved in 83% of all procedures and were the sole provider for 51% of procedures, especially in rural communities (McAuliffe & Henry, 1998). In more recent times, NAs in advanced roles have provided important contributions to anesthesia care in response to the COVID-19 pandemic (Ouersighni & Ghazali, 2020) and in humanitarian settings (Kudsk-Iversen et al., 2020). The education and scope of practice of NAs varies across countries and does not consistently meet requirements for APN roles in all situations. A review of nurse anesthesia practice in the Group of Seven (G7) countries identified advanced NA roles requiring graduate education in the United States and France, while in the United Kingdom nurses complete postbasic education and function as anesthesia assistants (Tenedios et al., 2018). In Canada, Germany, Italy, and Japan the development of NAs has been stymied by physician resistance and the lack of funding for NA positions and education programs.

The International Federation of Nurse Anesthetists (IFNA) provides leadership to support the global development of NA through policy development, accreditation of education programs, a student journal, and conferences. Country profiles provided by the IFNA (2020) show that in addition to the United States and France, graduate education is required for the NA as an advanced role in Jamaica and Sweden. In other countries such as Cambodia, the Democratic Republic of Congo, Ghana, Indonesia, Switzerland, and Tunisia, NAs require a postbasic nursing diploma or certificate. The number of NAs in each of the IFNA (2020) profiled countries varies widely from 70 in Cambodia to over 49,000 in the United States, but in most cases they are the largest group of anesthesia care providers. In Ghana ($n = 700$), Indonesia ($n = 1700$), and Tunisia ($n = 1300$), NAs provide 70% to 90% of anesthesia care alone or under the supervision of an anesthesiologist or surgeon. In Switzerland about 50% of hospitals have one or more NAs working in dedicated pain services. In the United States NAs are the primary providers of anesthesia care in rural communities and for vulnerable low-income populations such as the unemployed, the uninsured, or those eligible for Medicaid (Liao et al., 2015).

Progress in establishing advanced NAs in China occurred in 2015 with the launch of a 21-month postbasic education program (Hu et al., 2017). South Korea has a 55-year history of NA practice provided by master's-prepared advanced practice nurses and hospital-trained registered nurses (Rayborn et al., 2017). However, the future of advanced NA roles in South Korea is in jeopardy due to the absence of a regulated scope of practice, legal pressures from the medical community, and declining enrollment and access to NA education programs. Similarly, in Brazil, Israel, and Spain, a regulatory framework for NAs does not exist and access to education is limited (Aaron & Andrews, 2016; Lemos & Peniche, 2016). Education programs in Nordic countries range from hospital-based training to master's degrees, but they have similar entry requirements (i.e., registered nurse with 1 or 2 years of work experience), and four out of the five countries have a protected title of NA (Jeon et al., 2015).

Nurse Practitioner

Recent guidelines published by the ICN (2020) aim to distinguish the similarities and differences between NP and CNS roles from an international perspective. Variability in how APN roles were defined across countries and overlap in CNS and NP activities contributed to lack of clarity and role confusion. The ICN defines the NP as an

> *advanced practice nurse who integrates clinical skills associated with nursing and medicine in order to assess, diagnose, and manage patients in primary healthcare settings (PHC) and acute care populations as well as ongoing care for populations with chronic illness. (p. 6)*

Key features distinguishing NPs are a population focus and an expanded scope of practice required for advanced health assessment, ordering diagnostic tests, communicating a diagnosis, prescribing treatments/medication, and performing procedures.

The NP role was first launched in the United States in 1965, followed by Canada and Jamaica in the mid-1970s, with the aim to improve people's health by increasing access to primary health care for vulnerable populations and those living in rural, remote, and underserved communities (Jamaica Association of Nurse Practitioners, 2016; Kaasalainen et al., 2010; Saver, 2015). In the 1980s, Canada and the United States introduced acute care NPs, starting with neonatal care, to address physician shortages and to meet the complex needs of acute and critically ill patients (Haut & Madden, 2015; Kilpatrick et al., 2010). Countries such as Australia (M. A. Carter et al., 2015), Ireland (Begley et al., 2010), the Netherlands (De Bruijn-Geraets et al., 2014), New Zealand (Gagan et al., 2014), Sweden (Jangland et al., 2016), Taiwan (Tsay et al., 2018), Thailand (Hanucharurnkul, 2007), and the United Kingdom (East et al., 2015) introduced NPs in the 1990s and early 2000s.

In most developed countries (e.g., Australia, Canada, Ireland, Jamaica, Sweden, Netherlands, New Zealand, United States) NPs are required to have a master's degree, but not all have regulatory policies in place to fully support an expanded scope of practice (Heale & Rieck-Buckley, 2015). In other countries the education and regulatory requirements for NPs are evolving and quite varied. As an example, Taiwan has over 7000 NPs who receive postbasic training by accredited hospitals (Tsay et al., 2018). Title protection for the NP has existed since 2000, while legislation to approve an expanded scope of practice followed much later in 2016.

Worldwide, NPs may represent the largest growing sector of healthcare professionals, with substantial increases over the last decade, particularly in developed countries. Between 2010 and 2019, the number of NPs in the United States tripled from 91,000 to over 290,000, accounting for 69% of all advanced practice nurses and 7.6% of the nursing workforce (American Association of Nurse Practitioners [AANP], 2020; Auerbach et al., 2020; Health Resources and Services Administration, 2019). Compared with their United States counterparts, other countries such as Australia ($n = 1883$), Canada ($n = 6159$), Ireland ($n = 220$), the Netherlands ($n = 4071$), and New Zealand ($n = 365$) have fewer NPs who make up a smaller proportion (<2%) of their nursing workforce, but they have also experienced significant growth in NPs (Australian Health Practitioner Regulation Agency, 2019; Canadian Institute for Health Information [CIHI], 2020; Dutch Nursing Association, 2020; Nursing Council of New Zealand, 2020). Although the number of NPs in Canada and the United States has increased, the loss of graduate programs specifically for neonatal NPs has resulted in a shortage of NPs in this area for both countries (Dalhousie University, 2017; Staebler et al., 2016).

In Canada and the United States, the majority of NPs (60% and 70%, respectively) work in primary care (AANP, 2020; CIHI, 2020). From 2016 to 2019, England had a 32% increase in the number of primary care NPs ($n = 3555$; Royal College of Nursing, 2020). Increases in primary care NPs have also occurred in Australia, Ireland, Netherlands, and New Zealand; however, in these and other countries (e.g., Singapore, Sweden, Taiwan), more NPs are in specialized and acute care (Freund et al., 2015; Jangland et al., 2016; Tsay et al., 2018; Woo et al., 2019).

Internationally, there is a high demand or interest in NPs to meet the health needs of aging populations and those with chronic conditions. The NP role has been examined for the frail elderly in Sweden and the United Kingdom (Goldenberg et al., 2016; Ljungbeck & Forss, 2017) and found to improve outcomes for elderly trauma patients in the United States (Bethea et al., 2019). In addition to NP roles for disaster nursing (Zak et al., 2020), authors from several countries have advocated for the expansion of NP roles in emergency care (Minotti et al., 2020; Tyler et al., 2018; Williams, 2017) and critical care for adult and pediatric populations (Davis et al., 2015; Gigli et al., 2018). Primary care NPs in several countries were found to increase access to care for at risk ethnic groups, those living in areas of socioeconomic disadvantage and rural communities, and the frail elderly (Grant et al., 2017). The breadth of demand for NPs is reflected in the wide variety of practice settings in which they work, including hospitals, outpatient clinics, group practices, public health, emergency departments, community health centers, homes, schools, social services, prisons, hospices, and long-term care (Bryant-Lukosius, Jokiniemi et al., 2018; Donald et al., 2013; Grant et al, 2017; Maten-Speksnijder et al., 2015).

The effectiveness of NPs is well established for varied patient populations in different practice settings. Several systematic reviews show that compared with standard care, NPs have similar or improved outcomes related to patient health, satisfaction with care, quality of care, and healthcare use (Donald et al., 2015; Martin-Misener et al., 2015; Stanik-Hutt et al., 2013).

Clinical Nurse Specialist

A persistent challenge for the international development of the CNS has been the lack of clarity and poor stakeholder understanding of the role. Variability in education requirements and inconsistent role definitions, role titles, and job descriptions within and across countries has led to confusion about CNS role aims and how it differs from other specialized and APN roles and master's-prepared nurses in other types of roles (Cooper et al., 2019; Dury et al., 2014; Leary et al., 2017; Mohr & Coke, 2018). Following an international consultation process, the ICN (2020) offered this definition of the CNS as

> *an advanced practice nurse who provides expert clinical advice and care based on established diagnoses in specialized clinical fields of practice along with a systems approach in practicing as a member of the healthcare team. (p. 6)*

Implicit in this definition is that CNS interventions are reliant on patients having a medical diagnosis as a way of distinguishing CNSs and NPs related to scope of practice. Unlike other types of APN roles, CNSs in most countries do not have an expanded scope of practice that includes medical activities such as diagnosing and prescribing. While it is true that CNSs care for patients diagnosed with medical conditions, this definition contrasts with the results of a synthesis of the international evidence indicating that clinical CNS interventions are not solely reliant on a medical diagnosis but rather are health oriented, with a focus on whole person and family care and patient empowerment to promote health, prevent illness and complications, and reduce symptoms (Bryant-Lukosius & Rietkoetter, 2020). An important finding of this synthesis was international agreement about the nature of CNS interventions (e.g., clinical, leadership, education/mentorship, consultation, research, scholarship) across three spheres of practice (i.e., patients, nurses/nursing practice, organizations/systems). Further, rather than siloed interventions focused on a single domain, it was the integration of CNS interventions across the three spheres that contributed to beneficial patient (quality of life, physical symptoms, psychological well-being, self-management, treatment adherence, satisfaction) and organizational (hospital length of stay and readmissions, healthcare costs) outcomes. These findings are consistent with the ICN (2020) definition emphasizing the systems impact of CNS roles.

Studies from several countries show that while there is overlap in CNS and NP activities, NPs spend more time than CNSs providing direct clinical care (Bryant-Lukosius, Jokiniemi et al., 2018; Carryer et al., 2018; Gardner et al., 2016). In contrast, master's-prepared CNSs spend more time in all other role domains (support of systems, education, research, and professional leadership) compared with specialized nurses in nonadvanced roles and NPs (Bryant-Lukosius, Jokiniemi et al., 2018). CNSs with a master's degree compared with those without also implement activities in all APN role domains and address healthcare problems at a systems level (Bryant-Lukosius, Jokiniemi et al., 2018; Kilpatrick et al., 2013). These findings support the ICN's (2020) guidance that a master's degree distinguishes CNSs from specialized nurses in nonadvanced roles.

The CNS role was introduced in the United States, Canada, and the United Kingdom in the 1960s and 1970s in response to the rising complexity and specialization of health care and the need for clinical expertise, education, and leadership to improve care delivery and patient outcomes, develop nursing practice, and support nurses at the point of care (Fulton, 2014; Kaasalainen et al., 2010; Leary et al., 2008). In the 1990s and 2000s, CNSs were further introduced in China, Hong Kong, Japan, New Zealand, the Republic of Korea, Taiwan, and Thailand (Kaur, 2014; Roberts et al., 2011; Tian et al., 2014; Wongkpratoom et al., 2010). The lack of title protection and registries to identify master's-prepared CNSs makes it difficult to assess trends or estimate the global CNS workforce. The United States has 70,000 CNSs, compared with 55,000 in the United Kingdom and less than 1000 in Canada (Bryant-Lukosius, Jokiniemi et al., 2018; National Association of Clinical Nurse Specialists [NACNS], 2018; Royal College of Nursing, 2012b).

CNSs work in a variety of specialty areas that may be defined by a condition (e.g., cancer, cardiovascular disease, intellectual disability), health needs (e.g., pain control, mental health), type of care (e.g., wound, organ transplant, or critical care), setting (e.g., community), or age (e.g., neonatology, gerontology; Doody et al., 2017; Goemaes et al., 2019; Kilpatrick et al., 2013; NACNS, 2019). Although CNSs were initially introduced in hospitals, the role has spread to provide care in outpatient, emergency department, home, community, and long-term care settings ICN (Kilpatrick et al., 2013; NACNS, 2019; Tian et al., 2014).

Similar to NPs, a high demand for CNSs is observed for older adults and those with chronic conditions. More CNSs work in geriatrics in Canada (19%) and the United States (42%) compared with other specialties (Kilpatrick et al., 2013; NACNS, 2019). In the United States 33% of CNSs work with primary care or family/all ages populations (NACNS, 2019) that likely have high numbers of older adults and those with chronic conditions. In New Zealand CNSs have been used in primary care to provide geriatric comprehensive assessment, management, and care coordination (King et al., 2018). Nurse leaders have advocated for better use of CNSs for patients with chronic conditions and those requiring palliative care (Hansen et al., 2019; Reed, 2020; Whittaker et al., 2017). Internationally, innovative CNS roles are being introduced for populations with varied chronic conditions like diabetes (Lawler et al., 2019), cancer (Fleure & Sara, 2020), multiple sclerosis (Meehan & Doody, 2020), and arthritis (Wang et al., 2018).

Positive patient health (e.g., survival rates) and health system (e.g., quality of care) outcomes resulting from CNS roles that complement or substitute for other providers are consistently reported in systematic reviews (Bryant-Lukosius & Rietkoetter, 2020; Salamanca-Balen et al., 2018).

Nurse Consultant

The NC role exists in Australia, the United Kingdom, and Hong Kong. NCs were introduced to retain experienced nurses in clinical practice by broadening the career path (Cashin et al., 2015; Gerrish et al., 2013; Lee et al., 2013) and to improve the quality of care and outcomes for patients (Kennedy et al., 2011). The role was first introduced in Australia in 1986 and was modeled after the CNS role in the United States and the United Kingdom (O'Baugh et al., 2007). Three grade levels differentiate increasing NC responsibilities across five domains (clinical service and consultancy, clinical leadership, research, education, and clinical service planning), incremental work experience as a registered nurse (5–7 years) and specialty experience (0–5 years), and postbasic registration qualifications (New South Wales Department of Health, 2011). NC education in Australia is variable, ranging from a hospital certificate to a master's degree (Baldwin et al., 2013). In the United Kingdom, the NC role was introduced in 1999 and requires master's education and specialty experience. Role domains (direct care, professional leadership and consultancy, education and training, and service development) are similar to Australian NC roles (Gerrish et al., 2013). The NC sits near the top of the nursing career framework (eighth out of nine levels) in the United Kingdom (Royal College of Nursing, 2012a), and since 2000 the number of mental health NCs in the workforce has risen by about 4% (Brimblecombe et al., 2019). In Hong Kong, the NC role was introduced in 2009 with similar requirements, including master's education and 8 years of experience in one of five clinical specialties (diabetes, renal, wound/stoma, psychiatry, and continence; Lee et al., 2013). Role domains include clinical practice, academics, research, and leadership.

Studies show that NCs manage complex patient and healthcare situations (Franks, 2014; Jannings et al., 2010; Lee et al., 2013) and positively impact patient, health provider, organization, and systems outcomes (Cashin et al., 2015; Gerrish et al., 2013; Kennedy et al., 2011; Wong et al., 2017). These areas of impact are similar to those reported for CNSs in the United States (Lewandowski & Adamle, 2009). Similarities between the NC and CNS roles in Canada, New Zealand, and the United States have been noted (Carryer et al., 2018; Jokiniemi et al., 2012).

Emerging and New Frontiers for Future Role Development

There has been trendsetting growth in APN role development in Europe over the last 15 years. Most often in European countries such as Belgium and Germany, APN roles are similar to the CNS role, have been predominately introduced into specialized or hospital-based settings, and may not be formally recognized or have regulatory policies in place to support an expanded scope of practice (Goemaes et al., 2019; Prommersberger, 2020). In France, legislation for the regulation of advanced practice nurses with an expanded scope of practice for patients with chronic stable conditions was established in 2016 and graduates of APN-specific programs are now entering the workforce (Debout, 2018). In Sweden new graduate programs have facilitated the introduction of acute care NPs for surgical care (Jangland et al., 2016) and specialist advanced practice nurses to address healthcare needs in northern regions of the country (Bergström & Lindh, 2018), and new APN roles have been created to improve the coordination of cancer care (Westman et al., 2019). APN roles and education programs are also emerging or established in other Nordic countries, including Denmark, Finland, Iceland, and Norway (Henni et al., 2019; Oddsdóttir & Sveinsdóttir, 2011; Pill et al., 2012; Wisur-Hokkanen et al., 2015). The profile by Krista Jokiniemi describes the CNS role in Finland (Exemplar 5.1). In Spain, the advanced nurse specialist has been defined for midwifery, mental health, occupational health, geriatrics, pediatrics, and family/community nursing (Gonzalez Jurado, 2015), along with APN competencies for research and evidence-based practice, clinical and professional leadership, and care management (Sastre-Fullana et al., 2014). Innovative roles are also emerging to meet the needs of patients with complex comorbid conditions (del Rio Camara et al., 2015). In Switzerland, work has taken place to define (Morin et al., 2013), regulate (Swiss Association for Nursing Science, 2012), and evaluate APN roles (Bryant-Lukosius et al., 2016). The number

EXEMPLAR 5.1
PROFILE ON EMERGING ADVANCED PRACTICE NURSING (APN) ROLES IN FINLAND

Krista Jokiniemi, Postdoctoral Fellow, University of Eastern Finland, Kuopio, Finland, and McMaster University, Hamilton, Canada

Advanced roles for nurses emerged in Finland at the beginning of the 21st century with the introduction of the clinical nurse specialist (CNS) role. Other established roles include the nurse-midwife (NM), nurse anesthetist (NA), and, more recently, the nurse practitioner (NP). Although there is a long history of specialist nursing practice and education in Finland, the concept of the advanced practice nurse at the national level is fairly new. There are no uniform national education programs, legislative or regulatory mechanisms, or protected titles in place for APN roles. As an example, NMs and NAs complete specialty education programs but do not require a master's degree. Close to 100 CNSs work across the country in inpatient and outpatient units, clinics, and primary care. CNSs operate in four distinct, yet interrelated role spheres of patient, nursing, organization, and scholarship. The main goal of CNSs is to improve the quality of care, support staff and interprofessional teams in care provision, and foster the advancement of clinical nursing through scholarship. Competencies for the CNS have been developed and validated within the context of Scandinavian countries. The number of NPs in Finland is not known, but close to 400 NPs have completed university programs. The work of NPs combines clinical expertise and multidisciplinary cooperation with a comprehensive and patient-oriented approach to assess patients' needs for care as well as treat and monitor certain common health problems and conditions. The development of NP competencies is now underway. Strengthening the APN role is high on the healthcare agenda in Finland. Healthcare administrators have recognized the value of these roles for improving nursing practice, promoting evidence-based practices, strengthening the image of nursing, and increasing nursing recruitment and retention. To support the effective implementation of APN roles, it will be imperative to utilize validated competency descriptions to implement APN roles, develop education curricula, and inform evaluations to demonstrate their effectiveness.

of Swiss APN education programs has increased along with graduates working with varied patient populations, such as community-dwelling older adults (Imhof et al., 2012), victims of violence (Romain-Glassey et al., 2014), and adult patients with cancer and other chronic conditions (Bovero et al., 2018; Kocher & Spichiger, 2014; Müller-Staub et al., 2015; Serena et al., 2015). Recently APN roles have been introduced in Swiss primary care settings (Gysin et al., 2019).

Since the mid-1970s, efforts to strengthen the nursing workforce, enhance nursing practice, and develop APN roles in Africa have occurred mainly in sub-Saharan countries where there is a tremendous need to improve population health and increase access to high-quality healthcare services (Christmals & Armstrong, 2019). Most countries in sub-Saharan Africa are of low or lower middle income, with limited resources to support expanded nursing education and to finance healthcare services. This, coupled with the lack of nursing governance and/or regulatory policies and stakeholder resistance, has contributed to delayed progress in nursing and APN role development even in higher-income countries (Chimezie & Ibe, 2019; Dlamini et al., 2020; East et al., 2014; ICN, 2020; Mboineki & Zhang, 2017). Over time, nurses and NMs have responded to address provider shortages, especially in primary care, by taking on medical tasks associated with an expanded scope of practice similar to that of APN roles in other countries but without the benefit of graduate education (Msuya et al., 2017; Ugochukwu et al., 2013).

A burst of recent activities in sub-Saharan Africa suggests the tide is changing and that new progress is being made to develop APN roles. Several initiatives to improve quality and access to postbasic education have led to expansion of the NA workforce in Kenya (Umutesi et al., 2019). In South Africa, competencies and government approval for master's-prepared advanced practice nurses in specialized roles (critical care, midwifery, nephrology, occupational health, ophthalmology, orthopedics, pediatrics, perioperative care, and primary care) have been established (South African Nursing Council, 2014a, 2014b). While the NP role is not yet recognized in South Africa, master's- and PhD-prepared psychiatric nurses providing independent services in private clinics have been reported (Temane et al., 2014). In addition, education programs have been enhanced or new programs have been launched to introduce specialized advanced practice nurses in Botswana, Kenya, Malawi, and Zambia

(Christmals & Armstrong, 2019; North et al., 2019) and NPs in Botswana, Eswatini, Ghana, and Tanzania (Christmals & Armstrong, 2019; Dlamini et al., 2020; ICN, 2020). Exemplar 5.2 provides a profile on the evolution of APN roles in Botswana.

In Middle Eastern countries, APN roles have been introduced to expand, heighten the profile of, and modernize nursing and midwifery workforces. To overcome a reliance on foreign-trained nurses, countries such as Jordan (Zahran et al., 2012), Qatar (Hamad Medical Corporation, 2015), and Saudi Arabia (Brownie et al., 2015) have launched graduate programs in critical care, maternal/newborn care, renal care, oncology, diabetes, and community health. Education programs for NMs, palliative care CNSs, and geriatric NPs have also been established in Israel (Aaron & Andrews, 2016; Collett et al., 2019; Yafa et al., 2016). Hibbert et al (2017) noted that although legislation and regulation do not exist, specialty-based APN and NC roles have been evolving in Saudi Arabia since the 1990s. National forums have taken place to promote APN role development, and a few Saudi nurses have received APN education in other countries to address specific service needs. The concept of APN is newer in the United Arab Emirates; however, a pilot to introduce NPs was felt to be successful and planning is underway to integrate APN roles into the health system (Behrens, 2018). Likewise, stakeholder engagement has occurred to establish a framework to further develop specialist nurses in advanced and non-advanced roles in Iran (Irajpour et al., 2019). CNSs and family NPs are also emerging in Oman (Al-Maqbali, 2014; Almukhaini et al., 2016). Exemplar 5.3 provides a profile of APN roles in Oman.

In Asia, new developments include the establishment of APN graduate programs in Singapore and China (Ayre & Bee, 2014; Wong et al., 2010), an NP graduate program in Japan (Fukuda et al., 2014), and NP programs offering a master's degree in critical care and a postgraduate diploma in primary health care in India (Olabode, 2016). A recent study involving countries in the Western Pacific Region led by Kim

EXEMPLAR 5.2

COUNTRY PROFILE OF THE FAMILY NURSE PRACTITIONER AND ADVANCED PRACTICE NURSE ROLE IN BOTSWANA

Mabedi Kgositau, Lecturer, University of Botswana and Deborah Gray, Adjunct Scholar, University of Botswana, Gaborone, Botswana

Several related factors led to the development of the family nurse practitioner (FNP) and other advanced nurse specialist (NS) roles in Botswana. Botswana is a largely rural, landlocked country in southern Africa with 2.5 million people spread across the country in small rural villages. The health system is dominated by the public health sector and is based on the primary healthcare model. Nurses make up a large proportion of the healthcare workforce and delivery of health care. Botswana is one of the few countries in Africa to establish the FNP role. FNPs provide care at all levels of the health system, mainly in outpatient departments, clinics, health posts, and mobile stops. The FNP role was introduced in response to the government's 1973 Rural Development Policy, which prompted the building of health facilities and the need for nurses in advanced roles to provide services in these facilities, found mostly in rural communities.

The first NP faculty and preceptors were trained in the United States and, on return, were tasked with developing an NP education program. The initial FNP program started at a diploma level in 1981 in one government training institution and was later increased to 2 years. A second FNP program was started in 2005 and has expanded to include advanced NS roles. The University of Botswana began a master's program for NSs in adult and community health in 1996 and now offers master's programs for several NS roles (community health, adult critical care, pediatrics, mental health, midwifery). The master's program for FNPs began in 2005. FNPs continue to be educated at both the diploma and master's levels. In 2019 the School of Nursing at the University of Botswana launched a partially online FNP program with the hope of enabling diploma-prepared FNPs and registered nurses to obtain advanced degrees. There are close to 500 diploma-prepared FNPs and less than 20 master's-prepared FNPs, who work mostly in hospitals, clinics, health training institutions, industries, and private organizations like banks and schools. There are two FNPs in private practice in the country. FNPs have prescriptive authority guided by the Drug and Related Substance Act, which allows nurses to prescribe according to their training and an essential drug list. Overall, there has been steady progress since 1973 to integrate FNPs into the healthcare system in Botswana. Nationally, the recognized need to educate nurses at a higher level has contributed to current efforts to promote master's degree education for FNPs.

EXEMPLAR 5.3

PROFILE ON ADVANCED PRACTICE NURSING (APN) ROLES IN THE SULTANATE OF OMAN

Salma Al-mukhaini, PhD Candidate, School of Nursing, Dalhousie University and Lecturer, Sultan Qaboos University, Muscat, Oman and Zeyana Al-ismaili, NP, College of Health Sciences, Muscat, Oman

Many driving forces have necessitated the development of APN roles in Oman, including the shortage of specialized physicians, emergence of communicable and chronic diseases, increased life expectancy, and the shifting of care from hospital settings to community. Between 2004 and 2011, multiple situational analyses conducted by WHO consultants in collaboration with the Ministry of Health revealed that the traditional roles of nurses in small health centers were extended to include minor diagnoses and treatment as a response to a shortage of physicians. Thus, in collaboration with the WHO, a national APN committee was formed and in 2016 the scope of practice, prescription, licensure, and regulations for APN roles were established. The Ministry of Health has initiated APN title protection legislation due to instances of inappropriate APN title use. In 2016 the NP role was piloted for the first time in the North Al-Khuwair Primary Health Center and the Pediatric Accident and Emergency at the Royal Hospital. In 2017 two certified Adult–Gerontology NPs joined an outpatient clinic at the Royal Hospital and North Alkhuwair Primary Health Center. These NPs are internationally trained since the APN master's program in Oman was just launched in 2016 at Sultan Qaboos University.

APN roles are also found in inpatient settings. Various titles are used to describe APN roles, including CNS. The educational preparation of advanced practice nurses in inpatient settings varies from diploma to master's education. Those without master's education are considered qualified based on their work experience and on-the-job training. While in recent years, considerable progress has been made to introduce APN roles in Oman, further efforts are needed to promote the optimal implementation and integration of these roles within the healthcare system.

and colleagues (2019) highlights progress in APN role development in Asia. The use of varied definitions of APN roles across countries was a challenge for this study, but 10 out of 18 participating countries (Australia, China, Fiji, Hong Kong, Japan, Korea, New Zealand, Philippines, Solomon Islands, Vanuatu) reported having APN roles, with the NM ($n = 8$), CNS or specialist nurses ($n = 8$), and NP ($n = 6$) being the most common. In most countries, regulatory policies were in place for NMs and NPs but not for CNSs. Most often NMs and CNSs required a bachelor's degree or a postgraduate diploma or certificate, while NPs were more likely to require a master's degree. The demand for APN roles in higher-income countries (China, Hong Kong, Japan, and Korea) focused on chronic disease management, geriatrics, and mental health, whereas in lower-income countries (Philippines, Solomon Islands, Vanuatu), APN roles were needed for critical care, maternal care, and infection control. The profile by Frances Kam Yuet Wong describes APN role development in China (Exemplar 5.4).

The next frontier for introducing APN roles is Latin America, where few such roles exist (Bryant-Lukosius, Valaitis et al., 2017). Since 2015, numerous activities have laid the foundation to introduce APN roles into primary healthcare settings. With support from the regional nurse advisor of the Pan American Health Organization (PAHO) and from WHO Collaborating Centres in Primary Health Care in the United States and Canada, meetings have occurred to plan the introduction of APN roles (PAHO & School of Nursing, McMaster University, 2015; PAHO & University of Michigan, 2016), develop APN role competencies (Cassiani et al., 2018; Honig et al., 2019), and establish a framework for three proposed APN roles (NP, case manager, and obstetric nurse; PAHO, 2018). Primary healthcare reform, access to health care, and universal healthcare coverage are the policy drivers for APN roles in the region. Countries best positioned to introduce APN roles are those with existing graduate nursing education programs like Argentina, Brazil, Chile, Colombia, Mexico, Panama, and Peru (PAHO, 2018). Exemplar 5.5 provides a profile of APN role development in Chile.

Another priority on the new frontier will be the global expansion of innovative, sustainable, and cost-effective APN-led models of care. Such models will be essential for achieving sustainable development goals and improving global health through increased access to universal health coverage and access to care for high needs populations (WHO, 2020). In higher-income countries, APN-led models of care have demonstrated

EXEMPLAR 5.4
PROFILE ON ADVANCED PRACTICE NURSING (APN) ROLE DEVELOPMENT IN CHINA

Frances Kam Yuet Wong, Professor, The Hong Kong Polytechnic University, Hunghum, Hong Kong, China SAR

China is a vast country consisting of 23 provinces, five autonomous regions, four municipalities, and two Special Administrative Regions (Hong Kong and Macau). Factors facilitating the introduction of APN roles include the national strategy to develop "Healthy China"; the national strategy to develop nursing, which highlights the importance of specialization in nursing practice; and elevation of the status of nursing from a second-class to first-class subject in 2011. With this change, nursing is more autonomous and university departments of nursing can admit postgraduate students. Many schools work closely with clinical sectors to introduce clinical master's degree programs that prepare advanced practice nurses to meet health service needs. There are now at least 85 clinical master's programs across the country, including an NP program established in 2017 in Beijing. A challenge to introducing APN roles is the shortage of nurses. As of 2018, there were 4.1 million nurses in Mainland China, with a ratio of 2.94 nurses to 1000 population. This ratio is very low compared with other developed countries. Although there is a plan to increase the number of nurses, the sheer inadequacy in number will hamper the development of nursing at an advanced level. Another challenge is that structures to support APN roles (e.g., education, competencies) are not well established in the remote areas and less developed cities. Efforts are now underway by the Chinese Nurses Association to set up national standards and education requirements for different areas of specialty-based practice.

The Guangdong Province illustrates progress in APN role development in China by leveraging the expertise of neighboring nurse leaders in Hong Kong. From 2004 to 2005 the Hong Kong Polytechnic University provided a consultant course in collaboration with Nanfong Medical University to prepare advanced practice nurses in four specialty areas. From 2006 to 2011, 614 nurses were sent to Hong Kong for APN education in 13 different specialties. Guangdong now has a critical mass of advanced practice nurses to provide services and impact patient care. In 2017 the central Chinese government introduced a strategic initiative to connect Hong Kong and Macau with nine mainland cities to form the Greater Bay Area. This initiative provided impetus for further APN role development in this area. In 2018 the Hong Kong Academy of Nursing supported a certification assessment process to endorse 29 Guangdong nurses working in six specialty areas, benchmarking with standards set for advanced practice nurses in Hong Kong. The Guangdong nurses proved to possess the required competencies, making an impact on patient care, service delivery at the systems level, and the profession that is comparable with advanced practice nurses elsewhere.

EXEMPLAR 5.5
PROFILE ON ADVANCED PRACTICE NURSING (APN) ROLES IN CHILE

Maria Consuelo Cerón Mackay, Director of the School of Nursing, Los Andes University, Santiago, Chile

The development of APN roles in Chile began in the late 1990s, when the School of Nursing of Universidad de los Andes recognized the need to develop clinical master's programs. At that time, most graduate programs focused on developing nurses for an academic career. In 2001 a faculty member was sent to study in an APN program at New York University. In return, her commitment was to establish a master's program. The curriculum from New York University was used as a reference point, particularly for the CNS role, because it was most suitable for Chilean healthcare needs in hospitals. The APN master's program was launched in 2011. It is a 2-year program, with the first year focused on theoretical courses and the second year on clinical practice involving physician tutors. While recruitment to the program is low, faculty are sharing their APN education experiences at national conferences and other Latin American countries. The invitation to participate at the 2015 APN Summit organized by PAHO and the School of Nursing at McMaster University stimulated the process to implement the NP role. Main accomplishments included establishing a network among 11 Chilean schools and developing partnerships with nursing organizations, PAHO-Chile, and the Ministry of Health to implement the NP role in primary health care. As a result of these partnerships, schools of nursing participated in a Ministry of Health Advisory Commission on Cancer Care and successfully advocated for the inclusion of oncology APN roles in the National Cancer Plan. A committee involving nursing faculty and clinical nurses in oncology has worked to develop competencies, scope of practice, and education curricula for this new role. The next challenge is to establish the legal framework for APN roles to ensure safe practice.

promising results for increasing access to care, improving health outcomes, and reducing costs, but widespread use of these models is lacking (Casey et al., 2017). Examples of innovative APN-led models in high areas of need relate to mental health (Gillis et al., 2019; Rogers et al., 2016), hospitalized older adults (Hurlock-Chorostecki & Acorn, 2017), cancer and other chronic conditions (Moore, 2018; Wang et al., 2018), and palliative care (Salamanca-Balen et al., 2018). Further spread and increased integration of effective APN-led models of care within healthcare systems is required across developed and developing countries. Future models of APN-led care will also include increased use of technology (WHO, 2020). Technology (e.g., home monitoring, telehealth, videoconferencing, web-based interventions) use in models of care involving advanced practice nurses is emerging (Grant et al., 2017; Mooney et al., 2017; Penny et al., 2018; Romp & Cecil, 2017) and recently heightened as a result of the global COVID-19 pandemic. Postpandemic, the use of virtual models of APN-led care will continue to grow to improve timely access to care.

In summary, APN role development has occurred mainly in high-income countries. The evolution and expansion of APN roles is now taking place in upper-middle-income (e.g., Botswana, China) and lower-middle-income (e.g., India, Kenya) countries and may spread to low-income countries such as those in sub-Saharan Africa. APN roles are needed to strengthen the nursing and midwifery workforce, improve quality of care, reduce healthcare costs, and address health inequities through increased access to care for underserved populations. Areas of need relate to maternal–child care, chronic disease prevention, specialized management of complex and chronic conditions, and aging populations. A high demand for APN roles in primary care in most countries is expected to continue due to shortages of physicians (WHO, 2020).

FACILITATING THE INTRODUCTION AND INTEGRATION OF ADVANCED PRACTICE NURSING ROLES

Contextual factors (e.g., sociopolitical, economic, geographic) influence the introduction, optimal utilization, and full integration of APN roles within healthcare systems, with barriers often representing the absent mirror versions of facilitators (DiCenso et al., 2010). Table 5.1 highlights key facilitating factors, including pan-approaches and collaboration, funding and payment arrangements, systematic approaches to role planning, and the use and generation of evidence. Levels of engagement (international, national, and organizational) for successful APN role introduction and integration are examined for each factor.

Pan-Approaches and Collaboration

Pan-approaches are activities that span across jurisdictions. At the international level this may include activities involving more than one country and at the national level activities that cut across regions within a country. National and international collaboration related to human resource policies and priorities, legislation and regulation, and competency development and education are strategic for jump-starting the introduction and development of APN roles. Pan-approaches

TABLE 5.1

Facilitating Factors for the Introduction and Integration of Advanced Practice Nursing Roles

Facilitating Factors	International	National or Regional	Organization
Pan-approaches and collaboration			
Human resource policies and priorities	X	X	
Regulation	X	X	
Education and mentorship	X	X	X
Funding and payment arrangements			
To support the introduction of innovative advanced practice nursing roles and new models of care		X	X
Systematic approaches to role planning		X	X
Use and generation of evidence	X	X	X

at the international level that foster mutual learning and sharing of intellectual capital and resources across countries will be essential for the development of APN roles in lower-income countries (WHO, 2020). The growing importance of international pan-approaches for APN role development is illustrated in recent models outlining strategies for culturally relevant and successful international partnerships for NMs and NAs (Hu et al., 2019; Spies et al., 2017).

Human Resource Policies and Priorities

At the international level, policy priorities of the United Nations and the WHO have played a critical role in raising the profile of and triggering actions for APN role development. For example, United Nations (2012) and WHO (2010) priorities to improve global health influenced the PAHO 52nd Directing Council's (2013) resolution on Human Resources for Health calling for the introduction of APN roles for primary health care in Latin America and the Caribbean (Cassiani & Zug, 2014). This resolution laid the foundation for APN role development and partnerships between the PAHO, regional and international schools of nursing, and WHO collaborating centers. An output of these partnerships has been the relatively rapid process to introduce APN roles in Chile (Aguirre-Boza et al., 2019). The recent WHO (2020) report on the world's nursing provides compelling recommendations for strengthening the global nursing workforce that echo the facilitators outlined in Table 5.1 related to regulation, education, funding arrangements, and the use of evidence for systematic workforce planning. At national and international levels, leveraging the WHO (2020) recommendations to guide policies and actions will be important for the continued evolution of APN roles.

A powerful example offering a template for international nursing and APN association leadership in health policy and human resource planning is the collaboration between the ICM, the United Nations, and the WHO to improve the global midwifery workforce (Day-Stirk et al., 2014; UNFPA, 2011, 2014; WHO, 2015a). Through collaboration, midwifery workforce indicators and targets were agreed upon and implemented at national levels, resulting in a detailed data set used to evaluate and compare the impact of workforce policies and initiatives across countries. Early results showed improvement in educating and expanding the number of midwifery providers and in maternal–child health outcomes UNFPA, (2014). The midwifery example is notable because of its success in workforce development in low- and middle-income countries where health needs are the greatest and where few APN roles exist. The ICM (2015) emphasized the essential role of national midwifery associations in workforce policy and decision making. Similarly, a brief developed for the ICN provides guidance on how national nursing associations can provide leadership to promote APN role development (Bryant-Lukosius & Martin-Misener, 2016). A stronger role for nurses, including those in APN roles, in international organizations such as the WHO is also needed to inform human resource policy priorities and implementation strategies (Wong et al., 2015).

At the national level, healthcare contexts related to needs, policies, organization of services, the workforce, economics, and the societal role of women influence APN roles (Heale & Rieck-Buckley, 2015; Liu et al., 2015). In most countries, the integration of APN roles within health systems is a slow and complex process occurring over many years and often decades. An important role of national associations and nurse leaders is to formalize and guide a strategic process based on an analysis of existing healthcare policies (Officer et al., 2019; Schober et al., 2016). Through policy analysis, priorities and levers to facilitate APN role introduction or expansion and strategies to address policy barriers to successful implementation can be identified. At national and regional levels, ongoing analysis is important for assessing the impact of policy changes on APN roles. For example, in Kentucky the loosening of policies requiring physician oversight did not improve access to NAs due to other influential factors related to socioeconomics, organizational policies, and types of hospital (Feyereisen et al., 2020). National practice pattern studies can also facilitate role integration by providing information to define APN roles, identify implementation barriers, and assess deployment in relation to policies and priorities for improving health (Brimblecombe et al., 2019; DiCenso et al., 2010; Gardner et al., 2016).

The introduction of APN roles may be advantaged in countries with centralized healthcare governance and national health policies aligned with the roles. One example is Ghana, where national health human resource policies since 1995 have led to a steady increase in midwives (Matthews & Campbell, 2015). Qatar's National Cancer Strategy (2011–2016), with the goal for all cancer patients to be cared for by a CNS (Qatar Supreme Council of Health, 2011), quickly led to the introduction of the role (Oxford Business Group, 2014). A systematic approach to introduce NM and NP roles occurred in Ireland, where the national health ministry worked with the national nursing council to deploy roles focused on priorities for healthcare reform (Begley et al., 2010). By 2009 and within 8 years, Ireland introduced over 120 NPs, accounting for 0.2% of the nursing workforce (Delamaire & Lafortune, 2010). This is quite an accomplishment compared with Canada, with just 1600 NPs in 2008 making up 0.6% of the nursing workforce after 40 years of development. A second strategic launch in Ireland is now underway to deploy 700 new NPs for underserved populations (Ireland Department of Health, 2019). Since 2008, the number of NPs in Canada has increased sharply to over 6000 (CIHI, 2020). However, responsibility for health care lies with 13 provinces and territories, resulting in disparate deployment, with over 56% of NPs working in one province.

Regulation

The regulation of nursing is usually tied to health laws protecting public safety and promotes high-quality care by defining the scope and standards of practice, licensure, credentials, and educational requirements of the profession (ICN, 2013). Internationally, the regulatory requirements for APN roles are variable or absent in many countries (Carney, 2015; Heale & Rieck-Buckley, 2015; Maier, 2015). The WHO (2020) has called for countries to improve nursing regulation by ensuring the least restrictive policies while at the same time maintaining protection of the public. Legislative and regulatory policies embracing optimal scope of practice and full role autonomy without restrictions (e.g., physician supervision for practice or prescriptions) facilitate NM and NP recruitment and retention and increased access to care, especially for rural and vulnerable populations (Kuo et al., 2013; Ranchoff & Declercq, 2020; Xue et al., 2016). Restrictive scope of practice regulations inhibit innovation and the introduction of new models of care involving APN roles, reduce productivity, and increase the costs of healthcare services (Ritter et al., 2018). Regulatory policies offering title protection and standardized education and competencies have been found to improve NP role clarity and implementation (Lowe et al., 2011). Conversely, the lack of regulation for CNS and other APN roles contributes to poor role clarity, variability in how roles are operationalized, and an inability to monitor their workforce contributions and negatively impact role integration and sustainability (East et al., 2015; Kilpatrick et al., 2013).

Reports of pan-approaches at the international level to improve APN regulation are few and would be an asset for guiding role introduction in low-income countries and those with new or emerging roles. The importance of international collaboration is illustrated by the Global Midwifery Twinning project involving the Royal College of Midwives in the United Kingdom and midwifery associations in Nepal, Cambodia, and Uganda (Ireland et al., 2015). The project was successful in building the capacity of midwives to lead and advocate for stronger midwifery associations, education, and regulation in these countries. International variability in APN role titling and credentials restricts the mobility of nurses across countries to address service needs (Scanlon, Bryant-Lukosius et al., 2019). ICN (2020) guidance on APN, developed with input from international stakeholders, is a positive step toward international agreement on the credentialing of CNS and NP roles.

At national levels, pan-approaches to legislation and regulation in support of APN roles have been successful in Canada, the United States, New Zealand, and Wales for obtaining greater consistency in these policies, improving role understanding and implementation, and creating ways to monitor deployment across jurisdictions (Bryant-Lukosius, Martin-Misener et al., 2018; Goudreau, 2014; Kooienga & Carryer, 2015; National Council of State Boards of Nursing, 2008; Ryley & Middleton, 2015). In many countries, establishing a nursing regulatory framework will be an essential step in defining requirements for advanced practice. Ben Natan et al. (2013) found that the Israeli public was in favor of expanding nurses' scope of practice and authority. Engaging the public in the discourse may be an effective strategy to strengthen legislative and regulatory policies supportive of APN roles.

Competency Development, Education, and Mentorship

Competencies are the knowledge, skills, judgment, and attributes required by advanced practice nurses to provide safe, ethical practice (Canadian Nurses Association [CNA], 2010). They are informed by a collective understanding of the APN role and provide the basis for entry-to-practice requirements and APN education curricula. In 2008 the ICN outlined competencies for the advanced practice nurse, and this has been an important resource for national nursing associations to develop competencies for their country and to lobby for these requirements (DiCenso et al., 2010). However, varied national interpretations of what an advanced practice nurse is have led to a perceived lack of role clarity internationally (Dowling et al., 2013). The evolution of and the need for competency guidance are demonstrated by activities in several countries to establish or refine competencies in order to define and clarify APN roles and strengthen role implementation (CNA, 2015, 2019; Cassiani et al., 2018; Chang et al., 2012; Jokiniemi & Miettinen, 2020; Lin et al., 2015; Maijala et al., 2015; Nieminen et al., 2011).

A growing body of evidence from studies examining APN roles across countries suggests that international convergence on defining and understanding APN roles may be occurring. Sastre-Fullana et al. (2014) conducted a review of APN competency frameworks and found agreement on 17 competencies across six types of APN roles in 26 countries. Research, clinical and professional leadership, mentoring and coaching, and expert clinical judgment were common role domains in 16 of 29 countries. Jokiniemi et al. (2012) found similar domains for CNS and NC roles in the United States, Australia, and Finland. The Advanced Practice Nurse Role Delineation (APRD) tool developed in the United States has been used in different countries to examine APN role activities in five domains (direct care, support of systems, education, research, professional leadership) based on the Strong model (Bryant-Lukosius, Jokiniemi et al., 2018; Carryer et al., 2018; Gardner et al., 2016). Consistent findings demonstrate the ability of the APRD tool to discern different types of advanced and nonadvanced nursing roles. In addition, a visual analysis of mixed APN documents (e.g., policies, competencies, standards, role descriptions) from 19 countries found that 32% of the data could be mapped to the domains of the Strong model (Sastre-Fullana et al., 2021). The results of these studies can be used to inform APN competency development at national and international levels.

At the international level, pan-initiatives may facilitate the consistency and quality of APN education across countries. For example, in addition to standards for practice and education, the International Federation of Nurse Anesthetists developed an approval process for schools, now completed by 14 education programs in nine countries (Horton et al., 2014). A similar international accreditation program has been developed and pilot tested in two countries for midwifery education programs (Nove et al., 2018). The Bologna process aims to standardize all professional education requirements across Europe. This process has accelerated the professionalization of nursing and creation of baccalaureate and master's education programs necessary to develop APN roles (Collins & Hewer, 2014).

At national levels, health policies, population health needs, and social factors influence the level and types of APN education (Liu et al., 2015). Thus it is not surprising that a recent study found substantive variability in admission criteria, curricular content, clinical requirements, and teaching methods for NP programs across six countries (Jeffery et al., 2020). In many countries, APN role development is limited by a lack of graduate and specialty-based education programs and master's-prepared faculty with APN experience (Bryant-Lukosius, Martin-Misener, et al., 2018; Goh et al., 2019; Heale & Rieck-Buckley, 2015). There are numerous examples of partnerships between countries with emerging APN roles and schools of nursing in countries with established roles to address these education gaps. One such case is in Qatar, where the government partnered with the University of Calgary in Canada to develop undergraduate and graduate nursing education programs (Oxford Business Group, 2014). Partnerships with foreign funding agencies and universities have been influential in the development of APN roles and education programs in sub-Saharan Africa (Christmals & Armstrong, 2019). ICN (2020) guidance strongly supports a master's degree in nursing as the minimum education requirement for APN roles. There is limited research on APN education, but a few studies suggest that master's-prepared nurses implement their roles in a manner more consistent with APN standards of practice compared with non-master's-prepared nurses (Bryant-Lukosius, Jokiniemi et al., 2018; Kilpatrick et al., 2013). The leveling of APN education has become somewhat contentious with the requirement of the doctorate of nursing practice for APRNs in the United States (Fullerton et al., 2019; Ketefian & Redman, 2015). This is not an attainable goal in many countries where basic nursing education is being developed or where resources for graduate education are limited. At national levels it is important to keep in mind that a good fit between APN curricula and practice needs is key for optimal role implementation (Martin-Misener et al., 2010).

A growing area of international concern expressed by new graduates of APN education programs is that they feel overwhelmed and lack confidence and experience to fully implement their roles (Dover et al., 2019; Faraz, 2019; MacLellan et al., 2017; Officer et al., 2019; Tracy, 2017). Several factors contribute to this concern, including the increasing number of younger APN graduates with less clinical experience and the challenging demands of these complex roles. Inadequate preparation of new APN graduates has important implications for successful APN role implementation, job satisfaction, and retention. In response to this issue, many healthcare organizations are stepping up to provide transition supports such as fellowships (Keefe Marcoux et al., 2019), internships (Bruwer & Little, 2020), mentorship (Moss & Jackson, 2019), and communities of practice (Gullick & West, 2015). Further research is required to determine the effectiveness of these strategies for improving APN role transition and implementation for new graduates (Speight et al., 2019). At organizational levels, academic-clinical practice partnerships to provide mentorship and continuing education for advanced practice nurses can help build their confidence and strengthen skills in underdeveloped areas such as research (Bryant-Lukosius, 2015; Harbman et al., 2016).

Funding and Reimbursement Arrangements

Funding at national/regional and organizational levels is essential to introduce and expand the supply of advanced practice nurses to meet demands for health care. In the United States, funding from the 2010 Patient Protection and Affordable Care Act increased the number of APRNs providing primary care (Lathrop & Hodnicki, 2014). In Canada, allocation of specific government funding in the province of Ontario for NPs in primary, palliative, and long-term care enabled role expansion in these high-need areas (Bryant-Lukosius, Martin-Misener, et al., 2018). In the absence of targeted funding in the same province, similar expansion has not occurred for CNSs, acute care NPs, or NPs in anesthesia care, and in some cases positions were lost. In other provinces, the lack of dedicated funding has been a barrier to the introduction and sustainability of NP roles in primary care (Hunter et al., 2016). At an organizational level, advanced practice nurses are most often an operational cost as salaried employees. External funds or reallocated existing funds are required by organizations to introduce, maintain, or expand APN roles and may be difficult to obtain in challenging economic conditions (Gagan et al., 2014). Results of systematic reviews examining APN outcomes demonstrate that advanced practice nurses may reduce healthcare inefficiencies in 5 out of 10 areas identified by the WHO (Bryant-Lukosius, Valaitis et al., 2017). Using similar data to create a sound business case may help healthcare organizations identify efficiencies and cost savings that can be gained by the innovative use of APN roles and applied to offset salary costs. A study conducted in South Korea found that healthcare consumers would be willing to pay for family education and counseling services provided by critical care advanced practice nurses and that the fee they would pay was very consistent with existing national health insurance billing codes (Ko et al., 2019). These findings have created the opportunity for nurse leaders to advocate for the inclusion of APN services within these billing codes.

Increasingly, funders are looking to implement different reimbursement models to improve quality of care and reduce healthcare costs, but little is known about how these models impact APN roles, especially outside of North America. As an example, Shurson and Gregg (2019) found an absence of research examining NPs related to pay-for-performance models. Fee-for-service reimbursement models for advanced practice nurses exist in the United States and in Australia for primary care NPs (Carter et al., 2015). In the United States, pediatric and family NPs, NMs, and, to a lesser extent NAs and CNSs, can bill Medicaid and third-party payers such as insurance companies (American

Nurses Association, 2016). Such models provide economic flexibility to increase access to care and introduce new services involving APN roles, especially for high-risk, low-income, and underserved populations (Barnes et al., 2017) and may partially explain differences among countries in the number of NPs making up the nursing workforce. Compared with other countries with established roles, the United States has a significantly larger proportion of NPs in the nursing workforce (Maier et al., 2016). The recruitment of advanced practice nurses is also enhanced when policies ensure that they are reimbursed at the same funding level as physicians (Barnes et al., 2017).

How advanced practice nurses work may also be influenced by reimbursement policies. For example, more NPs working in community centers receiving all-inclusive fees for visits paid by Medicare had their own patient panel, compared with NPs in other settings reimbursed by Medicare at 85% of a physician fee (Poghosyan et al., 2017). Physician support is key for optimal NP role implementation and can be fostered by mitigating the impact of NPs on physician income. Reimbursement models not reliant on physician fee-for-service reimbursement and that support collaboration with NPs are advantageous in that regard (DiCenso et al., 2010). Flexible compensation models that enabled NAs to be self-directed in choosing work locations and areas of practice were also found to stimulate NA recruitment and retention and led to savings in human resource costs (Dunworth, 2020).

Systematic Approaches to Role Planning

APN roles have similar characteristics to complex interventions due to their multiple interacting competencies, responsibilities for addressing difficult healthcare problems, and multidimensional actions to improve outcomes for a variety of groups (e.g., patients, families, providers, teams, organizations, health systems; Bryant-Lukosius, Martin-Misener, et al., 2017). At national and regional levels, several factors (e.g., competencies, education, regulation, legislation, funding) are required to introduce and successfully implement all aspects of these complex roles. Other factors at organizational levels such as structures and processes are necessary to fully operationalize APN roles and expertise. Worldwide, numerous studies indicate that these factors are often not in place, resulting in serious challenges to job satisfaction and the recruitment and retention of advanced practice nurses, and APN role effectiveness, impact, and sustainability (Andregard & Jangland, 2014; Fernandez et al., 2017; Higgins et al., 2014; Officer et al., 2019; Sangster-Gormley et al., 2011; Steinke et al., 2017). These consistent findings pinpoint the critical need for the use of more systematic approaches to APN role planning and implementation at jurisdictional and organizational levels.

One such approach is the PEPPA (Participatory, Evidence-Based, Patient-Focused Process for Advanced Practice Nursing) framework, offering a nine-step participatory, evidence-based, patient-focused, process for APN role development, implementation, and evaluation (Bryant-Lukosius & DiCenso, 2004). PEPPA incorporates principles for effective health human resource planning and has been used successfully to introduce APN and other provider roles in over 20 countries (Boyko et al., 2016). The framework can be used by decision makers, researchers, educators, and nurses at international, national, regional, organizational, practice setting, or team levels to address APN role barriers related to role clarity, use of APN expertise, scope of practice, supportive practice environments, and evaluation. For example, at an international policy level, PEPPA was used to develop a plan for implementing APN roles in Latin America and the Caribbean (Oldenburger et al., 2017) and further applied at a national level to introduce the roles in Chile (Aguirre-Boza et al., 2019).

Involving stakeholders (e.g., patients, policymakers, managers, providers) early in the process is essential for successful APN role implementation. Many studies identify that key stakeholders, including the public, often lack a clear understanding of APN roles and how they can effectively contribute to the delivery of healthcare services (Casey et al., 2019; Craswell & Dwyer, 2019; Officer et al., 2019; Schober et al., 2016). A major strength of PEPPA is the use of stakeholder engagement strategies to determine the need for and define the role, obtain role acceptance and support, and anticipate and resolve implementation barriers (Bryant-Lukosius, Martin-Misener et al., 2017). For example, Dlamini et al., (2020) engaged multilevel stakeholders (policy, practice, community) though the first five steps of the framework to develop a contextually relevant family NP program in Eswatini.

At regional and organizational levels, the leadership and resources provided by healthcare administrators are pivotal for effective APN role implementation (Carter et al., 2010; Elliott et al., 2016; Heale et al., 2014). Healthcare leaders can use PEPPA to guide the role; planning and introduction process and to establish structures (e.g., policies, job descriptions) and supports (e.g., mentorship) to facilitate APN role implementation within practice settings, programs, and teams (Bryant-Lukosius, Martin-Misener et al., 2017). Processes such as recruitment/retention and orientation strategies and decentralized leadership structures that integrate APN roles; create forums for collaboration among advanced practice nurses; and build, utilize, and profile their leadership expertise at multiple levels can foster the successful implementation of these roles (Bourque et al., 2019; Fischer-Cartlidge et al., 2019; Hurlock-Chorostecki & McCallum, 2016).

Use and Generation of Evidence

Linked with poor planning and the lack of systematic approaches to introducing APN roles is the fact that existing evidence is often not used to inform this process and that influential stakeholders (e.g., government policymakers, healthcare administrators, healthcare team members, and the public) at all health system levels (international, national, organizational) do not have a good understanding of the roles (Andregard & Jangland, 2014; DiCenso et al., 2010; Schober et al., 2016; Wisur-Hokkanen et al., 2015). To address these issues, PEPPA promotes the use of existing data for making decisions at each step of APN role development, and it is through this process that stakeholders become more knowledgeable and accepting of the roles. Other strategies are also required to engage and inform stakeholders. Conducting a stakeholder analysis is beneficial for identifying the levels of support, influence, and priorities of decision makers (Bryant-Lukosius, 2009; Schober et al., 2016). APN champions can then be identified and leveraged to deliver evidence-based messages that are tailored to address the varied information needs of different stakeholders. Using multiple strategies to deliver tailored information in person and electronically, and in concise formats such as briefing notes, facilitates receipt of key messages by busy decision makers (Carter et al., 2014; Kilpatrick et al., 2015). The INP/APNN is a special interest group of the ICN that supports APN role development by providing information and creating forums, such as a biannual conference, for information sharing and networking (ICN, 2016). Network committees focus on practice, education, policy, and research and facilitate international surveys to examine APN roles (Heale & Rieck-Buckley, 2015; Steinke et al., 2017).

Numerous systematic reviews of randomized controlled trials conducted over the past 35 years demonstrate the effectiveness of APN roles, especially in high-income countries (Bryant-Lukosius, Carter, et al., 2015; Bryant-Lukosius, Cosby et al., 2015; Donald et al., 2013, 2015; Johantgen et al., 2012; Kilpatrick et al., 2014; Martin-Misener et al., 2015; Morilla-Herrera et al., 2016; Stanik-Hutt et al., 2013; Swan et al., 2015; Tsiachristas et al., 2015). However, many of the studies included in these systematic reviews reflect groundbreaking evaluations conducted in the 1990s, and few were published prior to 2010 (Bryant-Lukosius & Rietkoetter, 2020). Thus the current synthesized evidence about APN roles may not be relevant to healthcare systems of today and related advances in treatment and technology. Further research is needed on the cost-effectiveness of APN roles (Marshall et al., 2015), and guidelines to facilitate economic evaluations of these roles are being developed (Lopatina et al., 2017). The need for better research evidence on the effectiveness of nursing and APN roles, especially in lower-income countries, has been highlighted by the WHO (2020). Priority gaps to be addressed relate to nurse-led interventions focused on the social determinants of health, climate change, and complex emergency situations. The lack of country-specific (Bryant-Lukosius et al., 2016) and role-specific (Brimblecombe et al., 2019) data about effectiveness also hinders the introduction and sustainability of APN roles. In addition, improved data management systems at international, national, and organizational levels are also required to capture up-to-date health human resource data. Agreement on indicators and targets for health systems integration for all types of APN roles will be essential to ensure their adequate supply and optimal deployment.

To support contemporary evaluations and the generation of meaningful data for effective decision making about APN roles at national, organizational, setting, and team levels, the PEPPA framework has been enhanced (Bryant-Lukosius et al., 2016). Called

PEPPA-Plus, the framework provides guidance and tools to address the information needs of different decision makers across three stages of APN role development (introduction, implementation, and long-term sustainability). So far, international use of PEPPA-Plus has occurred to evaluate APN roles in Canada (Rickards & Hamilton, 2020) and Switzerland (Gysin et al., 2019; Kobleder et al., 2018; Serena et al., 2017).

NEXT STEPS IN THE GLOBAL EVOLUTION OF ADVANCED PRACTICE NURSING ROLES

Improving human resources for health will continue to be a global priority as outlined by the WHO's (2016 *Health Workforce 2030 Strategic Plan* and its report on the *State of the World's Nursing* (WHO, 2020). Recommendations for both reports outline priorities for investments in the health workforce, needs-based workforce planning, improved access to and quality of education, and optimizing provider scopes of practice that will benefit the global development of APN roles. Thus the next decade will provide exciting opportunities to expand the contribution of APN roles for improving global health. At the international level, nursing organizations and leaders can employ a variety of strategies to support the global development of APN roles, especially in countries where the roles do not exist or are just emerging. These strategies are summarized in Box 5.1. Strategies that nursing organizations and leaders can use to support APN role development at country levels are summarized in Box 5.2.

BOX 5.1

International-Level Strategies to Support the Global Development of Advanced Practice Nursing Roles

- Leverage and share expertise and resources for APN education, practice, and policy across countries
- Improve role clarity by working toward greater consensus on role definitions and terminology, including delineation of specialized roles at an advanced level
- Support policies that build capacity and prevent the outmigration of nursing leaders, educators, researchers, and advanced practice nurses from countries where APN roles are just getting started

Adapted from Bryant-Lukosius & Martin-Misener, 2016; Dury et al., 2014; Kooienga & Carryer, 2015; Nardi & Diallo, 2014; National Nursing Centres Consortium, 2014.

BOX 5.2

Country-Level Strategies to Support Advanced Practice Nursing Role Development

- Focus efforts on placing nurses at high-level policy decision-making tables to advocate for the APN role
- Advocate for systematic and evidence-based approaches to role development, implementation, and evaluation
- Connect with key stakeholders around shared policy concerns to create conditions for healthcare organization and system transformational change
- Build consensus among stakeholders on health systems solutions that utilize APN roles
- Establish a knowledge translation plan to promote stakeholder awareness and understanding of APN roles and their benefits and to reduce barriers to role implementation
- Create communities of practice to develop advanced practice nurses

Adapted from Bryant-Lukosius & Martin-Misener, 2016; National Nursing Centres Consortium, 2014.

CONCLUSION

To date, high-income countries have benefited the most from the introduction and expansion of APN roles. Despite growing evidence of APN role effectiveness for improving health outcomes, increasing access and quality of care, and reducing the unnecessary use of costly acute care services, the overall integration of APN roles within healthcare systems is limited in most countries. Over the next decade, policy priorities to improve global health by strengthening the development and use of nursing expertise will create new prospects to expand the introduction of APN roles. Successful health system integration of the next generation of APN roles will require pan-approaches, including international collaboration, greater attention to the use of systematic approaches, and collection and use of good data to identify implementation barriers and monitor role deployment and impact.

KEY SUMMARY POINTS

- There has been tremendous growth in the introduction of APN roles over the last decade. Population health needs for increased access to primary health care, care for the elderly, and chronic disease prevention and management will further drive role expansion.
- APN roles are an important strategy for developing and strengthening the nursing workforce to meet population health and health service needs.
- Systematic approaches to APN role development are essential for optimal role implementation and impact on outcomes.
- At international and national levels, ways to collect better APN role workforce data are needed to ensure an adequate supply of advanced practice nurses and their optimal deployment to areas of greatest need.

REFERENCES

Aaron, E. M., & Andrews, C. (2016). Integration of advanced practice providers into the Israeli healthcare system. *Israel Journal of Health Policy Research, 5*(1), 1–18.

Aguirre-Boza, F., Cerón Mackay, M. C., Pulcini, J., & Bryant-Lukosius, D. (2019). Implementation strategy for advanced practice nursing in primary health care in Chile. *Acta Paulista de Enfermagen, 32*(2), 120–128.

Al-Maqbali, M. R. (2014). In *Establishing the nurse practitioner role in Oman. Presentation at the Clute International Academic Conference* March 16-18, 2014.

Almukhaini, S. J., Donesky, D., & Scruth, E. A. (2016). Oman: The emergence of the clinical nurse specialist. *Clinical Nurse Specialist: The Journal for Advanced Nursing Practice, 30*(2), 71–73.

American Association of Nurse Practitioners (AANP). (2020). *NP facts.* https://storage.aanp.org/www/documents/NPFacts__080420.pdf

American College of Nurse-Midwives. (2019). *Essential facts about midwives.* https://www.midwife.org/acnm/files/cclibraryfiles/filename/000000007531/EssentialFactsAboutMidwives-UPDATED.pdf

American Nurses Association (ANA). (2016). *Medicaid coverage of advanced practice nursing.* http://www.nursingworld.org/DocumentVault/GOVA/Federal/Federal-Issues/MedicaidReimbursement%20.aspx

Andregard, A., & Jangland, E. (2014). The tortuous journey of introducing the nurse practitioner as the new member of the healthcare team: A meta-synthesis. *Scandinavian Journal of Caring Sciences, 29*, 3–14.

APRN Joint Dialogue Group. (2008). *Consensus Model for APRN regulation: Licensure, accreditation, certification & education.* http://www.aacn.nche.edu/education-resources/APRNReport.pdf

Auerbach, D. I., Buerhaus, P. I., & Staiger, D. O. (2020). Implications of the rapid growth of the nurse practitioner workforce in the US. *Health Affairs, 39*(2), 273–279.

Australian Health Practitioner Regulation Agency. (2019). *Annual report 2019/19. Our national scheme for a safer healthcare.* https://www.ahpra.gov.au/Publications/Annual-reports/Annual-Report-2019.aspx

Ayre, T. C., & Bee, T. S. (2014). Advanced practice nursing in Singapore. *Proceedings of Singapore Healthcare, 23*(4), 269–270.

Baldwin, R., Duffield, C. M., Fry, M., Roche, M., Stasa, H., & Solman, A. (2013). The role and functions of clinical nurse consultants, an Australian advanced practice role: A descriptive exploratory cohort study. *International Journal of Nursing Studies, 50*(3), 326–334.

Barnawi, N., Richter, S., & Habib, F. (2013). Midwifery and midwives: A historical analysis. *Journal of Research in Nursing and Midwifery, 2*(8), 114–121.

Barnes, H., Maier, C. B., Sarik, Altares, D., Germack, H., D., Aiken, L. H., & McHugh, M. D (2017). Effects of regulation and payment policies on nurse practitioners' clinical practices. *Medical Care Research and Review, 74*(4), 431–451.

Begley, C., Murphy, K., Higgins, A., Elliott, N., Lalor, J., Sheerin, F., Coyne, I., Comiskey, C., Normand, C., Casey, C., Dowling, M., Devane, D., Cooney, A., Farrelly, F., Brennan, M., Meskell, P., & MacNeela, P. (2010). *Evaluation of clinical nurse and midwife specialist and advanced nurse and midwife practitioner roles in Ireland (SCAPE): Final report.* Dublin, Ireland: National Council for the Professional Development of Nursing and Midwifery. https://nursing-midwifery.tcd.ie/assets/research/pdf/SCAPE_Final_Report_13th_May.pdf

Behrens, S. A. (2018). International nursing: Constructing an advanced practice registered nurse practice model in the UAE. Using innovation to address cultural implications and challenges in an international enterprise. *Nursing Administration Quarterly, 42*(1), 83–90.

Ben Natan, M., Dmitriev, Y., Shubovich, O., & Sharon, I. (2013). Views of the Israeli public on expanding the authority of nurses. *Journal of Nursing Management, 21*(2), 351–358.

Bergström, P., & Lindh, V. (2018). Developing the role of Swedish advance practice nurse through a blended learning master's program: Consequences of knowledge and organization. *Nurse Education and Practice, 28*, 196–201

Bethea, A., Samanta, D., White, T., Payne, N., & Hardway, J. (2019). Nurse practitioners' role in improving service for elderly trauma patients. *Journal of Trauma Nursing, 26*(4), 174–179.

Bourque, H., Gunn, K., & MacLeod, M. (2019). A pathway for implementing the nurse practitioner workforce in a rural and remote health region. *Canadian Journal of Nursing Leadership, 33*(2), 44–53.

Bovero, M., Giacomo, C., Ansari, M., & Roulin, M. J. (2018). Role of advanced nurse practitioners in the care pathway for children diagnosed with leukemia. *European Journal of Oncology Nursing, 36*, 68–74.

Boyko, J., Carter, N., & Bryant-Lukosius, D. (2016). Assessing the spread and uptake of a framework for introducing and evaluating advanced practice nursing roles. *Worldviews on Evidence-based Nursing, 13*, 277–284.

Brimblecombe, N., Nolan, F., Khoo, M. E., Culloty, L., O'Connor, K., & McGregor-Johnson, L. (2019). The nurse consultant in mental health services: A national mixed methods study of an advanced practice role. *Journal of Psychiatric and Menth Health Nursing, 26*(5-6), 117–130.

Brownie, S. M., Hunter, L. H., Aqtash, S., & Day, G. E. (2015). Establishing policy foundations and regulatory systems to enhance nursing practice in the United Arab Emirates. *Policy, Politics and Nursing Practice, 16*(1–2), 38–50.

Bruwer, L., & Little, L. (2020). Development of a clinical nurse specialist internship for master's graduate students to improve role transition. *Clinical Nurse Specialist, 34*(4), 178–181.

Bryant-Lukosius, D. (2009). *Designing innovative cancer services and advanced practice nursing roles: Toolkit*: Cancer Care Ontario. https://www.cancercare.on.ca/cms/one.aspx?pageId=9387

Bryant-Lukosius, D. (2015). Mentorship: A navigation strategy for promoting oncology nurse engagement in research. *Canadian Oncology Nursing Journal, 23*(3), 1–4.

Bryant-Lukosius, D., Carter, N., Reid, K., Donald, F., Martin-Misener, R., Kilpatrick, K., Harbman, P., Kaasalainen, S., Marshall, D., Charbonneau-Smith, R., & DiCenso, A. (2015). The clinical effectiveness and cost-effectiveness of clinical nurse specialist-led hospital to home transitional care: A systematic review. *Journal of Evaluation of Clinical Practice, 21*, 763–781.

Bryant-Lukosius, D., Cosby, R., Bakker, D., Earle, C., & Burkoski, V. (2015). *Practice guideline on the effective use of advanced practice nurses in the delivery of adult cancer services in Ontario*: Cancer Care Ontario. https://www.cancercare.on.ca/common/pages/UserFile.aspx?fileId=340702

Bryant-Lukosius, D., & DiCenso, A. (2004). A framework for the introduction and evaluation of advanced practice nursing roles. *Journal of Advanced Nursing, 48*(5), 530–540.

Bryant-Lukosius, D., Jokiniemi, K., Martin-Misener, R., Roussel, J., Carr, M., Kilpatrick, K., Tranmer, J., & Rietkoetter, S. (2018). *Clarifying the contributions of specialized nursing roles in Canada: Results of a national study.* Panel presentation. In *Canadian Nurses Association Conference*, June 20.

Bryant-Lukosius, D., & Martin-Misener, M. (2016). *Advanced practice nursing: An essential component of country level human resources for health.* Policy brief for the International Council of Nurses. http://www.icn.ch/images/stories/documents/pillars/sew/HRH/ICN_Policy_Brief_6.pdf

Bryant-Lukosius, D., Martin-Misener, R., Roussel, J., Carter, N., Kilpatrick, K., & Brousseau, L. (2018). Policy and the integration of advanced practice nursing roles in Canada: Are we making progress? In K. A. Goudreau, & M. Smolenski (Eds.), *Health policy and advanced practice nursing, impact and implications* (2nd ed.) (pp. 357–374). Springer.

Bryant-Lukosius, D., Martin-Misener, M., Tranmer, D., Donald, F., Brousseau, L., & DiCenso, A. (2017). Resources to facilitate advanced practice nurse outcome research. In R. M. Kleinpell (Ed.), *Outcome assessment in advanced practice nursing* (4th ed.) (pp. 227–249). Springer.

Bryant-Lukosius, D., & Rietkoetter, S. (2020). Nurse-sensitive outcomes. In J. S. Fulton, K. A. Goudreau, & K. L. Swartzel (Eds.), *Foundations of clinical nurse specialist practice* (3rd ed.) (pp. 45–69). Springer.

Bryant-Lukosius, D., Spichiger, E., Martin, J., Stoll, H., Degen Kellerhals, S., Fliedner, M., Grossmann, F., Henry, M., Herrmann, L., Koller, A., Schwendimann, R., Ulrich, A., Weibel, L., Callens, B., & De Geest, S. (2016). Framework for evaluating the impact of advanced practice nursing roles. *Journal of Nursing Scholarship, 48*(2), 201–209.

Bryant-Lukosius, D., Valaitis, R., Martin-Misener, R., Donald, F., Peña, L. M., & Brousseau, L. (2017). Advanced practice nursing: A strategy for achieving universal health coverage and universal access to health. *Revista Latino-Americana de Enfermagem, 25* Article e2826.

Canadian Institute for Health Information (CIHI). (2020). Nursing in Canada, 2019. *A lens on supply and workforce.* https://www.cihi.ca/en/nursing-in-canada-2019

Canadian Nurses Association (CNA). (2010). *Canadian registered nurse examination prep guide.* https://www.cna-aiic.ca/-/media/cna/page-content/pdf-en/crne_bulletin_june_2009_e.pdf?la=en&hash=33736321FCA6417611350D9ACF1C536180E5A728

Canadian Nurses Association. (2015). *Pan-Canadian core competency profile for clinical nurse specialists.* https://cnaaiic.ca/~/media/cna/files/en/clinical_nurse_specialists_convention_handout_e.pdf

Canadian Nurses Association. (2019). Advanced practice nursing. A pan-Canadian framework. https://www.cna-aiic.ca/-/media/cna/page content/pdf en/apn a pan canadian framework.pdf

Carney, M. (2015). Regulation of advanced nurse practice: Its existence and regulatory dimensions from an international perspective. *Journal of Nursing Management, 24*, 105–114.

Carryer, J., Wilkinson, J., Towers, A., & Gardner, G. (2018). Delineating advanced practice nursing in New Zealand: A national survey. *International Nursing Review, 65*(1), 24–32.

Carter, M. A., Owen-Williams, E., & Della, P. (2015). Meeting Australia's emerging primary care needs by nurse practitioners. *The Journal for Nurse Practitioners, 11*(6), 647–652.

Carter, N., Dobbins, M., Peachey, G., Hoxby, H., Ireland, S., Akhtar-Danes, N., & DiCenso, A. (2014). Knowledge transfer and dissemination of advanced practice nursing information and research to acute-care administrators. *Canadian Journal of Nursing Research, 46*(2), 10–27.

Carter, N., Martin-Misener, R., Kilpatrick, K., Kaasalainen, S., Donald, F., Bryant-Lukosius, D., Harbman, P., Bourgeault, I., & DiCenso, A. (2010). The role of nursing leadership in integrating clinical nurse specialists and nurse practitioners in healthcare delivery in Canada. *Canadian Journal of Nursing Leadership, 23*, 167–188. Special issue.

Casey, M., O'Connor, L., Cashin, A., Fealy, G., Smith, R., O'Brien, D., Stokes, D., McNamara, M., O'Leary, D., & Glasgow, M. E. (2019). Enablers and challenges to advanced nursing and midwifery practice roles. *Journal of Nursing Management, 27*(2), 271–277.

Casey, M., O'Connor, L., Cashin, A., Smith, R., O'Brien, D., Nicholson, E., O'Leary, D., Fealy, G., McNamara, M., Glasgow, M. E., Stokes, D., & Egan, C. (2017). An overview of the outcomes and impact of specialist and advanced nursing and midwifery practice on quality of care, cost, and access to services: A narrative review. *Nurse Education Today, 56*, 35–59.

Cashin, A., Stasa, H., Gullick, J., Conway, R., & Buckley, T. (2015). Clarifying clinical nurse consultant work in Australia: A phenomenological study. *Collegian (Royal College of Nursing, Australia), 22*, 405–412.

Cassiani, S. H. B., Aguirre-Boza, F., Hoyos, M. C., Barreto, M. F. C., Peña, L. M., Mackay, M. C. C., & Silva F. A. M. (2018). Competencies for training advanced practice nurses in primary health care. *Acta Paulista de Enfermagem, 31*(6), 572–584.

Cassiani, S. H., & Zug, K. E. (2014). Promoting the advanced nursing practice role in Latin America. *Revista Brasileira de Enfermagem, 67*(5), 673–674.

Chang, I. W., Shyu, Y. I., Tsay, P. K., & Tang, W. R. (2012). Comparison of nurse practitioners' perceptions of required competencies and self-evaluated competencies in Taiwan. *Journal of Clinical Nursing, 21*, 2679–2689.

Chimezie, R. O., & Ibe, S. N. (2019). Advanced practice nursing in Nigerian healthcare: Prospects and challenges. *Journal of Social Change, 11*(1), 61–74.

Christmals, C. D., & Armstrong, S. J. (2019). The essence, opportunities, and threats to advanced practice nursing in Sub-Saharan Africa: A scoping review. *Heliyon, 5*(10). Article e02531. https://doi.org/10.1016/j.heliyon.2019.e02531

Collett, D., Feder, S., Aaron, E., Haron, Y., & Schulman-Green, D. (2019). Palliative care advanced practice nursing in Israel: Bridging creation and implementation. *International Nursing Review, 67*, 136–144.

Collins, S., & Hewer, I. (2014). The impact of the Bologna process on nursing higher education in Europe: A review. *International Journal of Nursing Studies, 51*, 150–156.

Cooper, M. A., McDowell, J., & Raeside. L., the ANP-CNS Group. (2019). The similarities and differences between advanced nurse practitioners and clinical nurse specialists. *British Journal of Nursing, 28*(20), 1308–1314.

Craswell, A., & Dwyer, T. (2019). Reasons for choosing or refusing care from a nurse practitioner: Results from a national population-based survey. *Journal of Advanced Nursing, 75*(12), 3668–3676.

Dalhousie University, School of Nursing. (2017). *A national education forum for a sustainable neonatal nurse practitioner workforce.* Meeting report.

Davis, J., Lynch, F., Nyman, A., & Riphagen, S. (2015). The role and scope of retrieval nurse practitioners in the UK. *Nursing in Critical Care, 21*(4), 243–251.

Day-Stirk, F., McConville, F., Campbell, J., Laski, L., Guerra-Arias, M., ten Hoope-Bender, P., Michel-Schuldt, M., & de Bernis, L. (2014). Delivering the evidence to improve the health of women and newborns: State of the world's midwifery, report 2014. *Reproductive Health, 11*, 89.

DeBout, C. (2018). Advanced practice nurse in France. *Soins, 63*(824), 59–65. https://doi.org/10.1016/j.soin.2018.03.001

De Bruijn-Geraets, D. P., Van Eijk-Hustings, Y. J. L., & Vrijhoef, H. J. M. (2014). Evaluating newly acquired authority of nursing practitioners and physician assistants for reserved medical procedures in the Netherlands: A study protocol. *Journal of Advanced Nursing, 70*(11), 2673–2682.

del Rio Camara, M., Nuño Solinis, R., Chueca Ajuria, A., Abos Mendizabal, G., Cidoncha Morena, R., González Llinares, M., Peña González, M. L., Sánchez Martin, I., & de Lorenzo Urien, E. (2015). Advanced nursing roles and integrated care: A pilot study in the Basque country. *International Journal of Integrated Care, 15*, 1–3. Annual Conf Suppl.

Delamaire, M. L., & Lafortune, G. (2010). *Nurses in advanced roles: Description and evaluation of practices in 13 developed countries.* Organisation for Economic Co-operation and Development.

DiCenso, A., Bryant-Lukosius, D., Martin-Misener, R., Donald, F., Abelson, J., Bourgeault, I., Kilpatrick, K., Carter, N., Kaasalainen, S., & Harbman, P. (2010). Factors enabling advanced practice nursing role integration in Canada. *Canadian Journal of Nursing Leadership, 23*. Special edition, 211–338.

Dlamini, C. P., Khumalo, T., Nkwanyana, N., Mathunjwa-Dlamini, T. R., Macera, L., Nsibandze, B. S., Kaplan, L., & Stuart-Shor, E. M. (2020). Developing and implementing the family nurse practitioner role in Eswatini: Implications for education, practice, and policy. *Annals of Global Health, 86*(1), 1–10.

Donald, F., Kilpatrick, K., Carter, N., Bryant-Lukosius, D., Martin-Misener, R., Kaasalainen, S., Harbman, P., Marshall, D., & DiCenso, A. (2015). Hospital to community transitional care by nurse practitioners: A systematic review of cost-effectiveness. *International Journal of Nursing Studies, 52*(1), 436–451.

Donald, F., Martin-Misener, R., Carter, N., Donald, E., Kaasalainen, S., Wickson-Griffiths, A., Lloyd, M., Akhtar-Danesh, N., & DiCenso, A. (2013). A systematic review of the effectiveness of advanced practice nurses in long-term care. *Journal of Advanced Nursing, 69*(10), 2148–2161. https://doi.org/10.1111/jan.12140

Doody, O., Slevin, E., & Taggart, L. (2017). Activities of intellectual disability clinical nurse specialists in Ireland. *Clinical Nurse Specialist, 31*(2), 89–96.

Dover, N., Lee, G. A., Raleigh, M., Baker, E. J., Starodub, R., Bench, S., & Garry, B (2019). A rapid review of educational preparedness of advanced clinical practitioners. *Journal of Advanced Nursing, 75*(12), 3210–3218.

Dowling, M., Beauchesne, M., Farrelly, F., & Murphy, K. (2013). Advanced practice nursing: A concept analysis. *International Journal of Nursing Practice, 19*, 131–140.

Dunworth, B. A. (2020). Sustained value of implementation of a flexibility-based compensation structure for nurse anesthetists in a large multihospital healthcare system. *American Association of Nurse Anesthetists Journal, 88*(1), 66–70.

Dury, C., Hall, C., Danan, J. L., Mondoux, J., Aguiar Barbieri-Figueiredo, M. C., Costa, M. A., & Debout, C. (2014). Specialist nurse in Europe: Education, regulation and role. *International Nursing Review, 61*, 454–462.

Dutch Nursing Association. (2020). *About the nurse practitioner in the Netherlands.* https://venvnvs.nl/venvnvs/information-in-english/

East, L. A., Arudo, J., Loefler, M., & Evans, C. M. (2014). Exploring the potential for advanced nursing practice role development in Kenya: A qualitative study. *BMC Nursing, 13*(1), 1–11.

East, L. A., Knowles, K., Pettman, M., & Fisher, L. (2015). Advanced level nursing in England: Organizational challenges and opportunities. *Journal of Nursing Management, 23*, 1011–1019.

Elliott, N., Begley, C., Sheaf, G., & Higgins, A. (2016). Barriers and enablers to advanced practitioners' ability to enact their leadership role: A scoping review. *International Journal of Nursing Studies, 60*, 24–45.

Faraz, A. (2019). Facilitators and barriers to the novice nurse practitioner workforce transition in primary care. *Journal of the American Association of Nurse Practitioners, 31*(6), 364–370.

Fernandez, R. S., Sheppard-Law, S., & Manning, V. (2017). Determining the key drivers and mitigating factors that influence the role of the nurse and/or midwife consultant: A cross-sectional survey. *Contemporary Nurse, 53*(3), 302–312.

Feyereisen, S. L., Puro, N., & McConnell, W. (2020). Addressing provider shortages in rural America: The role of state opt-out policy adoptions in promoting hospital anesthesia provision. *The Journal of Rural Health, 37*(4), 684–691. https://doi.org/10.1111/jrh.12487

Fischer-Cartlidge, E., Houlihan, N., & Brownie, K. (2019). Building a renowned clinical nurse specialist team. *Clinical Nurse Specialist, 33*(6), 266–272.

Fleure, L., & Sara, S. (2020). An exploration of the role of the prostate cancer specialist nurse from two international perspectives. *Seminars in Oncology Nursing, 36*(4), Article 151043. https://doi.org/10.1016/j.soncn.2020.151043

Franks, H. (2014). The contribution of nurse consultants in England to the public health leadership agenda. *Journal of Clinical Nursing, 23*, 3434–3448.

Freund, T., Everett, C., Griffiths, P., Hudon, C., Maccarella, L., & Laurant, M. (2015). Skill mix, roles and remuneration in the primary care workforce: Who are the healthcare professionals in the primary care teams across the world? *International Journal of Nursing Studies, 52*, 727–743.

Fukuda, H., Miyauchi, S., Tonai, M., Ono, M., Magilvy, J. K., & Murashima, S. (2014). The first nurse practitioner graduate program in Japan. *International Nursing Review, 61*, 487–490.

Fullerton, J. T., Schuiling, K. D., & Sipe, T. A (2019). The doctorate of nursing practice and entry into midwifery practice: Issues for consideration and debate. *Nursing Education in Practice, 36*, 97–100.

Fulton, J. (2014). Evolution of the clinical nurse specialist role and practice in the United States. In J. S. Fulton, B. L. Lyon, & K. A. Goudreau (Eds.), *Foundations of clinical nurse specialist practice* (2nd ed.) (pp. 3–15). Springer.

Gagan, M. J., Boyd, M., Wysocki, K., & Williams, D. J. (2014). The first decade of nurse practitioners in New Zealand: A survey of an evolving practice. *Journal of the American Association of Nurse Practitioners, 26*, 612–619.

Gardner, G., Duffield, C., Doubrovsky, A., & Adams, M. (2016). Identifying advanced practice: A national survey of a nursing workforce. *International Journal of Nursing Studies, 55*, 60–70.

Gerrish, K., McDonnell, A., & Kennedy, F. (2013). The development of a framework for evaluating the impact of nurse consultant roles in the UK. *Journal of Advanced Nursing, 69*(10), 2295–2308.

Gigli, K. H., Dietrich, M. S., Buerhaus, P. I., & Minnick, A. F. (2018). Regulation of pediatric intensive care unit nurse practitioner practice: A national survey. *Journal of the American Association of Nurse Practitioners, 30*(1), 17–26.

Gillis, B. D., Holley, S. L., Leming-Lee, T. S., & Parish, A. L. (2019). Implementation of a perinatal depression care bundle in a nurse-managed midwifery practice. *Nursing for Women's Health, 23*(4), 288–298.

Goemaes, R., Lernout, E., Goossens, S., Decoene, E., Verhaeghe, S., Beeckman, D., & Van Hecke, A. (2019). Time use of advanced practice nurses in hospitals: A cross-sectional study. *Journal of Advanced Nursing, 75*(12), 3588–3601.

Goh, H. S., Tang, M. L., Lee, C. N., & Liaw, S. Y. (2019). The development of Singapore nurse education system – challenges, opportunities, and implications. *International Nursing Review, 66*(4), 467–473.

Goldenberg, S. E., Cooper, J., Blundell, A., Gordon, A. L., Masud, T., & Moorchilot, R. (2016). Development of a curriculum for advanced nurse practitioners working with older people with frailty in the acute hospital through a modified Delphi process. *Age and Ageing, 45*(1), 48–53.

Gonzalez Jurado, M. A. (2015). In *Advanced practice nursing in Spain. Presentation at the Pan American Health Organization meeting, Universal Access to Health and Universal Health Coverage: Advanced Practice Nursing Summit, at McMaster University*. April 15-17, 2015. http://fhs.mcmaster.ca/globalhealthoffice/documents/AdvancedPracticeNurseinSpain.pdf

Goudreau, K. A. (2014). Unit 1—Introduction to health policy from an advanced practice perspective. Implications for practice: The Consensus Model for APRN Regulation. In K. A. Goudreau, & M. Smolenski (Eds.), *Health policy and advanced practice nursing: Impact and policy implications* (pp. 57–64). Springer.

Grant, J., Lines, L., Darbyshire, P., & Parry, Y. (2017). How do nurse practitioners work in primary health care settings? A scoping review. *International Journal of Nursing Studies, 75*, 51–57.

Gullick, J. G., & West, S. H. (2015). Building research capacity and productivity among advanced practice nurses: An evaluation of the community of practice model. *Journal of Advanced Nursing, 72*(3), 605–619.

Gysin, S., Sottas, B., Odermatt, M., & Essig, S. (2019). Advanced practice nurses' and general practitioners' first experiences with introducing the advanced practice nurse role to Swiss primary care: A qualitative study. *BMC Family Practice, 20*(1), 1–11. https://doi.org/10.1186/s12875-019-1055-z

Hamad Medical Corporation. (2015). *HMC welcomes first set of Qatar-trained clinical nurse specialists*. http://www.hamad.qa

Hansen, M. P., Saunders, M. M., Kollauf, C. R., & Santiago-Rotchford, L. (2019). Clinical nurse specialists: Leaders in managing patients with chronic conditions. *Nursing Economics, 37*(2), 103–109.

Hanucharurnkul, S. (2007). Nurses in primary care and the nurse practitioner role in Thailand. *Contemporary Nurse, 26*, 83–91.

Harbman, P., Bryant-Lukosius, D., Martin-Misener, R., Carter, N., Covell, C. L., Gibbins, S., Kilpatrick, K., McKinlay, J., Rawson, K., Sherifali, D., Tranmer, J., & Valaitis, R. (2016). Partners in research: Building academic-practice partnerships to educate and mentor advanced practice nurses. *Journal of Evaluation in Clinical Practice, 23*, 382–390.

Haut, C., & Madden, M. (2015). Hiring appropriate providers for different populations: Acute care nurse practitioners. *Critical Care Nurse, 35*(3), e1–e8.

Heale, R., Dickieson, P., Carter, L., & Wenghofer, E. F. (2014). Nurse practitioners' perceptions of interprofessional team functioning with implications for nurse managers. *Journal of Nursing Management, 22*, 924–930.

Heale, R., & Rieck-Buckley, C. (2015). An international perspective of advanced practice nursing regulation. *International Nursing Review, 62*(3), 421–429.

Health Resources and Services Administration, National Center for Health Workforce Analysis, United States Government. (2019). *Brief summary results from the 2018 national sample survey of registered nurses.* https://bhw.hrsa.gov/sites/default/files/bhw/health-workforce-analysis/nssrn-summary-report.pdf

Henni, S. H., Kirkevold, M., Antypas, K., & Foss, C. (2019). The integration of new nurse practitioners into care of older adults: A survey study. *Journal of Clinical Nursing, 28*, 2911–2923.

Hibbert, D., Aboshaiqah, A. E., Sienko, K. A., Forestell, D., Harb, A. W., Yousuf, S. A., Kelley, P. W., Brennan, P. F., Serrant, L., & Leary, A. (2017). Advancing nursing practice: The emergence of the role of advanced practice nurse in Saudi Arabia. *Annals of Saudi Medicine, 37*(1), 72–78.

Higgins, A., Begley, C., Lalor, J., Coyne, I., Murphy, K., & Elliott, N. (2014). Factors influencing advanced practitioners' ability to enact leadership: A case study within Irish healthcare. *Journal of Nursing Management, 22*, 894–905.

Honig, J., Doyle-Lindrud, S., & Dohrn, J. (2019). Moving towards universal health coverage: Advanced practice nurse competencies. *Revista Latino-Americana de Enfermagem*, 27. Article e3132. https://doi.org/10.1590/1518-8345.2901.3132

Horton, B. J., Anang, S. P., Riesen, M., Yang, H. J., & Bjorkelund, K. B. (2014). International Federation of Nurse Anesthetists' anesthesia program approval process. *International Nursing Review, 61*, 285–289.

Hu, J., Fallacaro, J. D., Jiang, L., Wu, J., Jiang, H., Shi, Z., & Ruan, H. (2017). IFNA approved Chinese anaesthesia nurse education program: A Delhi method. *Nurse Education Today, 56*, 6–12. September.

Hu, J., Yang, Y., Fallacaro, M. D., Wands, B., Wright, S., Zhou, Y., & Ruan, H. (2019). Building an international partnership to develop advanced practice nurses in anesthesia settings: Using a theory-driven approach. *Journal of Transcultural Nursing, 30*(5), 521–529.

Hunter, K. F., Murphy, R. S., Babb, M., & Vallee, C. (2016). Benefits and challenges faced by a nurse practitioner working in an interprofessional setting in rural Alberta. *Canadian Journal of Nursing Leadership, 29*(3), 61–70.

Hurlock-Chorostecki, C., & Acorn, M. (2017). Diffusing innovative roles within Ontario hospitals: Implement the nurse practitioner as the most responsible provider. *Nursing Leadership, 30*(4), 60–66.

Hurlock-Chorostecki, C., & McCallum, J. (2016). Nurse practitioner role value in hospitals: New strategies for hospital leaders. *Canadian Journal of Nursing Leadership, 29*(3), 82–92.

Imhof, L., Naef, R., Wallhagen, M., Schwarz, J., & Mahrer-Imhof, R. (2012). Effects of an advanced practice nurse in-home health consultation program for community-dwelling persons aged 80 and older. *Journal of the American Geriatrics Society, 60*(12), 2223–2231.

International Confederation of Midwives (ICM). (2015). *The involvement of midwives associations in the development and management of the midwifery workforce.* Survey of ICM members associations. Report.

International Confederation of Midwives (ICM). (2019). Essential competencies for basic midwifery practice. 2019. *Update.* https://www.internationalmidwives.org/assets/files/general-files/2019/10/icm-competencies-en-print-october-2019_final_18-oct-5db05248843e8.pdf

International Council of Nurses (ICN). (2013). *Nursing regulation.* Position statement. http://www.icn.ch

International Council of Nurses (ICN). (2016). *Aims and objectives.* ICN International Nurse Practitioner/Advanced Practice Nurse Network. http://international.aanp.org/About/Aims

International Council of Nurses (ICN). (2020). *Guidelines on advanced practice nursing 2020.* https://www.icn.ch/system/files/documents/2020-04/ICN_APN%20Report_EN_WEB.pdf

International Federation of Nurse Anesthetists (IFNA). (2020). *Country information.* https://ifna.site/about-ifna/country-members-info/

Irajpour, A., Khorasani, P., Bagheri, M., Eshaghian, A., Ziaee, E. S., Saberi, Z., & Afshar, A. (2019). The framework for developing nursing specialist roles in the health care system of Iran. *Nursing Outlook, 68*(1), 45–54.

Ireland Department of Health. (2019). A policy on the development of graduate to advanced nursing and midwifery practice. https://assets.gov.ie/19260/f49c5ea1a19843b0aae20151aeaf694d.pdf

Ireland, J., van Teijlingen, E., & Kemp, J. (2015). Twinning in Nepal: The Royal College of Midwives UK and the Midwifery Society of Nepal working in partnership. *Journal of Asian Midwives, 2*(1), 26–33.

Jamaica Association of Nurse Practitioners. (2016). History of nurse practitioners in Jamaica. http://www.jamaicanursepractitioners.org/home/about-us.html

Jangland, E., Yngman Uhlin, P., & Arakelian, E. (2016). Between two roles – Experiences of newly trained nurse practitioners in surgical care in Sweden: A qualitative study using repeated interviews. *Nurse Education in Practice, 21*, 93–99.

Jannings, W., Underwood, E., Almer, M., & Luxford, B. (2010). How useful is the expert practitioner role of the clinical nurse consultant to the generalist community nurse? *Australian Journal of Advanced Nursing, 28*(2), 33–40.

Jeffery, N., Donald, F., Martin-Misener, R., Bryant-Lukosius, D., Johnsen, E. A., Egilsdottir, H. Ö., Honig, J., Strand, H., Jokiniemi, K., Carter, N., Roodbol, P., & Rietkoetter, S. (2020). A comparative analysis of teaching and evaluation methods in nurse practitioner education programs in Australia, Canada, Finland, Norway, the Netherlands and US. *International Journal of Nursing Education Scholarship, 17*(1), 1–9. https://doi.org/10.1515/ijnes-2019-0047

Jeon, Y., Lahtinen, P., Meretoja, R., & Leino-Kilpi, H. (2015). Anaesthesia nursing education in the Nordic countries: Literature review. *Nurse Education Today, 35*, 680–688.

Johantgen, M., Fountain, L., Zangaro, G., Newhouse, R., Stanik-Hut, J., & White, K. (2012). Comparison of labor and delivery care provided by certified nurse-midwives and physicians: A systematic review. *Women's Health Issues, 22*(1), e73–e81.

Jokiniemi, K., & Miettinen, M. (2020). Specialist nurses' role domains and competencies in specialized medical healthcare: A qualitative descriptive study. *International Journal of Caring Sciences, 13*(1), 171–179.

Jokiniemi, K., Pietila, A. M., Kylma, J., & Haatainen, K. (2012). Advanced nursing roles: A systematic review. *Nursing and Health Sciences, 14*, 421–431.

Kaasalainen, S., Martin-Misener, R., Kilpatrick, K., Harbman, P., Bryant-Lukosius, D., Donald, F., Carter, N., & DiCenso, A. (2010). An historical overview of the development of advanced practice nursing roles in Canada. *Canadian Journal of Nursing Leadership, 23* (special edition), 35–60.

Kaur, B. (2014). Challenges and opportunities of advanced practice nursing in Hong Kong. In *2nd Annual Worldwide Nursing Conference proceedings*, Open University of Hong Kong Press. 52–56.

Keefe Marcoux, K., Dickson, S., & Clarkson, K. (2019). Advancing the practice of nursing through specialty fellowship development of pediatric nurse practitioners. *Journal of the American Association of Nurse Practitioners, 31*(10), 598–602.

Kennedy, F., McDonnell, A., Gerrish, K., Howarth, A., Pollard, C., & Redman, J. (2011). Evaluation of the impact of nurse consultant roles in the United Kingdom: A mixed method systematic literature review. *Journal of Advanced Nursing, 68*(4), 721–741.

Ketefian, S., & Redman, R. W. (2015). A critical examination of developments of nursing doctoral education in the United States. *Revista Latino-Americana de Enfermagem, 23*(3), 363–371.

Kilpatrick, K., Carter, N., Bryant-Lukosius, D., Charbonneau-Smith, R., & DiCenso, A. (2015). Development of evidence briefs to transfer knowledge above advanced practice nursing roles in providers, policy-makers and administrators. *Canadian Journal of Nursing Leadership, 28*(1), 11–23.

Kilpatrick, K., DiCenso, A., Bryant-Lukosius, D., Ritchie, J. A., Martin-Misener, R., & Carter, N. (2013). Practice patterns and perceived impact of clinical nurse specialist roles in Canada: Results of a national survey. *International Journal of Nursing Studies, 50*, 1524–1536.

Kilpatrick, K., Harbman, P., Carter, N., Martin-Misener, R., Bryant-Lukosius, D., Donald, F., Kaasalainen, S., Bourgeault, I., & DiCenso, A. (2010). The acute care nurse practitioner role in Canada. *Canadian Journal of Nursing Leadership, 23*, 114–139. Special Edition.

Kilpatrick, K., Kaasalainen, S., Donald, F., Reid, K., Carter, N., Bryant-Lukosius, D., Martin-Misener, R., Harbman, P., Marshall, D. A., Charbonneau-Smith, R., & DiCenso, A. (2014). The effectiveness and cost effectiveness of clinical nurse specialists in outpatient roles: A systematic review. *Journal of Evaluation in Clinical Practice, 20*, 1106–1123.

Kim, S., Lee, T. W., Kim, G. S., Choi, M., Jang, Y., & Baek, S., Project Team for the WHO Collaborating Centres in the Western Pacific Region. (2019). *Study on nurses in advanced roles as a strategy for equitable access to health care in the Western Pacific Region. Final Report*. South Korea: Yonsei University College of Nursing.

King, A., Boyd, M. L., Dagley, L., & Raphael, D. (2018). Implementation of a gerontology nurse specialist role in primary health care: Health professional and older adult perspectives. *Journal of Clinical Nursing, 27*(3-4), 807–818.

Ko, C. M., Koh, C. K., & Kwon, S. (2019). Willingness to pay for family education and counselling services provided by critical care advanced practice nurses. *International Journal of Nursing Practice, 25*(6). Article e12782. https://doi.org/10.1111/ijn.12782

Kobleder, A., Mayer, H., & Senn, B. (2018). Advanced practice nursing in gynaecological oncology – Development of an evidence-based concept for Austria and Switzerland. *Supportive Care in Cancer, 26*(2), 539–5364. Suppl.

Kocher, A., & Spichiger, E. (2014). Supporting self-management for patients with systematic sclerosis—the development of a new role for an advanced practice nurse. *Annals of the Rheumatic Diseases, 73*, 1214.

Kooienga, S. A., & Carryer, J. B. (2015). Globalization advancing primary health care nurse practitioner practice. *The Journal for Nurse Practitioners, 11*(8), 804–811.

Kozhimannil, K. B., Henning-Smith, C., & Hung, P. (2016). The practice of midwifery in rural US hospitals. *Journal of Midwifery & Women's Health, 61*(4), 411–418.

Kudsk-Iversen, S., Trelles, M., Bakebaanista, E. N., Hagabimana, L., Momen, A., Helmand, R., Victor, C. S., Shah, K., Masu, A., Kendall, J., Edgecombe, H., & English, M. (2020). Anaesthesia care providers employed in humanitarian settings by Médecins Sans Frontières: A retrospective observational study of 173084 surgical cases over 10 years. *BMJ Open, 10*. Article e034891. https://bmjopen.bmj.com/content/bmjopen/10/3/e034891.full.pdf

Kuo, Y. F., Loresto, F. L., Rounds, L. R., & Goodwin, J. S. (2013). States with the least restrictive regulations experienced the largest increase in patients seen by nurse practitioners. *Health Affairs, 32*(7), 1236–1243.

Lathrop, B., & Hodnicki, D. R. (2014). The Affordable Care Act: Primary care and the Doctor of Nursing Practice nurse. *The Online Journal of Issues in Nursing, 19*(2), 1–14.

Lawler, J., Trevatt, P., Elliot, C., & Leary, A. (2019). Does the diabetes specialist nursing workforce impact the experiences and outcomes of people with diabetes? A hermeneutic review of the evidence. *Human Resources for Health, 17*(1), 1–9. https://doi.org/10.1186/s12960-019-0401-5

Leary, A., Crouch, H., Lezard, A., Rawcliffe, C., Boden, L., & Richardson, A. (2008). Dimensions of clinical nurse specialist work in the UK. *Nursing Standard, 23*(15), 40 44.

Leary, A., Maclaine, K., Trevatt, P., Radford, M., & Punshon, G. (2017). Variation in job titles within the nursing workforce. *Journal of Clinical Nursing, 26*(23-24), 4945–4950.

Lee, D., Choi, K., Chan, C., Chair, S., Chan, D., Fung, S. Y., & Chan, E. L. (2013). The impact on patient health and service outcomes of introducing nursing consultants: A historical matched controlled study. *BMC Health Services Research, 13*(1), 1–9.

Lemos, C., & Peniche, A. (2016). Nursing care in the anesthetic procedure: An integrative review. *Revista da Escola de Enfermagem da USP, 50*(1), 154–162.

Lewandowski, W., & Adamle, K. (2009). Substantive areas of clinical nurse specialist practice. *Clinical Nurse Specialist, 23*(2), 73–90.

Liao, C. J., Quraishi, J. A., & Jordan, L. M. (2015). Geographical imbalance of anesthesia providers and its impact on the uninsured and vulnerable populations. *Nursing Economics, 33*(5), 263–270.

Lin, L. C., Lee, S., Ueng, S. W., & Tang, W. R. (2015). Reliability and validity of the Nurse Practitioners' Roles and Competencies Scale. *Journal of Clinical Nursing, 25*, 99–108.

Liu, Y., Rodcumdee, B., Jiang, P., & Sha, L. Y. (2015). Nursing education in the United States, Thailand, and China: Literature review. *Journal of Nursing Education and Practice, 5*(7), 100–108.

Ljungbeck, B., & Forss, K. S. (2017). Advanced nurse practitioners in municipal healthcare as a way to meet the growing healthcare needs of the frail elderly: A qualitative interview study with managers, doctors, and specialist nurses. *BMC Nursing, 16*(1), 1–9. https://doi.org/10.1186/s12912-017-0258-7

Lopatina, E., Donald, F., Martin-Misener, R., Kilpatrick, K., Bryant-Lukosius, D., Carter, N., Reid, K., & Marshall, D. A. (2017). Economic evaluation of nurse practitioner and clinical nurse specialist roles: A methodological review. *International Journal of Nursing Studies, 72*, 71–82.

Lowe, G., Plummer, V., O'Brien, A. P., & Boyd, L. (2011). Time to clarify the value of advanced practice nursing roles in health care. *Journal of Advanced Nursing, 68*(3), 677–685.

MacLellan, L., Higgins, I., & Levett-Jones, T. (2017). An exploration of the factors that influence nurse practitioner transition in Australia: A story of turmoil, tenacity, and triumph. *Journal of the American Association of Nurse Practitioners, 29*(3), 149–156.

Maier, C. B. (2015). The role of governance in implementing task-shifting from physicians to nurses in advanced roles in Europe, US, Canada, New Zealand and Australia. *Health Policy, 119*, 1627–1635.

Maier, C. B., Barnes, H., Aiken, L. H., & Busse, R. (2016). Descriptive, cross-country analysis of the nurse practitioner workforce in six countries: Size, growth, physician substitution potential. *BMJ Open, 6* Article e011901.

Maijala, V., Tossavainen, K., & Turunen, H. (2015). Identifying nurse practitioners' required case management competencies in health promotion practice in municipal public primary health care. A two-stage modified Delphi study. *Journal of Clinical Nursing, 24*(17–18), 2554–2561.

Marshall, D., Donald, F., Lacny, C., Reid, K., Bryant-Lukosius, D., Carter, N., Charbonneau-Smith, R., Harbman, P., Kaasalainen, S., Kilpatrick, K., Martin-Misener, R., & DiCenso, A. (2015). Assessing the quality of economic evaluations of clinical nurse specialists and nurse practitioners: A systematic review of cost-effectiveness. *NursingPlus Open, 1*, 11–17.

Martin-Misener, R., Bryant-Lukosius, D., Harbman, P., Donald, F., Kaasalainen, S., & Carter, N. (2010). Education of advanced practice nurses in Canada. *Canadian Journal of Nursing Leadership, 23*, 61–87. Special Issue.

Martin-Misener, R., Harbman, P., Donald, F., Reid, K., Kilpatrick, K., Carter, N., Bryant-Lukosius, D., Kaasalainen, S., Marshall, D. A., Charbonneau-Smith, R., & DiCenso, A. (2015). Cost-effectiveness of nurse practitioners in ambulatory care: Systematic review. *BMJ Open, 5*. Article e007167. http://bmjopen.bmj.com/cgi/content/full/bmjopen-2014-007167?ijkey=uzaooKIc7lMSWrv&keytype=ref

Maten-Speksnijder, A. T., Pool, A., Grypdonck, M., Meurs, P., & van Staa, A. (2015). Driven by ambitions: The nurse practitioner role transition in Dutch hospital care. *Journal of Nursing Scholarship, 47*(6), 544–554.

Matthews, J. D., & Campbell, J. (2015). Joining hands for health workforce improvements. Ghana hosts consultation on new global health workforce strategy. *World Health Organization*. http://www.who.int/workforcealliance/media/news/2015/hrh-improvements_ghana-consult/en/

Mboineki, J. F., & Zhang, W. (2017). Healthcare provider views on transitioning from task shifting to advanced practice nursing in Tanzania. *Nursing Research, 67*(1), 49–54.

McAuliffe, M., & Henry, B. (1996). Countries where anesthesia is administered by nurses. *Journal of the American Association of Nurse Anesthetists, 64*(5), 469–479.

McAuliffe, M., & Henry, B. (1998). Survey of nurse anesthesia practice, education, and regulation in 96 countries. *Journal of the American Association of Nurse Anesthetists, 66*(3), 273–286.

Meehan, M., & Doody, O. (2020). The role of the clinical nurse specialist multiple sclerosis, the patients' and families' and carers' perspective: An integrative review. *Multiple Sclerosis and Related Disorders, 39*, 1–15. https://doi.org/10.1016/j.msard.2019.101918

Minotti, B., Blättler-Remund, T., Sieber, R., & Tabakovic, S. (2020). Nurse practitioners in emergency medicine: The Swiss experience. *European Journal of Emergency Medicine, 27*(1), 7–8.

Mohr, L. D., & Coke, L. A. (2018). Distinguishing the clinical nurse specialist from other graduate nursing roles. *Clinical Nurse Specialist, 32*(3), 139–151.

Mooney, K. H., Beck, S. L., Wong, B., Dunson, W., Wujcik, D., Whisenant, M., & Donaldson, G. (2017). Automated home monitoring and management of patient reported symptoms during chemotherapy: Results of the symptom care at home RCT. *Cancer Medicine, 6*(3), 537–546.

Moore, L. (2018). Nurse-led cancer care clinics: An economic assessment of breast and urology clinics. *Cancer Nursing Practice, 17*(1), 34–41.

Morilla-Herrera, J. C., Garcia-Mayor, S., Martín-Santos, F. J., Kaknani Uttumchandani, S., Leon Campos, Á., Caro Bautista, J., & Morales-Asencio, J. M. (2016). A systematic review of the effectiveness and roles of advanced practice nursing in older people. *International Journal of Nursing Studies, 53*, 290–307.

Morin, D., Ramelet, A. S., & Shaha, M. (2013). Advanced nursing practice: Vision in Switzerland. *Recherche En Soins Infirmiers, 115*, 49–58.

Moss, C., & Jackson, J. (2019). Mentoring new graduate nurse practitioners. *Neonatal Network, 38*(3), Article 151159.

Msuya, M., Blood-Siegfried, J., Chugulu, J., Kidayi, P., Sumaye, J., Machange, R., Mtuya, C. C., & Pereira, K. (2017). Descriptive study of nursing scope of practice in rural medically underserved areas of Africa, South of the Sahara. *International Journal of Africa Nursing Sciences, 6*, 74–82.

Müller-Staub, M., Zigan, N., Händler-Schuster, D., Probst, S., Monego, R., & Imhof, L. (2015). Being cared for and caring: Living with multiple chronic disease (Leila)—A qualitative study about APN contributions to integrated care [in German]. *Pflege, 28*(2), 79–91.

Nardi, D. A., & Diallo, R. (2014). Global trends and issues in APN practice: Engage in the change. *Journal of Professional Nursing, 30*(3), 228–232.

National Association of Clinical Nurse Specialists (NACNS). (2018). *Unlocking the mystery of the clinical nurse specialist*. https://nacns.org/wp-content/uploads/2018/04/Fact-or-Fiction-FINAL-4-23-18.pdf

National Association of Clinical Nurse Specialists (NACNS). (2019). *Key findings from the 2018 clinical nurse specialist census*. https://nacns.org/professional-resources/practice-and-cns-role/cns-census/

National Council of State Boards of Nursing. (2008). *Consensus model for APRN regulation: Licensure, accreditation, certification and education.* https://www.ncsbn.org/Consensus_Model_Report.pdf

National Nursing Centres Consortium. (2014). *International advanced practice nursing symposium.* http://www.nncc.us/images_specific/pdf/GlobalAPNSymposiumFINAL.pdf

New South Wales Department of Health. (2011). *Clinical nurse consultants—domains and functions.* http://www.health.nsw.gov.au/

Nieminen, A. L., Mannevaara, B., & Fagerstrom, L. (2011). Advanced practice nurses' scope of practice: A qualitative study of advanced clinical competencies. *Scandinavian Journal of Caring Sciences, 25*(4), 661–670.

North, N., Shung-King, M., & Coetzee, M. (2019). The children's nursing workforce in Kenya, Malawi, Uganda, South Africa and Zambia: Generating an initial indication of the extent of the workforce and training activity. *Human Resources for Health, 17*(1), 1–9. https://doi.org/10.1186/s12960-019-0366-4

Nove, A., Pairman, S., Bohle, L. F., Garg, S., Moyo, N. T., Michel-Schuldt, M., Hoffmann, A., & Castro., G. (2018). The development of a global midwifery education accreditation programme. *Global Health Action, 11*(1). Article 1489604. https://doi.org/10.1080/16549716.2018.1489604

Nursing Council of New Zealand. (2020). *The New Zealand workforce. A profile of nurse practitioners, registered nurses, and enrolled nurses.* https://www.nursingcouncil.org.nz/Public/Publications/Workforce_Statistics/NCNZ/publications-section/Workforce_statistics.aspx?hkey=3f3f39c4-c909-4d1d-b87f-e6270b531145

O'Baugh, J., Wilkes, L., Vaughan, K., & O'Donohue, R. (2007). The role and scope of the clinical nurse consultant in Wentworth area health service, New South Wales, Australia. *Journal of Nursing Management, 16*, 12–21.

Oddsdottir, E., & Sveinsdottir, H. (2011). The content of the work of clinical nurse specialists described by use of daily activity diaries. *Journal of Clinical Nursing, 20*, 1393–1404.

Officer, T., Cumming, J., & McBride-Henry, K. (2019). Successfully developing advanced practitioner roles: Policy and practice mechanisms. *Journal of Health Organization and Management, 33*(1), 63–77.

Olabode, I. (2016). India launches nurse practitioner courses and "live register" for nurses. *Nursing Arena Forum.* http://nursesarena.com/new/india

Oldenburger, D., Cassiani, S. H., Bryant-Lukosius, D., Valaitis, R., Baumann, A., Pulcini, J., & Martin-Misener, R. (2017). Implementation strategy for advanced practice nursing in primary health care in Latin America and the Caribbean. *Pan American Journal of Public Health, 41*, e40. https://doi.org/10.26633/rpsp.2017.40

Ouersighni, A., & Ghazali, D. A. (2020). Contribution of certified registered nurse anaesthetists to the management of the COVID-19 pandemic health crisis. *Intensive & Critical Care Nursing, May 26*. 102888. https://doi.org/10.1016/j.iccn.2020.102888

Oxford Business Group. (2014). *Gradual overhaul: As Qatar's population ages, a state-led transformation is underway.* London, UK: Oxford Business Group. http://www.oxfordbusinessgroup.com

Pan American Health Organization. (2018). *Expanding the roles of nurses in primary care.* https://iris.paho.org/handle/10665.2/34958

Pan American Health Organization and School of Nursing, McMaster University. (2015). *Universal access to health and universal health coverage: Advanced practice nursing summit.* https://www.salud.gob.sv/archivos/enfermeria/PAHO_Advanced_Practice_Nursing_Summit_Hamilton_CA.pdf

Pan American Health Organization and University of Michigan. (2016). *Report on developing advanced practice nursing competencies in Latin America to contribute to universal health.* Ann Arbor, MI: Collaborating Center for Primary Health Care, School of Nursing, University of Michigan.

Pan American Health Organization, 52nd Directing Council. (2013). *Resolution CD52.R13. Human resources for health: Increasing access to qualified health workers in primary health care-based health systems.*

Patient Protection and Affordable Care Act, 42 U.S.C. § 18001. (2010).

Penny, R. A., Bradford, N. K., & Langbecker, D. (2018). Registered nurse and midwife experiences of using videoconferencing in practice: A systematic review of qualitative studies. *Journal of Clinical Nursing, 27*, e739–e752.

Pill, K., Kolback, R., Ottmann, G., & Rasmussen, B. (2012). The impact of the expanded nursing practice on professional identity in Denmark. *Clinical Nurse Specialist, 26*(6), 329–335.

Poghosyan, L., Liu, J., & Norful., A. A. (2017). Nurse practitioners as primary care providers with their own patient panels and organizational structures: A cross-sectional study. *International Journal of Nursing Studies, 74*, 1–7.

Prommersberger, M. (2020). Advanced nursing practice: The German experience. *European Journal of Emergency Medicine, 27*(1), 11–12.

Qatar Supreme Council of Health. (2011). *National cancer strategy. The path to excellence.* http://www.nhsq.info/app/media/878

Ranchoff, B. L., & Declercq, E. R. (2020). The scope of midwifery practice regulations and the availability of the certified nurse-midwifery and certified midwifery workforce, 2012-2016. *Journal of Midwifery & Women's Health, 65*(1), 119–130.

Rayborn, M., Jeong, G., Hayden, S., & Park, S. (2017). The future of certified registered nurse anesthetist practice in South Korea: Fading into the sunset or breaking a new dawn? *American Association of Nurse Anesthetists Journal, 85*(5), 361–368.

Reed, S. (2020). President's message: The CNS in the post-acute care setting. *Clinical Nurse Specialist, 34*(4), 139–140.

Renfrew, M. J., McFadden, A., Bastos, M. H., Campbell, J., Channon, A. A., Cheung, N. F., Silva, D. R., Downe, S., Powell Kennedy, H., Malata, A., McCormick, F., Wick, L., & Declercq, E. (2014). Midwifery and quality care: Findings from a new evidence-informed framework for maternal and newborn care. *Lancet, 384*, 1129–1145.

Rickards, T., & Hamilton, S. (2020). Patient experiences of primary care provided by nurse practitioners in New Brunswick, Canada. *Journal for Nurse Practitioners, 16*(4), 299–304.

Ritter, A. Z., Bowles, K. H., O'Sullivan, A. L., Brooks Carthon, M., & Fairman, J. A. (2018). A policy analysis of legally required supervision of nurse practitioners and other health professionals. *Nursing Outlook, 66*(6), 551–559.

Roberts, J., Floyd, S., & Thompson, S. (2011). The clinical nurse specialist in New Zealand: How is the role defined? *Nursing Praxis in New Zealand, 27*(2), 24–35.

Rogers, E. S., Maru, M., Kash-MacDonald, M., Archer-Williams, M., Hashemi, L., & Boardman, J. (2016). A randomized clinical trial investigating the effect of a healthcare access model for individuals with severe psychiatric disabilities. *Community Mental Health Journal, 52*(6), 667–674.

Romain-Glassey, N., Ninane, F., de Puy, J., Abt, M., Mangin, P., & Morin, D. (2014). The emergence of forensic nursing and advanced nursing practice in Switzerland: An innovative case study consultation. *Journal of Forensic Nursing, 10*(3), 144–152.

Romp, C. R., & Cecil, M. J. (2017). Remote clinical nurse specialist: Making a difference from a distance. *Issues in Advanced Practice, 28*(4), 314–318.

Royal College of Nursing. (2012a). *A competence framework for orthopaedic and trauma practitioners.*

Royal College of Nursing. (2012b). *Fact sheet: Specialist nursing in the UK.* https://www.rcn.org.uk/-/media/royal-college-of-nursing/documents/policies-and-briefings/uk-wide/policies/2013/0413.pdf

Royal College of Nursing. (2020). *The UK nursing labour market review 2019.* https://www.rcn.org.uk/-/media/royal-college-of-nursing/documents/publications/2020/april/009-135.pdf?la=en#:~:text=The%20RCN%20Labour%20Market%20Review,across%20the%20four%20UK%20countries.&text=This%20year's%20LMR%20observes%20that,the%20following%20challenges%20and%20pressures

Ryley, N., & Middleton, C. (2015). Framework for advanced nursing, midwifery and allied health professional practice in Wales: The implementation process. *Journal of Nursing Management, 24*, E70–E76.

Salamanca-Balen, N., Seymour, J., Caswell, G., Whynes, D., & Tod, A. (2018). The costs, resource use and cost-effectiveness of clinical nurse specialist interventions for patients with palliative care needs: A systematic review of international evidence. *Palliative Medicine, 32*(2), 447–465.

Sangster-Gormley, E., Martin-Misener, R., Downe-Wamboldt, B., & DiCenso, A. (2011). Factors affecting nurse practitioner role implementation in Canadian practice settings: An integrative review. *Journal of Advanced Nursing, 67*(6), 1178–1190.

Sastre-Fullana, P., De Pedro-Gømez, J. E., Bennasar-Veny, M., Serrano-Gallardo, P., & Morales-Asencio, J. M. (2014). Competency frameworks for advanced practice nursing: A literature review. *International Nursing Review, 61*, 534–542.

Sastre-Fullana, P., Gray, D. C., Cashin, A., Bryant-Lukosius, D., Schumann, L., Geese, F., Rae, B., Duff, E., & Bird, B. (2021). Visual analysis of global comparative mapping of the practice domains of the nurse practitioner/advanced practice nursing role in respondent countries. *Journal of the American Association of Nurse Practitioners, 33*(7), 496–505. https://doi.org/10.1097/jxx.0000000000000458

Saver, C. (2015). 50 years of NP excellence. *The Nurse Practitioner, 40*(5), 15–21.

Scanlon, A., Bryant-Lukosius, D., Lehwaldt, D., Wilkinson, J., & Honig, J. (2019). International transferability of nurse practitioner credentials in five countries. *Journal for Nurse Practitioners, 15*(7), 487–491.

Scanlon, A., Murphy, M., Smolowitz, J., & Lewis, V. (2019). Low- and lower middle-income countries advanced practice nurses: An integrative review. *International Nursing Review, 67*, 19–34.

Schober, M., Gerrish, K., & McDonnell, A. (2016). Development of a conceptual policy framework for advanced practice nursing: An ethnographic study. *Journal of Advanced Nursing, 72*, 1313–1324

Serena, A., Castellani, P., Fucina, N., Griesser, A. C., Jeanmonod, J., Peters, S., & Eicher, M. (2015). The role of advanced nursing in lung cancer: A framework based development. *European Journal of Oncology Nursing, 19*(6), 740–746.

Serena, A., Dwyer, A., Peters, S., & Eicher, M. (2017). Feasibility of advanced practice nursing in lung cancer consultations during early treatment: A phase II study. *European Journal of Oncology Nursing, 29*, 106–114. https://doi.org/10.1016/j.ejon.2017.05.007

Shurson, L., & Gregg, S. R. (2019). Relationships of pay-for-performance and provider pay. *Journal of the American Association of Nurse Practitioners, 1(33)*, 11–19. https://doi.org/10.1097/jxx.0000000000000343

South African Nursing Council. (2014a). *Competencies for advanced practice nurses.* https://www.sanc.co.za/professional_practice.htm

South African Nursing Council. (2014b). *Notice relating to the creation of categories of practitioners in terms of section 31(2) of the Nursing Act, 2005.* https://www.sanc.co.za/reg_chg.htm

Speight, C., Firnhaber, G., Scott, E., & Wei, H. (2019). Strategies to promote the professional transition of new graduate nurse practitioners: A systematic review. *Nursing Forum, 54*(4), 557–564.

Spies, L. A., Garner, S. L., Faucher, M. A., Hastings-Tolsma, M., Riley, C., Millenbruch, J., Prater, L., & Conroy, S. F. (2017). A model for upscaling global partnerships and building nurse and midwifery capacity. *International Nursing Review, 64*(3), 331–344.

Staebler, S., Meier, S. R., Bagweil, G., & Conway-Orgel, M. (2016). The future of neonatal advanced practice nurse practice: White paper. *Advances in Neonatal Care, 16*(1), 8–14.

Stanik-Hutt, J., Newhouse, R. P., White, K. M., Johantgen, M., Bass, E. B., Zangaro, G., Wilson, R., Fountain, L., Steinwachs, D. M., Heindel, L., & Weiner, J. P. (2013). The quality and effectiveness of care provided by nurse practitioners. *The Journal for Nurse Practitioners, 9*(8), 492–500. e13.

Steinke, M. K., Rogers, M., Lehwaldt, D., & Lamarche, K. (2017). An examination of advanced practice nurses' job satisfaction internationally. *International Nursing Review, 65*(2), 162–172.

Swan, M., Ferguson, S., Chang, A., Larson, E., & Smaldone, A. (2015). Quality of primary care provided by advanced practice nurses: A systematic review. *International Journal for Quality in Health Care, 27*(5), 396–404.

Swiss Association for Nursing Science. (2012). *Key issues on the regulation advanced practice nurses.* http://www.pflegeforschung-vfp.ch/download/58/page/23766_dl_2012%2010%2010%20%20def%20eckpunkte%20anp%20d%20x.pdf

Temane, A. M., Poggenpoel, M., & Myburgh, C. P. (2014). Advanced psychiatric nurse practitioners' ideas and needs for supervision in private practice in South Africa. *Curationis, 37*(1) Article #1161.

Tenedios, C., O'Leary, S., Capocci, M., & Desai, S. P. (2018). Nurse anaesthesia practice in the G7 countries (Canada, France, Germany, Italy, Japan, the United Kingdom, and the United States of America. *European Journal of Anaesthesiology, 35*(3), 158–164.

Tian, X., Lian, J., Yi, L., Ma, L., Wang, Y., & Cao, H. (2014). Current status of clinical nursing specialists and the demands of osteoporosis specialized nurses in Mainland China. *International Journal of Nursing Sciences, 1*(3), 306–313.

Tracy, A. (2017). Perceptions of certified registered nurse anesthetists on factors affecting their transition from student. *American Association of Nurse Anesthetists' Journal, 85*(6), 438–444.

Tsay, S. L., Tsay, S. F., Ke, C. Y., Chen, C. M., & Tung, H. H. (2018). Analysis of nurse practitioner scope of practice in Taiwan using the Longest policy cycle model. *Journal of the American Association of Nurse Practitioners, 31*(3), 198–205.

Tsiachristas, A., Wallenburg, I., Bond, C. M., Elliot, R. F., Busse, R., van Exel, J., Rutten-van Mölken, M. P., & de Bont, A. MONROS Team. (2015). Costs and effects of new professional roles: Evidence from a literature review. *Health Policy, 119*(9), 1176–1187.

Tyler, D. O., Hoyt, K. S., Dowling Evans, D., Schumann, L., Ramirez, E., Wilbeck, J., & Agan, D. (2018). Emergency nurse practitioner practice analysis: Report and implications of the findings. *Journal of the American Association of Nurse Practitioners, 30*(10), 560–569.

Ugochukwu, C. G., Uys, L. R., Karani, A. K., Okoronkwo, I. L., & Diop, B. N. (2013). Roles of nurses in sub-Saharan African region. *International Journal of Nursing and Midwifery, 5*(7), 117–131.

Umutesi, G., McEvoy, M. D., Starnes, J. R., Sileshi, B., Atieli, H. E., Onyango, K., & Newton, M. W. (2019). Safe anesthesia care in western Kenya: A preliminary assessment of the impact of nurse anesthetists at multiple levels of government hospitals. *Anesthesia and Analgesia, 129*(5), 1387–1393.

United Nations. (2012). *Agenda item 123. Global health and foreign policy. A/67/L36. 67th United Nations General Assembly*. New York City: New York, USA.

United Nations Population Fund (UNFPA). (2011). *The state of the world's midwifery. Delivering health, saving lives*. http://www.unfpa.org/sites/default/files/pub-pdf/en_SOWMR_Full.pdf

United Nations Population Fund (UNFPA). (2014). *The State of the World's Midwifery. A Universal Pathway. A Woman's Right to Health*. vhttp://www.unfpa.org/sowmy.

Wang, J., Zou, X., Cong, L., & Liu, H. (2018). Clinical effectiveness and cost-effectiveness of nurse-led care in Chinese patients with rheumatoid arthritis: A randomized trial comparing with rheumatologist-led care. *International Journal of Nursing Practice, 24*. Article e12605. https://doi.org/10.1111/ijn.12605

Westman, B., Ullgren, H., Olofsson, A., & Sharp, L. (2019). Patient-reported perceptions of care after the introduction of a new advanced practice cancer nursing role in Sweden. *European Journal of Oncology Nursing, 41*, 41–48.

Whittaker, A., Hill, A., & Leary, A. (2017). Developing the next generation of specialist cancer nurses. *Cancer Nursing Practice, 16*(9), 25–30.

Williams, K. (2017). Advanced practitioners in emergency care: A literature review. *Emergency Nurse, 25*(4), 36–41.

Wisur-Hokkanen, C., Glasberg, G., Makela, C., & Fagerstrom, L. (2015). Experiences of working as an advanced practice nurse in Finland—the substance of advanced nursing practice and promoting and inhibiting factors. *Scandinavian Journal of Caring Sciences, 29*, 793–802.

Wong, F. K. Y., Lau, A. T. Y., Ng, R., Wong, E. W. Y., Wong, S. M., Kan, E. C. Y., Liu, E., & Bryant-Lukosius, D. (2017). An exploratory study on exemplary practice of nurse consultants. *Journal of Nursing Scholarship, 49*(5), 548–556.

Wong, F. K. Y., Liu, H., Wang, H., Anderson, D., Seib, C., & Molasiotis, A. (2015). Global nursing issues and development: Analysis of World Health Organization documents. *Journal of Nursing Scholarship, 47*(6), 574–583.

Wong, F. K. Y., Peng, G., Kan, E. C., Li, Y., Lau, A. T., Zhang, L., Leung, A. F., Liu, X., Leung, V. O., Chen, W., & Li, M. (2010). Description and evaluation of an initiative to develop advanced practice nurses in mainland China. *Nurse Education Today, 30*, 344–349.

Wongkpratoom, S., Srisuphan, W., Senaratana, W., Nantachiapan, P., & Sritanyarat, W. (2010). Role development of advanced practice nurses in Thailand. *Pacific Rim International Journal of Nursing Research, 14*(2), 162–177.

Woo, B. F. Y., Zhou, W., Lim, T. W., & Tam, W. W. S. (2019). Practice patterns and role perception of advanced practice nurses: A nationwide cross-sectional study. *Journal of Nursing Management, 27*, 992–1004.

World Health Organization. (2010). *Strategic directions for strengthening nursing and midwifery services 2011-2015*. http://www.who.int/hrh/resources/nmsd/en/

World Health Organization (WHO). (2012). *Progress report on nursing and midwifery 2008-2012*. http://www.who.int/hrh/nursing_midwifery/NursingMidwiferyProgressReport.pdf

World Health Organization (WHO). (2015a). *Health workforce? Does the world have enough midwives?* http://www.who.int/maternal_child_adolescent/news_events/news/2015/role-of-midwives/en/

World Health Organization (WHO). (2015b). *Progress report on nursing and midwifery 2013-2015*. http://www.who.int/hrh/nursing_midwifery/nursing-midwifery_report_13-15.pdf?ua=1

World Health Organization (WHO). (2016). *Health workforce 2030: A global strategy on human resources for health*. Draft for the 69th World Health Assembly. http://www.who.int/hrh/resources/16059_Global_strategyWorkforce2030.pdf

World Health Organization (WHO). (2020). *State of the world's nursing 2020: Investing in education, jobs, and leadership*. https://www.who.int/publications/i/item/nursing-report-2020

Xue, Y., Ye, Z., Brewer, C., & Spetz, J. (2016). Impact of state nurse practitioner scope-of-practice regulation on health care delivery: Systematic review. *Nursing Outlook, 64*, 71–85.

Yafa, H., Dorit, R., & Shoshana, R. (2016). Gerontological nurse practitioners (GNPs) for the first time in Israel: Physicians' and nurses' attitudes. *Journal of the American Association of Nurse Practitioners, 28*(8), 415–422.

Zahran, Z., Curtis, P., Lloyd-Jones, M., & Blackett, T. (2012). Jordanian perspectives on advanced nursing practice: An ethnography. *International Nursing Review, 59*(2), 222–229.

Zak, C., Wood, L. K., Adelman, D. S., & Fant, C. (2020). The personal and professional responsibilities of NPs in disaster response. *The Nurse Practitioner, 45*(5), 34–40.

PART II

Competencies of Advanced Practice Nursing

6 DIRECT CLINICAL PRACTICE

MARY FRAN TRACY ■ NANCY P. BLUMENTHAL

"There is nothing so stable as change."
~ Bob Dylan

CHAPTER CONTENTS

DIRECT CARE VERSUS INDIRECT CARE ACTIVITIES 169
SIX CHARACTERISTICS OF DIRECT CLINICAL CARE PROVIDED BY ADVANCED PRACTICE NURSES 172
USE OF A HOLISTIC PERSPECTIVE 173
Holism Described 173
Holism and Health Assessment 173
Nursing Model or Medical Model 175
FORMATION OF THERAPEUTIC PARTNERSHIPS WITH PATIENTS 176
Implicit Bias 179
Communication With Patients 179
Shared Decision Making 179
Cultural Influences on Partnerships 180
Therapeutic Partnerships With Noncommunicative Patients 181
EXPERT CLINICAL PERFORMANCE 182
Clinical Thinking 182
Ethical Reasoning 186
Skillful Performance 187
USE OF REFLECTIVE PRACTICE 190
USE OF EVIDENCE AS A GUIDE TO PRACTICE 191
Evidence-Based Practice 192
Theory-Based Practice 193
DIVERSE APPROACHES TO HEALTH AND ILLNESS MANAGEMENT 194
Interpersonal Interventions 194
Therapeutic Assessments and Interventions 194
Individualized Interventions 197
Complementary Therapies 197
Clinical Prevention 198
MANAGEMENT OF COMPLEX SITUATIONS 200
HELPING PATIENTS MANAGE CHRONIC ILLNESSES 202
DIRECT CARE AND INFORMATION MANAGEMENT 203
CONCLUSION 204
KEY SUMMARY POINTS 205

Direct care is the central competency of advanced practice nursing. This competency informs and shapes the execution of the other five competencies. Direct care is essential for a number of reasons. To collaborate and lead clinical staff and programs effectively, an advanced practice registered nurse (APRN) must have clinical credibility. With the deep clinical and systems understanding that APRNs possess, they facilitate the care processes that ensure positive outcomes for individuals and groups of patients. Advanced practice occurs within a healthcare system that is constantly changing—changing delivery models, reimbursement structures, regulatory requirements, technology, and population-based management. The challenge that many APRNs face is how to highlight and maintain the characteristics of their care that have helped patients achieve positive health outcomes and afforded APRN care a unique niche in the healthcare marketplace. Characteristics such as the use of a holistic perspective and formation of therapeutic partnerships with patients to co-implement individualized health care are challenged by cost containment strategies that emphasize standardization of care to achieve population-based outcome targets. Conversely, characteristics of APRN care such as health promotion, fostering self-care, and patient education add value because they result in an appropriate use of healthcare resources and sustain quality.

This chapter describes the direct clinical practice of APRNs and helps readers understand how it differs from the practice of nurses who are experts by experience, describes strategies for balancing direct care with other competencies, and describes strategies for retaining a direct care focus. The six characteristics of APRN direct care practice are identified.

DIRECT CARE VERSUS INDIRECT CARE ACTIVITIES

Direct care is the central APRN competency (see Chapter 3). The APRN is using advanced clinical judgment, systems thinking, and accountability in providing evidence-based care at a more advanced level than the care provided by the expert registered nurse (RN). The APRN is prepared to assist individuals through complex healthcare situations by the use of advanced communication, promotion of self-care management, counseling, and coordination of care (American Association of Colleges of Nursing [AACN], 2021). Although an expert RN may, at times, demonstrate components of care that are at an advanced level, it is care that is gained through experience and is exemplary (not expected) at that level. *The Essentials: Core Competencies for Professional Nursing Education* delineates that APRN-level care is demonstrated through advanced, refined assessment skills and implementation and evaluation of practice interventions based on integrated knowledge from a number of sciences, such as biophysical, psychosocial, behavioral, cultural, economic, and nursing science (AACN, 2021). Graduate-level APRN education provides a foundation for the evolution of practice over time necessitated by health care and patients. This advanced level of practice is an expected competency of all APRNs, not an exemplary skill that is intermittently or inconsistently displayed by staff or expert nurses.

For the purposes of this chapter, the terms *direct care* and *direct clinical practice* refer to the activities and functions that APRNs perform within the patient–nurse interface. Depending on the focus of an APRN's practice, the patient may, and often does, include family members and significant others. The activities that occur in this interface or as direct follow-up are unique because they are interpersonally and physically co-enacted with a particular patient for the purpose of promoting that patient's health or well-being. Many important processes transpire at this point of care (Box 6.1).

Advanced practice nursing activities occurring before and adjacent to the patient–nurse interface have a great influence on the direct care that occurs; however, they are not performed with an individual patient or their main purpose is tangential to or supportive of the direct care of the patient. Activities such as collaboration with, consultation to, and mentoring of staff may all be occurring in relation to the direct care interface. It is often difficult to separate out these

BOX 6.1

Examples of Processes That Occur at the Point of Care

- The patient-provider therapeutic partnership is established.
- Health problems become mutually understood through information gathering and effective communication.
- Health, recovery, or palliative goals are expressed by the patient.
- Management and treatment options are explored.
- Physical acts of diagnosis, monitoring, treatment, and pharmacologic and nonpharmacologic therapy are performed.
- Education, support, guidance and coaching, and comfort are provided.
- Decisions regarding future actions to be taken by each party are made.
- Future contact is planned.

indirect care interventions, which are equally necessary for adequate fulfillment of the APRN role and care of the patient (Box 6.2). For example, when an APRN consults with another provider regarding the nature of a patient's condition or the care that should be recommended to a patient, the APRN is engaging in advanced clinical practice, but it is not direct care. Even though the APRN is accountable for the consultation, the primary purpose of that contact is to acquire information and understanding to use in formulating recommendations for the patient's direct care provider. Thus according to the definition of direct care used in this chapter, the APRN is engaged in clinical practice but they are not providing direct care to the patient. The direct care role of the clinical nurse specialist (CNS) may not be as apparent to observers as it is for a nurse practitioner (NP), certified registered nurse anesthetist (CRNA), and certified nurse-midwife (CNM) because the CNS frequently shifts from direct to indirect activities depending on the situation and the providers involved. For the CNS, these shifts may occur during one patient encounter, and certainly across a day. Most APRNs will have a role in ensuring that others are providing quality and safe care through indirect practice (Exemplar 6.1).

APRN roles tend to diverge when comparing the amount of time spent in each of the direct care activities. Clinical nurse specialists have consistently reported spending the majority of their time in the nurse/nursing personnel and organization/systems spheres rather than direct patient care (National Association of Clinical Nurse Specialists, 2017, 2019, 2021). A research study by Oddsdottir and Sveinsdottir (2011) demonstrated that CNSs spend most of their time in education and expert practice in the institutional domain; the authors recommended that the focus for CNSs needs to be on direct practice in the client/family domain. This finding is consistent with other studies reporting that NPs and CNMs spend a majority of their time on individual patient care and less time on teaching, administration, and research (Kleinpell et al., 2018; Reuter-Rice et al., 2016; Van Hecke et al., 2019). This may change with time as CNSs are more consistently prepared similarly to other APRNs in advanced physical assessment and pharmacology. There is no set formula as to how much time in direct care is "enough" or appropriate; however, direct care is a core competency and APRNs functioning in a clinical practice should spend at least some time over the balance of their role in direct care activities.

This delineation of direct and indirect practice is not intended to denigrate clinical activities that occur outside the patient–nurse interface—quite the contrary. These clinical activities and functions should be recognized as influencing what happens in the interface and as having a significant impact on patient outcomes. Because these other clinical activities significantly affect patient outcomes, they must be valued by the nursing community and healthcare systems. In the current environment of cost containment and technological development, all activities that enhance patients' health, recovery, and adjustment are critical components of care delivered by APRNs. Becker et al. (2020), based on a practice analysis of adult–gerontology CNSs and adult–gerontology CNPs, found that APRNs engage in a range of strategic activities, an excellent characterization of the direct and indirect but adjacent actions that make up the clinical practice of APRNs as depicted in exemplars throughout the chapter.

Researchers are beginning to understand the specific activities that constitute the direct care component of various advanced practice nursing roles. However, it is difficult to make generalizations about these activities because the APRNs in the studies noted previously had

BOX 6.2

Examples of Advanced Practice Nurse Indirect Care Activities

- Consultation with other healthcare providers (e.g., physicians, nurses, pharmacists)
- Discharge planning
- Care coordination
- Communication with insurance organizations
- Education of bedside nurses
- Unit rounds
- Researching evidence-based care guidelines
- Leading quality-of-care initiatives
- Support staff supervision
- Billing and coding
- Compliance monitoring
- Budget development and implementation

EXEMPLAR 6.1
DIRECT AND INDIRECT CARE PROVIDED BY ADVANCED PRACTICE NURSES[a]

Direct Care

The care of patients with pulmonary hypertension is commonly managed in the outpatient environment. When those receiving continuous prostacyclin infusion therapy via tunneled central line come back to the hospital for treatment or testing, M.P., the cardiovascular clinical nurse specialist, completes a physical assessment of the patient's current condition and response to therapy.

Standard medical assessment of patient response to changes in prostacyclin therapy includes magnetic resonance imaging (MRI). Because the home infusion pump that delivers the medication cannot be taken into the MRI environment, and because disruption of the infusion can lead to significant complications (including rebound pulmonary hypertension), M.P. works directly with the patient to identify the safest method to continue therapy during the scan. After collecting information about the patient's medication, dose, and pump type, M.P. interviews the patient to assess how the patient is feeling in response to current therapy; the longest period of time the patient has gone without the infusion medication; and how they tolerated the pause in therapy. The plan for continuing therapy during the MRI is established based on this data collection.

If the patient's infusion pump can function when adequate lengths of tubing are added to the basic infusion set to reach into the MRI area, leaving the pump outside the magnetic field, then M.P. works with the patient to either pre-prime the additional tubing at home or in the preparation area of MRI. Review of the plan for the study and answering the patient's questions and concerns with expertise ease the patient's concerns about undergoing the test.

If the patient's pump will not function appropriately with additional lengths of tubing, M.P. collaborates with a pharmacist experienced in the use of intravenous prostacyclins. M.P. and the pharmacist establish an appropriate concentration of medication to be used during the test, calculate the rate needed to achieve the same dose as the patient has been receiving at home, and order both the medications to use during the test and a syringe of medication in the same concentration as the home concentration to use in repriming the patient's central line. After reviewing with the patient the steps to be taken, M.P. helps the patient to convert to the hospital-based infusion prior to the MRI and then assists with conversion back to the home pump at the end of the study. Using advanced assessment skills, M.P. assesses the patient's tolerance of these transitions as well as any side effects they may experience during the transitions.

Advanced clinical assessment and planning skills are critical in managing patients in this population. Complex care planning, early identification of complications if they occur, and the ability to safely resolve those issues exemplify the importance of the advanced practice registered nurse's role in care of this very challenging patient population.

Indirect Care

The medical intensive care unit acute care nurse practitioner (ACNP) was approached by an experienced staff nurse who was struggling to develop an interpersonal relationship with the family of a complex, critically ill patient. The family was very anxious and was having difficulty synthesizing the information that the staff nurse was trying to provide to them.

Rather than intervene directly with the family, the ACNP recognized that this would be a good opportunity for the staff nurse to develop and expand her skills at interpersonal relationship building. The ACNP explored with the nurse the interventions that she had already attempted and reviewed with her the literature regarding family stressors in critical care, family needs, and the goal of assessing and addressing what the family perceives as their educational and care needs. Armed with this information, the nurse felt comfortable in working with the family to assess their priority educational and psychosocial needs to obtain the resources and information they needed.

The ACNP could have intervened by establishing a direct relationship with the family, which would have been providing direct care. In this case, however, she determined that it was more important to assist the staff nurse in the development of the relationship as a growth opportunity and to help the nurse form an ongoing partnership with the family, with whom she would be interacting on a continuing basis.

[a]The author gratefully acknowledges Michael Petty, PhD, RN, APRN, CNS, for use of his direct care exemplar.

different roles and worked in different settings, with different populations. Different classification schemas were used to categorize APRN actions. For example, in some studies, investigators used the term *activities* to classify APRN actions; in others, the term *interventions* was used. The variability in terminology and definitions makes it difficult to compare results across APRN roles, settings, and populations. Nevertheless, a review of these studies yields some insights into the extent and nature of direct care activities in APRN roles.

Many direct care activities performed are similar across APRN roles, and preparation of all APRNs must include the "three Ps"—advanced *p*athophysiology, advanced health and *p*hysical assessment, and advanced *p*harmacology (AACN, 2021). Additional direct care activities that are similar across roles include patient and family education and counseling, ordering laboratory tests and medications, and performing procedures (Becker et al., 2006; Verger et al., 2005). Reuter-Rice et al. (2016) surveyed pediatric critical care NPs regarding their direct care activities, which included physical assessments, patient and family teaching, and performing procedures such as venipuncture, intravenous line insertions, lumbar punctures, feeding tube placements, endotracheal intubations, and central line placements. CNMs reported expansion of their direct care procedures to include first-assisting during cesarean sections and performing endometrial biopsies (Holland & Holland, 2007). CNSs and administrators need to have an ongoing understanding of the direct care components of the CNS role. With increasing complexity and diversity of the role, there can be a propensity to have CNSs perform less and less expert direct care of patients, which is the main characteristic of APRN practice (Lewandowski & Adamle, 2009).

Regardless of the population being cared for, surveillance was a key direct care activity of APRNs identified in studies (Brooten et al., 2003, 2007; Hughes et al., 2002). *Surveillance* is described as watching for physical and emotional signs and symptoms and monitoring dressing and wound care, laboratory results, medications, nutrition, response to treatment, and caregiving and parenting. Thus surveillance refers to an APRN's vigilant assessment of patient status, the rapid diagnosis of subtle or emergent conditions, and quick intervention to prevent or reverse a potentially negative outcome. Nursing surveillance can have a particularly important impact on the patient safety indicator of failure-to-rescue—situations in which providers fail to notice symptoms or respond adequately or swiftly to deteriorating clinical signs, resulting in patient death from preventable complications. Failure-to-rescue has been linked to nursing surveillance; for example, the higher the nursing surveillance, as defined by staffing ratios or by the frequency of checking on patients, the lower the number of cases of failure-to-rescue (Aiken et al., 2002; Burke et al., 2020; Clarke & Aiken, 2003; Lasater et al., 2021). Burke et al. (2020) conducted a systematic review of root causes of failure-to-rescue and strategies that would mitigate or prevent it. A key finding pertinent to APRNs is that a "nursing" style of communication (e.g., patient-centered, creating partnerships, open to patient expression, attuned to emotional and social environments) resulted in improved outcomes compared with a "biomedical" communication style (e.g., patriarchal, authoritative, focus on signs and symptoms). This nursing communication style may also benefit APRNs in these situations as they can "speak" the language of both nursing and medicine, communicating concerns to interdisciplinary team members, and engage in an appropriate reaction to the situation. In summary, direct care activities make up a large part of what most APRNs do, although there is considerable variation in which activities are performed and how much time is devoted to the direct care function across roles, settings, and patient populations.

SIX CHARACTERISTICS OF DIRECT CLINICAL CARE PROVIDED BY ADVANCED PRACTICE NURSES

APRNs function in many roles and settings and with different populations. Despite such variability in role implementation, there is a similarity in the components of direct care provided. Characteristics of advanced practice nursing care extend across advanced practice roles, healthcare settings, and populations of patients. These six characteristics are as follows:

- Use of a holistic perspective
- Formation of therapeutic partnerships with patients
- Expert clinical performance
- Use of reflective practice
- Use of evidence as a guide to practice
- Use of diverse approaches to health and illness management.

Accumulating evidence supports these features of APRN practice as having positive influences on patient outcomes (Newhouse et al., 2011). Throughout this chapter, the empirical evidence cited about APRN practice is illustrative and not based on a systematic review of research.

The six characteristics of APRN direct care practice have their roots in the traditional values of the nursing profession. These values are defined in nursing's social contract with society, as outlined by the American Nurses Association (ANA, 2010):

- People manifest an essential unity of mind, body, and spirit.
- People's experiences are contextually and culturally defined.
- Health and illness are human experiences. The presence of illness does not preclude health, nor does optimal health preclude illness.
- The relationship between the nurse and patient occurs within the context of the values and beliefs of the patient and nurse.
- Public policy and the healthcare delivery system influence the health and well-being of society and professional nursing.
- Individual responsibility and interprofessional involvement are essential.

Nurses in advanced practice roles often have a deep commitment to the values on which these characteristics rest and are able to advocate persuasively and incorporate these values in daily practice. The expanded scope of practice of APRN roles often enables APRNs to fully enact these characteristics in their interactions with patients. An overview of strategies for enacting these characteristics is provided in Box 6.3.

USE OF A HOLISTIC PERSPECTIVE

Holism Described

Holism has a variety of meanings. A broad view is that holism involves a deep understanding of each patient as a complex and unique person who is embedded in a temporally unfolding life. The holistic perspective recognizes the multiple dimensions of each person—physiologic, social, psychological, emotional, cognitive, functional, quality of life, personal happiness, well-being, and spiritual (National Academies of Science, Engineering, and Medicine [NASEM], 2021)—and that the relationships among these dimensions result in a whole that is greater than the sum of the parts. People are in constant interaction with themselves, others, the environment, and universe and exhibit maximum well-being when all parts are balanced and in harmony (Erickson, 2007); this state of well-being can exist whether there are physical disorders or not.

This comprehensive and integrated view of human life and health is considered in the healthcare encounter within the context of the full range of factors influencing patients' experiences (Box 6.4). Clearly, high-tech care environments with many healthcare providers, each focused on a particular aspect of a patient's condition and treatment, require coordinators who have a comprehensive and integrated appreciation of the patient and their experience of care as a whole. APRNs' capacity to keep the pieces together and promote continuity of care in a way that focuses on the unique individual is undoubtedly why many clinical programs have an APRN member or coordinator (see "Management of Complex Situations" later). Interprofessional team members caring for older adults view the APRN as a leader in facilitating holistic care (Cowley et al., 2016). For example, APRNs practicing in palliative care demonstrate practice at an advanced level by combining holistic care with treatment interventions to ameliorate symptoms, all while they are evaluating the care from a system context in terms of appropriate use of resources (George, 2016). The Shuler Nurse Practitioner Practice Model is based on a holistic understanding of human health and illness in older adults that integrates medical and nursing perspectives (Shuler et al., 2001; see Chapter 2).

Holism and Health Assessment

When working with a relatively healthy person, the APRN seeks to understand the person's life goals, functional interests, and health risks to preserve quality of life in the future. In contrast, when working with an ill patient, the APRN is interested in what the person views as problems, how they are responding to problems, and what the problems and responses mean to the individual in terms of daily living and life goals. Holism is an integral foundation to nursing's patient-centered care (AACN, 2021). In assessing patients, APRNs understand the interactions between body–brain–mind–spirit not only of the patients themselves but how those interactions occur between patients and other individuals, their communities, and their environment (Smith, 2019). Eriksson et al. (2018) reported that patients recognize the practice of APRNs in treating them as whole persons rather than focusing solely on their health problem. This was achieved through APRN approaches that were respectful and flexible,

BOX 6.3

Characteristics of Advanced Direct Care Practice and Strategies for Enacting Them

USE OF A HOLISTIC PERSPECTIVE

- Take into account the complexity of human life.
- Recognize and address how social determinants of health affect people and their health.
- Consider the profound effects of illness, aging, hospitalization, and stress.
- Consider how symptoms, illness, and treatment affect quality of life.
- Focus on functional abilities and requirements.

FORMATION OF THERAPEUTIC PARTNERSHIPS WITH PATIENTS

- Use a conversational style to conduct healthcare encounters.
- Optimize therapeutic use of self.
- Encourage the patient, and family as appropriate, to actively engage as partners in decision making.
- Look for cultural influences on healthcare discourse.
- Listen to the indirect voices of patients who are noncommunicative.
- Advocate the patient's perspective and concerns to others.

EXPERT CLINICAL PERFORMANCE

- Acquire specialized knowledge.
- Seek out supervision when performing a new skill.
- Invest in deeply understanding the patient situations in which you are involved.
- Generate and test alternative lines of reasoning.
- Trust your hunches—check them out.
- Be aware of when you are time-pressured and likely to make thinking errors.
- Consider multiple aspects of the patient's situation when you are deciding how to treat.
- Make sure that you know how to use technical equipment safely.
- Make sure that you know how to interpret data produced by monitoring devices.
- Pay attention to how you move and touch patients during care.
- Anticipate ethical conflicts.
- Acquire technology-related skills for accessing and managing patient data and practice information.

USE OF REFLECTIVE PRACTICE

- Explore your personal values, belief systems, and behaviors.
- Identify your basic assumptions about health care, the advanced practice registered nurse role, and the rights and responsibilities of patients.
- Consider how your implicit biases affect your judgments.
- Talk to colleagues and your teachers about your clinical experiences.
- Consider use of a journal to document experiences.
- Assess your current skill and comfort in reflection.

USE OF EVIDENCE AS A GUIDE FOR PRACTICE

- Learn how to search healthcare databases for studies related to specific clinical topics.
- Read research reports related to your field of practice.
- Seek out systematic revision of research and evidence-based clinical guidelines.
- Acquire skills in appraising the various forms of evidence.
- Work with colleagues to consider evidence-based improvements in care.

DIVERSE APPROACHES TO AND INTERVENTIONS FOR HEALTH AND ILLNESS MANAGEMENT

- Use interpersonal interventions to guide and coach patients.
- Acquire proficiency in new ways of treating and helping patients.
- Help patients maintain health and capitalize on their strengths and resources.
- Provide preventive services appropriate to your field of practice.
- Coordinate services among care sites and multiple providers.
- Acquire knowledge about complementary therapies.

BOX 6.4

Factors to Consider When Helping the Patient Holistically

- Patient's view of their health or illness.
- Patterns of physical symptoms and amount of distress they cause.
- Effect of physical symptoms on the patient's daily functioning and quality of life
- Symptom management approaches that are acceptable to the patient.
- Life changes that could affect the patient's physical or psychological well-being (e.g., relationship changes, job change, intrafamily conflict, retirement, death of a loved one).
- Social determinants of health and context of the patient's life, including the nuclear family unit, social support, job responsibilities, financial situation, health insurance coverage, responsibilities for the care of others (e.g., children, chronically ill spouse or partner, older parents).
- Spiritual and life values (e.g., independence, religion, beliefs about life, acceptance of fate).

conveying trust and safety (Eriksson et al., 2018). In today's world, it is imperative that this holistic approach consider social determinants of health that can greatly impact the health of individuals (NASEM, 2021). APRNs must incorporate screening for social needs into their care and engage appropriate interdisciplinary colleagues as part of a holistic care plan in patients with increasingly complex needs (NASEM, 2021). Faculty also engage students by role-modeling the provision of holistic care from a nursing perspective (Brykczynski, 2012; Kinchen, 2019). This includes nurse practitioner curricula that incorporate values such as knowledge of the patient's physical condition and listening to and being present with patients while partnering in the creation of a care plan (Kinchen, 2019). APRNs partner with patients to define health, identify their values, and guide their care by their preferences (NASEM, 2021).

The ability to function in daily activities and relationships is an important consideration for patients when they evaluate their health, so it is an appropriate and essential focus for holistic, person-centered assessment. Most functional assessment formats focus on the following: (1) how patients view their health or quality of life; (2) how they accomplish self-care and household or job responsibilities; (3) the social, physical, financial, environmental, and spiritual factors that augment or tax their functioning; and (4) the strategies that they and their families use to cope with the stresses and problems in their lives.

In pediatrics, measures of functional status have been developed, such as one for children with asthma (Centers for Disease Control and Prevention, 2013). In adults, APRNs may choose to use a disease- or problem-focused tool such as measurement of functional status in patients with heart failure (Rector et al., 2006), of symptom distress in patients with cancer (Chen & Lin, 2007; Cleeland et al., 2000), or of function and disability in geriatric patients (Denkinger et al., 2009) or a widely used general measure such as the Short Form-36 Health Survey, which measures overall health, functional status, and well-being in adults and is available in several languages (Ware & Sherbourne, 1992).

Nursing Model or Medical Model

As APRNs have taken on responsibilities that were formerly in the purview of physicians, some have expressed concern that APRNs are being asked to function within a medical model of practice rather than within a holistic nursing model. This concern is raised when APRNs function as substitutes for physicians. However, there is evidence that a nursing orientation is an enduring component of APRN practice, even when medical management is part of the role (Brykczynski, 2012; Cowley et al., 2016; George, 2016; Mason et al., 2015; Box 6.5). Activities described in these studies clearly reflect a nursing-focused practice.

Statements from professional organizations indicate that APRNs value both their nursing orientation and their medical functions. For example, the description of APRNs in the ANA's nursing social policy statement includes strong endorsement of specialized and expanded knowledge and skills within the context of holistic values (ANA, 2010). On the theoretical front, several models of advanced practice blend nursing and medical orientations (see "Shuler's Model of NP Practice" and "Dunphy and Winland-Brown's Circle of Caring: A Transformative, Collaborative Model" in Chapter 2).

BOX 6.5

Nursing-Focused Advanced Practice Interventions

- Partnering with patients in their own care
- Patient education
- Guidance and coaching
- Care planning and care coordination
- Physical and occupational therapy referrals
- Use of communication skills
- Promotion of continuity of care
- Teaching of nursing staff
- Advance directive discussions
- Wellness and health promotion initiatives

FORMATION OF THERAPEUTIC PARTNERSHIPS WITH PATIENTS

The Institute of Medicine (IOM, 2001) has recommended patient-centered care as the foundation of safe, effective, and efficient health care. The person-centered, holistic perspective of nursing and, by extension, advanced practice nursing serves as the foundation for the types of relationships that they co-create with patients. APRNs are well prepared to develop therapeutic relationships as the cornerstone of patient-centered care (Esmaeili et al., 2014; Kitson et al., 2012). The Gallup Poll has consistently reported that the public views nurses as the most trusted professionals (Saad, 2020). The skill of APRNs to develop therapeutic relationships with individual patients can influence broader public perceptions.

The development and maintenance of therapeutic relationships with patients and families is a key criterion in *The Essentials: Core Competencies for Professional Nursing Education*, which is specific and foundational to advanced practice nursing (AACN, 2021). Studies have shown that APRNs form collaborative relationships with patients. In research of an APRN-directed transitional care model (Bradway et al., 2012), the authors found that a mutually trusting relationship between the APRN, the cognitively impaired patient, and the caregiver was key to providing the caregivers with the confidence and information they needed to optimally care for their loved one. This personal relationship and the availability of the APRN outside routine visits led to the avoidance of potentially negative outcomes. The APRNs utilized their advanced skills in tailoring information to improve caregiver skills and knowledge in these complex patient cases. Bissonette et al. (2013) also found that an APRN-led collaborative team led to fewer emergency department visits and hospital admissions in kidney transplant recipients. In addition, Drennan et al. (2011) found that patients were satisfied with their relationships with nurses and midwives, including the consultation process, patient education, medication advice, and the patient's intent to comply with provider advice.

By virtue of recent advances in technology and necessary restrictions imposed by COVID-19, telehealth has quickly emerged as a forum for care delivery. Videoconferencing, emailing, and communicating via patient portals on smartphones and home computers have all become elements of therapeutic encounters (Arends et al., 2021). While telehealth has the potential to increase access to care, it presents challenges to the establishment of therapeutic rapport. In this setting, the traditional bedside manner is supplanted by the APRN's "telepresence." Attention to how the patient perceives the APRN in a telehealth clinical encounter requires a professional background and attire, privacy and the absence of distractions, eye contact with camera, and the ability to multitask with note taking and chart review on the computer (Finkelstein, 2020).

APRNs' therapeutic use of self contributes to the optimization of a therapeutic relationship with patient and family. Therapeutic use of self involves APRN awareness of personal feelings, attitudes, and values and how that awareness influences the patient–provider relationship (Warner, 2006). This increased awareness on the part of the APRN helps increase empathy, allowing the APRN to engage more deeply with patients while maintaining appropriate boundaries to uphold objectivity (Warner, 2006). Therapeutic use of self also entails awareness regarding how one's own attributes are perceived by patients and caregivers. The APRN must consider the meaning of these perceptions to the patient and how they inform the patient's engagement in the therapeutic relationship (Younas & Quennell, 2019). See Exemplar 6.2 for an example from a patient perspective when a therapeutic partnership is not established.

EXEMPLAR 6.2

A CAUTIONARY TALE: THE FOUNDER OF THE FIRST NURSE PRACTITIONER (NP) PROGRAM ON DISAPPOINTING NP ENCOUNTERS

Dr. Eileen O'Grady interviewed Dr. Loretta Ford, the founder of the NP role, on February 16, 2016. The following discussion captures a not-so-exemplary experience she had seeing an NP who did not meet her needs or appear to be practicing even the most basic nursing skills. This is presented as a cautionary tale about how patients can experience APRNs who do not embody the six competencies.

Dr. O'Grady: I'd like to start with an incident you had a few years ago, seeing an NP who fell short of meeting your needs.

Dr. Ford: I ended up with a NP from the cardiologists' office. [The cardiologist] called himself the electrician of the cardiac team because he puts in the pacemakers. I began to have tachycardia attacks that were unusual, so I made an appointment but the cardiologist was busy, so they said I could see the NP. So, I said, "Fine!" That was good. I was on some medications and I felt they needed to be changed but when I checked them out, I was taking the maximum dose, so I didn't want to increase it until I had some information about it. So, I went to see the NP. I hadn't seen her before and she came in and said her name; when I go to any health service I never tell them who I am or what my background is or anything. I'm careful not to use any technical language that might give me away. Right away there didn't seem to be any interest in me as a person, and so of course I didn't say anything. I didn't want to give it away, but I also didn't offer anything. First of all, there was no history of any kind taken, not even a nursing history. There was no asking. She was looking at the computer more than at me and asking the computer "Now, is this unusual, this recent event?" or "What triggered it?" She never asked what I thought might trigger it. So from there on, it lacked human interaction. I could see no evidence of whether she cared or not or whether or not there was any nursing presence at all. I didn't feel that there was any caring or compassion, it was purely technical. As a matter of fact, the NP was not as caring as my primary care physician. There was no sense of coordination, and in the end she said, "Well, I'll have to go and check with the cardiologist about new medication or different medication." And that ended the visit. So, I didn't feel that nursing was there at all. I didn't think it was even good medicine myself, but I'm used to having a primary care physician who is an excellent clinician and a good teacher. So, I was disappointed, and I was never really sure if my primary care physician was consulted. I don't want any special treatment.

Dr. O'Grady: So, the founder of the NP role has to do her own care coordination and sees an NP who does not appear to inhabit any of nursing's core values. What needs went unmet in that exchange?

Dr. Ford: Well, I'd like some human interaction, that the NP would indeed acknowledge that I was in the room instead of the computer. Now this is, in a way, an isolated incident, but it was repeated when my husband was in a rehabilitation center. The NP talked a little bit to me, but not much, and not to my husband, who didn't hear well anyway. So, it wasn't too different in that situation either. When I talk to my colleagues around the country, they have reported the same thing in terms of their experiences, so I don't know that this an isolated incident, but it seems to be the experience of nurses as patients around the country.Secondly, my daughter has been cared for by another NP, and it's been phenomenally good. The coordination was excellent, the caring and communication for her worked out beautifully because she's finally had somebody to listen to her. So, you don't want to condemn all the NPs from my experience, but it's interesting how variable it is and I don't know if its preparation or system problems. But certainly there's no legal restriction against practicing basic nursing care, the possibilities of nursing are so vast, in terms of patient care.

Dr. O'Grady: But this failure that you and your colleagues have experienced. What would you say is driving that? Where is the failure?

Dr. Ford: Well, I think there are failures in the systems controls. Some of the states are racing to the bottom as far as legal authorization for APRNs is concerned. But that shouldn't keep people from practicing basic nursing skills: caring, compassion, care coordination, teaching, and learning. After all, those nurses, many of them are practicing with specialists and know a great deal, and they ought to use that in teaching patients. None of us experienced that, those of us who haven't had a good experience seeing NPs as nurse patients. On the other hand, I think the system has failed because in a sense the rewards are not there either. Rewards that they sometimes experience is when they identify an unusual disease entity. It is a system that doesn't reward NPs with recognition, respect, or remuneration.Then, of course, you have to ask about their preparation. A lot of people don't know the history of the NP; they're not interested in history, they're interested in what's going on today and tomorrow. And, of course, once you take history out of the curriculum, you "integrate" it. Well, I say that integration means it's out of the curriculum. Because all they know about is Florence Nightingale, but they don't know all of the things that Florence Nightingale encompassed as basic tenants of nursing.

Dr. O'Grady: So, given this disappointing NP experience, does your vision for the nurse practitioner future differ from what it was in the 1960s?

Dr. Ford: It does, because frankly the role has been increasingly medicalized. In that sense, the system is changing in prevention and promotion. We had four elements really: prevention, promotion, preservation, and protection. Henry [Silver] and I had many discussions about the language that we were

Continued

EXEMPLAR 6.2
A CAUTIONARY TALE: THE FOUNDER OF THE FIRST NURSE PRACTITIONER (NP) PROGRAM ON DISAPPOINTING NP ENCOUNTERS—cont'd

using. We didn't call it physical exam; I insisted we call it physical assessment, because that is a nursing word. We have to keep nursing in the language and in concept and to use the forward-looking concept of interdependence. So that nurses were independent in nursing but not independent in teams. Everyone was interdependent in the team care. But the elements of nursing came right out of nursing. Because if you read the early literature, nursing was developing as a profession, and NPs needed to be independent in nursing, that it's health and wellness oriented and that the involvement of the patient as a member of the team is vital. That the nurse and the patient and others on the team were actually partners, and that's where many of the teaching elements came in. So it was built on what the profession was saying at the time, and we even used the nursing process; assessment, implementation, evaluation was part of what we were doing. And when we went to the state boards, we laid it out. That was the goal.

Dr. O'Grady: So how is your vision different today than it was in the 1960s for the future?

Dr. Ford: I think, for example, we're talking about nurses substituting for the primary care deficits of medicine. Well, I don't see that! I see them as being able to offer services to patients, regardless of their disease entity, with regards to health and wellness. How they cope with their illness, prevention. I mean, it was built on primary, secondary, and tertiary prevention of caring. And that could include adjusting medications; it has always involved medications but not to the extent it does today. You know, we have made the cardinal error of developing legal authority by going after it task, by task, by task. It was the worst strategy and I never agreed with that because every time you turned around, we were running to the legislature to order equipment, to give certain scheduled drugs. Next thing you know, we'll be asking the legislature to allow us to pluck eyebrows, and that's ridiculous! So we've in some way painted ourselves into a corner by these efforts. I've realized that creating one role (like the NP) was not going to change the system. The system was so strongly medically controlled. It's always one of these three things: power, control, and money. And you see them being played out every time, in every element, in every state: power, control, and money.

Dr. O'Grady: So, what could you say to a graduate student who's reading this book and doesn't want to become the NP who is not really assessing anything, not really being caring, not connecting. What would you say to that NP when working in this metric-driven delivery system, that doesn't value these other things, these nursing things? What could the NP do?

Dr. Ford: Well, in the first place, I think the NP ought to select the place of employment very carefully and negotiate ahead of time what she has to offer and find out what they don't have and say: "I cannot do what you don't have. You don't have physicians; you want physicians? Don't ask me. That's not what I do. Let me tell you what I do." In that way, in Colorado, by the way, there is a good example of this. I worked with a man who was a specialist and the best that ever happened is that I was a generalist in both pediatrics and family care (because I was a public health nurse). And we were a perfect match because he did what he did in medicine and I did all the family work and all kinds of things that made a difference in the outcome of the patients' wellness and health and living. So, you don't need to be a specialist duplicate of what the specialist is. You need to be doing the thing that you can do best as a nurse. This doesn't mean that you shouldn't know a lot about what the specialist does and what the treatments are and be able to adjust them to meet that patient's particular environment and experience. So it seems to me that you need to negotiate ahead of time, in terms of what you can and can't do and won't do—not because you can't do them but because they're not where you want to spend your time.

Dr. O'Grady: So, it almost sounds like staying in your lane. Doing what you do really well.

Dr. Ford: Well, that will change. Because things change. For example, the technology is changing so rapidly today that we have to change with it, or we have to invent it. We should not be flippant all the time of these inventions. And it doesn't need to be technology but technology that we have at hand. Different ways and things to think about asking: "Why are we doing this? Do we really need to do it, or does it matter?" I think we're in a time warp in a sense.

Dr. O'Grady: So before we end, is there anything parting that you'd say about this whole incident or incidents that you've had with your husband and the NPs? Is there any parting advice or solution?

Dr. Ford: Well, I think reflective practice has yet to come into being, so you must look at what you're doing every day and how you're spending the day. And it must include reflection on the interactions you are having with patients. Really know what a professional model of nursing is and talk with others about it. Really talk with and listen to the patients. The listening has gone out the window you know.

Dr. O'Grady: Well, I'm writing the policy chapter and we are seeing the lay of the land and scope of practice for APRNs is moving at such a glacial place. The Affordable Care Act has largely decentralized decision making, and so the governance of delivery systems will dictate how APRNs get paid and how they're involved. So, there are just many more tables to be at. It's harder to influence because it's a one-by-one.

Dr. Ford: Well, there's no doubt that there's going to be some changes in the air, but as I say, it's power, control, and money. But I'm sure that when I'd talk about independent practice, I'd sure talk about it in terms of the statutory authority. Because the states—anything, in fact, that raises such flags—and no one is independent; we're all interdependent.

Implicit Bias

An essential element of self-awareness is the identification of one's biases, conscious or unconscious, in favor of or against people with a characteristic that distinguishes them from societal norms (e.g., race, ethnicity, religion, sexual orientation, gender identification, socioeconomic status, disabilities, stigmatized diagnoses). In recent years, the concepts of implicit, or unconscious, bias and mitigating strategies have been recognized and well described. Implicit bias among healthcare providers has contributed to healthcare disparities (The Joint Commission, 2016) and is in direct conflict with the first tenet of the ANA code of ethics: "The nurse practices with compassion and respect for the inherent dignity, worth, and unique attributes of every person" (ANA, 2016, p. 1). It is essential that the APRN recognize and mitigate this in order to provide optimal patient-centered care. Narayan (2019) summarized several strategies that the APRN can employ to protect the therapeutic encounter from this type of sabotage. These strategies include counterstereotypic imaging, emotional regulation, habit replacement, individuation, increasing opportunities for engagement, partnership building, and mindfulness.

Communication With Patients

A foundation of good communication with patients is essential to developing a therapeutic relationship. Research has shown that good communication between the APRN and patients can increase patient satisfaction, establish trust, increase adherence to a treatment plan, and improve patient outcomes (Bentley et al., 2016; Burley, 2011; Kinder, 2016; Persson et al., 2011).

The ability to adapt communication styles is a needed skill of APRNs (McCourt, 2006) and can result in patients reporting that they have more knowledge, confidence, and control of their own care (Esmaeili et al., 2014). Communication is a skill that is necessary for an APRN to maintain a therapeutic relationship with a patient while also supporting them in effective decision making. The APRN needs to use an approach that incorporates verbal and nonverbal behaviors exhibited by the patient while being careful to maintain professional boundaries (Elliott, 2010). Considerations include language primacy, health literacy, and patient preferences for learning modalities.

Developing good communication skills takes ongoing practice throughout the APRN's career. Options for doing this include using standardized patients and simulation laboratories with feedback, which have been shown to improve APRN students' interpersonal and communication skills (Defenbaugh & Chikotas, 2016; Kesten et al., 2015). Reflective practice, discussed later in this chapter, is essential to the development of communication skills.

One critical aspect of communication is listening. Listening has been described as being fully present with the patient to garner patient details, increase the level of trust in the relationship, and improve patient compliance (Browning & Waite, 2010). Listening takes as much concerted effort to perform optimally as verbal communication. Key to good listening is the ability on the APRN's part to avoid being distracted by personal thoughts, forming instant judgments, and formulating a reply while the patient is still speaking and telling their story. In addition, the APRN must become aware of how individual expectations, experiences, and cultural paradigms can result in biases and misperceptions when working with patients (Browning & Waite, 2010). Reflective listening techniques can be useful when APRNs convey to patients that they have been heard and understood without judgment and can assist patients in exploring their personal situations more fully (Resnicow & McMaster, 2012). These techniques include taking patient statements and restating, rephrasing, reframing, and reflecting thoughts, feelings, and emotional undertones back to the patient (Miller, 2010). Maintaining eye contact is an important nonverbal indication of attention and can be challenging in settings where the clinician's documentation and data review are performed on an electronic device. APRNs must maintain an awareness of their own body language and facial expressions while listening to the patient or reviewing data in front of the patient.

Shared Decision Making

In addition to eliciting information that increases understanding of the patient's illness experience, APRNs encourage patients to participate in decisions regarding how their health and illness should be managed. There is a continuum of patient involvement in making decisions for their own health care. At one end of the continuum are patients who want to be fully engaged in a partnership with providers in making decisions, whereas at the other end of the continuum are patients who want to rely entirely on family members or care providers to receive information about the patient's condition and make all treatment decisions. This may include patients who are overwhelmed, sicker, or cognitively impaired or who have cultural beliefs that lead them to defer decisions to others. In addition, the patient's wishes for autonomy may be influenced by severity or complexity of illness, literacy level, or cultural factors. In general, patients express interest in wanting to be more involved in care planning and treatment decisions, and it has been demonstrated that with increased involvement, particularly in patients with chronic illness, there are improvements in individual care and outcomes and improved adherence to recommended regimens (Houlihan, 2015; Kitson et al., 2012; Kullberg et al., 2015). No matter where the patient falls on this continuum, it is still incumbent on the provider to establish a collaborative partnership to ensure that regardless of whom the patient wants to make decisions, it is done in congruence with the patient's beliefs and values (Esmaeili et al., 2014; Greaney & O'Mathuna, 2017).

APRNs should understand each patient's preference for participation in decision making and be sensitive to the fact that patients' preferences may change over time as they get to know the provider better and as different types of health problems arise. Once the patient's preference has been elicited, providers should tailor their communication and decision-making style to the patient's preference. Many patients have not had prior healthcare experiences in which shared decision making was a possibility but, when offered the opportunity, many choose it. Taking a more active role may require some help from the provider, such as explaining how it would work and which responsibilities are the patient's and which are the provider's. Providers can encourage patients to bring up issues by asking open-ended questions such as "How have you been?" and focused but open questions such as "How are things going at home?" Patients can be encouraged to participate in decision making by offering them explicit opportunities in the form of questions such as "Does one of those approaches sound better to you than the other?" Gradually, patients approached in this way will learn that healthcare encounters will be organized around their concerns, not around a series of questions asked by the provider, and that they should feel safe to express their concerns and preferences.

Open, honest, and thorough communication is foundational to a shared decision-making philosophy. It is important to begin by understanding the patient's knowledge base and insight (e.g., experience with the condition, medical background, awareness of others with similar condition) as well as how the patient typically gathers health information (Clarke et al., 2017) The APRN can redirect patients to sources of information that are medically accurate to avoid the dangers of misinformation that are widely available. It is helpful for the APRN to explain to patients how to communicate between encounters. With the advent of electronic health records have come patient portals through which patients can communicate with providers to ask questions or provide updates to their health. Some issues may indicate an after-hours call to an on-call provider, whereas others may be less urgent. It is important to empower the patient with clear expectations early in the therapeutic relationship.

APRNs must be cognizant of their own personal beliefs and value systems in a partnership in which they are coaching patients in decision making (see Chapter 8). Although they are uniquely prepared to facilitate the holistic management of the physical, psychosocial, and spiritual aspects of care in these particular situations, APRNs may be involved in interactions in which it is difficult for them to help patients make decisions. Implicit bias may result in undue or unintentional influence by the APRN on a patient's decision in emotionally charged situations. Bringing one's own beliefs and values to consciousness prior to a discussion focused on patient decision making, reflecting on one's own cognitive and affective responses to such discussions, and debriefing with a colleague can help APRNs maintain a therapeutic approach (or determine when it is appropriate for another clinician to become involved).

Cultural Influences on Partnerships

The *Essentials* identifies the need for APRNs to synthesize and incorporate principles of cultural diversity into preventive and therapeutic interventions for individuals and populations (AACN, 2021). The preparation of APRNs in the area of cultural competence and culturally appropriate care is key because the demographics of nurses, including APRNs, do not match the overall demographics of the US population (NASEM, 2021). Diversifying the nursing workforce (e.g., in terms of race, ethnicity, gender) has been identified as a pressing priority (NASEM, 2016, 2021).

Another important factor affecting whether and how persons want to participate in healthcare decision making is their cultural background. Recognizing and respecting the cultural identification of patients is essential to building meaningful partnerships. Cultural groups form along lines of racial, national origin, religious, professional, organizational, sexual orientation, and age group identification. It is important to include questions about the patient's identity or affinity as an element of the initial assessment in order to avoid making assumptions about cultural beliefs simply based on characteristics or attributes. These beliefs are learned by avoiding presumptions, asking the patient open-ended questions, and responding in a way that makes the patient feel understood.

Interactions that are complicated by cultural misunderstandings can result in incomplete or inaccurate assessments and even in misdiagnoses and suboptimal outcomes (Barakzai et al., 2007; Nokes, 2011). The APRN needs to individualize care based on an assessment of the cultural influences on the perception of illness, the reporting of symptoms, and the patient's desired level of autonomy. Otherwise, differences in perceptions can cause confusion, misunderstandings, and even conflicts that disrupt the patient–provider relationship and discourse. Moreover, cultural influences often complicate attempts to resolve misunderstandings because different cultural groups approach conflict negotiation differently. In every encounter, the APRN should expect that the patient may have values that are different in some ways from their own and must make a special effort to ensure that the care being given meets the patient's needs and is acceptable to them (Escallier & Fullerton, 2009). As a clinical leader, the APRN must ensure that cultural biases of the members of the care team are not imposed on the patient.

Therapeutic Partnerships With Noncommunicative Patients

Some patients are not able to enter fully into partnership with APRNs because they are too young, have compromised cognitive capacity, or are unconscious. Examples of clinical populations who may be unable to participate fully in shared decision making are listed in Box 6.6.

Although these patients may have limited ability to speak for themselves, they are not entirely without opinion or voice. Situations in which patients will experience temporary alterations in cognition or verbal ability can often be anticipated. For example, in planned perioperative situations in which general anesthesia and intubation will be used, the CRNA has the opportunity to dialogue with the patient prior to the procedure. This creates a shared relationship in which the patient can feel comforted and confident about the upcoming procedure (Rudolfsson et al., 2007). The CRNA can prepare patients for the period when communication will be a challenge and propose alternative methods for communication. In addition, the CRNA can discuss patients' preferences for handling possible events beforehand to elicit patient wishes.

In the absence of a prior dialogue, seasoned clinicians who work with noncommunicative patients learn to pay close attention to how patients respond to what happens to them. Facial expressions, body movement, and physiologic parameters are used to ascertain what causes the patient discomfort and what helps alleviate it. In a study of persons who had experienced and recovered from unconsciousness (Lawrence, 1995), 27% of the patients reported being able to hear, understand, and respond emotionally while they were

BOX 6.6

Patient Populations Unable to Participate Fully in Partnership

- Infants and preverbal children
- Anesthetized patients
- Unconscious or comatose patients
- People in severe pain
- Patients receiving medications that impair cognition
- People with dementia
- People with psychiatric conditions that seriously impair rational thought
- People with conditions that render them incapable of speech and conversation
- People with congenital or acquired cognitive limitations

unconscious. These findings suggest that nurses should communicate with unconscious patients by providing them with interventions such as reassurance, bodily care, pain relief, explanations, and comforting touch.

There are tools that can be used for patients who are conscious but unable to communicate. Unfortunately, many nurses are not adequately educated in using alternative methods of communication and, if they are, they may not be familiar or comfortable with the particular method required for an individual patient (Markor & Hazan, 2012; Thompson & McKeever, 2014). Other barriers include not having access to communication devices and time pressures that may not allow providers to engage adequately in a process that could take more time.

Other sources of information about patients who are unable to communicate or respond physically should also be identified. Loved ones and caregivers may offer insights regarding patient environmental preferences (e.g., favorite music, audiobooks, television), personal comfort measures, medical and social history, and personality attributes. All of these are ways of building a partnership with a noncommunicative patient. Advance directives, healthcare proxy documents, and organ donation cards are other sources of information regarding patients' wishes. Thus noncommunicative patients are not without voices, but hearing their preferences does require presence and attentiveness and establishing a relationship. Box 6.7 summarizes options for the APRN when engaging with noncommunicative patients.

BOX 6.7

Techniques for Communicating With Noncommunicative Patients

- Maintain verbal interactions and eye contact with patient throughout care.
- Explain procedures.
- Monitor tone of voice to avoid inadvertently relaying emotional subcontext to the actual words used.
- Use appropriate touch for reassurance.
- Use other communication devices such as alphabet and word boards, writing, computers, and electronic communication devices.
- Use other sources of information for patient's likes and dislikes—family, primary care providers, friends.
- Use physiologic cues—grimacing, frowning, turning away from touch, relaxing facial muscles, blood pressure and heart rate responses—as appropriate to evaluate patient responses to care and treatments.

EXPERT CLINICAL PERFORMANCE

Few studies have clearly differentiated between the advanced skills of the APRN and the foundational practice of the RN. The expert performance of an APRN encompasses clinical thinking and skills. An expert's clinical judgment is characterized by the ability to make fine distinctions among features of a particular condition that were not possible during beginning practice. Benner's (1984) studies of expert clinical judgment, although not with APRN participants, inform this discussion of APRNs' clinical expertise. Tanner (2006) reviewed the literature regarding clinical judgment and found that it requires three main categories of knowledge. The first is scientific and theoretical knowledge that is widely applicable. The second is knowledge based on experience that fills in gaps and assists in the prompt identification of clinical issues. The final category is knowledge that is individualized to the patient, based on an interpersonal connection. Clinical judgment involves application of skills to the situation (Tanner, 2006; Victor-Chmil, 2013).

Clinical Thinking

APRNs' specialized knowledge accrues from a variety of sources, including graduate and continuing education, clinical experience, professional reading and meetings, reflection, mentoring, and exchange of information and ideas with colleagues within and outside nursing. Maintaining familiarity with current scientific developments is an essential responsibility of the APRN (Albarqouni et al., 2018; IOM, 2011). The integration of knowledge from these sources provides a foundation for the expert clinical thinking that is associated with advanced direct care practice. As the APRN gains experience, formalized knowledge and experiential knowledge are integrated and iterative. Illness trajectories and presentations of prior patients make an impression and come to mind when a patient with a similar problem is seen later (Benner, 1984). The expert also remembers which interventions worked and did not work in certain situations. Eventually, the expert's clinical knowledge consists of a complex network of memorable cases, prototypic images, research findings, thinking strategies, moral values, maxims, probabilities, behavioral responses, associations, illness trajectories and timetables, and therapeutic information. Thus experts have extensive, varied, and complex knowledge networks upon which to draw to help them understand clinical situations and events. These networks are composed of internal and external resources. The APRN may mentally review internal resources such as educational knowledge, typical cases, and previously experienced cases when confronted with a complex or challenging patient. However, the APRN is also cognizant of when internal resources are no longer adequate and knows when to refer to external resources for consultation, more data, or guidance. Throughout the assessment, the APRN is using pattern recognition, deductive reasoning, and inductive reasoning to reach a differential diagnosis (Scordo, 2014).

Clinical reasoning brings together the clinical knowledge of the provider with specific observations, perceptions, events, and facts from the situation at hand to produce an understanding of what is occurring (Victor-Chmil, 2013). Sometimes, the understanding is arrived at by using cognitive processes to consider evidence and alternative explanations logically. At other times, the insight or understanding arrives intuitively—that is, through direct apprehension without recourse to deliberate reasoning (Benner et al., 1996; Tanner, 2006). In these situations, APRNs can use reflective practice to sort through the intuition to understand the components better and identify new insights. With experience, they can then repackage these insights and incorporate them into their experiential learning to use the information in the next relevant case prospectively and deliberately. Clinical reasoning can be improved through use of tools such as external verbalization ("thinking aloud"), algorithms, and reflective journaling (Victor-Chmil, 2013).

APRN experts have the ability to scan a situation rapidly (e.g., past records, patient's appearance, the patient's unexpressed concern or discomfort) and identify salient and relevant information. The APRN is able to suspend judgment purposefully about personal strongly held beliefs that may be proposed by others, such as "he's a difficult patient" or "she's just drug seeking." The ability to do this ensures as much objectivity as possible when caring for patients. For example, research has shown that expert CNSs are able to transcend the labeling of a "difficult patient" to engage in problem resolution through the use of patient respect, communication skills, and increased self-efficacy (Wolf & Robinson-Smith, 2007). Relying heavily on their perceptions, observations, and assessment skills, APRNs quickly activate one or several lines of reasoning regarding what might be occurring. They then conduct a more focused assessment to determine which one best explains the situation at hand. These lines of reasoning can be informal personal theories about the specific patient situation; this formulation draws from personal knowledge of the particular patient, personal knowledge acquired from previous experiences, and formalized domain-specific knowledge (Tanner, 2006). In implementing the solutions, these lines of reasoning can be tested by performing a clinical intervention and noting how the patient responds (de Sá Tinôco et al., 2021). Throughout this process, the APRN may be teaching and role-modeling with staff to assist in staff nurse self-awareness and reflection. A novice APRN may need to work through the situation in a formal, logical way and be more deliberate about the use of formal educational knowledge, enriching it over time with experiential knowledge (Richards et al., 2020; Tanner, 2006).

It has been shown that the values and underlying knowledge a nurse brings to a situation also have a profound influence on their assessment of the patient. Results of one study demonstrated that a nurse's beliefs about older adults can affect how a nurse assesses the older confused patient and can affect prioritization of that patient's needs (Dahlke & Phinney, 2008). If not self-aware, these potential values and perspectives may be manifested as implicit bias and impede the APRN's ability to make accurate diagnoses, impact determination of appropriate treatment plans, and alter the ability of the APRN to appropriately role model optimal care of patients for other interprofessional team members.

Through organized and methodical assessment, the APRN arrives at a diagnosis and/or intervention with a degree of confidence in their clinical inferences. At other times, however, there is uncertainty and lack of understanding regarding the situation. The uncertainty may pertain to information the patient provides, the diagnosis, the best approach to management, or how the patient is responding. When there is ambiguity, experts often break into conscious problem solving or "detective-like thinking" and questioning (Benner et al., 1996; Benner et al., 2011, p. 42) to try to determine what is going on.

Familiarity with the individual patient can be critical to perceptive and accurate clinical reasoning. Recognition of the patient's patterns of responses enables experienced nurses to detect subtle changes in a patient's condition over time (Tanner, 2006; Tanner et al., 1993). The extent to which any nurse knows a patient may be associated with that nurse's ability to do the following:

- Recognize that risk factors are present.
- Detect early indicators of a problem (e.g., a subtle change in pattern).
- Take timely preventive action.
- Recognize nonfitting and atypical data.

Nonfitting data suggest to experts that they need to generate new or additional hypotheses because the current observations and parameters do not fully explain the clinical picture as it has been or as it should be. For example, when faced with a nonfitting sign or symptom, the nurse may generate alternative hypotheses pertaining to the onset of a complication or worsening of the disease process.

Thinking Errors

The clinical acumen of APRNs and the inferences, hypotheses, and lines of reasoning that they generate are highly dependable. However, as practice becomes repetitive, APRNs may develop routine responses and then run the risk of making certain types of thinking errors (Scordo, 2014). *Errors of expectancy* occur when data collection is abbreviated or not methodical, resulting in an incorrect assumption. A set of circumstances in the clinician's experience or patient's presentation may predispose the clinician to disregard data and prematurely establish an incorrect diagnosis. For example, the NP who over several years has seen an older woman for problems associated with chronic pulmonary disease may fail to consider that the most recent onset of shortness of breath and fatigue could be related to worsening aortic stenosis; the NP has come to expect pulmonary disease, not cardiac disease. Or a patient presenting with nausea and vomiting during flu season may be treated for gastroenteritis, although appendicitis is the actual condition (Scordo, 2014).

Erroneous conclusions are also more likely when the situation is ambiguous—that is, when the meaning or reliability of the data is unclear, the interpretation of the data is not clear-cut, the best approach to treatment is debatable, or one cannot say for sure whether the patient is responding well to treatment (Brykczynski, 1991). To avoid errors in these types of situations, experts often revert to the use of maxims (a succinct metaphor for a general truth) to guide their thinking (Brykczynski, 1989). One of the maxims that NPs use to deal with uncertain diagnoses is "When you hear hoofbeats in Kansas, think horses, not zebras." This reminds clinicians who are about to make a diagnosis that occurs infrequently to consider the incidence of the condition in the population. Thus an older adult with respiratory problems seen in a suburban office in the United States is more likely to have pneumonia than tuberculosis. In this setting, clinical data for tuberculosis should be convincing if that diagnosis is proposed.

Poor judgment can also result from tunnel vision, overgeneralization, influence by a recent dramatic experience, premature closure (Croskerry, 2003), and fixation on certain problems to the exclusion of others (Benner et al., 2011). Faulty thinking is not the only source of error in clinical decision making. Others include inaccurate observations, misinterpretation of the meaning of data, a sketchy knowledge of the particular situation, and a faulty or outdated model of the disease, condition, or response.

It is important that APRNs recognize the potential for and avoid leaping to conclusions and making snap judgments. It can become easy to allow biases to lead to premature diagnoses without fully listening to or assessing patients. The expert APRN has learned to scan data constantly and look for deviations. The ability to differentiate effectively between significant and insignificant data is needed to have safe practice. Box 6.8 presents actions that APRNs can take to prevent thinking errors.

Time Pressures

Regardless of setting, all practitioners worry about the effect that time pressures have on the accuracy and

BOX 6.8

Actions to Use to Avoid Thinking Errors

- Listen fully to patients' concerns and descriptions of their problems.
- Develop and utilize a systematic approach.
- Listen to input from other providers as to their assessments and perspectives.
- Use a diagnostic "time-out" to review the situation with fresh eyes.
- Pay attention to intuition that points to an incongruence in data; what cannot be explained?
- Avoid reliance on knowledge derived solely from rote memorization or repetition, but critically think through the source of knowing and how it relates to the individual patient.
- Remain constantly open to reevaluation of working diagnoses and treatments; avoid premature closure.
- Be aware of personal biases and assumptions.
- Continually evaluate what is "critical" data in each patient case.

completeness of their clinical thinking and decision making. A galvanizing report on errors and patient safety cited studies in which between 3% and 46% of hospitalized patients in the United States were harmed by error or negligence (Kohn et al., 2000; Leape, 2021). More recently it has been estimated that more than 5 million deaths occur annually across the globe from defects in healthcare quality (NASEM, 2018). A heavy workload is associated with feelings of pressure, being rushed, cognitive overload, and fatigue, adding to already burdened clinicians; these feelings clearly contribute to unsafe acts and omissions in care (Kohn et al., 2000). Time pressures have been shown to lead to worsening diagnostic accuracy in physicians (Al Qahtani et al., 2016). Evidence also comes from studies of nurse staffing in hospitals in which fewer hours of nursing care per patient per day and less care provided by RNs were associated with poorer patient outcomes (Aiken et al., 2011; Blegen et al., 2011; Needleman et al., 2011). Effectively addressing the issues of time pressures and insufficient hours of nursing care requires culture change, process redesign, and appropriate use of technology. The patient safety movement has led to a variety of efforts aimed at preventing errors—root cause analysis of sentinel events, improved work processes, redesign of delivery systems, use of technological aids, communication training, human factors analysis, and team building. All of these factors can have significant direct and indirect effects on workload, fatigue, and time available for direct patient care.

The effects of a heavy workload on patient outcomes in nonhospital settings are less well understood; thus actions to address this issue have received less attention. However, as lengths of visits or contact times are decreased or the number of patients that practitioners are expected to see in a day is increased, it is logical to assume that the number of errors in clinical thinking will increase. Each contact requires the practitioner to reset his or her clinical reasoning process by closing out one thinking project and starting on an entirely new one. This resetting, which is done back to back often during a day, is cognitively and physically demanding. How these performance expectations affect clinical reasoning accuracy is unknown.

Moreover, time pressures often get compounded by hassles, which come in the form of interruptions, noise in the environment, missing supplies, increasing time needed to interact with technology, and system glitches that make clinical data or even whole charts unavailable to providers. These hassles likely interfere with providers' ability to concentrate on what the patient is saying and disrupt their efforts to make clinical sense of a patient's account. In many settings, providers are required to multitask. They start a task but must attend to another before completing the original one. This clearly increases the risks of failure to obtain needed information, broken lines of thought, technological missteps, omissions in care, and failure to respond to patients' requests for service (Cornell et al., 2011; Harrington et al., 2011; Sittig & Singh, 2012).

Studies of emergency department physicians and NPs have demonstrated that their workflow patterns have frequent interruptions, which can result in shortcuts, failure to return to the original task, increased perceptions of stress, and a potential for commission of errors (Burley, 2011; Chisholm et al., 2011; Westbrook et al., 2010). While the emergency department may be an extreme example of a multitasking environment, other settings also impose interruptions at a very high rate. An experienced APRN may be more skilled at focusing on and prioritizing tasks and quickly dismissing interruptions and extraneous information. The novice APRN, conversely, may take longer to perform tasks (allowing for more interruptions) and may need more assistance with consultations or accessing resources (Phillips, 2005). As time pressures for clinicians increase, organizational efforts to monitor for errors and potential errors and seek correction when there are system weaknesses are actions that APRNs owe patients and themselves as providers functioning in busy environments.

Many patients are sensitive to the pace with which staff and providers greet them, talk with them, and do things, particularly those activities that involve verbal interaction and physical contact. Some patients respond to the fast-paced talk and hurried movements of providers by not bringing up some of the questions that they had intended to ask. Others may just get flustered and forget to mention important information; still others may become hostile and withhold information. Thus errors in the form of information omission by the patient enter the clinical reasoning and decision-making process.

In summary, clinical thinking is a complex task. It involves drawing on knowledge in memory and attending to multiple sources of situational input, some of which are difficult to interpret. Often, multiple clinical issues must be addressed during a patient encounter. These complexities make clinical thinking a challenging task, even under the best of circumstances. *Situational awareness*—perceptions of the current environment in which the APRN is functioning—can make the APRN more cognizant of the potential for error and improve diligence to the thought process at critical junctures, such as when writing orders, when performing procedures, or during handoffs to other clinicians (Anzai et al., 2021; Phillips, 2005).

Ethical Reasoning

Clinical reasoning is inextricably linked to ethical reasoning. Clinical reasoning generates possibilities of what *could* be done in a situation, whereas ethical reasoning adds the dimension of what *should* be done in the situation (see Chapter 11). Advances in healthcare and medical technology have increasingly resulted in gaps between care that is medically possible and care that is in the best interest of the patient. These gaps may be most notable when making decisions regarding withdrawing or limiting care, when dealing with reproductive technology or human genetics, and when cost must figure into clinical treatment decisions. These situations are at high risk for becoming ethically problematic.

The literature regarding how to resolve ethical issues is extensive. One approach is to incorporate preventive or prospective ethical considerations into clinical thinking and decision making (Epstein, 2012). Rather than waiting until a conflict arises, this approach places an emphasis on preventing ethical conflicts from developing by shaping the process of clinical care so that potential value conflicts are anticipated and discussed before outright conflict occurs. APRNs can use this approach during routine encounters with patients. For example, during an encounter with a healthy patient, an APRN may be able to say, "I'd like to discuss an important issue with you while you're well so I will know how to best help you if certain situations should come up in the future." Such issues could include pain management, advance directives, or organ donation. In addition to emphasizing early communication among the patient, significant others, and the healthcare provider(s) about values, preventive ethics requires explicit critical reflection on the institutional factors that lead to conflict (Epstein, 2012). An additional aspect of preventive ethics is an effort to create and preserve trust and understanding among providers, as well as between providers and patients (and their families). Thus the use of preventive ethics can be considered proactive in that it requires providers to consider how the routine processes of care foster or prevent conflicts from occurring or, at the very least, ensure that such issues are identified at an early stage. The preventive approach has the potential to avoid conflicts because clinicians integrate ethical reasoning into clinical reasoning at an earlier point in time than when a traditional, conflict-based ethics approach is used.

The concept of moral distress is being recognized increasingly as an issue for all nurses, including APRNs. *Moral distress* is defined as knowing what the ethically appropriate action should be but encountering barriers that discourage the provider from carrying out the action (Epstein et al., 2019; Rushton et al., 2017). This results in internal conflict that is not resolved and can have devastating effects on the APRN (Morley et al., 2019; see Chapter 11).

The American Association of Critical-Care Nurses (2004) has developed a model to address moral distress. APRNs can use this "four As" model to understand and work toward the resolution of distressing situations:

- Ask—explore and understand where the distress is coming from.
- Affirm—confirm the distress and consider one's professional obligations.
- Assess—use self-awareness, reflection, and evaluation to assess barriers, opportunities, and potential consequences in preparation for action.
- Action—put into place actions that will initiate resolving the distress, anticipating setbacks and ways to cope with them.

Such situations can be daunting but can also be opportunities for an APRN to reflect upon their own beliefs and values. Fostering the development of moral resilience is important for APRNs and those who support their practice (Rushton, 2016; Stutzer & Bylone, 2018).

Skillful Performance

Although the healthcare professions place high value on knowledge and expert clinical reasoning, it is important to keep in mind that the public values skillful performance in physical examinations, delivery of treatments, diagnostic procedures, and comfort care. Most graduate schools require students to perform a specific set of procedural skills recommended by a national specialty organization before they complete their program. However, there is little research about how APRNs acquire competency in new or expanded procedural skills once they are in practice. Presumably, competency of APRNs to perform specific procedures and treatments is initially ensured through the processes that agencies use to credential and grant privileges to APRNs. After that, the responsibility for acquiring new competencies lies with the individual APRN and employing agency. When an APRN or agency recognizes that patients would receive better care if the APRN could perform a new procedure, an agreement should be reached regarding exactly which new procedure the APRN will perform, the conditions under which the procedure will be done, how the APRN will acquire the necessary skill, and how supervision will be provided during the learning period. The APRN must also be aware that refinement of the technical component is only a piece of the procedure. They must also understand indications, contraindications, complications, and consequences of performing the procedures (Hravnak et al., 2005). Documented evidence that formal training has occurred is sometimes required for regulatory purposes.

The types of skills nurses have performed have evolved over time. For example, it used to be within the physician's scope of practice (and outside the nurse's) to measure blood pressure and administer chemotherapy. With the advent of each of the APRN roles, APRNs have acquired new performance skills when indicated for the comfort, convenience, safety, and satisfaction of patients. It is key for APRNs to be cognizant of the scope of their role, regulatory requirements of the states, and the reasonableness of acquiring the skill.

Advanced Physical Assessment

Discussion continues about what actually constitutes advanced physical assessment in the differentiation between RN and APRN practice. In one survey, 99 APRNs, physician assistants, and their corresponding preceptor physicians were asked to rank the importance of 87 competencies as an advanced skill (Davidson et al., 2004). All skills were ranked fairly high as being necessary for advanced practice care. Skills ranked highest as advanced skills were cardiac assessments, such as rhythm interpretation, and women's health skills, such as gynecologic and breast examinations. Competencies such as head, neck, and throat and skin assessment skills were rated lower on the advanced skill priority scale. The authors reported that higher-rated skills appeared to need more use of clinical judgment to interpret or differentially diagnose compared with lower-rated skills, which tended to be more demonstration or technical skills.

Another component of advanced assessment is the use of evidence in assessing and formulating a diagnosis (Munro, 2004). APRNs should be skilled at understanding and using the concepts of sensitivity, specificity, and the kappa statistic (i.e., interrater reliability) to differentiate the likelihood of presence or absence of disease based on physical signs and the reliability of that finding. The increased use of technology does not preclude the importance of the physical assessment in reaching an accurate diagnosis (Munro, 2004). Using advanced practice nurses as specialized standardized patients in simulations can facilitate improved clinical reasoning in APRN students (Payne, 2015; Turrise et al., 2017).

Patient Education

Patient education is a central and well-documented function of all nurses in any setting, and evidence of its effectiveness has been well established (Redman, 2004). Teaching and counseling are significant clinical activities in nurse-midwifery (Holland & Holland, 2007) and CNS practice (Parry et al., 2006). There are several examples of the role of NPs in patient education to promote adherence to treatment regimens and provide healthcare information to improve outcomes and quality of life (Hahn, 2014; McAfee, 2012; Whitehead et al., 2014). APRNs must understand the basic principles of patient education and the specific educational needs of their clinical populations. The teach-back method is especially helpful in ensuring understanding by the patient of the content the APRN is teaching (Agency for Healthcare Research and Quality [AHRQ], 2015). APRNs must be aware of the current evidence in their specialties and be responsible for knowing the theoretical and scientific bases for patient teaching and coaching in their specialties and practice settings.

The APRN may be charged with the development and implementation of patient education materials or programs in their practice setting. There are many strategies that may be employed. For example, the APRN might lead a self-management group for patients with a chronic condition, using motivational interviewing. Other activities could include evaluating and adapting existing patient education materials to meet the needs of patients with lower literacy levels or evaluating the reliability and appropriateness of health information on the Internet. APRNs should be aware of the health information resources likely to be used by their patient populations and be able to advise patients as to which websites are reliable and regularly updated.

In today's technology-accessible world, consumers are increasingly using the Internet as a primary source of healthcare information. Patients use the Internet to access information and educate themselves about their health and diseases. Patients may actually come to appointments knowing more about their disease than the APRN expects. Although this can be disconcerting, it is important to recognize this as information-seeking behavior and capitalize on the opportunity to work with the patients to help them gain the information they need (Cutilli, 2006). Patients vary widely in terms of how much information they want and how they want it presented. Allowing them to make choices about how and what they learn should help prevent content overload and enhance the relevancy of the information given, resulting in better retention and application. Along similar lines, technology can be designed to allow patients to acquire information that is most important to them and to help them sort out their values, priorities, and preferences in their specific situation (Lin & Effken, 2010; Ryan et al., 2009). It is apparent that technology-assisted learning and decision-making tools will become increasingly more acceptable.

It will be important for APRNs to help consumers differentiate among websites that are reputable and offer valid information and those that may not have solid evidence. The Internet is also now used for patients with similar or rare diseases to connect with each other as support in a way that might never have been possible before the advent and ease of use of the Internet. APRNs can also direct patients to state health department websites as excellent sites for accessing helpful information, such as immunization schedules, tobacco cessation tools, and information on diabetes care, sexually transmitted diseases, tuberculosis, and newborn screening.

In the United States only 12% of adults have adequate health literacy to be able to navigate the healthcare system (AHRQ, 2016; Box 6.9). Assessment of functional health literacy must be done sensitively. Years of education completed may not be an adequate indicator of reading and computational literacy. In addition, people with higher levels of education who experience a new diagnosis or other stresses may be unable to process complex information and consequently may benefit from the use of limited-literacy

BOX 6.9

Red Flags for Low Literacy

- Frequently missed appointments
- Incomplete registration forms
- Nonadherence with medication
- Unable to name medications, explain purpose or dosing
- Identifies pills by looking at them, not reading label
- Unable to give coherent, sequential history
- Asks fewer questions
- Lack of follow-through on tests or referrals

From *Health Literacy: Hidden Barriers and Practical Strategies*, by Agency for Healthcare Research and Quality, 2015, www.ahrq.gov/professionals/quality-patient-safety/quality-resources/tools/literacy-toolkit/tool3a/index.html.

materials (AHRQ, 2016). A variety of tools are available to assist clinicians in assessing patient literacy (Baker et al., 1999; Davis et al., 1993; Sand-Jecklin & Coyle, 2014). APRNs involved in developing programmatic approaches to patient education must ascertain that materials are appropriate to the literacy level of participants in educational programs. Educational materials should use plain language (National Institutes of Health, 2012; Stableford & Mettger, 2007); plain language text is accessible, engaging, and reader friendly. Stableford and Mettger (2007) noted that reading levels alone are insufficient to determine whether text was prepared using plain language principles.

Numerous resources exist to help APRNs improve their abilities to assess health literacy and prepare useful, readable instructional materials. The Harvard T.H. Chan School of Public Health (2019) website is particularly useful; it includes information regarding the problem of health literacy and its effects on health, as well as links to numerous resources.

Adverse Events and Performance Errors

Since the publication of *To Err Is Human* (Kohn et al., 2000), medical errors have been prominent in the public eye, as well as a focus of reform for healthcare institutions. Ideally, institutions and care providers should focus on improving the reliability of complicated systems to prevent failures or quickly identify, redesign, and rectify failures that do occur. Improving reliability ensures that care is consistently and appropriately provided. Traditionally, institutions and providers have been reluctant to be forthcoming with patients when errors or near misses have occurred. That stance is slowly changing with the movement toward increasing transparency in care and a focus on addressing system dysfunction to improve patient safety. In 2002 the National Quality Forum (NQF) first identified a list of adverse medical events that healthcare systems should work to prevent and publicly report when they occur to encourage public access to information about healthcare performance (NQF, 2008). This list was updated in 2008 and 2011. The 29 events are categorized into seven main areas: surgical or invasive procedure events, product or device events, patient protection events, care management events, environmental events, radiologic events, and potential criminal events (NQF, 2011). The Centers for Medicare & Medicaid Services is now denying payment for some of these publicly reported events, and it is anticipated that additional events will continue to be identified for denial of payment. There are increasing resources available in clinics and healthcare settings to try to prevent adverse events, including computer-generated alerts for ordering medications and laboratory tests; interdisciplinary colleagues, such as pharmacists and dietitians; electronic resources to access and verify recommendations and practice guidelines; appropriate steps in patient identification; and optimal team communication techniques (White, 2012). It is critical that APRNs consistently use safety protocols and be involved in decisions related to their development (Armstrong, 2019).

These changes are relevant to APRNs as they relate to direct care and the potential to be involved in "never," near miss, or medical error situations. The APRN must be cognizant of the institution's or practice group's policies related to appropriate actions when errors occur and what is required to be reported publicly based on federal and state regulations. APRNs may find themselves involved in these situations as a result of the issues already discussed, such as thinking errors and time pressures. APRNs involved as providers in these types of events should anticipate the need to readily inform the patient and family of the event. Honest, open communication and sensitivity will help preserve trust and support ongoing care. When errors in care happen, patients expect to receive an explanation and an apology; doing so may help preserve a trusting relationship and at least ameliorate anxiety, fear, and confusion (Leape, 2012).

A consensus group of Harvard hospitals (Massachusetts Coalition for the Prevention of Medical Errors, 2006) has recommended four steps for communicating about adverse events:

1. Tell the patient what happened immediately but leave details of how and why for later when a thorough review has occurred.
2. Take responsibility for the incident.
3. Apologize and communicate remorse.
4. Inform the patient and family what will be done to prevent similar events.

APRNs should take advantage of training and educational opportunities on how to communicate bad news and ways to promote safety. In addition, APRNs involved in incidents should recognize the need for their own emotional support following medical errors and be aware of the resources available to them.

USE OF REFLECTIVE PRACTICE

To continually grow and develop, APRNs must be reflective practitioners. APRNs may be familiar with multiple methods of learning—didactic, small-group projects, clinical experiences with preceptors—but may be less familiar with this method of learning, which will be useful to them throughout their careers. Reflective practice is a way to take the experiences a practitioner has (positive or negative) and explore them for the purpose of eliciting meaning, critically analyzing, synthesizing, and using learning to improve practice (Gee et al., 2018; Health Education England, 2021; Johns, 2017; O'Brien & Graham, 2020; Schön, 1992). The goal is to turn experience into personal knowledge by seeking insights that are not available with superficial recall (Kumar, 2011; Rolfe, 1997; Schön, 1992). Research findings have shown that reflective practice by students is a valuable learning method, may increase self-confidence as a practitioner, and may improve clinical decision making (O'Brien & Graham, 2020; Raterink, 2016).

Forms of clinical supervision are frequently used in mental health nursing but can be useful in other specialties as well. Barron and White (2009) described clinical supervision in this realm as a relationship between a more experienced and a more novice nurse in which the expected outcome is to assist the less-experienced nurse in the professional development of knowledge, skills, and autonomy. In these cases, clinical supervision may be used as a debriefing with a trusted and more-experienced colleague of a situation that has been complex, intense, or characterized by uncertainty. Gee et al. (2018) reported that clinical supervision is useful in determining boundaries, builds confidence, and provides peer support, interaction, and cohesion. Experienced APRNs can also use self-reflection to enhance learning and ongoing improvement in even routine, frequently used clinical skills (Ingram, 2017).

Silverman and Hutchinson (2019) found that providing mental health consultations to nurses and midwives providing direct care for pregnant persons from marginalized families contributed to the care providers focusing on the centrality of the patient–provider relationship. It can improve self-reflection, which can support their ability to explore their own values, motivation, and biases. This is important in being able to counteract structural impediments that promote issues of inequity and reproductive oppression/injustice (Silverman & Hutchinson, 2019).

Reflection is not just a retrospective activity; it may occur prospectively or concurrently while providing care. Retrospective reflection occurs when an APRN takes the opportunity to consider how a situation could have been handled differently. Prospective reflection may occur when an APRN prepares to enter a difficult or uncertain clinical situation; one draws on experience and scientific knowledge to plan an approach and anticipates possible reactions or outcomes. Reflection can also occur concurrently. Concurrent reflection is termed *reflection-in-action* and can promote flexibility and adaptation of interventions to suit the situation. Reflection-in-action may be the goal of a more expert practitioner who has honed the skill of reflection (Benner et al., 2011). Although Benner's work was done with bedside staff nurses, it may be applicable to APRNs as well. Several models have been proposed to gain expertise in reflective practice (Brubakken et al., 2011; Johns, 2017; Kim, 1999), although they use similar processes to guide the practitioner through the reflective process. Deliberate self-reflection allows the APRN to anticipate alternative possibilities, remain flexible in challenging and changing situations, and strategically integrate the results of self-reflection with best practices to match interventions to patient and family needs.

Strengthening skills in self-reflection can be done in a number of ways for the APRN—through solitary self-evaluation, with a supervisor or teacher, or in small groups of supportive colleagues. Learning from guided group reflection provides students a foundation for ongoing reflection throughout their careers (O'Brien & Graham, 2020). With experience, the APRN may be asked to be the mentor in guiding others through a self-reflective process. Regardless of which model is used for reflection, the following guidelines can be considered:

- If reflection occurs in a small group, participants must feel safe to express thoughts, emotions, and thinking processes without fear of judgment.
- Practitioners need to gain self-awareness of personal values, beliefs, and behaviors.
- Practitioners need to develop the skills to articulate a situation with objective and subjective details.
- Critical debriefing and analysis are used to identify practitioner goals in the situation, extent of knowledge that was present or missing, feelings on the part of the practitioner and patient, consequences of actions, and which alternative options existed.
- Knowledge gained through this process can be integrated with current knowledge to change interventions in a current situation or improve approaches in future situations.
- Evaluation of this reflective process supports masterful practice and creates lasting improvements in practice.

There are several barriers to using reflection in daily practice. Lack of time may result in care and interventions becoming routine. The use of a reflective practice process will require dedicated time. If not thoughtfully arranged, it may seem to be extraneous and a "nice thing to do" rather than a necessary component to the APRN role. Acknowledging that one does not always know the right answer can be difficult for an APRN who is trying to establish a practice and role. In addition, reflection may elicit emotions that may be painful or difficult to deal with. It takes experience and skill to use reflection, which is particularly important when an APRN is very involved in a situation. Novice APRNs may need guidance in performing reflection to assist in ascertaining meaning and making connections that otherwise might be missed (Johns, 2017). Reflective practice discussions are more than official surveillance with supervisors involved and can be developed and incorporated into one's practice as a means to demonstrate professional accountability for practice and a source of lifelong learning. Knowledge from reflection informs future clinical decision making, especially in those situations for which no benchmarks or best practice guidelines exist.

USE OF EVIDENCE AS A GUIDE TO PRACTICE

An important form of knowledge that must be brought to bear on clinical decision making, for individuals and for populations, is the ever-increasing volume of evidence. For the nursing profession, the use of evidence as a basis for practice is more than the latest trend (see Chapter 10). The profession has been intensively exploring and considering issues regarding the use of research since the early 1970s. Historically, CNSs have led efforts in many agencies to move toward research-based practice (DePalma, 2004; Hanson, 2015; Mackay, 1998; Obrecht et al., 2014; Patterson et al., 2017; Stetler et al., 1995). They have brought research findings to the attention of the nursing staff and interprofessional teams and worked to develop the research appraisal skills of nursing staffs. With the advent of the doctorate of nursing practice, evidence-based practice skills are seen as central to APRNs' role competency and a differentiating component to the PhD-prepared nurse, who is specifically prepared to conduct research (see Chapter 10).

Identifying and locating evidence and research findings is becoming easier with improved technology and categorization. However, clinicians often do not have sufficient experience in the use of various search engines available to retrieve information from databases. APRNs could benefit from education on simple tools that could greatly increase the efficiency of their searches. APRNs in all settings engaging in an evidence-based practice project would be well served by developing a relationship with a health sciences librarian who can assist with searches, save time, and prevent the omission of relevant evidence. (McKeown & Ross-White, 2019; McTavish, 2017).

Evidence-Based Practice

It would be ideal to have all healthcare delivery based on research. However, in reality, there frequently may be no research on which to base decisions. Sackett (1998) defined *evidence-based practice* as the explicit and judicious integration of best evidence with clinical expertise and patient values. Using only external evidence to make practice decisions is as unacceptable as using only individual clinical expertise.

When designing care for a population of patients, the APRN should consider all forms of objective evidence, including quality improvement data, data from internal databases, expert opinion panels, consensus statements, national guidelines data from benchmarking partners, and data from state and national databases (e.g., the Centers for Disease Control and Prevention). Agency-specific information, collected to pinpoint the nature of a problem, is particularly useful evidence that should be combined with the more general knowledge gained from research evidence (see Chapter 10).

The process and extent of quality improvement (QI) have advanced significantly in the past few years with APRNs as QI leaders in their healthcare settings. Use of improved QI methods and tools and a national focus on the need to make significant changes in the care of patients provide nurses with the opportunity to identify patient care issues, evaluate the problem, and implement potential solutions in a more rapid fashion than ever before. APRNs can use QI methods such as the plan–do–study–act process and tools (Institute for Healthcare Improvement, 2021) and the lean principles (Lean Enterprise Institute, 2021) to lead and facilitate teams in improving care. Although QI data do not have broad generalizability and the rigor of formal research, they can provide evidence for significant improvements that the APRN can implement on a daily local basis.

With the increasing bombardment of evidence available in the literature and via the Internet, APRNs must develop a plan to stay abreast of and evaluate the mass of information. Examples of how an APRN can do this include reading primary research reports and summaries of research findings on a regular basis, evaluating the soundness of the methods, and adjusting or fine-tuning their own practice on the basis of credible findings. This is the form of research use in which every professional nurse should engage. It is part of maintaining competence in one's area of clinical practice.

Additionally, APRNs can subscribe to listservs, such as those from the AHRQ, that send timely summaries of emerging evidence and new national guidelines. Alternatively, an APRN could join or form an interprofessional group that meets monthly to discuss research reports on topics of mutual interest. By developing an organized process to keep track of topics for inquiry, APRNs can make the most efficient use of resources to explore the evidence related to the questions of interest.

Evidence-based practice is a more systematic, rigorous, and precise way of translating research findings into practice. The evidence-based practice process is used in an organization to design a standard of care for a population of patients. This process is more formal because evidence-based care will be widely used as a guide to care; therefore the scientific conclusions on which it is based must be as free of bias and error as possible. In general terms, the process involves four steps: (1) locating, evaluating, and summarizing the science; (2) translating the science into clinical recommendations; (3) strategically implementing the recommendations; and (4) measuring and reporting their impact. The recommendations may take the form of a clinical practice guideline, decision algorithm, clinical protocol, or changes in policies or procedures.

Clinical Practice Guidelines

Evidence-based clinical practice guidelines can be useful decision-making and planning aids for clinicians. Many guidelines have been developed in close association with providers, are based on systematic and thorough reviews of research, and have attained a balance between optimal care and economic reality. However, clinical guidelines are also used to ensure quality, limit variation of care, and control resource use. Distinct from policies, clinical practice guidelines are based on research that is evaluated and summarized by a credible panel, inside or outside the system, to ensure that the guidelines serve to incorporate science into practice and contain costs. APRNs and the multidisciplinary team members involved in the care of patients with the condition that the guideline addresses should have the opportunity to adapt guidelines produced by others. Proposed guidelines should be reviewed and deliberated in advance to avoid situations in which the care of the individual becomes the focus of a dilemma. In addition, clinicians should acknowledge that, although the guidelines may serve most patients well, some patients will require treatment and interventions not recommended in the guidelines. An explicit method for advocating for individual needs should be available to clinicians. Guidelines can be found through organizations such as the AHRQ (www.ahrq.gov) and the National Comprehensive Cancer Network as well as professional organizations such as the American Heart Association. Clinicians should review published guidelines carefully and be familiar with the criteria each organization uses to grade the strength of the evidence used to make care recommendations. It is important that APRNs be part of teams that are developing new guidelines for practice and that they advocate for interdisciplinary review of practice recommendations. Colleagues within medicine, nursing, physical therapy, respiratory therapy, occupational and vocational therapy, social work, and nutrition all have expertise to contribute to the development of evidence-based clinical practice guidelines.

Theory-Based Practice

The preceding discussion of evidence-based practice recognizes how research evidence informs practice but ignores the role of theory. APRNs are becoming comfortable with the idea of research as a guide to practice, yet the idea of theory-based practice is less familiar. It should not be, because, contrary to common perception, theory can be a practical tool. Theory often brings together research findings in a way that helps practice be more purposeful, systematic, and comprehensive. In an integrative review, Younas and Quennell (2019) found that nursing theories have been used to guide practice in both Eastern and Western countries.

Historically, most discussions of theory-based practice addressed the use of conceptual models of nursing to guide care (Bonamy et al., 1995; Hawkins et al., 1993; Laschinger & Duff, 1991; Sappington & Kelley, 1996). Huynh and colleagues (2021) have reiterated that nursing theoretical models are "essential and relevant to the ongoing innovations in oncology nursing care" (p. 474). Recently, emphasis has shifted to middle-range theories, which guide practice more specifically. Middle-range theories typically address a particular patient experience (e.g., living with rheumatoid arthritis) or problem (e.g., managing chronic pain); thus their range of applicability is relatively narrow (Smith & Liehr, 2018). However, this narrow range allows them to be developed to address specific issues encountered in clinical practice. Another approach to developing theories that are more specific to clinical situations is to generate a middle-range theory from one of the broader conceptual models. For example, Whittemore and Roy (2002) developed a middle-range theory describing adaptation to diabetes mellitus based on the concepts and theoretical statements of the broader Roy adaptation model. Middle-range theories have a structure of ideas and concepts that are more focused than general nursing theories and are more directly applicable to nursing practice (Smith & Liehr, 2018).

Smith and Liehr (2018) have delineated middle-range theories that have the potential for impact on clinical nursing practice. The list in Box 6.10 provides a sampling of the middle-range theories currently available to practicing nurses, and the reader can see that the topics of the theories are substantively specific, although some are more specific than others. An APRN in a

BOX 6.10

Middle-Range Theories

- Uncertainty in illness
- Theory of meaning
- Self-transcendence
- Symptom management
- Unpleasant symptoms
- Self-efficacy
- Story theory
- Self-reliance
- Cultural marginality
- Caregiving dynamics
- Moral reckoning

From *Middle Range Theory for Nursing*, 4th ed., by M. J. Smith and P. R. Liehr (Eds.), 2018, Springer.

particular field may find that only one or two of these theories are applicable to their area of practice. However, as middle-range theories are developed for other topics, APRNs will be able to use several of these types of theories to guide different aspects of practice.

DIVERSE APPROACHES TO HEALTH AND ILLNESS MANAGEMENT

APRNs' holistic approach to care and their commitment to using evidence as a basis for care contribute to how they help patients. APRNs use a variety of interventions to effect change in the health status or quality of life of an individual or family and tailor their recommendations, approaches, and treatment to individual patients. Interpersonal interventions that are psychosocial in nature are frequently termed *support interventions*. Support interventions are distinct from educational interventions. Coaching uses a combination of support and educational strategies (see Chapter 8). There are also discrete physical actions, which are frequently categorized as nonpharmacologic and pharmacologic interventions. Skilled clinicians craft interventions specific to the patient that are a combination of various types as they seek to alleviate, prevent, or manage specific physical symptoms, conditions, or problems.

Interpersonal Interventions

Support is not a discrete intervention; it is a composite of interpersonal interventions based on the patient's unique psychological and informational needs. Supportive interpersonal interventions include providing reassurance, giving information, coaching, affirming, providing anticipatory guidance, guiding decision making, listening actively, expressing understanding, and being fully present. Each of these interventions can be described in terms of the circumstances for which it is indicated. For example, reassurance is indicated when a patient is experiencing uncertainty, distress, or lack of confidence; active listening is indicated when a patient has a strong need to tell their story. The actions that constitute these interventions are not mutually exclusive. For example, giving factual information can be reassuring, instructional, guiding, or all of these things at the same time.

In practice, these interpersonal interventions are blended and may be subtle. APRNs interact with patients in ways that intermingle the conceptually separate interventions. This crafting of support evolves as the APRN talks with patients; infers their worries, fears, and concerns; learns about their expectations and goals; and acts to alleviate their distress. A patient may experience the interaction as mere conversation with the APRN or as a feeling of being understood. However, support is a complex nursing intervention that is strategically crafted and purposefully administered, and that often makes a difference in how the patient feels and acts (Exemplar 6.3).

Therapeutic Assessments and Interventions

The nursing process (featured in Table 6.1) is a systematic approach to care used by nurses, including the APRN (Sanford, 2020). Beginning with assessment, the APRN seeks first to understand the nature of a patient's condition and response to that condition. Environmental, physiologic, psychosocial, and spiritual factors are considered part of the APRN's assessment. Once data are collected, a list of possible diagnoses is established and ranked in order of likelihood. This is referred to as a *differential diagnosis*. The APRN considers both medical diagnoses and nursing diagnoses in the differential diagnosis. Diagnostic testing is then conducted in order to rule out, confirm, and/or stage a diagnosis or to evaluate response to treatment.

The decision about how or whether to treat a particular condition is based on the provider's determination of risk and benefit. There is often pressure from patients to do something. In this phase of the nursing process, the APRN considers planning and implementation, based upon the following five types of information:

- The degree of certainty about the diagnosis, condition, or symptom
- What is known about the effectiveness of the various treatment alternatives
- What is known about the risks of the treatment alternatives
- The clinician's comfort with a particular treatment or intervention
- The patient's preference for a certain type of treatment or management

In addition, there are resources available with recommendations on when not to provide an intervention because the intervention may risk adverse effects

EXEMPLAR 6.3
AN INTERPERSONAL INTERVENTION[a]

J.E. is a certified nurse-midwife (CNM) in a joint CNM–obstetricians/gynecologists (OB/GYNs) practice model. The seven CNMs have an independent nurse-midwife patient panel. Consultants for the CNM practice are with the seven OB/GYNs in the shared clinical office space. Patients have access to both services at the initiation of care.

Patient care is coordinated and maintained in the respective patient panels. There is a formal process for patients to be seen by the alternative groups in the practice because patients are not allowed to alternate between CNM and OB/GYN provider patient panels. Transfers of care for patients who wish to have CNM care and are considered low risk are accepted in the same manner as transfers to the OB/GYNs of patients who develop high-risk complications outside the scope of the CNM practice.

J.E. has an appointment to see a couple in their early 30s who are expecting their first child. In this group CNM practice, he has met Jan and Steve once previously in this pregnancy. They are very excited about the upcoming birth because they are now 37 weeks and 5 days pregnant. Jan and Steve have prepared themselves with childbirth education classes and have hired a doula to assist them in the birthing process.

J.E. reviews the record and notes that Jan has had no complications during this pregnancy. Accurate dating has been established by an early ultrasound, which corresponds with Jan's last menstrual period and estimated due date. Vital signs today are normal and the patient voiced no concerns to the medical assistant who did the initial intake for this routine, scheduled prenatal visit.

J.E. interviews Jan, who reports she feels well and has no concerns. Jan states that she has had more issues becoming comfortable—at night with increased hip pain, having to get up and urinate frequently, with the baby moving, and with itching. J.E. asks more about the itching and Jan relates that she has been noticing it more in the last few weeks but hadn't mentioned it before. She had looked up itching in pregnancy on the Internet and discussed it with her doula, who told her that this itching (pruritic urticarial papules and plaques of pregnancy [PUPPP]) seems pretty common in pregnancy. J.E. asks Jan more questions about the itching, and she states that it is primarily on the palms of her hands and soles of her feet and only scratching seems to help. Steve relates it is getting so bad lately it's like "watching a dog with an unrelenting scratch." Jan states that she has tried Benadryl a couple of times but it didn't help.

J.E. performs a physical examination, which reveals some minor stretch marks but no notable trunk rash, as would be expected with PUPPP. There are some excoriated marks on Jan's palms because she has been rubbing her hands during the interview.

J.E. recognizes that this does not appear to be a typical PUPPP presentation and believes that the itching may be a symptom of intrahepatic cholestasis of pregnancy (ICP), a potentially serious complication. J.E. relays his thoughts to Jan and Steve and tells them that he is going to order additional blood tests. He orders a complete blood count (CBC), liver function tests, and total bile acid tests.

The laboratory results reveal a normal CBC but an elevated total bile acid level of 27.6 μmol/L (normal range, 0–7.0 μmol/L) and alanine aminotransferase level of 104 IU/L (normal range, 0–50 IU/L). These results confirm that the itching is related to ICP, which puts Jan at an increased risk of intrauterine fetal demise (IUFD). With confirmation laboratory data and a term pregnancy, J.E. calls Jan and informs her of the diagnosis and the need for induction of labor because of the increased risk of IUFD. She is upset and wants to have a direct conversation in the clinic to discuss if induction is really necessary.

J.E. sees Jan and Steve in the clinic and provides answers to their many questions about ICP. They want to discuss alternatives to induction because they had planned for a low-intervention, spontaneous labor and delivery. J.E. reviews with the couple that ICP is associated with a substantial risk of IUFD. This risk increases as a pregnancy approaches term. He explains that induction is considered the best option with a term pregnancy because routine antepartum testing such as ultrasound or electronic fetal monitoring (EFM) is used to evaluate for a placental insufficiency disease process and does not have the specificity to predict an increased risk of IUFD in ICP. J.E. also explains that the elevated bile acids in the amniotic fluid can cause the fetus to experience a sudden cardiac death because of effects on the umbilical artery and/or the electrical activity in the fetal heart. J.E. reviews other treatment options with the couple. Using ursodiol has been effective at decreasing the level of bile acids in the maternal system in preterm pregnancies, but its use to extend pregnancies to spontaneous labor is not recommended because the risk for IUFD still remains, even with decreased maternal bile acids at or beyond term. J.E. also informs Jan that the elevated levels of bile acid are caused by a genetic enzyme deficiency that she has and are not related to anything she did or did not do during her pregnancy.

Jan is crying out of fear and disappointment. J.E. reviews the couple's birth plan with them, pointing out that the desires they had expressed in their birth plan do not have to be revised at this time because of the need for induction. Although constant EFM with induction is required, the use of telemetry will not affect Jan's movement while she is in labor, nor will the use of hydrotherapy as an alternative to pharmaceutical pain management.

Continued

EXEMPLAR 6.3
AN INTERPERSONAL INTERVENTION—cont'd

Jan and Steve agree with the plan of induction after this consultation and arrive at the hospital with their doula, Rita. After the initiation of induction, J.E. uses this early labor period to discuss and educate Rita privately on the rationale for induction and the pathophysiology of ICP. J.E. recognizes that educating Rita is important so she can use this information with her future clients. J.E. also knows that as a member of a childbirth cooperative group, Rita is in a place to inform and instruct her doula peers that the subjective signs of increased itching of the palms of the hands and soles of the feet can be indicative of ICP, and they can advise future clients of doulas to notify their healthcare providers about these findings.

Emily is born to Jan and Steve at 7 pounds, 5 ounces, with an 8/9 Apgar score via normal spontaneous vaginal delivery after a 16-hour labor and delivery hospitalization for induction with prostaglandins and Pitocin. Jan's maternal itching is resolved and total bile acid and liver function test results are returning to normal 48 hours postpartum. Baby and mother are discharged, with no additional follow-up needed for ICP, except for the increased risk of recurrence in future pregnancies.

[a]The author gratefully acknowledges John Eads, MSN, APRN, CNM, for use of his exemplar.

TABLE 6.1
The Nursing Process

Nursing Process Component	Corresponding Activities
Assessment	The nurse gathers information about the patient's psychological, physiologic, sociologic, and spiritual status. This is done through patient interviews, physical examinations, patient and family history, and general observation.
Diagnosis	The nurse makes an educated judgment about potential or actual patient health problems. Multiple diagnoses are sometimes made for a single patient. These include present problems and risks of future problems.
Planning	Nurse and patient agree on diagnoses. A plan of action is then developed. Each problem is assigned a clear, measurable goal. Nurses refer to standardized terms and measurements for tracking patient wellness.
Implementing	Nurse follows through on plans of action, which are specific to each patient. Actions include monitoring, direct care, performance of technical procedures, educating and instructing patients and family, and referring or contacting patient for follow-up.
Evaluating	Nurse evaluates whether goals for wellness have been met. Possible outcomes are improvement in patient condition, stabilized patient condition, or the patient's condition deteriorated. If the patient has shown no improvement or wellness goals have not been met, the process begins again from the first step.

Adapted from "Always a Nurse: A Professional for a Lifetime," by Sanford, 2020, *Nursing Administration Quarterly, 44*(1), 9.

or has no evidence to support that its use would positively impact the condition or outcome (American Board of Internal Medicine Foundation, 2021).

The most clear-cut situation is when the condition is readily diagnosed, a particular treatment is known to be highly effective, the treatment can be expected to be low in risk for the particular patient, and the clinician and patient are comfortable with the treatment. Unfortunately, many therapeutic decisions are not so clear-cut. In these cases, the weight of factors in support of a particular treatment and the weight of those against treatment or in support of another treatment are balanced. Regardless of the choice of intervention, the APRN completes the iterative cycle of the nursing process by evaluating the patient's response to care and then adjusts as indicated on the basis of an ongoing assessment.

When prescribing or recommending medications, APRNs consider the patient's health literacy and agency, financial status and payor formularies, the patient's previous experience with similar medications, ease of taking the medication, how many other medications the patient is taking, how often the medications must be taken, the side effect profiles of the drugs being considered, and potential drug and disease interactions. A systematic review of nurses as prescribers has shown that APRNs tend to prescribe similar or lower total numbers of medications overall compared with physicians, clinical parameters are the same or better for patients treated by prescribing APRNs, and quality of care is similar or better, with similar or improved patient satisfaction (Kapu, 2021; Kapu et al., 2017; Reed, 2021; Van Ruth et al., 2008).

Beyond prescribing medications, the treatment and management interventions that APRNs perform include a wide variety of self-care modalities and low-tech, nonpharmacologic modalities (Hahn, 2014; Hannon, 2013; Morilla-Herrera et al., 2016). In addition, surveillance, teaching, guidance, counseling, and case management are interventions used more often than procedural interventions (Brooten et al., 2003). The frequency with which the various categories of interventions are used varies with patient populations. The repertoire of interventions used by individual APRNs depends on the problems experienced by the population of patients with whom they work. APRNs working in inpatient settings, for example, use therapeutic interventions different from those used by APRNs who provide primary care or deliver care in the outpatient or home setting. The interventions that an individual APRN uses also depend on the influences of colleagues, practice setting, and reimbursement system. Nevertheless, APRNs must make an ongoing effort to extend and refine their repertoire beyond the interventions learned during graduate education. This is the foundation of evidence-based practice discussed earlier in this chapter.

Individualized Interventions

One goal of treatment decision making is to choose from several possible interventions and to use the one that will have the highest probability of achieving the outcomes the patient most desires. That probability is increased by particularizing the treatment or action to the individual patient (Benner et al., 1996). Particularizing requires that the recommendation or action take into consideration the following:

- Acceptability of the treatment to the patient
- What has worked for the patient in the past
- Patient's motivation and ability to use or follow the treatment (self-care)
- Likelihood that the patient will continue to use the treatment, even if side effects are experienced
- Financial burden of the treatment
- Health literacy of the patient

Individualizing nursing care—that is, tailoring care to the unique characteristics of the person and their situation—produces the best patient outcomes. In contrast, standardization of care and control of wide variation are important to quality control and cost containment. Clearly, a blending of the two perspectives is required to produce care that is effective for an individual and congruent with available resources. This can be accomplished by adopting evidence-based standards and guidelines to provide a framework for care while acknowledging that at the point of care (i.e., in the patient–provider interface), interventions and management may need to be tailored to reflect the patient's unique situation and needs.

In establishing a treatment plan, it is useful for the APRN to appreciate the distinction among the concepts of patient adherence, patient compliance, and patient–provider concordance (Fawcett, 2020; Rae, 2021). Because the science of nursing emphasizes person-centered care, APRNs strive to promote patient autonomy and partnership with the healthcare team. The term *adherence* represents the actions a patient must take to follow a prescribed regimen in order to meet goals established by the provider. *Compliance* is similar in that the patient follows a prescribed regimen but differs in the fact that the goals of treatment are established collaboratively with the provider. *Concordance* requires that both the treatment plan and the goals of care be determined collaboratively between the patient and the provider. The latter equalizes the perceived power differential in the therapeutic relationship and is a standard to which the APRN strives. Concordance requires a thorough understanding of the patient's personhood.

Complementary Therapies

The extent of public use of complementary and alternative therapies was well documented in the 1990s by Eisenberg and colleagues when they reported that approximately 33% of Americans were using at least one unconventional therapy (Clarke et al., 2015; Eisenberg, et al., 1993, 1998). Use of complementary therapies has been further supported in the most recent National Health Interview Survey, which demonstrated increase in use of yoga and meditation by adults and children and increases in use of chiropractors by adults (Black et al., 2018; Clarke et al., 2018). Many patients use complementary therapies (i.e., non-mainstream, non-Western therapies) in conjunction with conventional medical services; when complementary therapies are purposefully coordinated with conventional therapies in a treatment plan, the term *integrative therapies* is used. Jou and Johnson (2016) noted that patients often fail to disclose use of complementary therapies to their primary care providers because the provider does not explicitly ask or because the patient does not believe the provider needs the information.

The effectiveness and safety of complementary therapies vary widely. Some have been scientifically studied (e.g., relaxation, guided imagery, glucosamine and chondroitin for osteoarthritis), whereas others have not undergone scientific review for safety and efficacy and therefore, for those therapies ingested, do not have approval by the United States Food and Drug Administration. Of concern is that some may interact with other medications that the patient is receiving (National Center for Complementary and Integrative Health, 2021). Another issue specific to dietary supplements and herbal therapy is the lack of control over ingredients (National Center for Complementary and Integrative Health, 2021). Providers are caught between the desire of patients to use complementary therapies and reservations about their safety, often in the face of insufficient scientific evidence.

APRNs are incorporating complementary therapies into their practices in a variety of ways, albeit with some caution (Brykczynski, 2012; Maloni, 2013; Steefel et al., 2013; Yu, 2014). APRNs have expressed interest in being able to provide complementary therapies for patients, even if it means expanding their scope of practice (Patterson et al., 2003). They are increasing their engagement in these therapies, are more willing to ask patients about complementary and alternative therapy practices, and are counseling patients on appropriate use. Many APRNs report a need to increase their own knowledge about complementary therapies to incorporate it fully into care (Hajbaghery & Mokhtari, 2018). An expert complementary therapies provider is a valuable resource to APRNs considering integrative care. In summary, because patients are using these therapies, APRNs have a responsibility to understand the implications of their use.

Clinical Prevention

Population-Based Data to Inform Practice

The hallmark of the APRN role that differentiates it from other advanced nursing roles is the nature of the direct care that the APRN provides to patients. Although this is a key component of the role, it is expected that APRNs also use a prevention and population health focus (AACN, 2021). *Prevention* refers to the health promotion and risk reduction components of individual health care that are learned as a result of population data. APRNs are considered to be leaders in achieving national health goals for individuals and populations.

Healthy People, an initiative of the US Department of Health and Human Services, is a public health blueprint that aims to promote health and prevent disease by prioritizing areas for intervention. The latest iteration, Healthy People 2030, was released in August 2020. Healthy People 2030 contains 355 specific objectives and raises awareness about gaps between actual and optimal health status. It is the fifth iteration of the Healthy People strategy for 10-year national objectives and targets for improving the health of all Americans. The website (http://www.healthypeople.gov) is a great resource for APRNs and patients to access basic healthcare information (Office of Disease Prevention and Health Promotion, 2017).

APRNs can use population trends to inform direct care and improve the assessments and interventions used at the direct care interface. Central to acknowledging social determinants of health, population data are frequently based on the diseases and conditions prevalent in the geographic setting in which the APRN practices, including the following:

- COVID-19 vaccine access and hesitancy in ethnic minority groups
- Monitoring for metabolic syndrome in the southeast United States
- Assessing for asthma in Virginia
- Surveillance for neurologic disorders in Minnesota

- Cognizance of altitude-based disorders in mountain states
- High suspicion for tuberculosis in homeless patients with pulmonary symptoms who live in densely populated urban settings

Aggregated, individual clinical outcomes are also useful for the evaluation of program and practice effectiveness. By requiring that care be administered and individual outcomes be documented in standardized ways, the healthcare system can conduct programmatic evaluations of clinical outcomes. Population-based evaluations can also be used by APRNs to evaluate and improve the care they provide. Such evaluations can help answer questions such as the following:

- "Is the specific care I (we) provide patients the best way of managing their health or illness?"
- "Are my (our) patients doing as well as similar patients who are cared for by other providers?"

Conducting such an evaluation involves the following: (1) identifying groups of patients (i.e., populations) who have high costs of care, less than optimal outcomes, or both; (2) monitoring and analyzing variances in outcomes and costs; (3) examining processes of care to determine how management of the condition could be improved; and (4) incorporating management methods found to be effective in research or best practice networks. For example, population data in New Mexico have revealed a high mortality rate from alcoholism, prompting the state to invest more in alcoholism prevention programs and emphasize a sharper clinical focus on substance abuse.

Evaluation of the degree to which desirable outcomes are attained enables healthcare systems to compare their effectiveness with that of a comparable system or to evaluate the relative effectiveness of a new program or process of care. These types of evaluations and comparisons can lead to the identification of best practice methods at the healthcare system level. Use of services, readmission rates, complication rates, average total cost per case, and mortality rates are examples of population outcomes used in various types of evaluations and comparisons.

Preventive Services in Primary Care

Health promotion and disease prevention interventions are tools that APRNs in primary care regularly use to help people achieve and maintain a high quality of life. These preventive services include the following:

- Counseling regarding personal health practices that can protect a person from disease or promote screening for the presence of disease
- Immunization to prevent specific diseases
- Chemoprevention (e.g., use of aspirin for prevention of cardiovascular events).

Discernment is needed in the use of these interventions because time and effort can be wasted if their use is not based on current scientific knowledge and tailored to the individual person or community. Conflicting information from lay websites, media sources, and non-peer-reviewed sources detract from many of the preventive recommendations that are based on current science. The US Preventive Services Task Force (https://www.uspreventiveservicestaskforce.org) and the Canadian Task Force on Preventive Health Care (http://canadiantaskforce.ca) provide specific preventive guidelines for many health conditions. These include valuable summaries of the state of the science for each recommendation.

An important point made in the early document *Guide to Clinical Preventive Services* (US Preventive Services Task Force, 1996) is that primary prevention in the form of counseling aimed at changing health-related behavior may be more effective than diagnostic screening and testing. Many healthy people, as well as those who have had a recent health scare, are receptive to—even eager for—information and guidance about how to stay healthy and avoid age-related disabilities. However, other people who engage in one or several unhealthy behaviors can be defensive and resistant to talking about their risks and how behavior changes could reduce risks. Introducing behavior change issues with unreceptive people requires a high level of interpersonal skill and a good sense of timing. An APRN must consider that it is possible that no healthcare provider has previously attempted to discuss the problem (e.g., smoking, lack of exercise, alcohol abuse) with the person, even though signs of a problem have existed for a long time.

Talking about the risks of the current behavior and benefits of the behavior change is not enough. To be effective, counseling regarding these issues should also include a discussion of how the person perceives the burden of changing a personal behavior—that is, what would be lost and what would be required to make the change? The provider must first make the patient feel understood and must elicit how much effort will be required, what would give the individual the confidence to change, and which forms of self-help assistance are acceptable to the individual. Then and only then can a specific recommendation about a strategy or program be made. Theoretical models that can be useful in planning a behavior change program or protocol include the Transtheoretical Model (Cancer Prevention Research Center, University of Rhode Island, 2017) and the Health Belief Model (Resource Center for Adolescent Pregnancy Prevention, 2017). Both models include provider strategies for building a person's *self-efficacy*—confidence in one's ability to take action.

Clinicians also have at their disposal a wide array of screening tools, some of which are better with certain populations or age groups than others. Staying current with the latest screening recommendations in one's area of practice ensures that care is provided in a way that is scientific and cost-effective.

Preventive Services in Hospitals and Home Care

The preventive services provided in inpatient and home care settings are somewhat different from those provided in primary care. Many of the actions and assessments performed on behalf of acutely ill patients are aimed at early detection and prevention of problems related to treatment, disease progression, self-care deficits, or the hospital environment itself. Complications typically result from a complex set of factors, such as inadequate delivery systems or failure to assess patients for risk of complications common to their condition. Nurses assist patients by preventing adverse events and complications, including adverse medication reactions, unexpected physiologic decline, poor communication, pressure injuries, and death. As noted earlier, this function is also termed *surveillance* or *rescuing* (as in rescuing from a bad course of events or death).

In the home setting, APRNs serve as advisors and partners. In addition to assessment and surveillance, guidance and coaching are particularly important. The patient may be new to the role of partner in this setting (Holman & Lorig, 2004). APRNs work with patients to prioritize measures that might prevent rehospitalizations. Interventions may include teaching about reportable signs and symptoms, guidance on how to communicate with their providers, and assistance in making connections between behaviors and situations in the home that directly affect health status.

MANAGEMENT OF COMPLEX SITUATIONS

APRNs' direct care often involves the management and coordination of complex situations. Many illustrations of this advanced practice nursing feature may be found in the chapters on specific advanced practice nursing roles (see Chapters 12 through 16). In some settings, APRNs have been designated as the providers responsible for coordination of complex follow-up care (Bradway et al., 2012; Looman et al., 2013; Morilla-Herrera et al., 2016). APRNs manage diverse and complex patient conditions and care requirements, which include the following:

- Confusion in older hospitalized patients
- Frail older adults
- Pain in patients who are chronically or terminally ill
- Acute pain
- High-risk pregnant women
- Long-term mechanical ventilation
- Heart failure patients
- Neurosurgical patients
- Pediatric and adult palliative care
- Critically ill neonates
- Transplant recipients

Many APRNs have been called in for consultation when there is a need for skilled communication, advocacy, or coordination of the various providers' plans—or some combination thereof (Exemplar 6.4). The patient's condition may not be improving as expected or communication between the healthcare team and the patient and family may be strained. In assessing the situation, the APRN talks with the patient and family to become familiar with their concerns and objectives and then brokers a new plan of care that reflects the patient's and family's needs and preferences, as well as the clinical objectives of the involved providers. The agreed-on plan must also be consistent with the care authorized by the third-party payers for the patient, or a special agreement must be negotiated. This brokering

EXEMPLAR 6.4
MANAGEMENT OF COMPLEX PATIENT SITUATIONS[a]

C.M. is a diabetes clinical nurse specialist with 20 years of experience. She works in an 800-bed academic medical center, where she is accountable for overall outcomes of glycemic control in the inpatient setting. She is also responsible for evaluating, treating, and educating patients with complex diabetes needs.

C.M. has been asked to consult on and write treatment recommendations for a 30-year-old Somali woman. Before seeing the patient, C.M. reviewed the chart to ascertain patient history and information. The patient was diagnosed with type 2 diabetes mellitus (DM) 11 years ago and had been on oral hypoglycemic agents, although not well controlled. She has been managed by multiple providers over the years. The patient was not married and had two sons, 13 and 17 years of age; both have been diagnosed with type 1 DM.

Documentation in the chart indicated that the patient had been admitted to the hospital in diabetic ketoacidosis (DKA) caused by presumed nonadherence to her regimen. The healthcare team had initiated an insulin infusion but had not initiated the DKA protocol and had been having difficulty getting the patient's glucose level in the target range.

When C.M. entered the patient's room, she saw an African woman with truncal obesity, a puffy face, acne, and facial hair. The patient did not make eye contact and appeared standoffish. The patient was reluctant to answer questions. C.M. recognized the need to proceed thoughtfully in developing a relationship with the patient to establish trust. C.M. also realized that multiple visits would be required to fully ascertain the extent of needs for this complex patient. From C.M.'s experience and knowledge base, she knew that the symptomatology of DM in the African population is different from the typical presentation of DM in Caucasians. Type 1 DM symptoms in the African population may not be as severe on initial presentation and may not reflect ketosis; therefore this population can be misdiagnosed with type 2 DM and started on oral agents when they actually have type 1 DM and should be treated with insulin. C.M. suspected that this might have been the case with this patient. In addition, on first glance, C.M. immediately suspected that the patient had other endocrine issues (e.g., adrenal dysfunction or polycystic ovary syndrome) because of the presence of puffy face, acne, and facial hair.

C.M. decided the priority for this initial visit was to focus on the physical care aspects while clarifying the diagnosis and prescribing appropriate treatment to control the patient's glucose. She performed a physical examination and ordered the following diagnostic tests:

- C-peptide and antibodies (to differentiate between types 1 and 2 DM)
- Fasting cortisol
- Adrenocorticotropic hormone stimulation test
- Estradiol–androgen panel
- 24-hour urine
- Endocrinologist consult
- Initiation of standardized DKA protocol

C.M. returned the following day with the intent to explore knowledge and psychosocial areas with the patient. Again, the patient was wary in her interaction but started to have better eye contact. C.M. started by asking about the patient's psychosocial situation and determined that the patient was making ends meet financially. However, there were income issues, and C.M. determined that a social work referral was in order. The patient described having a good relationship with her sons and acknowledged an extensive family support system in the community. She identified herself as a Christian, not a Muslim, as most people assumed.

C.M. then started to inquire about the physical signs she had noticed on the previous visit by asking how long the patient had had acne and facial hair. At that point, the patient started to cry and stated that C.M. was the first person to have ever asked her about it. They were clearly distressing symptoms for the patient, and she relayed that she had tried multiple over-the-counter products to try to resolve the acne but without success. C.M. shared with the patient what she suspected might be happening with other endocrine issues and reassured her that if that were the case, prescription dermatology creams and hormone therapies would help resolve the symptoms. It was at this point that the patient realized that C.M. was committed to helping her and a therapeutic relationship began to develop. The patient was now more receptive to allowing a full knowledge assessment.

C.M. discovered that the patient understood DM well and knew how to count carbohydrates and how to use that information when planning meals. Although the patient spoke English well, C.M. discovered that the patient could not read English and had some visual disturbances. What had been labeled as nonadherence was actually an inability to read and see healthcare instructions. When C.M. reviewed the diagnostic test results, it was determined that the patient had Cushing's syndrome, polycystic ovary syndrome, and type 1 DM, rather than type 2. Over the following days, in educational sessions with C.M., the patient quickly gained knowledge about insulin and how to administer it, and she became proficient at using a magnifier to read the insulin syringe. C.M. developed instructional tools that did not require the ability to read complicated English. Whenever the patient's sons were present, they were included in the teaching.

The patient was eventually discharged to home with new knowledge of insulin and type 1 DM management, as well as information about her new diagnoses and medications,

Continued

EXEMPLAR 6.4
MANAGEMENT OF COMPLEX PATIENT SITUATIONS—cont'd

ongoing support from external social services, and referral to a physician group that could manage the health needs of the entire family and provide continuity of care over time.

HIGHLIGHTS OF ADVANCED PRACTICE NURSING CARE OF A COMPLEX PATIENT

This case exemplifies the role that an APRN can play in making accurate diagnoses and optimizing care for a complex patient. C.M. exhibited the following:

- Use of evidence and knowledge of unique population-based data applied to an individual patient, which resulted in prompt correction of a diabetes misdiagnosis
- Expert clinical assessment and intervention skills that identified new endocrine diagnoses and assisted in rapid correction of glycemic control
- Holistic approach to care, incorporating cultural assessment, psychosocial needs, and barriers to knowledge
- Individualized interventions to meet patient needs
- Interpersonal approach that allowed for rapid development of a trusting therapeutic relationship with a patient who was traditionally wary of healthcare providers who had consistently misidentified her as noncompliant.

[a]The author gratefully acknowledges Carol Manchester, MSN, APRN, CNS, BC-ADM, CDE, for the use of her exemplar.

requires a thoughtful, thorough nursing assessment; a broad clinical knowledge regarding the objectives of various providers; interpersonal skill in dealing with the results of misunderstandings; diplomacy to encourage stakeholders to see each other's points of view; and a commitment to keeping the patient's needs at the center of what is being done.

HELPING PATIENTS MANAGE CHRONIC ILLNESSES

Another type of complex situation that APRNs manage effectively is chronic illness. Chronic diseases such as multiple sclerosis, cognitive degeneration, psoriasis, heart failure, chronic lung disease, cancer, acquired immunodeficiency syndrome, and organ failure with subsequent transplantation affect individuals and families in profound ways. Most chronic illnesses are characterized by a great deal of uncertainty—uncertainty about the future life course, effectiveness of treatment, chances of leading a happy life, bodily functions, medical bills, and intimate relationships (Clayton et al., 2018). The unique perceptions that the patient can experience with uncertainty in chronic illness have led to the proposal of a new model integrating the two concepts: the health change trajectory model (Christensen, 2015). Given the distinct characteristics of advanced practice nursing, APRNs are positioned and well prepared to provide care in this complex situation to persons with chronic conditions and their families.

The US Department of Health and Human Services has issued proposed rules for healthcare providers and systems based on the Patient Protection and Affordable Care Act (2010). to improve the coordination of patient care, particularly those with chronic or complex illnesses, through the establishment of accountable care organizations (US Department of Health and Human Services, 2011). Although the details of any specific legislative efforts will certainly change with time, the essential foundation of an accountable care organization's effort is to place patients at the center of their care, maintain quality standards of care, and lower healthcare costs.

APRNs who see chronically ill patients in a primary care or specialty setting improve care by coordinating the services patients receive from multiple providers. Chronic illnesses often affect several body systems or have numerous sequelae. Thus persons who are chronically ill often receive care from a primary care provider and several other clinicians, including physicians and APRN specialists, social workers, physical therapists, and dietitians. In 1995, Burton identified that without coordination, families coping with chronic illness can find themselves in an "agency maze" (p. 457). Unfortunately, this vivid phrase captures a persisting phenomenon describing the confusing experiences that ensue when the agencies and providers rendering care to a family do not communicate with one another. Families do not know where to go for help and, as a result, many resort to a trial-and-error approach to get what they need. They often suffer the negative effects of misinformation, repetitive intake interviews, denial of service, conflicting approaches, and unsolved problems. A resource-savvy APRN can often assess these situations and intervene to reduce stress, improve communication, and benefit patients and families. By contacting other providers to develop a coordinated management plan and by linking patients with suitable agencies, the APRN can do much to relieve the burdens of chronic illness on a family.

Among the reasons that APRNs are successful in providing care to persons with chronic illness is their advocacy of patient self-care. It has been proposed that the key to self-care by patients with chronic illness is to provide self-management education and support in conjunction with traditional patient education (McGowan, 2012). Self-management education is aimed at promoting confidence to carry out new behaviors, teaching the identification and solving of problems, and setting patient-directed, short-term goals (Lorig et al., 2003; McGowan, 2012). Many self-management educational interventions for those with chronic conditions are designed to bolster patients' sense of self-efficacy related to coping with their condition and gaining control over the impact of the disease on their lives. This can include engaging patients in shared decision making, promoting healthy lifestyles, and monitoring of symptoms (McGowan, 2012), all of which APRNs are skilled at providing and supporting.

Through the use of diverse approaches and individualized, interpersonal, and therapeutic interventions, APRNs have the skills and resources to partner in managing populations throughout the care continuum, from preventive care to the most complex care required by patients with a chronic condition. This is important in view of the increasing complexity of patients' health problems in today's society.

DIRECT CARE AND INFORMATION MANAGEMENT

Health care is an information-rich environment. It has been said that healthcare encounters occur essentially for the exchange of information—between the patient and care provider and among care providers themselves (IOM, 2001). With the adoption of information technology (IT), healthcare information management has become increasingly complex. Inadequate resources and difficulty in accessing information at the time it is needed complicate the situation further (IOM, 2001). The IOM report recommended that government, healthcare leaders, and vendors work collaboratively to build an information infrastructure quickly to eliminate handwritten clinical data. With the implementation of the Affordable Care Act, the HHS has made recommendations to encourage widespread implementation of electronic systems and databases to facilitate access to seamless and accessible healthcare information for everyone (US Department of Health and Human Services, 2010). Although there is still much to do, it is believed that appropriate use of these systems will decrease errors in prescribing and dosing, increase appropriate use of best practice guidelines, reduce redundancy, improve access to information for patients and providers, and improve quality of care. The direct care practice of APRNs is directly influenced by these changes as increasing numbers of healthcare systems and clinics implement electronic health records and databases.

The *Essentials* task force recognized the increasing importance of information systems for APRN practice and education. The *Essentials* require that APRNs be prepared to participate in design, selection, and evaluation of systems used for outcomes and quality improvement (AACN, 2021). This includes leadership in the area of legal and ethical issues related to information systems and knowledge about how to evaluate consumer sources of information available through technology. Borycki et al. (2017) outlined additional nursing informatics competencies required of multiple levels of nurses. With rapid changes in technology, it will be an ongoing challenge throughout an APRN's career to lead in this area.

There is an expectation of increasing competence in the use of technology. Wilbright et al. (2006) surveyed 454 nursing staff at all role levels in their self-reported skill in 11 key areas of computer use. Although the APRNs reported excellent to good skills at entering orders and accessing laboratory results, they rated their skills as fair or poor in 5 of 11 areas that were deemed essential to their role. If APRNs struggle with the need for increasingly complex technology skills, it will be difficult for them to use tools and their time optimally to care for their patients.

Well-functioning information systems can ease the workload of the APRN by optimizing the management of extensive data. However, meaningful IT needs more development to overcome challenges that clinicians face on a daily basis in their use of IT, such as workflow disruptions; lack of interfaces between systems; workarounds, in which providers subvert the IT to get the job done; and inappropriate use of order entry warning alerts (Magrabi et al., 2010, 2012; Palojoki et al., 2016). Computer technology can actually require increased staff time when used for complex order entry and clinical documentation.

Healthcare institutions and private practices are rapidly implementing information systems across the country, so it is likely that APRNs will work in an environment in which a system is being implemented or upgraded. APRNs can have an impact on how these systems function to make them user-friendly and efficient at the direct care interface. Although APRNs may feel they have neither the time, inclination, nor expertise to participate in these implementations, user input is imperative and ultimately affects direct care.

As information systems are implemented, APRNs need to be cognizant of the potential for at least a temporary increase in errors, reduced charge capture, incomplete or difficult-to-access information, and increased time for routine tasks. Implementation of these systems is a major undertaking because it takes time to re-equilibrate workflow and organizational skills, regardless of APRN experience. When information systems are well implemented and used, the APRN will be able to use and view data in new ways to improve patient care.

The expansion of technology can lead to a corresponding increase in the number of tools and amount of data that are available for use—both within and external to the healthcare setting. Examples include email or video communication with patients rather than telephone calls or office visits, patient use of "apps" to assist healthy self-care, patient use of personal fitness devices that record activity levels and calories expended, data that can be downloaded and transmitted from mobile invasive technology to maintain life, the practice of telehealth for routine or specialty patient care, and the use of computers to assist in oncology protocol care decisions (e.g., Watson for Oncology: https://www.ibm.com/watson/health/oncology-and-genomics/oncology/). One commonality throughout these examples is the need to determine when and how to use these data to make patient care decisions (Harrington, 2017). There will be a need for robust analytics to obtain meaning from these data, and APRNs must partner with informaticists and be at the table when determining strategy regarding when and how to use analytics (Harrington, 2016a). The goal is to integrate technology with practice for value-added benefit (Harrington, 2016b). Although information systems and electronic resources can be great tools in the APRN's repertoire, the APRN must be constantly aware that these technologies bring with them their own pitfalls by intruding on the patient relationship and creating a potential for errors (Harrington, 2014). APRNs can play important roles in evaluating proposed technology and information management systems and the impact they have on APRN practice and patient care.

CONCLUSION

The central competency of advanced practice nursing is direct care, regardless of the specific role of the CNS, NP, CRNA, or CNM. APRNs are currently providing direct healthcare services that affect patients' healthcare outcomes positively and that are qualitatively different from those provided by other healthcare professionals. Of importance, these services are valued by the public and are cost-effective. APRNs can offer this essential care through the use of the six characteristics that comprise APRN direct care: use of a holistic perspective, formation of therapeutic partnerships with patients, expert clinical performance, use of reflective practice, use of evidence as a guide to practice, and use of diverse approaches to health and illness management. Their mastery accomplishes several goals, including differentiation of practice at an advanced level and context for the development of other competencies, such as guidance, coaching, and collaboration. Together, these characteristics form a solid foundation for providing scientifically based, person-centered, and outcome-validated healthcare. Research supports each of these claims and hence substantiates the nursing profession's and public's confidence in the care provided by APRNs. As APRNs continue to expand the scope and settings of their practice, it will be imperative that these six characteristics continue to be substantiated by solid research in each of the roles. In addition, research will be important in documenting the optimal so-called nurse dose of APRN intervention as we continue to face challenges in caring for culturally diverse, aging, and chronically ill populations.

KEY SUMMARY POINTS

- Direct care is the central APRN competency.
- The six characteristics of direct care are use of a holistic perspective, formation of therapeutic partnerships with patients, expert clinical performance, use of reflective practice, use of evidence as a guide to practice, and use of diverse approaches to health and illness management.
- It is imperative that APRNs use these six characteristics in their direct care practice through a lens of social determinants of health and systemic inequities and injustice.
- While APRNs provide many strategic functions throughout and over the course of their role, time needs to continue to be spent in direct clinical care with patients in order to maintain differentiation between the APRN role and other doctorate of nursing practice–prepared non-APRN roles.
- Mastery of these six characteristics of direct care delineates the differentiation of practice at an advanced level and sets the foundation for attaining skill in the other APRN competencies.

REFERENCES

Agency for Healthcare Research and Quality [AHRQ]. (2015). Health literacy: Hidden barriers and practical strategies. Retrieved from www.ahrq.org/professionals/quality-patient-safety/quality-resources/tools/literacy-toolkit/tool3a/index.html

Agency for Healthcare Research and Quality [AHRQ]. (2016). AHRQ health literacy universal precautions toolkit. Retrieved from https://www.ahrq.gov/professionals/quality-patient-safety/quality-resources/tools/literacy-toolkit/index.html

Aiken, L. H., Cimiotti, J. P., Sloane, D. M., Smith, H. L., Flynn, L., & Neff, D. F. (2011). Effects of nurse staffing and nurse education on patient deaths in hospitals with different nurse work environments. *Medical Care, 49*(12), 1047–1053.

Aiken, L. H., Clarke, S. P., Sloane, D. M., Sochalski, J., & Silber, J. H. (2002). Hospital nurse staffing and patient mortality, nurse burnout, and job dissatisfaction. *Journal of the American Medical Association, 288*, 1987–1993.

Albarqouni, L., Glasziou, P., & Hoffmann, T. (2018). Completeness of the reporting of evidence-based practice educational interventions: A review. *Medical Education, 52*(2), 161–170.

Al Qahtani, D. A., Rotgans, J. I., Manneded, S., Al Alwan, I., Mazzoub, M. E., Altayeb, F. M., Mohamedani, M. A., & Schmidt, H. G. (2016). Does time pressure have a negative effect on diagnostic accuracy? *Academic Medicine: Journal of the Association of American Medical Colleges, 91*(5), 710–716

American Association of Colleges of Nursing (AACN). (2021). The essentials: Core competencies for professional nursing education. https://www.aacnnursing.org/Portals/42/AcademicNursing/pdf/Essentials-2021.pdf

American Association of Critical-Care Nurses. (2004). The 4A's to rise above moral distress. http://www.aacn.org/wd/practice/docs/4as_to_rise_above_moral_distress.pdf

American Board of Internal Medicine Foundation. (2021). Choosing wisely. http://abimfoundation.org/what-we-do/choosing-wisely

American Nurses Association (ANA). (2010). *Nursing's social policy statement.*

American Nurses Association (ANA). (2016). *Code of ethics with interpretive statements* (2nd ed). American Nurses Association.

Anzai, T., Yamauchi, T., Ozawa, H., & Takahashi, K. (2021). A generalized structural equation model approach to long working hours and near-misses among healthcare professionals in Japan. *International Journal of Environmental Research and Public Health, 18*(13), 7154.

Arends, R., Gibson, N., Marckstadt, S., Britson, V., Nissen, M. K., & Voss, J. (2021). Enhancing the nurse practitioner curriculum to improve telehealth competency. *Journal of the American Association of Nurse Practitioners, 33*(5), 391–397.

Armstrong, G. (2019). Quality and safety education for nurses teamwork and collaboration competency: Empowering nurses. *The Journal of Continuing Education in Nursing, 50*(6), 252–255.

Baker, D. W., Williams, M. V., Parker, R. M., Gazmararian, J. A., & Nurss, J. (1999). Development of a brief test to measure functional health literacy. *Patient Education and Counseling, 38*, 33–42.

Barakzai, M. D., Gregory, J., & Fraser, D. (2007). The effect of culture on symptom reporting: Hispanics and irritable bowel syndrome. *Journal of the American Academy of Nurse Practitioners, 19*, 261–267.

Barron, A. M., & White, P. A. (2009). Consultation. In A. B. Hamric, J. A. Spross, & C. M. Hanson (Eds.), *Advanced practice nursing. An integrative approach* (4th ed.) (pp. 191–216). St. Louis: Elsevier.

Becker, D., Dechant, L., McNamara, L. J., Konick-McMahon, J., Noe, C. A., Thomas, K., & Fabrey, L. J. (2020). Practice-analysis: Adult-gerontology acute care nurse practitioner and clinical nurse specialist. *American Journal of Critical Care, 29*(2), e19–e30.

Becker, D., Kaplow, R., Muenzen, P. M., & Hartigan, C. (2006). Activities performed by acute and critical care advanced practitioners: American Association of Critical-Care Nurses study of practice. *American Journal of Critical Care, 15*, 130–148.

Benner, P. A. (1984). *From novice to expert: Excellence and power in clinical practice.* Addison-Wesley.

Benner, P. A., Hooper-Kyriakidis, P., & Stannard, D. (2011). *Clinical wisdom and interventions in acute and critical care: A thinking-in-action approach.* 2nd ed. Springer.

Benner, P. A., Tanner, C. A., & Chesla, C. A. (1996). *Expertise in nursing practice: Caring, clinical judgment, and ethics.* Springer-Verlag.

Bentley, M., Stirling, C., Robinson, A., & Minstrell, M. (2016). The nurse practitioner–client therapeutic encounter: An integrative review of interaction in aged and primary care settings. *Journal of Advanced Nursing, 72*(9), 1991–2002.

Bissonette, J., Woodend, K., Davies, B., Stacey, D., & Knoll, G. A. (2013). Evaluation of a collaborative chronic care approach to improve outcomes in kidney transplant recipients. *Clinical Transplantation, 27*, 232–238.

Black, L. I., Barnes, P. M., Clarke, T. C., Stussman, B. J., & Nahin, R. L. (2018). Use of yoga, meditation and chiropractors among US children aged 4–17 years. *NCHS Data Brief*(324).

Blegen, M. A., Goode, C. J., Spetz, J., Vaughn, T., & Park, S. H. (2011). Nurse staffing effects on patients: Safety-net and non-safety-net hospitals. *Medical Care, 49*, 406–414.

Bonamy, C., Schultz, P., Graham, K., & Hampton, M. (1995). The use of theory-based practice in the Department of Veterans' Affairs Medical Centers. *Journal of Nursing Staff Development, 11*, 27–30.

Borycki, E. M., Cummings, E., Kushniruk, A. W., & Saranto, K. (2017). Integrating health information technology safety into nursing informatics competencies. *Studies in Health Technology and Informatics, 232*, 222–228.

Bradway, C., Trotta, R., Bixby, M. D., McPartland, E., Wollman, M. C., Kapustka, H., McCauley, K., & Naylor, M. D. (2012). A qualitative analysis of an advanced practice nurse–directed transitional care model intervention. *The Gerontologist, 52*(3), 394–407.

Brooten, D., Youngblut, J. M., Deatrick, J., Naylor, M., & York, R. (2003). Patient problems, advanced practice nurse (APRN) interventions, time and contacts among five patient groups. *Journal of Nursing Scholarship, 35*, 73–79.

Brooten, D., Youngblut, J. M., Donahue, D., Hamilton, M., Hannan, J., & Neff, D. F. (2007). Women with high-risk pregnancies: Problems and APRN interventions. *Journal of Nursing Scholarship, 39*, 349–357.

Browning, S., & Waite, R. (2010). The gift of listening: JUST listening strategies. *Nursing Forum, 45*, 150–158.

Brubakken, K., Grant, S., Johnson, M. K., & Kollauf, C. (2011). Reflective practice: A framework for case manager development. *Professional Case Management, 16*, 170–179.

Brykczynski, K. A. (1989). An interpretive study describing the clinical judgment of nurse practitioners. *Scholarly Inquiry for Nursing Practice, 3*, 75–104.

Brykczynski, K. A. (1991). Judgment strategies for coping with ambiguous clinical situations encountered in primary family care. *Journal of the American Academy of Nurse Practitioners, 3*, 79–84.

Brykczynski, K. A. (2012). Clarifying, affirming, and preserving the nurse in nurse practitioner education and practice. *Journal of the American Association of Nurse Practitioners, 24*(9), 554–564.

Burke, J. R., Downey, C., & Almoudaris, A. M. (2020). Failure to rescue deteriorating patients: A systematic review of root causes and improvement strategies. *Journal of Patient Safety, 18*(1), e140–e155.

Burley, D. (2011). Better communication in the emergency department. *Emergency Nurse, 19*, 32–36.

Burton, D. (1995). Agency maze. In I. M Lubkin (Ed.), *Chronic illness: Impact and interventions* (3rd ed.) (pp. 457–480). Boston: Jones & Bartlett.

Cancer Prevention Research Center, University of Rhode Island. (2017). *Transtheoretical model: stages of change*. Retrieved from http://web.uri.edu/cprc/transtheoretical-model-stages-of-change/

Centers for Disease Control and Prevention. (2013). 2011–2012 National survey of children's health. Retrieved from http://www.cdc.gov/nchs/slaits/nsch.htm

Chen, M. L., & Lin, C. C. (2007). Cancer symptom clusters: A validation study. *Journal of Pain and Symptom Management, 34*, 590–599.

Chisholm, C. D., Weaver, C. S., Whenmouth, L., & Giles, B. (2011). A task analysis of emergency physicians activities in academic and community settings. *Annals of Emergency Medicine, 58*, 117–122.

Christensen, D. (2015). The Health Change Trajectory Model: An integrated model of health change. *Advances in Nursing Science, 38*, 55–67.

Clarke, S., Ells, C., Thombs, B. D., & Clarke, D. (2017). Defining elements of patient-centered care for therapeutic relationships: A literature review of common themes. *European Journal for Person Centered Healthcare, 5*(3), 362–372.

Clarke, S. P., & Aiken, L. H. (2003). Failure to rescue: Needless deaths are prime examples of the need for more nurses at the bedside. *American Journal of Nursing, 103*, 42–47.

Clarke, T. C., Barnes, P. M., Black, L. I., Stussman, B. J., & Nahin, R. L. (2018). Use of yoga, meditation, and chiropractors among US adults aged 18 and over. *NCHS Data Brief*(325).

Clarke, T. C., Black, L. I., Stussman, B. J., Barnes, P. M., & Nahin, R. L. (2015). Trends in the use of complementary health approaches among adults: United States, 2002–2012. *National Health Statistics Reports*(79), 1–16.

Clayton, M. F., Dean, M., & Mishel, M. (2018). Theories of uncertainty in illness. In M. J. Smith, & P. R. Liehr (Eds.), *Middle range theory of nursing* (pp. 48–81). Springer Publishing.

Cleeland, C. S., Mendoza, T. R., Wang, X. S., Chou, C., Harle, M. T., Morrissey, M., & Engstrom, M. C. (2000). Assessing symptom distress in cancer patients: The M.D. Anderson Symptom Inventory. *Cancer, 89*, 1634–1646.

Cornell, P., Riordan, M., Townsend-Gervis, M., & Mobley, R. (2011). Barriers to critical thinking: Workflow interruptions and task switching among nurses. *Journal of Nursing Administration, 41*, 407–414.

Cowley, A., Cooper, J., & Goldberg, S. (2016). Experiences of the advanced practice nurse practitioner role in acute care. *Nursing Older People, 28*(4), 31–36.

Croskerry, P. (2003). Cognitive forcing strategies in clinical decision-making. *Annals of Emergency Medicine, 41*, 110–121.

Cutilli, C. C. (2006). Accessing and evaluating the Internet for patient and family education. *Orthopaedic Nursing, 25*, 333–338.

Dahlke, S., & Phinney, A. (2008). Caring for hospitalized older adults at risk for delirium. *Journal of Gerontological Nursing, 34*, 41–47.

Davidson, L. J., Bennett, S. E., Hamera, E. K., & Raines, B. K. (2004). What constitutes advanced assessment? *Journal of Nursing Education, 43*, 421–425.

Davis, T. C., Long, S. W., Jackson, R. H., Mayeaux, E. J., George, R. B., Murphy, P. W., & Crouch, M. A. (1993). Rapid estimate of adult literacy in medicine: A shortened screening instrument. *Family Medicine, 25*, 391–395.

de Sá Tinôco, J. D., Enders, B. C., Sonenberg, A., & de Carvalho Lira, A. L. B. (2021). Virtual clinical simulation in nursing education: A concept analysis. *International Journal of Nursing Education Scholarship, 18*(1), 1–13.

Defenbaugh, N., & Chikotas, N. E. (2016). The outcome of interprofessional education: Integrating communication studies into a standardized patient experience for advanced practice nursing students. *Nurse Education in Practice, 16*(1), 176–181.

Denkinger, M. D., Igl, W., Coll-Planas, L., Bleicher, J., Nikolaus, T., & Jamour, M. (2009). Evaluation of the short form of the late-life function and disability instrument in geriatric inpatients—validity, responsiveness, and sensitivity to change. *Journal of the American Geriatrics Society, 57*, 309–314.

DePalma, J. A. (2004). Advanced practice nurses' research competencies: Competency I—using evidence in practice. *Home Health Care Management and Practice, 16*, 124–126.

Drennan, J., Naughton, C., Allen, D., Hyde, A., O'Boyle, K., Felle, P., Treacy, M. P., & Butler, M. (2011). Patients' level of satisfaction and self reports of intention to comply following consultation with nurses and midwives with prescriptive authority: A cross-sectional survey. *International Journal of Nursing Studies, 48*, 808–817.

Eisenberg, D. M., Davis, R. B., Ettner, S. L., Appel, S., Von Rampay, M., & Kessler, R. C. (1998). Trends in alternative medicine in the United States, 1990–1997: Results of a follow-up national survey. *JAMA: The Journal of the American Medical Association, 280*, 1569–1575.

Eisenberg, D. M., Kessler, R., Foster, C., Norlock, F., Calkings, D., & Delbanco, T. (1993). Unconventional medicine in the United States. *New England Journal of Medicine, 328*, 246–252.

Elliott, N. (2010). Mutual intacting. A grounded theory study of clinical judgment practice issues. *Journal of Advanced Nursing, 66*, 2711–2721.

Epstein, E. G. (2012). Preventive ethics in the intensive care unit. *AACN Advanced Critical Care, 23*, 217–224.

Epstein, E. G., Whitehead, P. B., Prompahakul, C., Thacker, L. R., & Hamric, A. B. (2019). Enhancing understanding of moral distress: the measure of moral distress for health care professionals. *AJOB Empirical Bioethics, 10*(2), 113–124.

Erickson, H. L. (2007). Philosophy and theory of holism. *Nursing Clinics of North America, 42*, 139–163.

Eriksson, I., Lindblad, M., Möller, U., & Gillsjö, C. (2018). Holistic health care: Patients' experiences of health care provided by an advanced practice nurse. *International Journal of Nursing Practice, 24*(1), e12603.

Escallier, L. A., & Fullerton, J. T. (2009). Process and outcomes evaluation of retention strategies within a nursing workforce diversity project. *Journal of Nursing Education, 48*, 488–494.

Esmaeili, M., Cheraghi, M. A., & Salsali, M. (2014). Cardiac patients' perception of patient-centered care: A qualitative study. *British Association of Critical Care Nurses, 21*(2), 97–104.

Fawcett, J. (2020). Thoughts about meanings of compliance, adherence, and concordance. *Nursing Science Quarterly, 33*(4), 358–360.

Finkelstein, J. B., Nelson, C. P., & Estrada, C. R. (2020). Ramping up telemedicine in pediatric urology—Tips for using a new modality. *Journal of Pediatric Urology, 16*(3), 288–289.

Gee, C., Andreyev, J., & Muls, A. (2018). Developing advanced clinical practice skills in gastrointestinal consequences in cancer treatment. *British Journal of Nursing, 27*(5), 237–247.

George, T. (2016). Role of the advanced practice nurse in palliative care. *International Journal of Palliative Nursing, 22*(3), 137–140.

Greaney, A. M., & O'Mathúna, D. P (2017). Patient autonomy in nursing and healthcare contexts. In P. A. Scott (Ed.), *Key concepts and issues in nursing ethics* (pp. 83–99). Springer.

Hahn, J. E. (2014). Using nursing intervention classification in an advanced practice registered nurse–led preventive model of adults aging with developmental disabilities. *Journal of Nursing Scholarship, 46*(5), 304–313.

Hajbaghery, M. A., & Mokhtari, R. (2018). Complementary and alternative medicine and holistic nursing care: The necessity for curriculum revision. *Journal of Complementary Medicine, 5*(4), 13–14.

Hannon, J. (2013). APN telephone follow up to low-income first time mothers. *Journal of Clinical Nursing, 22*(1–2), 262–270.

Hanson, M. D. (2015). Role of the clinical nurse specialist in the journey to Magnet recognition. *AACN Advanced Critical Care, 26*(1), 50–57.

Harrington, L. (2014). Health information technology safety: The perfect storms. *AACN Advanced Critical Care, 25*(2), 91–93.

Harrington, L. (2016a). Analytics 1.0, 2.0, 3.0. *AACN Advanced Critical Care, 27*(2), 141–144.

Harrington, L. (2016b). Going digital: What does it really mean for nursing? *AACN Advanced Critical Care, 27*(4), 358–361.

Harrington, L. (2017). Closing the science–practice gap with technology: From evidence-based practice to practice-based evidence. *AACN Advanced Critical Care, 28*, 12 15.

Harrington, L., Kennerly, D., & Johnson, C. (2011). Safety issues related to the electronic medical record (EMR): Synthesis of the literature from the last decade, 2000–2009. *Journal of Healthcare Management, 56*(1), 31–44.

Harvard T.H. Chan School of Public Health. (2019). Health literacy studies. www.hsph.harvard.edu/healthliteracy

Hawkins, J. W., Thibodeau, J. A., Utley-Smith, Q. E., Igou, J. F., & Johnson, E. E. (1993). Using a conceptual model for practice in a nursing wellness centre for seniors. *Perspectives, 17*, 11–16.

Health Education England. (2021). South west updates. *Quarterly Faculty Update*, June 2021. https://advanced practice.hee.nhs.uk/south-west-updates/

Holland, M. L., & Holland, E. S. (2007). Survey of Connecticut nurse-midwives. *Journal of Midwifery & Women's Health, 52*, 106–115.

Holman, H., & Lorig, K. (2004). Patient self-management: A key to effectiveness and efficiency in care of chronic disease. *Public Health Reports, 119*, 239–243.

Houlihan, N. G. (2015). Patient satisfaction with information sharing. *Oncology Nursing Forum, 42*(2), 423–424.

Hravnak, M., Tuite, P., & Baldisseri, M. (2005). Expanding acute care nurse practitioner and clinical nurse specialist education: Invasive procedure training and human simulation in critical care. *AACN Clinical Issues, 16*, 89–104.

Hughes, L. C., Robinson, L., Cooley, M. E., Nuamah, I., Grobe, S. J., & McCorkle, R. (2002). Describing an episode of home nursing care for elderly postsurgical cancer patients. *Nursing Research, 51*, 110–118.

Huynh, P., Williams, J., Darcy, K. S., Sherinsky, A., English, A., Heye, D., Joseph, S., & Ross, L. (2021). Theory-informed models and application to nursing practice. *Clinical Journal of Oncology Nursing, 25*(4), 474–478.

Ingram, S. (2017). Taking a comprehensive health history: Learning through practice and reflection. *British Journal of Nursing, 26*(18), 1033–1037.

Institute for Healthcare Improvement. (2021). Plan–do–study–act (PDSA) worksheet. http://www.ihi.org/resources/Pages/Tools/PlanDoStudyActWorksheet.aspx

Institute of Medicine (US) Committee on Quality of Health Care in America. (2001). *Crossing the quality chasm: A new health system for the 21st century*. Washington (DC): National Academies Press (US) PMID: 25057539.

Institute of Medicine (US) Committee on the Robert Wood Johnson Foundation. (2011). *The future of nursing: Leading change, advancing health*: National Academies Press.

Johns, C. (2017). *Becoming a reflective practitioner* (5th ed.). Wiley-Blackwell.

The Joint Commission. (2016). Implicit bias in health care. *Quick Safety, 23*, 1–4. https://www.jointcommission.org/-/media/deprecated-unorganized/imported-assets/tjc/system-folders/joint-commission-online/quick_safety_issue_23_apr_2016pdf.pdf?db=web&hash=A5852411BCA02D1A918284EBAA775988

Jou, J., & Johnson, P. J. (2016). Nondisclosure of complementary and alternative medicine use to primary care physicians: Findings from the 2012 National Health Interview Survey. *JAMA Internal Medicine, 176*(4), 545–546.

Kapu, A. (2021). Origin and outcomes of acute care nurse practitioner practice. *The Journal of Nursing Administration, 51*(1), 4–5.

Kapu, A., Sicoutris, C., Broyhill, B., D'Agostino, R., & Kleinpell, R. (2017). Measuring outcomes in advanced practice nursing: Practice-specific quality metrics. In R. Kleinpell (Ed.), *Outcome assessment in advanced practice nursing* (4th ed.) (pp. 1–18). Springer Publishing Company.

Kesten, K. S., Brown, H. F., & Meeker, M. C. (2015). Assessment of APRN student competency using simulation: A pilot study. *Nursing Education Perspectives, 36*(5), 332–334.

Kim, H. S. (1999). Critical reflective inquiry for knowledge development in nursing practice. *Journal of Advanced Nursing, 29*, 1205–1212.

Kinchen, E. (2019). Holistic nursing values in nurse practitioner education. *International Journal of Nursing Education and Scholarship, 16*(1), 1–10.

Kinder, F. D. (2016). Parents' perception of satisfaction with pediatric nurse practitioners' care and parental intent to adhere to recommended healthcare regimen. *Pediatric Nursing, 42*(3), 138–144.

Kitson, A., Marshall, A., Bassett, K., & Keitz, K. (2012). What are the core elements of patient-centered care? A narrative review and synthesis of the literature from health policy, medicine, and nursing. *Journal of Advanced Nursing, 69*, 4–15.

Kleinpell, R., Cook, M. L., & Padden, D. L. (2018). American Association of Nurse Practitioners national nurse practitioner sample survey: Update on acute care nurse practitioner practice. *Journal of the American Association of Nurse Practitioners, 30*(3), 140–149.

Kohn, L. T., Corrigan, J. M., & Donaldson, M. S. (2000). *To err is human: Building a safer health system*. National Academy Press.

Kullberg, A., Sharp, L., Johansson, H., & Bergermar, M. (2015). Information exchange in oncological inpatient care—patient satisfaction, participation, and safety. *European Journal of Oncology Nursing, 19*, 142–147.

Kumar, K. (2011). Living out reflective practice. *Journal of Christian Nursing, 28*, 139–143.

Lasater, K. B., McHugh, M., Rosenbaum, P. R., Aiken, L. H., Smith, H., Reiten, J. G., Niknam, B. A., Hill, A. S., Hochman, L. L., Jain, S., & Silber, J. H. (2021). Valuing hospital investments in nursing: Multistate matched-cohort study of surgery patients. *BMJ Qual Safety, 30*, 46–55.

Laschinger, H. K., & Duff, V. (1991). Attitudes of practicing nurses towards theory-based nursing practice. *Canadian Journal of Nursing Administration, 4*, 6–10.

Lawrence, M. (1995). The unconscious experience. *American Journal of Critical Care, 4*, 227–232.

Lean Enterprise Institute. (2021). *Principles of lean*. www.lean.org/WhatsLean/Principles.cfm

Leape, L. L. (2012). Apology for errors: Whose responsibility? *Frontiers of Health Services Management, 28*(3), 3–12.

Leape, L. L. (2021). *Making healthcare safe: The story of the patient safety movement*. Springer Nature.

Lewandowski, W., & Adamle, K. (2009). Substantive areas of clinical nurse specialist practice. A comprehensive review of the literature. *Clinical Nurse Specialist, 23*, 73–90.

Lin, Z. C., & Effken, J. A. (2010). Effects of a tailored web-based educational intervention on women's perceptions of and intentions to obtain mammography. *Journal of Clinical Nursing, 19*(9–10), 1261–1269.

Looman, W. S., Presler, E., Erickson, M. M., Garwick, A. W., Cady, R. G., Kelly, A. M., & Stanley, M. (2013). Care coordination for children with complex special health care needs: The value of the advanced practice nurses' enhanced scope of knowledge and practice. *Journal of Pediatric Health Care, 27*(4), 293–303.

Lorig, K., Ritter, P. L., & Gonzalez, V. (2003). Hispanic chronic disease self-management: A randomized community-based outcome trial. *Nursing Research, 52*, 361–369.

Mackay, M. H. (1998). Research utilization and the CNS: Confronting the issues. *Clinical Nurse Specialist, 12*, 232–237.

Magrabi, F., Ong, M. S., Runciman, W., & Coiera, E. (2010). An analysis of computer-related patient safety incidents to inform the development of a classification. *Journal of the American Medical Informatics Association, 17*, 663–670.

Magrabi, F., Ong, M. S., Runciman, W., & Coiera, E. (2012). Using FDA reports to inform a classification for health information technology safety problems. *Journal of the American Medical Informatics Association, 19*(1), 45–53.

Maloni, H. W. (2013). Multiple sclerosis: Managing patients in primary care. *Nurse Practitioner, 38*(4), 24–35.

Markor, M., & Hazan, A. (2012). Advances in communication technology: Implications for new nursing skills. *Journal of Pediatric Nursing, 27*(5), 591–593.

Mason, D. J., Jones, D. A., Roy, C., Sullivan, C. G., & Wood, L. J. (2015). Commonalities of nurse-designed models of health care. *Nursing Outlook, 63*(5), 540–553.

Massachusetts Coalition for the Prevention of Medical Errors. (2006). When things go wrong: Responding to adverse events. http://www.macoalition.org/documents/respondingToAdverseEvents.pdf

McAfee, J. L. (2012). Developing an advanced practice nurse–led liver clinic. *Gastroenterology Nursing, 35*, 215–224.

McCourt, C. (2006). Supporting choice and control? Communication and interaction between midwives and women at the antenatal booking visit. *Social Science and Medicine, 62*, 1307–1318.

McGowan, P. T. (2012). Self-management education and support in chronic disease management. *Primary Care: Clinics in Office Practice, 39*(2), 307–325.

McKeown, S., & Ross-White, A. (2019). Building capacity for librarian support and addressing collaboration challenges by formalizing library systematic review services. *Journal of the Medical Library Association, 107*(3), 411–419.

McTavish, J. (2017). Negotiating concepts of evidence-based practice in the provision of good service for nursing and allied health professionals. *Health Information and Libraries Journal, 34*(1), 45–57.

Miller, N. H. (2010). Motivational interviewing as a prelude to coaching in health care settings. *Journal of Cardiovascular Nursing, 25*, 247–251.

Morilla-Herrera, J. C., Garcia-Mayor, S., Martín-Santos, F. J., Kaknani Uttumchandani, S., Leon Campos, Á., Caro Bautista. J., & Morales-Asencio, J. M. (2016). A systematic review of the effectiveness and roles of advanced practice nursing in older people. *International Journal of Nursing Studies, 53*, 290–307.

Morley, G., Ives, J., Bradbury-Jones, C., & Irvine, F. (2019). What is "moral distress"? A narrative synthesis of the literature. *Nursing Ethics, 26*(3), 646–662.

Munro, N. (2004). Evidence-based assessment: No more pride or prejudice. *AACN Clinical Issues, 15*, 501–505.

Narayan, M. C. (2019). Addressing implicit bias in nursing: A review. *American Journal of Nursing, 119*(7), 36–43.

National Academies of Sciences, Engineering, and Medicine. (2016). *Assessing progress on the Institute of Medicine report, The Future of Nursing*. The National Academies Press.

National Academies of Sciences, Engineering and Medicine. (2018). *Crossing the quality chasm: Improving health care worldwide*. The National Academies Press.

National Academies of Sciences, Engineering, and Medicine. (2021). *The future of nursing 2020–2030: Charting a path to achieve health equity*. The National Academies Press.

National Association of Clinical Nurse Specialists. (2017). Key findings from the 2016 clinical nurse specialists census. https://nacns.org/resources/cns-census/

National Association of Clinical Nurse Specialists. (2019). Key findings from the 2018 clinical nurse specialists census. https://nacns.org/resources/cns-census/

National Association of Clinical Nurse Specialists. (2021). The role of the CNS: Findings from the 2020 census. https://nacns.org/resources/cns-census/

National Center for Complementary and Integrative Health. (2021). *Safe use of complementary health products and practices*. http://nccih.nih.gov/health/safety

National Institutes of Health. (2012). Plain language. www.nih.gov/clearcommunication/plainlanguage.htm

National Quality Forum. (2008). *Serious reportable events*. www.qualityforum.org/Publications/2008/10/Serious_Reportable_Events.aspx

National Quality Forum. (2011). Serious reportable events in health care—2011 update. A consensus report. www.qualityforum.org/Publications/2011/12/Serious_Reportable_Events_in_Healthcare_2011.aspx

Needleman, J., Buerhaus, P., Pankratz, V. S., Leibsno, C. L., Stevens, S. R., & Harris, M. (2011). Nurse staffing and inpatient hospital mortality. *New England Journal of Medicine, 364*, 1037–1045.

Newhouse, R. P., Stanik-Hutt, J., White, K. M., Johantgen, M., Bass, E. B., Zangaro, G., Wilson, R. F., Fountain, L., Steinwachs, D. M., Heindel, L., & Weiner, J. P. (2011). Advanced practice nurse outcomes 1990–2008: A systematic review. *Nursing Economics, 29*(5), 230–250.

Nokes, K. M. (2011). Symptom disclosure by older HIV-infected persons. *Journal of the Association of Nurses in AIDS Care, 22*(3), 186–192.

Obrecht, J. A., Van Hull Vincent, C., & Ryan, C. S. (2014). Implementation of evidence based practice for a pediatric pain assessment instrument. *Clinical Nurse Specialist, 28*(2), 97–104.

O'Brien, B. O., & Graham, M. M. (2020). BSc nursing and midwifery students' experiences of guided group reflection in fostering personal and professional development: Part 2. *Nursing Education and Practice, 48*, 1–6.

Oddsdottir, E. J., & Sveinsdottir, H. (2011). Content of the work of clinical nurse specialists described by use of daily activity diaries. *Journal of Clinical Nursing, 20*, 1393–1404.

Office of Disease Prevention and Health Promotion. (2017). *Healthy People 2020*. http://www.healthypeople.gov/2020

Palojoki, S., Mäkelä, M., Lehtonen, L., & Saranto, K. (2016). An analysis of electronic health record–related patient safety incidents. *Health Informatics Journal, 23*(2), 135–145.

Parry, C., Kramer, H. M., & Coleman, E. A. (2006). A qualitative exploration of a patient-centered coaching intervention to improve care transitions in chronically ill older adults. *Home Health Care Services Quarterly, 25*, 39–53.

Patient Protection and Affordable Care Act, 42 U.S.C. § 18001. (2010).

Patterson, A. E., Mason, T. M., & Duncan, P. (2017). Enhancing a culture of inquiry. The role of a clinical nurse specialist in supporting the adoption of evidence. *Journal of Nursing Administration, 47*(3), 154–158.

Patterson, C., Kaczorowski, J., Arthur, H., Smith, K., & Mills, D. A. (2003). Complementary therapy practice: Defining the role of advanced nurse practitioners. *Journal of Clinical Nursing, 12*, 816–823.

Payne, L. K. (2015). Using specialized standardized patients to improve differential diagnosis. *Nurse Practitioner, 40*(6), 50–54.

Persson, M., Hornsten, A., Wirkvist, A., & Mogren, I. (2011). Mission impossible? Midwives' experiences counseling pregnant women with gestational diabetes mellitus. *Patient Education and Counseling, 84*, 78–83.

Phillips, J. (2005). Neuroscience critical care: The role of the advanced practice nurse in patient safety. *AACN Clinical Issues, 16*, 581–592.

Rae, B. (2021). Obedience to collaboration: compliance, adherence and concordance. *Journal of Prescribing Practice, 3*(6), 235–240.

Raterink, G. (2016). Reflective journaling for critical thinking development in advanced practice registered nurse students. *Journal of Nursing Education, 55*(2), 101–104.

Rector, T. S., Anand, I. S., & Cohn, J. N. (2006). Relationships between clinical assessments and patients' perceptions of the effects of heart failure on their quality of life. *Journal of Cardiac Failure, 12*, 87–92.

Redman, B. K. (2004). *Advances in patient education*. New York: Springer.

Reed, S. M. (2021). President's message: Publishing the evidence of CNS outcomes. *Clinical Nurse Specialist, 35*(1), 1–5.

Resnicow, K., & McMaster, F. (2012). Motivational interviewing: Moving from why to how with autonomy support. *International Journal of Behavioral Nutrition and Physical Activity, 9(1)*, 1–9.

Resource Center for Adolescent Pregnancy Prevention. (2017). Theories & approaches: Health belief model (HBM). http://recapp.etr.org/recapp/index.cfm?fuseaction=pages.theoriesdetail&PageID=13

Reuter-Rice, K., Madden, M. A., Gutknecht, S., & Foerster, A. (2016). Acute care pediatric nurse practitioner: The 2014 practice analysis. *Journal of Pediatric Health Care, 30*(3), 241–257.

Richards, J. B., Hayes, M. M., & Schwartzstein, R. M. (2020). Teaching clinical reasoning and critical thinking: from cognitive theory to practical application. *Chest, 158*(4), 1617–1628.

Rolfe, G. (1997). Beyond expertise: Theory, practice, and the reflexive practitioner. *Journal of Clinical Nursing, 6*, 93–97.

Rudolfsson, G., von Post, I., & Eriksson, K. (2007). The perioperative dialogue. Holistic nursing in practice. *Holistic Nursing Practice, 21*, 292–298.

Rushton, C. H. (2016). Moral resilience: A capacity for navigating moral distress in critical care. *AACN Advanced Critical Care, 27*(1), 111–119.

Rushton, C. H., Schoonover-Shoffner, K., & Kennedy, M. S. (2017). A collaborative state of the science initiative: Transforming moral distress into moral resilience in nursing. *American Journal of Nursing, 117*(2), 52–56.

Ryan, P., Pumilia, N. J., Henak, B., & Chang, T. (2009). Development and performance usability testing of a theory-based, computerized, tailored intervention. *CIN: Computers, Informatics, Nursing, 27*(5), 288–298.

Saad, L. (2020). US ethics ratings rise for medical workers and teachers. Gallup. https://news.gallup.com/poll/328136/ethics-ratings-rise-medical-workers-teachers.aspx

Sackett, D. L. (1998). Evidence-based medicine. *Spine, 23*, 1085–1086.

Sand-Jecklin, S., & Coyle, S. (2014). Efficiently assessing patient health literacy: The BHLS instrument. *Clinical Nursing Research, 23*(6), 581–600.

Sanford, K. D. (2020). Always a nurse: A professional for a lifetime. *Nursing Administration Quarterly, 44*(1), 4–11.

Sappington, J., & Kelley, J. H. (1996). Modeling and role-modeling theory: A case of holistic care. *Journal of Holistic Nursing, 14*, 130–141.

Schön, D. A. (1992). *The reflective practitioner: How professionals think in action* (2nd ed.). San Francisco: Jossey-Bass.

Scordo, K. A. (2014). Differential diagnosis: Correctly putting the pieces of the puzzle together. *AACN Advanced Critical Care, 25*(3), 230–236.

Shuler, P. A., Huebscher, R., & Hallock, J. (2001). Providing wholistic health care for the elderly: Utilization of the Shuler Nurse Practitioner Practice Model. *Journal of the American Academy of Nurse Practitioners, 13*, 297–303.

Silverman, M. E., & Hutchinson, M. S. (2019). Reflective capacity: an antidote to structural racism cultivated through mental health midwifery students' consultation. *Infant and Mental Health Journal, 40*, 742–756.

Sittig, D. F., & Singh, H. (2012). Electronic health records and national patient-safety goals. *The New England Journal of Medicine, 367*(19), 1854–1860.

Smith, M. C. (2019). Regenerating nursing's disciplinary perspective. *Advances in Nursing Science, 42*(1), 3–16.

Smith, M. J., & Liehr, P. R. (2018). *Middle range theory for nursing* (4th ed.). Springer.

Stableford, S., & Mettger, W. (2007). Plain language: A strategic response to the health literacy challenge. *Journal of Public Health Policy, 28*, 71–93.

Steefel, L., Hyatt, J., & Heider, G. (2013). Talking about CAMs for menopause. *Nurse Practitioner, 38*(8), 48–53.

Stetler, C. B., Bautista, C., Vernale-Hannon, C., & Foster, J. (1995). Enhancing research utilization by clinical nurse specialists. *Nursing Clinics of North America, 30*, 457–473.

Stutzer, K., & Bylone, M. (2018). Building moral resilience. *Critical Care Nurse, 38*(1), 77–89.

Tanner, C. A. (2006). Thinking like a nurse: A research-based model of clinical judgment in nursing. *Journal of Nursing Education, 45*, 204–211.

Tanner, C. A., Benner, P., Chesla, C., & Gordon, D. R. (1993). The phenomenology of knowing a patient. *Image–the Journal of Nursing Scholarship, 25*, 273–280.

Thompson, J., & McKeever, M. (2014). Improving support for patients with aphasia. *Nursing Times, 110*(25), 18–20.

Turrise, S. L., O'Donnell, S. M., Arms, T., Kuiper, R., & Pesut, D. J. (2017). Clinical reasoning: Optimizing teaching and learning in nursing education. https://sigma.nursing.repository.org/handle/10755/623235

US Department of Health and Human Services. (2011). *Affordable Care Act to improve quality of care for people with Medicare*. www.hhs.gov/news/press/2011pres/03/20110331a.html

US Department of Health and Human Services, Office of the National Coordination for Health Information Technology.

(2010). Electronic eligibility and enrollment. http://healthit.hhs.gov/portal/server.pt?open=512&mode=2&objID=316

US Preventive Services Task Force. (1996). *Guide to clinical preventive services*. In *Report of the US Preventive Services Task Force* (2nd ed.). Baltimore: Williams & Wilkins.

Van Hecke, A., Goemaes, R., Verhaegh, S., Beyers, S. W., Decoene, E., & Beckham, D. (2019). Leadership in nursing and midwifery: Activities and associated competencies of advanced practice nurses and midwives. *Journal of Nursing Management, 27*, 1261–1274.

Van Ruth, L. M., Mistiaen, P., & Francke, A. L. (2008). Effects of nurse prescribing of medications: A systematic review. http://www.ispub.com/journal/the-internet-journal-of-healthcare-administration/volume-5-number-2/effects-of-nurse-prescribing-of-medication-a-systematic-review.html

Verger, J. T., Marcoux, K. K., Madden, M. A., Bojko, T., & Barnsteiner, J. H. (2005). Nurse practitioners in pediatric critical care: Results of a national survey. *AACN Clinical Issues, 16*, 396–408.

Victor-Chmil, J. (2013). Critical thinking versus clinical reasoning versus clinical judgment: Differential diagnosis. *Nurse Educator, 38*(1), 34–36.

Ware, J. E., & Sherbourne, C. D. (1992). The MOS 36-item short form health survey (SF-36): I. Conceptual framework and item selection. *Medical Care, 30*, 473–483.

Warner, H. (2006). Caring for a child with disabilities: Part 2. The child/family/nurse relationship. *Paediatric Nursing, 18*, 38–43.

Westbrook, J. I., Woods, A., Rob, M. I., Dunsmuir, W. T. M., & Day, R. O. (2010). Association of interruptions with an increased risk and severity of medication administration errors. *Archives of Internal Medicine, 170*, 683–690.

White, C. S. (2012). Advanced practice prescribing: Issues and strategies in preventing medication error. *Journal of Nursing Law, 14*, 120–127.

Whitehead, D., Zucker, S. B., & Stone, J. (2014). Tobacco cessation education for advanced practice nurses. *Nurse Educator, 39*(5), 252–255.

Whittemore, R., & Roy, C. (2002). Adapting to diabetes mellitus: A theory synthesis. *Nursing Science Quarterly, 15*, 311–317.

Wilbright, W. A., Haun, D. E., Romano, T., Krutzfeldt, T., Fontenot, C. E., & Nolan, T. E. (2006). Computer use in an urban university hospital: Technology ahead of literacy. *Computers, Informatics, Nursing: CIN, 24*, 37–43.

Wolf, Z. R., & Robinson-Smith, G. (2007). Strategies used by clinical nurse specialists in "difficult" clinician–patient situations. *Clinical Nurse Specialist, 21*, 74–84.

Younas, A., & Quennell, S. (2019). Usefulness of nursing theory–guided practice: An integrative review. *Scandinavian Journal of Caring Sciences, 33*, 540–555.

Yu, A. (2014). Complementary and alternative treatments for primary dysmenorrhea in adolescents. *The Nurse Practitioner, 39*(11), 1–12.

7 GUIDANCE AND COACHING

EILEEN T. O'GRADY ■ JEAN E. JOHNSON

"Always bear in mind that your own resolution to succeed is more important than any other."

~ Abraham Lincoln

CHAPTER CONTENTS

WHY GUIDANCE AND COACHING? 213
Patient Engagement 213
Burden of Chronic Illness 214
GUIDANCE AND COACHING DEFINITIONS 214
Guidance 215
Coaching 215
THEORIES AND RESEARCH SUPPORTING APRN GUIDANCE AND COACHING 217
Nightingale's Environmental Theory 217
Middle Range Theory of Integrative Nurse Coaching 217
Transtheoretical Model 218
Watson's Model of Caring 219
Positive Psychology 219
Growth Mindset 219
Self-Determination Theory 220
Transitions in Health and Illness 220
BUILDING RELATIONSHIPS FOR APRN GUIDANCE AND COACHING 223
Presence 223
Communication 224
Nonjudgmental (Suspending Judgment) 225
Empathy and Compassion 226
Managing Conflict 227
Partnership 227
DETERMINING PATIENT READINESS FOR CHANGE 228
Patient Readiness 228
THE "FOUR *As*" OF THE COACHING PROCESS 233
Agenda Setting 233
Awareness Raising 234
Actions and Goal Setting 235
Accountability 235
APRN PRACTICE PRINCIPLES FOR SUCCESSFUL GUIDANCE AND COACHING 235
Ask Questions 235
Ask Permission 236
Build on Strengths 236
Support Small Changes 237
Be Curious 237
Challenge 237
Get to the Feelings 238
BUILDING COACHING INTO PRACTICE 238
CONCLUSION 239
KEY SUMMARY POINTS 239

This chapter defines *guidance* and *coaching* as advanced practice registered nurse (APRN) competencies that are at the heart of nursing and are an effective means to engage patients in change leading to healthier lives. Since researchers first identified the teaching–coaching function of expert nurses and APRNs, guidance and coaching by APRNs have been researched and integrated into APRN competencies and described through case studies and other writings about APRN practice (Benner, 1984; Benner et al.,

1999; Fenton & Brykczynski, 1993; Hayes & Kalmakis, 2007; Ross et al., 2018).

The American Association of Colleges of Nursing (AACN) *The Essentials: Core Competencies for Professional Nursing Education* (2021) have re-envisioned a model of nursing education that is built on 10 domains of nursing practice and incorporates four spheres of knowledge:

> *1) disease prevention/promotion of health and well-being, which includes the promotion of physical and mental health in all patients as well as management of minor acute and intermittent care needs of generally healthy patients; 2) chronic disease care, which includes management of chronic diseases and prevention of negative sequela; 3) regenerative or restorative care, which includes critical/trauma care, complex acute care, acute exacerbations of chronic conditions, and treatment of physiologically unstable patients that generally requires care in a mega-acute care institution; and, 4) hospice/palliative/supportive care which includes end-of-life care as well as palliative and supportive care for individuals in long term care or those with disabling conditions, complex chronic disease states, and those requiring rehabilitative care.*
>
> *(AACN, 2021, p. 6).*

The *Essentials* identify competencies and the sub-competencies address the advanced and entry-level nursing education. There is a strong focus in the updated *Essentials* on patient-centered care and the emphasis on communication that strongly supports guidance and coaching competencies for APRNs throughout the domains.

This chapter will include guidance and coaching competency-building to effectively engage and build trust in the APRN–patient relationship. The theoretical and research basis of guidance and coaching provides the foundation for relationship competencies that include communication, presence, nonjudgmental thinking, empathy, partnership mindset, and conflict management skills (Johnson et al., 2022). Situations appropriate for guiding patients and those appropriate for coaching patients are emphasized. Foundational skills of the coaching methodology are discussed, and guidance and coaching skills will be contrasted. Integrative health care, often linked with guidance and coaching, is not fully covered in this chapter; rather, a thorough discussion explores the relational skills needed across all four APRN roles. (See Chapter 6 for a discussion of integrative therapies in APRN practice.)

WHY GUIDANCE AND COACHING?

Guidance and coaching are effective in facilitating behavior change for patients to lead healthier lives. APRNs are most likely to use both guidance and coaching as an integrated model to help patients gather the motivation necessary to engage in change. The "why" of guidance and coaching is to engage patients in their own care, to prevent and/or effectively manage chronic illness, and to keep patients as functional and healthy as possible throughout their life. Nursing care looks at the whole person in the context of their life. Guiding and coaching patients through important transitions and in the pursuit of behavior change or well-being is done through a whole-person lens.

Patient Engagement

There are many reasons why people are becoming more engaged in their health care: the ease of information access through the Internet, the shifting of costs of care to consumers, the heightened awareness of healthy behaviors leading to longer health spans, and an aging population with chronic illness insisting on living with the highest degree of independence and functionality possible. Patient experience surveys focus on how patients feel about the care they receive, and for acute care institutions, payment add-ons or decrements depend on those patient experience results. Hibbard and Greene (2013) have shown that patients activated to engage in their care have better outcomes and lower costs.

Guiding and coaching patients requires patient activation and empowerment by placing the responsibility of the *pursuit* of health where it rightly belongs—with the patient. Information technology has advanced to support the activation and empowerment of patients by giving them critical health information. The Patient Protection and Affordable Care Act of 2010 in the United States provided the structures and requirements to make data about quality of care publicly available and enhanced patient-centered care through client-centered medical homes and healthcare financing models that empower patients. Health systems are continuing to design care that engages patients in their treatment, develops their abilities to manage their health and lowers their modifiable risks, helps them express concerns and preferences regarding treatment, empowers them to ask questions about treatment options, and builds strategic patient–provider partnerships through shared decision making (Chen et al., 2016). Recognizing patients as the source of control for their health requires building confidence, trust, and partnerships with patients rather than having healthcare providers simply tell patients what they need to do.

Burden of Chronic Illness

The current biomedical model of care does not work for lifestyle-related diseases. In the United States, 6 in 19 people have one chronic disease and 4 in 10 have two or more chronic illnesses (Centers for Disease Control [CDC], 2020). Heart disease, cancer, respiratory illness, and diabetes account for 71% of deaths worldwide (World Health Organization [WHO], 2020a). These diseases are costly and are the lead driver of healthcare costs that are amenable to prevention. These diseases are caused by four behaviors: tobacco, inactivity, poor nutrition, and excessive alcohol use (CDC, 2020). Helping patients change these behaviors will greatly decrease untold suffering, early mortality, and disability.

A startling statistic that represents opportunity for behavior change is the number of people who are obese tripled between 1975 and 2016, with over 340 million children and adolescents aged 5 to 19 overweight or obese in 2016 (WHO, 2020b). Of great concern is the 2019 estimate that 38.2 million children under the age of 5 were overweight or obese (WHO, 2020b). Overweight and obesity are generally preventable and present an impending disaster for worldwide health, for society, and for the global macroeconomy.

Chronic disease in the United States is estimated to cost $3.7 trillion a year, including direct and indirect costs, with a gross domestic product (GDP) of $21 trillion. This accounts for almost 20% of the US GDP (O'Neill-Hayes & Gillian, 2020). It is estimated that global GDP could increase 8% by 2040 if chronic illness were reduced through innovation and prevention of illness (Remes et al. 2020). Chronic illnesses cause billions of dollars in losses of national income and push millions of people below the poverty line each year. In the United States alone, chronic diseases attributable to lifestyle factors are responsible for 7 of 10 deaths each year, and they account for an estimated 90% of our nation's healthcare costs, which in 2019 was $3.8 trillion (before the COVID-19 pandemic; Centers for Medicare & Medicaid Services, 2020). In addition, the increasing burden of preventable chronic diseases globally has made very clear the vulnerability of those with a chronic condition to COVID-19 and other acute health emergencies that have arisen (Institute for Health Metrics and Evaluation, 2020).

As every APRN knows, lifestyle factors and behaviors can be modified to lessen the risk of chronic illness. People can reduce their chances of getting a chronic disease or improve their health and quality of life if they already have a chronic disease by making healthy choices. Liu et al. (2016) found that only 6.3% of US adults engaged in all five key health behaviors that can reduce their risk of chronic diseases: (1) avoiding alcohol consumption or only drinking in moderation, (2) exercising regularly, (3) getting enough sleep, (4) maintaining a healthy body weight, and (5) not smoking. These findings, based on nearly 400,000 adults aged 21 and older, showed that 1% failed to engage in any of the five health behaviors; 24% engaged in four, 35% engaged in three, and 24% engaged in two. As APRNs use their expertise to sharply focus on patients' lifestyles, their value in the healthcare marketplace will be more fully realized.

GUIDANCE AND COACHING DEFINITIONS

Guidance and coaching are relational approaches that focus on helping a person create change in their life to advance individual autonomy, well-being, and goal attainment. *Guidance* is the act of providing information and direction, and *coaching* is an inquiry process to help patients set and achieve their own goals by using powerful questions rather than telling them what they need to do. APRNs are in a unique position to integrate these two approaches so that the focus is on the patient's goals and APRNs provide targeted and highly individualized information for patients to make informed decisions. Understanding and integrating into practice the characteristics of guidance and coaching comprise a key APRN competency that is built on having trust and rapport with patients.

Guidance

Guidance is a broad term that means the provision of help, instruction, or assistance, and there are several forms of guidance. The distinguishing feature of guidance compared with coaching is that guidance requires the provision of advice or education, whereas coaching is an inquiry, an excavation of answers from a person. To guide is to advise, or show the way to others, so guidance can be considered the act of providing expert counsel by leading, directing, or advising. *To guide* also means to assist a person to travel through or reach a destination in an unfamiliar area. Guidance is best used in situations when a person has a perceived knowledge deficit in an area for which expert APRN knowledge can fill the void. When providing guidance, the APRN is serving as a knowledge source for the patient. Guidance can include laying out, simplifying, or integrating the options for a patient to make a healthcare decision. It is imperative that the APRN determine the patient's level of knowledge before launching into guidance. Asking patients what they know about their condition is an important skill to respectfully build on what they know and make APRN guidance more powerful and effective. What follows are some common forms of guidance.

Anticipatory Guidance

Anticipatory guidance and teaching are particular types of guidance aimed at helping patients and families know what to expect. Anticipating common problems or symptoms and what to do about them can go a long way in reducing unnecessary care, promoting self-efficacy and reducing a patient's anxiety. Anticipatory guidance is when the APRN informs the patient a priori about an expected health process that is likely to occur. For example, when a patient sustains a cervical hyperextension injury (whiplash) after a car accident and a fracture has been ruled out, the APRN informs the patient that the muscles surrounding the neck will become far more painful within 48 hours. She or he may explain that torticollis may ensue and that this is normal, temporary, and to be expected. The APRN offers remedies and guidelines on when to seek more assessment. Another example of anticipatory guidance is when a woman experiences a miscarriage and the APRN lets the patient know to expect very heavy blood loss that may alarm her. The APRN provides guidelines about when to seek additional care, offers reassurance, and anticipates that the patient may experience intense feelings of loss and grief.

Patient Education

Patient empowerment can be achieved by teaching patients about their illnesses/conditions and by guiding them to be more involved in decisions related to ongoing care and treatment. The WHO (2016) defines patient education more broadly as any combination of learning experiences designed to help individuals and communities improve their health by increasing their knowledge or influencing their attitudes. The goal of patient education is to produce change and promote self-care. Clinicians have long held the myth that if the patient is provided with the right information, the patient will see the wisdom of making change in their life to be healthier and simply follow the recommendations.

For APRNs it is essential to determine what a person wants to learn *before* launching into a teaching or "telling" expert role. Patients often come with an array of information from available websites and other sources. As information has become so readily available, patients are looking for customized wisdom and a broker of information to cut through the large amount of confusing, often conflicting, sources of knowledge. They want to know what information applies to them and how should they use it. (See Chapter 6 for further discussion of patient education.)

Coaching

Coaching is a broad umbrella term that encompasses different approaches, philosophies, techniques, and disciplines. Coaching is defined by the International Coaching Federation (ICF, 2020) as "partnering with clients in a thought-provoking and creative process that inspires them to maximize their personal and professional potential." For APRNs this definition also extends to a health potential. The ICF (2020) identified four main domains of a coach's responsibility which could apply to APRN practice:

1. Engages in foundational work that is based on ethical principles and a coaching mindset that is flexible, open, curious, and client centered.

2. Cocreates a relationship that is based on agreement about the relationship, plans, goals, and client accountability and creates trust and safety and maintains presence with the client.
3. Communicates effectively using deep listening and evokes client awareness.
4. Cultivates learning and growth.

The ICF definition and components of coaching provide significant leeway in the development of different philosophic approaches to coaching. Although there are common principles, there are different philosophies and schools of thought in the coaching sphere. One example is motivational coaching, based on a focused approach to explore and ignite motivation for change and address ambivalence. Another is integrative coaching, developed at Duke University to help patients make changes to lead healthier lives (Duke Integrative Health, 2020). Integrative coaching is intended to address the gap between medical recommendations and the patient's success in implementing the recommendations. Each of these approaches has commonalities, including working toward change that is defined by the patient. In addition, there are different foci of coaching, such as health and wellness, executive, life transition, end of life, and attention deficit/hyperactivity coaching, to name a few. A meta-analysis on coaching by Sonesh et al. (2015) found wide-ranging impacts of coaching, including that coaching is an effective way to change patient behaviors and improve leadership skills, job performance, and skill development. Specific findings concluded that coaching:

- Improves personal and work attitudes, including self-efficacy, commitment to the organization, and reducing stress.
- Elicits a strong bond, which in turn facilitates joint goal setting and may be the mechanism through which goals are reached.

In addition, systematic reviews related to the more prevalent chronic conditions such as weight loss, type 2 diabetes, chronic obstructive lung disease, and cardiac risk factor reduction found health coaching reduces hospitalization and improves healthy behaviors (An & Song, 2020; Perez-Cueto, 2019; Long et al., 2019; Pirbaglou et al., 2018).

Coaching is based on a relationship in which the *individual identifies their goals*. It is founded on the recognition that the person seeking coaching is mentally healthy and has internal resources to deploy toward attaining their goals. The role of the coach is to work with that person in accomplishing those goals. The coach helps individuals clarify, define, reflect, and move forward. Coaching can be thought of as leading change from behind as well as walking with the patient (McLean, 2019). This concept clearly puts the individual in charge while the coach fully engages with the patient. A coaching partnership can last from a "spot" coaching session of one time to interactions over several years.

There is considerable discussion within coaching as to how much advice-giving should be offered. Because coaching is considered a partnership with a coach asking powerful questions, the APRN must trust that the person has their own answers that are true and right for them. However, working with patients to make change is different in that providers have specific health-related information that patients need and want. Providing that information is providing guidance within a coaching context. Combining coaching with guidance is essential to a complete provider–patient relationship. Table 7.1 differentiates guidance and coaching. It is important to note that coaching is neither counseling nor mentoring. The American Counseling Association defines counseling as "a professional relationship that empowers diverse individuals, families, and groups to accomplish mental health, wellness, education, and career goals" (Kaplan et al., 2014, p. 368). Counseling

TABLE 7.1

Elements of Guidance and Coaching Competencies

Guidance	Coaching
Expert APRN has higher authority gradient	Power is shared
APRN is the expert	Patient is the expert/has the answers
Provides advice	Seeks understanding
Fixes problems	Builds on strengths
Expertise is valued	Curiosity is valued
Telling	Asking
Teaching	Inquiring
Anticipates	Explores
APRN leads/sets agenda	Patient leads/sets agenda

can be a very long-term relationship focused on helping individuals address their problems. Counseling is generally focused on psychological, social, or performance issues. The key distinction is that counseling is intended to "fix" a problem through gaining insight and advice from the counselor. Counseling as a technique operates from a problem-based approach as well as building on a person's strengths. Psychiatric mental health nurse practitioners use all three modalities: counseling, coaching, and guidance.

Background of Nurse Coaching

Nurse coaching is aimed at working with individuals to promote their maximal health potential by integrating the skills of nursing and coaching. Professional nurse coaching can be defined as "a skilled, purposeful, results-oriented, and structured relationship-centered interaction with clients provided by a registered nurse for the purpose of promoting achievement of client goals" (Dossey et al., 2015, p. 3). Although this definition is specific to nursing and nursing care, it is consistent with the intent of the ICF definition. The American Holistic Nurses Credentialing Corporation (2020) has created momentum to integrate coaching into all registered nurse programs through the International Nurse Coaching Association (INCA), providing educational opportunities to become a nurse coach and certification as a coach. The texts *The Art and Science of Nursing Coaching: The Providers Guide to the Nursing Scope and Competencies* (Dossey et al., 2013), published by the American Nurses Association (ANA), and *Nurse Coaching: Integrative Approaches for Health and Well-being* (Dossey et al., 2015) provided the framework for the work of INCA. These works have been endorsed by the American Holistic Nurses Association.

Coaching has been explicitly integrated into several APRN practices, although the extent of APRN coaching is unknown. For example, Hayes and Kalmakis (2007) asserted that coaching is a critical component of a holistic care approach for nurse practitioners. Most midwives say that their practice incorporates coaching throughout the mother's pregnancy and delivery (Rafferty & Fairbrother, 2015; Exemplar 7.1). There has long been the concept of a "labor coach" within midwifery. Clinical nurse specialists have worked within the areas of both consultant and coach (Goudreau, 2021). As coaches, they have worked with patients and family members to manage multiple chronic illnesses, especially around care transitions or a specific disease. Many clinical nurse specialists have roles that incorporate coaching when working with nurses to develop skills. A Certified Registered Nurse Anesthetist uses coaching to customize and personalize pain management or anesthesia to meet the patient's stated goals and needs.

THEORIES AND RESEARCH SUPPORTING APRN GUIDANCE AND COACHING

There are numerous evidence-based theories and frameworks that inform the APRN guidance and coaching competency. These are deeply rooted in Florence Nightingale's environmental theory and the science of human caring, which broadens and deepens the therapeutic use of self. In fact, the importance of the APRN-patient therapeutic relationship is foundational to the APRN guidance and coaching competency. Although there are many theories and models, we will note those that are important to informing and developing the APRN guidance and coaching competency.

Nightingale's Environmental Theory

Florence Nightingale's *Notes on Nursing: What It Is and What It Is Not* (1860) makes a strong link between a person's environment and their health. Working with a person to manage their environment is the fundamental role of nursing, and as we experience a chronic illness epidemic in modern times, this observation still holds true. In fact, Nightingale built the foundation of nursing as a distinct profession on her observation that external factors associated with patients' surroundings greatly affect their lives, their development, and their biologic and physiologic processes (Nightingale, 1860). This seminal conceptual thinking lies at the heart of modern APRN guidance and coaching.

Middle Range Theory of Integrative Nurse Coaching

A theoretical framework for nurse coaching has been developed by Dossey et al. (2015). They defined an integrative nurse coaching framework as "a distinct nursing role that places clients/patients at the center and assists them in establishing health goals, creating

EXEMPLAR 7.1
BEING A MIDWIFE AND FAMILY NURSE PRACTITIONER IS BEING A COACH[a]

Dawn Lovelace, DNP, RN, CNM, FNP, is both a certified nurse-midwife (CNM) and a family nurse practitioner (FNP) who believes coaching is integral to her practice. She lives in Grand Coulee, Washington, an area with 1000 people in the town and 10,000 people in the 20-square-mile service area surrounding the town. She and several colleagues worked to build a full-scope health service with her focus on developing maternity care services that did not exist. She was on call 24/7 for births, saw patients 4 days a week in clinic, provided emergency room coverage, and saw patients in the hospital and nursing home. The practice has added more clinicians and is now a medical home.

Dr. Lovelace says that coaching has always been part of "being" a midwife and FNP, and she has a strong commitment to helping people be as healthy as possible. As a midwife, she helps women prepare for and meet their goals for the birth as well as becoming a parent. The beauty of coaching pregnant women is that she has 9 months and often much longer to engage in a coaching relationship. Coaching has been part of the very deep and long value she has had. It is integral to her personal belief system. She starts where the person is, helps her evolve based on her reproductive life plan, and determines how to help get her there. For Dr. Lovelace, it is difficult to tease out what is coaching because it is so embedded within the role. She describes how being with women outside the hospital setting helps one truly be present with them. She knows she is present when she loses track of time and is in the "zone" or "flow." She has used the transformative power of pregnancy and birth knowing that this is a time of life when people want to grow and that tapping into that desire is easy.

When asked what she likes best about coaching, Dr. Lovelace says she has seen so many amazing outcomes of coaching. She described working with a 14-year-old pregnant girl who was heavily involved in drugs. Dr. Lovelace's coaching went beyond the birthing process as she worked with the young woman to get her life together. Despite every roadblock conceivable, that young woman is now in college and is an effective parent. She also described another young girl who came for birth control and who was going from house to house sleeping on sofas. This young woman is now a nurse practitioner, and when she recently saw Dr. Lovelace, she said that it was really important that Dr. Lovelace treated her like a human being and saw the potential in her.

When asked what she would say to her students about integrating coaching into their practice, Dr. Lovelace quickly said, "Start where the person is. Accept them where they are. We all have people we don't like, but we need to accept them and don't ever write anyone off." In asking how she would advise students to be able to be present with patients, Dr. Lovelace said, "It takes work and self-evaluation, you need to know your prejudices and beliefs. We have off days in which we don't listen, but we need to keep working at deep listening. Helping people figure out how to change their lives—that is what matters. You have to be committed to having coaching being part of your practice and value it."

[a]The author gratefully acknowledges Dawn Lovelace, DNP, CNM, FNP for use of her exemplar.

change in lifestyle behaviors for health promotion and disease management, and implementing integrative modalities as appropriate" (Dossey et al., 2015, p. 29). The authors identified five components of this model: "(1) Self-development (Self-reflection, Self-assessment, Self-evaluation, and Self-care); (2) Integral Perspectives and Change; (3) Integrative Lifestyle Health and Well-being; (4) Awareness and Choice; and (5) Listening with HEART (Healing, Energy, Awareness, Resiliency, and Transformation)" (Dossey et al., 2015, p. 29). Based on this theoretical framework, the ANA published a guide to nurse coaching competencies (Dossey et al., 2013). This model is patient directed, with the coach facilitating learning and decision making.

Transtheoretical Model

The transtheoretical model is an integration of several hundred psychotherapy and behavior change theories; hence the term *trans* (Prochaska et al., 2002). Using smokers as research subjects, Prochaska et al. (2002) learned that behavior change unfolds through a series of sequenced stages of change, which were not delineated in any of the existing multitude of theories. The transtheoretical model has been used successfully in many maladaptive lifestyle behaviors such as alcohol and substance abuse, eating disorders, anxiety/panic disorders, obesity, sedentary lifestyles, high-risk sexual behavior, and nonadherent medication use. This model is highly relevant to the APRN, who can tailor the intervention to the patient's specific stage of change to maximize the likelihood that the patient will proceed through a needed change process. Providing specific knowledge about disease trajectories or prevention strategies and advice is overused and often counterproductive when it comes to motivating patients toward sustained lifestyle change. A thorough discussion on readiness for change and application of this theory is provided later in this chapter in Determining Patients Readiness for Change.

Watson's Model of Caring

The theoretical framework for Watson's model of caring is based on loving kindness. Her work has focused on the science of caring and moving from *carative* to *caritas* ("love"); that is, the process of relating to others in an authentically present way, going beyond the ego (Watson, 2020). The APRN would go beyond self-interest and ego to fully and spiritually integrate body, mind, and spirit. This model provides a strong feelings-based approach to coaching, recognizing the openness of spirit to another person as essential in a therapeutic relationship. Honoring and respecting the patient's values, history, beliefs, autonomy, goals, and being are foundational in this model. It also requires self-reflection for the APRN to reach deep love and respect in a relationship. This includes, for example, being present to and supportive of the expression of positive and negative feelings, the creative use of self and using *all* ways of knowing, and assisting with basic needs with intentional caring consciousness (Watson, 2020). *Ways of knowing* are how knowledge comes to us and can include, for example, our experiences, senses, logic and reason, language, emotions, and imagination.

Positive Psychology

Positive psychology is the scientific study of the strengths that enable people to thrive. The field is founded on the belief that people want to lead meaningful and fulfilling lives, to cultivate what is best within themselves, and to enhance their experiences of love, work, and play (Positive Psychology Center, 2021). There are many notable positive psychologists, including Carl Rogers, Alfred Adler, Abraham Maslow, and Martin Seligman (2011) who built on their work and found five dimensions that lead to a flourishing life or a high degree of well-being. The five dimensions (PERMA) are as follows: **Positive emotions** are emotions that feel good. People who are flourishing feel positive emotions in a 3:1 ratio to negative emotions. These are not positive or optimistic thoughts; they are deeper full-body feelings of connection to others, to meaningful work or the feeling one gets with important accomplishments. **Engagement,** also known as *flow* is the state of being completely absorbed in an activity. It is the sweet spot between stress and boredom. People in this state are entirely absorbed in what they are doing and lose track of time while doing it. If a person is angry, anxious or depressed they are completely barred from this state. When people engage in these kinds of activities regularly they are able to withstand the hardships of life more effectively. **Relationships** are strong in people who are flourishing because other people matter and very little in life is positive that is solitary. People who are flourishing tend to have strong and positive relationships of many kinds from acquaintances all the way up to intimacy. **Meaning and purpose** is evident in those who flourish because what they do and what they engage in matters to them. They also feel that they belong to something that is larger than themselves. People who are flourishing have a strong sense of **achievement** that they've been practicing a craft, hobby or their work for years and have achieved some level of mastery in what they do (Seligman, 2011).

These dimensions can be cultivated to build one's capacity to flourish. The five dimensions of positive psychology are directly applicable to the APRN interacting with a wide range of people. In looking at the dimension of positive emotions as an example, Fredrickson (2001, 2020) significantly contributed to our understanding of how positive emotions can broaden a person's momentary thought–action choices, which builds their enduring personal resources. This "broadening and building" suggests that the capacity to experience positive emotions may be a fundamental human strength central to human well-being. The APRN can facilitate a person's positive psychology, especially in a guidance and coaching interaction, by promoting any or all of the five dimensions of well-being.

Growth Mindset

Dweck (2017), in her study of mindset and its impact on achievement, found that there are two types of belief systems. One is a *growth mindset* in which the individual believes they can learn and practice and achieve success. In addition, there is the belief that people with a growth mindset have a high degree of resilience. People with a *fixed mindset* believe they are endowed with talents that are fixed; they focus on documenting and defending their talent rather than developing skills. People with fixed mindsets delink talent from effort, acting on the belief that talent is a fixed, immutable entity. Fostering a growth mindset in the clinical space can create motivation and productivity, leading to improved outcomes. Guiding patients to shift from a hunger for approval (fixed mindset) to a passion for learning (growth mindset) by the tiniest degree can have a profound impact on nearly every aspect of life (Dweck, 2017).

Self-Determination Theory

Ryan and Deci (2006) provided a framework for the understanding of human motivation and conditions that either promote or thwart it. The theory purports that there are two forms of motivation, intrinsic and extrinsic, and that all humans are motivated both by rewards (outside of ourselves) and by our interests, curiosity, and abiding values (inside). This framework offers three conditions that are associated with the level of a person's motivation for engagement (Fig. 7.1). These three psychological needs have a robust impact on wellness (Ryan & Deci, 2006).

This framework is directly applicable to the APRN guidance and coaching competency because the APRN can promote the environment that supports competence, autonomy, and human relatedness (Exemplar 7.2). When these three needs are satisfied, enhanced self-motivation and health follow; when thwarted, motivation and well-being are diminished. Placing high value on positive regard, warmth, and giving patients as much psychological freedom as possible will lead to more engaged patients and better health outcomes (Ryan & Deci, 2000).

Transitions in Health and Illness

Guidance and coaching assists patients with a variety of life experiences in order to reduce healthcare costs and increase quality of care (Naylor et al., 2011). Early

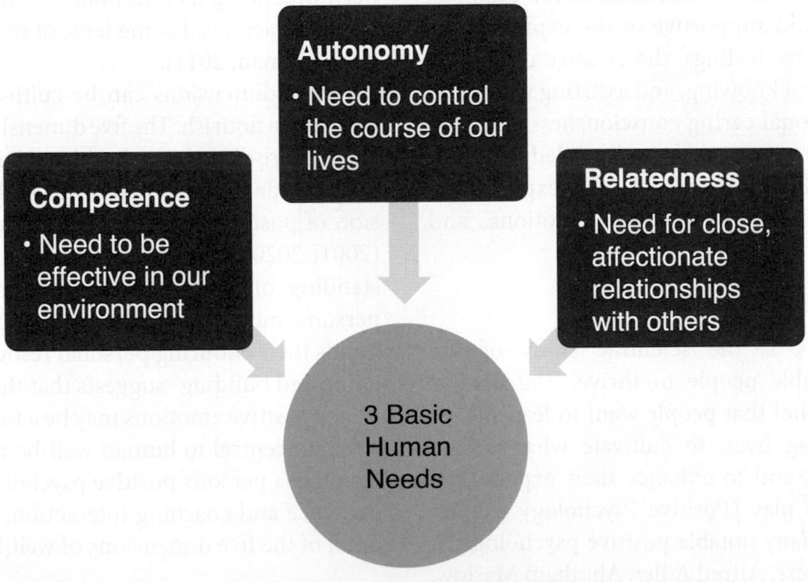

Fig. 7.1 ■ Self-determination theory posits that all humans have three central areas of motivation: competence, autonomy, and relatedness.

work by Schumacher and Meleis (1994) remains relevant to the APRN guidance and coaching competency and contemporary interventions, often delivered by APRNs, designed to ensure smooth transitions for patients as they move across settings (e.g., Aging and Disability Resource Centers, 2011; Coleman & Berenson, 2004; Coleman & Boult, 2003).

Schumacher and Meleis (1994) defined the term *transition* as a passage from one life phase, condition, or status to another: "Transition refers to both the process and outcome of complex person-environment interactions. It may involve more than one person and is embedded in the context and the situation" (Chick & Meleis, 1986, pp. 239–240).

Transitions have been characterized according to type, conditions, and universal properties. Schumacher and Meleis (1994) proposed four types of transitions: developmental, health and illness, situational, and organizational. *Developmental transitions* are those that reflect life cycle transitions, such as adolescence, parenthood, and aging. *Health and illness transitions* require not only adapting to an illness but more broadly reducing risk factors to prevent illness, changing unhealthy lifestyle behaviors, and numerous

EXEMPLAR 7.2

APRN GUIDANCE AND COACHING TO REVERSE METABOLIC SYNDROME

TS was a 68-year-old male presenting to primary care with metabolic syndrome: Important markers are all elevated and outside of normal range. Elevated triglycerides (250), blood pressure (158/90), fasting glucose (136), hemoglobin A1c (6.4), BMI (27), and weight was 244 lb on a 5'8" frame with a 42-inch waist	Objective presentation
TS was concerned because his cardiologist told him he "would be dead in 5 years if he did not change." The nurse practitioner (NP) sensed he was fearful about his future and began asking him what was working well in his life. He had a loving wife who also had many of the same health conditions and grandkids to whom he was devoted. He enjoyed his retired life, traveling in his RV, and eating out often at buffets in casinos. He ate a standard American diet (SAD), including nutrient-poor, highly processed food, excess sugar, and refined carbohydrates. He spent evenings in front of the TV, eating sweets that he described as far more than a serving. He did not regularly exercise. He did not feel ready to die.	Powerful questions Strong personal motivator identified
The NP asked what would be most useful with the 20 minutes they had together, what would be most helpful to him now, and what he wanted to get out of their time together. He said he needed help with what he was eating, and he knew the nighttime snacking was a bad habit.	Agenda setting
On further questioning, it seemed that TS may have a food addiction. He was largely oblivious to the quantity he was ingesting in the evenings, reporting that he was often unaware when he had eaten a whole box of cookies. This would take him by surprise as he intended to only have a few. The NP explained to TS that addiction was a loss of control over a substance, a feeling of powerlessness. Once ingested, it sets off a physical craving and mental obsession and the person loses their sense of agency. If addicted, one is unable to stop despite all of the negative consequences. As the NP explained this craving phenomenon, TS nodded his head vigorously, acknowledging this is what happened to him. He could not cut down as he had tried for years to do so.	Guidance

Continued

EXEMPLAR 7.2

APRN GUIDANCE AND COACHING TO REVERSE METABOLIC SYNDROME—cont'd

Once TS recognized that he was powerless over sugar once in his body, he became clear that he wanted to stop being controlled by junk food. He recognized that his health and his life depended on him directly addressing this problem and that it was not just a "bad habit." It would kill him. He saw that he would soon be on insulin. He was able to see the pattern of his nighttime eating every night: overeat–repent–repeat. This awareness led him to ask how he could interrupt this pattern. The NP asked him what he was not willing to give up. He said he liked his black coffee in the morning; other than that, he was willing to try anything.	Awareness raising Stage of change: Late contemplation Shifting to preparation stage of change: he is seeking specific advice
He accepted a 30-day challenge to eliminate all added/processed sugar and junk food. The NP explained how he may fight uncomfortable cravings for the first 3 days, and after that, the cravings would reduce or vanish. He agreed to switch all of his meals to proteins, vegetables, and whole unprocessed grains. The NP noticed the way he loved and cared for his family and suggested he find ways to apply that same devotion to his lifestyle change. The NP asked him when he was ready and he said, "Today." He was advised to set a date after his home was purged of junk food and he was able to acquire the foods and a plan for how he would eat going forward. He would need to have delicious, nutritious foods in abundance available to him before he initiated change. He was asked about obstacles and challenges, and he felt he could stop going to the casino buffets and instead eat meals at home. He was worried about cravings and not having desserts. The NP suggested some food substitutes for times he felt intense cravings, which crest and dissipate. He said he wanted to drop 65 pounds.	A challenge was offered (and was accepted) Using strengths in new ways Anticipatory guidance In preparation stage of change Action and goal setting
He agreed to use his brother for accountability. He sent a picture of each meal to his brother. He agreed to call the NP with questions or if a setback lasted more than 2 days. He was told to expect setbacks, but as soon as one occurred, to get back on the meal plan the next meal. He would follow up in 1 month.	Accountability
At the 1-month follow up appointment, TS had lost 15 pounds; his blood pressure was reduced, and he was feeling much better. He was off processed food and was eating "real food" at every meal. The nighttime binging, while difficult in the beginning, had stopped. He and his wife began evening walks and he was surprised by how much he enjoyed it. The NP offered many ideas on adding variety to his diet, how to order carry-out, and how to manage snacking.	Patient is in the action stage of change Specific advice is offered and received
The NP continued to see the patient monthly and discussed his personal motivator (i.e., extending his health span), as well as his obstacles and challenges at every visit. She explained plateaus and how to stay on course despite what appears to be a stall. She offered practical solutions and encouraged him to continue. Eight months later, he had lost 65 pounds. His metabolic syndrome had nearly reversed itself and he had a fasting glucose of 88.	Through the action stage of change, the patient continued to gain more awareness about his food addiction and destructive eating patterns. The NP offered action advice, anticipatory guidance, and practical tools for eating nutrient-dense foods. Action stage of change moved into maintenance.

other clinical phenomena. *Situational transitions* are most likely to include changes in educational, work, and family roles. These can also result from changes in intangible or tangible structures or resources (e.g., loss of a relationship or financial reversals; Schumacher & Meleis, 1994). *Organizational transitions* are those that occur in the environment: within agencies, between agencies, or in society. They reflect changes in structures and resources at a system level.

Developmental, health and illness, and situational transitions are the most likely to lead to clinical encounters requiring guidance and coaching. Successful outcomes of guidance and coaching related to transitions include subjective well-being, role mastery, and well-being of relationships, all components of quality of life (Schumacher & Meleis, 1994).

This description of transitions as a focus for APRNs underscores the need for and the importance of incorporating guidance and coaching into the APRN–patient therapeutic partnerships.

BUILDING RELATIONSHIPS FOR APRN GUIDANCE AND COACHING

In order to effectively work with patients to create healthy life changes, APRNs will engage in both guidance and coaching. Effectiveness of guiding and coaching is based on the quality of the relationship between the APRN and patient. Trust is essential to the relationship, and Johnson et al. (2021) have identified six competencies critical to building a trusting relationship; being present, communicating effectively, being nonjudgmental, being empathic and compassionate, managing conflict, and partnering with patients. Even though the competencies noted in this section are part of basic nursing care, the following discussion of skills is described within the context of APRN guidance and coaching. Note that there is considerable interaction among the skills—they are interdependent and should be part of every APRN toolbox.

Presence

How well honed is your ability to be present? Thich Nhat Hah (2015), a Buddhist philosopher, said, "The most precious gift we can give others is our presence." In a guiding or coaching relationship, presence is not only a gift but a prerequisite to being a full partner. The ICF defines coaching presence as the "ability to be fully conscious and create [a] spontaneous relationship with the client, employing a style that is open, flexible and confident" (ICF, 2016). This definition uses the words "fully conscious"; others may use the words "fully aware" or "mindful." Some people equate the words "mindful" and "presence." A definition of *mindfulness* noted by Kabat-Zinn (2017, para. 2) is "mindfulness means to purposefully pay attention in the present moment with a sense of acceptance and nonjudgment." The commonality of both definitions is paying attention and being fully conscious. Presence requires mindfulness and mindfulness requires presence.

There are two common pitfalls to being present that relate to APRNs: external distractions/interruptions and the well-honed ability to anticipate what the patient needs. We are often physically present, but our minds tend to jump from one thought to another. When we are with a patient, we may be thinking about the patient we just saw, our frustration with one of our colleagues, or getting our child to basketball practice. When we take the time to be aware of what we think during a patient visit, we may be astounded by how many thoughts unrelated to the patient enter our mind.

In addition to the challenges of our work environment, we have deeply rooted ways of thinking as nurses and APRNs to anticipate patient problems. (See Chapter 6 for a discussion on thinking errors in practice.) We have been taught that we need to have answers for problems so we can fix a problem and thereby fix a patient. We think ahead of what we hear from the patient. Once we start anticipating, we have stopped being present. We need to slow our thinking and follow what the patient is saying. This is a fundamental challenge to the APRN: the art of coaching is to develop the ability to set aside distractions—including jumping ahead in problem solving, which often leads to misdiagnosis and care that is not patient-centered—and engage fully in the moment with the patient.

Presence can be enhanced through practice with the following tools:

- Review patient information before seeing the patient, not when you are initially with the patient.

- Situate yourself at eye level when possible, to maximize eye contact.
- Recognize the patient's feelings—without this recognition, trust will be limited.
- If looking at or entering data into a device, invite the patient to look at the data with you.
- Use the STOP method that was developed by Jon Kabat-Zinn (2020, para. 3) to refocus and be present:
  - **S: Stop.** Stop what you are doing and pause momentarily.
  - **T: Take a breath.** Take a deep breath or several. Deep breathing can anchor you to the present moment.
  - **O: Observe.** Notice what is happening both outside and inside of yourself. Where has your mind gone? What do you feel? What are you doing?
  - **P: Proceed.** Continue doing what you were doing or, using the information gained during this check-in, change course.

Communication

Communication encompasses all forms, including verbal (words and tone), written, and body language. Synthesis of all forms of communication must be used by the APRN to determine a patient's health status. This includes what the patient understands, how they want to engage, and their style of communication. Of all of the skills that are inherent to effective communication, the most important is listening. We listen every day. It is part of our ability as human beings (as long as our hearing is anatomically and physiologically intact). However, how often are we thinking of other things when someone is talking to us? Are we looking at the patient or at the computer screen to review lab results? We intend to give our attention to the patients we serve, but there is so much work to do and so many patients to see. Every aspect of guidance and coaching has to do with highly skilled listening: listening for energy, what the person wants or needs, resistance, choices made, and how choices move toward or away from goals. Coaching in particular requires that patients do most of the talking, with the APRN doing most of the listening. We cannot adequately guide patients or do anticipatory teaching without knowing what the person already understands.

Rachel Naomi Remen (1996) is a pioneer of relationship-centered care and noted, "The most basic and powerful way to connect with another person is to listen. Just listen. Perhaps the most important thing we give to each other is our attention" (p. 143). Listening is a foundational skill to both guidance and coaching and in any relationship. Listening is the process of understanding others and establishing trust in the relationship. Trust is the foundation of the APRN–patient therapeutic relationship. We can only understand a person's level of health literacy if we listen deeply.

There are several different taxonomies of listening. A useful classification described by Whitworth and colleagues (2007) includes three levels of listening (Fig. 7.2). The level 1 listener is tuned out, either ignoring the person talking or pretending to listen. This level is also referred to as *internal listening*, where the listening is all about the listener. Level 2 listening is selective, with the listener sometimes focusing but at times being distracted by his own inner dialogue. Level 2 listening has a sharper focus on the other person than level 1. In level 3, the APRN becomes a mirror in which the information is reflected back. This listening is collaborative, empathic, and clarifying. The APRN is unattached to their agenda and own interests. Level 3 is empathic listening, representing the highest level, in which the listener gives time and attention to listening and gives their full self. Empathic listening is not only hearing what is said but also understanding the words, emotions, and meaning. It is considered "deep" listening or listening with the heart. Deep listening is hearing what is *not* said and includes tone of voice and nonverbal expressions. It is a global form of listening, in which one is using all of the senses to listen, noticing gestures, the action, inaction, and interaction. It requires the APRN to be very open and softly focused without an agenda or judgment of any kind. Level 3 listening is often described as a force field with invisible radio waves in which only the skilled listener can receive the information, often unobservable to the untrained listener (Whitworth et al., 2007). Guiding and coaching require level 3 listening in order to fully engage with the patient's baseline knowledge, goals, actions,

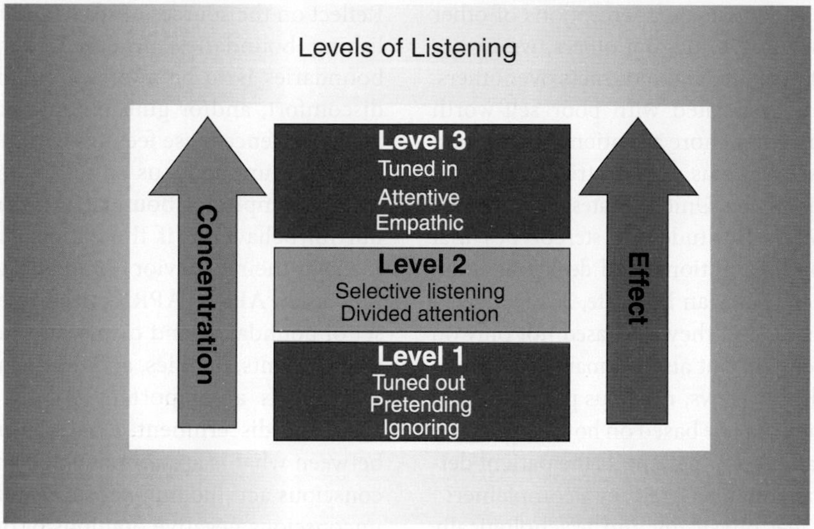

Fig. 7.2 ■ **Levels of listening.**

and emotions. Suggestions for levels 2 and 3 listening are the following:

- Stop talking!
- Relax for a minute prior to engaging with a patient by deep breathing, visualizing a pleasant memory that triggers relaxation.
- Review the health record prior to beginning a dialogue.
- Remove distractions and potential interruptions and clear your head of intruding thoughts.
- Listen for the tone of the conversation as well as the words.
- Acknowledge what is said by reflecting and probing further.
- Ask powerful questions (Table 7.2).

Literature reflecting the benefits of deep listening includes patient satisfaction with care, enhanced patient engagement in care planning, and improved health outcomes (Wentlandt et al., 2016). Listening is the most critical skill for APRNs, as discussed in Chapter 6. There is no guidance or coaching without deep listening.

Nonjudgmental (Suspending Judgment)

Being completely accepting toward another person, without reservations, is a concept developed by the psychologist Carl Rogers. He proposed that each individual has vast resources to marshal for self-understanding and self-directed behavior, but an interpersonal climate of positive regard was necessary to facilitate this (C. Rogers, 1961). It is about accepting a person as they are without judgment and is the basis for patient-centered therapy.

Being judgmental means that we are unusually harsh or critical in disapproving, blaming, or finding fault in others. Often judgmentalism is steeped in our biases and closed-mindedness. When we hold negative

TABLE 7.2

Powerful Questions
If your life depended on taking action, what would you do?
What's the takeaway from this?
What are three other possibilities?
If you could wave a magic wand, what would you do?
What resources do you need?
How could you use your strengths in this situation?
How will you know when you have achieved success?
What would happen if you don't do anything?
What is this costing you? ... What else is it costing you?
If you say "yes" to this [change], what are you saying "no" to?
What is the hardest part for you?
What does success look like to you?

opinions of others, it distorts our perceptions of other people and of ourselves. By judging others, we garner distorted feelings of power or righteousness over others. Being judgmental is associated with poor self-worth and self-esteem. Currently, more attention is being paid to implicit (unconscious) bias as a contributing factor in health disparities in the United States. One definition of *implicit bias* is "attitudes or stereotypes that affect our understanding, actions, and decisions in an unconscious manner" (Kirwan Institute, 2015). Everyone has implicit biases, and they are based not only on race, ethnicity, or religion but also on manner of dress, weight, gender, political views, religious practices, and other issues. And they may be based on how we perceive the behavior of a patient *as a* patient. Is the patient deferential? Are they personable? Are they a complainer?

A patient must feel physically and psychologically safe from being judged in order to fully engage in a relationship. We often take for granted that people seek health care and trust APRNs to do the best for them simply because we are credentialed healthcare providers. However, they often feel that they must "please us" rather than being honest about their concerns. Pleasing a provider is deeply rooted in patient behavior. Patients want their APRN to like them, so they may be afraid that the APRN will be angry or judgmental of them if they are challenging or have not adhered to a treatment plan, so they may tell APRNs what they think we want to hear. We often give subtle messages of greater acceptance when patients are "compliant" and of nonacceptance if they are not.

Suspending judgment does not mean we have to like every patient. Mearns (1994) noted that liking someone is based on shared values and complementary needs and is therefore conditional. However, it is especially important to be nonjudgmental for all patients and particularly for those we find most frustrating. Being nonjudgmental includes setting boundaries by creating clarity of expectations in the relationship. The concept of *boundary awareness* in coaching is founded on the initial work of Kerr and Bowen (1988) on self-differentiation within the context of family. In an APRN coaching relationship, there is a fine line between boundaries that are too tight and those that are too loose, and it can be a significant challenge to maintain a balance. To be more aware of boundaries, pay attention to situations in which you feel stressed. Reflect on the sources of stress and how you are establishing boundaries. Another exercise in clarifying boundaries is to be aware of feelings of resentment, discomfort, and/or guilt (Gionta & Guerra, 2015). If you experience these feelings within a patient relationship, it is time to focus on setting or resetting boundaries. Examples of boundaries include not tolerating hurtful behaviors (if the patient has the capacity to manage their behavior) or being treated disrespectfully as an APRN. APRNs need to establish their own set of boundaries and clarify and maintain them with their patients, families, and healthcare team.

There is an important difference between judgment and discernment. *Discernment* is differentiating between what is appropriate or inappropriate and is a conscious act. Judgmentalism is holding strong, often unconscious negative opinions of others involving little knowledge and fast thinking. If we are judging, it is nearly impossible to be truly helpful. TOME is a tool to practice being nonjudgmental:

- **Notice Triggers.** Notice what triggers judgments and why. Understanding the triggers will enhance awareness of making judgments about patients.
- **Observe like a reporter.** Look at your patients in as neutral a manner as possible. Look at them without placing your value set on them and explore their values and the meaning of health and/or illness to them.
- **Meditate.** Meditation is a way of being aware of thoughts and questioning their origins and impact on patients.
- **Extend empathy.** Every patient wants to be understood and have their APRN understand their situation and how they feel about their health or illness. Conveying empathy through acknowledging the patient's feelings helps patients move through the change cycle.

Empathy and Compassion

Carl Rogers built on Maslow's hierarchy of needs by adding that in order for a person to "grow," they need acceptance, genuineness, and empathy. Rogers believed that each person can achieve their deepest desires in life and achieve self-actualization but that empathy helps foster that growth, just as a seed needs soil and water. His greatest contribution was likely in his study of accurate empathy and its role in the growth of humans. He described *empathy* as an underappreciated way of being and posited that accurate empathy is "being one with the patient in the here and now, being highly sensitive to their experience and their world" (C. Rogers, 1961, p. 34). He stressed that listening is not a passive endeavor, because active listening can bring about changes in people's attitudes toward themselves. People who experience accurate empathy and are listened to in this way become more emotionally mature, more open, and less defensive (C. Rogers, 1961). There is increasing recognition and evidence that provider–patient relationships, the quality of their communications, and accurate empathy influence quality, safety, and health outcomes (Price et al., 2014).

Trzeciak et al. (2019) suggested in their book *Compassionomics* that empathy precedes compassion, that first you need to have empathy—the feeling of truly understanding another person—and then compassion, the action that results from empathy. In working with patients to create change, empathy and compassion are essential. Although empathy is woven into basic nursing, as we get pressed for time with interruptions, technology intrusions, and demands of patients, exhibiting empathy requires constant vigilance.

Although we accept empathy as an emotional state, there is growing understanding of the neurophysiology of empathy. Research beginning in the mid-1990s has identified neural networks of mirror neurons that may explain the capacity for empathy (Rizzolatti & Craighero, 2004). Mirror neurons are activated by both the action of an individual and the observation of a similar action performed by another (Lamm & Majdandzic, 2015; Preston & de Waal, 2002). It appears that mirror neural pathways extend to multiple structures in the brain based on the stimuli producing the effect. A possible explanation for empathy is that when we are listening to and looking at a patient, our mirror neurons are activated as if we are experiencing what the patient is doing or experiencing. With ongoing research into mirror neurons, there is great promise to better understand the neural activation that forms and supports relationships and how feelings are experienced. To expand empathy and compassion:

- Audio-record a visit with a patient and reflect on the content of the visit.
- Practice reflecting back to the patient your understanding of the feelings the patient may be experiencing. Be present and listen.
- Acknowledge the emotional content of what the patient is saying.
- Ask the patient how you can help them.

Managing Conflict

Conflicts may result from differences in ideas and values and when certain needs are not met. This could be the case if a patient feels disrespected in some way, frequently because of feeling not listened to or cared about. Conflict can range from a minor annoyance to significant hostility about some aspect of the patient visit. Examples include patients feeling a loss of control or when a treatment has not worked, they are not feeling understood/listened to, and/or they are fearful about their future. While preventing conflict with patients is preferable to managing a conflict, there will always be some conflict to manage in a healthcare situation. Suggestions for managing healthy conflict include:

- **Take a deep breath before responding**. This will be calming and provide a moment to recognize the situation.
- **Never meet a feeling with a fact**. Acknowledge the patient's feelings. This all-important step deescalates highly charged encounters. Until intense emotions are acknowledged, there is little that will be accomplished in a patient visit. For example, if a patient comes into an exam room angrily saying that they were treated rudely by the receptionist, the APN must first recognize and notice that they are upset. By validating the patient's feelings first, the conversation can move to a constructive dialogue.
- **Ask questions to understand the patient's emotional landscape**. Asking about how they are doing or feeling makes the well-being of the patient the priority (within a realistic boundary).
- **Maintain a respectful stance with the patient while working through the conflict.**
- **Make sure they feel heard and understood**. Provide a summary of the conflict and agreements to the patient before the patient leaves.

Partnership

There has been much written about the importance of APRNs creating healthcare partnerships with patients.

APRNs are keenly aware of the potential power gradient between themselves and patients. However, each patient knows themselves better than any provider, including their fears, behaviors, and healthcare concerns. When partnering with patients, APRNs must see the patient as a full partner and expert on *themselves*. This approach greatly reduces the power gradient, with the patient having self-knowledge and APRNs having healthcare expertise. In addition, patients are becoming more knowledgeable, with healthcare expertise available online and with communities such as "Patients Like Me" that provide a forum for people to support each other with shared disease experiences and provide resources to manage their lives. The extent of the partnership also depends on the needs of the patients. For instance, individuals with an ear infection may simply want a limited interaction to confirm a diagnosis and get treatment. However, patients with a chronic or life-threatening illness will want to have a partnership to understand the diagnostics and treatment options. The nature of the partnership will differ with patients having differing expectations and capabilities for partnering. To foster a partnership relationship, consider these practices:

- Create a safe environment.
- Recognize and respect patient preferences. Ask questions such as:
  - What is most important to you at this moment?
  - What are your life goals?
  - What do you value most?
  - Convey your understanding of the patient's concerns.
- Set goals that are patient driven.
- Create a plan that is the result of shared decision-making.

DETERMINING PATIENT READINESS FOR CHANGE

Guidance and coaching are the basis for promoting change in patients (Exemplar 7.3). The transtheoretical model of change noted above describes the change process that includes assessing the readiness of the patient to engage in change, preparation to make the change, taking action, and finally maintaining the change (Prochaska et al., 2002; Fig. 7.3).

Patient Readiness

In order to be coached, the patient must be functionally able, creative, and resourceful. Therefore most people in the general population are appropriate to receive/participate in coaching. If an APRN is considering using coaching, patients must first be deemed well enough to imagine a better future for themselves. Consequently, coaching will not be productive with people who cannot envision a different future. Explicitly, those who are severely mentally ill, psychotic, manic, severely depressed, suicidal, inebriated, obtunded, demented, or high or who are in a severe emotional state such as acute grief or trauma are not appropriate to engage in a coaching partnership. People with mental illness or in an acute intense emotional state are best engaged with empathy and guidance. A simple way to determine whether a person is coachable is to ask the individual to describe their life in the future, if everything went as well as it possibly could for them. If the person cannot articulate an answer, the APRN should not enter into a coaching dialogue but instead work with them to be able to envision a future healthier life.

After rapport has been established and some degree of empathy expressed, the APRN must determine the person's readiness for change. The person's stage of change in any given self-defeating lifestyle must be documented in the health record for the entire healthcare team to use and build on, measure progress, and guide interventions. Staging people is a necessary first step to any coaching encounter because it drives skilled conversations. Taking the time to assess where the person is in the change process and their willingness to be coached on any issue sets the stage for a deeper, more meaningful, and more effective encounter.

Resistance

When people are resistant, they are saying they will not change, they have no plans to change in the near future, or they are wholly not interested in changing. The main task for the APRN in working with people who are resistant to change is to help them *feel understood*. These interactions need not take a great deal of time, and the patient should leave the APRN with the feeling of being understood, that the APRN "gets me." The challenge for the APRN is to see how the self-defeating patient activity serves a larger purpose in the

EXEMPLAR 7.3

PATIENT SEEKING COACHING FOR OBESITY, PREDIABETES, AND MIGRAINE PAIN

DEBORAH MCELLIGOTT, DNP, HWNC-BC

Setting: Nurse practitioner (NP) private coaching practice.

Issue: Marie's Narrative: Marie is a 35-year-old female who comes to the office to see what a "coaching session" entails. She has a history of migraines, obesity, prediabetes, and fatigue. She is married, works full time, and has two children under the age of 7. Her migraine pain ranges from 5 to 8 (on a scale of 1–10), with nausea and occasional vomiting. The symptoms are worse with stress and relieved by her "additional migraine medication" and lying down but followed by a day of fatigue and dull level 2 to 4 pain. The frequency ranges from three times a week to once a month, with no identifiable pattern. Marie has seen multiple specialists over the last 20 years, including her primary care physician, neurologist, pain specialist, allergist, and chiropractor. Her laboratory values are normal with the exception of an elevated hemoglobin A1c (5.7%). Her body mass index was 30 and her body fat was 42%.

SESSION 1

Marie scheduled a 1-hour appointment with the NP for a coaching session after reading an article linking lifestyle to migraines. The NP prepared for the appointment by reviewing the questionnaires Marie completed online and then doing a brief centering exercise before Marie entered the room. During the introductions, the NP described the coaching process and asked Marie what she was hoping for (eliciting the agenda). She described her need to lose weight in order to have the energy to care for her family and complete her responsibilities at work. She was fearful of diabetes because she has a family history (personal motivators). Although she has had migraines for 15 years, her increased responsibilities have made coping with them more difficult (awareness raised about the link to stress). The NP reflected that Marie did have a lot on her plate. Marie was clearly ready to make changes but didn't know where to begin (moving from contemplation to preparation).

The NP asked if she could share what others in her situation have done and Marie was interested. The NP shared that some patients have found a relationship between food, stress, and headaches, receiving some relief by following an elimination food plan. Marie said she tried everything—she had been to an allergist, nutritionist, Weight Watchers. She did lose some weight, but her headaches didn't improve (resistance emerging).

The NP recognized the success Marie had in the past and focused on her strengths. Marie acknowledged that she did feel lighter and had more energy with the weight loss. But her most recent attempt at Weight Watchers failed and her migraines didn't decrease. She was willing to try anything.

The NP asked if she could review the elimination food plan (a chart of healthy foods to eat while eliminating dairy and gluten) and a food log planner (chart to log food, activity, migraine, sleep, bowel movement, and stress) with her and Marie agreed. The NP identified that the purpose for the tracking was for Marie to be able to identify any patterns that existed. Marie said she had done all these things in the past but not together. She said she would do this, that she was ready to try, and would "complete the log sheet each day and eat only the foods on the chart for 2 weeks."

The NP asked how confident she was that she could do this (on a scale of 1–10) and Marie replied 5. She felt it was easy enough but that stress either at work or at home may trigger her to eat the wrong food. The NP asked what would make it a 7. Marie replied that if she could control her stress, she would be more confident in her plan. On questioning, Marie preferred to run to reduce stress but identified that running is not an option at work or when caring for the kids, so she eats. The NP asked whether Marie wanted to try a short meditation and she agreed. After a 5-minute practice, Marie replied that she felt relaxed and was confident that she could incorporate this into her plan—she said she almost felt like she had had a nap. At the end of the session, Marie agreed to log her food, eliminate dairy and gluten (for 1 week), and do 5 minutes of meditation 4 days a week (actions/goal setting). She was going to be accountable to the NP and come back in 1 week to review the plan and see if patterns emerged. Her new confidence level rose to a 7 out of 10.

SESSIONS 2 TO 7

Marie returned for weekly visits. On week 2 she had only one migraine, improved sleep, and success with her meditation—she logged everything on her weekly log sheet and noted an extremely busy day prior to her migraine. Over the next 3 weeks she continued on the elimination plan as her energy increased and her cravings for sugar decreased. The NP explored her next goals and Marie wanted to decrease her migraine medications. The NP asked her to speak to her neurologist before she made any medication changes. Marie also wanted to begin an exercise plan—she already belonged to a gym and set a goal to exercise three times a week for 30 minutes prior to going to work. The NP asked if she would begin to reintroduce dairy or gluten but Marie did not want to. She continued on the elimination plan with an occasional "cheat day."

SESSION 8

By week 8 Marie had been successful in meeting her activity goal, food goal, meditation, and food log. She decreased her migraine medication to half the dose, had an average

Continued

EXEMPLAR 7.3
PATIENT SEEKING COACHING FOR OBESITY, PREDIABETES, AND MIGRAINE PAIN—cont'd

of two migraines a month, and didn't need any additional medication to control them. She felt better, her clothes were looser, and people noticed a difference in her appearance, even though she had only lost 1 pound. She became aware that she was building muscle. The NP summarized all of the changes she had made as they compared her initial evaluations to the most recent one, seeing a dramatic decrease in symptoms. Her A1c was 5.6%. She was less stressed and had more energy. She was determined to stay on her routine and was comfortable introducing small amounts of gluten on special occasions. Marie continues to follow up with her medical team, feeling empowered by her efforts.

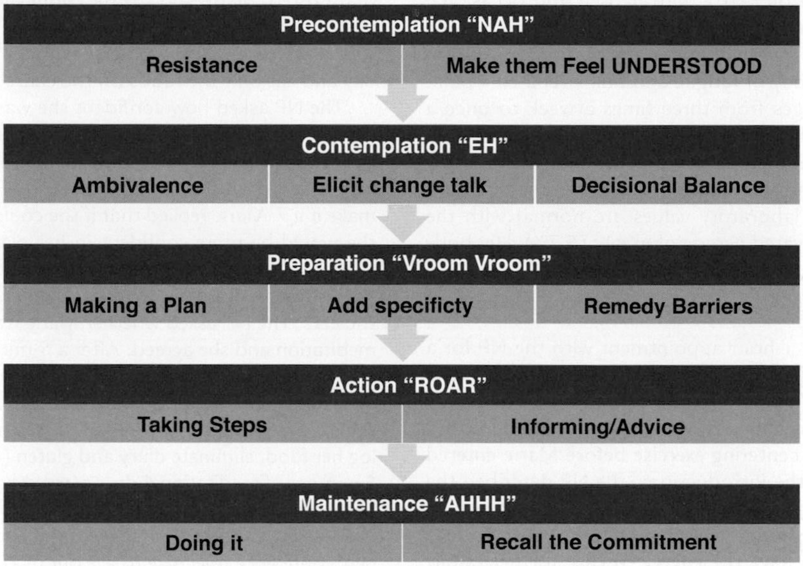

Fig. 7.3 Stages of change.

patient's life and to offer a partnership statement for the future, such as "I can see how smoking makes you feel like you are making your own decisions in your life and how important that is to you. If you ever want to quit, come back and I can work with you to quit." Specific advice at this stage can drive resisters deeper into resistance; therefore it is harmful to offer advice and suggestions to patients in resistance.

Motivational Interviewing

Motivational interviewing (MI) is a way of communicating with patients to help them get past their resistance or ambivalence and move forward with change (Exemplar 7.4). By skillfully approaching those in resistance and contemplation with nonjudgmentalism and the freedom to choose how they want to live, we create an environment for them to be less defensive and more reflective. It is based on the early work of Miller and Rollnick (2013) from their experience working with individuals who had a drinking problem. The most recent definition:

> *MI is a collaborative, goal-oriented style of communication with particular attention to the language of change. It is designed to strengthen personal motivation for and commitment to a specific goal by eliciting and exploring the person's own reasons for change within an atmosphere of acceptance and compassion.*
>
> ***(Miller & Rollnick, 2013, p. 29)***

MI may be especially useful in working with patients who have mixed feelings about making a change, who

EXEMPLAR 7.4

MOTIVATIONAL INTERVIEWING FOR DIABETES[a]

APRN/Client Interaction	APRN Coaching Skill
AM is a 40-year-old female. Presents for annual health review. Weight 271.4, elevated BMI 42.5, BP 139/88, fasting glucose 157, and triglycerides 547.	Objective data
AM has not been successfully consistent controlling her blood glucose since first being diagnosed with type 2 Diabetes 6 years ago. Her Hb A1c 5.1% 6 months ago was normal and is now elevated at 8.8%. She conveys that she got engaged 5 months ago, which is when she feels she started to gain weight. While she prefers to eat a healthier diet, her fiancé, also a diabetic, does not like "diet food." He prefers "meat and potatoes."	
APRN: Tell me, how I can be most helpful to you with our time together?	Agenda setting/powerful question
AM: Well, I knew my blood sugar wasn't going to be good. But I didn't know it would be that high. Honestly, it scares me a little bit. I know I should do better, but it's just easier to cook what he likes. I guess I need to figure out how to get my sugars down.	Ambivalence
APRN: You want to make him happy, even though you know it's not always in your best interest.	Reflective listening
AM: Yeah, I don't like it, but it's just easier with all the wedding planning. I'm not sure I can take on anything else right now.	Some resistance
APRN: It sounds like you value your relationship with your fiancé, and you want to make him happy, but that means putting your own health on the back burner.	
AM: I guess so.	
APRN: That must be frustrating for you, to feel torn about your own health and wanting to please your fiancé.	Uncovering discrepancy Expressing empathy
AM: It is. I'm just not sure what to do about it.	
APRN: What scares you about the numbers?	
AM: I've struggled for a long time with my diabetes, and I seem to go back and forth between doing really well, and then as soon as it gets hard, I give up. I'm afraid it's going to keep getting worse until I end up on insulin like my dad. And I don't want that to happen.	
APRN: Why would that be a bad thing?	
AM: It would make me feel like I failed myself. My dad's super overweight and not healthy.	Excavating a personal motivator
APRN: You're worried that if you stay on this trajectory, you're going to end up really unhealthy, and that'll make you feel like a failure. How do you want to feel?	Evoking change talk
AM: I want to feel like I'm in control of my health and that I'm paying attention to my diabetes.	Reflective listening
APRN: If you could make one move in that direction, what would it be?	Evoking change talk
AM: I think I should probably start by having a conversation with my fiancé about our health and that we need to eat better.	Raising awareness
APRN: Assuming he's on board, what would you do differently?	Powerful question/forwarding the action
AM: I'd probably start by cutting back on the amount of bread and pasta we eat.	
APRN: How will you do that?	
AM: Maybe just have one or two nights a week when I make those things, and I just won't eat much of it. I'll make sure I have something I like that's healthier too.	
APRN: So, you're talking about doing two things. You want to have a conversation with your fiancé about the importance of eating healthier to avoid the health consequence if you don't do that. And you want to limit the carb heavy meals to two nights a week. Can we try to get a little more specific about that? When do you plan to have the discussion?	Preparation/planning

Continued

EXEMPLAR 7.4
MOTIVATIONAL INTERVIEWING FOR DIABETES—cont'd

APRN/Client Interaction	APRN Coaching Skill
AM: We're having date night on Saturday, so I'll talk to him then.	Goal setting
APRN: And what about the meals? How will you go about limiting those carb heavy meals?	Identify obstacles
AM: Well, I can't speak for him yet, but I'll make sure I only eat those on the weekends.	
APRN: How do you want to be accountable in talking to your fiancé and limiting carb heavy meals to the weekends?	Accountability
AM: Hmmm ... I think if I share this with my sister—she will help me, she has been very worried about my health, so I will ask her to help me keep my promises to myself.	
APRN: Sounds great. I will see you back in 1 month for another fasting glucose and if things don't go as we planned, please come and see me sooner.	Supporting self-efficacy Partnership statement
AM: Yes, that would be helpful, I think. I really do want to get back on track.	

[a]The author gratefully acknowledges Eva Schmidt, APRN, FNP-BC, CHWC, for use of her motivational interviewing exemplar.

have a low level of confidence, who don't want to make a change, or for whom change is not important (Motivational Interviewing Network of Trainers, 2019). MI incorporates four fundamental processes that describe the back-and-forth and flow of a conversation. These processes are as follows:

- **Engaging**: This is the foundation of MI. The goal is to establish a productive working relationship through careful listening to understand and accurately reflect the person's experience and perspective while affirming strengths and supporting autonomy.
- **Focusing**: In this process an agenda is negotiated that draws on both the patient and APRN's expertise to agree on a shared purpose, which gives the APRN permission to move into a directional conversation about change.
- **Evoking**: In this process the APRN gently explores and helps the person to build their own "why" of change through eliciting their ideas and motivations. Ambivalence is normalized, explored without judgment, and, as a result, may be resolved. This process requires skillful attention to the person's talk about change.
- **Planning**: Planning explores the "how" of change, where the APRN supports the person to consolidate commitment to change and develop a plan based on the person's own insights and expertise.

Contemplation

APRNs most often see patients when they are in the contemplation phase. It is the place of ambivalence, where they both want to change but do not want to. They have one foot on the gas pedal and one on the brake. Advice at this stage can be harmful. Instead, the APRN can inquire about their personal motivators and bring forth the emotional conflict the person is experiencing. The APRN should approach the person in ambivalence with a neutral stance, without pushing. To determine their readiness for change, use questions such as "Why is this important? Why now? What if you did nothing and stay on this course—what is your future like in 10 years?" These powerful questions can move the person to identify personal motivators. The key task in this stage is to arouse emotions and encourage people to start talking about their ambivalence. These questions elicit change-talk in the patient.

Preparation

Once a patient moves to the preparation phase, they are ready to make a change. The ambivalence has dissolved. The task of the APRN is to identify barriers and develop remedies for these obstacles in partnership with the patient. With many life changes, it is important to set a start date and prepare the environment for change, such as finding an exercise partner or identifying impulse control techniques. Suggestions, gently offered, can be helpful in this stage as long as the

APRN has no strong ownership in the person's willingness to adopt a specific suggestion.

Action

Action is when the patient is actively engaged in making a lifestyle change. This stage is one in which direct advice and guidance is most helpful. Brainstorming on strategies to overcome obstacles and conversations on what to do in the event of a short-term lapse (a one-time reemergence of an unwanted behavior) or relapse (fully reverting back to prior behavior) are important. A common technique is to create "if … then" scenarios. For example, if a patient was working to reverse their type 2 diabetes and was excluding sugar from their diet, they might craft a plan that *if* they ingest sugar, *then* they get right back to avoiding sugar at the next meal. Anticipating setbacks and having remedies planned for lapses and relapses are crucial during the action stage (Krebs et al., 2018).

Maintenance

Maintenance often requires the APRN to acknowledge the patient's success and to ask about how the patient holds themselves accountable, how they manage lapses, and what they would do if a relapse occurred. When a patient experiences a full relapse, they revert to consistently exhibiting old behaviors. The APRN must determine where the patient is in the cycle of change again (e.g., are they in resistance vs. contemplation, or are they back in action?). It is important for the APRN to approach change as a process and to be aware that having setbacks can be common for some people.

THE "FOUR *As*" OF THE COACHING PROCESS

According to J. Rogers (2016), coaching is a partnership of equals whose aim is to achieve speedy, increased, and sustainable effectiveness through focused learning on some aspect of the patient's life. Coaching raises awareness and identifies choices, with the APRN and patient working from the patient's agenda. Together they have the sole aim of closing the gap between performance and potential. A crucial first step is asking permission from each person prior to initiating a coaching conversation. For example, "You seem to be having a hard time taking your Lasix regularly. May I do some coaching with you on this?" Initiating a coaching and guiding conversation hands control almost entirely over to the patient.

Coaching with guidance is a mindset that is integrated into every encounter with a patient or family member. Generally, there is a four-step sequenced coaching methodology—agenda setting, awareness raising, actions and goal setting, and accountability—with each step building on the previous step (Fig. 7.4 and Table 7.3).

Agenda Setting

Agenda setting, and the broader coaching methodology, requires handing over control and the choice of topic to the patient. The APRN elicits the agenda (the topic the patient wants to discuss) from the patient and the APRN and patient work together to address the patient's agenda. Guidance can be useful in this stage by providing factual information that the patient can use in creating their agenda. For example, the APRN may say, "You have a lot of things going on with you and we have 15 minutes together today. What would be most useful for you to have accomplished with our time together?" *Allow for silence,* because this is a powerful question in and of itself. The patient may struggle with that question, and the APRN may need to ask more probing questions; however, the agenda must be specific, measurable, and within the patient's control. Agendas cannot be centered around feelings

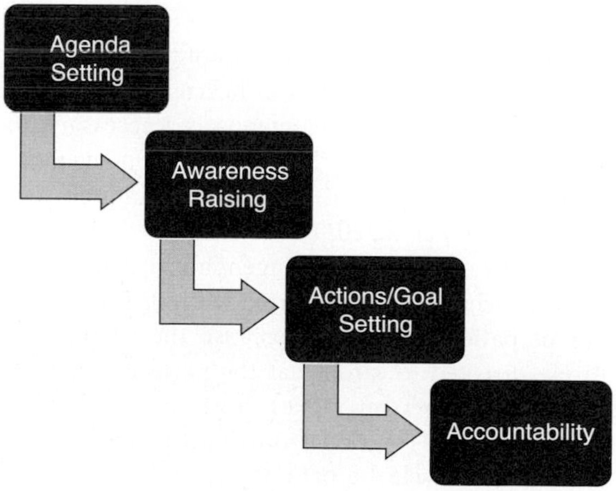

Fig. 7.4 ■ The "Four *As*" of the coaching process.

TABLE 7.3

Coaching Phases, APRN Skills, and Examples of Questions for Patients

Coaching Phase	APRN Skill	Powerful Questions
Agenda elicited	Excavate what is most meaningful Clarify needs	What is most important/meaningful/helpful to you at this time? What do you need from our time together?
Awareness raised	Ask powerful questions Shift consciousness Let the person do most of the talking Explore assumptions with curiosity Promote "generative moments"	What are you **not** willing to give up? If you say "yes" to *X*, what do you say "no" to? What is working well in this situation? Who do you need to become to make it happen? What do you want to see happen? What do you want to be held accountable for? What do you most value about yourself? What would your life be like if you were not [name limitation]? What is your deepest desire for yourself?
Actions/goal setting	Link raised awareness to specific goals to forward into action Brainstorm Determine self-efficacy Challenge whether the person could do more (gently and once)	What do you want to do and when do you want to do it? On a scale of 1–10, how successful do you think you will be? What is going to get in your way? What is the remedy to that obstacle? Can I challenge you to ... (do more)?
Accountability	Help person use resources, not pursue goals alone Partner with supportive others Use technology Confirm agenda met	How do you want to be accountable? What will you do if you go off your plan? What is your "when-then" plan? Did you get what you needed today?

or the actions of others. Acceptable agendas could include, "I need a plan for managing sugar cravings" or "I want to be able to manage the colostomy myself," and unacceptable agendas are "I want to feel better" or "I want my wife to have more concern about my pain." Eliciting and clarifying the agenda is a necessary and important step in the coaching process. If no agenda is determined by the patient, then no coaching can occur (Kimsey-House et al., 2011).

Focusing on the patient's agenda is a sharp departure from what is typically provided by APRNs in the form of patient education because the encounter is entirely directed toward what the patient wants. The decisions each person makes, no matter how small, lead them toward (or away from) a life that is healthier. Thus at some level, the patient agenda is wrapped in the person's fundamental values and truth.

Awareness Raising

Awareness raising requires challenging the patient's mindset and assumptions about an issue with which they are struggling. It requires skillful inquiry in which the APRN adopts a highly curious approach to understand what and how the patient thinks about an issue. Awareness is raised by asking powerful questions (Table 7.2) that have likely never been asked of the patient and require deep reflection. This phase of coaching generally is the most time consuming. It can also be useful to incorporate guidance in the form of providing the patient information about their health concerns or interests as well as information about their health status. As the APRN builds coaching skills, it can be helpful to have five powerful questions that are used regularly to begin an inquiry. During the awareness phase, the APRN is using deep listening skills, watching for nonverbal messages. The APRN may become aware of the moment in which the patient has a major insight or makes new connections. The APRN can identify when awareness has been raised because there may be more silence and the patient will begin to identify changes they want to make.

Actions and Goal Setting

The APRN asks the patient what they want to do and when they want to do it. Goals flow directly from the awareness raised, which arouses emotions, and the patient has a higher degree of self-efficacy in pursuing the goal(s). If the patient seems stuck on developing a solution, the APRN can set up a brainstorming exercise in which the patient and APRN take turns coming up with a list of ideas/solutions. The key competency in brainstorming is to not allow the patient to judge the ideas until they are all laid out. Once the goals or actions are determined, the APRN must determine *self-efficacy* (the belief a person has in themselves to complete a task). The APRN asks, "On a scale of 1 to 10, how successful are you likely to be in doing this (10 = success)?" If the chosen number is less than 7, the goal must be modified. That is, the goal must be made less ambitious so that the patient has a self-efficacy score of at least a 7 in order for the patient to be positioned for success. Guidance may be useful here to help the patient define manageable goals and actions by providing information related to specific goals such as realistic lab measures for cholesterol or specific products available for smoking cessation.

Success breeds success, so as any adult embarks on a change process, it is important to have early successes. During this phase of the coaching, the APRN is letting the patient talk. The APRN may need to ask clarifying questions to make the patient's goal more specific. If the APRN has a sense the patient could do more, they can *challenge* the patient. This skill is only used during the goal-setting phase and when the APRN thinks the patient could do more. For example, if the patient commits to ambulating down the hall once a day, the APRN can challenge them to do so three times a day. The patient will respond to the challenge in one of three ways: (1) agree to it, (2) reject it, or (3) modify it. It is crucial that the APRN accepts fully however the patient responds and challenges the patient no further.

Accountability

The final step in the coaching method is determined by the APRN asking, "How do you want to hold yourself accountable?" Ideally, it is best for the patient to rely on their own resources to achieve accountability, such as relatives, coworkers, or apps. The APRN could offer themselves as a way to hold a patient accountable, but it must not present *any* burden to the APRN. Accountability could be in the form of an email, text, or follow-up visit. It is important in this phase to have the patient outline a plan if the goals are not being met; this may include developing "when–then" strategies such as "When a week goes by and I haven't done what I said I would, I will reschedule with you" (J. Rogers, 2016).

APRN PRACTICE PRINCIPLES FOR SUCCESSFUL GUIDANCE AND COACHING

Within the guiding and coaching process there are several important principles to keep in mind (Table 7.4). The following considerations are helpful, skillful ways for APRNs to approach patients by consistently bringing these principles to patient relationships.

Ask Questions

Perhaps the most important single change an APRN can do to move toward a coaching and guiding mindset is pause when you are going to tell a patient to do something. Do a self-check about whether it is an opportunity for coaching and ask a question instead. For example, replace "I see you are short of breath and that you need to take your diuretic every day" with "I see you are short of breath, and maybe uncomfortable. How

TABLE 7.4

Practice Principles for Guidance and Coaching
Ask questions
Ask permission
Build on strengths
Support small changes
Be curious
Challenge
Get to the feelings

can I best be helpful to you today?" In order to more fully engage patients in their self-care, asking questions places the patient in the driver's seat, where they belong. It creates a psychological spaciousness for patients to feel and claim a sense of agency over their own care.

Ask Permission

Although nursing is a wonderful blend of science, technology, and caring, nurses have a strong drive to make people better, whatever the specific situation. APRNs have embraced the idea of holistic health care and are empathic with patients, but there continues to be an attitude that providers know what is best for patients. Integrating coaching into practice requires a culture shift and a change in personal philosophy and approach to caring for patients. To effectively integrate coaching into personal beliefs as well as the practice culture, there are many small actions that can support more effective APRN encounters. This can be difficult as the APRN is a clinical expert and knows the population so well, making it hard to resist telling others what and how to do things.

A crucial first step is asking permission from each person prior to initiating a coaching conversation. Asking permission, such as "Is it okay for me to explore this with you further?" is a way of respecting boundaries. Asking permission also demonstrates to the person that they have a choice and power in the relationship (Kimsey-House et al., 2011). If the patient decides against coaching, the APRN should move to providing guidance.

Build on Strengths

There is increasing recognition that building on patient strengths is a way for patients to gain confidence in their ability to change. The tendency in the past has been to focus on what is broken or not working or what an individual does not do well. This has supported the idea that the health issues a patient has are the result of not doing something or not doing something correctly, and that gap needs to be addressed. Rather than fixing what is broken, building on strengths can make the broken parts desiccate and shrink. For example, if a person has a great *appreciation for excellence* in their profession, that inherent skill can be applied to a weight loss journey by raising the quality of food they are ingesting or using *love of learning* to experiment with different strategies to manage their stress. An interprofessional summit was convened to identify that a major change that must occur in care delivery is to build on patient strengths to assist patients to achieve their goals (Swartwout et al., 2016).

The recent focus on building strengths is based on seminal research by Peterson and Seligman (2004), who demonstrated the benefit of assessing and using people's strengths in making and sustaining change in a person's life. There are years of research showing the benefits of building on strengths (VIA Institute on Character, 2016). The Classification of Strengths is an important tool that has been used in a growing body of evidence since the mid-1990s (Peterson & Park, 2009). This classification has six "virtues": wisdom and knowledge, courage, humanity, justice, temperance, and transcendence. In addition, there are 24 characteristics within the overall classification (Table 7.5). Although the research has not been specific to health care, there are clearly applications to health promotion by assessing and then building on patients' strengths for a healthier future.

Building on strengths has become an approach broadly used in health coaching. Confidence gained from building on strengths helps individuals not only to deploy those strengths toward achieving their goals but to also work on areas to be developed. Often

TABLE 7.5

The Classification of Human Strengths

Values in Action Classification of Strengths

6 Virtues	24 Characteristics
Wisdom and knowledge	Creativity, curiosity, judgment, love of learning, perspective
Courage	Bravery, perseverance, honesty, zest
Humanity	Love, kindness, social intelligence
Justice	Teamwork, fairness, leadership
Temperance	Forgiveness, humility, prudence, self-regulation
Transcendence	Appreciation of beauty and excellence, gratitude, hope, humor, spirituality

From *Character Strengths and Virtues: A Handbook and Classification*, by Peterson and M. Seligman, 2004, APA Press, p. 29-30.

people do not recognize their strengths, and the initial work of the APRN is to help the patient identify their strengths. There are strengths assessments available online that have strong validity profiles. One example is the VIA Survey of Character Strengths, which can be found at http://www.viacharacter.org/www/Character-Strengths-Survey. If there is no formal values in action (VIA) assessment, the APRN can help the patient recognize their strengths to build on by asking:

- "Tell me about a challenge that you feel you successfully managed."
- "What would your friends and family say were the best parts about you?"
- "What strengths helped you be successful?"
- "How would you describe your strengths to create the change you want to make?"

APRNs can incorporate strength finding into any visit. Identifying strengths could take place during the history or physical examination. APRNs already respect, value, and engage with each patient, and identifying and building on their strengths will help in the APRN efforts to build capacity to relate well to patients.

Support Small Changes

Although big change is often desired, small changes are what create forward movement. Nearly everyone at some time has intentions to lead a healthier life by making adjustments in lifestyle. Each New Year, millions of resolutions fall by the wayside because we try to take big leaps to change behaviors and then realize a big leap is too difficult.

When coaching a patient, there is a tendency by both APRN and patient to jump to big interventions. Well-intentioned patients may want to initiate major interventions to manage their health, but they overestimate the change they can realistically make and sustain in their lives. Overestimating the ability to make lifestyle changes can then be demoralizing when the changes are not successful. Often, a patient will commit to making a change in order to please the APRN but cannot follow through.

Having patients consider small changes may produce bigger and more lasting results. According to Seligman (2011), humans are more likely to achieve their goals if they have early success. A person trying to lose a few pounds may believe that a strict diet is mandatory, requiring considerable changes, such as how food is purchased and prepared, who does the preparation, limiting food intake, and changing social patterns to adhere to the diet. However, as a coach, you can work with your patient to make a small change, such as taking a walk to add exercise or decreasing the amount of liquid low-nutrient calories. Small changes are part of a larger process of change. Patients can be coached to do one intervention, and once that is integrated into their lives, additional small changes can be added. These small changes can add up to major lifestyle changes.

Although small changes can have a big impact and are a useful start for lifestyle change, there may be patients who need to decide on a big change in their lives, such as having bariatric surgery to achieve weight loss or leaving a toxic relationship.

Be Curious

Perhaps one of the most useful coaching tools is to be curious (Sherman, 2019). Curiosity provides the foundation for asking great questions. Patients nearly always give clues as to what is on their minds but may not be direct. One should follow up with questions such as "I wonder what … means to you?" or "I am curious about what you just said that. …" These very simple questions based on curiosity often net a rich conversation and help bring out issues that are important to patients. In a time-constrained environment, APRNs may feel inhibited from opening any doors to topics that they may not be able to pursue with patients. However, not opening the door deprives patients of opening up about what is really important to them, and opportunities to positively impact their life are missed.

Challenge

Are you comfortable challenging a patient? The APRN coach must be willing to challenge a patient in order to help move the patient forward. While it is important to maintain a good working relationship, wanting to be liked may interfere with the effectiveness of challenging a patient's view or with interpretation of situations, beliefs, or values. Patients often get "stuck," and respectfully challenging them to think differently or see themselves or their situation differently can get them "unstuck" (Moore & Tschannen-Moran, 2010). Challenging patients is a way of deepening awareness and forwarding action by making a request or suspending a belief. For example, a challenge might be, “Could I challenge you to 30 days with no sugar?” or “What would it be like to approach this situation without any fear or anxiety, instead cultivating calm confidence?” One useful way of maintaining an effective APRN therapeutic relationship while challenging the patient is to inquire about feedback. Ask the patient if the conversation was useful, what part was most helpful, and what created discomfort. When challenging, make sure patients know that you are fully with them on their journey and that the point of the journey is to create change.

Get to the Feelings

Change happens when people understand and incorporate the need for change at an emotional level. Although knowledge of data is helpful, it is usually only a starting point, because the knowledge alone usually does not create transformative change. In coaching patients, it is important to get to the emotional meaning of their issues (Stober & Grant, 2006). Naming emotional feelings is a driver for motivation to change. Exploring feelings related to change links mindfulness and contemplation to taking action.

Getting to the feelings requires awareness of the APRN’s comfort level with range of feelings for both yourself and the patient, including anxiety, fear, sadness, and anger, in order to give patients the opportunity to talk about their feelings. If a patient senses your discomfort with anxiety, they will not talk about it. Transformational change for patients occurs at the emotional level, and the APRN coach will only be able to support this by recognizing and accepting their own feelings in order to accept those of the patient. A patient with newly diagnosed breast cancer or who is having unexpected triplets will have a range of feelings, and if the APRN is not comfortable with the patient’s feelings, the patient will feel inhibited to share those feelings.

A universal response to change—even change we believe we should make—is resistance. We create reasons for or exceptions to why we cannot change, such as, “It’s too hard,” “I don’t really like/need/want to do this,” or “I’ve tried before and failed.” A major reason for resistance to change is simply fear—fear of not being successful, fear of what other people may think, and many other types of fears. As an APRN, having a trusting relationship with your patients can help them name and understand their fears and other feelings about change.

Getting to the feelings has boundaries. This does not mean getting to feelings that relate to psychopathology or feelings related to issues that require counseling. Naming/identifying feelings should not be focused on the past, such as on past relationships with family members, but on the present and future. It is about getting to the feelings related to the present circumstances creating the need for change, the change process itself, and the potential outcome. The following statements can be used to get to feelings:

- “Tell me about how you feel when you think about (or talk about). …”
- “Knowing how you feel about … is important to me.”

To get a better understanding of one’s own feelings when interacting with a patient, use root cause analysis. Create some mental space (between patients) and keep asking yourself why you were experiencing your feelings. This can take you to a deep level toward understanding your feelings. It is also useful to pay attention to triggers. When you note a particular feeling while guiding or coaching, reflect on what might have contributed to that feeling. Being aware of your physical (somatic) responses to different emotional situations will help you make adjustments in being effective with your patients. Somatic sensations will let you know when you are getting into uncomfortable emotional territory. Some people may feel a physical tenseness, while others may clench their teeth or cross their arms. Whatever the reaction may be, it is important to be aware of the somatic feeling in order to make adjustments, such as taking deep breaths or mentally calming yourself for effective APRN guidance and coaching. A technique that may be useful to enhance somatic awareness is using Silsbee’s (2018) “body scan” approach. Starting with the feet and, moving up your body, scan for physical responses to a situation. This can be done quickly—in a few seconds.

BUILDING COACHING INTO PRACTICE

Although building coaching into APRN practice is largely based on integrating the skills and mindset of coaching as a way of relating to patients, there are small things that the APRN can do to integrate coaching into practice. Some examples of building coaching into the structure and process of care include:

- Collect information from patients while they are in the waiting room or waiting in the examination room that is related to their goals for the visit. Questions on an intake form could include:
  - What are your current goals for maintaining or managing your health?
  - How committed are you (1–10, 10 = *highly committed*) to pursuing these goals?
  - What makes these goals important to you now?
  - What would you like to leave the visit with today?
- Focus on the *patient's* goals and ask what would be useful from the APRN to move toward achieving those goals.
- Establish a section in the medical record that summarizes the patient's goals, actions, and follow-up plan. If using an electronic health record, negotiate with the service provider to integrate this information into the record.
- Create a safe and welcoming environment in the examination rooms using pictures, soft colors, and other visuals that are comforting.

APRNs may be concerned that coaching will require additional time. Coaching is an effective modality in approaching behavior change. Given that chronic diseases due to lifestyle are a worldwide epidemic, the APRN must have the capacity to skillfully and meaningfully engage with patents on lifestyle change. Simply telling people what to do is not effective and lacks an evidence base. New innovative models must be created by the APRN such as group coaching visits (in person or online) or building patient reflection into visits such as having them write a "best future life" paragraph while they are waiting (it's a year from now and everything with your health has gone very well. You have reached your goals and are living the best life you could possibly imagine. Write a paragraph about what that would be.). There are several useful resources that include sample coaching contracts, exercises to practice skills, and other useful materials (Donna & Wheeler, 2009; Dossey et al., 2015).

CONCLUSION

Guidance and coaching are effective, rewarding, and critical skills to bring to patient care. APRNs are providers who have already integrated the value of patient-centered care, and guidance and coaching bring the focus of care to the patient's goals, preferences, and abilities. Guidance is different from coaching in that it is directive, values patient education, and relies on the APRN as the expert. Coaching is focused on goals established by the patient and assists the patient in understanding and uses their capacity to achieve those goals. Although many APRNs have built guidance and coaching into their practice, there is a need to have all APRNs examine their mental model of interacting with patients to build on the guidance and coaching processes and skills to better partner with patients to help them create healthy change. Guidance and coaching are necessary skills for all APRNs.

KEY SUMMARY POINTS

- Guidance and coaching require deep listening and strong empathic skills.
- All patients must be assessed for appropriateness of guidance and/or coaching.
- Guidance requires exploring what the patient already knows.
- Patients must be assessed for readiness to change before the coaching methodology is used.
- Integrating guidance and coaching is integral to patient-centered care.
- Although there is broad agreement that patient-centered care is important, developing ways to support it has been challenging.
- Integrating coaching with guidance establishes the patient as the center of care and as a full partner and source of control.

REFERENCES

Aging and Disability Resource Centers. (2011). Evidence-based care transitions models side-by-side. http://www.communitysolutions.com/assets/2012_Institute_Presentations/caretransitionsmodels6modelsfeb2011v5526116hill051812.pdf

American Association of Colleges of Nursing. (2021). The Essentials: Core competencies for professional nursing education. https://www.aacnnursing.org/Education-Resources/AACN-Essentials

American Holistic Nurses Credentialing Corporation. (2020). Professional nurse coach role: Core essentials. https://www.ahncc.org/wp-content/uploads/2021/01/FINAL-REVISED-NC-Core-Essentials-DOC-12-30-2020.pdf

An, S, & Song, R (2020). Effects of health coaching on behavioral modification among adults with cardiovascular risk factors: Systematic review and meta-analysis. *Patient Education and Counseling, 103*(10), 2029–2038. https://www.sciencedirect.com/science/article/pii/S0738399120302378?casa_token=Wmk8T9QVQOAAAAAA:TRC5RsYmVU_fR4X1l2IEmGbyFfLgUWu9MASd-CB6OJ-mmRd0ckBgvDaHKvQ9kgsUOUSsyV3ZH0w

Benner, P. (1984). *From novice to expert: Excellence and power in clinical nursing practice*. Addison-Wesley.

Benner, P., Hooper-Kyriakidis, P., & Stannard, D. (1999). *Clinical wisdom and interventions in critical care: A thinking-in-action approach*: WB Saunders.

Centers for Disease Control and Prevention. (2020). About Chronic Disease. https://www.cdc.gov/chronicdisease/about/index.htm

Centers for Medicare & Medicaid Services. (2020). National Health Expenditures 2019 Highlights. https://www.cms.gov/files/document/highlights.pdf

Chen, J., Mullins, C. D., Novak, P., & Thomas, S. B. (2016). Personalized strategies to activate and empower patients in health care and reduce health disparities. *Health Education & Behavior, 43*(1), 25–34.

Chick, N., & Meleis, A. (1986). Transitions: A nursing concern. In P. Chinn (Ed.), *Nursing research methodology: Issues and implementation* (pp. 237–258). Aspen.

Coleman, E. A., & Berenson, R. A. (2004). Lost in transition: Challenges and opportunities for improving the quality of transitional care. *Annals of Internal Medicine, 140*, 533–536.

Coleman, E. A., & Boult, C. (2003). Improving the quality of transitional care for persons with complex care needs: Position statement of The American Geriatrics Society Health Care Systems Committee. *Journal of the American Geriatrics Society, 51*, 556–557.

Donna, G., & Wheeler, M. (2009). *Coaching in nursing: An introduction. International Council of Nursing and The Honor Society of Nursing*. Sigma Theta Tau.

Dossey, B. M., Hess, D. R., Southard, M. E., Schaub, B. G., Luck, S., & Bark, L. (2013). *The art and science of nursing coaching: The providers guide to the coaching scope and competencies*. American Nurses Association. http://www.utb.edu/vpaa/nursing/ce/Documents/CoachingandMentoringWorkbook.pdf

Dossey, B. M., Luck, S., & Schaub, B. G. (2015). *Nurse coaching: Integrative approaches for health and wellbeing*. International Nurse Coach Association.

Duke Integrative Health. (2020). Integrative Health Coaching. https://dukeintegrativemedicine.org/patient-care/individual-services/integrative-health-coaching/

Dweck, C. (2017). *Mindset: Changing the way you think to fulfill your potential* (6th ed). Robinson.

Fenton, M. V., & Brykczynski, K. A. (1993). Qualitative distinctions and similarities in the practice of clinical nurse specialists and nurse practitioners. *Journal of Professional Nursing, 9*(6), 313–326.

Fredrickson, B. (2001). The role of positive emotions in positive psychology: The broaden-and-build theory of positive emotions. *American Psychologist, 56*(3), 218–226.

Fredrickson, B. (2020). Barbara Fredrickson. https://www.pursuit-of-happiness.org/history-of-happiness/barb-fredrickson/

Gionta, D., & Guerra, D. (2015). How successful people set boundaries at work. http://www.inc.com/dana-gionta-dan-guerra/how-to-manage-boundaries-at-work.html

Goudreau, K. A. (2021). Patient-centered teaching and coaching: The clinical nurse specialist role. In J. S. Fulton, K. A. Goudreau, & K. L. Swartzell (Eds.), *Foundations of clinical nurse specialist practice* (3rd ed.) (pp. 329–343). Springer Publishing Company. doi:10.1891/9780826129673.0018

Hayes, E., & Kalmakis, K. A. (2007). From the sidelines: Coaching as a nurse practitioner strategy for improving health outcomes. *Journal of the American Academy of Nurse Practitioners, 19*(11), 555–562.

Hibbard, J., & Greene, J. (2013). What the evidence shows about patient activation: Better health outcomes and care experiences; fewer data on costs. *Health Affairs, 32*(2), 207–214. doi:10.1377/hlthaff.2012.1061. PMID: 23381511.

Institute for Health Metrics and Evaluation. (2020). Latest global disease estimates reveal perfect storm of rising chronic diseases and public health failures fueling COVID-19 pandemic. http://www.healthdata.org/news-release/lancet-latest-global-disease-estimates-reveal-perfect-storm-rising-chronic-diseases-and

International Coach Federation. (2016). Updated ICF core competencies. https://coachfederation.org/core-competencies

International Coach Federation. (2020). ICF definition of coaching. https://coachfederation.org/about#:~:text=ICF% 20defines%20coaching%20as%20partnering, their%20personal%20 and%20professional%20potential

Johnson, J. E., O'Grady, E. T., & Coetzee, M. (2022). *Intentional therapeutic relationships: Advancing caring in health care*. DesTech Publications Inc.

Kabat-Zinn, J. (2017). Definition of mindfulness. https://www.mindful.org/jon-kabat-zinn-defining-mindfulness/

Kabat-Zinn, J. (2020). Mindfulness STOP skill. https://cogbtherapy.com/mindfulness-meditation-blog/mindfulness-stop-skill#:~:text=Jon%20Kabat%2DZinn%2C%20a%20prominent,STOP%20skill%2C%20or%20STOP%20Acronym

Kaplan, D. M., Tarvydas, V. M., & Gladding, S. T. (2014). 20/20: A vision for the future of counseling: The new consensus definition of counseling. *Journal of Counseling and Development, 92*, 366–372.

Kerr, M. E., & Bowen, M. (1988). *Family evaluation: An approach based on Bowen theory*. Norton.

Kimsey-House, H., Kimsey-House, K., Sandahl, P., & Whitworth, L. (2011). Co-active coaching. In *Changing business, transforming lives* (3rd ed.). Nicholas Brealey Publishing.

Kirwan Institute. (2015). Defining implicit bias. http://kirwaninstitute.osu.edu/researchandstrategicinitiatives/#implicitbias

Krebs, P., Norcross, J., Nicholson, J., & Prochaska, J. (2018). Stages of change and psychotherapy outcomes; A review and a meta analysis. *Journal of Clinical Psychology*, 1–16. doi:10.1002/jclp.22683

Lamm, C., & Majdandzic, J. (2015). The role of shared neural activations, mirror neurons, and morality in empathy: A critical comment. *Neuroscience Research, 90*, 15–24.

Liu, Y., Croft, J. B., Wheaton, A. G., Kanny, D., Cunningham, T. J., Lu, H., Onufrak, S., Malarcher, A., Greenlunf, K., & Giles, W. (2016). Clustering of five health-related behaviors for chronic disease prevention among adults, United States, 2013. *Preventing Chronic Disease, 13*, Article 160054. doi:10.5888/pcd13.160054

Long, H., Howells, K, Peters, S, & Blakemore, A. (2019). Does health coaching improve health-related quality of life and reduce hospital admissions in people with chronic obstructive pulmonary disease? A systematic review and meta-analysis. *British Journal of Health Psychology, 24*(3), 515–546. https://bpspsychub.onlinelibrary.wiley.com/doi/full/10.1111/bjhp.12366

McLean, P. (2019). *Self as Coach, Self as Leader*. Wiley.

Mearns, D. (1994). *Developing person-centered counseling*: Sage.

Miller, W. R., & Rollnick, S. (2013). *Motivational interviewing: Helping people to change* (3rd ed.). Guilford Press.

Moore, M., & Tschannen-Moran, B. (2010). Coaching behavior change. *Coaching Psychology Manual, 33*, 51.

Motivational Interviewing Network of Trainers. (2019). Understanding motivational Interviewing. https://motivationalinterviewing.org/sites/default/files/understanding_mi_aug_2019.pdf

Naylor, M. D., Aiken, L. H., Kurtzman, E. T., Olds, D. M., & Hirschman, K. B. (2011). The importance of transitional care in achieving health reform. *Health Affairs, 30*, 746–754.

Nightingale, F. (1860). *Notes on nursing: What it is and what it is not*. Harrison.

O'Neill-Hayes, T., & Gillian, S. (2020). Chronic disease in the United States: A worsening health and economic crises. *American Action Forum*. https://www.americanactionforum.org/research/chronic-disease-in-the-united-states-a-worsening-health-and-economic-crisis/#:~:text=When%20including%20indirect%20costs%20associated,the%20country's%20gross%20domestic%20product

Patient Protection and Affordable Care Act of 2010, Pub. L. No. 111-148, 124 Stat. 119. (2010). https://www.congress.gov/111/plaws/publ148/PLAW-111publ148.pdf

Perez-Cueto, F. J. (2019). An umbrella review of systematic reviews on food choice and nutrition published between 2017 and 2019. *Nutrients, 11*(10), 2398.

Peterson, C., & Park, N. (2009). Classifying and measuring strengths of character. In S. J. Lopez, & C. R. Snyder (Eds.), *Oxford handbook of positive psychology* (2nd ed.) (pp. 25–33). Oxford University Press.

Peterson, C., & Seligman, M. (2004). *Character strengths and virtues: A handbook and classification*. APA Press. Oxford University Press.

Pirbaglou, M., Katz, J., Motamed, M., Pludwinski, S., Walker, K., & Ritvo, P. (2018). Personal health coaching as a type 2 diabetes mellitus self-management strategy: A systematic review and meta analysis of randomized controlled trials. *American Journal of Health Promotion, 32*(7), 1613–1626. https://journals.sagepub.com/doi/pdf/10.1177/0890117118758234

Positive Psychology Center. (2021). Mission. https://ppc.sas.upenn.edu/our-mission

Preston, S. D., & de Waal, F. B. (2002). Empathy: Its ultimate and proximate bases. *The Behavioral and Brain Sciences, 25*, 1–20. discussion 20-71.

Price, R. A., Elliott, M. N., Zaslavsky, A. M., Hays, R. D., Lehrman, W. G., Rybowski, L., Edgeman-Levitan, S., & Cleary, P. (2014). Examining the role of patient experience surveys in measuring health care quality. *Medical Care Research and Review, 71*(5), 522–554. doi:10.1177/1077558714541480

Prochaska, J., Redding, C., & Evers, K. (2002). The transtheoretical model and stages of change. In K. Glanz, B. Rimer, & K. Viswanath (Eds.), *Health behavior and health education* (3rd ed.) (pp. 99–120). Jossey-Bass.

Rafferty, R., & Fairbrother, G. (2015). Factors influencing how senior nurses and midwives acquire and integrate coaching skills into routine practice: A grounded theory study. *Journal of Advanced Nursing, 71*(6), 1249–1259. doi:10.1111/jan.12607

Remen, R. (1996). *Kitchen table wisdom*: Riverhead Books.

Remes, J., Linzer, K., Singhal, S., Dewhurst, M., Dash, P., Woetzel, J., Smit, S., Evers, M., Rutter, K., & Ramdorai, A. (2020). *Prioritizing health: A prescription for prosperity*. McKinsey & Company. https://www.mckinsey.com/industries/healthcare-systems-and-services/our-insights/prioritizing-health-a-prescription-for-prosperity

Rizzolatti, G., & Craighero, L. (2004). The mirror-neuron system. *Annual Review of Neuroscience, 27*(1), 169–192.

Rogers, C. (1961). *On becoming a person*. Houghton Mifflin Company.

Rogers, J. (2016). *Coaching skills: The definitive guide to being a coach* (4th ed.). Open University Press.

Ross, A., Brooks, A. T., Yang, L., Touchton-Leonard, K., Raju, S., & Bevans, M. (2018 May). Results of a national survey of certified nurse coaches with implications for advanced practice nurses. *Journal of the American Association of Nurse Practitioners, 30*(5), 251–261. doi:10.1097/JXX.0000000000000041 PMID: 29757841.

Ryan, R. M., & Deci, E. (2000). Self-determination theory and the facilitation of intrinsic motivation, social development and well-being. *American Psychologist, 55*(1), 68–78.

Ryan, R. M., & Deci, E. L. (2006). Self-regulation and the problem of human autonomy: Does psychology need choice, self-determination, and will? *Journal of Personality, 74*, 1557–1585.

Schumacher, K., & Meleis, A. (1994). Transitions: A central concept in nursing. *Journal of Nursing Scholarship, 26*, 119–127.

Seligman, M. E. P. (2011). *Flourish: A visionary new understanding of happiness and well-being*. Free Press.

Sherman, T. (2019). Quick coaching tools-being curious. https://www.tsp-uk.co.uk/leadership-coaching/carrying-out-the-coaching/quick-coaching-tools-being-curious/

Silsbee, D. (2018). *Presence-based coaching: Complexity practice for clarity, resilience and results that matter*. Yes! Global, Inc.

Sonesh, S., Coultas, C., Lacerenza, C., Marlow, S., Benishek, L., & Salas, E. (2015). The power of coaching: A meta-analytic investigation. *Coaching: An International Journal of Theory, Research and Practice, 8*(2), 73–95.

Stober, D., & Grant, A. (2006). *Evidence-based coaching*. John Wiley & Sons.

Swartwout, E., Drenkard, K., McGuinn, K., Grant, S., & El-Zein, A. (2016). Patient and Family Engagement Summit: Needed changes in clinical practice. *Journal of Nursing Administration, 46*(3 Suppl.), S11–S18.

Thich Nhat, H. (2015). *How to love*. Parallex Press.

Trzeciak, S., Mazzarelli, A., & Booker, C. (2019). *Compassionomics: The revolutionary scientific evidence that caring makes a difference*. Studer Group.

VIA Institute on Character. (2016). *Character strengths research: Breaking new ground*. https://www.viacharacter.org/www/Research/Character-Strengths-Research

Watson, J. (2020). The theory of human caring. https://www.watson-caringscience.org/jean-bio/caring-science-theory/

Wentlandt, K., Seccareccia, D., Kevork, N., Workentin, K., Blacker, S., Grossman, D., & Zimmerman, C. (2016). Quality of care and satisfaction with care on palliative care units. *Journal of Pain and Symptom Management, 51*(2), 184–192. doi:10.1016/j.jpainsymman.2015.10.006

Whitworth, L., Kimsey-House, K., Kimsey-House, H., Sandahl, P., & Whitworth, L. (2007). *Co-active coaching: New skills for coaching people towards success*. Davies-Black.

World Health Organization. (2016). Patient engagement. https://apps.who.int/iris/bitstream/handle/10665/252269/9789241511629-eng.pdf

World Health Organization. (2020a). Noncommunicable diseases: Key facts. https://www.who.int/news-room/fact-sheets/detail/noncommunicable-diseases

World Health Organization. (2020b). Obesity and overweight: Key facts. https://www.who.int/news-room/fact-sheets/detail/obesity-and-overweight

8

EVIDENCE-BASED PRACTICE

MIKEL GRAY ■ TERRAN W. SIMS

"I think you can change your belief, but sometimes your behavior takes a lot longer."

~ Tara Westover

CHAPTER CONTENTS

APRNS AND THE DNP 244

EVIDENCE-BASED PRACTICE AND THE APRN 245

- Identifying Evidence 245
- Resources for Evidence-Based Practice, 248
- Quality Improvement Projects: Evaluating EBP 250

GENERATING EVIDENCE: HISTORICAL PERSPECTIVE 252

STEPS OF THE EVIDENCE-BASED PROCESS 253

- Step 1: Formulate a Measurable Clinical Question 253
- Step 2: Search the Literature for Relevant Studies 254
- Step 3: Critically Appraise and Extract Evidence 259
- Step 4: Implement Useful Findings in Clinical Decision Making 268

FROM POLICY TO PRACTICE: TIPS FOR ACHIEVING MEANINGFUL CHANGES IN PRACTICE BASED ON CURRENT BEST EVIDENCE 268

- Stakeholder Engagement 271
- Organizational Support 271
- Clinical Leadership Support 272
- Evidence-Based Practice Innovation: Feedback 273

FUTURE PERSPECTIVES 273

CONCLUSION 274

KEY SUMMARY POINTS 274

Evidence-based practice (EBP) is the dominant approach for clinical decision making in the 21st century and a core competency of advanced practice registered nurse (APRN) practice (American Association of Colleges of Nursing [AACN], 2021a). The primary purpose of this chapter is to review principles of EBP and how the APRN incorporates these principles into practice. It also describes the four fundamental steps of the evidence-based process and identifies resources for EBP, including individual research studies, systematic or scoping reviews, best practice statements, and clinical practice guidelines.

EBP is defined as the conscientious, explicit, and judicious use of research-based evidence when making decisions about the care of individual patients (Sackett et al., 1996). Current best evidence is drawn from *research* produced by nurses and others comprising the interdisciplinary team providing care to individual patients, groups of patients, or communities. *Nursing research* is defined as a systematic inquiry that generates new knowledge about issues of importance to the nursing profession; individual studies may focus on clinical practice, education, administration, and informatics (Polit & Beck, 2021). Although all such research contributes to knowledge, *current best evidence* entails the application of research findings from studies that evaluate interventions or assessments used by nurses and other care providers to improve patient outcomes. For the APRN, much of this research will be generated by nurses. Nevertheless, the APRN will frequently draw upon research produced by multiple members of the interdisciplinary team delivering care in the 21st century. Further, the APRN will apply these findings to evidence-based clinical decision making as an individual provider or as a member of a team charged with constructing, revising, or applying evidence-based policies in a healthcare facility or system.

Advanced practice nursing has evolved significantly since its inception in the 20th century. Entry into APRN practice now occurs following completion of a master's or doctoral degree. All APRNs are educated to seek out and apply current best evidence, a core component of EBP. In addition, the APRN may be involved with generation of original research, acting as a data collector or a member of a multisite clinical trial. The APRN also may participate in and lead quality improvement projects that collect and analyze data from a specific unit, facility, or multisite health system in order to evaluate and improve care processes in a patient care unit, facility, or health system.

The APRN who wishes to play a more active or lead role in generating original research may complete a doctoral program with a research focus. Most research-based doctoral programs in the United States lead to a doctor of philosophy (PhD) degree (AACN, 2021b). These programs prepare nurses for a research-intensive career; coursework leading to a PhD focuses on theory and metatheory, research methodology, and statistical analysis of findings needed to produce new knowledge for the advancement of nursing. Having completed a research doctorate, the PhD-prepared APRN may act as principal investigator or coinvestigator of studies with other nurse researchers. In addition, the PhD-prepared nurse may act as a member of an interdisciplinary team designing a research project, overseeing data collection, analyzing findings, and disseminating these findings via the professional literature. Many PhD-prepared nurses will function primarily in a faculty role, whereas others engage in clinical practice based on knowledge and training as an APRN.

APRNS AND THE DNP

Many APRN students are now electing to complete a practice-focused doctorate degree, the doctor of nursing practice (DNP). The DNP-prepared APRN is ideally prepared for advanced practice and receives additional education enabling them to synthesize existing research findings essential for EBP, use data from increasingly sophisticated databases linked to electronic medical record systems and national databases, and participate in the formation and implementation of policies and procedures on a facility-wide or health system–wide basis. In addition, this individual may participate in the generation of original research as a data collector or clinical consultant to a research team charged with designing a particular study. The DNP-prepared APRN is also prepared to design, lead, and participate in quality improvement projects that analyze practice- and care-related processes. Quality improvement projects evaluate practice processes within a specific unit, clinic, facility, service, or community in order to change (improve) patient-centered outcomes, whereas a formal research study is designed to generate new knowledge (Gregory, 2015). The DNP-prepared APRN also may synthesize findings from multiple studies via a systematic or scoping literature review that analyzes pooled data, differentiates evidence-based from best practice–based assessments or interventions, and identifies gaps in research. The DNP-prepared APRN is also well qualified to lead or participate in nursing or interdisciplinary groups charged with creating clinical guidelines that combine evidence-based and best practice statements to guide clinical decision making and interventions.

Whereas the role of the APRN in EBP is well established, the role of the master's- or DNP-prepared APRN in generating original research continues to evolve. The role of DNP-prepared APRNs in research, in particular, is evolving rapidly. As these individuals move through their careers and gain expertise, they are likely to form strategic and productive alliances within transdisciplinary groups in order to expand current best evidence in multiple areas of care and explore novel methodological approaches for generating evidence such as real-world clinical trials and analysis of data from large electronic databases to more fully understand the processes of nursing and interdisciplinary clinical practice (Kneipp et al., 2014). The AACN (2015) has published a valuable white paper concerning the role of the DNP in generation of new knowledge that provides initial expert opinion concerning this new level of APRN education and practice; nevertheless, additional time is needed to determine the DNP's optimal involvement in the generation and synthesis of evidence.

EVIDENCE-BASED PRACTICE AND THE APRN

EBP is the dominant approach for clinical decision making and a core competency for APRNs (AACN, 2021a; Stiffler & Cullen, 2010; see Chapter 3). The AACN has defined essentials of master's and doctoral education in nursing (AACN, 2021a). All APRNs are expected to translate current best evidence into practice. The master's-prepared APRN is expected to integrate policies and seek evidence for every aspect of practice; this skill requires application of EBP principles to clinical decision making and professional practice. Education within a DNP program builds on these skills by developing the student's competencies to use analytic methods to appraise existing literature and other forms of evidence (such as abstracts or grey literature[a]) to determine best practices, design and implement processes to evaluate practice outcomes, develop practice patterns that influence these outcomes, and compare practice within an individual unit, facility, or health system to national benchmarks. The DNP-prepared APRN is also able to use information technologies in order to collect data related to current nursing practice patterns and outcomes, analyze these data, and play a leadership role in designing and implementing quality improvement initiatives and projects within a local unit, facility, or regional or national health system.

Although components tend to overlap, three levels of this core competency for APRN practice are (1) interpretation and use of EBP principles in individual clinical decision making; (2) interpretation and use of EBP principles to determine policies, standards, and procedures for patient care; and (3) use of EBP to evaluate clinical practice.

[a]Grey literature includes documents that are protected by intellectual property rights and of sufficient quality to be collected and preserved by libraries and institutional repositories, but they are not controlled by commercial publishers and have not gone through external peer review.

Identifying Evidence

Historically, a formal, four-step process for identifying and determining EBP has been defined that continues to be the dominant model for EBP. The four steps of this model are (1) formulation of a clinical question, (2) identification and retrieval of pertinent research findings based on literature review, (3) critical appraisal and extraction of data from pertinent studies, and (4) clinical decision making based on results of this process (Sackett et al., 2000). This four-step process acts as a template for incorporating current best evidence in practice and is the foundation for the growing number of clinical practice guidelines and related EBP resources.

Principles of EBP are used to guide clinical decision making for individual patients, creating policies and procedures that influence practice on a facility- or health system–wide level, and determining policies for delivering care to large groups (Gerrish et al., 2011; Stiffler & Cullen, 2010). Despite widespread acceptance of the concept of EBP, adoption of current best evidence in daily practice is limited. For example, a study of adherence to the American College of Cardiology and American Heart Association Guidelines for perioperative assessment of patients with hip fractures found that more than 90% of clinicians overscreened patients for cardiovascular comorbidities, resulting in delays in surgery, increased risk for perioperative complications, and early mortality (Smeets et al., 2020). Similarly, a random sample of 850 children from 28 school-based health centers in six states found that, despite recommendations from a multidisciplinary expert panel of physicians, nurses, nutritionists, psychologists, and epidemiologists, body mass index was not calculated on 27% of children's health records and blood pressure was not documented on 68.5% of records (Gance-Cleveland et al., 2015). Additional analysis revealed that only half (51.7%) of obese children were identified based on recommended screening procedures. A number of factors are thought to influence clinician acceptance and application of this problem-solving approach to direct patient care, including a lack of knowledge of the principles of

EBP. This chapter defines EBP, differentiates it from concepts of research and quality improvement, and defines three levels of advanced practice nurse competency related to EBP (Table 8.1):

Level I: use of evidence in individual APRN practice
Level II: use of evidence to change practice
Level III: use of evidence to evaluate practice

Exemplars 8.1, 8.2, and 8.3 provide examples of each of these EBP-related competencies.

The term *evidence-based practice* represents a blending of several related concepts, including evidence-based nursing and evidence-based medicine. The original term, *evidence-based medicine*, traces its historical roots to a strategy for educating medical students developed by the faculty at McMaster Medical School in Hamilton, Ontario (Rosenberg & Donald, 1995). Evidence-based nursing is defined as the process that nurses use to make clinical decisions using the best available research evidence, their clinical expertise, and patient preferences (DiCenso et al., 2002). The explicit inclusion of patient preference and clinical expertise is a unique nursing contribution subsequently included in physician-based descriptions of EBP and it is particularly significant for APRNs as a reflection of the holistic approach central to nursing practice that informs clinical decision making.

EBP offers several advantages compared with previous models of clinical decision making. For example, tradition-based practice is based on clinical and anecdotal experience, combined with received wisdom, often provided by instructors or experts. By substituting a standard of current best evidence, EBP encourages the APRN to update and refine clinical practice continually as newer evidence is generated and published.

EBP also offers distinctive advantages compared with rationale-based clinical decision making. Rationale-based clinical decision making relies on identifying a rational explanation for an intervention (Gray, 2002). This form of clinical decision making relies on application of knowledge from the underlying disease process or in research performed using nonhuman subjects or materials (in vitro or in vivo studies). Although these types of studies are enormously valuable to our overall understanding of health, disease, and the reasons that interventions exert a particular effect, EBP is limited to studies that directly measure the efficacy or effectiveness of a particular intervention, the predictive power

TABLE 8.1

Overview of Evidence-Based Practice Competencies and Levels

Competency	Fundamental Level	Expanded Level
Level I: Interpretation and use of research and other evidence in clinical decision making	Incorporate evidence-based practice (EBP) principles and processes into individual clinical practice.	Create and incorporate EBP practices and principles on a unit, clinic, department, facility, healthcare system, national, or international level. The advanced practice registered nurse (APRN) may serve as member of interdisciplinary team formulating policies and procedures on a unit-wide, facility-wide, or health system–wide level. The APRN may function as member of an expert panel that formulates best practice, evidence-based, or blended practice guidelines intended for use on a national or global level.
Level II: Use of evidence to change practice	Incorporate best practice changes according to EBP principles into own practice or act as mentor to front-line staff incorporating change.	Design and implement a process for changing practice beyond the scope of individual practice on a unit, clinic, facility, healthcare system, or national basis.
Level III: Use of evidence to evaluate practice	Identify benchmarks for evaluating own practice or participate in evaluation of practice among front-line nursing and other clinical staff.	Design and implement a process to evaluate pertinent outcomes of practice beyond the scope of individual practice (e.g., generic nursing practice, group APRN practice, interdisciplinary team practice, facility-wide or healthcare system–wide practice).

EXEMPLAR 8.1

LEVEL I: INTERPRETATION AND USE OF EVIDENCE-BASED PRACTICE IN INDIVIDUAL CLINICAL DECISION MAKING

The most basic level of evidence-based practice (EBP) competency is the application of the four steps for clinical decision making in an individual patient. This proficiency requires more than formulation of a clinical question and identification of pertinent studies needed to determine best available evidence. The advanced practice registered nurse (APRN) must combine knowledge of best evidence with an assessment of individual patient factors likely to affect treatment effects, such as the presence of comorbid conditions, psychosocial and cultural factors such as locus of control, preference and impact on quality of life, and cost considerations.

Example: As an APRN in a urology department, I am often asked by patients and physician colleagues whether cranberry juice or supplements (including cranberry capsules) should be prescribed to prevent urinary tract infection (UTI). This persistent query led me to formulate a clinical question, "Are cranberry juice or cranberry products effective in the prevention or management of urinary tract infection?" A systematic literature review based on current best evidence available in 2002 suggested that regular consumption of cranberry juice reduces the incidence of UTIs in community-dwelling women and residents of long-term facilities but does not reduce the risk in patients who undergo intermittent or indwelling catheterization (Gray, 2002). The findings of this systematic review were further supported by a recent randomized controlled trial (RCT) that evaluated a 6-week course of cranberry juice versus placebo capsules in 106 women following gynecologic surgery. Analysis revealed a lower incidence of UTI in women allocated to active cranberry tablets; this difference persisted after adjusting for likely confounding variables, including intermittent self-catheterization (Foxman et al., 2015).

However, additional evidence has emerged that influences these conclusions. Specifically, two RCTs published in 2011 and 2012 found that cranberry juice was no more effective than antimicrobial therapy or cranberry-flavored placebo drink for preventing UTI (Barbosa-Cesnik et al., 2011; Stapleton et al., 2012). On initial consideration, this evidence appeared to support discontinuing recommendations of consumption of cranberry juice for women seeking to prevent recurrent UTIs. However, additional evaluation of findings from one of the studies, a study using a placebo group (Barbosa-Cesnik et al., 2011), revealed that both groups experienced a considerably lower incidence of UTIs than anticipated. In a subsequent interview with one of the investigators, the researchers acknowledged a possibility that the placebo-flavored drink might have contained some of the ingredients hypothesized to exert an antimicrobial effect in the urine (Larson, 2010). In addition, I considered the fact that consumption of cranberry juice twice daily is not associated with any known harmful side effects. I also considered the fact that cranberry juice is relatively inexpensive compared with dietary supplement cranberry capsules. Considering all of these factors, cranberry juice is preferred as a natural means for preventing UTIs among many women in my practice.

This example of basing individual clinical decisions on an EBP process illustrates several important points. It points out the importance of remaining abreast of emerging evidence and the real possibility that newer evidence may significantly alter our understanding of the benefits or harmful effects associated with a specific intervention. In addition, this case illustrates the role of patient preference in clinical decision making. Clinical experience strongly suggests that a significant proportion of women prefer nonpharmacologic interventions for preventing UTIs, and regular consumption of cranberry juice tends to increase overall fluid intake and provide possibly beneficial effects without associated adverse side effects. Therefore given the absence of harm, low direct cost, and mixed evidence concerning efficacy of this preventive intervention, I discuss consumption of cranberry juice with women as a possibly effective intervention that is free from harmful side effects. I also counsel women to consider engaging in other behavioral interventions for the prevention of UTIs, including adequate daily fluid intake based on recommendations from the Institute of Medicine, daily consumption of a dietary source of the probiotic *Lactobacillus*, and consideration of avoiding use of a diaphragm and vaginal spermicide as birth control strategies (Salvatore et al., 2011).

This case also illustrates the time-consuming and rigorous demands of basing individual clinical decisions on the EBP process. Fortunately, APRNs have access to various evidence-based resources such as the Cochrane Database of Systematic Reviews and the systematic reviews available at the US Preventive Services Task Force web page.

In addition to these resources, a growing number of professional societies have generated evidence-based clinical practice guidelines that address measurable clinical questions with thorough and extensive systematic reviews of existing evidence to formulate clinical recommendations covering comparatively broad topics such as heart failure, diabetes mellitus, chronic obstructive pulmonary disease, breast cancer, end-stage renal disease, osteoporosis, and other topics of special interest to APRN practice. In addition to searching the resources of the appropriate professional association's web page, the National Clearinghouse of Practice Guidelines, operated by the Agency for Healthcare Research and Quality, houses a large collection of evidence-based clinical practice guidelines that can be accessed at http://www.guideline.gov.

EXEMPLAR 8.2
LEVEL II: INTERPRETATION AND USE OF EVIDENCE-BASED PRACTICE TO CREATE POLICIES FOR PATIENT CARE

For many advanced practice registered nurses, the growing demand to formulate evidence-based policies and protocols needed to prevent the growing list of "never events" provides an opportunity to master the second competency level, interpretation and use of evidence-based practice (EBP) to create policies for patient care.

Example: Fineout-Overholt et al. (2010a, 2010b, 2010c) have described the EBP process needed to answer a clinical question about whether a rapid response team affects the number of cardiac arrests and unplanned intensive care unit admissions in hospitalized adults. Based on this question, the authors described the process used to search the evidence for pertinent studies, code and extract data from these studies using a standardized protocol, and synthesize data to implement policies needed to launch a rapid response team at their facility. Based on this process, the team concluded that there is sufficient evidence to justify developing policies and committing the resources needed to form a rapid response team at their facility. In addition to providing an example of the EBP described in this chapter, this series of articles describes the processes required to implement such a program. Although a detailed discussion of this translation from research-based evidence to clinical practice is beyond the scope of this chapter, the authors identified and briefly reviewed essential components of this step in the implementation process, including engaging stakeholders in their facility; securing administrative support; preparing a campaign to launch the rapid response team, including staff education and changes in care protocols; and measuring outcomes following implementation of the practice change.

of diagnostic studies, and the presence and severity of adverse side effects.

Resources for Evidence-Based Practice

As described earlier in this chapter, EBP relies on identification and application of current best evidence in clinical decision making and formulating policies or guidelines that guide practice. The four-step process used to identify current best evidence remains valid, but it is time-consuming. Therefore APRNs and other providers rely on published documents that use the EBP process to guide practice. These principle sources used by APRNs and other care providers are clinical practice guidelines, algorithms, consensus statements for best practice, position statements, and practice alerts (Joshi et al., 2019). Clinical practice guidelines are written using a structured and validated methodology; the essential steps of this method are identification of appropriate studies pertinent to the aims of the guideline, extraction and synthesis of pertinent study findings, and grading the evidence gleaned from these studies. For example, the National Comprehensive Cancer Network provides multiple guidelines for treatment of various cancers (https://www.nccn.org/professionals/physician_gls/default.aspx). This process is followed by development and grading the strength of recommendations for practice. In an ideal setting, clinical practice guidelines are solely based on findings of multiple studies examining an intervention or assessment. Another principle source for APRNs are algorithms, or flowcharts designed to guide a clinician through clinical decision-making processes in a stepwise manner. They provide a useful alternative or supplement to clinical practice guidelines when the APRN is faced with a complex or multistep decision-making process requiring multiple assessments leading to a variety of interventions or intervention bundles. Similar to clinical practice guidelines, the decisions advocated in algorithms are ideally based on current best evidence. For example, the Wound Ostomy Continence Society has a growing library of clinical practice algorithms designed specifically for first line and advanced practice nurses (https://www.wocn.org/learning-center/clinical-tools/).

Because evidence is frequently lacking or incomplete in a particular area of care, many clinical decisions rely on best judgment. In this case the APRN should seek out best practice recommendations. Similar to evidence-based clinical practice guidelines, best practice recommendations are based on a structured process designed to reflect the collective opinion of a panel of clinicians with expertise and experience in a particular area of practice (Murphy et al., 1998). Essential components of this process include creation of a panel that shares expertise in the area of practice. The panel should be diverse in terms of professional background and geographic location

EXEMPLAR 8.3

LEVEL III: EVALUATION OF EVIDENCE-BASED PRACTICE TO DETERMINE STANDARDS OF CARE

Participation in an interdisciplinary team to evaluate and determine standards of care using evidence-based practice (EBP) is the third and most advanced level of the EBP competency for advanced practice registered nurse (APRN) practice. Generation of an evidence-based clinical practice guideline entails identification of a number of clinically measurable questions required for establishing and evaluating clinical practice in a broad area of patient care, along with an extensive systematic review of pertinent studies. This often encompasses major assessment strategies related to the management of a particular disorder and first-line and alternative interventions for management.

Example: A professional nursing society charged a task force of three APRNs with clinical expertise in chronic wound care with development and validation of an evidence-based algorithm for use of compression for prevention and treatment of chronic venous insufficiency (CVI) and venous leg ulcers (VLUs; Ratliff et al., 2016). The task force began this task by identifying pertinent clinical questions, an appropriate theoretical framework for clinical decision making in patients with CVI and/or VLUs, and an exploratory literature review. The nursing society committee worked with a PhD-prepared APRN consultant with experience in literature review and generation of evidence-based guidelines for clinical practice, including algorithms. Patient population/Problem, Intervention, Comparison, and Outcome (PICO)-formatted questions were generated by the three-member task force and a literature review was initiated. It soon became apparent that the algorithm must combine evidence-based decisional nodes with clinical decision points that lack sufficient evidence to be deemed evidence based. Based on this initial review, the task force elected to complete a scoping review that focused on current clinical practice guidelines and research specifically focusing on a single aspect of CVI and VLU prevention and treatment: compression. This search revealed eight clinical practice guidelines; each recommended compression as part of a bundle of interventions for prevention and management of CVI and VLUs, but none provided adequate guidance concerning when to select a specific type of compression (stockings, bandages, intermittent pneumatic compression devices) or best practices for donning and removing compression devices. Based on these initial findings, a second phase of the literature review was completed that included studies in adult patients that compared one or more types of compression or evaluated techniques for aiding patients or lay caregivers in donning or removing compression devices. This two-step scoping literature review was used to develop a draft algorithm that incorporated evidence-based interventions and interventions lacking adequate clinical evidence, along with evidence-based statements supporting the algorithm and best practice statements linked to clinical decisions not supported by adequate research-based evidence.

A multidisciplinary team that represented all regions of the United States was assembled that reviewed and critiqued the algorithm and reached consensus on best practice statements supporting the algorithm. This panel comprised APRNs; specialty practice nurses in wound, ostomy, and continence vascular care; physical therapists; physicians; and basic science researchers in the area of compression devices. Under the direction of this multidisciplinary group, the algorithm was modified, including addition of supplemental materials deemed necessary for adaptation of the algorithm by clinicians with limited experience and knowledge in management of CVI and VLUs. It was also adapted into an electronic format for ease of use in multiple care settings. This second draft of the algorithm was submitted to content validation by a second and separate multidisciplinary group that was composed of APRNs, specialty practice nurses, physicians, and physical therapists. The resulting guideline has been downloaded by more than 7000 providers in North America, including APRNs, specialty practice nurses, vascular surgeons, and physicians and physical therapists specializing in chronic wound care. The construction and validation of this algorithm demonstrates how a small task force of APRNs consulted with a PhD-prepared APRN to design PICO-based questions and complete a scoping literature review that combined evidence-based decisions with best practice decisions essential to construction of a clinically relevant and pragmatic algorithm guiding APRNs, specialty practice and front-line nurses, physicians, and physical therapists in selecting, applying, and reapplying compression for prevention and management of VLUs in adult patients with CVI. Research concerning the influence of this algorithm in two settings, long-term care and home care, is ongoing.

and free of financial relationships likely to unduly influence their opinion. Best practice statements are usually generated by a task force or individual panelists and discussed by the entire panel. Statements are accepted only after one or more rounds of discussion including all panelists and anonymous voting resulting in acceptance of the statement by a majority of panelists (statements are usually accepted only if agreed upon by 75% or more of panelists). For example, the American Association of Critical-Care

Nurses TeleICU Nursing Consensus Statement provides consensus-based best practice recommendations for the rapidly evolving delivery of telehealth interventions in the critical care setting (https://www.aacn.org/nursing-excellence/standards/aacn-teleicu-nursing-consensus-statement).

In addition to seeking out pertinent clinical practice guidelines or algorithms, the APRN should identify other EBP resources including position statements or practice alerts. A position statement is a document that describes a dilemma in clinical practice, presents strengths and limitations of alternatives in clinical decision making related to the dilemma, and provides a rationale for the position advocated by the authors. Position statements are frequently generated by professional societies. A clinical practice alert is a brief document developed in response to a rapidly evolving clinical issue that requires immediate action. Such alerts frequently rely on best practice statements or sparse evidence when clinicians face a rapidly evolving change in practice. For example, the coronavirus pandemic led to generation of multiple practice alerts related to prolonged positioning for patients with severe acute respiratory syndrome coronavirus 2 (SARs-CoV-2) and prevention of skin damage related to use of personal protective equipment (Davis & Beeson, 2020; Ghelichkhani & Esmaeili, 2020; Wound Ostomy and Continence Nurses Society Board of Directors Task Force, 2020).

Because the proportion of clinical practice supported by robust evidence is limited, both clinical practice guidelines and algorithms often represent a combination of recommendations for practice that are based on variable levels of supporting evidence and best practice recommendations. The APRN should be alert to the level of evidence supporting a recommendation for practice and opportunities for evaluating the safety and efficacy of an intervention supported by consensus-based best practice statements or limited evidence.

Quality Improvement Projects: Evaluating EBP

A quality improvement (QI) project is a systematic activity that generates outcome data in order to achieve rapid improvements in healthcare delivery in a specific setting (Arndt & Netsch, 2012; Shirey et al., 2011; US Department of Health and Human Services, Health Resources and Services Administration, 2011; Table 8.2). The data generated during a QI project are designed to improve specific outcomes within a local facility, clinic, or community. Unlike the data generated by a research study, the results of a QI project can only be generalized to the specific patient population that comprised the project setting.

Despite these differences, the APRN should remember that research, EPB, and QI projects share a common goal: improvement of patient care. For example, an acute care APRN observed that the use of restraints in her facility's five intensive care units (ICUs) was subject to scrutiny. In this case the APRN should evaluate the facility's policies and each unit's practice related to use of patient restraints and compare their findings to national benchmarks. Questions guiding this evaluation include:

- What is current best evidence related to use of restraints in critically ill patients?
- Are there clinical practice or best practice guidelines suggesting strategies to maintain patient safety and reduce the use of restraints and their potential complications?
- How does restraint use in the ICUs in my facility compare to national benchmarks?

A review of the literature suggests that the use of restraints can have negative patient outcomes that must be balanced by strong beliefs that their use prevents other adverse outcomes. The chief benefit of restraint use is preventing patient harm during specific interventions such as those related to the use of mechanical ventilation (Rose et al., 2016; Van der Kooi et al., 2015). Potential harms from the use of restraints include increased agitation, inadvertent removal of devices (chest tubes, nasogastric tubes, endotracheal tubes), and falls. A clinical practice guideline suggests benefit in reducing use of both pharmacologic and physical restraints (Maccioli et al., 2003). Recommendations included information about the least restrictive options, risk versus benefit consideration, and identification of alternatives. Patients need to be reevaluated in a timely fashion for any complications and to reassess the continued need for restraints and alternatives to be considered. This guideline also made recommendations for the use of pharmacologic mitigation to limit restraint use (sedatives, analgesics, and

TABLE 8.2

Evidence-Based Practice, Research, and Quality Improvement: Understanding the Similarities and Differences

	Evidence-Based Practice	Research Study	Quality Improvement Project
Overall goal	Apply current best evidence to clinical decision making for individual patient, facility, or large group	Produce generalizable new knowledge	Enhance quality of care delivery by evaluating the effect of specific action plan on local unit, clinic, facility, or health system
Methodology for generating results	Systematic review with ordinal ranking of strength of evidence and/or meta-analysis Scoping literature review (study) may be combined with consensus-based expert opinion for identifying best practice documents when evidence is lacking	Various methods employed: Randomized controlled trial Comparison cohort study Prospective cohort study Retrospective comparison control study Qualitative study	Various models used; most common include: CHRONIC CARE model (Problem Solving, Decision Making, Resource Utilization, Taking Action, Counseling, Community Resources) Lean model PDSA (Plan–Do–Study–Act) model (also referred to as Model for Improvement) Focus–Analyze–Develop–Execute–Evaluate (FADE) model Six Sigma model (DMAIC: Define, Measure, Analyze, Improve, Control)
Unit of study	Individual studies, systematic review with pooled analysis of multiple studies	Varies, typically aggregate (sample) of individual patients, families, communities	Varies, typically one or more units within facility, individual facility, or individual health system
Does involvement of human subjects require institutional review board review and approval?	Not indicated; evidence-based practice is the study of studies and application in daily practice	Always indicated when study has any involvement of human subjects	May be indicated if project involves evaluation of novel or nonstandard care (intervention) of patients
Tangible product (may or may not be published or made available to public)	Individual clinical judgment Policy for care on individual unit/clinic, facility-wide or health system–wide Protocol for care delivery Clinical practice guideline	Research report, may be initially presented as abstract or poster at scientific meeting; ultimate goal is to publish as research report in peer-reviewed scholarly journal	Internal report to health system leadership and/or administration; may be published as quality improvement report in peer-reviewed scholarly journal

neuroleptics) but cautioned against their use as chemical restraint.

In order to address this complex issue, Mitchell et al. (2018) completed a QI project designed to reduce use of restraints in five ICUs while avoiding potential negative outcomes related to reductions in their use. The authors also compared restraint use in their facility to a national benchmark established by the National Database of Nursing Quality Indicators (NDNQI). A collaborative team was developed to improve cross-unit communication, identify barriers to best care, review evidence-based practice, and work toward reduced restraint use in patient care. The group met regularly over several months to examine baseline data related to restraint data for each ICU. They designed and distributed a survey to identify attitudes toward current practices and guide their educational efforts. Barriers to change were identified, including the lack of awareness by some staff regarding benchmark standards. Members of the QI team provided a structured educational program for staff related to restraint use and identified key informal leaders in each ICU who acted as clinical champions for reducing restraint use. Outcomes of this QI project included a reduction in the use of physical restraints commensurate with the NDNQI national benchmark for their use.

In this case the APRN team used existing EBP sources (clinical practice guideline and national benchmark) to identify a need for improvement in care processes. Process steps included review of current policies and deficiencies, identification of local barriers to practice innovation, construction of an intervention bundle for restraint use, focused education and product changes if indicated, measurement and comparison of data before and following implementation of the QI program, and transparent reports to all stakeholders.

GENERATING EVIDENCE: HISTORICAL PERSPECTIVE

Although the meaning of the term *evidence* may appear transparent on initial consideration, a more careful analysis of the historical roots of evidence generation in health care is needed. The Oxford English Dictionary Online (2020) defines evidence as an object or document that serves as proof. The objects or documents acceptable for use as evidence vary for each discipline or profession; historians seek out original documents or artifacts, and lawyers have developed a complex system for identifying evidence codified with federal, state, or other rules of evidence documents. Within the context of EBP, evidence is limited to research findings evaluating the efficacy and safety of an intervention or the predictive power of a diagnostic procedure. Although the search for evidence can be traced back more than 2000 years, definitions for what constitutes sufficient evidence to reach these conclusions have evolved over time.

Despite a growing number of study designs used to evaluate the effectiveness of various interventions, diagnostic procedures, and intervention bundles, the randomized controlled trial (RCT) remains the gold standard research design for generating evidence (Sackett, 2015; Turner, 2012). The RCT is based on three critical elements: (1) manipulation of an experimental intervention; (2) comparison of the group receiving the experimental intervention to a control or comparison group that receives a placebo, sham device, or standard intervention based on ethical considerations; and (3) random allocation of subjects to an intervention or comparison/control group. Random allocation, advocated since the early 1930s, is an essential element of an RCT because it is the most effective technique for spreading potentially confounding factors evenly among treatment and control groups (Hill, 1937). The trial comparing streptomycin with standard care at the time (bed rest) is usually cited as the world's first large-scale RCT ("Streptomycin Treatment," 1948). Randomization was achieved using a closed envelope system and subjects were blinded to treatment group. However, at least one trial was completed and published before this landmark study. Amberson et al. (1931) compared the antibiotic sanocrysin for treatment of pulmonary tuberculosis with a placebo. In addition to random allocation of subjects by flipping a coin, they blinded physician data collectors to group assignment to minimize bias, another important design feature of the modern RCT.

Based on this historical legacy and guided by the pioneering efforts of Archibald Cochrane, current best evidence is now defined as individual and collective findings from studies evaluating the efficacy and safety of an active or preventive intervention or the predictive accuracy of an assessment (Gray et al., 2004; van Rijswijk & Gray, 2012). These studies must directly evaluate the effect of an intervention; compare the intervention with a placebo, standard care, or a sham device; and document adverse side effects associated with the intervention. Studies used to establish current best evidence must be executed in human (rather than animal) subjects and must measure the most direct outcome of treatment, rather than relying on interim outcomes based on convenience. For example, a study of the efficacy of a topical wound therapy should measure wound closure rather than concluding efficacy based on the percentage of wound closure completed at a convenient or arbitrary point after the initiation of treatment (van Rijswijk & Gray, 2012).

This definition of current best evidence raises a corollary question: What criteria must be fulfilled to deem an intervention is "evidence based"? At least two major regulatory groups, the US Food and Drug

Administration (FDA) and the European Medicines Agency (EMA), have established specific criteria for labeling an intervention as evidence based (Cormier, 2011). For a drug to receive an indication for clinical use, the FDA requires results from two well-designed RCTs with consistent results, both of which must compare the agent with a placebo- or sham-based control group; EMA criteria are broadly similar (EMA, 2000).

Although these groups provide well-defined criteria for defining an intervention (administration of a drug) as evidence based, achieving this level of evidence is work-intensive and enormously costly. For example, the approximate cost of achieving a new drug indication has risen sharply over the past decade and may be as high as $2.5 billion (Mullin, 2014). The impact of this on APRN practice is profound; for example, a study of primary care practice found that only 18% of recommendations are based on high-level patient-oriented evidence, whereas half are based on expert opinion, usual care, or rationale-based decisions based on disease-oriented evidence (Ebell et al., 2017).

STEPS OF THE EVIDENCE-BASED PROCESS

As discussed earlier, the predominant model for EBP contains four well-defined steps. Other models have been described, but this chapter is based on this four-step model.

Step 1: Formulate a Measurable Clinical Question

Clinical decision making using the EBP process begins with formulation of a measurable clinical question. Questions arise from various sources. For example, many APRNs will formulate their first clinical questions as part of an EBP process when planning their final scholarly project as part of a DNP degree. Individual clinical APRN or staff nurse practice provides another rich source for clinical questions. Queries may arise when the APRN is faced with a questionably effective intervention or when managing an uncommon or rare disorder that is not addressed in major clinical practice guidelines. APRNs often serve on multidisciplinary committees that may be charged with developing a policy or protocol for presenting or managing a particular clinical challenge. For example, the growing list of "never events" (National Quality Forum, 2021) presents an ongoing challenge to APRNs practicing in the acute and critical care settings, who are often charged with designing facility-wide prevention programs for conditions such as catheter-associated urinary tract infections, surgical site infections, and central line–associated bloodstream infections.

Results of several studies suggest that application of the PICO (Problem, Intervention, Comparison, and Outcome) model aids nurses in formulating clinically relevant and measurable questions and assists in efficiently searching the literature for available evidence (Balakas & Sparks, 2010; Fineout-Overholt & Stillwell, 2019; Hastings & Fisher, 2014; LaRue et al., 2009; Table 8.3).

The *P* in PICO indicates *population* (Hastings & Fisher, 2014), although the *P* is sometimes expanded to include the *primary problem* (Balakas & Sparks, 2010). This element of the formula alerts the APRN to define the population to be studied and the nature of the problem to be scrutinized. The population may comprise a smaller group of patients receiving care, such as patients with an indwelling urinary catheter, but it often incorporates much larger populations, such as all patients with diabetes mellitus. Identification of the primary problem is closely tied to the population

TABLE 8.3

PICO(T) Model for Generating EBP Clinical Questions

Component	Definition
P	*Patient/population*—identify the population of interest *Problem*—identify the primary problem
I	*Intervention*—identify the intervention(s) to be considered
C	*Comparison*—identify to what the intervention will be compared
O	*Outcome*—identify the goal of the intervention(s)
T[a]	*Time*—time frame for measuring outcomes

[a]Optional.

Adapted from Fineout-Overholt, E., & Stillwell, S. B. (2019). Asking compelling clinical questions. In B. M. Melnyk & E. Fineout-Overholt (Eds.). *Evidence-based practice in nursing and healthcare: A guide to best practice*. (4th ed.). p. 33–54. Wolters Kluwer.

under scrutiny. Examples of primary problems may be a disease such as sinusitis, a disorder such as chronic osteoarthritis, or a predisposition to a potentially preventable condition such as a pressure injury.

The *I* in the PICO model represents the main *intervention* to be considered. In many cases, an APRN will examine a single intervention, such as the efficacy of telemedicine encounters in the presence of a pandemic such as COVID-19, or a traditional intervention, such as structured education for patients with newly diagnosed diabetes mellitus (Evans, 2010). In contrast, the APRN may examine an intervention bundle. For example, Moore et al. (2019) implemented a nurse-driven protocol embedded within the electronic medical record designed to improve rapid response to evolving sepsis. The bundled intervention, a modified version of DART (detect, act, reassess, titrate) comprised regular use of a sepsis screening tool, measurement of lactate and blood cultures, administration of fluids and antibiotics, reevaluation of lactate after 6 hours, and reassessment of volume status after fluid bolus.

Nayan et al. (2011) faced a similar challenge when studying whether smoking cessation rates were higher in oncology patients who receive smoking cessation interventions compared with usual care. Their initial search identified a meta-analysis of eight RCTs that detected no differences in self-reported cessation rates compared with usual care. However, subclassifying smoking interventions into pharmacologic, behavioral, and combined interventions suggested that cessation protocols that combine pharmacologic and behavioral interventions appeared to increase cessation rates compared with usual care or single-intervention protocols.

The *C* in the PICO model indicates the *comparison* to the intervention undergoing scrutiny. The *C* may indicate a placebo or sham device, though it frequently indicates standard or usual care when employment of a placebo or sham intervention falls below standard of care. It is essential that the APRN specifically define the intervention(s) that comprise standard care and ensure that the studies retrieved enable adequate differentiation of this standard from the intervention under scrutiny.

The *O* in PICO indicates the *outcome*, or intended goal of the intervention. When determining the outcome used to define efficacy, it is important to identify and evaluate the most direct indication of clinical effectiveness and avoid indirect outcomes that are often more easily measured. In prevention studies, the most direct outcome is generally a reduction in the incidence of the disease or disorder under scrutiny. For example, an APRN evaluating the effect of a prevention protocol on surgical site infection should base conclusions of efficacy on incidence rates, rather than interim outcomes. Examples of interim outcomes to be avoided include studies that only report a change in nurse knowledge after education or self-reported changes in practice.

A final element, *T*, indicating *time*, may be added to the PICO conceptual framework. The time frame is meant to indicate the relevant observation period for outcomes; it may be short, such as the first 24 to 48 hours following surgery, or long, such as years to decades following the onset of a chronic condition such as dementia or diabetes mellitus (Balakas & Sparks, 2010; Hastings & Fisher, 2014; Milnes et al., 2015).

Step 2: Search the Literature for Relevant Studies

Evidence-based clinical decision making relies on identifying research-based evidence. Therefore it is essential for the APRN to develop expertise in searching the literature to identify and retrieve appropriate studies. Fortunately, the development of modern electronic databases has revolutionized our ability to search the literature rapidly. A number of electronic databases are now available to the APRN (Table 8.4). Although full access to many databases requires a paid subscription, APRNs may be able to access these electronic databases via their facility-based subscription. Specifically, the vast majority of health system, university, and college libraries maintain institutional subscriptions to Ovid, ensuring access to multiple electronic databases such as MEDLINE or CINAHL. In addition, access to PubMed is available without charge on the Internet.

MEDLINE and PubMed

Administered by the National Library of Medicine, MEDLINE is the world's largest electronic database of health-related research and literature (National Library of Medicine, 2021). There are articles from a number of professions, including medicine, nursing, dentistry, veterinary medicine, and associated disciplines such

TABLE 8.4

Examples of Electronic Databases for Identifying and Retrieving Pertinent Research

Name	Description	URL
MEDLINE	Largest online database for nursing, medical, and allied health journals	https://www.nlm.nih.gov/bsd/pmresources.html
PubMed	Freely accessible online version of MEDLINE database; lacks the robust Boolean features of MEDLINE	http://www.ncbi.nlm.nih.gov/sites/entrez?db=PubMed
Cumulative Index to Nursing and Allied Health Literature (CINAHL)	Largest database for nursing and allied health literature; includes multiple nursing journals not indexed in the MEDLINE database	http://www.ebscohost.com/biomedical-libraries/the-cinahl-database
Education Resource Information Center (ERIC)	Linked to more than 320,000 articles from 1966 to the present; focuses on educational literature, including undergraduate and graduate nursing	http://www.eric.ed.gov/
PsycINFO	Contains more than 3 million resources dating back to 1888; excellent resource for the APRN who specializes in providing mental health care	http://www.apa.org/pubs/databases/psycinfo/index.aspx
Web of Science	Includes journals in the basic and clinical sciences drawn from approximately 9300 journals with impact factors; administered by Clarivate Analytics	https://apps.webofknowledge.com/WOS_GeneralSearch_input.do?product=WOS&search_mode=GeneralSearch&SID=1AtDcGoWCHV3rnpT4ub&preferencesSaved=

as physiology, pharmacology, and molecular biology. More than 5200 journals are indexed in approximately 40 languages (National Library of Medicine, 2021). The MEDLINE database is primarily organized around MESH (*me*dical *s*ubject *h*eading) terms. Entering a MESH term, such as "coronary artery disease" or "osteoporosis," will trigger a number of subheads that are potentially useful to identify evidence for answering a clinical question, such as "diagnosis," "drug therapy," "diet therapy," and "nursing." The MEDLINE database may also be searched using various keywords that are not official MESH terms; these searches retrieve articles that include the keyword in its title, abstract, or a list of identifying keywords, but they will not provide the subheads available when a MESH term is accessed. The MEDLINE database includes articles published in 39 languages; 91% are printed in English and 83% of those published in other languages have English-language abstracts, greatly increasing access for English-speaking searchers.

MEDLINE has robust Boolean functions, allowing the APRN to focus or narrow a search by combining two or more MESH terms or keywords using the functions "AND," "OR," and "NOT." For example, an APRN might pose a question about the effectiveness of administering an angiotensin-converting enzyme inhibitor for the prevention of mortality and disease progression in patients with heart failure. In this case the APRN might initially select the MESH term "heart failure" along with the MESH term "angiotensin-converting enzyme inhibitors." By using the "AND" Boolean function, the database will retrieve articles that merge the intervention (angiotensin-converting enzyme inhibitor agents) with the primary patient problem under scrutiny (heart failure).

A second Boolean function, "OR," allows the searcher to retrieve articles that contain either of two keywords or MESH terms. This function is useful when terms that are recently coined or historically relevant differ from the corresponding MESH term. For example, an APRN may be seeking information about patients who experience chronic lower urinary tract pain not associated with bacterial infection. The MESH term for this condition is "interstitial cystitis." However, a more recent term (bladder pain syndrome) has been increasingly used to describe this condition (Hanno et al., 2014); combining the MESH term "interstitial cystitis" with the keyword "bladder pain syndrome" retrieves more citations than entering either term alone.

A third Boolean function, "NOT," allows the APRN to limit a search by eliminating articles that do not address the intervention, assessment, or patient population under scrutiny. For example, an APRN interested in prevention of central line infections might enter the MESH term "indwelling catheters," which will retrieve studies focusing on infections associated with multiple types of catheters, including urinary and peritoneal dialysis catheters. Use of the "NOT" Boolean function will enable the APRN to eliminate articles about various types of catheters not pertinent to a clinical question focusing on hospital-acquired central line infections.

The MEDLINE database allows searches via multiple alternative fields, including author, journal, publication type (e.g., review article), language, experimental approach (human, in vivo, or in vitro), gender, age range, and publication year. These options are useful for focusing searches based on the parameters specified in the clinical question.

The PubMed web page (http://www.ncbi.nlm.nih.gov/pubmed) provides free access to the MEDLINE database. The basic search engine will retrieve articles based on keywords. Clinicians searching PubMed can click on an advanced search icon and access a site that allows a combination of keywords or keyword and author or journal using the Boolean function "AND." However, the PubMed database does not have the robust search functions characteristic of MEDLINE. In addition, although a limited number of articles can be downloaded directly from the PubMed site, access to most articles is restricted to the complete citation and abstract.

Cumulative Index for Nursing and Allied Health Literature

The Cumulative Index for Nursing and Allied Health Literature (CINAHL) is an electronic database containing more than 2.6 million elements from approximately 3000 nursing and allied health journals and books. Similar to MEDLINE, the CINAHL database is available online as a subscription service typically accessed as part of an EBSCO Information Services subscription maintained by larger healthcare facilities and universities. Articles can be searched using keywords; the CINAHL database also contains the Boolean features "AND," "OR," and "NOT" and multiple search fields similar to those described for MEDLINE. CINAHL also indexes doctoral dissertations, an important source for grey literature (unpublished documents) in the field of nursing.

Online Evidence-Based Resources

In addition to retrieving individual research reports from electronic databases such as MEDLINE and CINAHL, the APRN should search online evidence-based databases such as the Cochrane Library and PubMed Health. The Cochrane Library is part of the Cochrane Collaboration; it is administered by a nonprofit organization, and reviews are generated by more than 28,000 volunteers from across the globe (Cochrane Collaboration, 2021). The Cochrane Library contains multiple resources for identifying current best evidence, including the Cochrane Database of Systematic Reviews and the Cochrane Central Register of Controlled Trials. The Database of Systematic Reviews contains more than 5000 systematic literature reviews based on clinical questions covering almost every specialty practice area in contemporary health care. Whenever possible, these reviews include a meta-analysis of data pooled from comparable studies. The systematic reviews can be accessed by multiple search fields, including keywords found in the title or abstract and author. Systematic reviews can be retrieved as a summary, standard report, or full report. A plain language summary provides a brief synopsis of the review's main findings. A standard report provides more detailed information, including a structured abstract of the review, plain language summary, background, objectives, methods, results, and discussion, along with reference lists for included and excluded studies. Systematic reviews are also available as a full report that incorporates all the elements of the standard report plus a detailed summary of all analyses generated for the review.

The plain language summary is useful as a quick reference when the APRN is only interested in a succinct summary of the main findings of a systematic review; this document may also be shared with a patient or family with a college-level education who may wish to know more about evidence supporting a particular intervention or assessment strategy. The full summary provides the more detailed information necessary when the APRN is evaluating current best evidence for individual decision making or generation of recommendations for practice. The detailed report also may be used for this purpose; study of this longer version is especially recommended for the novice APRN who is learning to synthesize evidence for clinical decision making or generating evidence-based documents such as a plan for a scholarly project.

Other online resources include the Joanna Briggs Institute, Essential Evidence Plus, and PubMed Health. The Joanna Briggs Institute is an international collaboration of nurses and other allied healthcare professionals, including the Cochrane Nursing Care Field and Cochrane Qualitative Research Methods Group, that provides evidence-based resources for nursing (Joanna Briggs Institute, n.d.). Essential Evidence Plus is a subscription service administered by Wiley-Blackwell Publishers (Essential Evidence Plus, 2021) that enables users to access multiple electronic databases, including the Cochrane Library, to obtain evidence-based resources and information. An individual or institutional subscription to Essential Evidence Plus also provides access to POEMS (*P*atient-*O*riented *E*vidence that *M*atters). POEMS includes regularly updated synopses of evidence from individual studies and an archive of more than 3000 previously posted summaries. They may be downloaded online, downloaded to a smartphone, or viewed via podcast.

PubMed Health is an electronic database for evidence-based resources administered by the National Center for Biotechnology Information, US National Library of Medicine (http://www.ncbi.nlm.nih.gov/pubmedhealth). This electronic database includes reviews of clinical effectiveness research; reviews are available in brief reports designed for use by consumers, along with full reports designed for use by clinicians such as APRNs. In addition to its link to the extensive MEDLINE/PubMed database, PubMed Health is linked to evidence-based resources from the Cochrane Library, the Agency for Healthcare Research and Quality (AHRQ), the National Cancer Institute, the National Institute for Health and Clinical Excellence (NICE) guidelines program, and the National Institute for Health Research, Health Technology Assessment Program. Table 8.5 summarizes additional online resources for EBP.

TABLE 8.5

Additional Online Resources for Evidence-Based Practice

Name	Description	URL
Clinical Practice Guidelines		
Agency for Healthcare Research and Quality (AHRQ)	Evidence report topics, technical reviews, and clinical guidelines	https://www.ahrq.gov/
Institute for Healthcare Improvement	List of published articles about developing and using evidence-based protocols	http://www.ihi.org/
General Sites With Links to Other EBP Sites		
National Association of Clinical Nurse Specialists	Provides resources for evidence-based practice	https://nacns.org/professional-resources/research/ebp-resources/
Centre for Evidence-Based Healthcare	Lists of reviews and evidence research reports	https://nottingham.ac.uk/research/groups/cebhc/index.aspx
Centre for Evidence-Based Medicine (CEBM)	Links to evidence-based resources, tools, continuing education, and discussion groups	http://www.cebm.net/
Joanna Briggs Institute	Privately owned evidence-based practice site with some free resources and subscription pages	https://jbi.global
Essential Evidence Plus	Subscription service administered by Wiley-Blackwell Publishers	https://www.essentialevidenceplus.com/
Advanced Practice Nursing	Subscription site for evidence-based resources	http://www.enursescribe.com/evidencebased.html
Registered Nurses Association of Ontario	Repository of best practice guidelines focusing on front-line nursing practice	http://rnao.ca/bpg/

Clinical Practice Guidelines

Searches of electronic databases should also incorporate the identification and retrieval of existing clinical practice guidelines or best practice documents. Clinical practice guidelines may be enormously helpful to the APRN because they represent a systematic review of existing evidence based on measurable clinical questions and recommendations for management of the disease, disorder, or condition (Fletcher, 2008). Identification and incorporation of appropriate guidelines is also important to APRNs because these documents are increasingly being viewed as a standard of care among clinicians, especially given the widespread acceptance of EBP principles. In addition to increasing scrutiny by clinicians, courts within the United States have begun to grapple with the issue of clinical practice guidelines and their relationship to the *legal* definition of a *standard of care*. The current legal definition for standard of care for physicians is "that which a minimally competent physician in the same field would do under similar circumstances" (Moffett & Moore, 2011, p. 111). Legal precedents concerning use of these documents continues to evolve; nevertheless, multiple courts have ruled that guidelines may be used as learned treatises to lend credence to or impeach an expert witness, to defend a clinician for using recommendations with the document as a standard of care, and to suggest that the clinician failed to deliver standard of care by not following guideline recommendations (Moffett & Moore, 2011; Taylor, 2014). The evolving use of practice guidelines provides another powerful rationale for the inclusion of EBP principles as a core competency for APRNs.

The APRN should also search for best practice documents pertaining to the clinical question under scrutiny. As noted earlier, best practice guidelines are a synthesis of expert and clinical opinions when higher levels of evidence are not available to guide clinical decision making (Triano, 2008). Although these documents do not provide the systematic review and evidence-based recommendations of care incorporated into a clinical practice guideline, they can provide an excellent source of current knowledge of a specific intervention or assessment technique. In addition to housing clinical practice guidelines, the National Guideline Clearinghouse indexes best practice documents produced within the past 5 years (https://www.thecommunityguide.org/resources/national-guideline-clearinghouse). The Registered Nurses' Association of Ontario (RNAO) is another excellent resource for best practice guidelines that affect multiple areas of nursing care, including many areas pertinent to advanced practice nursing (http://rnao.ca/bpg/).

Strategies for Searching Electronic Databases

Because of their robust size and ability to identify potential resources in a matter of seconds to minutes, any hunt for best current evidence begins with a search of more than one electronic database. Searching multiple databases is strongly suggested because limited evidence has shown that searching a single database is likely to miss meaningful research compared with searches of multiple databases (Bramer et al., 2016). Findings of an RCT indicate that the efficiency of a literature search is improved when a medical librarian is consulted (Gardois et al., 2011). Several factors probably contribute to incomplete retrieval of pertinent studies when relying solely on searches of electronic databases. Challenges related to keywords are postulated to be a primary cause of incomplete retrieval. Many conditions and interventions are referred to by multiple names, and these terms evolve over time. For example, the chronic wound currently referred to as a "pressure injury" (Edsberg et al., 2016) was historically labeled a "bed sore," a term that was later changed to "decubitus ulcer," "pressure sore" or "pressure ulcer." Nevertheless, pressure ulcer remains the official MESH term as of July 2021. In addition to this limitation, electronic databases typically identify keywords for search purposes from the title, abstract, and a short list of key terms provided by the author and/or publisher. Although authors and publishers share the goal of maximizing the number of times an article is cited in subsequent peer-reviewed publications, even subtle changes in narrative or selection of less widely used terms limit the likelihood that a particular study report will be identified in subsequent searches.

In addition, electronic databases are heavily weighted toward published documents. Publication bias is defined as the tendency for studies with provocative results to achieve favorable peer review and acceptance for publication compared with research reporting negative results (M. B. Smith, 1956). In the current era of blended print, electronic, and open access sources of healthcare research, publication bias arises from multiple sources; specifically, articles are more likely to be published if they report positive findings or provocative findings likely to attract lay media attention (Song et al., 2013). The magnitude of this effect is hypothesized to be substantial (Guyatt et al., 2011). For example, Sutton et al. (2000) carried out meta-analyses of 48 systematic reviews and reported that 20% were found to have omitted or missed studies reporting negative results.

Electronic databases are also limited by the relative paucity of grey literature, which is especially significant in nursing research. The term *grey literature* is defined as unpublished results of studies as abstracts or short reports in conference proceedings or journal supplements. Sparse research suggests that the magnitude of nursing studies that remain unpublished despite completion is substantial. For example, Hicks (1995) reported that only 16 of a group of 161 British nurses who completed a study and presented results at a professional conference submitted their findings for publication in a peer-reviewed journal, and only 14 were ultimately published (9%).

Several strategies can be used to increase the proportion of pertinent studies identified during a literature search. They include ancestry searches, searching grey literature sources, consulting experts in the field, and using Internet-based search engines. Ancestry searches are completed by reviewing the reference list of individual research reports, review articles, or systematic reviews identified during a literature search (Melnyk & Fineout-Overholt, 2010). Weak evidence suggests that ancestry searches may reveal multiple studies that are missed during electronic database searches (Horsley et al., 2011). Identifying pertinent grey literature sources remains a challenge. Hand searches of one or more peer-reviewed journals that publish research abstracts in a supplement to or regular issue of the society's official journal or abstracts made available to conference attendees in a written or electronic format may serve as a rich source of pertinent studies. Although these sources may identify multiple potentially pertinent studies, they typically contain limited details of the study design and analyses of findings, thus limiting their value as evidence-based resources. In contrast, the CINAHL, PsycINFO, and ERIC databases index doctoral theses and dissertations that provide intensely reviewed and detailed reports of graduate students' supervised research.

Internet-based search engines, such as Google or Google Scholar, are an increasingly robust source of published and unpublished studies. They are particularly useful when attempting to retrieve full reprints of older articles not yet incorporated into the major electronic databases. Nevertheless, considerable caution must be used when relying on unpublished information from the Internet, especially if the source material has not undergone peer review. An evaluation of the coverage, recall, and precision of search strategies used in 120 systematic reviews found that Google Scholar lacked the full coverage needed for performing a systematic review (Bramer et al., 2016; Gehanno et al., 2013). Consulting with an experienced researcher or clinical experts in a particular field can also lead to identification of pertinent studies (Godin et al., 2015).

Access to published literature continues to evolve; Plan S arose from a coalition of industry, universities, and other stakeholders to ensure that all published research funded by public or private grants is published in open access journals, on open access platforms, or made immediately available through open access repositories without embargo (Dal-Re, 2019). The motivation and context for this group have not been made public but are speculated to include increased control for larger search engines and databases and the corporations that control these powerful search engines and data repositories. Such a plan would revolutionize access to research-based publications, but its effect on nonfunded research (particularly important to nursing and advanced practice nursing) is of considerable concern.

Step 3: Critically Appraise and Extract Evidence

While a careful search of the literature using the strategies described will retrieve pertinent studies, it will also retrieve many publications that do not qualify as current best evidence. Therefore the APRN must critically appraise the various documents for their contribution to current best evidence, extract pertinent data, and set aside findings that do not address the clinical question under scrutiny. This process begins with separation of individual research reports and systematic reviews summarizing research findings from secondary sources, such as integrative review articles or editorials, via a title search. An integrative review is a comprehensive discussion of research, expert opinion, and theoretical knowledge about a topic (Cronin & George 2020). Although the integrative review typically includes studies that may provide valuable sources of evidence when subjected to an ancestry search, it is ultimately a synthesis of knowledge about a given topic, rather than an evidence-based review of studies. Similarly, opinion-based articles such as editorials are eliminated because they report expert opinion rather than original research.

Evidence Pyramid

After eliminating articles that do not report or systematically review original data, the remaining studies are usually evaluated based on a pyramid of evidence (Bracke et al., 2008; Fig. 8.1). The pyramid provides a taxonomy for ranking a study's contribution to current best evidence. The base of this pyramid comprises laboratory-based studies using animals (in vivo model), tissue samples, cell lines, or chemical media (in vitro models). While these studies are typically well designed and apply much more rigid controls than those used in clinical research, they are eliminated because their findings do not yield evidence about efficacy, safety, or predictive power in *human* subjects treated in a clinical setting.

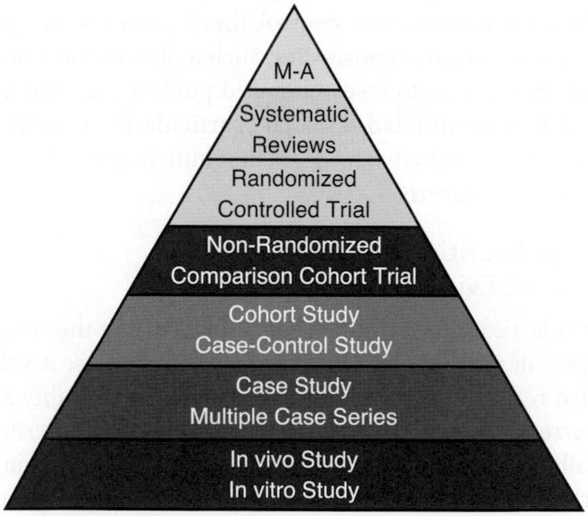

Fig. 8.1 ■ Pyramid illustrating levels of evidence used to evaluate efficacy of an intervention. *M-A*, Meta-analysis.

The second rung up from the base of the evidence pyramid is typically occupied by individual or multiple case series. A case study is a detailed description of results when an individual patient, family, inpatient care unit, long-term care facility, healthcare system, or community is subjected to an intervention or intervention bundle (Polit & Beck, 2021). Multiple case series summarize results from more than one patient or community. The results of case studies and multiple case series can be used to demonstrate that an intervention is feasible, offers an attractive alternative to usual care, can be applied safely in a selected patient or patients, and merits further investigation to determine efficacy. However, individual case studies or multiple case series do not compare the intervention of interest with a control or standard care, and their results cannot be used to reach conclusions about efficacy, effectiveness, or predictive power. The APRN must remain aware that findings from these designs tend to favor positive effects of the intervention.

The higher rungs of the evidence pyramid are occupied by the RCT, nonrandomized comparison cohort trials, and cohort or case-control studies. Results of one or more studies employing these designs are typically used to determine current best evidence. The nonrandomized comparison cohort trial shares certain similarities with the RCT; it compares outcomes from at least two groups, including one cohort that is exposed to an experimental intervention and a second group exposed to usual care, a sham device, or placebo (Polit & Beck, 2021). However, this study design uses nonrandomly selected groups because of ethical, financial, or other considerations. This lack of random group assignment creates potential bias in group membership likely to influence study findings.

A cohort study is a prospective, observational design in which a large sample is identified and followed over time to determine which participants will develop a disease or disorder under scrutiny (Polit & Beck, 2021). A cohort study allows researchers to identify new (incident) cases and temporal relationships between preventive interventions or constitutional factors and incidence. While the cohort study provides valuable results, data collection requires an extended observation period, resulting in a comparatively high likelihood of subject dropout and significant cost.

The case-control study provides a less expensive but less robust alternative to the cohort study. It requires comparison of two groups, one with the condition under study and the other free from the condition at a single point in time. The cohort study prospectively identifies cases from persons who remain free of the disorder of interest, and the nonrandomized comparison cohort study relies on identification of two groups, those with a condition (cases) and a second group without the condition (controls). Selection of this second group (controls) is especially difficult and often acts as a source of bias within this retrospective design (Polit & Beck, 2021). These study designs differ from that of the RCT because they are observational rather than interventional in nature. Study findings can be used to identify relationships between the presence of a given factor and the likelihood of the condition being studied, but they cannot be used to establish a cause-and-effect relationship between the associated factor and disease or disorder that is needed to determine efficacy.

The nested case-control study is a newer hybrid research design that blends elements of cohort and case-control studies. In this design, the researcher prospectively or retrospectively identifies cases (participants with a disease or disorder) and compares them to controls (participants who have not developed the condition at the time of disease occurrence in the case participants; Biesheuvel et al., 2008). Advantages of the nested control include the ability to analyze subgroups from a larger cohort and to generate new studies from vulnerable populations within a larger cohort while reducing selection bias compared with a traditional case-control study.

The most powerful study design is the RCT, which is considered the gold standard for measuring the efficacy of an intervention or predictive power of an assessment strategy (Sackett, 2015; Turner, 2012). *Efficacy* is defined as the likelihood that an intervention will achieve the desired outcome in a group of subjects based on evaluation in a research setting that controls for random effects produced by extrinsic factors. The concept of efficacy must be differentiated from *effectiveness*, which is defined as the effect of a specific intervention when administered to a particular patient at a given point during the course of an illness or condition.

Several types of RCTs are commonly reported in the healthcare literature (Chow & Liu, 2014). The parallel design RCT assigns subjects randomly allocated to an experimental group to a control group exposed to a placebo, sham device, or standard intervention. A crossover RCT is characterized by random assignment of subjects to an experimental or control group, followed by crossing the subject over to the alternative group after a washout period designed to remove (wash away) initial exposure effect. Although the crossover RCT requires fewer subjects and less cost than the parallel group design, it carries the potential for contamination of findings caused by residual effects when subjects are crossed over. The factorial RCT compares two or more experimental interventions with a control group treated with a placebo, sham, or usual care. Because the RCT is the most powerful study design, it should be routinely included when reviewing the literature for current best evidence.

Systematic Reviews and Meta-Analyses

Even though the RCT is considered the most powerful individual research design, the highest rung of the evidence pyramid is typically occupied by systematic reviews with meta-analyses (see Fig. 8.1). This design is placed at the apex of the evidence pyramid because it pools data from multiple studies to determine the effect created by a specific intervention. A systematic review uses a structured methodology to comprehensively seek out, select, appraise, and analyze studies based on a measurable clinical question (Holly et al., 2017). The methods used for generating a systematic review are comparable to those used to identify current best evidence for clinical decision making, and the rise of EBP closely parallels the recent explosion of systematic reviews published in the professional literature.

While the benefits of meta-analysis are apparent, studies must be carefully analyzed before completing this type of statistical analysis. This evaluation is based on data extraction and consideration of the sample populations of the various studies, experimental intervention, study methods, and outcome variables used to determine treatment effect. The outcomes of a meta-analysis based on a dichotomous (nominal) outcome measure are usually expressed as an odds ratio, relative risk, or absolute risk reduction, depending on the nature of the clinical question. The results of a meta-analysis based on a continuous outcome variable will be based on the weighted mean difference and standardized mean difference, usually referred to as *effect size*. The precision of the magnitude of the effect size is expressed by the accompanying confidence interval.

The evidence pyramid is useful for the APRN engaging in EBP because it provides a taxonomy for categorizing studies based on their potential contribution to current best evidence needed to answer a clinical question. Nevertheless, research design alone cannot be used to judge the quality of individual studies or their contribution to current best evidence (Holly et al., 2017). As discussed earlier, RCTs provide an excellent design for evaluating interventions such as a drug or behavioral therapy, but their expense limits the number of available studies. Rather, systematic reviews often pool findings from nonrandomized trials or observational studies such as cohort or case-control studies. In addition, the quality of one or more RCTs may be less than optimal. Ogilvie et al. (2005) evaluated systematic reviews of the efficacy of psychosocial interventions and observed that including RCTs alone is likely to miss pertinent evidence because these interventions are embedded with physical interventions.

Critical Appraisal

Individual Studies. After eliminating studies that do not evaluate clinical outcomes, the APRN must evaluate the quality of individual studies by identifying sources of potential bias (Higgins & Green, 2011). In selected circumstances, this evaluation may be used to eliminate studies that do not meet criteria for meta-analysis or contain sufficient flaws that severely compromise the generalizability of findings. However, studies must not be eliminated because they report negative findings or based on design alone. Although no standardized form for evaluating study quality exists, several models have been developed that provide a useful framework for evaluating bias within individual studies. Melnyk and Fineout-Overholt (2010) have advocated for a Critical Appraisal Guide for Quantitative Studies (Table 8.6). Alternatively, the CONSORT (Consolidated Standards of Reporting Trials) criteria for improving reporting the results of RCTs and the STROBE (Strengthening Reporting of Observational Studies in Epidemiology) criteria for reporting the results of observational epidemiologic studies can be adapted to enable assessment of bias within individual studies (Moher et al., 2001; von Elm et al., 2007). Fig. 8.2 is the form used by the Cochrane Collaboration. It is based on a three-level ranking (0–2), where a score of 2 indicates the criterion was clearly met, a score of 1 indicates it was partially met, and a score of 0 indicates it was not met. Tables 8.7 and 8.8 summarize criteria for an initial evaluation of study quality adapted from the CONSORT and STROBE statements, respectively (Moher et al., 2001; von Elm et al., 2007). While

TABLE 8.6
Critical Appraisal Guide for Quantitative Studies

Question	Evaluation Criteria
Why was the study done?	Does the study include clearly stated research questions, aims, hypotheses, or purpose statements?
What is the sample size?	Did the study enroll enough subjects to allow statistical analysis so that results did not occur by chance?
Are the instruments used to measure major variables valid and reliable?	Were the outcome measures of the study clearly defined? Were instruments used to measure these outcomes valid and reliable?
How were data analyzed?	What statistical tests were used to determine whether the study purpose was achieved?
Were there any untoward events during the study?	Did subjects withdraw before completing the study; if so, why did they withdraw?
How do results fit with previous research in this area?	Did the researchers base their work on a thorough literature review?
What does this research mean for clinical practice?	Is the study purpose an important clinical issue?

Adapted from *Evidence-Based Practice in Nursing and Healthcare: A Guide to Best Practice*, by B. M. Melnyk and E. Fineout-Overholt, 2010, Wolters-Kluwer.

Review:
Quality Assessment Tool
Study ID #__ Raters initials: __ Date__

	Scoring	Score	Query	A/B/C
A: Was the assigned treatment adequately concealed prior to allocation?	2 = Method did not allow disclosure of assignment 1 = Small but possible chance of disclosure of assignment or unclear 0 = quasirandomized or open list/tables Clearly yes = A Not sure = B Clearly no = C			
B: Were the outcomes of patients who withdrew described and included in the analysis (intention to treat)?	2 = withdrawals well described and accounted for in analysis 1 = withdrawals described and analysis not possible 0 = no mention, inadequate mention or obvious differences and no adjustment			
C: Were the outcome assessors blinded to treatment status?	2 = effective action taken to blind assessors 1 = small or moderate chance of unblinding of assessors 0 = not mentioned or not possible			
D: Were the treatment and control group comparable at entry?	2 = good comparability of groups, or confounding adjusted for in analysis 1 = confounding small; mentioned but not adjusted for 0 = large potential for confounding, or not discussed			
E. Were the subjects blind to the assignment status after allocation?	2 = effective action taken to blind subjects 1 = Small or moderate chance of unblinding of subjects 0 = not possible, or not mentioned (unless double-blind) or possible but not done			
F. Were the treatment providers blind to assignment status?	2 = effective action taken to blind treatment providers 1 = Small or moderate chance of unblinding of treatment providers			

Fig. 8.2 ■ **Individual study quality assessment tool.** (From "Study Quality Guide: Guide for Review Authors on Assessing Study Quality," by Cochrane Collaboration, 2013, https://cccrg.cochrane.org/sites/cccrg.cochrane.org/files/public/uploads/StudyQualityGuide_May%202013.pdf)

	0 = not possible, or not mentioned (unless double-blind) or possible but not done		
G: Were care programs, other than the trial options, identical?	2 = care programs clearly identical 1 = clear but trivial differences 0 = not mentioned, or clear and important differences in care programs		
H. Were the inclusion and exclusion criteria clearly defined?	2 = clearly defined 1 = inadequately defined 0 = not defined		
I. Were the interventions clearly defined?	2 = clearly defined 1 = inadequately defined 0 = not defined		
J. Were the outcome measures used clearly defined?	2 = clearly defined 1 = inadequately defined 0 = not defined		
	Outcome 1:		
	Outcome 2:		
	Outcome 3:		
	Outcome 4:		
	Outcome 5:		
K. Were diagnostic tests used in outcome assessment clinically useful?	2 = optimal 1 = adequate 0 = not defined, not adequate		
	Outcome 1:		
	Outcome 2:		
	Outcome 3:		
	Outcome 4:		
	Outcome 5:		
L. Was the surveillance active, and of clinically appropriate duration?	2 = optimal 1 = adequate 0 = not defined, not adequate		
	Outcome 1:		
	Outcome 2:		
	Outcome 3:		
	Outcome 4:		
	Outcome 5:		

Fig. 8.2 ■ **cont'd**

these statements were designed to assess quality of an individual study, they can be easily adapted for evaluating studies included in a scoping or systematic review.

Appraisal of Systematic Reviews and Meta-Analyses. Few instruments have been developed and validated for the evaluation of potential bias in systematic reviews with or without meta-analysis of pooled data. A technical report prepared for the AHRQ identified more than 20 guidelines for evaluating the quality of systematic reviews, but only 2 were considered high quality (West et al., 2002). Nevertheless, this report identified common factors that should be incorporated into any evaluation of the quality of systematic review; they included presence of a clear clinical question, methods for searching the literature and extracting data, and recommendations for practice or policy based on identified evidence (Table 8.9).

TABLE 8.7

Evaluating Quality of the Randomized Controlled Trial and Nonrandomized Comparison Cohort Trial

Criterion Section of the Research Report	Evidence That Criterion Was Met
Study purpose (introduction and background)	The purpose of the study is clearly stated. A rationale for the study is clearly stated and supported by appropriate literature.
Study participants (methods)	Inclusion and exclusion criteria for study participants are described, along with the study setting.
Study aims (methods)	Measurable research aims, questions, or hypotheses. These statements include measurable study outcomes consistent with the stated purpose of the study.
Sample size (methods)	The authors describe how the sample size was determined. Ideally, sample size is based on a power analysis to determine the number of subjects needed to determine group differences. The sample size recruited may be slightly larger than the minimum group size suggested by the power analysis to account for subjects who withdraw prior to completion of data collection.
Random allocation (methods)	Methods used to achieve random allocation are described, the success of randomization may be illustrated in a table comparing demographic and key clinical characteristics between experimental and control groups, and inferential analysis should identify no significant differences between groups. Procedures for group selection in the nonrandomized comparison cohort trial are described. Absence of randomization in group assignment is clearly acknowledged, and a table comparing demographic and key clinical characteristics of intervention and comparison group is provided.
Blinding (methods)	Study participants and data collectors are blinded to group assignment whenever feasible; blinding is not feasible for multiple nursing interventions, such as education or counseling.
Statistical methods (methods)	Appropriate statistical methods are used to compare primary and secondary outcomes. Descriptive statistics and inferential statistical analyses are based on considerations of level of measurement (nominal, ordinal, or continuous) and distribution of data. Multivariate analyses are used when multiple outcome measures are analyzed. Intention to treat analysis is used, when indicated.
Participant flow (methods and results)	Study procedures are thoroughly described in the methods section; a diagram of participant flow may be placed in the results section. The number of subjects who do not complete data collection is stated, and reasons for early study withdrawal are clearly stated. Ideally, the proportion of patients who do not complete the study is ≤15%.
Outcomes (results)	Outcomes based on research questions or aims are stated for each group and the precision of the outcomes is measured using a 95% confidence interval.
Adverse events	Adverse events are reported, along with their impact on study completion.
Generalizability	Results are interpreted in the context of current evidence along with limitations of the study, including potential sources of bias. Limitations associated with multiple analyses are discussed.

Adapted from "The CONSORT Statement: Revised Recommendations for Improving the Quality of Reports of Parallel-Group Randomized Trials," by D. Moher, K. F. Schulz, D. Altman, and CONSORT Group, 2001, *JAMA, 285,* 42.

The APRN should evaluate the systematic review for sources of potential bias associated with study retrieval. Common sources are time-, language-, and geography-related bias, as well as publication bias (discussed in *Strategies for Searching Electronic Databases*; Campbell et al., 2015).

Time-related bias may be created when systematic reviewers limit the time frame for study inclusion.

TABLE 8.8

Evaluating Quality of Observational Studies: Adapted From the STROBE Statement

Criterion Section of the Research Report	Evidence That Criterion Was Met
Study purpose (introduction and background)	The purpose of the study is clearly stated. A rationale for the study is clearly stated and supported by appropriate literature.
Study participants (methods)	Eligibility criteria for study participation and follow-up criteria are clearly described for the cohort study. Criteria for cases and controls are described for the case-control study; criteria used to match cases and controls are clearly described.
Study outcomes (methods)	Outcome variables are clearly defined, along with confounding factors and potential associated (predictive) factors. Diagnostic criteria for differentiating cases and controls are clearly described for cohort and case-control studies.
Bias (methods)	Potential sources of bias are acknowledged.
Statistical methods (methods)	Appropriate statistical methods are used to analyze primary and secondary outcome measures. Descriptive statistics and inferential statistical analyses are based on considerations of level of measurement (nominal, ordinal, or continuous) and distribution of data. Multivariate analyses are used when multiple outcome measures are analyzed. An explanation of methods used to control for confounding factors and how missing data were managed is provided.
Participants (results)	Demographic and pertinent clinical characteristics of cases and controls are described.
Outcome data (results)	For the cohort study, a report of incidence or summary measures over time should be reported. For the case-control study, outcomes of variables potentially associated with likelihood of status as a case or control subject are reported. Association between outcome as a case or control should be based on multivariate analysis when multiple factors are analyzed.
Generalizability (discussion)	Key findings are presented based on study questions or aims. Limitations of the study are clearly acknowledged, including sources of bias and inability to determine cause and effect based on the presence of statistically significant associations. Limitations associated with multiple inferential analyses are acknowledged.

Adapted from "Strengthening the Reporting of Observational Studies in Epidemiology (STROBE) Statement: Guidelines for Reporting Observational Studies," by E. von Elm, D. G. Altman, M. Egger, S. J. Pocock, P. C. Gøtzsche, J. P. Vandenbroucke, and STROBE Initiative, 2007, *BMJ, 335*, 869–870.

Ideally, decisions about time frames in a systematic review should include the latest publications available at the time the review was conducted and extend backward to a *meaningful* point in time. This meaningful point may be based on a landmark event, such as passage of legislation, development of a novel intervention or diagnostic technology, or approval of a drug for use. Gaps in the timeline must be avoided.

Language-related bias is also common in systematic reviews. Although English is the predominant language of science (Meneghini & Packer, 2007), and most articles in MEDLINE and CINAHL are published in English, many studies are only published in other languages. The potential for language-related bias associated with the use of English language–only sources should be acknowledged in the methods section or discussion of a systematic review.

Risk of Bias in Systematic Studies (ROBIS) is a validated instrument specifically developed for assessment of bias in systematic reviews. It was designed to reflect the domain-based structure used by the Cochrane Collaboration when identifying bias in individual studies (Whiting et al., 2016). The instrument is divided into three phases. In the first phase, the user is prompted to evaluate whether the systematic review adequately adhered to the stated inclusion and exclusion criteria;

TABLE 8.9

Criteria for Evaluation of a Systematic Review, With or Without a Meta-Analysis

Criterion	Evidence That Criterion Was Met
Study question	A clearly defined clinical question is provided; the question should define the patient population and problem, intervention or assessment strategy under scrutiny, comparison treatment, and outcomes indicating intervention effect or predictive power of the assessment strategy.
Inclusion or exclusion criteria	Search methods are clearly described. Techniques used to identify studies include electronic database searches along with techniques to increase the efficiency of the search, such as ancestry search, consultation with experts in the field of inquiry, web engine searches, trial registries, and conference proceedings. Inclusion and exclusion criteria for studies are clearly stated. Potential sources of bias in selection criteria (time-, language-, and geography-related) are acknowledged and minimized.
Data extraction	The process for data extraction from individual studies is clearly described. A standardized protocol for data extraction is included in the methods section of the systematic review. This protocol specifies persons involved in data extraction and procedures for coding data, ranking study quality, building consensus about data extraction, and resolving conflicts in individual study coding. Incorporation of an independent coder is used to measure reliability (interrater agreement rates) similar to that used for reporting original data when multiple data collectors participate in a research protocol. Interrater agreement rates should vary from 75% to 100%. A persuasive rationale for excluding studies based on methodological quality is provided and excluded studies are clearly identified. The process used to weight evidence (e.g., results of meta-analysis, ranking of evidence) is clearly defined. The process for determining study quality, including weighting of the study for purposes of evidence ranking or meta-analysis, is clearly explained. Evidence ranking is based on consensus among authors, and a process for resolving disagreements concerning quality rankings via consensus is clearly described.
Recommendations for clinical practice	Recommendations for clinical practice are supported by evidence extracted from the systematic review. The strength of recommendations should be specified and the process for determining strength of recommendation clearly explained. Ideally, evidence ranking and determination of strength of recommendations for clinical practice are based on validated and published ranking systems.

Adapted from Appraising the Quality of Systematic Reviews. FOCUS Technical Brief No. 17, by R. W. Schlosser, 2007, p. 2-6 http://ktdrr.org/ktlibrary/articles_pubs/ncddrwork/focus/focus17/Focus17.pdf; and Systems to Rate the Strength of Scientific Evidence. Evidence Report–Technology Assessment No. 47. AHRQ Publication 02-E016, by S. West King, V., Carey, T. S., Lohr, K. N., McKoy, N., Sutton, S. F., & Lux, L, 2002, Agency for Healthcare Research and Quality. https://www.ncbi.nlm.nih.gov/books/NBK11930/#A86942

whether these criteria were clearly stated, mutually exclusive, and unambiguous; and whether these criteria appeared appropriate for the question(s) or aim(s) of the systematic review. The second phase includes an evaluation of the techniques used to identify and retrieve studies, such as use of more than one electronic database, selection of multiple search terms, restrictions based on language or publication format, and efforts to minimize errors in study selection. It also prompts users to evaluate the methods used to synthesize findings, extract data, and present findings using appropriate outcomes such as risk, effect size, and sensitivity analyses or funnel plots. Phase 3 prompts users to evaluate the methods used to detect sources of potential bias within individual studies and their relevance to the clinical question. It also prompts users to evaluate whether the authors of the systematic review summarized findings based on statistical significance alone. Access to this instrument, along with guidance for its use, is available at http://www.bristol.ac.uk/social-community-medicine/projects/robis/.

Data Extraction

Data extraction requires more than simply retrieving studies and basing a clinical decision on a generalized impression of findings. Instead, the APRN should use a consistent process to extract only pertinent outcomes based on criteria determined in the clinical question posed in Step 1. To ensure consistency, study review and data extraction should follow a predetermined protocol, just as original research adheres to established study procedures. The process used to extract data varies based on the nature of the clinical question. For example, the protocol used in a systematic review of a specific intervention differs from a review of a diagnostic test. The Cochrane Collaboration (http://bjmt.cochrane.org/resources-developing-review) provides excellent resources for creating a standardized protocol for data extraction (Fig. 8.3). The web page also provides a standardized form designed to aid the clinician when extracting data from RCTs comparing the effects of multiple interventions.

Step 4: Implement Useful Findings in Clinical Decision Making

Implementing useful findings is a deceptively complex process. This process occurs on multiple levels, including clinical decision making when caring for an individual patient, creation and implementation of policies on a facility- or community-wide level, and creation of evidence-based clinical practice guidelines designed to set standards of care on a national or global level. Clinical decision making is based on evidence of the intervention's predictive power or efficacy, consideration of physical and psychosocial factors influencing effectiveness when applied to an individual patient, and knowledge of its direct cost or economic impact (van Rijswijk & Gray, 2012). For example, while a new drug may prove effective in a Phase 3 pivotal trial, its inclusion in a clinical practice guideline also must address its comparative effectiveness to existing agents with similar pharmacologic actions, its adverse side effects, and cost. The increased cost associated with a new drug may be justified if it proves more effective than existing agents or is associated with a lower risk of adverse side effects.

The process of implementing findings from an EBP document requires generation of recommendations for clinical practice. The strength of these recommendations varies according to the strength of the underlying evidence. Similar to classification systems used to grade evidence, more than 60 taxonomies for grading the strength of practice recommendations are available (Garcia et al., 2010). Widely used systems include the Strength of Recommendation for Treatment taxonomy (SORT) scale; United States Preventative Services Task Force (USPSTF) recommendations; Grading of Recommendations Assessment, Development and Evaluation (GRADE) scales; UK National Institute for Health and Care Excellence (NICE) scale; Center for Preventive Medicine scale; and Scottish Intercollegiate Guideline Network (SIGN) taxonomy. Garcia et al. (2010) compared the effect of evidence-based clinical decision making for a child with diarrhea using four scales (NICE, GRADE, Centre for Evidence-Based Medicine [CEBM], and SIGN scales) in a group of 216 novice physicians (pediatric residents). A significant number of physicians changed their recommendation for management in an index case after reviewing these guidelines. Of the four, the GRADE scale was found to exert the greatest influence on clinical decision making.

The GRADE scale was developed by a group of clinicians who ranked the strength of clinical recommendations based on current best evidence using a four-point scale (Atkins et al., 2004; Brozek et al., 2009). The highest grade indicates benefits that clearly outweigh potential for harm, the second level indicates that benefits of treatment must be carefully weighed against potential adverse sides effects, the third level indicates that balance between benefit and harm cannot be clearly distinguished based on best available evidence, and the lowest grade level indicates that the best available evidence suggests the intervention is likely to produce more harm than benefit (Box 8.1).

A second ranking system will be familiar to many APRNs practicing in North America. The US Preventive Services Task Force (USPSTF) uses an ordinal scale with grades ranging from A to D and a fifth category labeled I (Trinite et al., 2009). Similar to the rankings advocated by the GRADE Working Group, recommendations for practice are linked to the direction, magnitude, and balance between benefit and harm. Table 8.10 summarizes the Task Force scale for recommendations for clinical practice.

FROM POLICY TO PRACTICE: TIPS FOR ACHIEVING MEANINGFUL CHANGES IN PRACTICE BASED ON CURRENT BEST EVIDENCE

Although the EBP process is effective for identifying current best evidence, completion of the process does not guarantee meaningful changes in the behavior of clinicians essential to achieve desired clinical outcomes. In contrast, evidence strongly suggests that merely

{Review name}- Basic information for study ID: ....

Method

Randomisation	Blinding	Intention to treat - Loss to Follow-up

Participants

N	Age	Sex	Type of injury:
Country	Hospital	Period of Study	Other participants (not review?)

Inclusion criteria	Exclusion Criteria

Interventions

Intervention (including description, when started, frequency, duration & when stopped etc)

Overall length of follow-up:

Outcomes

Outcomes	Tick if available	How measured	When done

Notes - see over **Reviewer:**

Fig. 8.3 Data extraction form of individual studies comparing two groups. (From Ryan, R., Hill, S., Prictor, M., & McKenzie, J; Cochrane Consumers and Communication Review Group.(2013). Study quality guide. https://cccrg.cochrane.org/sites/cccrg.cochrane.org/files/public/uploads/StudyQualityGuide_May%202013.pdf)

BOX 8.1

Grade Scale

1. High evidence indicates that additional research is unlikely to change confidence of the direction or magnitude of the effect size associated with a specific intervention.
2. Moderate evidence indicates that additional research may significantly influence the magnitude of treatment effect.
3. Low evidence indicates that new research may affect the direction and magnitude of treatment effect.
4. Very low evidence indicates insufficient evidence to determine treatment effect.

introducing a new policy is unlikely to lead to meaningful or sustained changes in practice (Ryan, 2017). Many EBP innovations lead to short-term adoption by a limited number of clinicians (Stetler, 2003). To overcome this problem, the APRN must be aware of successful strategies to design and implement a structured program for translating current best evidence into meaningful and sustained changes in practice. Rogers' diffusion of innovation theory provides a useful framework (Rogers, 2003). This theoretical framework describes four stages that an individual clinician or group will experience when evaluating and deciding to adopt or reject a practice innovation. The first phase, described as the knowledge stage, occurs when clinicians are made aware of the innovation and its potential impact on practice and patient outcomes. Typically, the innovation is introduced through continuing education activities, announcement of a practice innovation, or informal communication from colleagues or informal clinical leaders. Historically, many clinicians believed that simply introducing a practice innovation is sufficient to ensure a sustained practice change, but research utilization studies have repeatedly proven this assumption false (Rogers, 2003; Stetler, 2003).

The second stage is based on persuasion. During this stage, clinicians will form a favorable or unfavorable attitude toward the practice innovation. Although the decision-making process is highly individualized, formation of a positive attitude is primarily determined by two major factors: the perceived benefit of the innovation on patient outcomes and the investment required to alter practice. Such considerations are particularly relevant when an EBP innovation comprises an intervention bundle. For example, current best

TABLE 8.10

US Preventive Services Task Force Scale for Strength of Recommendations for Clinical Practice

Rank	Description	Recommendation for Practice
A	The service[a] is recommended and supported by evidence of substantial benefit.	The APRN should offer or provide this service when indicated.
B	The action is recommended and supported by strong evidence of moderate benefit associated with the service or moderate-level evidence suggesting moderate to substantial benefit from the service.	The APRN should offer or provide this service when indicated.
C	Evidence suggests that the service provides only a small benefit.	The APRN should offer or provide this service only when other considerations support offering or providing this service.
D	Evidence demonstrates no benefit from the service or potential harm outweighs the service.	The APRN should discourage use of the service.
I	Current evidence is insufficient to assess the balance between harm and benefit of the service.	The APRN should counsel patients about the uncertainty of the balance between benefit and harm before offering or providing this service.

[a]*Service* is defined as an intervention, intervention bundle, or assessment strategy.

From "The US Preventive Services Task Force: An Evidence-Based Prevention Resource for Nurse Practitioners," by T. Trinite, C. L. Cherry, and L. Marion, 2009, *Journal of the American Academy of Nurse Practitioners, 21,* 303.

evidence indicates that prevention of facility-acquired pressure injuries is based on a number of preventive interventions, including risk assessment using a validated instrument (National Pressure Injury Advisory Panel et al., 2019). Various pressure injury risk instruments have been validated, but the Braden Scale for Pressure Sore Risk is predominant in North America (Bolton, 2007). This predominance is not based on its predictive power alone; instead, it is based on a combination of its predictive power and its parsimony.

The third phase (decision stage) occurs when individual clinicians reach a decision whether to support (accept) or oppose (reject) the innovation (Rogers, 2003). Historically, adoption was based on the judgment of a single decision maker, but the rise of EBP and interdisciplinary care teams has led to a more transparent separation of individual decision making from adoption of a practice innovation.

The final stage of innovation diffusion is adoption into daily clinical practice. Similar to the other stages, successful adoption requires more willingness to integrate the innovation into practice. It also requires adapting or restructuring the practice environment in a manner that enables clinicians to change practice. In order to facilitate adoption of an innovation, the APRN should consider the following factors: (1) its relative advantages, (2) its compatibility with current practice patterns, (3) the degree to which the innovation can be adapted on a trial basis, and (4) the degree to which results of the innovation can be observed (Rogers, 2003). Additional factors that favor adoption include support from organizational administration, clinical leadership at the inpatient unit or facility level, and manipulation of the practice environment to enhance adoption.

The degree to which a practice innovation can be adopted on a trial basis can also enhance the likelihood of its successful and sustained adoption (Rogers, 2003). For example, implementation of a facility-acquired pressure injury prevention program might include risk assessment using the Braden Scale for Predicting Pressure Sore Risk. In this case, integration of the Braden Scale into the hospital's electronic medical record, combined with an online training program, allows nurses to familiarize themselves with use of the instrument prior to officially adopting this assessment into routine practice (Magnan & Maklebust, 2008, 2009).

Adoption of an EBP innovation is also enhanced by the degree to which results are observable. Meaningful feedback has traditionally been reserved for administrators or select clinical leaders. However, we assert that front-line clinicians must be included in this feedback loop if they are to adopt practice changes on a sustained basis.

The process of implementing EBP in the APRN's local facility must be individualized based on existing practice patterns, staffing and resources of the facility, and its organizational culture (Carlson et al., 2012). Key elements needed for achieving a successful and sustained change in practice patterns are (1) identification of an interdisciplinary team of stakeholders to plan and implement the practice innovation, (2) support from the organization's administration, (3) a clinical leadership structure that supports EBP principles, and (4) feedback data for monitoring improvement and rewarding clinician stakeholders.

Stakeholder Engagement

Formation of an interdisciplinary team is essential to the implementation of a successful and sustained EBP innovation (Powell et al., 2012). This group should include key clinical leaders who will be affected by the proposed practice innovation, such as clinical nursing leaders, physicians, and other clinicians (e.g., physical or occupational therapists, case managers). This group will be most directly responsible for identifying current best evidence or using available resources, such as clinical guidelines, to guide practice innovation. The interdisciplinary team should also take primary responsibility for determining how the practice innovation should be incorporated into existing practice patterns based on analysis of local barriers and facilitators to implementation. Although evidence is limited, Weiner et al. (2008) have provided a detailed description of strategies that have proven effective for assessing organizational culture and barriers or facilitators likely to influence introduction of an EBP innovation. The core group should also design strategies to gain administrative support and support from key clinical leaders. An APRN is often the coordinator or leader of this interdisciplinary team.

Organizational Support

In some cases, administrative personnel may approach the APRN concerning the need for a practice innovation based on regulatory changes, such as the identification and promulgation of "never events" by the National Quality Forum and Centers for Medicare and Medicaid Services in 2008 (Drake-Land, 2008). However, clinical experience strongly suggests that most EBP innovations are initiated by a clinician seeking to improve patient care outcomes. Ensuring administrative support involves more than merely informing administrative personnel of an intention to change organizational practice based on EBP principles (Brindle et al., 2015). Instead, the APRN must work with key stakeholders to formulate a proposal that provides key administrative personnel with knowledge of the rationale for the recommended practice innovation, its anticipated impact on patient outcomes and associated costs, and the extent of needed resources, which will vary depending on the practice innovation proposed. Essential resources usually include a commitment to clinical leaders and staff education about the proposed innovation, alterations to the electronic health record, disposable supplies or durable medical equipment needed to implement the practice change, and a system for measuring outcomes and providing staff and stakeholders with meaningful feedback.

Clinical Leadership Support

The presence of a corporate culture and clinical leadership structure that supports EBP principles may be the single most important factor influencing the adoption of EBP innovations (Creehan et al., 2016; Rapp et al., 2010). Rapp et al. (2010) evaluated barriers to the implementation of EBP initiatives and observed that the behavior of clinical supervisors forms a substantial barrier to statewide EBP innovation projects. Specifically, they found that although clinical leaders did not oppose the use of EBP principles for clinical decision making, they did not set expectations among front-line clinicians, relying instead on informal methods of practice adoption. Although this approach may not act as a barrier to select clinicians who share an inherent interest in EBP and practice innovation, it ultimately favors maintenance of the status quo rather than organizational adoption of EBP principles and practice innovations.

Fortunately, several strategies have been identified to avoid this potential barrier to the adoption of EBP innovations. Obtaining Magnet status is a strategy for promoting an organizational environment that promotes EBP in nursing practice. Magnet status from the American Nurses Credentialing Center requires the integration of EBP principles into nursing care (Reigle et al., 2008). Although obtaining Magnet status is a major undertaking that goes well beyond the implementation of a single EBP innovation, it has been shown to aid facilities when transforming an organizational culture to one that promotes these principles.

Involvement of clinical leadership facilitates unit- or facility-based adoption of EBP practice innovations. Clinical leaders, such as the clinical nurse specialist, may act as facility-wide leaders for EBP changes by working with an interdisciplinary team evaluating policies and procedures for care delivery. The clinical nurse specialist also may act as mentor and educator for unit- or clinic-based champions, which has been shown to facilitate adoption of EBP innovations in multiple healthcare settings (Taggart et al., 2012; Yevchak et al., 2014). The unit- or clinic-based champion is a clinician who practices on the unit and acts as a mentor to front-line staff nurses and others to implement EBP innovations. Selection of effective champions is critical; Rogers (2003) noted that group adoption of innovation occurs in a stepwise manner, with some individuals acting as early adopters, followed by the majority who adopt the innovation based on the actions of early adopters, followed by a second minority of individuals (late adopters) who change practice only after it becomes apparent that the innovation is inevitable. Clinicians who are early adopters and are recognized as informal practice leaders are ideal champions.

Research has identified several strategies that enhance the effectiveness of unit-based champions (Taggart et al., 2012; Yevchak et al., 2014). These include scheduling time for them to receive education for their enhanced role and to meet with clinical experts and unit managers as their role is delineated. Production and distribution of easily accessible educational materials for staff, including online information, pocket cards, and traditional education sessions tailored to staff with varying work hours, have also been shown to enhance the effectiveness of unit-based champions on daily practice. The APRN can enhance the effectiveness of unit champions by participating in clinical rounds and case presentations and being available for consultation as needed.

Evidence-Based Practice Innovation: Feedback

As noted earlier, generating objective and meaningful outcomes when engaging in an EBP change is essential to determine its impact on clinical outcomes and cost. Feedback should be easily interpretable to all stakeholders and provided on a regular basis to promote sustained changes. For example, feedback may include regular reporting of facility-wide pertinent clinical outcomes, such as reduction in surgical site infections or indwelling urinary catheter days, or it may include individual provider or unit outcomes. While the value of providing feedback as a means of engaging clinical staff in an EBP innovation seems apparent, evidence concerning its impact is mixed. For example, a study of a structured monthly feedback program on a ventilator care prevention bundle in two urban critical care units found no effect on adherence after 1 year (Lawrence & Fulbrook, 2012). Similarly, researchers conducted a cluster RCT that analyzed the impact of a monthly versus quarterly feedback strategy on nursing shifts (the unit of analysis for this cluster RCT) in 24 Dutch intensive care units (de Vos et al., 2015). No differences in adherence to evidence-based guideline standards were found when the structured feedback intervention was compared with standard feedback. Whether these results reflect the lack of efficacy of any structured feedback program versus lack of effect owing to the nature of the feedback is not clear. Additional research is needed before recommendations concerning routine feedback for front-line clinicians participating in an EBP innovation can be made.

FUTURE PERSPECTIVES

The identification and evaluation of studies to identify current best evidence is based on a hierarchy that identifies the RCT as the most powerful study design for generating evidence, along with systematic reviews and meta-analyses of pooled data from multiple RCTs to reach conclusions about the strength of evidence. Although the RCT remains the best research design for evaluating the efficacy of an intervention, it does not necessarily follow that determination of efficacy indicates that an intervention will prove effective when applied in daily clinical practice as opposed to the rigidly controlled clinical trial setting (van Rijswijk & Gray, 2012). In addition, evaluations of current best evidence do not incorporate other real-world factors that influence treatment effectiveness when applied to the management of individual patients, such as patient preference and the impact of cost. In order to address these gaps, clinicians, researchers, and policymakers are working together to look at sources of real-world data as complementary to data generated from traditional research designs.

For example, in 2010, Congress allocated funds for development and generation of comparative effectiveness studies that seek to measure clinical effectiveness based on considerations of treatment effect, patient preference, and resource allocation (Patient Protection and Affordable Care Act, 2010; US Department of Health and Human Services, Health Resources and Services Administration, 2011). At the same time, the National Institutes of Health formed the Patient-Centered Outcomes Research Institute (PCORI), which was charged with generating research to help patients and providers make more informed decisions about their own care. The Institute continues to fund comparative effectiveness studies. This approach differs from traditional EBP processes because it relies on data collected under real-world conditions rather than the highly controlled environment of the RCT (AHRQ, 2016). Alternatives to traditional EBP sources also include real-world clinical trials and health sciences research. The essential components of a well-designed, real-world trial continue to evolve, but basic principles include comparison of existing options for treatment, enrolling participants with few inclusion and exclusion criteria, minimal or no manipulation of treatment interventions outside individual clinical judgment, and consideration of treatment effect, cost, and patient preference (Curtis et al., 2019). Health services research is generated by an interdisciplinary or transdisciplinary research team that investigates how social factors, financing systems, organizational structures, technologies, and individual behaviors affect access to health care (Aubin et al., 2019).

In addition, electronic databases are a rich source of real-world data stored in national repositories. An increasing number of robust databases exist that can be used to investigate clinical outcomes in large groups of patients; they include the Minimum Data

Set (MDS); Health Outcome and Assessment Information Set (OASIS); Surveillance, Epidemiology, and End Results Program (SEER); and the NDNQI (Yang et al., 2020). Key steps when mining data from these databases are (1) construct a clear research question or aim, (2) identify a database, (3) formulate a plan for extracting pertinent data, and (4) analyze and present findings based on the original aim or research question (A. K. Smith et al., 2011).

Though robust, access to these databases is limited. For the APRN seeking to answer questions within a particular facility or health system, the electronic health record (EHR) is an underutilized resource that is more easily accessible, is less expensive, and requires less time to analyze than the much larger national databases. Researchers have used EHRs to conduct epidemiologic investigations, cross-sectional studies within a given hospital, and longitudinal studies of patients managed in a health system (Casey et al., 2016). In addition, data from the EHR can form the bases of quality improvement projects. More work is needed to develop techniques for data extraction from this rich source, and further software development is needed to enhance clinicians' abilities to use these data to improve care outcomes.

CONCLUSION

EBP involves the generation of a clinically measurable question, identification of pertinent research findings, extraction of essential data, and implementation of findings. Intimate knowledge of this process is critical for the APRN to master three core levels of the EBP competency: application to individual clinical decision making, formulating policies for patient care in a local facility, and evaluating evidence in order to establish standards of care via clinical practice guidelines. These competencies are increasingly essential as the APRN functions as a team member, leader, and decision maker within an interdisciplinary healthcare team.

KEY SUMMARY POINTS

- Evidence-based practice is a core competency of advanced practice nursing.
- Evidence-based clinical decision making arises from a four-step process beginning with identification of a pertinent clinical question, systematic literature review, extraction of pertinent data, and implementation of findings into clinical practice.
- The APRN is well prepared to synthesize existing research findings needed to translate current best evidence into clinical practice on an individual, unit-wide, facility-wide, or health system–wide basis.
- Translating current best evidence into clinical practice requires more than simply introducing new policies or procedures in order to achieve meaningful or sustained changes in clinical practice.
- Formation of an interdisciplinary team of key stakeholders, clinical support, and clinical leadership on a facility-wide level from an APRN and others, along with unit-based support from clinical champions, are essential for achieving sustained changes in clinical practice.

REFERENCES

Agency for Healthcare Research and Quality. (2016). What is comparative effectiveness research? Retrieved from http://effectivehealthcare.ahrq.gov/index.cfm/what-is-comparative-effectiveness-research1/

Amberson, J., McMahon, B., & Pinner, M. (1931). A clinical trial of sanocrysin in pulmonary tuberculosis. *American Review of Tuberculosis, 21*, 401–435.

American Association of Colleges of Nursing. (2015). The Doctor of Nursing Practice: Current issues and clarifying recommendations. Report from the task force on the implementation of the DNP. https://moodle.selu.edu/moodle/pluginfile.php/1126669/mod_resource/content/2/AACN%20DNP%20White%20Paper.pdf

American Association of Colleges of Nursing. (2021a). The Essentials: Core competencies for professional nursing education. American Association of Colleges of Nursing.

American Association of Colleges of Nursing. (2021b). PhD in nursing. https://www.aacnnursing.org/News-Information/Research-Data-Center/PhD

Arndt, J. V., & Netsch, D. S. (2012). Research study or quality improvement project? *Journal of Wound, Ostomy, and Continence Nursing, 39*, 371–375.

Atkins, D., Best, D., Briss, P. A., Eccles, M., Falck-Ytter, Y., Flottorp, S., Guyatt, G. H., Harbour, R. T., Haugh, M. C., Henry, D., Hill, S., Jaeschke, R., Leng, G., Liberati, A., Magrini, N., Mason, J., Middleton, P., Mrukowicz, J., O'Connell, D., … Zaza, S. (2004). Grading quality of evidence and strength of recommendations. *BMJ (Clinical Research Ed.), 328*, 1490.

Aubin, D., Hebert, M., & Eurich, D. (2019). The importance of measuring the impact of patient-oriented research. *CMAJ Canadian Medical Association Journal, 191*(31), E860–E864.

Balakas, K., & Sparks, L. (2010). Teaching research and evidence-based practice using a service-learning approach. *Journal of Nursing Education, 49*, 691–695.

Barbosa-Cesnik, C., Brown, M. B., Buxton, M., Zhang, L., DeBusscher, J., & Foxman, B. (2011). Cranberry juice fails to prevent recurrent urinary tract infection: Results from a randomized placebo-controlled trial. *Clinical Infectious Disease, 52*, 23–30.

Biesheuvel, C. J., Vergouwe, Y., Oudega, R., Hoes, A. W., Grobbee, D. E., & Moons, K. G. M. (2008). Advantages of the nested case-control design in diagnostic research. *BMC Medical Research Methodology, 8*, 48. https://doi.org/10.1186/1471-2288-8-48

Bolton, L. (2007). Evidence-based report card. Operational definition of moist wound healing. *Journal of Wound, Ostomy, and Continence Nursing, 34*, 23–29.

Bracke, P. J., Howse, D. K., & Keim, S. M. (2008). Evidence-based medicine search: A customizable federated search engine. *Journal of the Medical Library Association, 96*, 108–113.

Bramer, W. M., Giustini, D., & Kramer, B. M. (2016). Comparing the coverage, recall, and precision of searches for 120 systematic reviews in Embase, MEDLINE, and Google Scholar: a prospective study. *Systematic Reviews, 5*(1), 1–7.

Brindle, C. T., Creehan, S., Black, J., & Zimmerman, D. (2015). The VCU Pressure Ulcer Summit: Collaboration to operationalize hospital-acquired pressure ulcer prevention best practice recommendations. *Journal of Wound, Ostomy, and Continence Nursing, 42*(4), 331–337.

Brozek, J. L., Akl, E. E., Alonso-Coello, P., Lang, D., Jaeschke, R., Williams, J. W., Phillips, B., Leigermann, M., Lethaby, A., Bousquet, J., Guyatt, G. H., & Schunemann, H. J. (2009). Grading quality of evidence and strength of recommendations in clinical practice guidelines. Part 1 of 3. An overview of the GRADE approach and grading quality of evidence about interventions. *Allergy, 64*, 669–677.

Campbell, J. M., Klugar, M., Ding, S., Carmody, D. P., Harkonsen, S. J., Jadotte, Y. T., White, S., & Munn, Z. (2015). Diagnostic test accuracy: Methods for systematic review and meta-analysis. *International Journal of Evidence Based Health Care, 13*(3), 154–162.

Carlson, L., Rapp, C. A., & Eichler, M. S. (2012). The experts rate: Supervisory behaviors that impact the implementation of evidence-based practices. *Community Mental Health Journal, 48*, 179–186.

Casey, J. A., Schwartz, B. S., Stewart, W. F., & Adler, N. E. (2016). Using electronic health records for population health research: A review of methods and applications. *Annual Reviews of Public Health, 37*, 61–81.

Chow, S. C., & Liu, J. P. (2014). *Design and analysis of randomized controlled trials: Concepts and methodologies*. John Wiley & Sons, Inc.

Cochrane Collaboration. (2021). About the Cochrane Library. http://www.cochranelibrary.com/about/about-the-cochrane-library.html

Cormier, J. W. (2011). Advancing FDA's regulatory science through weight of evidence evaluations. *Journal of Contemporary Health Law and Policy, 28*, 1–22.

Creehan, S., Cuddigan, J., Gonzalez, D., Nix, D., Padula, W., Pontieri-Lewis, J., Walden, C., Wells, B., & Wheeler, R. (2016). The VCU Pressure Ulcer Summit—Developing centers for pressure ulcer prevention excellence: A framework for sustainability. *Journal of Wound, Ostomy, and Continence Nursing, 43*(2), 121–128.

Cronin, M. A., & George, E. (2020). The why and how of the integrative review. *Organizational Research Methods*, 1–25. https://doi.org/10.1177/1094428120935507

Curtis, J. R., Foster, P. J., & Saag, K. G. (2019). Tools and methods for real-world evidence generation: Pragmatic trials, electronic consent, and data linkages. *Rheumatic Diseases Clinics of North America, 45*(2), 275–289.

Dal-Re, R. (2019). Plan S: Funders are committed to open access to scientific publication. *European Journal of Clinical Investigation, 49*(6), e13100.

Davis, C. R., & Beeson, T. (2020). Mitigating pressure injury challenges when placing patients in a prone position: A view from here. *Journal of Wound, Ostomy, and Continence Nursing, 47*(4), 326–327.

de Vos, M. L., van der Veer, S. N., Wouterse, B., Graafmans, W. C., Wilco, C., Peek, N., de Keizer, N. F., Jager, K. J., Westert, G. P., & van der Voort, P. H. (2015). A multifaceted feedback strategy alone does not improve the adherence to organizational guideline-based standards: A cluster randomized trial in intensive care. *Implementation Science, 10*(1), 1–9.

DiCenso, A., Cullum, N., & Ciliska, D. (2002). Implementing evidence-based nursing: Misconceptions. *Evidence-Based Nursing, 5*, 4–5.

Drake-Land, B. (2008). CMS never events. https://downloads.cms.gov/cmsgov/archived-downloads/smdl/downloads/smd073108.pdf

Ebell, M. H., Sokol, R., Lee, A., Simons, C., & Early, J. (2017). How good is the evidence to support primary care practice? *Evidence-Based Medicine, 22*(3), 88–92.

Edsberg, L. E., Black., J. M., Golberg., M., McNichol., L., Moore., L., & Sieggreen, M. (2016). Revised national pressure ulcer advisory panel pressure injury staging system: Revised pressure injury staging system. *Journal of Wound, Ostomy and Continence Nursing, 43*(6), 585–597.

Essential Evidence Plus. (2021). Browse our databases and interactive tools. https://www.essentialevidenceplus.com/#accept

European Medicines Agency. (2000). Points to consider on switching between superiority and non-inferiority. http://www.emea.europa.eu/docs/en_GB/document_library/Scientific_guideline/2009/09/WC500003658.pdf

Evans, M. M. (2010). Evidence-based practice protocol to improve glucose control in individuals with type-2 diabetes mellitus. *Medical-Surgical Nursing, 19*, 317–322.

Fineout-Overholt, E., Melnyk, B. M., Stillwell, S. B., & Williamson, K. M. (2010a). Evidence-based practice: Step by step. Critical appraisal of the evidence: Part I. *American Journal of Nursing, 110*, 47–52.

Fineout-Overholt, E., Melnyk, B. M., Stillwell, S. B., & Williamson, K. M. (2010b). Evidence-based practice: Step by step. Critical appraisal of the evidence: Part II. *American Journal of Nursing, 110*, 41–48.

Fineout-Overholt, E., Melnyk, B. M., Stillwell, S. B., & Williamson, K. M. (2010c). Evidence-based practice: Step by step. Critical appraisal of the evidence: Part III. *American Journal of Nursing, 110*, 43–51.

Fineout-Overholt, E., & Stillwell, S. B. (2019). Asking compelling clinical questions. In B. M. Melnyk & E. Fineout-Overholt (Eds.). *Evidence-based practice in nursing and healthcare: A guide to best practice*. (4th ed.). p. 33–54. Wolters Kluwer.

Fletcher, R. H. (2008). Clinical practice guidelines. http://www.themgo.com/content/CIguidelines.pdf

Foxman, B., Cronenwett, A. E., Spino, C., Berger, M. B., & Morgan, D. M. (2015). Cranberry juice capsules and urinary tract infection after surgery: Results of a randomized trial. *American Journal of Obstetrics & Gynecology, 213*, 194.e1–194.e8.

Gance-Cleveland, B., Aldrich, H., Schmeige, S., Coursen, C., Dandreaux, D., & Gilbert, L. (2015). Clinician adherence to childhood overweight and obesity recommendations by race/ethnicity of the child. *Journal for Specialists in Pediatric Nursing, 20*, 115–122.

Garcia, C. A. C., Alvarado, K. P. P., & Gaxiola, G. P. (2010). Grading recommendations in clinical practice guidelines: Randomized experimental evaluation of four different systems. *Archives of Disease in Childhood, 96*, 723–728.

Gardois, P., Calabrese, P., Colomib, N., Deplano, A., Lingua, C., Longo, F., Villanacci, M. C., Miniero, R., & Piga, A. (2011). Effectiveness of bibliographic searches performed by pediatric residents and interns assisted by librarians. A randomized controlled trial. *Health Information and Libraries Journal, 28*, 273–284.

Gehanno, J. F., Rollin, L., & Darmoni, S. (2013). Is the overage of Google Scholar enough to be used alone for systematic reviews? *BMC Medical Information and Decision Making, 13*(1), 1–5.

Gerrish, K., Nolan, M., McDonnell, A., Tod, A., Kirshbaum, M., & Guillame, L. (2011). Factors influencing advanced practice nurses' ability to promote evidence-based practice among frontline nurses. *Worldviews on Evidence-Based Nursing, 9*, 30–39.

Ghelichkhani, P., & Esmaeili, M. (2020). Prone position in management of COVID-19 patients: A commentary. *Archives of Academic Emergency Medicine, 8*(1), e48.

Godin, K., Stapleton, J., Kirkpatrick, S. I., Hanning, R. M., & Leatherdale, S. T. (2015). Applying systematic review search methods to the grey literature: A case study examining guidelines for school breakfast programs in Canada. *Systematic Reviews, 4*(1), 1–10.

Gray, M. (2002). Are cranberry juice or cranberry products effective for prevention or management of urinary tract infections? *Journal of Wound, Ostomy, and Continence Nursing, 29*, 122–126.

Gray, M., Beitz, J., Colwell, J., Bliss, D. Z., Engberg, S., Evans, E., Gallagher, J., Moore, K. N., & Pieper, B. (2004). Evidence-based nursing practice II. Advanced concepts for WOC nursing practice. *Journal of Wound, Ostomy, and Continence Nursing, 31*, 53–61.

Gregory, K. (2015). Differentiating between research and quality improvement. *Journal of Perinatal & Neonatal Nursing, 29*(2), 100–102.

Guyatt, G. H., Oxman, A. D., Montori, V., Vist, G., Kunz, R., Brozek, J., Alonso-Coello, P., Djulbegovic, B., Atkins, D., Falck-Ytter, Y., & Williams Jr., J. W. (2011). GRADE Guidelines 5. Rating the quality of evidence—Publication bias. *Journal of Clinical Epidemiology, 64*, 1277–1282.

Hanno, P. M., Burks, D. A., Clemens, J. Q., Dmochowski, R. R., Erickson, D., FitzGerald, M. P., Forrest, J. B., Gordon, B., Gray, M., Mayer, R. D., Moldwin, R., Newman, D. K., Nyberg Jr., L., Payne, C. K., Wesselmann, U., & Faraday, M. M. (2014). American Urological Association (AUA) guideline diagnosis and treatment of interstitial cystitis/bladder pain syndrome. http://www.auanet.org/documents/education/clinical-guidance/IC-Bladder-Pain-Syndrome-Revised.pdf

Hastings, C., & Fisher, C. A. (2014). Searching for proof: Creating and using an actionable PICO question. *Nursing Management, 45*(8), 9–12.

Hicks, C. (1995). The shortfall of published research: A study of nurses' research and publication activities. *Advanced Nursing, 21*, 594–604.

Higgins, J. P. T., & Green, S. (2011). Cochrane handbook for systematic reviews of interventions, version 5.1.0. http://handbook.cochrane.org/

Hill, A. B. (1937). Principles of medical statistics. I. The aim of the statistical method. *Lancet, 1*, 41–43.

Holly, C., Salmond, S., & Saimbert, M. (2017). *Comprehensive systematic review for advanced practice nursing*. Springer.

Horsley, T., Dingwall, O., & Sampson, M. (2011). Checking reference lists to find additional studies for systematic reviews. *The Cochrane Database of Systematic Reviews*, (*8*), MR000026.

Joanna Briggs Institute. (n.d.). JBI collaboration. https://jbi.global/about-jbi

Joshi, G. P., Benzon, H. T., Gan, T. J., & Vetter, T. R. (2019). Consistent definitions of clinical practice guidelines, consensus statements, position statements, and practice alerts. *Anesthesia & Analgesia, 129*(6), 1767–1770.

Kneipp, S. M., Gilleskie, D., Sheely, A., Schwartz, T., Gilmore, R. M., & Atkinson, D. (2014). Nurse scientists overcoming challenges to lead transdisciplinary research teams. *Nursing Outlook, 62*(5), 352–361.

Larson, N. F. (2010). Cranberry juice may not prevent urinary tract infection. http://www.medscape.com/viewarticle/734360

LaRue, E. M., Draus, P., & Klem, M. L. (2009). A description of a Web-based educational tool for understanding PICO framework in evidence-based practice with a citation ranking system. *Computers, Informatics, Nursing, 27*, 44–49.

Lawrence, P., & Fulbrook, P. (2012). Effect of feedback on ventilator care bundle compliance: Before and after study. *Nursing in Critical Care, 17*, 293–301.

Maccioli, G. A., Dorman, T., Broan, B. R., Mazuski, J. E., McLean, B. A., Kuszaj, J. M., Rosenbaum, S. H., Frankel, L. R., Devlin, J. W., Govert, J. A., Smith, B., & Peruzzi, W. T. (2003). Clinical practice guidelines for the maintenance of patient physical safety in the intensive care unit: Use of restraining therapies—American College of Critical Care Medicine Task Force 2001–2002. *Critical Care Medicine, 31*(11), 2665–2676.

Magnan, M. A., & Maklebust, J. (2008). The effect of Web-based Braden Scale training on the reliability and precision of Braden Scale pressure ulcer risk assessments. *Journal of Wound, Ostomy, and Continence, 35*, 199–208.

Magnan, M. A., & Maklebust, J. (2009). The effect of web-based Braden Scale training on the reliability of Braden Subscale ratings. *Journal of Wound, Ostomy & Continence Nursing, 36*, 51–59.

Melnyk, B. M., & Fineout-Overholt, E. (2010). *Evidence-based practice in nursing and healthcare: A guide to best practice*. Wolters-Kluwer.

Meneghini, R., & Packer, A. L. (2007). Is there science beyond English? Initiatives to increase the quality and visibility of non-English publications might help to break down language barriers in scientific communication. *EMBO Reports, 8*, 112–116.

Milnes, V., Gonzalez, A., & Amos, V. (2015). Aprepitant: A new modality for the prevention of postoperative vomiting: An evidence-based review. *Journal of Perianesthesia Nursing, 30*(5), 406–417.

Mitchell, D. A., Panchsin, T., & Seckel, M. A. (2018). Reducing use of restraints in intensive care units: A quality improvement project. *Critical Care Nurse, 38*(4), e8–e16.

Moffett, P., & Moore, G. (2011). The standard of care: Legal history and definitions: The bad and good news. *Western Journal of Emergency Medicine, 12*(1), 109–112.

Moher, D., Schulz, K. F., & Altman, D. CONSORT Group (Consolidated Standards of Reporting Trials). (2001). The CONSORT statement: Revised recommendations for improving the quality of reports of parallel-group randomized trials. *The Journal of the American Medical Association, 285*, 1987–1991.

Moore, W. R., Vermuelen, A., Taylor, R., Kihara, D., & Wahome, E. (2019). Improving 3-hour sepsis bundled care outcomes: Implementation of a nurse-driven sepsis protocol in the emergency department. *Journal of Emergency Nursing, 54*(6), 690–698.

Mullin, R. (2014). Tufts study finds big rise in cost of drug development. *Chemical & Engineering News*. http://cen.acs.org/articles/92/web/2014/11/Tufts-Study-Finds-Big-Rise.html

Murphy, M. K., Black, N. A., Lamping, D. L., McKee, C. M., Sanderson, C. F., Askham, J., & Marteau, T. (1998). Consensus development methods, and their use in clinical guideline development. *Health Technol Assessment, 2*, 1–88.

National Library of Medicine. (2021). *MEDLINE: Overview*. https://www.nlm.nih.gov/medline/medline_overview.html

National Pressure Injury Advisory Panel European Pressure Ulcer Advisory Panel, and Pan Pacific Pressure Injury Alliance. (2019). *Prevention and treatment of pressure ulcers/injuries: Quick reference guide* (3rd ed.). file:///quick-reference-guide-version-04dec2019-secured.pdf

National Quality Forum. (2021). *Serious reportable events. Serious reportable events "aka" never events*. https://www.qualityforum.org/Topics/SREs/Serious_Reportable_Events.aspx

Nayan, S., Gupta, M. K., & Sommer, D. D. (2011). Evaluating smoking cessation interventions and cessation rates in cancer patients: A systematic review and meta-analysis. *ISRN Oncology, 2011*, Article 849023.

Ogilvie, D., Egan, M., Hamilton, V., & Petticrew, M. (2005). Systematic reviews of health effects of social interventions: 2. Best available evidence: How low should you go? *Journal of Epidemiology and Community Health, 59*, 886–892.

Oxford English Dictionary Online. (2020). Evidence. http://www.oed.com/view/Entry/65368?rskey=xSGaCx&result=1&isAdvanced=false#eid

Patient Protection and Affordable Care Act, 42 U.S.C. § 18001 (2010).

Polit, D. F., & Beck, C. T. (2021). *Nursing research: Generating and assessing evidence for nursing practice* (11th ed.). Wolters-Kluwer.

Powell, H. P., Doig, E., Hackley, B., Leslie, M. S., & Tillman, S. (2012). The midwifery two-step: A study on evidence-based midwifery practice. *Journal of Midwifery and Women's Health, 57*, 454–460.

Rapp, C. A., Etzel-Wise, D., Marty, D., Coffman, M., Corlson, L., Asher, D., Callaghan, J., & Holter, M. (2010). Barriers to evidence-based practice implementation: Results of a qualitative study. *Community Mental Health Journal, 46*, 112–118.

Ratliff, C. R., Yates, S., McNichol, L., & Gray, M. (2016). Compression for primary prevention, treatment, and prevention of recurrence of venous leg ulcers: An evidence-and consensus-based algorithm for care across the continuum. *Journal of Wound, Ostomy, and Continence Nursing, 43*, 347–364.

Reigle, B. S., Stevens, K. R., Belcher, J. V., Hugh, M. M., McGuire, E., & Mals, D. (2008). Evidence-based practice and the road to magnet status. *Journal of Nursing Administration, 38*, 97–102.

Rogers, E. M. (2003). *Diffusion of innovation* (5th ed.). Simon & Schuster.

Rose, L., Burry, L., Mallick, R., Luk, E, Cook, D., Fergusson, D., Dodek, P., Burns, K., Granton, J., Ferguson, N., & Devlin, J. W. (2016). Prevalence, risk factors, and outcomes associated with physical restraint use in mechanically ventilated patients. *J Critical Care, 31*(1), 31–35.

Rosenberg, W., & Donald, A. (1995). Evidence-based medicine: An approach to clinical problem-solving. *British Medical Journal, 310*, 1122–1126.

Ryan, M. A. (2017). Adherence to clinical practice guidelines. *Otolaryngology Head & Neck Surgery, 157*(4), 548–550.

Ryan, R., Hill, S., Prictor, M., & McKenzie, J; Cochrane Consumers and Communication Review Group. (2013). Study quality guide. https://cccrg.cochrane.org/sites/cccrg.cochrane.org/files/public/uploads/StudyQualityGuide_May%202013.pdf

Sackett, D. L. (2015). Why did the randomized clinical trial become the primary focus of my career? *Value in Health, 18*, 550–552.

Sackett, D. L., Rosenberg, W. M., Gray, J. A., Haynes, R. B., & Richardson, W. S. (1996). Evidence based medicine: What it is and what it isn't. *British Medical Journal, 312*, 71–72.

Sackett, D. L., Strauss, S. E., Richardson, W. S., Rosenberg, W., & Haynes, R. B. (2000). *Evidence-based medicine: How to practice and teach EBM* (2nd ed.). Churchill-Livingstone.

Salvatore, S., Salvatore, S., Cattoni, E., Siesto, G., Serati, M., Sorice, P., & Torella, M. (2011). Urinary tract infections in women. *European Journal of Obstetrics, Gynecology, and Reproductive Biology, 156*, 131–136.

Shirey, M. R., Hauck, S. L., Embree, K. L., Kinner, T. J., Schaar, G. L., Phillips, L. A., Ashby, S. R., Swenty, C. F., & McCool, I. A. (2011). Showcasing differences between quality improvement, evidence-based practice, and research. *Journal of Continuing Education in Nursing, 42*(2), 57–70.

Smeets, S. J. M., van Wunnik, B. P. W., Poeze, M., Smooter, G. D., & Verrruggen, J. P. A. M. (2020). Cardiac overscreening hip fracture patients. *Archives of Orthopedic and Trauma Surgery, 140*, 33–41.

Smith, A. K., Ayanian, J. Z., Covinsky, K. E., Landon, B. E., McCarthy, E. P., Wee, C. C., & Steinman, M. A. (2011). Conducting high-value secondary dataset analysis: Introductory guide and resources. *Journal of General Internal Medicine, 26*, 920–929. https://doi.org/10.1007/s11606-010-1621-5.

Smith, M. B. (1956). Editorial. *Journal of Abnormal and Social Psychology, 52*, 4.

Song, F., Hooper, L., & Loke, Y. K. (2013). Publication bias. What is it? How do we measure it? How do we avoid it? *Open Access Journal of Clinical Trials, 5*, 71–81.

Stapleton, A. E., Dziura, J., Hooton, T. M., Cox, M. E., Yarova-Yarovaya, Y., Chen, S., & Gupta, K. (2012). Recurrent urinary tract infection and urinary *Escherichia coli* in women ingesting cranberry juice daily: A randomized controlled trial. *Mayo Clinic Proceedings, 87*, 143–150.

Stetler, C. B. (2003). Role of the organization in translating research into evidence-based practice. *Outcomes Management, 7*, 97–103.

Stiffler, D., & Cullen, D. (2010). Evidence-based practice for nurse practitioner students: A competency-based teaching framework. *Journal of Professional Nursing, 26*, 272–277.

Streptomycin treatment of pulmonary tuberculosis. (1948). *British Medical Journal, 2*, 769–782.

Sutton, A. J., Duvall, S. J., Tweedie, R. L., Abrams, K. R., & Jones, D. R. (2000). Empirical assessment of effect of publication bias on meta-analyses. *BMJ (Clinical Research Ed.), 320*, 1574–1577.

Taggart, E., McKenna, L., Stoelting, J., Kirkbride, G., & Mottar, M. (2012). More than skin deep: Developing a hospital-wide Wound Ostomy Continence Unit Champion program. *Journal of Wound, Ostomy, and Continence Nursing, 39*, 385–390.

Taylor, C. (2014). The use of clinical practice guidelines in determining standard of care. *Journal of Legal Medicine, 35*(2), 273–290.

Triano, J. J. (2008). What constitutes evidence for best practice? *Journal of Manipulative and Physiological Therapeutics, 31*, 637–643.

Trinite, T., Cherry, C. L., & Marion, L. (2009). The US Preventive Services Task Force: An evidence-based prevention resource for nurse practitioners. *Journal of the American Academy of Nurse Practitioners, 21*, 301–306.

Turner, J. R. (2012). The 50th anniversary of the Kefauver-Harris amendments: Efficacy assessment and the randomized clinical trial. *Journal of Clinical Hypertension, 14*(11), 810–814.

US Department of Health and Human Services, Health Resources and Services Administration. (2011). Quality improvement. http://www.hrsa.gov/quality/toolbox/508pdfs/qualityimprovement.pdf

van der Kooi, A. W., Peelen, L. M., Raijmakers, R. J, Vroegop, R. L., Bakker, D. F., Tekatli, H., van den Boogaard, M., & Slooter, A. J. (2015). Use of physical restraints in Dutch intensive care units: A prospective multicenter study. *American Journal of Critical Care, 24*(6), 488–495.

van Rijswijk, L., & Gray, M. (2012). Evidence, research and clinical practice: A patient-centered framework for progress in wound care. *Journal of Wound, Ostomy, and Continence Nursing, 39*, 35–44.

von Elm, E., Altman, D. G., Egger, M., Pocock, S. J., Gøtzsche, P. C., & Vandenbroucke, J. P. (2007). The Strengthening the Reporting of Observational Studies in Epidemiology (STROBE) statement: Guidelines for reporting observational studies. *Bulletin of the World Health Organization, 85*, 867–872.

Weiner, B. J., Amick, H., & Lee, S. Y. (2008). Conceptualization and measurement of corporate readiness for change. A review of the literature in health services research and other fields. *Medical Care Research and Review, 65*, 379–436.

West, S., King, V., Carey, T. S., Lohr, K. N., McKoy, N., Sutton, S. F., & Lux, L. (2002). *Systems to rate the strength of scientific evidence.* Evidence report—Technology assessment No. 47. AHRQ Publication 02-E016. Agency for Healthcare Research and Quality.

Whiting, P., Savovic, J., Higgins, J. P. T., Caldwell, D. M., Reeves, B. C., Shea, B., Davies, P., Kleijnen, J., & Churchill, R. (2016). ROBIS: A new tool to assess risk of bias in systematic review was developed. *Journal of Clinical Epidemiology, 69*, 225–234.

Wound Ostomy Continence Nurses Society Board of Directors Task Force. (2020). Guidance for maintaining skin health when utilizing protective masks for prolong time intervals: A message from the WOCN Society. *Journal of Wound, Ostomy and Continence Nursing, 47*(4), 317–318.

Yang, J., Li, Y., Liu, Q., Li, L., Feng, A., Wang, T., Zheng, S., Xu, A., & Lyu, J. (2020). Brief introduction of medical database and data mining technology in big data era. *Journal of Evidence-Based Medicine, 13*(1), 57–69. https://doi.org/10.1111/jebm.12373

Yevchak, A. M., Fick, D. M., McDowell, J., Monroe, T., May, K., Grove, L., Kolanowski, A. M., Waller, J. L., & Inouye, S. K. (2014). Barriers and facilitators to implementing delirium rounds in a clinical trial across three diverse hospital settings. *Clinical Nursing Research, 23*, 201–215.

9 LEADERSHIP

LAURA REED ■ MICHAEL CARTER

"I think knowing what you cannot do is more important than knowing what you can."

~ Lucille Ball

CHAPTER CONTENTS

THE IMPORTANCE OF LEADERSHIP FOR APRNS 280
- Constantly Evolving Healthcare Systems 280
- Evolving Health Professional Education 281
- APRN Competencies 281

LEADERSHIP: DEFINITIONS, MODELS, AND CONCEPTS 282
- Leadership Models That Lead to Transformation 282
- Leadership Models That Address System Change and Innovation 285
- Concepts Related to Change 286

TYPES OF LEADERSHIP FOR APRNS 289
- Clinical Leadership 289
- Professional Leadership 290
- Systems Leadership 290
- Health Policy Leadership 292

CHARACTERISTICS OF APRN LEADERSHIP COMPETENCY 293
- Mentoring 293
- Empowering Others 295
- Innovation 295
- Political Activism 296

ATTRIBUTES OF EFFECTIVE APRN LEADERS 296
- Timing 296
- Self-Confidence and Risk-Taking 297
- Communication and Relationship Building 298
- Boundary Management: Balancing Professional and Personal Life 298
- Self-Management/Emotional Intelligence 299
- Moral Courage 300
- Respect for Cultural and Gender Diversity 301
- Global Awareness 302

DEVELOPING SKILLS AS APRN LEADERS 302
- Factors Influencing Leadership Development 302
- Personal Characteristics and Experiences 302
- Strategies for Acquiring Competency as a Leader 303

DEVELOPING LEADERSHIP IN THE HEALTH POLICY ARENA 303
- Using Professional Organizations to the Best Advantage 305
- Internships and Fellowships 305
- New Modes of Communication 305

OBSTACLES TO LEADERSHIP DEVELOPMENT AND EFFECTIVE LEADERSHIP 305
- Clinical Leadership Issues 305
- Professional and System Obstacles 306
- Dysfunctional Leadership Styles 306
- Horizontal Violence 306

STRATEGIES FOR IMPLEMENTING THE LEADERSHIP COMPETENCY 309
- Developing a Leadership Portfolio 309
- Promoting Collaboration Among APRN Groups 309
- Networking 310
- Effectively Working With Other Leaders to Advance Health Care 310
- Institutional Assessment Regarding Readiness for Change 310
- Followship 311

CONCLUSION 311

KEY SUMMARY POINTS 311

The purposes of this chapter are to describe the advanced practice registered nurse (APRN) leadership competency, provide useful literature and resources on leadership and change, describe characteristics of effective leaders, identify obstacles to effective leadership, and discuss strategies for developing leadership skills. This chapter will help APRNs define their need for leadership abilities and develop a plan for acquiring the necessary skills appropriate to their particular positions and professional goals.

THE IMPORTANCE OF LEADERSHIP FOR APRNS

The American Association of Colleges of Nursing (AACN, 2021) has identified that leadership is a core competency of APRNs. This competency may come as a surprise to some new APRNs in that they are often so focused primarily on understanding and applying the art and science of clinical practice that leadership seems like a distant concern. Yet APRNs quickly learn in clinical practice that care is provided in complex systems, and these systems require leadership to function effectively. APRNs have unique knowledge and clinical legitimacy that provide a strong basis for their leadership.

Healthcare systems are under constant redesign and transformation, and there is a continuing evolution in health professional education as well (AACN, 2021; Dreher et al., 2014). Interprofessional care among a variety of different clinicians has become more important to ensure quality outcomes, and leading these teams is very complex (Farrell et al., 2015). The unique leadership provided by APRNs occurs in the systems where they provide care. Clinical care is usually delivered at the individual patient level but is embedded within larger organizations. These larger care delivery organizations rely on leaders to improve safety, quality, and reliability and to evaluate the outcomes of care. In short, systems leaders must be able to identify the need for innovation and change and implement strategies to achieve them. In partnership with others, APRNs craft approaches to evaluate, reassess, and implement systems redesign and innovation.

APRNs provide leadership in several areas, ranging from taking a stand on behalf of an individual patient to advocating for a change in national health policy. Competency in leadership does not stand alone but interacts with other APRN competencies (AACN, 2021).

Constantly Evolving Healthcare Systems

The World Health Organization (2020b) has reasoned that everyone in the world should have access to the health services they need without being forced into poverty when paying for these services. This goal requires substantial changes in the health systems of many countries, including the United States, which is the only developed country in the world without universal health coverage. Other nations are experiencing similar evolution of their systems of care, and these changes are often related to the new types of healthcare problems seen in these countries, the organization of their healthcare systems, and the ways in which these countries pay for care.

The Institute of Medicine (IOM), subsequently named the National Academy of Medicine (NAM), released their groundbreaking *The Future of Nursing* report in the United States in 2011, and the subsequent work in 2021 in monitoring these changes highlights the important goals for APRNs to lead change and advance health (NAM, 2021). These reports contend that it is essential for nurses to be full partners and leaders in the transformation of health care.

The NAM has issued several reports over the years calling for radical redesign and transformation of the American healthcare system. Such changes do not occur quickly, in part because they require a significant rethinking of how care is delivered, the roles of patients and education of providers, effective channels for diffusing innovation, how health care is financed, where and how care is delivered, and which provider activities are valued and paid for (Hunter et al., 2013). The early IOM reports calling for transformation of the healthcare system are predicated on six national quality aims—safety, effectiveness, patient-centeredness, timeliness, efficiency, and equity (IOM, 2001). The NAM has long noted that patients throughout the health system are at high risk for the occurrence of adverse events, yet numerous institutional barriers to reporting these events still exist. One barrier has been the long-standing tendency toward naming and blaming individuals rather than exploring gaps in systems of

The authors acknowledge Charlene Hanson for contributions to earlier editions of this chapter.

care and organizational culture (Wagner et al., 2006). Leaders have come to realize that errors occur because of a continuum of reasons. APRN leaders can use the six quality aims to facilitate the evaluation of errors, near misses, and questionable behavior to determine root causes of situations in which employee behavior does not match organizational values. Causes for these situations can range from organizational culture to defective systems and processes to bad choices on the part of employees.

The Institute for Health Improvement (IHI) launched a campaign in 2001 to save 100,000 lives from medical errors (Berwick et al., 2006). This campaign was so successful, with an estimated 122,000 lives saved between January 2005 and June 2006, that a new goal was created to decrease mortality and morbidity in 5 million lives (IHI, 2012). More recently, the IHI has begun to focus more on new issues in leadership, including behaviors for leaders, a broad approach to transformation of organizations to pursue excellence, and organizational learning including the governance leaders, executive team, and point-of-care leaders (IHI, 2021).

Evolving Health Professional Education

Just as health care has been evolving throughout the world, so too has health professional education. These rapid changes call upon leadership in very different ways than in the past. Nurses have an intimate knowledge of person centered care and a unique opportunity to lead these new educational changes needed for future care (Marcellus et al., 2018). Part of these educational changes reflect the new or expanded competencies health professionals must have for future practice based on changes in the type of healthcare conditions being treated and emphasis being placed on patient quality, costs, access, and patient-centered care. The Josiah Macy Jr. Foundation (2021) has funded programs directed at how healthcare providers need to be trained to meet the needs of diverse populations in the United States. There continues to be substantial interest in expanding and improving interprofessional education. This approach to education is very complex in that health professionals come from different theoretical perspectives, educational programs may not be co-located, academic calendars are seldom synchronized, and faculty obligations often preclude working with other professions. Measuring the impact of interprofessional education on provider practice and the outcomes for patients has been very difficult. This may be attributed to the substantial length of time from when the professionals were in education until actual changes in patient outcomes could be measured. In addition, the system of care delivery is changing the way it is financed, and this can compound the measurement of outcomes from education alone.

APRN Competencies

In the AACN's (2021) *The Essentials: Core Competencies for Professional Nursing Education*, several specific competencies relate to leadership for APRNs. Core competencies developed by the National Association of Clinical Nurse Specialists (NACNS, 2019) address leadership requirements of clinical nurse specialists (CNSs), and those developed by the National Organization of Nurse Practitioner Faculties (NONPF, 2017) address nurse practitioners (NPs). Nurse practitioner leadership competencies are also in place for Canada (Canadian Nurses Association, 2010) and Australia (Nursing and Midwifery Board of Australia, 2021).

Earlier APRN education programs were focused primarily on learning to provide expert clinical care. This focus was necessary but is no longer sufficient for future practice. Health care has changed in many ways and continues to evolve. Practice today and for the future means that APRNs must possess the appropriate knowledge, skills, and abilities to address larger system issues in a way not expected in the past. APRNs have a social covenant with the society that they serve. New issues concerning the social determinants of health have emerged and must be understood by APRNs. Patients are living longer, and some of this extension of life includes periods of active dying. Many health conditions have no cure or hope of cure. Learning to diagnose and treat patients with acute and chronic health conditions is central for much of APRN practice, but the work does not stop there. Understanding the evolving structures, regulations, and ethos of care is mandatory for APRNs to deliver high-quality care with the greatest access for those in need and at the lowest costs. These changes in focus of care mean that APRNs must be able to seamlessly move from the individual recipient of the service to the much larger system context and then back. Leadership is often required to make these moves.

In summary, numerous contextual and educational factors that require APRN leadership have been identified in calls for the redesign and transformation of the healthcare system. Certain themes are apparent—in particular, patient-centeredness (see Chapter 6), teamwork (see Chapter 10), quality improvement, the use of information technology, and complexity. These factors are an appropriate part of graduate and continuing education so that APRNs acquire the knowledge and skills they need to lead effectively.

LEADERSHIP: DEFINITIONS, MODELS, AND CONCEPTS

Contemporary definitions of leadership generally fit into one of two categories: transformational leadership or situational leadership (Carlton et al., 2015). Transformational leadership is focused on the leader using influence processes to focus on system change usually at the system level (Bush, 2018). Situational leadership is focused on choosing the leadership style that best fits the goals and circumstances at a particular time (St. Thomas University, 2019). Both categories are built upon attributes of the leader that are learned and can be taught.

APRNs can draw on numerous models of leadership and change processes to inform their leadership development. Most leadership models are predicated on leaders having an ability to understand themselves. Leadership grows out of personal characteristics that can be learned and are associated with successful leadership. One model of self-awareness is the emotional awareness model created by Goleman (2005), who proposed that there are four core skills that lead to improved leadership effectiveness: self-awareness, self-management, social awareness, and relationship management. Most important is that successful leaders understand the importance of self-regulation in their relationships.

Leadership Models That Lead to Transformation

Vernon (2015) asserted that transformational leaders constantly ask themselves and their team questions about what the goal is, how to try things differently, and what the costs of maintaining the status quo are. This form of leadership transforms the team by leading to changes in values, attitudes, perceptions, and/or behaviors on the part of leaders and followers and lays the groundwork for further positive change. Thus transformational leadership occurs when people interact in ways that inspire higher levels of motivation and morality among participants. One may question how leaders accomplish this. Transformational leaders analyze a situation to understand the particular leadership needs and goals; they then use this information, together with their interpersonal skills, to motivate, stimulate, share with, conciliate, and satisfy their followers in an interdependent interactional exchange. DePree (2011) defined leadership as an art form in which the leader does what is required in the most effective and humane way. The definition by DePree proposes that contemporary leadership may be viewed as a process of moving self and others toward a shared vision that becomes a shared reality. Successful transformational leadership is relational, driven by a common goal or purpose, and satisfies the needs of the leader and followers. Further, a transformational leadership style is often associated with effective change agents. Schwartz et al. (2011) studied the effects of transformational leadership on the Magnet designation for hospitals and reported that transformational leadership led to the change needed to obtain and maintain Magnet status. Other authors who have described a transformational approach to leadership include Wang et al. (2012), who studied transformational leadership with Chinese nurses. Transformational leadership was associated with job satisfaction in nurses.

Many different models of leadership are available (Table 9.1). One model that is frequently used is the work of Stephen Covey, who authored and presented an exemplar in 1989.

The Seven Habits of Highly Effective People

In his seminal work, Stephen Covey (1989) presented personal and interdependent characteristics that foster acquisition of leadership skills (Box 9.1). In creating a personal view of leadership, Covey suggested that the most effective way to keep the end in mind is to create a personal mission statement that becomes a standard to live by as one progresses from independence to interdependence. In Covey's model, interdependence is achieved only after one has defined and integrated this

TABLE 9.1
Useful Models of Transformational Leadership and Change

Author	Title	Relevant Concepts	APRN Use
Senge	The Fifth Discipline (1990, 2006)	Describes five actions or processes that characterize effective teams and organizations that manage change well: Personal mastery Awareness of mental models Shared vision Team learning Systems thinking	APRNs can use these concepts to identify: Personal leadership goals Strengths and needs of the teams and organizations with whom they work Strategies to enhance team development and collaboration
Covey	The Seven Habits of Highly Effective People (1989) The 8th Habit (2004) Leading in the Knowledge Worker Age (2006)	Development of a personal mission statement to live by as one develops independence and interdependence. The eight habits that foster acquisition of leadership skills are as follows: Be proactive. Take the initiative; choose your response. Begin with the end in mind. Define success. Put first things first; personally manage yourself. Think win-win, with a willingness to cooperate. Seek first to understand and then to be understood. Synergize; the whole is greater than the sum of its parts. Sharpen the saw; renew your physical, mental, spiritual, and social dimensions. Find your voice and inspire others to find theirs.	APRNs can use these characteristics to: Acquire leadership skills Attain interdependence by fully incorporating one's personal mission statement into practice Use influence and inspiration as a creative catalyst for change
Nelson et al.	Microsystems in Health Care: Learning From High-Performing Front-Line Clinical Units (2002)	Studied 20 varied microsystems; identified nine common success characteristics associated with delivery of high-quality, cost-efficient care: Leadership Culture Organizational support Patient focus Staff focus Interdependence of care team Information and information technology Process improvement Performance patterns	APRNs can use these characteristics to assess one's system and identify gaps in and opportunities for leadership.
Massoud et al.	A Framework for Spread (2006)	Model evolved by the Institute for Healthcare Improvement to understand phases of successful system change. Key elements: Prepare for spread Establish aim for spread Develop an initial spread plan Execute and refine plan	APRNs can use ideas for each phase of spread. Also useful for: Understanding the importance of leadership in planning for spread Detailing elements of the aim and initial plan for spread (addresses the who, what, when, where)

Continued

TABLE 9.1
Useful Models of Transformational Leadership and Change—cont'd

Author	Title	Relevant Concepts	APRN Use
Cooperrider et al.	Appreciative Inquiry Handbook (2008)	Uses a 4D cycle to seek positive attributes to build on through conversations and relationship building rather than focusing on problem areas: Discovery Dream Design Destiny	APRNs can use these concepts to: Motivate and inspire colleagues to excellence in practice Develop partnerships to capitalize on positive attributes of individual team members to solve complex problems in health care

BOX 9.1

Covey's Eight Habits of Highly Successful People

- Be proactive.
- Begin with the end in mind.
- Put first things first.
- Think win–win.
- Seek first to understand and then to be understood.
- Synergize.
- Sharpen the saw.
- Find your voice and inspire others to find theirs.

Adapted from Covey, S. (1989). *The seven habits of highly effective people: Powerful lessons in personal change*. Simon & Schuster; Covey, S. (2004). *The 8th habit. From effectiveness to greatness*. Free Press; and Covey, S. (2006). Leading in the knowledge worker age. *Leader to Leader Journal, 41*, 11–15.

personal mission or standard into their practice. Covey described attributes of those who lead from a philosophy of interdependence: listening twice as much as you speak, remaining trustworthy by never compromising honesty, maintaining a positive attitude, and keeping a sense of humor. Interdependence allows one to hear and understand the other person's viewpoint, leading to a synergistic or win–win level of communication. In 2004 Covey expanded on this leadership model by proposing an eighth habit—leaders must find their voice and help others to find theirs. He noted that leaders at any level can use their inspiration and influence to overcome negativity and use creativity to move the organization to greatness; this type of leader can be a catalyst for change. Covey (2006) also developed leadership ideas that incorporate managing people in the information age. A key concept in this update is that leaders must be aware that the manners in which they lead will influence the choices that followers make.

Situational Leadership

The term *situational leadership* is defined as the interaction between an individual's leadership style and the features of the environment or situation in which they are operating. Leadership styles are not fixed and may vary based on the issues being addressed or on the environment. Situational leadership depends on particular circumstances, with leaders and followers assuming interchangeable roles according to environmental demands (Huber, 2014). The role of follower is important because APRNs occasionally will find themselves in both roles. Leaders must have followers, and followers must have leaders. Therefore successful leaders must learn to follow and also allow others to lead. DePree (2011) expanded on this idea and used the term *roving leadership* to describe a participatory process in which leadership in a particular situation may shift among the team members. This notion of leadership is relevant because the work of APRNs in collaborative healthcare teams requires the roles of leader and follower to be interchangeable depending on the complex needs of the patient.

Servant Leadership

Servant leadership was first introduced by Robert Greenleaf in 1970. He suggested that the best leaders were servants first and were driven by their desire to

BOX 9.2

Ten Key Principles of Servant Leadership

- Listening and understanding
- Empathizing and accepting
- Healing
- Awareness and perception
- Persuasion (hallmark of servant leadership)
- Conceptualization
- Foresight (the core ethic of leadership)
- Stewardship
- Commitment to the growth of people
- Building community (knowledge)

Adapted from Tatsumi, C. L. (2019). The nurse as servant leader: Guiding others in caring advocacy. *Beginnings, 39*(4), 6–14.

serve others. He identified 10 key principles as guides for those practicing servant leadership. These principles are listed in Box 9.2 (Tatsumi, 2019). Servant leaders possess certain qualities such as being a visionary, listening, investing in others, sharing power, and building community through strategic relationships (Mustard, 2020). These qualities are common to nursing, therefore causing this leadership style to increase in popularity among nursing leadership. Servant leadership has been viewed by some as a passive form of leadership, but it actually leads to the enhancement of interprofessional practice, improved patient satisfaction, and improved nursing satisfaction. A great servant leader creates a work environment that encourages all employees to be involved in decision making, therefore lending to the overall success of the organization (Fahlberg & Toomey, 2016; Savel & Munro, 2017).

Leadership Models That Address System Change and Innovation

Change is a constant in today's clinical environments. Efforts to transform the healthcare system are generally focused in three areas: diffusion of innovation, clinician behavior change, and patient behavior change. The reality is that change is often messy and not always welcome even when it seems straightforward. An integrative review of diffusion and dissemination of innovations revealed why redesign and transformation are messy—they are exceedingly complex (Kwamie, 2015). For example, an NP was very concerned about how long it was taking patients to schedule return visits. The booking system was controlled by the larger healthcare organization and was not easily adapted to a specific purpose. In addition, all of the providers wanted to keep all slots filled for the next 2 weeks, so double-booking was common, resulting in some clinic times being overloaded. Office staff had no authority to override the system, and billing staff could not determine whether a particular insurance plan would pay for more frequent visits. Making any change in scheduling involved the information technology staff, the office staff, the billing staff, and the clinicians—any one of whom could stop the change.

Clinical microsystems are the front-line units in which patients and providers interface and are the foundation for providing safe and high-quality care within large organizations. Thus transforming care at the front-line unit is essential to optimizing care throughout the continuum.

APRNs practice at the patient–provider interface, and their leadership can contribute greatly to the optimization of other successful characteristics. APRNs are skilled at creating cohesive teams, identifying and advocating patient and staff needs, leading performance improvement efforts at the front-line interface, and contributing to a positive organizational culture.

One helpful model for understanding leadership in complex organizations is the complexity theory. Henry (2014) contended that complexity theory is focused on understanding the ways in which individuals are free to act in interconnected but unpredictable ways. This means that one person's actions can lead to changes in the context for others in the organization. Some theories of leadership and management are built upon the assumption that individuals and organizations are logical and predictable in the ways they function. The complexity theory holds that some actions are not predictable in a linear manner and evolve more organically.

APRNs who are learning to lead change may find the use of the complexity theory helpful. Clancy et al. (2008) provided insights when multiple providers, new technology competition, and complex information systems are involved.

Spread of Innovation

Massoud et al. (2006) developed a model to address the difficulty in spreading effective, evidence-based innovation beyond the immediate environment. Diffusion within and among healthcare organizations is key with today's goal of implementing best practices throughout health care. Founded on Rogers' (2003) definition of diffusion, this framework for spread is based on four main components—preparing for spread, establishing an aim for spread, developing an initial spread plan, and executing or refining the spread plan. Leadership is essential in preparing a plan to spread innovation. As leaders, APRNs must take an active role in ensuring the innovation is evidence-based throughout all aspects of the spread plan. During the development of the spread plan, the leader oversees the project and may take an active role in developing the plan. Finally, the APRN leader needs to ensure collection and use of information about the effectiveness of the plan, supporting course correction as needed.

Several common themes emerge when considering models of leadership and change. Effective leadership requires sound knowledge of oneself and one's organization regarding values, strengths, and weaknesses, as well as expert communication and relationship-building skills and the ability to think and act strategically.

Appreciative Inquiry

Appreciative inquiry (AI) is a leadership model that seeks to find positives through appreciative conversations and relationship building (Cooperrider et al., 2008). Rather than focusing on a problem, this model encourages focusing on what is working well and what the organization does well and then broadens and builds on the strengths. This model is predicated on the belief that when we expand what we do best, problems seem to fall away or are outgrown. Leading through positive interactions results in people working together toward a shared vision and preferred future without being weighed down by problems. Leaders using this leadership model are open to inquiry without having a preconceived outcome in mind; rather, they facilitate a search for shared meaning and build and expand on what is working well. For example, faculty in an APRN graduate program wanted to create a doctor of nursing practice (DNP) program but encountered quality concerns about some of their existing master of science in nursing options. Through an AI process, the faculty decided to build a DNP program based solely on the certified registered nurse anesthetist (CRNA) role because that was their strongest offering at the time. Moreover, through this process, they decided to phase out two of their master of science in nursing options because they were not up to the same level of quality. Over time, the CRNA program was recognized as one of the nation's top programs. So, rather than investing solely in "fixing what's broken," the AI model directs resources and visioning to an organization's greatest strengths. This leadership model uses a 4D cycle:

- *D*iscovery—an exploration of what is; finding organizational strengths and processes that work well
- *D*ream—imagining what could be; envisioning innovations that would work even better for the organization's future
- *D*esign—determining what should be; planning and prioritizing those processes
- *D*estiny—creating what should be; implementing the design

AI uses a positive perspective that can be motivational and inspirational for employees, with the goal of increasing exceptional performance. This model can work well for APRNs who are skilled in developing partnerships. Although evidence for the effectiveness of this leadership model is limited, there is enough evidence to support further rigorous research (Jones, 2010). The consequences of leading with an emphasis on defects are that the process lacks vision, places attention on yesterday's causes, and can lead to narrow and fragmented solutions. The AI model shifts from asking, "What is the biggest problem?" to asking, "What possibilities exist that we have not yet considered?" This approach quickly leads individuals to a shared purpose and vision.

Concepts Related to Change

Change refers to the various types of initiatives aimed at improving the quality and safety of practice, whether by revising policies or helping clinicians master new knowledge and change behavior. In other words, change is seen as any clinical or systems effort to encourage the adoption and diffusion of innovation, including quality improvement, product rollouts, clinician education, and skill development. Change is viewed as a process so that it does not have a discrete beginning and end but, instead, appears to be a series of continuous transitions that overlap one another. This means that the ability to bring about change must be woven into the fabric of the everyday life and work of APRNs. As with patient assessment to effect individual behavior change, APRNs must be skilled at assessing and reassessing their organizations and the complex forces that drive the healthcare system to be effective change agents. Systems innovation requires leadership that is continuous and flexible and demands ongoing attention to and redefinition of appropriate strategies (Kwamie, 2015; Shirey, 2015).

Opinion Leadership

One way that change can be initiated is through the use of opinion leadership (Anderson & Titler, 2014). Opinion leaders are clinicians who are identified by their colleagues as likeable, trustworthy, and influential (Flodgren et al., 2019). Clinicians are likely to listen to the opinion leader and make a change in practice based on what has been learned from the opinion leader. Shirey (2008) pointed out that there are several elements of being the opinion leader, including being knowledgeable, respected, trusted, and well connected within the organization; in addition, opinion leaders must also be generous with their time and advice. APRNs become opinion leaders because they are recognized for their astute clinical decision-making and influence of others. They are sought out by others, and when APRN opinion leaders speak, others listen. Thus a staff nurse may ask a CNS wound care specialist to examine a wound and provide treatment advice. Colleagues are eager to try the new information when an NP returns from a conference and shares what was learned. CRNAs are consulted for their opinion on airway management. These examples suggest the importance of attending to environmental cues when change is planned. Unfortunately, there is very limited evidence on the effectiveness of opinion leaders concerning change. This may be because there have been few studies of this model of leadership.

Driving and Restraining Forces

Driving and restraining forces are useful concepts for APRNs planning for change, including managing the intended and unintended consequences of change. For example, the movement toward multistate licensure has gained momentum as APRNs extend their practices across state lines (Young et al., 2012). These forces can serve as driving or restraining influences for APRNs depending on different policies and procedures for reimbursement and prescriptive authority within states. As multistate licensure for APRNs evolves, telehealth may be considered a driving force, and states' rights may be a restraining force. For example, a psychiatric/mental health NP in one state may wish to use telehealth methods to treat patients in an adjoining state to save patients the time and expense of driving to therapy sessions. Some states allow for this under the RN license but do not allow for this under the APRN approval. The APRN would have to seek and obtain recognition from the board of nursing in the state where the patient is located. There may be very different rules in the two states about physician collaboration or supervision, scope of practice, and prescription rules, and these could be a restraining force for extending this practice. The unintended consequence of these rules and regulations could be to restrict care by APRNs for rural residents.

Understanding driving and restraining forces helps in analyzing the organizational settings in which APRNs work. For example, an organizational assessment of these various forces is useful in determining an institution's level of commitment to diversity.

At times, physicians have been both driving and restraining forces for change. Experienced APRNs know that one of the challenges in system redesign and transformation has been engaging physicians in the work of improving quality as a team member. Berwick (2016) argued that there is now a new era in health care that calls for an end to the protectionism seen earlier. Further, he pointed out that better care, better health, and lower costs can be brought about by working with others to improve care in a transparent way. APRNs and physicians are stakeholders who can lead together to offset professional prerogative and greed while listening to the voices of the people served.

Pace of Change

A major concern is the rapidity with which change occurs in the healthcare industry. Even when one develops detailed plans for a change, events may occur that reshape the process and progress so that what gets implemented may not be the same as the original proposal. As the rapidity of change increases, the time frame to accomplish change strategies shortens. This phenomenon makes change more difficult for individuals and organizations to manage. Consequently, many of the traditional models still being used to implement change will not be successful.

Planned versus unplanned change is based predominantly on issues of time—time to plan for and think through the desired change, time to orient and allow stakeholders to become comfortable with the proposed change, and time to educate and allow the change process to occur. Many required changes in health care do not have sufficient time to allow the proposed change to naturally evolve. Transformational leadership may offer the best hope for survival in rapid change situations.

Whether healthcare organizations can sustain fast-paced change is not clear unless there is a commitment to the culture of change. This commitment assists and supports adaptation to new systems and ways of knowing and doing. A culture of change requires several components, including learning about change and change strategies, encouraging dialogue, valuing collaboration and differences, and being committed to enacting change. In a classic work, O'Connell (1999) proposed strategies for promoting a culture of change within an organization (Box 9.3).

BOX 9.3

O'Connell's Strategies That Promote a Culture of Change

- Maintain momentum toward change.
- Emphasize managerial support in the process of changing workflow and practice patterns.
- Encourage the question "why" and exercise tolerance for the results.
- Emphasize the importance of personal concerns and address them.
- Find new and different ways to demonstrate administrative support.

Adapted from O'Connell, C. (1999). A culture of change or a change of culture. *Nursing Administration Quarterly, 23*, 65–68.

APRNs can use one or more of the models of leadership described here to assess their systems. Knowing where one's system is in terms of readiness for change and identifying the forces that will support or restrain adoption of an innovation can help the APRN design strategies that will work. It is also helpful to consider the techniques used for implementing change, such as building alliances, creating a shared vision, being assertive, negotiating conflict, and managing transitions as they relate to providing a positive culture for change. As leaders, APRNs can use their skills to translate the need for and perspectives on change among clinicians, patients, families, and administrators. In addition, APRN leaders must be prepared to identify when it is not in an organization's best interest to pursue a change based on context, environment, inadequate problem solving, or unresolved barriers. Repetitive, rapid change can take a toll on engagement and productivity and potentially on patient safety, particularly if implications and consequences are not thoroughly considered. Most important, leaders must understand the personal implications of change if a culture of change is to be realized. Box 9.4 provides a

BOX 9.4

Leadership Strategies for Moving Through Change

- Spark a passion; believe in what you are doing; shine a light on activities that inspire and excite.
- Understand the organizational culture.
- Create a vision.
- Get the right people involved.
- Hand the work over to the champions of change.
- Let values serve as the compass for where you are headed.
- Change people first; organizations evolve.
- Seek and provide opportunities for professional renewal and regeneration.
- Maintain a healthy balance.

Adapted from Kerfoot, K., & Chaffee, M. W. (2007). Ten keys to unlock policy change in the workplace. In D. J. Mason, J. K. Leavitt, & M. W. Chaffee (Eds.), *Policy and politics in nursing and health care* (pp. 482–484). Saunders; and Kerfoot, K. (2005). On leadership: Building confident organizations by filling buckets, building infrastructures, and shining the flashlight. *Dermatology Nursing, 17*, 154–156.

useful set of strategies for APRN leaders who are helping their organizations and colleagues work through change transitions.

TYPES OF LEADERSHIP FOR APRNS

Some APRNs are not comfortable with the idea of being leaders. This may be because they see leadership as outside of their goal of caring for their patients. However, upon a more careful view, leadership is understood to be necessary to bring about the kinds of things that ensure good patient care. APRN leadership competency can be conceptualized as occurring in four primary areas: in clinical practice with patients and staff, within professional organizations, within healthcare systems, and in health policymaking arenas. The extent to which individual APRNs choose to lead in each of these areas depends on patients' needs; personal characteristics, interests, and commitments of the APRN; institutional or organizational priorities and opportunities; and priority health policy issues in nursing as a whole and within one's specialty. These four areas have substantial overlap. For example, developing clinical leadership skills will enable the APRN to be more effective at the policy level, as clinical expertise informs policymaking.

Clinical Leadership

Clinical leadership focuses on the needs and goals of the patient and family and ensures that quality patient care is achieved. Clinical leadership is a foundational component to attaining and maintaining a productive environment in which safe and excellent care that employs best practices is provided. This leadership occurs when APRNs acquire and apply knowledge about how to build appropriate working relationships with healthcare team members, how to instill confidence in patients and colleagues, and how to problem-solve as part of a team (Bally, 2007). APRN leaders propose and implement change strategies that improve patient care. Some clinical leadership skills are part of the competency of collaboration (see Chapter 10). The most common clinical leadership roles APRNs fulfill are those of advocate (for patient, family, staff, or colleagues), group leader, and systems leader. APRNs may advocate for a particular patient or family, as when an acute care nurse practitioner (ACNP) discusses with the attending surgeon the need for the patient to have a clear understanding of the potential adverse effects of an elective surgery. While the surgeon may have concluded that the patient and family fully understand the potential outcomes of the surgery, the ACNP may have discovered that there was a broad misunderstanding by the patient and family. Presenting talks or writing articles on clinical topics are other ways of expressing clinical leadership and influencing others. One important aspect of clinical leadership is that the APRN steps up, ensuring the best clinical outcome for any particular patient.

Group leadership may be informal, as when an APRN agrees to coordinate multiple referrals for a patient with complex care needs or has expertise in a particular clinical problem, such as pain management, skin care, or screening for cervical cancer, and assumes a team leadership role reflecting this expertise. APRNs may also have more formal leadership responsibilities; for example, an APRN may lead a weekly team meeting or agree to convene a group and lead the development of a new practice protocol to bring care into line with newly released standards of care. One function of the APRN leader is to motivate colleagues and facilitate their use of new knowledge and/or the adoption of new practices with the goal of improved patient outcomes.

APRNs often exercise leadership to ensure that clinical problems are addressed by administrative leaders at a systems level. This type of leadership requires that APRNs move between the clinical and administrative arenas, interpreting the needs of one to the other. Advancing clinical excellence requires financial, creative, and political skills to promote innovative care with others (Younger, 2020). Having these additional skills improves the success of this form of clinical leadership and the compelling translation of ideas between distinct, sometimes competing perspectives. APRNs recognize the clinical problems related to their specialty that require attention or intervention from the larger (macro) system of which they are a part. For example, when a CNS called a patient to learn why he had not kept his appointment at the heart failure clinic, she learned that the patient could not find parking nearby because of hospital construction, did not know that a shuttle would take him from the satellite lot to the clinic, and did not have the energy to walk from the satellite lot. The CNS knew that this could be a problem for other clinic patients and worked with administrators to make sure patients had knowledge of and access to the resources that were needed and available. The CNS understood the clinical implications (patients might experience more complications requiring readmission) and systems implications (e.g., lower care quality, increased risks for patients, higher costs, missed appointments) of construction-related missed appointments for her patient population.

APRNs who lead patient care teams effectively find that their interprofessional leadership skills are in demand. For example, one APRN who was successful in leading a quality improvement initiative to improve care of patients with asthma who were admitted to the hospital was later invited to chair a national task force of healthcare professionals developing practice guidelines for the treatment of asthma. The ability to provide clinical interprofessional leadership requires a firm grasp of clinical and professional issues while responding to the challenges of other disciplines and the larger society. It necessitates a deep respect for other clinicians and the creation of a safe and welcoming place for all voices to be heard. APRNs develop the attributes needed to lead in other domains as they build on a solid foundation of strong clinical leadership.

Professional Leadership

Active participation and leadership are particularly important and exercised in professional organizations. Novice APRNs may begin by seeking membership on a committee of a local, state, or national nursing or interprofessional organization. These organizations are built on the voluntary contributions of their members and rely on members to achieve the organization's goals. As APRNs become more experienced, they may seek opportunities to apply the leadership skills they have learned in their work to their professional organizations. Most APRNs are members of one or more nursing and interprofessional organizations. These memberships provide a myriad of leadership opportunities, including organizing continuing education offerings, presenting at national conferences, chairing a committee, and running for the board of directors. In these situations, APRNs exercise more choice as to whether and when they will participate in leadership activities than they do in their usual work roles.

Professional leadership often begins locally and proceeds to state, national, and international levels. Novice APRNs can acquire leadership skills and experience by becoming involved in the leadership and committee work of local advanced practice nursing coalitions and organizations and progressing into state and regional leadership roles as they develop their style, strengths, and network as APRN leaders. The ability to place APRN leaders in key local, state, and national positions is critical to the visibility and credibility of APRNs and to the establishment of their place within nursing and the larger healthcare community. In addition to informal leadership development opportunities, there are formal programs in which APRNs can develop the skills to lead in positions such as board membership (Carlson et al., 2011).

Systems Leadership

Systems leadership means leading at the organizational or delivery system level—a skill that requires a multidimensional understanding of systems. Systems leadership often requires a "big picture" view and understanding elements in care delivery far beyond nursing. Within healthcare organizations, APRNs may lead clinical teams, chair committees, chair or serve as members of boards, manage projects, and direct other initiatives aimed at improving patient care as well as the clinical practice of nurses and other professionals. Systems leadership overlaps professional situations in which leaders are elected or appointed to positions within defined organizations and groups. For example, APRNs may identify an increase in the rate of patient falls and lead a task force to evaluate the problem and design corrective interventions. A critical care CNS or ACNP may initiate interprofessional rounds to monitor patients on mechanical ventilation and gather data on clinical variables such as complication rate and time to weaning. APRNs may be asked to participate in or lead standing or ad hoc interprofessional committees such as credentialing, ethics, institutional review boards, or pharmacy and therapeutics committees. APRNs may be asked by administrators to participate in organizational reengineering or other activities aimed at improving the environment in which others practice.

APRNs must be aware that the characteristics of successful entrepreneurs are desirable and valued in systems leaders. The term *entrepreneurial leadership* refers to leaders who go outside of traditional employment systems to create new opportunities to exercise their unique abilities (Bagheri & Akbari, 2018). When these leaders use the entrepreneurial skills of innovation and risk-taking and assume responsibility for achieving specific targets in an organization, they are termed *intrapreneurs*. Because this leadership style is consistent with the call for healthcare system redesign, it is worth reviewing characteristics associated with entrepreneurial leadership. Shirey (2007a) stated that nurse entrepreneurs have a desire to make a difference and see opportunities in situations in which others see barriers or challenges. Blanchard et al. (2007) developed tools for leaders to assess their entrepreneurial strengths and identified attributes of entrepreneurs, including being resourceful, purposeful, a risk-taker, a problem-solver, innovative, communicative, and determined. Universities that prepare APRNs are offering coursework on innovation, entrepreneurship, and innovative thinking to prepare entrepreneurial and intrapreneurial APRN leaders (Shirey, 2007b). APRNs frequently underestimate their transferable skills, which can be used in entrepreneurial or intrapreneurial opportunities (Shirey, 2009). Recognition of these skills will assist intrapreneurial APRNs to build a case for how their services can assist the organization in achieving innovative clinical excellence (Shirey, 2007a). Entrepreneurial leadership skills are illustrated in Exemplar 9.1, which also illustrates the evolving nature of advanced practice nursing leadership and how it can expand in breadth over time to lead national and international policy. Note that Dr. Bednash moved from staff nurse to NP to leader of one of the premier national organizations in nursing education. She credits her NP education with providing her the basis for her international leadership.

Willingness to Name Difficult Organizational Problems

A common human characteristic in organizations is to operate around the periphery of problems and not in the heart of them. Rare is the leader who directly acknowledges and names dysfunctional activities that are deeply embedded in organizations. A key role of APRNs is to name the problem without implying blame. This approach to leadership brings a problem into the light without the burden of having to solve it. In this way, the APRN is inviting others into the conversation for a better understanding of barriers to collaborative practice and state-of-the-art, patient-centered care. For example, if office staff think that they do not have the authority to make scheduling and patient flow work better, the APRN can name this problem and invite members of the organization to explore it further. The willingness for APRNs to enter into these courageous conversations is a key skill set for effective leadership. When there are high-stakes issues with high emotions, it is tempting to focus instead on peripheral issues.

In another example, a primary care practice grappled for some time with a significant number of patient and staff complaints about waiting times to see a physician who was excellent but slow. She was always behind in her appointment times and could not keep pace with the demands of primary care. This created conflict in the waiting room and with support staff, as patients frequently waited more than 2 hours to be seen for a scheduled appointment. Sometimes patients left without being treated after they had been checked in. The APRN who recently joined the practice was able to name the problem and the impact on the entire system, including paying overtime for medical assistants to work late. This naming of a problem that had been going on for years greatly relieved the organization. Once the problem and its dimensions were defined, the physician became aware of the impact that these long waits had on the entire office as well as on her patients. The team determined an approach that would allow this particular physician to have longer appointments and booked some vacant slots to allow for catch up. The manner in which the APRN raised the quality concerns made it safe because it was always in the context of patient care.

APRNs can enter these conversations by naming troubling dynamics or environmental threats. A patient's problem cannot be resolved without having dimensions of that problem clearly defined. The same holds true for organizational leadership and the need to foster more collaboration and unity at the systems level. This type of acknowledgment of issues and willingness to name problems without having to solve them is a powerful way for APRNs to model true leadership.

EXEMPLAR 9.1
APRN LEADERSHIP IN ACTION[a]

Dr. Geraldine "Polly" Bednash attributes much of her rise to national and international leadership to her preparation as a nurse practitioner. Her childhood was spent in San Antonio, Texas, which was primarily a small military town at the time with strong Latin American roots. She fondly recalls making tamales with family and going to the market with her grandmother to acquire the needed ingredients to help treat family illnesses. She did not grow up with the idea of becoming a nurse but selected this when she entered the university. Money was tight, so she worked throughout her time in school. She enrolled in the Army Nurse Corps for the last 2 years of school and immediately entered service after graduation. She met her husband while serving as a Nurse Corp officer in Vietnam. She and her husband moved to New York after her Army service, and she assumed a position as a faculty member at a diploma nursing school in the New York area.

Later, her husband's company moved them to the Washington, DC, area, but there she quickly discovered that her baccalaureate degree would not garner her a faculty position. She obtained her master's degree in medical–surgical nursing at Catholic University and again assumed a faculty position in nursing education.

She was accepted into the Robert Wood Johnson Foundation program to prepare nursing faculty to become nurse practitioners. She describes becoming a nurse practitioner in the early 1980s as "eye-opening" and "ground-breaking." In this new role, she was expected to be a risk-taker, to be on top of her game, and to have good working relationships with physicians and other healthcare professionals. She credits this education with forming the foundation for much of her future success as a national and international leader in nursing. Nurse practitioners diagnosed and treated patients but also considered the cultural and economic issues related to their care. As an independent practitioner she was required to understand the needs of the individual within the context of the larger system. This was not a part of traditional hospital nursing practice at the time. She went on to complete her PhD at the University of Maryland and transitioned her career to policy leadership.

For 3 years, Dr. Bednash was director of government affairs of the American Association of Colleges of Nursing (AACN), and she was then selected to be executive director. She led that organization through its dramatic evolution as one of the nation's most important voices for nursing education, practice, and research. Her leadership at the AACN is credited with establishing the association as the national voice for baccalaureate and graduate nursing education. Dr. Bednash was the driving force behind expanding the AACN's reach and influence in all healthcare and higher education circles as well as in the US Congress and with the administration. She mobilized support for the AACN's signature initiatives, including the creation and ongoing revision of the *Essentials* documents, the establishment of the Commission on Collegiate Nursing Education, the advancement of the practice doctorate, and the development of the clinical nurse leader role and the Commission on Nurse Certification. In addition, Dr. Bednash spearheaded dozens of grant-funded initiatives, including the End-of-Life Nursing Consortium and the New Careers in Nursing Program.

Like many leaders, Dr. Bednash credits a number of individuals who helped her along the way. These include internationally renowned leaders in nursing and health care who provided support, words of wisdom, and encouragement at important times in her life. For example, when a patient experienced an adverse effect from a medication Dr. Bednash had prescribed, it was a physician colleague who helped her to understand that sometimes the work of nurse practitioners may place patients in harm's way and that she must learn from this event to help other patients.

She has devoted a good deal of her leadership experience to mentoring, coaching, and assisting others who aspire to leadership. The unique nature of her work as the head of a nursing organization that served many nursing schools meant that she had to be judicious in the selection of individuals to assist. Most of the people for whom she has served as a mentor are in professions other than nursing. In recognition of her years of outstanding work, the American Academy of Nursing designated her a Living Legend in 2019, their most prestigious honor.

Her suggestions for advance practice registered nurses (APRNs) who are building competence in leadership is to always be open to the advice of those around you, even if you are not sure at the time you want to hear that advice. She also encourages APRNs to cultivate colleagues who will tell it like it is rather than rapidly agreeing with your position. Last, always strive for transparency in your leadership work.

[a]The author gratefully acknowledges Geraldine (Polly) Bednash, PhD, RN, FAAN, Nurse Practitioner for use of her exemplar.

Health Policy Leadership

Some APRNs may not see themselves as being particularly interested in or talented at political advocacy. However, all APRNs have a vested interest in policymaking that affects their patients' care, healthcare funding, national priorities in health, and state and local policies related to the health of the community they serve. Understanding and leading in health policy have become increasingly important, as more laws and regulations are being enacted with implications for APRN practice. APRNs should be aware of and must often respond to local, state, and national policymaking efforts likely to affect these laws and regulations. Organizations that define competencies for APRNs also have competencies related to health policy. Leadership in health policy requires an ability to analyze healthcare systems, an understanding of the personal qualities associated with effective leadership, and the skill to use this knowledge strategically.

Across these four domains of leadership, APRNs use their clinical expertise, team building, and collaborative skills to build community around shared values such as patient-centeredness and commitment to quality. To exert leadership in health policy, APRNs are expected to remain informed about current and emerging issues in health care such as changes in federal and state regulations concerning scope of practice and nursing education funding proposals. APRNs are also expected to understand the broad elements of government so that there can be timely and effective contact with policymakers to ensure that the APRNs' patients will be well represented in any proposed changes in laws or regulation. The APRN may not passively allow changes to happen but is expected to actively participate in discussion and actions for policy change. This policy work can combine leadership in clinical care, professional activities, and systems leadership.

CHARACTERISTICS OF APRN LEADERSHIP COMPETENCY

Three defining characteristics of APRN leadership—mentoring, empowering others, and innovation—are listed, along with their core elements, in Table 9.2. These are discussed separately here to assist in understanding the differences among them. However, there is considerable overlap in the knowledge and skills needed for each characteristic. APRNs often focus on developing clinical leadership first because the new clinical work can be time-consuming. As APRNs gain more confidence in their advanced clinical abilities, they tend to expand their leadership in

TABLE 9.2 Characteristics and Core Elements of the Leadership Competency	
Defining Characteristic	**Core Elements (Knowledge and Skills)**
Mentoring	Shared vision
	Seeks mentors and serves as a mentor
	Willing to share power
	Empowering self and others
	Self-reflection
Empowering Others	Educate to empower through increasing the individual's knowledge base
	Use inspiration, motivation, and encouragement
	Provide structure that offers protection and security as one moves into new territory
	Provide resources to support others' growth and development
	Give the support and direction necessary for change toward empowerment
	Foster actualization, empowering others to evoke change
Innovation	Knowledge of models of leadership and change
	Systems thinking
	Systems assessment skills
	Flexibility
	Risk-taking
	Expert communication
	Credibility
	Change agent

additional domains such as mentoring and empowering others.

Mentoring

A key element of APRN leadership competency is mentoring others. The ability to help others grow and encourage them toward developing their full potential requires competent, caring leaders who are interested in the success and well-being of others. Mentoring also ensures the development of future nurse leaders (McCloughen et al., 2009). Mentoring bridges the gap between professional education and the experiences of the subsequent working world (Barker & Kelley, 2020). Guiding and coaching, leading by example, and role modeling with awareness and attentiveness to the needs and concerns of followers are basic characteristics of successful leaders. The ideas behind colloquial phrases like "taking someone under your wing" or "giving a colleague a leg up" are grounded in the mentoring process. Mentors are competent and self-confident, having qualities that epitomize success in their own careers and having the ability and desire to help others succeed. Other characteristics of successful mentors include inspiring others, being confident, being committed to the development of others, and having a willingness to share. Mentors take on responsibility for the development of protégé skills, such as flexibility, adaptability, judgment, and creativity (McCloughen et al., 2009). Protégés are viewed as individuals who express a desire to learn, are committed to the long course of events, and are open to the process of trial and error. Successful protégés have high self-esteem, can self-monitor, and are resilient risk takers (Tourigny & Pulich, 2005). The reward for the mentor is to step back and enjoy the success and achievements of the protégé. APRNs who have had the benefit of mentoring report that it affected the progression of their career and enriched their leadership development (McCloughen et al., 2009).

Two types of mentoring are described in the literature. *Formal mentoring* has the approval and support of an organization with objectives, a selection process, and a mentoring contract. Mentors are chosen from the ranks of experienced clinicians and provide exposure to clinical situations that offer opportunities to demonstrate competence, coaching, and role modeling and afford protection in controversial situations (Tourigny & Pulich, 2005). Many professional organizations, such as Sigma Theta Tau International and the National Organization of Nurse Practitioner Faculties, offer formal mentoring programs and often make information available on the organizations' websites. *Informal mentoring* is a relationship that is unstructured and mutually beneficial; the experiences usually last longer and are self-selected (Tourigny & Pulich, 2005). Good mentors foster growth rather than dependency and instill the internal strengths to enable protégés to traverse rough spots in their career development. Mentors lead protégés on a journey of self-discovery and help them find the value they bring to the role and to nursing leadership (Vos, 2009). As mentoring relationships progress, protégés take on more freedom to try new behaviors and develop confidence in trying new skills, always with the knowledge that someone is behind them.

Mentoring relationships can be developed based on specific needs of the APRN protégé, such as writing for publication or developing professional presentation skills, or on the general development of career and leadership skills. Harrington (2011) reported that mentoring new NPs will accelerate their development as primary care providers. Finding a mentor in one's geographic location may not be feasible, depending on the skill to be developed. In today's technological world, however, APRN leaders can establish mentoring relationships at a distance that can be a rewarding experience as well. Use of conference calls, videoconferencing, social media, and networking at professional conferences can all be feasible means to support a distance mentoring relationship.

There are two parts to the APRN mentorship equation: APRNs who are seeking to be mentored by those they aspire to emulate and APRNs who can serve as mentors. Some APRN leaders are reluctant to serve as a mentor for a variety of reasons. However, Vance (2002) asserted that a chaotic healthcare environment makes mentoring support more important than ever. She suggested that mentors and protégés adopt a mentoring philosophy that encourages collaboration, not competition, with others. Novice APRNs are fortunate if they can find a mentoring relationship that lasts over time. The APRN mentor creates a safety net in which the protégé can expose vulnerabilities and be coached to develop confidence in new skills. Mentoring is a gift that allows new APRN leaders to emerge. Today, APRNs taking on large leadership roles engage executive coaches and, more often, paid executive coaches. There is a cadre of nurses who do executive coaching, and these relationships can be highly valuable because the mentor is safely outside of the organization. APRNs who take on new executive leadership positions can negotiate in their employment package for the organization to pay for executive coaching.

An interrelationship exists among the concepts of mentoring, organizational culture, and leadership. Watkins (2013) described organizational culture as the patterns of behavior of an organization where said patterns are dynamic and change over time. A positive organizational culture offers social support and a sense of well-being and empowerment that fosters the mentoring process (Harrington, 2011). Thus APRNs should seek opportunities to mentor or be mentored and articulate the benefits of mentoring activities to their organization.

Empowering Others

The term *empowerment* is best understood as giving power to others, and this is often done by encouraging others and giving them authority. APRNs operationalize empowerment by sharing power with others, including patients, as well as by enabling them to access or assert their own power. Empowerment as a leadership strategy is guided by the shared vision of the leader and follower and a willingness of the leader to delegate authority to others. Leaders who empower their followers greatly increase the influence of APRNs within nursing and beyond nursing's boundaries. In some ways, empowerment shares some characteristics with mentoring. There is a continuously developing reciprocal relationship between the two key players.

Empowerment requires more than just giving other permission to act on their own. Good leaders foster empowerment over time and encourage constituents to feel competent, responsible, independent, and authorized to act. Quast (2011) provides some useful ideas about empowerment that leaders can use. Fostering empowerment means that the leader provides the information needed to make decisions. Leaders help guide the creation of appropriate goals and objectives, and this can sometimes lead to mistakes. Learning to accept mistakes can be an important part of empowerment particularly when the leader celebrates successes and failures. Accepting mistakes can lead to the development of learning environments if the leader fosters this view.

For example, certified nurse-midwives (CNMs) empower pregnant women by putting them in control of the birthing process through education, mentoring, and providing resources for parenting that nurture self-esteem and enhance family structure. CNMs are quick to let others know that they do not deliver babies—mothers deliver babies and midwives assist. This changes the power gradient in such a way that the mother is no longer dependent or passive in the birthing process. Instead, she is the decision maker and in control. This is very different from the paternalistic and hierarchical relationships seen in many obstetric medical practices.

Innovation

As the prior discussion suggests, initiating and sustaining innovation are critical elements of the APRN leadership competency. Covey's (1989) work with interprofessional groups is instructive to APRNs who are learning innovation skills. Innovation requires the capacity of the person to envision a world that can be and not just a world that is. This can be difficult for some because such a vision requires stepping over boundaries, cultures, politics, personal likes, and other elements that we hold very closely. Change occurs at the system and personal levels, and one must deal with core values to change or to serve as an agent for change successfully. Covey contended that people have a changeless core inside them that they need if they themselves are to be able to change. Thus one key to the ability of people to change is a strong sense of who they are and what they value. Lasting change comes from the inside out. This observation is relevant to APRNs. First, APRNs need to identify their own core values to become effective in leading change. Second, Covey's insight can help APRNs who encounter resistance to change initiatives, especially when it is persistent. The resistance may come from the sense that a core value is being threatened.

There is an affective dimension to change. Although many people express an excitement at the prospect of change, some changes are difficult and painful, and any change contains an element of loss. Mastering emotional tension during change requires perseverance, patience, and compassion. At best, change can be described as challenging and invigorating. Lazarus and Fell (2011) suggested that it is important to close the gap in creativity and use innovation as a process to induce change in health care. To understand change in today's healthcare environment, APRNs must explore the dynamics of change and the culture in which it occurs.

APRNs generally consider several factors when they are proposing an innovation—the relevance of power and influence, stakeholders' concerns and interests, contextual factors, individuals' values, and the affective dimensions of change. Understanding these important factors is integral to APRN leadership competency.

Political Activism

Political activism and advocacy will become even more important as APRNs hone their skills for systems leadership and change. Many of the skills needed to navigate successfully in political waters are closely associated with good leadership. The core elements that define contemporary leadership, such as shared vision, systems thinking, and the ability to engage in high-level communication within the context of a changing environment, are all basic to political effectiveness. Again, change leading to care improvement is the common element that drives APRNs to advocate for advanced practice and patient issues. There is little room for discussion about whether APRNs should take on the mantles of policymaker and patient advocate as part of their leadership role. Working for social justice is seen as part of the ethical practice competency of APRNs (see Chapter 11). APRNs must position themselves strategically at the policy table to advocate for access to care and appropriate interventions for everyone. Great strides have been made in developing nurses' skill and acuity as policymakers (see Chapter 17). Rapidly evolving policy situations mean that APRNs are often faced with trial-by-fire learning when it comes to activism and advocacy. However, policy issues tend to wax and wane so that APRNs do not always have to be highly engaged and can at times monitor the situation. Identifying trusted mentors with whom to debrief and developing a plan of action can help APRNs develop the poise and skills needed to respond effectively in unexpected, chaotic, and tense political situations.

Although activism is frequently associated with advocacy in the political realm, activism can occur in the clinical and system environments as well. The same leadership skills apply in those settings when advocating for issues such as access to care, ethical decision making, and resolving injustice.

ATTRIBUTES OF EFFECTIVE APRN LEADERS

Several personal attributes foster successful leadership (Box 9.5). Effective leaders demonstrate these broad qualities because they are needed in the interprofessional context of today's health care. Nurses are called to exert their leadership expertise far beyond nursing circles. The history of advanced practice registered nursing (see Chapter 1) demonstrates that nurse leaders have always led outside the realm of organized nursing education and practice.

Timing

A good sense of timing may come easily to some, but for most people it requires painstaking development and practice. APRN leaders know when to act and when to hold back. They recognize the need for urgency at times as, for example, during an unexpected legislative vote in Congress; they also know to take the time to develop a carefully thought-out plan with deliberate strategy when a change in scope of practice is being considered. The notion of timing is apparent when APRNs use mandated change as an opportunity to introduce other changes. For example, institutions applying for accreditation by The Joint Commission (TJC) are expected to demonstrate compliance with TJC's current evidence-based standards for specific healthcare problems (TJC, 2020). Many institutions use these mandated changes to launch a variety of initiatives aimed at improving care management.

One example of timing took place during a legislative session in Tennessee. APRNs were seeking to have a joint Senate and House committee remove regulations that restricted NP practices to limited locations. During the committee meetings, an NP testified about the many challenges the restrictive language imposed on NPs in providing good care in rural and underserved communities. The chairman of the committee stated that if the NPs were "unshackled" from their communities, they would leave and that the existing rules kept the NP tied to the community. Clearly, this language offended nurses, patients, and communities, but this committee meeting was not the time to call the chairman out. Following the committee hearing, the press got wind of the statement with the help of some very astute nurses in the audience, and the public outrage over these insensitive comments was explosive. The news media reported that the chairman, who happened to be African American, should have recognized the inappropriateness of his statements, particularly in a southern and former slave state. The chairman subsequently met with the NP who testified before the committee, apologized for the language, and sponsored a new bill to revoke the restrictive language during the next session. The timing of the release of the chairman's comments by the media made all the difference in this situation.

Self-Confidence and Risk-Taking

Taking risks is inherent in the leadership process and is tied inextricably to self-confidence. The willingness to take a chance, try, and occasionally fail is the mark of a true leader. Risk-taking behaviors differentiate APRNs who will be recognized as leaders and change drivers from other capable nurses. By learning to take risks, APRNs enhance their leadership repertoire, allowing for more spontaneity and flexibility in response to conflict, resistance, anger, and other reactions to change and high-risk situations. *Motivation* is the desire to move forward and can also be viewed as a component of risk-taking. Wheatley (2005) affirmed that another component of risk-taking is the willingness to be disturbed. Certainty is more comfortable. Staying put is rarely as risky as taking the chance to move ahead. Risk-taking, however, should be differentiated from risky leadership behaviors. Taking good risks involves evaluating all types of evidence available at the time and making educated decisions based on that information. It also involves trying to anticipate consequences of actions, having a plan in place to evaluate the implementation, being willing to accept that the risk was unsuccessful, and learning from the experience. Risky behavior, on the other hand, involves making decisions impulsively without fully exploring available information or having a strategy to address unintended consequences.

Several of the key attributes in Box 9.5 incorporate some form of the word *willingness*. The abilities to be open, to learn, to change one's mind, to be willing to take what comes, and to work through differences are key to all levels of leadership. Leadership is about negotiation and interactions with others to reach common goals. To do this may mean failing and trying again and again to reach the desired outcome. This quality of personal hardiness—the ability to pick oneself up and start again—is seen repeatedly in biographies of successful leaders who have made change happen in difficult times.

BOX 9.5

Attributes of APRN Leaders

EXPERT COMMUNICATION SKILLS

- Articulate in speech and in writing
- Able to get own point across
- Uses excellent listening skills
- Desires to hear and understand another's point of view
- Stays connected to other people

COMMITMENT

- Gives of self personally and professionally
- Listens to own inner voice
- Balances professional and private life
- Plans ahead; makes change happen
- Engages in self-reflection

DEVELOPING ONE'S OWN STYLE

- Gets and stays involved
- Sets priorities
- Manages boundaries
- Uses technology
- Engages in lifelong learning
- Maintains a good sense of humor

RISK TAKING

- Gets involved at any level
- Demonstrates self-confidence and assertiveness
- Uses creative and big picture thinking
- Willing to fail and begin again
- Has an astute sense of timing
- Copes with change

WILLINGNESS TO COLLABORATE

- Respects cultural diversity
- Desires to build teams and alliances
- Shares power
- Willing to mentor

Adapted from Hanson, C., Boyle, J., Hatmaker, D., & Murray, J. (1999). *Finding your voice as a leader*. American Academy of Nursing.

Communication and Relationship Building

The relevance of communication skills and collegial relationships to quality health care has received attention (Castledine, 2008). APRNs who lead must be able to communicate effectively with others (see Chapter 10) and participate in the identification and resolution of clinical and ethical conflicts among team members (see Chapter 11). The successful leader must have the requisite communication skills to build the trust and cooperation necessary to negotiate difficult intraprofessional and interprofessional issues. The ability to understand another's viewpoint and respect opposing views is key to effective communication and ultimately to reaching a mutually satisfactory outcome. Covey (1989) suggested that leaders will need to understand and be understood by others. Good leaders listen and understand the other person's viewpoint before they speak. The charisma associated with many leaders is often simply outstanding listening and communication skills. The ability to influence a key power strategy used to gain the cooperation of others is an outcome of excellent communication. A second part of expert communication is relationship building. The art of building strong alliances and coalitions with others and staying connected with colleagues and groups is basic to the sense of community needed to lead effectively. Building relationships within the work environment can minimize the impact of organizational structures that hinder one's ability to collaborate and solve problems (Wheatley, 2005). These alliances are important, whether at the highest levels of international policymaking or at the local level when building a coalition to address a recurring patient issue. Building relationships is central to the effectiveness of a team who cares for patients. Not only must APRNs establish effective relationships with their coworkers but they are often in a position to strengthen relationships among other members of the team through role modeling and mediation.

Thought leaders use conversational leadership as a way to bring key groups together to raise critical questions and issues and gain collective intelligence leading to innovation and wise actions. Open conversations are one way in which leaders share what they know with colleagues and create new ways of knowing and doing. This type of open conversation may lead to having the courageous conversations that are sometimes needed to name a problem so that the communication can move forward. Building relationships is also central to another APRN communication skill: conflict negotiation. APRN students may come to their educational programs having been socialized to be silent or suppress their opinion in situations of conflict. Specific approaches to identifying conflicts and resolving them successfully have been identified and used successfully in business (Fisher et al., 2011) and in health care (Longo & Sherman, 2007). The website for the Conflict Resolution Network (www.crnhq.org) is a valuable resource on conflict negotiation.

Boundary Management: Balancing Professional and Personal Life

Managing boundaries refers to how APRNs deal with various aspects of practice within the professional and personal components of their lives. Sometimes APRNs are in the position of guarding the boundary, such as when they are approached to undertake a task that is not within their scope of practice. Productivity requirements mean that APRNs must be clear about the numbers and types of patients that they can care for on a given day. Often, managing boundaries means extending them—building a bridge that enables the APRN to partner with other groups or expanding a boundary as other patient or healthcare needs are identified. For example, although CRNAs may not need prescriptive authority in a given state, they assist other APRN colleagues in their quest for state prescriptive authority. Extending a boundary may also mean expanding one's scope of practice at an agency level so that patient needs can be better met. Boundaries in practice tend to be fluid and often situation dependent. For example, in some practices, family NPs treat patients in the emergency department of the hospital, whereas in other practices, only ACNPs treat patients in the emergency department. Pushing boundaries in practice is usually based on education and experience in a particular area. That may mean that the APRN will have to acquire new training or credentialing in an area or technique and then be supervised in performing this new skill before expanding the boundary in autonomous practice.

As boundary managers, APRNs recognize communications and behaviors that breach or enhance interpersonal relationships. APRN leaders also teach others how to collaborate with colleagues in other disciplines, build coalitions, and set limits while maintaining their own boundaries—a fine distinction but strategically important. For example, a CNM may negotiate the boundaries or responsibilities among the neonatologist, obstetrician, and nurse-midwifery staff. Clinical leadership and professional leadership require the negotiation of boundaries, regardless of whether the borders are drawn around professional roles, patient populations, or organizations.

Important to this discussion is the issue that APRNs are people with lives outside their work. They are often spouses, parents, grandparents, members of their religious communities, and members of their broader community. Each of these components of their lives will carry boundary requirements in addition to their professional boundaries. There are no easy answers as to how to manage boundary issues that arise between personal and professional demands. APRN leaders will find an almost constant interplay between personal and professional boundaries. Grant (2013) pointed out that asking for help results in a cascade of important assistance from family and colleagues. The successful APRN leader is quick to ask for help and use that help to achieve goals.

Self-Management/Emotional Intelligence

Most people know when they have overextended themselves; their bodies give clues such as fatigue, stress signals, feelings of frustration, and even physical illness. One of the challenging aspects of being a good leader is the provocative realization that one is being asked to play many important cutting-edge roles at the same time. These invitations are exciting and seductive because they open new opportunities and speak to the high regard that others have for the leader. For these reasons, it is easy for good leaders to overextend their activities well beyond manageable, realistic boundaries. The skills of being able to delegate tasks; say no and mentor others to take on some of the load; and enlarge the circle of leaders, strategists, and followers are integral to effective leadership. Unfortunately, the inability to set realistic personal boundaries can lead to stress, frustration, and burnout. Being a leader and competent APRN provider at the same time is not easy, but it is achievable. This skill requires APRNs to decline a request when competing responsibilities make it not possible to accept the request. Skillful practice with saying "no" uses the sandwich technique. It begins with saying the larger "yes"—what the APRN is currently reaching for in the practice or trying to accomplish—followed by a firm "no" and ends with a hopeful statement such as, "Perhaps I can help you find somebody else" or "Maybe I can help in the future." The goal is to leave the requester with a sense of respect and a better understanding of the APRN. The following is an example: "I am really trying to build the prenatal care outreach service to underserved women. So, I cannot serve on the hospital CEO search committee. Perhaps I can help you find another qualified CNM to serve."

The process of self-reflection is useful for APRNs to determine which personal and work characteristics seem to set off imbalances. Three strategies are useful and simple in concept but can be complicated in execution. First, expecting perfection is often a setup for imbalance. Keeping in mind the axiom "Perfect is the enemy of good" may help APRNs establish realistic expectations. Reframing the notion to "good enough for now" allows the leader to move along. Another strategy is for APRNs to examine what makes them say "yes" or "no." It is easy to think, "If I just do this one more thing, everything will be fine." One APRN kept a note on her phone reminding her either to decline something that would tip the scales to overcommitment or to buy time by asking, "Can I think about it and call you tomorrow?" One colleague avoids commitments that are large but far into the future; these are invitations for activities months or even years in the future. Such activities may not appear to threaten one's usual commitments and deadlines but, as the time to fulfill the commitment approaches, these commitments can become very threatening. The challenge for the APRN is to ensure that adequate time to plan for, develop, and organize the work is budgeted well in advance of the due date. The third strategy is to make appointments with oneself for important personal and professional activities. By putting these appointments into a calendar, APRNs can lessen the risk of giving away time that they need to maintain balance. Using "the three things rule" may be helpful; identifying the three most important things that must be done before any new commitments are made or started is an advisable approach to achieving effective self-management.

Moral Courage

The idea of patient advocacy is understood by most APRNs as being very important to caring for patients. But there are times that advocacy is not sufficient. What is called for is moral courage. *Moral courage* is the willingness to take the right action to ensure the patient receives the best care even when there are restraints that make the right action nearly impossible (Gallagher, 2011). The expectation of moral courage for APRNs is derived from the American Nurses Association's (ANA, 2015a) *Code of Ethics for Nurses* and is expected for all nurses, not just APRNs (Fahlberg, 2015).

A number of situations can arise that lead to moral distress and call for moral courage on the part of the APRN. Examples of situations that can lead to moral distress include conflicts with other providers, conflicts with employers, breaking bad news to patients and their families, challenging an impaired colleague, and ethical dilemmas that can emerge at the beginning or the end of life. These may require that APRNs step forward and provide their voice even when they feel discounted or threatened. Exhibiting moral courage can be difficult, but Lachman (2010) provided a model that can be helpful. This model is based on the acronym CODE and is defined as follows:

- **Courage** to take the right action
- **Obligations** to do what is right as defined by the ANA *Code of Ethics*
- **Danger management** by seeking and accepting the support to move beyond fear
- **Expression and action** to maintain moral integrity

Following the CODE model will require skills in assertiveness and negotiation strategies, including working with patients and families, colleagues, health systems, and oftentimes payers for health care. Learning these abilities for the APRN can be enhanced by support and role modeling by preceptors and mentors (Musto et al., 2015). Exemplar 9.2 demonstrates the use of moral courage by a CRNA.

EXEMPLAR 9.2

MORAL COURAGE

Elizabeth has been a certified registered nurse anesthetist (CRNA) for several years. She prides herself in the care she provides to her patients. She has learned to be assertive but tactful in dealing with organizational issues that had the potential to lead to less than optimal outcomes for care. These included noting some of the anesthesia equipment was not being properly cleaned between patients, short staffing in the post-anesthesia care unit, and dealing with stressful situations in the operating room. She works with a number of other CRNAs and anesthesiologists in a group practice in a medium-sized hospital.

Over the past month, she has been asked by the nurses in the post-anesthesia care unit to assist them with patient care issues that have arisen around the care provided by John, one of the anesthesiologists, who was a partner in her anesthesia group. The nurses were concerned that John's practice was not meeting current standards, and when they tried to talk to him about this, he became defensive. When they tried to gain support from nursing administration, they were told that John was a respected member of the staff and a major income earner for the hospital and that the nurses should not go further with this issue.

Elizabeth was reluctant to become involved, but she decided the time had come to demonstrate moral courage when she was asked to help rescue the third patient of John's. She scheduled a meeting with John to discuss these three cases. She knew she would need courage to take the right action, and she believed she had a moral obligation to do what was right. She believed that she should assess the potential risk of taking this action by discussing the situation with both the operating room supervisor and the chief of anesthesiology before meeting with John. During her meeting with John, he became very defensive and told her to mind her own business and she had no right to question his work. During this meeting, she noted his speech was slurred and he had difficulties forming complete sentences. She came away with a concern that John may have an impairment that was influencing his care provision. She again met with the chief of anesthesiology and operating room supervisor to report her concerns. The two managers invoked the hospital's random drug screen on John, and he tested positive for opiates. When he was confronted with this information, he initially denied he had a problem but subsequently agreed to stop practice, self-report to the medical board, and begin drug treatment.

This was a very difficult action for Elizabeth. She had been friends and colleagues with John for a number of years but believed this action was a necessary expression and action to maintain her moral integrity.

Respect for Cultural and Gender Diversity

Successful APRN leaders strive for cultural competence and value diversity in their work. These attributes require awareness of one's own biases—overt and unconscious—attitudes, and behaviors that surface at all levels of interaction and in all settings. Marcelin et al. (2019) argued that continued overt bias such as racism, misogyny, and transphobia/homophobia influence many interactions in health care today. Much more subtle is the issue of unconscious bias in which individuals are categorized quickly without much thought. The effects can be similar to overt bias but much more difficult to recognize because of the unconscious nature of the bias. The American Nurses Association (2015a) *Code of Ethics for Nurses With Interpretive Statements* very clearly speaks to the requirement that all nurses are to practice with respect for the unique attributes for every person. This directs that nurses attempt to understand the role of their unconscious bias in providing their care.

An APRN leader must serve as a role model by demonstrating respect for the cultural differences of individuals and constituencies in any given situation. When a systems framework is used for understanding a complex concept such as culturally competent leadership, four levels can be identified—societal, professional, organizational, and individual. For the APRN, the responsibility for culturally competent care includes all four of these levels. A useful aid for developing a sound respect for cultural diversity can be found in the Interprofessional Education Collaborative competencies developed in 2011 (Interprofessional Education Collaborative, 2011); (see Chapter 10, Box 10.2 for this resource). Culturally competent care is delivered with knowledge, sensitivity, and respect for the patient's and family's cultural background and practices. Cultural competence is an ongoing process that involves accepting and respecting differences (Giger et al., 2007). This definition is built on the assumption that care providers are aware of and sensitized to their own cultural backgrounds and that they are able to integrate this sensitivity into their delivery of care. The interactive nature of caregiving requires the authentic engagement of the provider with the patient to appreciate and respond to differences that may affect giving or receiving care. A good example of the challenge that culturally competent care presents was provided by Wheatley (2005). In this example, a group practice offered free car seats and training in their use to a group of parents, but no one took advantage of the gift. On debriefing, the providers learned that for this group of parents, using a car seat was an invitation to God to cause a car accident. Differences are issues for every person, and they become even more important when one becomes a leader and role model. Working with colleagues who are different provides APRNs with opportunities for soliciting information about others' experiences. Box 9.6 presents strategies for enhancing cultural awareness.

Gender can play an important component in leadership. Gender stereotypes can exert a strong influence similar to cultural stereotypes and can affect the way a leader is viewed and how the leader actually performs (Burgess et al., 2012). As with culture, successful leaders understand their own biases about gender, the role gender may play in the provision of care, and gender issues in team functioning.

BOX 9.6

Strategies to Achieve Cultural Competence

- Explore and learn about your own racial and ethnic culture and background.
- Explore and learn about the different racial and ethnic cultures most frequently encountered in your practice.
- Read ethnic newspapers, magazines, and books.
- Learn the language of a different culture. Become bilingual with the verbal and nonverbal behavior of the culture.
- Take advantage of training opportunities to increase your cultural awareness and sensitivity.
- Be able to identify personal biases and develop strategies to manage, eliminate, or sublimate those potentially damaging attitudes and behaviors.
- When faced with patient difficulties, consider whether implicit biases may be operating for you or your colleagues.

Adapted from Hanson, C. M., & Malone, B. (2000). Leadership: Empowerment, change agency, and activism. In A. B. Hamric, J. A. Spross, & C. M. Hanson (Eds.), *Advanced nursing practice: An integrative approach* (2nd ed., pp. 279–313). Saunders.

Global Awareness

The world is highly interconnected and interdependent; this affects APRN leaders because issues such as access to care, patient safety, and quality care are global issues that are not confined to any particular geographic region. There are workforce challenges throughout the world, natural and human catastrophes occur with regularity, and there are fewer barriers to interactions among countries (Abbott & Coenen, 2008; Carter et al., 2015). APRN leaders interface with a multicultural workforce in their immediate setting or through professional organizations, and often they are asked to lead multicultural teams (Nichols et al., 2011). APRNs may look to other countries for problem-solving ideas or may be asked for consultation in person or via technology from healthcare providers across the globe.

The sharing of new techniques, therapies, and knowledge resources is important in working together to address global issues such as the global chronic illness epidemic, infectious diseases, and common health crises (World Health Organization, 2020a). Nichols et al. (2011) identified global competencies for nurse leaders as outlined in Box 9.7. In addition, the group outlined areas for nurse leaders to consider in development of a worldview that includes sense of self and space, cultural dress, family relationships and decision making, values and beliefs, nutrition habits, and religious preferences (Nichols et al., 2011). Friedman (2006) termed this view *global citizenship* and suggested that individuals and groups in leadership positions have a responsibility to think and act as global citizens. Several organizations have a global perspective of their mission and can be accessed for resources:

- International Council of Nurses
- World Health Organization
- Sigma Theta Tau International
- Pan American Health Organization

BOX 9.7

Global Competencies for Nurse Leaders

Develop global mindset and worldview:
- Global environmental awareness
- Cultural adaptation
- Awareness of social, political, and economic trends

Understand needs of technology:
- Enhanced ability of communication and technology
- Create global networks
- Individuals can now drive change just as businesses used to drive change

Respect diversity and cultivate cross-cultural competencies:
- Institutional mergers and growth
- Multicultural workforce
- Multicultural patient populations

Adapted from Nichols, B., Shaffer, F., & Porter, C. (2011). Global nursing leadership: A practical guide. *Nursing Administration Quarterly, 35*, 354–359.

DEVELOPING SKILLS AS APRN LEADERS

There are formal and informal strategies that are useful when considering a leadership development plan. Students will need to have experiences in their educational program to help them develop leadership skills. These can occur in the classroom, clinical practice, and student leadership and health-related service projects. In general, lessons learned in one domain will apply to leadership situations in other domains. Health policy leadership is discussed separately because it has specific features that are somewhat different from the APRN's everyday leadership activities.

Factors Influencing Leadership Development

There may be a misconception that leadership is a trait that one is born with rather than a skill that is learned. Several resources are available that new APRNs can access to help them learn to be leaders. Zaccaro (2007) argued that with increases in conceptual and methodological resources, learned attributes are more likely to predict leadership than once was believed. Leadership represents complex patterns of behavior explained in part by multiple leader attributes (Zaccaro, 2007). This section explores leadership traits and attributes of leadership for APRNs.

Personal Characteristics and Experiences

In a classic work, Allen (1998) explored the primary factors and individual characteristics that influenced leadership development in nurse leaders. Self-confidence, traced to childhood and subsequent risk-taking behaviors, was reported as a critical factor. Feedback from significant others led to enhanced self-confidence over time. The nurse leaders also spoke about having innate qualities and tendencies of leaders, such as being extroverted or bossy and wanting to take charge, and about having roles as team captains and officers in organizations. They saw themselves as people who rise to the occasion. A third important factor was a progression of experiences and successes that were pivotal in moving them forward. Being at the right place at the right time and taking advantage of opportunities presented in those situations allowed them to grow as leaders. Closely aligned with this factor was the influence of people important to them, such as mentors, role models, faculty, and parents, who had the ability to encourage and provide opportunities for advancement. Personal life factors, such as time, family, health, and work schedules, influenced leadership development. For example, supportive spouses and relatives who assisted with family and home responsibilities and employers who were flexible were important to the leadership development process. Upon close examination, one can see that the leadership abilities grew out of a combination of education and learning opportunities and depended on the support of others. These same characteristics can be used by aspiring APRN leaders.

Zaccaro et al. (2004) developed a model that describes distal attributes, including personality, cognitive abilities, motives, and values, along with proximal attributes, including social appraisal skills, problem-solving skills, expertise, and tacit knowledge. In this model, the leader's operating environment influences the trajectory toward success, which supports the importance of organizational culture described by Watkins (2013; see "Mentoring" section earlier). Carroll (2005) identified six factors that were present in women leaders and nurse executives: personal integrity, strategic vision and action orientation, team-building and communication skills, management and technical competencies, people skills (collaboration, empowering others, valuing diversity), and personal survival skills. These factors share similarity with the attributes in Box 9.5.

Strategies for Acquiring Competency as a Leader

Formal educational opportunities in leadership are an expected part of APRN education. Opportunities to work with faculty and other mentors help students acquire leadership skills and further reinforce self-confidence as a leader. Seeking office while a student in local leadership positions or in professional organizations and serving on local and national coalitions are other good strategies for developing this competency (Sandrick, 2006). Also, leadership conferences that foster effective communication and interaction are beneficial. Exemplar 9.3 shows how students can practice their leadership development while in school.

Leadership skills are developed and enhanced over time and in many ways. Communication is one of the strengths often attributed to nurses; it is a skill that can be strengthened through practice. Staying connected is important for busy APRNs and can be achieved in a variety of ways, from social media and shared projects to attending conferences that allow for time to interact and problem-solve with colleagues about similar professional issues. A community of APRN leaders is important for faculty and students involved with raising the visibility of advanced practice nursing roles in their institutions and communities.

DEVELOPING LEADERSHIP IN THE HEALTH POLICY ARENA

Health policy issues affecting APRNs and their patients, including strategies for political advocacy, are explored in Chapter 17. The following section describes how APRNs can develop skills to influence health policy through creative leadership and political advocacy, whether by means of local grassroots endeavors or directly through top government involvement. The term *advocacy* is the act of pleading another person's cause and is multifaceted with diverse activities (Kendig, 2006); "the endpoint of advocacy is the health and welfare of the public" (Leavitt et al., 2007, p. 37). APRNs are being called on, both collectively and individually, to make their voices heard as governments struggle with budget constraints and difficult decisions about health policies, organization, and the funding of healthcare programs.

In the political arena, developing power and influence uses a number of leadership skills. Leadership strategies used by APRNs in the political arena include developing influence with policymakers, motivating colleagues to stay informed of current issues, and providing bridges to other leaders who have access to

EXEMPLAR 9.3

MENTORING AN ADVANCED PRACTICE NURSE STUDENT IN COMMUNITY LEADERSHIP

John was required to complete a course in the family nurse practitioner program focused on healthcare leadership. John was not too sure just why this was required since his primary goal was to graduate and open a practice in northeast Alaska where he would be providing care to Alaska Native people in a small village. This had been a long-term dream, and he had selected a very strong clinical program and an experienced Alaskan Native preceptor so he would be ready to begin providing care upon graduation. He was unclear about what leadership activities would be expected of him as a primary care provider. One of the assignments he had in the leadership course was to complete a community assessment of his future site of practice to determine areas in which he could lead change. John learned many things about his future practice site during this assignment.

The community where he would be in practice did not have a potable water supply. Untreated water was taken from a nearby stream during the summer months, but the stream was frozen during the long and very harsh winter. Ice could be melted for water but there was no assurance that the water would be clean enough for drinking. John also learned that the sewage system was a "honey bucket" self-haul system that was nearly impossible for the elderly to use and exposed children to raw sewage.

Working under the mentorship of his preceptor who lived in the village, John began to grasp the scope of the problem and quickly learned that substantial leadership would be required to bring an acceptable and affordable solution to the problems of potable water and sewage management. Solutions suitable for other climates just would not work in this community. Previous plans had failed because they did not fit the culture of the community, could not survive the harsh winter climate or spring floods from ice dams on the river, and were far too expensive for the small community to afford. John also learned that what he thought was a simple issue was a very large problem and would likely take many years to remedy. He was able to engage community elders to begin the process of finding long-term solutions. He had skills in grant writing that were very useful in securing funds to help with the planning. Most of his success was a result of the excellent mentorship he received from both his faculty member and his Alaskan Native preceptor. They gently guided him through the many complex areas related to this problem.

Following graduation and after beginning practice in the village, John has continued his leadership. A new drinking/washing water system is in place, but work continues on the community sewage system. His project in his leadership class has led to a longer-term role in leading his village to build other needed infrastructure.

important resources. The policy arena is made of a variety of rules, regulations, laws, court opinions, funding strategies, and other interrelated areas. There is often no one simple approach to this area. Mentoring APRNs to understand their power and influence in the health policy arena is a key role for the APRN leader. The developmental process for becoming a political activist begins early in life with an understanding of how government and the political systems work. Focused understanding often begins when health policy is introduced in the nursing curriculum (see Exemplar 9.3). These students are usually coached to understand the power inherent in policymaking, the power of politics to influence practice, and the ways in which they can influence the system, individually and collectively, to better their own practice and be high-level patient advocates. Faculty members keep students informed about key legislative issues and introduce them, through role modeling, to the role of political advocacy. Inviting APRN students to accompany faculty who are giving testimony at a legislative hearing is one way to model the advocacy role. Faculty may also be members of committees or boards that focus on policy issues, and students can accompany the faculty member in this work. Many professional organizations also offer tools on how to engage in the political process, such as the American Association of Nurse Anesthesiology (2020).

There is no question that influencing policy takes substantial commitment, time, and energy. Timing is an important consideration. APRNs ask themselves several personal and professional questions to determine the degree of involvement and level of sophistication at which advocacy is to be undertaken. Questions to be considered are included in Box 9.8.

APRNs will need to find an appropriate mentor once they have made a decision about the depth of involvement to which they can commit. There are numerous effective nurse leaders and advocates who are willing and able to move new advocates into positions to make positive changes in health policy. Opportunities for

BOX 9.8

Personal and Professional Questions to Determine the Degree of Involvement and Level of Sophistication

- What are my personal responsibilities related to wage earning, small children, dependent parents, single parenthood, health issues, school, and gaining initial competence as an APRN?
- How can I best serve the APRN community at this time?
- What data sources can I access that keep me informed and up-to-date?
- What learning opportunities will help me be an effective APRN advocate?
- How can I develop short-term and long-term plans for becoming a more politically astute advocate for myself, my patients, and nursing?
- What do I care deeply about?
- What am I able to commit to based on the responses to these questions?

input and influence exist at various levels of the legislative process (see Chapter 17).

Using Professional Organizations to the Best Advantage

For APRNs, close contact with their professional organizations is an important link for staying current of national and state policy agendas, finding a support network of like-minded colleagues, and accessing information about changes in credentialing and practice issues. This means being an active member of more than one affiliate organization to stay on the cutting edge of pertinent issues. Most APRNs are aligned with at least one nursing organization; those who aspire to an active role in influencing policy will need to have memberships in several. As new graduates move into diverse practice settings, they must align with the advanced practice nursing organizations that best meet their needs and offer the strongest support, choosing to engage actively in some and remaining on the periphery in others. Choosing the "right" organizations to belong to is based on one's particular needs, comfort level, specialty, and experience.

Internships and Fellowships

One excellent way to develop enhanced skills as an advanced practice nursing policy advocate is to apply for a national or state policy internship or fellowship. These appointments, which last from several days to 1 or 2 years, offer a wide range of health policy and political experiences that are targeted to novice and expert APRNs. For example, the Nurse in Washington Internship (NIWI), sponsored by the Nursing Organizations Alliance, is a 4-day internship that introduces nurses to policymaking in Washington, DC. This internship serves as an excellent beginning step in learning the APRN policy role. Federal fellowships and internships that link nurses to legislators or to the various branches of federal and state government are invaluable in assisting APRNs to understand how leaders are developed and how the system for setting health policy operates.

New Modes of Communication

The ability to communicate with others accurately, efficiently, and in a timely manner is a driving force in making effective change. There is substantial opportunity to share information and to engage with others at a distance. Time and distance are no longer serious obstacles to communication. The multiple modes of Internet access make virtual communication a reality.

OBSTACLES TO LEADERSHIP DEVELOPMENT AND EFFECTIVE LEADERSHIP

There are a number of areas in which leaders encounter obstacles to developing effective leadership. Some of these were touched on earlier, but there are other areas in which obstacles can arise in unanticipated ways.

Clinical Leadership Issues

APRNs can find that exerting clinical leadership can be challenging at times. Some health systems have archaic rules and regulations that can infect professional staff privileges and the ability for APRNs to lead. For example, some health systems do not credential APRNs as independent practitioners but rather as dependent practitioners. This means that records must be signed by another professional; admissions, transitions of care, and discharges are a challenge; and procedures or scope of practice can be restricted. The world of health care is changing, so the astute APRN will keep pushing the boundaries in this area. Sometimes these issues can be resolved by creativity. For example, in one state, there was a statewide regulation governing all hospitals that there must be a physician appointed to be the chief of the medical staff. The particular hospital wanted to appoint a CNM to be in charge of all clinical services offered by the hospital. This was done by appointing the CNM to the title of chief clinical officer and having the chief of the medical staff report to this position. This approach allowed the hospital to achieve its goal and to conform to state regulations.

Many rules and regulations that limit practice will fall away as new APRNs join the team and their unique expertise is valued. Some hospitals that claim that they do not credential APRNs do credential CRNAs to practice. They would have to close their surgical services if they did not do so. The day will come when the rest of the APRNs will be viewed as similarly valuable.

Professional and System Obstacles

There are several obstacles to achieving recognition as an APRN leader. Most of the obstacles result from conflict or competition among individuals, groups, or organizations. These obstacles can develop as the scopes of practice of various professionals overlap in clinical practice. A lack of legal empowerment to practice to the fullest extent of knowledge and skills has been a dominant barrier to the optimal practice of APRNs in recent years. CNMs and CRNAs have the longest track record in the United States of dealing with these issues and have earned many successes. Competition can be intraprofessional, as among APRN groups, and interprofessional, as among pharmacists, optometrists, physicians, and nurses. One approach to good leadership is to focus on bringing dignity to self and others rather than being liked; for most people, this is difficult because being accepted and liked by others is important.

Dysfunctional Leadership Styles

Leadership can be a lonely place, and successful leadership requires careful nurturing. Although good leaders are sought after and desired, we have all experienced the other side of the coin—a dysfunctional leader. There are a multitude of traits and styles that can be attributed to a dysfunctional leader, such as micromanager, passive–aggressive, narcissistic personality, conflict avoidant, a quest for personal power, and a game player. The dictatorial leader or the leader who is most interested in empire building is easily recognized. Dysfunctional leaders often have poor self-control, have no time for others, or fail to accept responsibility for their own actions. At its worst, dysfunctional leadership moves into the realm of horizontal violence.

Horizontal Violence

Horizontal violence, sometimes called *lateral violence* or *bullying*, is described as harmful, nonphysical actions carried out by one colleague toward another (Detwiler & Vaughn, 2020). This type of behavior is often seen among oppressed groups as a way for individuals to achieve a sense of power. Some of these behaviors are being overly critical, intentionally undermining another's actions, fighting among colleagues, and wrongfully blaming others. These behaviors leave one feeling humiliated, overwhelmed, and unsupported. Although there are many barriers to leading effectively and creating community, several constellations of behaviors that are particularly destructive have been identified. Nurses may be vulnerable to these destructive behaviors because of the profession's historical marginalization as being female and a relatively powerless group in health care. The culture of an organization as described earlier is also a factor in the development of these dysfunctional styles. These behaviors undermine successful APRN leadership. APRNs must avoid engaging in such behaviors and intervene quickly and assertively when they do occur. Four manifestations of horizontal violence in workplace culture limit the ability of APRNs to lead: the *star complex*, the *queen bee syndrome*, *failure to mentor* ("eating one's young"), and *bullying*. These behaviors are of particular concern because the profession needs to recruit and develop new nurses to help build satisfying careers and pass on this legacy to future generations of nurses. Faculty and preceptors need to be alert to the appearance of such toxic behaviors and assure that they will not be tolerated. Readers are referred to K. Anderson (2011), Longo and Smith (2011), and Detwiler and Vaughn (2020) for specific suggestions on strategies for communicating with students and colleagues who demonstrate these negative interpersonal styles.

Abandoning One's Nursing Identity: Star Complex

Effective APRN leaders are proud of their identity as a nurse. Those with a star complex deny or minimize their nursing identity when being identified as a nurse might diminish their influence. The star complex is a condition that is seen in some experienced APRNs or in APRNs who have not been well socialized into nursing as a profession. Individuals with a star complex are those whose sense of self and identity depend a great deal on the opinions of powerful others. Acknowledging or promoting their identity as nurses is seen to diminish their power or the opinions that powerful others hold about them. As an example, consider Janice, an expert APRN who provides superior patient-focused care. Physician colleagues consider her to be a partner in the delivery of care, but staff and other APRNs gave up consulting with her because her self-promotion often interfered with patient and colleague interactions. In a recent conversation, a well-respected physician colleague told her how impressed he was with her practice. "In fact," he stated, "you're really not a nurse. You're different from all the other nurses I know." Janice graciously accepted this compliment, knowing that stardom, although overdue, had finally arrived. She had ascended to the heights of provider status and crashed through the nursing ceiling into a zone beyond nursing. Clearly, Janice's understanding of herself as an APRN was dormant.

APRNs are particularly vulnerable to being seduced into believing that they are something other (more) than a nurse. Advanced practice nursing specialties that have expanded roles may seek the status of medicine. This vulnerability stems from the historical lack of recognition of nursing by physicians, other disciplines, and even other nurses; the need for approval; and a lack of personal mastery.

A primary strategy for the management of this obstacle is effective mentoring by a powerful APRN with a strong nursing identity. An additional essential strategy is to use clear and concise communication skills to provide an appropriate response to a colleague who believes that it is a compliment to be identified as other than a nurse. An appropriate response for Janice to have made would have been to say, "Thank you, but I'm proud to be an APRN. It is good that we can work together to help our patients." The existence of a star complex may represent a more fundamental problem for the APRN than good communication skills can address. The issue is whether the APRN truly desires to be identified as a nurse, performing at the boundaries of nursing practice and being accepted by other nurses as a valued member of the nursing profession. As APRNs are increasingly recognized as valued members of the healthcare team and as mentoring and empowerment become understood as core elements of leadership, star complex behavior will become less tolerated, unnecessary, and less frequent.

Hoarding or Misusing Power: Queen Bee Syndrome

An effective leader is generous, looking for opportunities to lift colleagues up by sharing opportunities, knowledge, and expertise and acknowledging the contributions of others. Queen bee syndrome refers to individuals who believe they have achieved a level of prominence by their own individual hard work, with little or no assistance from others, and that everyone else should do the same. These people hoard all the visible leadership tasks for themselves. Like those with a star complex, the effort to garner power is a theme. In this case, power derives not from powerful others but from the queen bee's own knowledge and expertise. Such APRNs are threatened by strong individuals and tend to denigrate them instead of sharing power. This type of leader prefers to be surrounded by servile individuals who will not challenge personal authority. For example, Rita, an experienced wound and ostomy APRN, makes sure that she sees every patient and that patients know she is the authority on wounds and ostomies. Staff nurses who are competent in these skills report that Rita undermines them with patients by saying that the care should have been done a certain way. Rita was not happy when the staff on a surgical unit, who had tried unsuccessfully to involve her in a unit project, conducted a quality improvement project during which both physicians and patients identified some service delivery issues relative to ostomy care. These staff members changed the way wound and ostomy services were managed.

The antidote to a queen bee syndrome is to use knowledge and expertise to move away from hoarding power and move toward collaborative, empowered leadership. Queen bee behavior is the antithesis of good leadership. Queen bees will have more difficulty remaining as leaders and keeping positions of power as APRNs become more confident in their leadership abilities and join the circle of leaders. All effective leaders empower others.

Failure to Mentor

Other distressing forms of horizontal violence can also occur regularly in the workplace. "Nurses eat their young" is an epithet that characterizes the experience of some novice nurses and APRNs, as well as some older, more experienced nurses (Baltimore, 2006). Nurses who advance in their profession may forget their roots and leave novice nurses behind or, worse, actively undermine their advancement. For example, nurses are often criticized by other nurses for continuing their education and moving into APRN roles. This denigration of important values and goals by colleagues is dispiriting and discouraging; it can also hamper nurses from moving forward in their careers. In another example, the orientation process for a new position may become a survival test to see whether the new APRN can survive without mentoring or a supportive network. Because perceived powerlessness is at the root of this behavior, an important antidote is empowerment. The common practice of mentoring, taking an active interest in another's career, apprenticing, and "giving a leg up" to the least experienced is not as common in nursing as it is in many other professions. Box 9.9 lists the behaviors that provide evidence that there has been a failure in mentorship (Baltimore, 2006; Longo & Sherman, 2007; Longo & Smith, 2011).

Bullying

Bullying is a severe form of horizontal violence attributed to oppressed group behavior. Plonien (2016) and the American Nurses Association (2015b) suggested that horizontal violence is a more complex phenomenon and includes those external to nursing who make up the organization's culture and add to stress in the work setting. Curran (2006) reported that there will be more career nurses vying for leadership positions and that forms of horizontal violence such as bullying will worsen. Bullying is not a one-time event but instead is subtle, deliberate, and ongoing behavior that accumulates over time and leaves the victim feeling hurt, vulnerable, and powerless (Anderson, 2011; Longo & Sherman, 2007).

BOX 9.9

Failure in Mentorship Behaviors

- Gossiping or bad-mouthing
- Criticizing
- Failure to give assistance when needed
- Setting up roadblocks by withholding information
- Bullying
- Scapegoating
- Undermining performance

Strategies to Overcome Horizontal Violence

Nursing leaders have an ethical obligation to become knowledgeable about horizontal violence and its impact on their team members. Many professional nursing organizations have adopted standards for healthy work environments. These standards include identifying, addressing, and eliminating disruptive behaviors in the workplace. It is the responsibility of a leader to educate the staff on horizontal violence and disruptive behaviors, empower everyone to report any witnessed negative behaviors, ensure there are formal processes in place to deal with the issue, and act quickly to address any issues that are brought forward (Longo & Sherman, 2007; Longo & Smith, 2011). A change in the culture of the organization as well as leadership is necessary to eliminate horizontal violence and create a positive work environment. Personal and organizational symptoms of horizontal violence are job dissatisfaction, increased stress levels, and physical and psychological illness. If the broader cause is a negative organizational culture, then the most effective leadership strategy to prevent its occurrence is to adopt a zero-tolerance policy and a shared set of values with the staff (Longo & Sherman, 2007; Longo & Smith, 2011) that support positive behaviors. For example, fostering mentoring opportunities and enhancing the transition of colleagues into new positions of leadership can create a positive culture that does not tolerate horizontal violence. Box 9.10 presents suggested leadership strategies to eliminate horizontal violence.

Carefronting is an innovative approach to dealing with horizonal violence (Sherman, 2012). This approach is different from conflict management in

BOX 9.10

Leadership Strategies to Stop Horizontal Violence

- Examine the organizational culture for symptoms of horizontal violence.
- Name the problem as horizontal violence when you see it.
- Educate staff to break the silence.
- Allow victims of horizontal violence to tell their stories.
- Enact a process for dealing with issues that occur.
- Provide training for conflict and anger management skills.
- Empower victims to defend themselves.
- Engage in self-reflection to ensure that your leadership style does not support horizontal violence.
- Encourage a culture of zero tolerance for horizontal violence.

Adapted from Longo, J., & Sherman, R. O. (2007). Leveling horizontal violence. *Nursing Management, 38*, 34–37, 50–51.

that the goal is to attain and maintain effective productive working relationships. Those interested in this approach can learn more by reviewing the reference.

STRATEGIES FOR IMPLEMENTING THE LEADERSHIP COMPETENCY

Developing a Leadership Portfolio

Throughout this chapter, definitions, attributes, and components of leadership and key strategies for developing competency in APRN leadership have been presented. These approaches will help new APRNs acquire leadership skills and can assist faculty in teaching these skills. Developing a leadership component as part of a professional portfolio is helpful to novice APRNs who desire to individualize continuing development of the leadership competency consistent with their personal vision, goals, timeline, and APRN role in the practice setting. An Australian study reported increased knowledge, skill sets, and outcomes in clinicians and leaders who used portfolios to enhance their effectiveness (Dadich, 2010). Falter (2003) suggested the use of a strategy map that includes vision, goals, and objectives that outline steps to achieve a particular strategy. Portfolios are designed to meet the needs of individual APRNs and should be consistent with clinical and personal interests and professional goals and provide a timeline that allows for personal and professional balance and boundary setting. Chapter 18 provides the elements of a marketing portfolio.

Promoting Collaboration Among APRN Groups

At different times, each subgroup of APRNs in America has emerged as a leader for the nursing profession. Psychiatric CNSs were early APRNs to enter private practice, despite the litigious climate in which they could be threatened with lawsuits for "practicing medicine." CNMs and CRNAs have led the way in using data effectively to justify their practice and attain appropriate scopes of practice. Early in their history, both groups began to record the results of their practices, showing the quality and suitability of their care (see Chapter 1). In the 1990s, NPs, with their flexible, community-based primary care practices, stood at the forefront of the changing healthcare delivery system. Although these subgroups of APRNs have made impressive strides, an obstacle to effective leadership has been the tendency for APRN specialty groups to separate and establish rigid boundaries that distinguish them from one another, thereby fragmenting APRN groups and blocking opportunities for the increased power that unity would bring.

The tension and fragmentation created by rigid boundaries require leaders who can transcend APRN roles and specialties. Consensus groups have developed at the national level to discuss policy issues in which the power of the collective numbers of all APRN groups speaking with one voice cannot be overemphasized (see Chapters 2, 10, and 20). An excellent example of professional collaboration among nurse leaders is the Consensus Model (Chapter 20). APRN organizations have joined to speak out collaboratively about state regulations regarding reimbursement, prescriptive authority, and managed care empanelment.

Each APRN, regardless of specialty, has the responsibility of moving toward an integrative and unified understanding of advanced practice nursing. Creating community in the current healthcare environment is particularly challenging because of the realignment of clinical decision making, changing scopes of practice for APRNs, and new roles that blur boundaries between and among providers.

An understanding of change, effective communication, coalition building, shared vision, and collaborative practice leads to the development of structures on which unity is built. These five building blocks form the foundation of interprofessional leadership and practice.

Networking

Networking is a valuable technique used by leaders to stay informed and connected regarding APRN issues. Networking is not a new strategy for APRN leaders. Formal networks take the form of committees, coalitions, and consortia of people who come together to share information, collaborate, and plan strategy regarding mutual issues. Formal networks open doors to new opportunities and provide shared resources that ensure a competitive edge in the organization. Informal networking is a strategy that takes place behind the scenes and allows for contact with APRNs and others who speak a similar language, share viewpoints, and offer support and feedback at critical times. The ability of APRNs to stay connected to important practice and education issues through networking is key to leadership competency. The most effective strategy for becoming an insider is networking with colleagues within the circle of APRN peers and with other healthcare providers who have a stake in the outcomes of a particular issue.

Effectively Working With Other Leaders to Advance Health Care

Other strategies also assist in the process of planning and implementing change. It is important to analyze the situation and explore the need for change. If change is warranted, one must craft an implementation plan that involves the key players. Box 9.4 lists leadership strategies that are useful for moving through these transitions. An important component of leadership during times of change is the ability to foster and encourage resilience in change recipients. Grafton et al. (2010) defined resilient people as being positive and self-assured in the face of life's complexities; having a focused, clear vision of what they want to achieve; and having the ability to be organized but flexible and proactive rather than reactive. Helping colleagues and followers develop resilience should be a major focus for APRN leaders who seek to facilitate the growth of their followers.

Institutional Assessment Regarding Readiness for Change

With the emphasis on evidence-based practice and the knowledge that evidence-based guidelines and therapies are underused, overused, or misused, APRNs have an important systems leadership role in improving care. This can be accomplished by leading and collaborating with nurses and interprofessional colleagues to ensure the adoption of best practices (Weaver et al., 2011). An institutional assessment of specific factors will help the APRN identify facilitators of and barriers to change. These data can then be used to design a plan for change in collaboration with others. Box 9.11 lists key assessment questions to consider.

BOX 9.11

Assessment Questions to Evaluate Readiness for Change

- What is the nature of the change (e.g., policy, procedure, new skill, behavior)?
- Is the issue significant? For all stakeholders or just one group?
- Is a national policy, guideline, or standard the focus of the change? Is it a mandate with which the agency must be in compliance?
- Is the change simple or complex? Will different stakeholders perceive its simplicity or complexity differently?
- Do you foresee major problems associated with change, such as an increase in errors or resistance on the part of a group?
- Will it be possible to address these major problems?
- Are there vested interests—who is likely to gain from the change, who will view the change as a loss (e.g., of power)?
- Are there opinion leaders who will promote the change? Do you anticipate strong opposition?
- Have you observed a gap between public statements and private actions (e.g., a colleague agrees to serve on a committee but never shows up or participates in the committee's work)?
- Are there resource implications? What are the costs (e.g., staffing, materials, lost revenue)?

Adapted from the University of York National Health Centre for Reviews and Dissemination (1999). Getting evidence into practice. *Effective Health Care Bulletin, 5*, 1–16.

Followship

As APRNs focus on developing their leadership skills, they discover the importance of being a good follower. Skill is necessary to recognize when one should be a follower rather than a leader—when another is more skilled or more appropriate to lead a particular situation or when it is appropriate to let others who are developing leadership skills take the lead on a project. Successful collaboration and teamwork require not just leadership but skilled followers as well. Expert followers know how to accept direction, be forthcoming with pertinent information that is valuable to the team, seek clarification, and provide appropriate constructive feedback.

CONCLUSION

The healthcare system is constantly evolving, and while this evolution can appear rather chaotic at times, most of the changes seen are the results of effective leadership. This means that the future is bright for APRNs as clinical, professional, health policy, and systems leaders. APRNs can exert their leadership influence in far-reaching ways, from the bedside and clinic to the highest political office. APRNs are also constantly evolving in various roles, and these changes have had substantial influence on the healthcare system as well as on the nursing profession itself. APRNs exercise leadership when they present ideas or dilemmas and offer solutions to colleagues or communities, whether through social media or at a national meeting. Small changes often lead to much larger changes, so APRNs should not underestimate the impact of leadership exercised with patients, colleagues, and administrators. APRNs can consider how they can lead, make a difference, and commit to doing so, knowing that they can redefine the scope of their leadership influence in response to opportunities or changing life circumstances. The dynamic, ever-changing environment of health care sets the stage for ceaseless opportunities for APRNs to innovate and lead.

Nursing practice is based on an interactive style that empowers patients and colleagues. This foundation holds APRN leaders in good stead as they move into the emerging interprofessional practices that are developing. APRNs can work toward identifying, clarifying, and demystifying the healthcare system of today, for within today's reality lies the basis of tomorrow's change. APRNs are poised to lead change as they operate at the boundary between today's healthcare system and that of tomorrow. The attributes, goals, and vision of APRN leaders put them at the forefront of the healthcare frontier.

KEY SUMMARY POINTS

- Leadership is a core APRN competency, requiring deep knowledge of the art and science and an emphasis on interpersonal skills.
- The healthcare system is evolving continuously, requiring APRNs to create mastery around change management.
- Effective leaders use mentors, mentor others, network, and learn how to follow.
- Effective leaders are able to understand and respect cultural and gender diversity as well as unconscious bias to lead effective organizations.
- APRNs can use a variety of different approaches to understand and mitigate dysfunctional leadership styles that impede care.

REFERENCES

Abbott, P. A., & Coenen, A. (2008). Globalization and advances in information and communication technologies: The impact on nursing and health. *Nursing Outlook, 56*, 38–246. doi:10.1016/j.outlook.2008.06.009

Allen, D. W. (1998). How nurses become leaders: Perceptions and beliefs about leadership development. *Journal of Nursing Administration, 28*, 15–20. doi:10.1097/00005110-199809000-00005

American Association of Colleges of Nursing (AACN). (2021). *The essentials: Core competencies for professional nursing education.* https://www.aacnnursing.org/Portals/42/Downloads/Essentials/Essentials-Draft-Document-10-20.pdf

American Association of Nurse Anesthesiology. (2020). *Federal government affairs.* https://www.aana.com/advocacy/federal-government-affairs

American Nurses Association. (2015a). *Code of ethics for nurses with interpretive statements.* https://www.nursingworld.org/practice-policy/nursing-excellence/ethics/code-of-ethics-for-nurses/

American Nurses Association. (2015b). *Position statement on incivility, bullying, and workplace violence.* https://www.nursingworld.org/~49d6e3/globalassets/practiceandpolicy/nursing-excellence/incivility-bullying-and-workplace-violence–ana-position-statement.pdf

Anderson, C. A., & Titler, M. G. (2014). Development and verification of an agent-based model of opinion leadership. *Implementation Science, 27*(9), 136. doi:10.1186/s13012-014-0136-6

Anderson, K. (2011). Workplace aggression and violence: Midwives and nurses say no. *Australian Nursing Journal, 19*(1), 26–29.

Bagheri, A., & Akbari, M. (2018). The impact of entrepreneurial leadership on nurses' innovation behavior. *Journal of Nursing Scholarship, 50*, 28–35. https://doi.org.ezproxy.uthsc.edu/10.1111/jnu.12354

Bally, J. M. (2007). The role of nursing leadership in creating a mentoring culture in acute care environments. *Nursing Economic$, 25*(3), 143–148.

Baltimore, J. (2006). Nurse collegiality: Fact or fiction. *Nursing Management, 37*(5), 28–36. doi:10.1097/00006247-200605000-00008

Barker, E., & Kelley, P. W. (2020). Mentoring. *Journal of the American Association of Nurse Practitioners, 32*(9), 621–625. doi:10.1097/JXX.0000000000000417

Berwick, D. M. (2016). Era 3 for medicine and health care. *The Journal of the American Medical Association, 315*(13), 1329–1330. doi:10.1001/jama.2016.1509

Berwick, D. M., Caulkins, D. R., McCannon, C. J., & Hackbarth, A. D. (2006). The 100,000 Lives Campaign: Setting a goal and a deadline for improving health care quality. *The Journal of the American Medical Association, 295*(3), 324–327. doi:10.1001/jama.295.3.324

Blanchard, K., Hutson, D., & Willis, E. (2007). *The one-minute entrepreneur: Discover your entrepreneurial strengths*. Executive Books.

Burgess, D. J., Joseph, A., van Ryn, M., & Carnes, M. (2012). Does stereotype threat affect women in academic medicine? *Academic Medicine: Journal of the Association of American Medical Colleges, 87*(4), 506–512. doi:10.1097/ACM.0b013e318248f718

Bush, T. (2018). Transformational leadership: Exploring common conceptions. *Educational Management Administration and Leadership, 46*(6), 883–887. doi:10.1177/1741143218795731

Canadian Nurses Association. (2010). *Canadian nurse practitioner core competency framework*. http://www.cno.org/globalassets/for/rnec/pdf/competencyframework_en.pdf

Carlson, E., Klakovich, M., Broscious, S., Delock, S., Roche-Dean, M., Hittle, K., Jumaa, M. O., Stewart, M. W., & Alston, P. (2011). Board leadership development: The key to effective nursing leadership. *Journal of Continuing Education in Nursing, 42*, 107–113. doi:10.3928/00220124-20101201-03

Carlton, E. L., Holsinger, J. W., Riddell, M. C., & Bush, H. (2015). Full-range public health leadership, part 2: Qualitative analysis and synthesis. *Frontiers in Public Health, 3*, 174. doi:10.3389/fpubh.2015.00174

Carroll, T. L. (2005). Leadership skills and attributes of women and nurse executives: Challenges for the 21st century. *Nursing Administration Quarterly, 29*, 146–153.

Carter, M., Owen-Williams, E., & Della, P. (2015). Meeting Australia's emerging primary care needs by nurse practitioners. *Journal for Nurse Practitioners, 11*(6), 647–652. doi:10.1891/1939-2095.8.1.13

Castledine, S. G. (2008). Dealing with difficult doctors. *British Journal of Nursing, 17*, 1305. doi:10.12968/bjon.2008.17.20.31651

Clancy, T., Effken, J., & Pesut, D. (2008). Applications of complex systems theory in nursing education, research, and practice. *Nursing Outlook, 56*(5), 248–256. doi:10.1016/j.outlook.2008.06.010

Cooperrider, D. L., Whitney, D., & Stavros, J. M. (2008). *Appreciative inquiry handbook* (2nd ed.). Berrett-Koehler.

Covey, S. (1989). *The seven habits of highly effective people: Powerful lessons in personal change*. Simon & Schuster.

Covey, S. (2004). *The 8th habit. From effectiveness to greatness*. Free Press.

Covey, S. (2006). Leading in the knowledge worker age. *Leader to Leader Journal, 41*, 11–15. doi:10.1002/ltl.184

Curran, C. (2006). Boomers: Bottlenecked, bored, and burned out. *Nursing Economic$, 24*(2), 57–59.

Dadich, A. (2010). From bench to bedside: Methods that help clinicians use evidence-based practice. *Australian Psychologist, 45*, 197–211. doi:10.1080/00050060903353004

DePree, M. (2011). *Leadership is an art*. Crown Business.

Detwiler, K. & Vaughn, N. (2020). What is lateral violence in nursing? https://www.relias.com/blog/what-is-lateral-violence-in-nursing

Dreher, M. C., Clinton, P., & Sperhac, A. (2014). Can the Institute of Medicine trump the dominant logic of nursing? Leading change in advanced practice education. *Journal of Professional Nursing, 30*(2), 104–109. doi:10.1016/j.profnurs.2013.09.004

Fahlberg, B. (2015). Moral courage: A step beyond patient advocacy. *Nursing, 45*(6), 13–14. doi:10.1097/01.NURSE.0000464991.63854.51

Fahlberg, B., & Toomey, R. (2016). Servant leadership: A model for emerging nurse leaders. *Nursing, 46*(10), 49–52. doi:10.1097/01.NURSE.0000494644.77680.2a

Falter, E. (2003). Successful leaders map and measure. *Nurse Leader, 1*, 40–42. 45.

Farrell, K., Payne, C., & Heye, M. (2015). Integrating interprofessional collaboration skills into the advanced practice registered nurses socialization process. *Journal of Professional Nursing, 31*(1), 5–10. doi:10.1016/j.profnurs.2014.05.006

Fisher, R., Ury, W., & Patton, B. (2011). *Getting to yes: How to negotiate an agreement without giving in* (2nd ed.). Penguin Putnam.

Flodgren, G., O'Brien, M. A., Parmelli, E., & Grimshaw, J. M. (2019). Local opinion leaders: effects on professional practice and healthcare outcomes. *The Cochrane Database of Systematic Reviews, 6*, Article CD000125. doi:10.1002/14651858.CD000125.pub5

Friedman, T. L. (2006). *The world is flat*. Farrar, Straus, & Giroux.

Gallagher, A. (2011). Moral distress and moral courage in everyday nursing practice. *Online Journal of Issues in Nursing, 16*(2), 8. doi:10.3912/OJIN.Vol16No02PPT03

Giger, J., Davidhizar, R., Purnell, L., Taylor-Harden, J., Phillips, J., & Strickland, O. (2007). Understanding cultural language to enhance cultural competence. *Nursing Outlook, 55*, 212–213.

Goleman, D. (2005). *Emotional intelligence: Why it can matter more than IQ*. Bantam Books.

Grafton, E., Gillespie, B., & Henderson, S. (2010). Resilience: The power within. *Oncology Nursing Forum, 37*, 698–705. doi:10.1188/10.ONF.698-705

Grant, A. (2013). *Give and take: A revolutionary approach to success*. Viking.

Harrington, S. (2011). Mentoring new nurse practitioners to accelerate their development as primary care providers. *Journal of the American Academy of Nurse Practitioners, 23*, 168–174. doi:10.1111/j.1745-7599.2011.00601.x

Henry, H. (2014). *Complexity theory in nursing*: Independent Nurse. http://www.independentnurse.co.uk/professional-article/complexity-theory-in-nursing/65669/

Huber, D. (2014). *Leadership and nursing care management* (5th ed.). Elsevier Saunders.

Hunter, T., Nelson, J., & Birmingham, J. (2013). Preventing readmissions through comprehensive discharge planning. *Professional Case Management, 18*(2), 56–63. doi:10.1097/NCM.0b013e31827de1ce

Institute for Healthcare Improvement (IHI). (2012). *Protecting 5 million lives*. http://www.ihi.org/offerings/Initiatives/PastStrategicInitiatives/5MillionLivesCampaign/Pages/default.aspx

Institute for Healthcare Improvement. (2021). *Improving health and health care worldwide: Leadership*. http://www.ihi.org/Topics/Leadership/Pages/default.aspx?utm_source=IHI_Homepage&utm_medium=Topics_Navigation

Institute of Medicine. (2001). *Crossing the quality chasm: A new health system for the 21st century*. National Academy Press.

Institute of Medicine (IOM). (2011). *The future of nursing: Leading change, advancing health*. National Academy Press.

Interprofessional Education Collaborative. (2011). *Core competencies for interprofessional collaborative practice: Report of an expert panel*. https://www.aacom.org/docs/default-source/insideome/ccrpt05-10-11.pdf?sfvrsn=77937f97_2

Jones, R. S. P. (2010). Appreciative inquiry: More than just a fad? *British Journal of Healthcare Management, 16*, 114–119. doi:10.12968/bjhc.2010.16.3.46818

Josiah Macy, Jr. Foundation. (2021). *Our priorities*. https://macyfoundation.org/our-priorities

Kendig, S. (2006). *Advocacy, action, and the allure of butter: A focus on policy*. www.medscape.com/viewarticle/523631

Kwamie, A. (2015). Balancing management and leadership in complex health systems: Comment on "Management Matters: A Leverage Point for Health Systems Strengthening in Global Health. *International Journal of Health Policy and Management, 4*, 849–851. doi:10.15171/ijhpm.2015.152

Lachman, V. (2010). Strategies necessary for moral courage. *The Online Journal of Issues in Nursing, 15*(3), 1. doi:10.3912/OJIN.Vol15No03Man03

Lazarus, I. R., & Fell, D. (2011). Innovation or stagnation: Crossing the creativity gap in healthcare. *Journal of Healthcare Management, 56*, 263–267. doi:10.1097/00115514-201111000-00003

Leavitt, J. K., Chaffee, M. W., & Vance, C. (2007). Learning the ropes of policy, politics, and advocacy. In D. J. Mason, J. K. Leavitt, & M. W. Chaffee (Eds.), *Policy and politics in nursing and health care* (5th ed.) (pp. 19–28). Saunders.

Longo, J., & Sherman, R. O. (2007). Leveling horizontal violence. *Nursing Management, 38*, 34–37. doi:10.1097/01.numa.0000262925.77680.e0. 50–51.

Longo, J., & Smith, M. (2011). A prescription for disruptions in care: Community building among nurses to address horizontal violence. *Advances in Nursing Science, 34*, 345–356. doi:10.1097/ANS.0b013e3182300e3e

Marcelin, J. R., Siraj, D. S., Victor, R., Kotadia, S., & Maldonado, Y. A. (2019). The impact of unconscious bias in healthcare: How to recognize and mitigate it. *Journal of Infectious Diseases*, 220 (Suppl. 2), S62–S73. doi:10.1093/infdis/jiz214

Marcellus, L., Duncan, S., MacKinnon, K., Jantzen, D., Siemens, J., Brennan, J., & Kassam, S. (2018). The role of education in developing leadership in nurses. *Nursing Leadership, 31*(4), 26–35. doi:10.12927/cjnl.2019.25758

Massoud, M. R., Nielsen, G. A., Nolan, K., Schall, M. W., & Sevin, C. (2006). *A framework for spread: From local improvements to system-wide change*. Institute for Healthcare Improvement. IHI Innovation Series White Paper. http://www.ihi.org/resources/Pages/IHIWhitePapers/AFrameworkforSpreadWhitePaper.aspx

McCloughen, A., O'Brien, L., & Jackson, D. (2009). Esteemed connection: Creating a mentoring relationship for nurse leadership. *Nursing Inquiry, 16*, 326–336. doi:10.1111/j.1440-1800.2009.00451.x

Mustard, R. W. (2020). Servant leadership in the Veterans Health Administration. *Nurse Leader, 18*(2), 178–180. doi:10.1016/j.mnl.2019.03.019

Musto, L., Rodney, P., & Vanderheide, R. (2015). Toward interventions to address moral distress: Navigating structure and agency. *Nursing Ethics, 22*(1), 91–102. doi:10.1177/0969733014534879.

National Academy of Medicine (NAM). (2021). *The future of nursing 2020-2030*. https://nam.edu/publications/the-future-of-nursing-2020-2030/

National Association of Clinical Nurse Specialists. (2019). *Statement on CNS practice and education (Online)*. https://portal.nacns.org/ItemDetail?iProductCode=STATEMENT_W&Category=WEB&WebsiteKey=cd0cefd9-bfa4-45cc-a6f8-1c4ea4450d93

National Organization of Nurse Practitioner Faculties. (2017). *Core competencies for nurse practitioners*. https://cdn.ymaws.com/www.nonpf.org/resource/resmgr/competencies/2017_NPCoreComps_with_Curric.pdf

Nelson, E. C., Batalden, P. B., Huber, T. P., Mohr, J. J., Godfrey, M. M., Headrick, L. A., & Wasson, J. H. (2002). Microsystems in health care: Part 1. Learning from high-performing front-line clinical units. *The Joint Commission Journal on Quality Improvement, 28*(9), 472–493.

Nichols, B., Shaffer, F., & Porter, C. (2011). Global nursing leadership: A practical guide. *Nursing Administration Quarterly, 35*, 354–359.

Nursing and Midwifery Board of Australia. (2021). *Australian nurse practitioner standards for practice*—Effective from 1 March 2021. https://www.nursingmidwiferyboard.gov.au/Codes-Guidelines-Statements/Professional-standards/nurse-practitioner-standards-of-practice.aspx

O'Connell, C. (1999). A culture of change or a change of culture. *Nursing Administration Quarterly, 23*, 65–68.

Plonien, C. (2016). Bullying in the workplace: A leadership perspective. *Association of Operating Room Nurses, 103*(1), 107–110. doi:10.1016/j.aorn.2015.11.014

Quast, L. (2011). *6 ways to empower others to succeed*. Forbes. http://www.forbes.com/sites/lisaquast/2011/02/28/6-ways-to-empower-others-to-succeed/#18b792493cc8

Rogers, E. M. (2003). *Diffusion of innovation* (5th ed.). Simon & Schuster.

Sandrick, K. (2006). The new political advocacy. *Trustee: The Journal for Hospital Governing Boards, 59*, 6–10.

Savel, R. H., & Munro, C. L. (2017). Servant leadership: The primacy of service. *American Journal of Critical Care, 26*(2), 97–99. doi:10.4037/ajcc2017356

Schwartz, D., Spencer, T., Wilson, B., & Wood, K. (2011). Transformational leadership: Implications for nursing leaders in facilities seeking Magnet designation. *AORN Journal, 93*, 737–748. doi:10.1016/j.aorn.2010.09.032

Senge, P. M. (1990). *The fifth discipline: The art and the practice of the learning organization*. Currency Doubleday.

Senge, P. M. (2006). *The fifth discipline: The art and the practice of the learning organization* (Revised edition). Currency Doubleday.

Sherman, R. O. (2012). Carefronting: An innovative approach to managing conflict. https://www.myamericannurse.com/carefronting-an-innovative-approach-to-managing-conflict/

Shirey, M. R. (2007a). An evidence-based understanding of entrepreneurship in nursing. *Clinical Nurse Specialist, 21*, 234–240. doi:10.1097/01.NUR.0000289748.00737.ef

Shirey, M. R. (2007b). AONE Leadership Perspectives. Competencies and tips for effective leadership: From novice to expert. *Journal of Nursing Administration, 37*, 167–170. doi:10.1097/01.NNA.0000266842.54308.38

Shirey, M. R. (2008). Influencers among us: A practical approach for leading change. *Clinical Nurse Specialist, 22*, 63–66. doi:10.1097/01.NUR.0000311670.26728.1f

Shirey, M. R. (2009). Transferable skills and entrepreneurial strategy. *Clinical Nurse Specialist, 23*, 128–130. doi:10.1097/NUR.0b013e3181a075a8

Shirey, M. R. (2015). Strategic agility for nursing leadership. *Journal of Nursing Administration, 45*(6), 305–308. doi:10.1097/NNA.0000000000000204

St. Thomas University (STU). (2019). *What is situational leadership®? How flexibility leads to success*. https://online.stu.edu/articles/education/what-is-situational-leadership.aspx

Tatsumi, C. L. (2019). The nurse as servant leader: Guiding others in caring advocacy. *Beginnings Magazine, 39*(4), 6–14.

The Joint Commission (TJC). (2020). *About the Joint Commission: Mission and vision statement*. https://www.jointcommission.org/about-us/#08ceda0dc745434fb6891232e0290e82_e39ab377a6ae-4acc99142664a6e4548e

Tourigny, L., & Pulich, M. (2005). A critical examination of formal and informal mentoring among nurses. *The Health Care Manager, 24*(1), 68–76. doi:10.1097/00126450-200501000-00011

University of York National Health Centre for Reviews and Dissemination. (1999). Getting evidence into practice. *Effective Health Care Bulletin, 5*, 1–16.

Vance, C. (2002). Mentoring at the edge of chaos. *Creative Nursing, 8*(7), 7–14. doi:10.1016/S1541-4612(03)70074-3

Vernon, A. (2015). Developing the 3 habits of transformational leaders. *Forbes*, 1–3. https://www.forbes.com/sites/yec/2015/08/27/developing-the-3-habits-of-transformational-leaders/?sh=39b0da986c99

Vos, T. C. (2009). Leadership begins with you. *Gerontology Nursing, 32*, 374–375. doi:10.1097/SGA.0b013e3181c5b5e3

Wagner, L. M., Capezuti, E., & Ouslander, J. G. (2006). Reporting near-miss events in nursing homes. *Nursing Outlook, 54*, 85–93. doi:10.1016/j.outlook.2006.01.003

Wang, X., Chontawan, R., & Nantsupawat, R. (2012). Transformational leadership: Effect on the job satisfaction of registered nurses in a hospital in China. *Journal of Advanced Nursing, 68*, 444–451. doi:10.1111/j.1365-2648.2011.05762.x

Watkins, M. D. (2013). What is organizational culture? And why should we care? *Harvard Business Review, 15*, 1–5. https://hbr.org/2013/05/what-is-organizational-culture

Weaver, S., Salas, E., & King, H. (2011). Twelve best practices for team training evaluation in healthcare. *Joint Commission Journal on Quality and Patient Safety, 37*, 341–349. doi:10.1016/s1553-7250(11)37044-4

Wheatley, M. J. (2005). *Finding our way: Leadership for uncertain times*. Berrett-Koehler.

World Health Organization. (2020a). *Collaborations and partnerships*. https://www.who.int/about/collaborations/en/

World Health Organization. (2020b). *Health financing*. https://www.who.int/health_financing/universal_coverage_definition/en/

Young, H., Siegel, E. O., McCormick, W. C., Fulmer, T., Harootyan, L. K., & Dorr, D. A. (2012). Interdisciplinary collaboration in geriatrics: Advancing health for older adults. *Nursing Outlook, 59*, 243–251. doi:10.1016/j.outlook.2011.05.006

Younger, S. J. (2020). Leveraging advanced practice nursing in complex health care systems. *Nursing Administration Quarterly, 44*(2), 127–135. doi:10.1097/NAQ.0000000000000408

Zaccaro, S. J. (2007). Trait-based perspectives of leadership. *The American Psychologist, 62*, 6–16. doi:10.1037/0003-066X.62.1.6

Zaccaro, S. J., Kemp, C., & Bader, P. (2004). Leader traits and attributes. In J. Antonakis, A. T. Cianciolo, & R. J. Sternberg (Eds.), *The nature of leadership* (pp. 101–124). Sage.

10 COLLABORATION

CINDI DABNEY ■ MICHAEL CARTER

"Five guys on the court working together can achieve more than five talented individuals who come and go as individuals."

~ Kareem Abdul-Jabbar

CHAPTER CONTENTS

DEFINITION OF COLLABORATION 316
Collaboration: What It Is 316
Collaboration: What It Is Not 316
Domains of Collaboration in Advanced Practice Registered Nursing 318
Types of Collaboration 319
Interprofessional Collaboration 320
CHARACTERISTICS OF EFFECTIVE COLLABORATION 320
Clinical Competence and Accountability 321
Common Purpose 321
Interpersonal Competence and Effective Communication 321
Trust and Mutual Respect 322
Recognizing and Valuing Diverse, Complementary Culture, Knowledge, and Skills 322
Humor 322
IMPACT OF COLLABORATION ON PATIENTS AND CLINICIANS 324
Evidence That Collaboration Works 324
Research Supporting Interprofessional Collaboration 325
Effects of Failure to Collaborate 326
IMPERATIVES FOR COLLABORATION 327
Ethical Imperative to Collaborate 327
Institutional Imperative to Collaborate 328
Research Imperative to Study Collaboration 329
CONTEXT OF COLLABORATION IN CONTEMPORARY HEALTH CARE 329
Incentives and Opportunities for Collaboration 329
Challenges to Collaboration 330
PROCESSES ASSOCIATED WITH EFFECTIVE COLLABORATION 332
Recurring Interactions 332
Effective Conflict Negotiation and Resolution Skills 333
Partnering and Team Building 333
IMPLEMENTING COLLABORATION 333
Assessment of Personal, Environmental, and Global Factors 334
STRATEGIES FOR SUCCESSFUL COLLABORATION 334
Individual Strategies 334
Team Strategies 335
Organizational Strategies 335
CONCLUSION 337
KEY SUMMARY POINTS 337

Advanced practice registered nurse (APRN) practice is highly complex and requires that the APRN be competent in collaboration. Collaboration takes place in a number of reciprocal relationships including the APRN, patient, families, other healthcare providers, and a number of others who are a part of the treatment experience. Patients assume that their healthcare providers communicate and collaborate effectively and become concerned when this does not occur. Patient dissatisfaction with care, unsatisfactory clinical outcomes, and clinician frustration can often be traced to a failure to collaborate among those caring for the patient. Collaboration depends on clinical and interpersonal expertise and is built on strong collegial relationships. The primary focus of this chapter is on collaboration among individuals and work groups. The goal is to explicate the values, behaviors, and processes that facilitate collaboration and thus improve patient care.

DEFINITION OF COLLABORATION

Collaboration: What It Is

The term *collaboration* often is used in health care and is a necessary part of teamwork and partnership. The collaborative combination of communication and interprofessional partnering has been described as having positive outcomes among healthcare professionals (Janotha et al., 2018). Collaboration is built upon sharing, teamwork, and respect, all of which are factors that develop over time. The conceptual definition of collaboration is a process by which nurses come together with patients and other healthcare members and form a team to solve a patient care or healthcare system problem with members of the team respectfully sharing knowledge and resources (Emich, 2018).

Defining collaboration as being interactive connotes the communicative and behavioral aspects of this competency. This definition implies teamwork and respect while sharing knowledge and resources. Working together to solve a patient care or healthcare system problem includes the notion that collaboration is a process that evolves over time. Functioning is a learned part of an interprofessional team and is not always inherent. Positive attitudes can influence behaviors that can enhance accession of collaborative expertise (Tamayo et al., 2017).

The ability to commit to interprofessional interaction over time requires that participants bring a set of characteristics and qualities to the situation. There are four desired competencies that promote interprofessional collaboration and are identified as follows: interprofessional communication, understanding each member's roles and responsibilities, teamwork, and understanding values and ethics of interprofessional practice (Interprofessional Education Collaborative [IPEC], 2016; Monahan et al., 2018). To interact authentically involves partners sharing the emotional satisfactions and frustrations of clinical work while also developing ways of supporting each other. A collaborative practice may include the interpersonal ups and downs that occur and the challenges of dealing with the same person(s) frequently over a number of issues. Successful collaboration requires engaging and managing conflict and having crucial conversations that are fundamental even if at times difficult.

Collaboration requires relationships that are productive for professionals, patients, and communities. Those in collaborative relationships may often experience disagreements. Therefore individuals in successful collaborative relationships develop strategies for dealing with disagreements that are mutually satisfactory and enhance the process. Collaboration demands a sophisticated level of communication. This means that collaboration cannot be mandated, legislated, or regulated.

Collaboration: What It Is Not

There are several forms of interaction that occur among clinicians, patients, families, and administrators in the complex processes that occur in care delivery. Collaboration is likely the most sophisticated and complicated among these forms. There are times that there can be confusion as to what collaboration is and what other forms of communication exist. These other forms do not meet the definition of collaboration used here.

Parallel Communication

Parallel communication is a form of functioning in which clinicians interact with a patient separately; they do not talk together before seeing a patient nor do they see the patient together. Parallel functioning of various interprofessional advanced practice roles can lead to competition rather than collaboration and ultimately create ineffective and expensive patient care models (McNamara et al., 2011). There is no expectation of joint interactions. For example, the staff registered nurse, medical student, attending physician, acute care nurse practitioner (ACNP), and certified registered nurse anesthetist (CRNA) all ask the patient the same questions about medications. In this example, multiple interactions are burdensome and frustrating for the patient. These types of interactions also may confuse the patient and yield fragmented information, leading to errors in clinical decision making. The patient expects that, at a minimum, information will be captured in the medical record and all those involved with care will read and understand this information. Repeated questions over the same topic can be interpreted by the patient and family as being a result of either the information not being recorded or the clinician failing to read the record.

Parallel Functioning

Parallel functioning occurs when providers care for patients, addressing the same clinical problem, but do not engage in any joint or collaborative planning. For example, nurses, physical therapists, and physicians document their interventions for pain in separate parts of the patient record but do not communicate about the case. In collaboration, interprofessional team members can use a tag team approach to gather valuable information that can be shared among the team to facilitate successful and efficient patient care plans (Haney et al., 2017). The effect of such interactions is equivalent to that of parallel communication.

One-Sided Compromise

Communication that demonstrates a one-sided compromise occurs when the APRN is overly agreeable, consistently yields to the other healthcare providers, and demonstrates a personal lack of responsibility in the care. This yielding results in compromised care and occurs when the APRN lacks the willingness or skill to engage in a collaborative negotiation. The development of one-sided relationships can be linked to insufficient knowledge sharing between professional teams that leads to a hierarchical structure of professional relationships with physicians that ultimately results in unclear treatment plans for patients (Busari et al., 2017).

Faux Collaboration

Faux collaboration occurs when persons in a position of authority believe that they are being collaborative because those around them are agreeing with the authority figure but not engaging in meaningful dialogue. This form of communication can be rather subtle and difficult for others to understand. Barriers of hierarchical vantage points and professional territorialism have caused interprofessional collaboration (IPC) to develop slowly in health care. The true nature of IPC requires shared leadership to achieve common goals that are beneficial for all team members (Goldsberry, 2018; Green & Johnson, 2015).

Information Exchange

Informing may be one-sided or two-sided and may or may not require action or decision making. If action is needed, the decision is unilateral and not a result of joint planning. Information exchange may be sufficient and exert a neutral or beneficial effect on care processes and outcomes. There is a risk of yielding a negative outcome if the situation requires joint planning and decision making. Communication is the key competency that healthcare professionals need for effective collaboration and consists of the individual's ability to participate in information exchange with other members of the healthcare team, patients, and their families (Frank et al., 2015).

Coordination

This form of communication lends structure to the encounter and may include actions to minimize duplication of effort but not interaction. For example, the Canadian Interprofessional Health Collaborative (CIHC, 2010) developed the Interprofessional Collaborative Practice (IPCP) model, which demonstrates how patients cared for in this framework benefit from the "one-stop shop" approach. IPCP allows the providers to devote more time to patients, which facilitates more thorough care. Calling the supplier to ensure that the patient receives durable medical equipment needed after an office visit is one way that the APRN may engage in coordination. This form of communication is usually one-sided and direct and may achieve the goal. However, it should not be confused with collaboration. Collaboration comes in the form of the IPCP model, allowing more time for communication among the team caring for the patient that leads to improved outcomes, not simply the mechanics of coordinating care (Selleck et al., 2017).

Consultation

The clinician who is caring for a patient seeks advice regarding a patient's concern but retains primary responsibility for care delivery. The certified nurse-midwife (CNM) may believe that there is a need for an evaluation and recommendation for treatment of a mother who is experiencing symptoms of depression and ask for a consultation by the psychiatric/mental health nurse practitioner. Consultation and collaboration allow women to receive the appropriate prenatal and intrapartum care based on their preferences and medical needs. The result is a recommendation to the CNM for treatment of the mother, but the CNM retains the responsibility of actually prescribing the intervention if the recommendation is determined to be appropriate.

Co-management

Two or more clinicians provide care, and each professional retains accountability and responsibility for defined aspects of care. This process usually arises from consultation in which a problem requires management that is outside the scope of practice of the referring clinician and the treatment will be continuing. Providers must be explicit with each other about their defined roles as they share joint responsibility related to all care management tasks (Norful et al., 2018). Co-management may also be a process used by interdisciplinary teams such as palliative care. The possibility may occur where co-management becomes parallel functioning.

Referral

A referral occurs when the APRN directs the patient to another clinician for the management of a particular problem or aspect of that patient's care when the problem is beyond the APRN's expertise. The nurse practitioner (NP) works with the patient and family through shared decisions to establish a mutually agreed-upon and evidence-based plan of care that encompasses ordering referrals centered on standards of professional care (American Association of Nurse Practitioners [AANP], 2019). For example, the APRN may determine that a patient could benefit from a course of physical therapy and a referral is initiated or, in another example, the APRN decides that the patient has appendicitis and requires surgery, so a referral to a surgeon is initiated.

Supervision

Some clinicians may confuse collaboration with supervision. Supervision occurs when one clinician delegates aspects of care to another clinician but retains full authority for the care. Authority and accountability for all aspects of the care, which include conducting the billing process, are retained by the supervisor. Collaboration is also meant to be mutually beneficial for all and accomplish common goals. This is the meaning of shared leadership that is the hallmark of IPC, not supervision. APRNs are autonomous practitioners; therefore supervision of them by other disciplines is not appropriate, nor is it appropriate for APRNs to supervise other disciplines. APRNs may supervise other nursing personnel regarding aspects of nursing care they provide.

With the exception of parallel communication, the processes just described require some level of interaction among providers but may not involve collaboration. Information exchange, coordination, consultation, co-management, and referral may be sufficient for particular situations to achieve clinical goals. Effective and timely communication is required among clinicians for these processes to work to benefit patients, minimize errors, and enhance quality.

Domains of Collaboration in Advanced Practice Registered Nursing

APRNs execute the collaboration competency in several domains—among individuals, work groups, and organizations. Competency in collaboration is often executed concurrently with other competencies and is also dynamic, shifting as the particulars of a situation change.

Collaboration With Individuals

Collaboration with patients, families, and colleagues in the delivery of direct care is the primary domain in which collaboration is practiced, for example, in forming partnerships with patients (see Chapter 6). APRNs aim to understand how the patient wants to interact, which, in turn, allows APRNs to collaborate with patients and families to mutually set and revise goals and determine barriers for outcomes. These activities are aimed at creating a common purpose, which is a hallmark of collaboration. When APRNs are involved in patient care and can function as a point of care for individual patients, they yield better outcomes. This is a strength they bring to IPC and is a missed benefit for patients if they are not involved as part of the team (Parker et al., 2013). APRNs also collaborate with individual clinicians. For example, the diabetes clinical nurse specialist (CNS) may collaborate with the cardiac CNS and a staff nurse to determine who will carry out each aspect of patient education for a patient. The collaborative process may include determining the order and timing of content to be taught. In this case the APRN is also executing direct care (interacting with the patient to assess learning needs) and coaching competencies (instructing patients on how to undergo lifestyle changes).

Collaboration With Teams and Groups

Another common domain in which APRNs implement collaboration is in their work with clinical teams and on departmental and institutional committees. These groups usually consist of individuals from multiple disciplines. One key function of collaborative competency is the facilitation of teamwork to ensure the delivery of effective, safe, high-quality care that will lead to positive outcomes. APRNs play key roles in facilitating and leading interdisciplinary teams, which ultimately require integrated collaboration of leadership competencies. APRNs often become more skilled in facilitating group collaboration with more experience. Sellick and colleagues (2017) described many advantages of APRNs functioning in teams and groups, including the ability to avoid repetition in errors and confusion because team members are able to speak directly to one other, helping to eliminate back-and-forth messaging. Team members are also able to learn from one other and develop an understanding of each other's roles, which in turn builds respect. Team and group approaches to care allow for immediate consultation and feedback that improves understanding of complex patient conditions and helps develop comprehensive treatment plans that lead to better health outcomes faster by eliminating the need for multiple appointments with different providers (Sellick et al., 2017).

Collaboration in the Organizational and Policy Arenas

In this domain, the focus of collaboration extends beyond the delivery of care to individuals and groups. APRNs are important in the development of our nation's healthcare policy. As demand grows for interprofessional healthcare services, the increasing numbers of APRNs will help meet these needs and influence health promotion policy (Bachynsky, 2020). The organizational and policy forces shaping clinical care require that even novice APRNs cultivate collaboration. Initiatives aimed at areas such as clarifying credentialing requirements, simplifying processes involved in practicing across state lines, and improving payment for APRNs require them to use their status as clinicians, citizens, and members of professional organizations to collaborate with organizational leaders and policymakers.

Collaboration in Global Arenas

Global or international collaboration is expanding as an essential domain for APRNs (American Association of Colleges of Nursing [AACN], 2020; Institute of Medicine [IOM], 2010; National Organization of Nurse Practitioner Faculties [NONPF], 2017; see Chapter 5). As traditional roles continue to shift and physicians become more specialized and less likely to care for patients in rural areas, APRNs are able to fill gaps and relieve shortages. These roles once reserved for physicians are being met by APRNs globally (Maier & Aiken, 2016).

Global communication and collaboration have been critical to successful living as well as working and economic success for many years (Friedman, 2005), and this is also true for health care. Evidence has shown that globalization is a part of practice. For instance, the APRN covering the emergency room at night may communicate with a radiologist in Australia about a diagnostic image that was sent electronically to be interpreted in real time, much like an APRN in critical care may collaborate with critical care physicians in Israel monitoring the electronic intensive care unit.

Types of Collaboration

Interprofessional collaboration leads to improved health care, which leads to increased demand for interprofessional collaboration. This increased demand is a global need and has led to recommendations for learning and education. The terminology used to describe collaboration among national and international health professions varies; therefore the various terms used to describe interprofessional collaboration require clarification. Several terms are used interchangeably, including *multidisciplinary*, *interdisciplinary*, and *transdisciplinary* and *interprofessional collaboration*. However, there seems to be no agreement on the use of terms to describe the collaboration among health professions. To promote understanding across various disciplines, standard definitions should be used for interprofessional collaboration, as described by Mahler and colleagues (2014). To address this issue, they clarified definitions of frequently used terms regarding interprofessional collaboration such as *multi-*, *inter-*, *trans-*, and *intra-* in the academic literature (Mahler et al., 2014). The prefix indicates the level and depth of interactions to which the term refers. The different prefixes describe the essence of the collaboration. For example, *multi-* indicates that various professions work parallel to each other but not necessarily together. *Intraprofessional* collaboration describes teamwork within a specific profession. This could be a description for a group of APRNs coming together for a common goal like governmental policy change. *Interprofessional* collaboration means different professions work together with varying degrees of overlap for the same objective. *Interdisciplinary* collaboration involves different scientific fields working together with some degree of intersection. *Transprofessional* collaboration, sometimes referred to as transdisciplinary collaboration, indicates separate professions may become interchangeable (Mahler et al., 2014). *Multidisciplinary* teams use the knowledge from different disciplines but these teams stay within their own boundaries.

Interprofessional Collaboration

Interprofessional collaboration has been central to the delivery of improved health care and is recognized as essential by top organizations like the World Health Organization (WHO) and the IOM (Goldsberry, 2018). Improving healthcare systems around the world to achieve reliability of care, safety, quality, efficiency, and cost-effectiveness requires that clinicians, teams, and administrators undertake important collaborative work.

Several forces have come together to foster interprofessional collaboration. The WHO and IOM have encouraged healthcare professionals to improve the delivery of health care by joining together through interprofessional collaboration (IOM, 2010; WHO, 2010). Additionally, the IOM report *The Future of Nursing* urged teamwork among healthcare providers (IOM, 2010). The need for collaboration among healthcare professionals led to the development of specific interprofessional competencies (IPEC, 2016).

The mere notion of distinct professions can automatically engender boundaries. Each group may be unique in its own special language, theories, and values, which can create territorialism, leading to conflict and additional separation from other professions (Bell et al., 2014; Green & Johnson, 2015). An understanding of this challenge can help APRNs and their colleagues approach opportunities for collaboration strategically and build and sustain clinical environments that support collaboration.

CHARACTERISTICS OF EFFECTIVE COLLABORATION

The definition of collaboration invites exploration of the characteristics that comprise a successful collaborative relationship. Personal and setting-specific attributes are pivotal to successful collaborations. Some characteristics of collaboration have long been recognized, but clinicians and organizations have often resisted adopting the necessary philosophy, commitment, and behaviors that accompany collaboration. Four characteristics of effective collaboration are development of role clarity, interprofessional trust and confidence, possessing the ability to overcome adversity and personal differences, and collective leadership. Members have a duty to perform their unique role, with the success of the team being the focus. Individuals must be confident in their own abilities to ensure team trust. The team as a whole deals with setbacks, and each member remains committed to the shared goal. Team members may not always get along with one another, but personal differences must be set aside for the success of the team. Lastly, the pressure to accomplish a goal is shared by the entire team, not placed solely on one individual (Bosch & Mansell, 2015). These early works highlight the core elements necessary for collaboration that are listed in Box 10.1.

Additionally, collaboration requires clinical competence, common purpose, and effective interpersonal and communication skills or, at a minimum, a willingness to learn them. Trust, mutual respect, and valuing each other's knowledge and skills are equally important but develop over time. For these characteristics to develop, prospective partners must approach encounters with a willingness to trust, commitment to respect each other, and assumption that the knowledge and skills of others

BOX 10.1

Essential Characteristics of Collaboration

- Clinical competence and accountability
- Common purpose
- Interpersonal competence and effective communication
- Trust
- Mutual respect
- Recognition and valuing of diverse, complementary knowledge and skills
- Humor

are valuable. These characteristics are necessary and fully realized only after many constructive and productive interactions. Finally, a sense of humor among team members often serves many functions in helping them stay committed to each other's collaborative practice.

Clinical Competence and Accountability

Clinical competence is perhaps the most fundamental characteristic underlying a successful collaborative experience among clinicians; without it, the trust and desire necessary to work together fail to develop. Trust and respect are built on the assurance that each participant is able to carry out their roles, function in a competent manner, and be accountable for practice. Clinical competence is a basic element of collaboration and has been supported by research (Bosque, 2011), yet stereotyped views of nursing and medical practice may interfere with collaborative efforts. These stereotypes may include physicians as having ultimate responsibility and nurses as having little responsibility.

Mutual trust and respect develop when collaborating clinicians can rely on each other's clinical competency. Contemporary leadership shifts among partners in a departure from the traditional "captain of the team" approach. Thus the person with the most expertise, interest, talent, or willingness to lead can respond to the particular demands of the situation or problem. The trust and respect among collaborators are such that they can count on the satisfactory resolution of the problem, even when they know as individuals that they might have approached the issue differently. This openness to shared leadership and alternative solutions allows partners to learn from each other.

Being accountable for practice enhances collaboration. APRNs model full partnership on caregiving teams when they share planning, decision making, problem solving, and goal setting for patient care (Clausen et al., 2012; IPEC, 2016).

Common Purpose

Collaboration is predicated on the notion of sharing a common purpose (Murray-Davis et al., 2011; Petri, 2010). Even if partners have not discussed the purposes and goals of their interactions, the organizations in which they work usually have explicit missions and goals. Goals can be the starting point for identifying the purposes of clinical collaboration. Common purposes may range from ensuring that an underserved patient gains access to preventive services, such as mammography, to a more ambitious quality improvement agenda to improve the management of patients with heart failure across settings.

One of the paradoxes of collaboration is that the partners are autonomous (self-governing, accountable) but interdependent, reflecting a reciprocal reliance on each other for support in carrying out their responsibilities. Recognizing their interdependence, team members can combine their individual skills to synthesize care plans that are more complex and comprehensive than what they could have created working alone. Like other characteristics, the common purpose that initially brought partners together may change over time. The situation that brought clinicians together may become secondary to the deep personal commitment to work together in ways that improve patient care and are interpersonally and professionally satisfying. In addition to a common purpose, partners who are guided by a shared vision of the possibilities inherent in collaboration, believe in the value of collaboration, and are committed to achieving the relationship's potential (Young et al., 2012) will most likely be able to develop interprofessional collaboration. Developing a shared vision permits partners to value each other's ideas, opinions, and actions.

Interpersonal Competence and Effective Communication

Interpersonal competence is the ability to communicate effectively with colleagues in a variety of situations, including uncomplicated, routine interactions; disagreements;

unique cultural value conflicts; and stressful situations. The key to demonstrating interpersonal competence is the ability to communicate openly, clearly, and convincingly in oral and written communications.

Transparency is the honest and open sharing of information and ideas among parties while recognizing issues that are present. Transparent communications are closely linked to accountability. Transparency engenders trust and thus is an underlying requisite for collaboration. After clinical competence, interpersonal competence and effective communication may be the most important characteristics needed for APRNs to establish collaborative relationships.

Assertiveness is a key element of interpersonal competence needed by all APRNs. Assertiveness may be a challenge for some and will have to be carefully exhibited. A range of qualities may be required for APRNs to be able to do the following: take risks, discuss disagreements in clinical judgment and agree to criteria for resolving such conflicts, be able to avoid a near-miss clinical situation such as an error in prescribing or interpreting clinical data, and admit that a mistake, miscommunication, or oversight has happened. Assertiveness is not sufficient in certain situations and environments and, in these cases, courage will be required to confront the problem.

Trust and Mutual Respect

Implicit in discussions of collaboration is the presence of mutual trust, respect, and personal integrity—qualities evidenced in the nature of interactions among partners. The development of trust and respect depends on clinical competence that often develops over time. This does not mean that novice APRNs cannot establish collaborative relationships. However, the environments in which APRN students and new graduates work must support their "novice hood" so that they can learn and mature clinically. Trust and assertiveness seem to act reciprocally in collaboration; as trust grows, so does the ability to communicate in difficult situations. Responding assertively in situations of risk and keeping the focus on the patient's welfare can enhance trust.

Respect for others' practice and knowledge is important to successful collaboration because it enhances shared decision making. Respect extends to acknowledgment and appreciation for each other's time and competing commitments.

Recognizing and Valuing Diverse, Complementary Culture, Knowledge, and Skills

High-quality patient care requires an interpersonal belief that the complementary knowledge other team members have will enhance one's own personal plan for patient care. Appreciation for the diverse and complementary knowledge each party brings to the work, commitment to quality and patient-centeredness, and a willingness to invest in the partnership or team are all necessary for collaboration to become the normative process in team interactions.

A lack of knowledge about another's discipline is a barrier to developing effective teamwork (Dumez, 2011). Team members must recognize and value the overlapping and diverse skills and knowledge that each discipline brings to the team (IPEC, 2011) so that mutual trust and respect can develop and deepen over time. Partners observe that patients benefit from their combined talents and efforts. They come to depend on each other to use good clinical judgment and to take appropriate actions.

Initially, collaborators have limited knowledge of each other as individuals and as professionals. Collaboration is a conscious, learned behavior that improves as team members learn to value and respect one another's practice and expertise (IPEC, 2011). The first step is to recognize these differing contributions. For example, medicine and nursing, although overlapping disciplines, are culturally distinct and have diverse goals for patient care. In many cases, they complement each other. These complementarities also extend to other disciplines. Collaboration is built on the respect and valuing of the contributions of each profession to the common goal of optimal healthcare delivery.

Humor

Humor is often a part of the collaborative process, yet data are sparse regarding the effectiveness of humor in improving collaboration. The work of APRNs is serious, but there seems to always be room for levity somewhere. A report by Ghaffari and associates (2015) suggested that nurses can influence the care delivered to patients and improve their well-being by using humor. Using humor to decrease stress and occupational burnout can be especially beneficial when there is a shortage of personnel.

Through understanding humor, there are valuable insights to patients' and nurses' mental, emotional, and physical health (Ghaffari et al., 2015). Positive and non-demeaning humor may be a creative way to facilitate communication and problem solving among members of different disciplines. Nir and Halperin (2018) suggested that humor can connect groups through highlighting their commonality, willingness to compromise, and ability to be vulnerable. These ideas can be applied to APRN practice to decrease distances and be more accessible to patients. Appropriate humor also may decrease defensiveness, invite openness, relieve tension, and deflect anger. It helps individuals keep perspective, acknowledge their lack of perfection, and reframe difficult situations. APRN students can be encouraged to observe how expert clinicians use humor to improve communication and defuse conflict situations. Humor can be a challenge at times, however. Humor is a complex cognitive experience usually designed to cause laughter, but these experiences are often very contextual. That means that some attempts at humor can be misinterpreted and invoke a negative response.

Although this list of characteristics of effective collaboration may seem daunting to the novice, a consistent commitment to and practice of collaboration can develop this competency over time in an APRN's practice. Exemplar 10.1 showcases the elements of collaboration in an individual practice. All health professionals need to recognize that investing the time and energy to build these relationships is an important component of clinical practice. The high levels of idea exchange and expertise that become possible when these characteristics unite is one of the greatest satisfactions of collaborative practice.

EXEMPLAR 10.1

ELEMENTS OF COLLABORATION IN ONE ADVANCED PRACTICE NURSE'S PRACTICE

Caesar M. is a family nurse practitioner who has a nursing home practice. He also volunteers one evening per week at a free clinic, serving people living in poverty and without insurance. Donna is a 35-year-old patient with Crohn's disease. Donna is married to a welder, and they have two children under 10 years of age. Donna had previously worked as a home health aide but had to stop because of her illness. She applied for disability coverage but was denied. The staff at the university medical center 75 miles away had initiated IV immune system suppression therapy. Donna was charged about $10,000 for each treatment, which occurred every 6 weeks. Donna's family income was $32,000 per year.

The company that produced the drug approved the free clinic to receive the medication without charge given Donna's family income. This medication had to be reconstituted by a pharmacist under a laminar-flow hood and administered IV over a 2-hour period. Once constituted, the medication was only viable for 4 hours. An additional complicating condition was that Donna had a history of extreme difficulty with IV access via peripheral veins.

Caesar knew that only through multiple collaborative arrangements would he be able to ensure that Donna would repeatedly receive this needed treatment. The free clinic lacked the necessary supplies, personnel, or equipment to administer the medication. Caesar's nursing home did have this ability. The owners, administrator, and director of nursing at the nursing home were approached and all agreed that this could be done in their facility at no charge to Donna.

The next issue was to collaborate on developing a plan to mix the medication. The director of pharmacy at the local critical access hospital agreed to mix the medications when needed as long as the clinic provided the medication. What was left was obtaining the free services of a surgeon to place an access port through which the IV medication could be administered. One of the volunteer ministers at the free clinic was married to a woman who was the clinic manager for a local surgeon. The surgeon was reluctant to offer the surgical placement for free, but he placed the port after substantial pressures from Caesar and the minister's wife/office manager.

Now the medication administration dance began. On the day of administration, Donna stopped by the clinic and obtained the medication vial. She took it to the hospital where the pharmacist reconstituted the drug under the hood and gave the IV bag to Donna. She brought this to the nursing home where Caesar met her, obtained an IV pump, and administered the medication through her port over 2 hours.

One year later, the state approved the Medicaid expansion under the Affordable Care Act. Donna received full insurance to cover her existing condition and was able to be treated at a facility that could take over all aspects of this care. This is an example of multiple collaborations that might be required to ensure treatment.

IMPACT OF COLLABORATION ON PATIENTS AND CLINICIANS

Building skills in collaboration is not easy. Common barriers to collaboration include equity and social justice, health disparities, and cultural sensitivity (Bachynsky, 2020). Other barriers to collaboration include innate hierarchical factors, gender and professional inequalities and boundaries, territorial behaviors, and attempted restrictions of full scope of practice (Goldsberry, 2018). Patients and each of the health professionals who provide care to the patient have their own history with these issues, and these are often not shared among the group but can form a backdrop of barriers to collaboration.

The benefits of collaboration among patients and providers have been documented over many years. Patients are sensitive to the relationships among caregivers and quickly recognize a lack of respect or trust among their providers. To begin to overcome professional and historical boundaries, IPC must be incorporated into the education of healthcare professionals. When these boundaries do not exist, professionals are comfortable sharing knowledge and working together as a team, as reported by Barwell et al. (2013). For interprofessional collaboration to work, there must be shared leadership and equitable power that focuses on building trust and working together for common goals facilitated by effective and respectful communication (Wilson, 2013). Collaboration requires an ability to transform competitive situations into opportunities for working together that are mutually beneficial and in which all parties can imagine the possibility of creating a win–win situation. In the past, this movement among providers was hampered by a lack of ability for the patient's information to flow with the patient. This has become easier with the use of electronic record systems with patient portals.

The impact of APRNs on disease management and care transition interventions indicates that there are positive outcomes for patients. Table 10.1 illustrates the types of patient and provider benefits that have been ascribed to collaboration. Collaboration competencies have been in place for APRNs for several years in the United States, Canada, and Australia (AACN, 2006; Creamer & Austin, 2017; NONPF, 2017; Nursing and Midwifery Board of Australia [NMBA], 2014).

TABLE 10.1
Benefits of Collaboration

Who Benefits?	Benefits
Patients	Improved quality of care
	Increased patient satisfaction
	Lower mortality rate
	Improved patient outcomes
	Patients feel more secure, cared for, and closer to healthcare providers
	Empowers patients and family to become team members
Providers	Improved trust and respect for caregivers
	Improved communication and clarity of message
	Increased sharing of responsibility
	Increased sharing of expertise
	Mutually satisfying problem solving
	Improved communications
	Increased personal satisfaction
	Increased quality of professional life
	Enhanced mutual trust and respect
	Bridges care–cure dichotomy
	Expanded horizons of providers
	Avoids redundant care and ensures coverage
	Empowers providers to influence health policy

Adapted from *Collaboration: A health care imperative* (pp. 26–27), by T. J. Sullivan, 1998, McGraw-Hill Health Professionals Division.

Evidence That Collaboration Works

Exemplar 10.2 provides an example of one way that collaboration can work. For the past decade, the Agency for Healthcare Research and Quality (AHRQ) has funded projects conducted by the National Committee for Quality Assurance (NCQA) focused on improving patient safety. Collaboration among health professionals has been a major focus of these studies. The critical element is collaboration among the health professionals treating the patient. The substantial amount of research that has been reported to date shows reductions in cost measures and a decrease in utilization, particularly in what are called patient-centered medical homes (NCQA, 2019).

The global literature, especially from Canada, shows similar findings (Global Confederation for Interprofessional Education & Collaborative Practice, 2020).

EXEMPLAR 10.2

COLLABORATION WORKS FOR PATIENTS AND CLINICIANS

Dr. C. is a psychiatric CNS at a large tertiary hospital that is part of a rapidly expanding health system. This system includes hospitals, clinics, rehab centers, and home health services and has been participating in new demonstration projects with the US Centers for Medicare & Medicaid. These projects are designed to improve the quality of care and decrease the overall costs of care. New for this health system is changing from a fee-for-service payment system to a global payment for the care received by the patient across settings. In the past, each element of care was paid for as the service was provided and there was little linkage among the various aspects of care. Dr. C has reviewed the past 3 months' data on readmission after discharge from the acute care hospital, because this is one of the key quality improvement measures. The new single electronic health record allows providers to follow the patient's care across different sites of care. What Dr. C. determined was that about 70% of the patients who were readmitted to the hospital had depression or anxiety identified during their acute care admission. Yet there was no evidence-based plan of care provided to deal with these problems. Based on this analysis, Dr. C. decided to build a collaborative pathway to ensure that patients who experience depression or anxiety during acute care hospitalization were identified and provided with appropriate treatment.

Dr. C. quickly discovered that there would be many providers involved in creating and delivering this plan. The first requirement was to ensure that all patients received appropriate screening for depression and anxiety. Dr. C. engaged the assistance of social work in helping select the screening tools that were best suited to this situation. Next, Dr. C. met with the manager of the hospitalist program. In this particular hospital, acute care nurse practitioners and internal medicine physicians provided hospitalist services. The nurse manager for critical care was also included, because the decision had to be made as to whether the screening would be done by nursing staff or by the hospitalists. The screening tools selected were such that they could be completed easily and accurately by the staff nurse who performs the admission assessment and included in the electronic record. Scores indicating the potential for depression or anxiety in the patient were automatically flagged by the record so that the hospitalists could request a consult by the psychiatric team for further analysis and recommendations for treatment. Evidence-based plans of care were then prescribed as appropriate by either the consultant or by the hospitalist.

Dr. C. led a formative evaluation as this new approach to screening, diagnosis, and treatment unfolded and was able to make modifications in the plan based on the information provided by all concerned, including the patients and families. Three months after implementation, Dr. C. conducted a summative evaluation of the program. What was found was that almost all patients were screened. Those who scored as being at risk for depression or anxiety were placed into a treatment pathway that continued across sites of care, and the readmissions to the hospital after discharge were reduced by 50%. Dr. C. continues to monitor the system and provide written reports to the key collaborators in a timely manner.

Important ideas about collaboration from leaders in other disciplines have also informed this discussion of collaboration.

Research Supporting Interprofessional Collaboration

Impact on Health Outcomes

Nurse practitioners have been shown to be effective in managing health conditions in primary care and have been shown to be cost-effective in prior research (Newhouse et al., 2011). Newhouse et al. (2011) reported that the outcomes of NP and CNM care were found to be equal to or in some cases better than outcomes for care provided by physicians alone. CNS care was found to help reduce hospital costs and length of hospital stay. When hospitals score poorly on outcome measures, it is very costly due to Centers for Medicare & Medicaid Services (CMS) reimbursement based on value rather than volume (CMS, 2019). Value measures place APRNs in the unique position to solidify their role as effective and efficient members of the healthcare team, because they are experts at coordination of care in hospital settings. There has been insufficient evidence to evaluate CRNA practices.

Some states in the United States do not provide APRNs full practice authority as autonomous practitioners. The opposition for APRN autonomy reasons that APRNs will not collaborate if not mandated by regulations. Evidence does not support this contention. Dillon and Gary (2017) reported that NPs fill an important need to improve primary care and in new areas in critical care. Dillon and Gary also found that NPs are more effective team members when they have full practice authority.

Effects of Physician and Advanced Practice Nurse Collaboration on Costs

Norful et al. (2018) reported that collaboration between nurse practitioners as a part of co-management increased patient access to care and promoted continuity of care. This was seen particularly in rural and medically underserved populations. The three elements that ensured strong collaboration were effective communication, mutual respect and trust, and a shared philosophy of care.

Souter et al. (2019) reported that midwifery care in a hospital-based labor and delivery setting with obstetrician collaboration is associated with decreased intervention and decreased cesarean and operative vaginal births. Of course, opposition from hospital systems can be expected as long as the United States pays hospitals based on complexity of care, as this becomes a serious loss of income for hospitals. King (2020) made observations beyond cost reduction, contending that midwifery–obstetrician collaborative practices complement and enhance the work of each other, breaking down silos.

One of the challenges of evaluating cost-effectiveness when it comes to clinical collaboration is to measure change over an appropriate time horizon. Relatively short collaborative interventions may be enough to change patient behaviors in ways that reduced important clinical markers but are insufficient to assess and measure the impact of complications and disease-related comorbidities on the disease trajectory over time. The use of a 1-year time frame is often insufficient to demonstrate sustained behavior change. Desborough (2012) reported that the first 12 months of a new NP practice likely represents a period of transition in which elements of the practice are defined. Desborough's position supports our conceptualization of collaboration as a process that evolves over time. Even so, evidence has suggested that organizationally supported teams, such as rapid response teams, can improve patient outcomes (AHRQ, 2019).

There are many fine examples of collaboration initiatives leading to positive changes in health care and collaborative interactions among the healthcare disciplines. Ongoing work by the National Academies of Sciences, Engineering and Medicine (2021) on the future of nursing continues to examine the current state of science and technology to inform an assessment of the capacity of nursing to meet future healthcare needs as a part of collaborative care. These efforts are encouraging, and it is likely that new positive strides will be fulfilled in preparing health professions students for collaborative practice.

Effects of Failure to Collaborate

Concerns about the quality of health care began to take on new importance in the United States and elsewhere during the latter part of the 20th century and continue today. Some time ago, the IOM (2000) highlighted that patients were not receiving the best care possible and that thousands were dying each year by errors in care delivery. The emerging approaches for improving the quality of health care were traced to the classic work of Deming (1982), who argued that organizations can increase quality and simultaneously reduce costs. The basic assumption of these new approaches to improving health care was that problems were not the fault of any particular individual clinician but were better understood as problems with systems of care delivery. The new idea to decrease errors and improve quality was that collaboration among providers, administrators, and patients would lead to improved quality, decrease injury and costs, and save lives. Failures of collaboration often resulted in harm to patients, including morbidity and mortality (Karam et al., 2017). This means that failure to collaborate not only results in poor working conditions for the professionals but can also result in harm and increased costs of care.

Balik and associates (2011) provided an in-depth analysis of research, studied organizations, and interviewed experts in hospital care to better understand how to improve care to patients and their families during hospitalization. One of the key drivers of quality care was respectful partnerships among providers and administrators, which is also one of the critical elements of quality collaboration. These researchers reported that quality care did not occur without this level of collaboration. Failure to collaborate results in poor quality care, increased costs often associated with high staff turnover, and harm to patients. These problems continue despite substantial effort. Anderson and Abrahamson (2017) reported that medical error was the third leading cause of death in the United States. While questions have arisen concerning their analytical methods, medical errors are a substantial cause of both morbidity and mortality. Most of these errors can be traced to a lack of collaboration among healthcare providers.

IMPERATIVES FOR COLLABORATION

Failure to collaborate in health care can result in harm to patients. Therefore organizations and clinicians have an obligation to collaborate under the moral requirement to do no harm. The effects of collaboration or its failure can be seen in how ethical and institutional dilemmas are resolved and how research is conducted.

Ethical Imperative to Collaborate

IPEC (2020) contends that all health professionals must assert the values and ethics of interprofessional practice by placing the needs and dignity of patients at the center of healthcare delivery and include a specific ethics domain and competencies (Box 10.2). Compassionate and ethical patient care that provides a healing

BOX 10.2

Interprofessional Collaborative Initiative Domains and Competencies

COMPETENCY DOMAIN 1: VALUES AND ETHICS FOR INTERPROFESSIONAL COLLABORATION

- Place patients and populations at center of care.
- Respect dignity and privacy of patients and confidentiality of team members.
- Embrace cultural diversity.
- Respect unique cultures, values, and roles.
- Work in cooperation with patients and providers and those who support care.
- Develop trusting relationships with patients, families, and team members.
- Demonstrate ethical conduct and quality care as a member of the team.
- Manage ethical dilemmas in interprofessional care situations.
- Act with honesty and integrity.
- Maintain personal and professional competence.

COMPETENCY 2: ROLES AND RESPONSIBILITIES FOR COLLABORATION

- Communicate role and responsibilities clearly to patients and professionals.
- Recognize skill, knowledge, and ability limitations.
- Engage with professionals who complement one's practice.
- Explain roles and responsibilities of other team members.
- Use the full scope of the knowledge, skills, and abilities of all team members.
- Communicate with the team to clarify roles and responsibilities.
- Forge interdependent relationships.
- Engage in continuous interprofessional development.
- Use unique and complementary abilities of all members to optimize care.

COMPETENCY 3: INTERPROFESSIONAL COMMUNICATION

- Choose effective communication tools to enhance team function.
- Communicate information to patients and team members, avoiding discipline-specific terminology.
- Express knowledge and opinions to team with confidence, respect, and clarity to ensure common understanding.
- Listen actively and encourage ideas and opinions of other team members.
- Give timely, sensitive, and instructive feedback to team members about their performance and respond respectively to feedback from others.
- Use respectful language in difficult situations or interprofessional conflict.
- Recognize one's own uniqueness and contributions to effective communication, conflict resolution, and positive working relationships.
- Consistently communicate the importance of patient-centered care.

COMPETENCY 4: INTERPROFESSIONAL TEAMWORK AND TEAM-BASED CARE

- Describe the process of team and role development and the role and practice of effective teams.

Continued

BOX 10.2

Interprofessional Collaborative Initiative Domains and Competencies—cont'd

- Develop consensus on ethical principles to guide all aspects of patient care and teamwork.
- Engage other health professionals in shared, patient-centered problem solving.
- Integrate knowledge and experience of other professions to inform care decisions while respecting patient and community values and priorities.
- Apply leadership practices that support collaborative practice.
- Engage self and others to manage disagreements constructively about values, roles, and goals of care.
- Share accountability with other professions, patients, and communities for relevant healthcare outcomes.
- Reflect on individual and team performance to improve individual and team performance.
- Use process improvement strategies to improve the effectiveness of interprofessional teamwork and practice.
- Use available evidence to inform effective teamwork and team-based practice.
- Perform effectively on teams and in different team roles in a variety of settings.

Adapted from Interprofessional Education Collaborative (2011). Core competencies of interprofessional collaborative practice. www.aacn.nche.edu/education/pdf/IPECreport.pdf

environment requires collaborative working relationships among all providers, including APRNs. Environments that foster collaboration may also create a more supportive context for addressing ethical issues.

Quality patient care requires collaboration, because it reinforces commitment to a common goal and reaffirms the central goal of patient welfare. Collaboration enhances shared knowledge, because all healthcare providers repeatedly educate each other about the patient. Collaboration also demonstrates that the manner in which care is delivered is as important as who delivers the care.

Institutional Imperative to Collaborate

The evidence that collaboration works has suggested that there are structural and interpersonal dimensions to collaboration. In essence, although institutional policies or standards do not guarantee collaboration, they can establish expectations for collaboration. These institutional expectations can provide a structure that facilitates interpersonal communication and relationship building (IOM, 2010; US Department of Health and Human Services [HHS], 2011). The mutual goals of quality patient care and the ethical imperative to collaborate are at the center of interprofessional efforts to provide care or resolve conflicts in approaches to care for patients. For example, institutions that apply for American Nurses' Credentialing Center (ANCC) Magnet status are expected to have a structure in place for interprofessional collaboration as one of the key characteristics (ANCC, 2020). The incentive for hospitals to move to Magnet status emphasizes nurse retention, quality, costs, and safety. Institutions that have applied for the Magnet credential must demonstrate that they meet five characteristics (ANCC, 2020). These criteria have been associated with the ability to attract and retain nurses. APRNs are usually intimately involved in efforts to seek Magnet status, such as leading quality improvement initiatives, facilitating professional development of staff, and contributing to the establishment of policies and procedures that shape an environment in which effective collaboration can occur.

Finally, incentives and mandates to reduce errors and increase the reliability of care by adopting evidence-based practices constitute another significant institutional imperative to foster collaboration. Improvements that result from such initiatives are often tied to payment for the organization.

An example of the institutional imperative to collaborate has been the development and progression of the doctor of nursing practice (DNP) degree. The national concerns about the quality and safety of health care informed the development of the DNP and helped form consensus among schools, faculty, and other stakeholders (AACN, 2004). The DNP *Essentials* (AACN, 2006) set collaboration as a core competency for this degree for APRNs. More recently the AACN has approved the updated *Essentials* that deals with all of professional nursing education (AACN, 2021). The document includes numerous mentions of the terms *collaboration* and *collaborative* in the competencies required for all nurses including DNP graduates. Examples that require collaborative competencies include the ability to create change in healthcare delivery systems, need to collaborate across settings to enhance population-based health care, and need for interprofessional collaboration to implement practice guidelines and peer review processes (AACN, 2021).

Research Imperative to Study Collaboration

There are many institutional pressures to collaborate and support collaboration research. For example, the AHRQ (n.d.) is an important resource for funding and disseminating the results of research on quality improvement, patient safety, adoption of evidence-based practices, and other issues associated with the delivery of safe and reliable health care. Manojlovich and colleagues (2014) stressed the need to build a better safety climate through improved interprofessional collaboration. In addition, the National Institutes of Health's (NIH, 2020) Common Fund continues to expect collaboration among clinical investigators and supports a number of collaborative practice initiatives.

The important contribution of collaboration among providers with different perspectives will require additional study. The results of these studies will have implications for APRNs, administrators, other clinicians, researchers, and others. Focused research will be needed to understand the collaborative climate, determine facilitators and barriers, and determine the contribution of strengthened relationships to the organization and to patients while building an organizational culture to better explicate the values of collaboration. APRNs, other clinicians, and administrators will require assistance from researchers to understand the structures and processes associated with collaboration and the extent to which collaboration affects patient and utilization outcomes and costs.

CONTEXT OF COLLABORATION IN CONTEMPORARY HEALTH CARE

The pressures on APRNs and others to improve quality, work more efficiently, and allow others to be involved in decisions about patient care could be expected to foster collaboration among clinicians. Paradoxically, these same factors may undermine collaboration. As APRNs practice autonomously and collaboratively, other clinicians have experienced concerns including the increasing supply of APRN providers, which seemingly could encroach on the autonomy of others and their willingness to collaborate. This sort of change can challenge the status quo and lead to fear about relinquishing authority and power, leading some individuals to withdraw from or sabotage efforts to collaborate. Thus the transition to a presumably more effective, accessible, and efficient healthcare system may actually undermine collaboration.

In addition, confusion about the scope of practice can be damaging to collaboration for all involved. According to Safriet (2002), other independent practitioners may ask themselves the following questions:

- What is in it for me to collaborate?
- What areas of my work do I get to expand because other providers can do things that I have traditionally done?

APRNs may be uncertain about how to proceed with collaboration; for example, when they are asked to assume responsibility for a new skill such as performing an invasive procedure. The reality is that regulatory initiatives and payment structures are rearranging collaborative relationships frequently. These changes are often at the heart of the tension associated with collaboration among players, as the roles and boundaries of disciplines have blurred and expanded.

Incentives and Opportunities for Collaboration

Efforts to reduce costs and improve quality of health care provide APRNs, other clinicians, and administrators with common goals toward which to work and opportunities for learning from each other. National interdisciplinary guidelines and standards of care are intended to reduce unwarranted and often expensive variations in health care. Many guidelines specify interdisciplinary collaboration as a critical component of effective care. Standards and guidelines developed and agreed on by interdisciplinary groups, whether at the local (office or institution), national, or international level, offer a starting point for jointly determining patient care goals, processes, and outcomes. Accreditation activities offer another opportunity to build collaborative relationships. The Joint

Commission (TJC, 2021) requires documentation that demonstrates collaborative, interdisciplinary practice to help providers develop stronger interdisciplinary approaches to care. The need for a highly coordinated system of chronic care management led the Health Sciences Institute (HSI) to promulgate interdisciplinary competencies (HSI, 2022). The goals for chronic illness care, which include promoting health and preventing disease, managing disease and disease impacts, and promoting consumer independence and life quality, are centered on a model in which all players are valued for their contributions and collaborative effort.

The move toward a more community-based health promotion and disease prevention model of care has also been creating new opportunities for collaborative practice in primary care (Bodenheimer, 2019). Also, telehealth and wide adoption of electronic health records offer creative opportunities for interaction. For these systems to work, APRNs and other clinicians must be involved in selecting, piloting, modifying, and implementing new technologies (see Chapter 22). From the selection of vendors to full deployment of the technology, the adoption of new technologies offers opportunities for clinicians to develop collaborative learning communities. In the current global market, innovative new alliances among advanced practice nursing groups and physician groups need to be developed and nurtured.

Challenges to Collaboration

Implementing effective collaborative professional relationships in the workplace can be challenging. These challenges can be characterized as professional, sociocultural, organizational, and regulatory. Part of the issue is that team members often see themselves primarily as representatives of their own discipline rather than as members of a collaborative team.

Disciplinary Challenges

The ways in which health professional education is conducted in the United States have long been an impediment to successful collaboration. Each profession is a culture with its own epistemology, values, knowledge, rules, and norms, and educational programs reflect this culture. Additionally, educational programs are conducted at a variety of colleges and universities where there may be little opportunity for shared learning. The basic epistemology that underlies each type of profession may be unique and, at times, may overlap other professions. This leads to differences in understanding what constitutes truth, goals of practice, and expected outcomes even when there is joint practice. One profession may firmly believe that they are the only one that has the whole picture for the patients. This can be seen by the continuing efforts to place CRNAs under physician supervision (see Chapter 16). There are similar issues seen at times for NPs, CNMs, and CNSs. Pharmacists may believe that they are the single authority for questions concerning medication. In an evaluation of the Hartford Foundation initiative to strengthen interdisciplinary team training in geriatrics (Reuben et al., 2004), faculty and students in advanced practice nursing, medicine, and social work were found to be influenced by disciplinary attitudes and cultural factors that were obstacles to teamwork, a phenomenon the authors termed *disciplinary split*. They observed that disciplinary heritage and a differential willingness to participate in teamwork characterized disciplinary split and constituted an obstacle to implementing effective interdisciplinary teamwork in geriatrics training.

The Robert Wood Johnson Foundation (RWJF) Partnerships for Training initiative (Rice et al., 2010; Young et al., 2012) identified many of the stresses inherent in building and sustaining interdisciplinary academic–community partnerships. Stresses encountered by participants as they developed partnerships centered on money, differing agendas, systems that were not integrated, varying philosophies, and long-held beliefs about how things should be done.

Collaboration at the community grassroots level is often easier to implement and maintain than at the professional organizational level. Although collaboration happens daily among practicing clinicians, collaboration may not exist at the national level, impeding efforts to move toward a coordinated healthcare system. The outdated positions espoused by some policymakers from all disciplines may be based on stereotyped beliefs about disciplinary roles and responsibilities rather than reflecting consideration of the issues or what is best for patients. These factors make it increasingly important for APRNs and other clinicians practicing at local levels who have learned the art of collaboration to take an active role in bringing their perspectives and experiences to policymaking at institutional, community, state, and national levels to foster collaboration. The AANP (2020) believes that a broader statutory definition of professional autonomy for APRNs than what is found in many states is necessary if the more complex autonomy of interdependent collaborators is to be exercised effectively.

Despite these existing challenges to collaboration, there is evidence of progress. The US Preventive Services Task Force, which is part of the AHRQ, comprises an interdisciplinary group of providers and researchers who develop, disperse, and revise evidence-based recommendations on screening and prevention for a variety of healthcare concerns (US Preventive Services Task Force, 2020).

Ineffective Communication and Team Dysfunction

Communication styles may also be a barrier to collaboration. Dysfunctional styles of interactions among healthcare professionals that particularly undermine collaboration include being difficult, bullying, or abusive. The term *disruptive behavior* has been used to include these and other intimidating behaviors. Clinicians whose behavior is disruptive display arrogance, rudeness, and poor communication (Longo & Smith, 2011). APRNs have a responsibility to recognize disruptive behavior as risks to collaboration and safe patient care and to develop a repertoire of interpersonal and system strategies with which to address these behaviors directly and promptly.

Lencioni (2005), a business consultant on team effectiveness, proposed one model of team dysfunction that has a practical use by APRNs. In this model, the first four of the five dysfunctions reflect the absence of key components of our definition of collaboration: (1) absence of trust, (2) fear of conflict, (3) lack of commitment, (4) avoidance of accountability, and (5) inattention to results. The fifth dysfunction, inattention to results, is consistent with the observation that efforts within health care to improve safety, reliability, and quality represent an opportunity to foster teamwork and collaboration by examining the processes and outcomes of care, attending to results.

Sociocultural Issues

Tradition, role, racial, and gender stereotypes are obstacles to collaboration (Rafferty et al., 2001). Safriet (1992) suggested that the field of medicine staked out broad professional territory early on and considered any movement into this turf by other clinicians, at any level, to be unacceptable. This can lead to challenges to successful collaboration.

Nursing remains a predominantly female profession and, despite the influx of women into medicine, pharmacy, and dentistry, gender role stereotypes still exist and affect collaboration. Gender stereotypes dominate how images of staff nurses in the media and APRNs are commonly portrayed on television. However, the rules are changing as all of health care becomes increasingly female.

Stereotypical images of APRNs influence how they are viewed by consumers, and this can be positive. Australia has had limited experience with NPs in primary care, so Parker and colleagues (2013) asked consumers in five states what they thought about receiving their primary care from NPs. Almost none of the consumers had any knowledge about what NPs were. The consumers indicated that they highly valued registered nurses and that NPs would be very acceptable for their primary care.

Organizational Challenges

Competitive situations arise that can interfere with collaboration. The patchwork of US federal and state policies, rules, and regulations along with organizational rules and policies concerning APRN practice can make collaboration difficult. This set of rules can also lead to unproductive competition among clinicians. For example, the intent of Medicare billing requirements was to foster cooperation among clinicians, but they also discourage collaborative relations between healthcare providers and may actually serve as disincentives. "Incident-to" billing (see Chapter 19) requires that patient care services provided by APRNs be directly supervised by physicians and offers reimbursement inequities, severely hampering a collaborative environment (CMS, 2019).

Regulatory Challenges

Legislation and regulations pose a number of challenges to the implementation of collaborative roles. In the early days of advanced practice nursing, the overlap in APRNs' and physicians' scopes of practice was often addressed by requiring physician supervision of aspects of APRN practice. An outcome of this early requirement was that physician supervision often appeared in the advanced practice nursing literature on collaboration and in state practice acts and regulations. In the past 40 years, there has been a slow but steady movement away from references to protocols and language requiring physician supervision toward emphasizing consultation, collaboration, peer review, and use of referral (AANP, 2019).

Eliminating regulatory barriers to full practice authority has been one of the pillars of the IOM work on the *Future of Nursing* (2010) and has been reiterated in the updated document (National Academies of Sciences, Engineering, and Medicine, 2021). Substantial work continues to remove these and other barriers for APRNs throughout the United States. Similar efforts are taking place in other countries as they discover that creating artificial barriers to full practice is counter to national goals of access to high-quality care for their people (Carter et al., 2015).

Adopting a multistate licensure compact for APRNs has become important to ensure that collaboration and continuity of care can occur (National Council of State Boards of Nursing [NCSBN], 2016). Consumers are consulting quality scorecards, licensing boards, websites, blogs, and other Internet resources to identify agencies and individual clinicians who provide the best health care.

Opportunities to create collaborative relationships can be lost during rapid changes in health care (Young et al., 2012). Furthermore, nurses and other clinicians who are confronting their own professional concerns may not fully appreciate the stresses that others experience in today's volatile market. This factor is a serious deterrent to collaborative relationships.

Collaboration within the APRN nursing community is also problematic at times. Overall, there are four dimensions of APRN regulation—licensure, accreditation, certification, and education. Often, language and policy barriers make it difficult for the groups responsible for each of these to collaborate. These groups have created a collaborative network that allows them to match their individual organizational priorities to the priorities for APRNs overall. Exemplar 10.3 describes this effort and illustrates how an initial failure to collaborate can turn into a win–win situation for all involved.

PROCESSES ASSOCIATED WITH EFFECTIVE COLLABORATION

Recurring Interactions

Establishing a trusting and collaborative relationship develops over time and depends on recurring, meaningful interactions (Alberto & Herth, 2009). Development of trust, in particular, takes place over time. This means that collaborative relationships are difficult to

EXEMPLAR 10.3

A LONG-TERM COLLABORATION FOR THE EDUCATION AND REGULATION OF ADVANCED PRACTICE REGISTERED NURSES

In the United States, the board of nursing in each state has the responsibility and authority to regulate nursing at the beginning and advanced levels. This usually includes titles that nurses can use for their profession. In the 1990s, there was a rapid proliferation of educational programs and certification processes of postgraduate educational programs, particularly for nurse practitioners. The National Council of State Boards of Nursing (NCSBN) was confronted with an array of different and potentially confusing set of credentials that varied from state to state. There had been a long history of practice by nurse anesthetists and nurse midwives, but these were regulated by the nursing board in some states and by the medical board in others. Multiple new nurse practitioner programs were developing and often in narrow areas such as pediatric oncology or palliative care.

Emerging from what had become a confusing system of education and requests for board of nursing recognition was the creation of the LACE consensus model for APRN regulation. LACE stands for Licensure, Accreditation, Certification, and Education. Over 70 nursing organizations participate in the consensus process for APRN regulation. The goal of this consensus process is to assist all state boards of nursing to adopt a common model of regulation for APRNs. This would allow movement among states much more seamlessly than currently exists. In most cases, the state legislatures and governors must pass legislation to meet the new standards for education and certification as well as recognition for independent practice and independent prescribing for all four roles of APRNs. This is a slow process with several different parts. Progress is being made each year to achieve this goal of common recognition.

Prior to this work, there were few examples of nationwide collaboration among nurse anesthetists, nurse midwives, nurse practitioners, and clinical nurse specialists; their certification groups; and the boards of nursing. This work continues today with regularly scheduled meetings and recognition of the consensus process.

develop in organizations where there is a high staff turnover or frequent rotation of clinicians, such as with house staff physicians. A series of less-complicated interactions that have been clinical or personal will contribute to the development of trust in collaborative relationships. Team members need recurring interactions to acquire an understanding of each other's backgrounds, roles, and functions and develop patterns of interaction that are constructive, productive, and supportive. Projects focused on quality and outcomes of care that involve joint collection and analysis of data build collegiality and foster collaboration. Membership on such interdisciplinary committees, such as pharmacy and therapeutics, performance improvement, institutional review boards, ethics, and others with a patient care focus, also fosters communication and collegiality.

Effective Conflict Negotiation and Resolution Skills

Conflict will arise as individuals, teams, and organizations work more closely together on their shared goals. Therefore APRNs must have some general approaches to conflict negotiation and resolution. Box 10.3 lists some key conflict resolution skills (Conflict Resolution Network, 2020). Extensive detail on these skills and how to apply them are available at https://www.crnhq.org/12-skill-summary/.

Partnering and Team Building

Healthcare leaders are examining ways to improve the functioning of teams (IPEC, 2020). Effective models of teamwork have been used in subspecialties in psychology and health care. APRNs can draw on the lessons learned in these fields to improve team functioning. Some of the processes that have been associated with effective team building and conflict negotiation are listed in Box 10.3. Partnering is often a long-term process over several years with different partners, as illustrated in Exemplar 10.3.

BOX 10.3

Conflict Resolution Network's 12 Skills Summary

- Win-win approach (how we can solve this as partners rather than opponents).
- Creative response (transform problems into creative opportunities).
- Empathy (develop communication tools to build rapport; use listening to clarify understanding).
- Appropriate assertiveness (apply strategies to attack the problem, not the person).
- Cooperative power (eliminate "power over" to build "power with" others).
- Managing emotions (express fear, anger, hurt, and frustration wisely to effect change).
- Willingness to resolve (name personal issues that cloud the picture).
- Mapping the conflict (define the issues needed to chart common needs and concerns).
- Development of options (design creative solutions together).
- Introduction to negotiation (plan and apply effective strategies to reach agreement).
- Introduction to mediation (help conflicting parties to move toward solutions).
- Broadening perspectives (evaluate the problem in the broader context).

Adapted from Conflict Resolution Network. (2020). 12 Skill summary: Conflict resolution skills. https://www.crnhq.org/12-skill-summary/

IMPLEMENTING COLLABORATION

There are times that APRNs may feel as though they are the only ones with an active commitment to collaboration. Collaboration may be difficult to accomplish because it is mediated by social processes such as attitudinal and cultural factors that are ingrained. Efforts to change the environment to one that is more collaborative involve proving oneself over and over and challenging colleagues' behaviors that restrain attempts to work together. These interpersonal demands, along with clinical demands, can be exhausting. Therefore APRNs should evaluate the potential for collaboration when seeking career opportunities. Questions about how clinicians work together, the degree of hierarchy, and the interpersonal climate and organizational structures that support collaboration should be a high priority. A realistic appraisal of collaboration is needed to determine whether APRNs can provide the standard and quality of care characteristic of advanced practice nursing and whether they can expect a reasonable level of job satisfaction.

Assessment of Personal, Environmental, and Global Factors

APRNs bring many personal attributes to a professional partnership. Assessment of their current attributes against the characteristics of collaboration listed in Box 10.4 can help beginning APRNs to determine the areas in most need of development.

In a classic work, Covey (1989) offered a perspective on moving toward a higher level of interdependence with colleagues. He portrayed interdependence as a higher level of performance than independence. Only individuals who have gained competence and confidence in their own expertise are able to move beyond autonomy and independence toward the higher synergistic level of collaboration. Collaboration appears to have a similar meaning as interdependence in Covey's work. This view is provocative when one considers the hierarchical context that often frames clinical collaboration. The notion that interdependence is the higher level of performance is supported in the evolution of advanced practice nursing. A number of clinical specialties are evolving to such a stage as disciplines mature and identify a shared interdisciplinary component to their work. For example, in the specialty of diabetes, advanced diabetes management involves interprofessional collaboration (Gucciardi et al., 2016) and is recognized by a certification examination open to a number of disciplines.

Self-assessment is one important component to consider when embarking on a new professional relationship or evaluating the success or failure of current or potential collaborative relationships. The self-directed questions in Box 10.4 may help individuals identify personal strengths and weaknesses. APRNs should also consider contextual factors in the systems in which they practice.

Administrative leadership plays a key role in the development of collaborative relationships among organizational members. Administrators who support team and interdisciplinary administrative models, and who are themselves good communicators, can do a great deal to increase the momentum of new collaborations. The common vision of quality patient care and provider satisfaction makes collaboration a worthy goal for APRNs and nursing administrators.

Global interactions require high levels of individual and organizational collaboration beyond what we can often envision. APRNs who recognize the need for global participation and collaboration at the personal, organizational, and systems levels are more likely to be successful.

BOX 10.4

Personal Strengths and Weaknesses Questionnaire

- Am I clear about my role in the partnership?
- What values do I bring to the relationship?
- What do I expect to gain or lose by collaborating?
- What do others expect of me?
- Do I feel good about my contribution to the team?
- Do I feel self-confident and competent in the collaborative relationship?
- Are there anxieties causing repeated friction that have not been addressed?
- Has serious thought been given to the boundaries of the collaborative relationship?

Adapted from Rider, E. (2002). Twelve strategies for effective communication and collaboration in medical teams. *British Medical Journal*, 325, S45.

STRATEGIES FOR SUCCESSFUL COLLABORATION

Individual Strategies

Box 10.5 lists strategies that promote collaboration (Rider, 2002). APRNs can examine their interactions for opportunities to implement these ideas and strengthen their interpersonal competence.

One strategy is for APRNs to promote their exemplary nursing practices to help other health professionals and consumers better understand the strengths of APRNs as healthcare providers (Pohl et al., 2010). Participating in interdisciplinary quality improvement initiatives and developing and evaluating evidence-based practice (EBP) guidelines (see Chapter 8) are other ways to engage with colleagues within and across

BOX 10.5

Strategies to Promote Effective Communication and Collaboration

- Be respectful and professional.
- Listen intently.
- Understand the other person's viewpoint before expressing your opinion.
- Model an attitude of collaboration and expect it.
- Identify the bottom line.
- Decide what is negotiable and nonnegotiable.
- Acknowledge the other person's thoughts and feelings.
- Pay attention to your own ideas and what you have to offer to the group.
- Be cooperative without losing integrity.
- Be direct.
- Identify common, shared goals and concerns.
- State your feelings using "I" statements.
- Do not take things personally.
- Learn to say, "I was wrong" or "You could be right."
- Do not feel pressure to agree instantly.
- Think about possible solutions before meeting and be willing to adapt if a more creative alternative is presented.
- Think of conflict negotiation and resolution as a helical process, not a linear one; recognize that negotiation may occur over several interactions.

disciplines. One way to share excellence in practice in grand rounds or a team conference is to include the opportunity for care team members to describe their own decision making about patients and suggest new strategies for care to the team.

Working together on joint projects is another excellent way to facilitate collaboration. Collaborative research and scholarly writing projects, as well as community service projects that tap into the strengths of various members, demonstrate the benefits of collaboration. These strategies move across lines from personal life to organizational settings and from education to practice arenas. More important, collaboratively developed practice guidelines improve communication and clarify clinicians' roles in patient treatment (US Preventive Services Task Force, 2020).

Team Strategies

Lencioni's field guide (2005) provided activities aimed at helping team members overcome the team dysfunctions described earlier, noting that there were two important questions team members must ask themselves:

- Are we really a team?
- Are we ready to do the heavy lifting that will be required to become a team?

A group of collaborators will be able to use the field guide to their advantage if they can respond affirmatively to both questions. The activities are aimed at helping teams address each of the five dysfunctions by helping them build trust, master conflict, achieve commitment, embrace accountability, and focus on results.

One serious challenge to collaboration is team members who are not interested in developing collaborative teams. In this type of situation, APRNs must step up and operate from a stance and expectation of collaboration; that is, APRNs should model collaboration in all interactions and expect the same from all other members of the team. Building a group of likeminded colleagues can also increase the momentum toward collaboration as the expected style of interaction within a team. APRNs should understand that collaboration is only beginning to be taught in health professions schools. Consequently, they must be prepared to teach this process to others.

Organizational Strategies

The numerous initiatives to improve safety and quality that have evolved from the IOM reports can help health administrators and leaders create organizational structures that facilitate collaboration while attending to important quality and safety goals. The Institute for Healthcare Improvement's (IHI) white papers, TJC, and Magnet requirements for evidence of interdisciplinary collaboration in patient care, toolkits for interdisciplinary education, and clinical and organizational toolkits to facilitate the adoption of EBP guidelines (e.g., from the Registered Nurses Association of Ontario, rnao.org) are all readily available. These toolkits often include assessments that can be performed to identify the location of the barriers and the opportunities for improvement. APRNs and other clinical colleagues and leaders can use these assessments to develop strategic plans for improving the collaborative environment. Clinicians may need professional development to enable them to collaborate depending on the results of the assessment.

Health professional organizations have endorsed the shift toward a collaborative model (NCSBN, 2016). As noted, there are some successful models of consensus building in some sectors of health care. These models, across disciplines, must be replicated more widely in health care if barriers to successful interprofessional collaboration are to be reduced.

Exemplar 10.4 is one example of how APRNs from different specialties can work together to alter a hospital policy. They pooled the expertise in their particular specialty and their knowledge of the political issues that often surround hospital-based work. They knew that if they wanted to make this change, the key players in the decision-making process would have to buy in to the idea. The usual pattern is not to change because past policy and procedures have been in place and there is substantial pressure not to change something that is viewed as working. The pull of the familiar was in place, yet it was not working for the mothers who wanted different options available to them.

EXEMPLAR 10.4

COLLABORATION IN QUALITY IMPROVEMENT: IMPROVED ANALGESIA AND ANESTHESIA OPTIONS DURING LABOR

Ms. Smith is a CNM who provides full-scope midwifery services to women who choose this approach for pregnancy and delivery. The birthing center at which Ms. Smith attends the delivery of her patients has a policy that women must choose no analgesia during labor and delivery or they must have an epidural. Many of the women were not happy with having only two choices. Also, the policy of the hospital was that women who selected epidural anesthesia had to have a fetal monitor and were confined to bed for labor. Some women believed that they might need some help with the discomfort of delivery but did not want to be confined to labor in bed as required if they selected traditional epidural anesthesia. Ms. Smith investigated this issue and found that the policy seems to have been developed in the past by a committee that consisted of obstetrics–gynecology physicians and anesthesiologists. The policy was approved by the medical staff. No mothers, CNMs, NPs, or CRNAs were part of the policymaking. There have been several advances in care since this policy was developed, and Ms. Smith wished to bring about a change to improve care to the mothers and their families.

In this particular facility, only anesthesia providers (physician or CRNA) were credentialed to administer any analgesic or anesthetic agents to mothers in labor, a practice touted as necessary for the quality of care for recipients of these agents. Ms. Smith did not believe that she would be able to alter this policy, nor did she really wish to do so. However, she wanted to provide an expanded set of options for her mothers. Although many of the mothers did not choose to receive any analgesia for labor or delivery, they wanted to have the option available prior to needing it.

Ms. Smith consulted with a CRNA colleague who specialized in obstetric anesthesia. They met and discussed a number of options and decided that there were types of epidural approaches that could allow the mother to continue to walk while in labor and therefore improve the likelihood of a normal vaginal birth. Also, additional approaches were added to the list of available agents. One was a handheld device that delivered inhaled nitrous oxide when the mother thought she needed it. The services of the pediatric nurse practitioner (PNP) were requested because the APRN believed that the substantial literature on the topic indicated that newborns have better outcomes if the mother does not receive a standard epidural and that normal vaginal birth could be encouraged.

This trio of APRNs crafted the new policy proposal; engaged support from the chair of obstetrics–gynecology, chair of pediatrics, chair of anesthesiology, and nursing supervisor; and advanced the change in policy to the medical staff committee. After a great deal of argument, discussion, and negotiation, the policy was changed and approved by the hospital board. Now, women can choose from a variety of approaches that best meet their wishes and particular situation. This group of APRNs knew that there were some parts of the policy that would not change, including the administration by anesthesia providers only. Also, all of the anesthesiologists and CRNAs who provided obstetric anesthesia were not equally adept at all of the new approaches, so the CRNA provided in-service education for them. The nursing staff of the birthing center needed additional training, and the CNM provided this education along with the CRNA. Although the change in policy was created to accommodate the wishes of the midwifery practice, the outcome was that all women who delivered in the facility now had options that improved their satisfaction and quality of care. In addition, all of the APRN caregivers believed that they had enhanced the labor experience of their maternity patients.

These APRNs all knew that in their facility, policy approval was the purview of the medical staff. They would have to be included to make this change. Also, the hospital was governed by strong department chairs in medicine and they would also have to agree. These APRNs well understood that science, although critically important, was not sufficient to bring about this change. All of the stakeholders had to be included. The APRNs knew which parts of the policy were open for negotiation and which were not and crafted their proposal cleverly. This change did not happen quickly; several months were required to gain the support of all of the key players. However, in the end, the women who used the birthing center were greatly advantaged by the collaborative efforts of all involved.

CONCLUSION

Many of the barriers to successful collaboration occur because of values, beliefs, and behaviors that have until recently gone unchallenged in society and in the organizations where nurses practice. Substantial additional change is needed if the conditions conducive to collaboration are to become the norm. Collaborative relationships not only are professionally satisfying but also improve access to care and patient outcomes. Although APRNs collaborate successfully with many individuals within and outside of nursing, they may find that one of their most important collaborative relationships—with physicians—may also be the most challenging. Despite the fact that there are many successful individual APRN–physician collaborative practices, including many with evidence demonstrating their beneficial effects on health care, tradition and stereotypes are often powerful negative influences on policymaking and in health care and professional organizations.

To meet the demands for cost-effectiveness and quality, clinicians from all disciplines have been meeting together to discuss the care they provide and to define ways to deliver it to maximize quality and minimize duplication of effort. These interactions foster the trust and respect required for mature collaboration. They enable collaborators to recognize their interdependence and value the input of others, thus creating a synergy that improves the quality of clinical decision making. Systems citizenship starts with seeing the systems we have shaped and that in turn shape us (Friedman, 2005). Collaboration becomes a priority as global interconnectedness enters our everyday interactions in the complex healthcare arena in which APRNs practice. In today's healthcare environment, collaboration may flourish, regardless of the barriers identified in this chapter.

KEY SUMMARY POINTS

- There is a need for a better understanding of the organizational structures, communication processes, and interactive styles that enable clinicians to collaborate in ways that benefit clinical processes and outcomes.
- APRNs can contribute to this understanding in several ways:
  - by documenting and analyzing their experiences with collaboration in published case studies;
  - by serving as preceptors for health science students and helping them develop the skills essential for collaboration; and
  - by working with researchers who are studying the characteristics and clinical implications of collaboration
- Effective collaboration must be at the heart of any redesign of the healthcare delivery system, whether that redesign occurs in a unit, in a clinic, within and between organizations, or globally.

REFERENCES

Agency for Healthcare Research and Quality (AHRQ). (n.d). *Defining the patient centered medical home.* https://pcmh.ahrq.gov/page/defining-pcmh

Agency for Healthcare Research and Quality. (2019). *Rapid response systems.* https://psnet.ahrq.gov/primer/rapid-response-systems

Alberto, J., & Herth, K. (2009). Interprofessional collaboration within faculty roles: Teaching, service, and research. *Online Journal of Issues in Nursing, 14*(2), 1–14. https://doi.org/10.3912/OJIN.Vol14No02PPT02

American Association of Colleges of Nursing. (2004). *AACN position statement on the practice doctorate in nursing.* https://www.aacnnursing.org/Portals/42/News/position-Statement/DNP.pdf

American Association of Colleges of Nursing. (2006). *The essentials of doctoral education for advanced nursing practice.* https://www.aacnnursing.org/Portals/42/Publications/DNPEssentials.pdf

American Association of Colleges of Nursing. (2021). *The essentials: Core competencies for professional nursing education.* https://www.aacnnursing.org/Education-Resources/AACN-Essentials

American Association of Nurse Practitioners. (2019). *Scope of practice for nurse practitioners.* https://www.aanp.org/advocacy/advocacy-resource/position-statements/scope-of-practice-for-nurse-practitioners

American Association of Nurse Practitioners. (2020). *State policy priorities*. https://www.aanp.org/advocacy/state/2020-state-policy-priorities

American Nurses Credentialing Center (ANCC). (2020). *Magnet recognition program*. https://www.nursingworld.org/organizational-programs/magnet/magnet-model/

Anderson, J. G., & Abrahamson, K. (2017). Your health care may kill you: Medical errors. *Studies in Health Technology and Informatics, 234*, 13–17.

Bachynsky, N. (2020). Implications for policy: The triple aim, quadruple aim, and interprofessional collaboration. *Nursing Forum, 55*, 54–64. https://doi.org/10.1111/nuf.12382

Balik, B., Conway, J., Zipperer, L., & Watson, J. (2011). *Achieving an exceptional patient and family experience of inpatient hospital care. IHI Innovation Series white paper*. Institute for Healthcare Improvement.

Barwell, J., Arnold, F., & Berry, H. (2013). How interprofessional learning improves care. *Nursing Times, 109(21)*, 14–16.

Bell, A., Michalec, B., & Arenson, C. (2014). The stalled progress of interprofessional collaboration: The role of gender. *Journal of Interprofessional Care, 28*(2), 98–102. http://doi.org/10.3109/1356180.2013.851073

Bodenheimer, T. (2019). Building powerful primary care teams. *Mayo Clinical Proceedings, 94(7)*, 1135–1137. http://doi.org/10.1016/j.mayocp.2019.05.017

Bosch, B., & Mansell, H. (2015). Interprofessional collaboration in health care: Lessons to be learned from competitive sports. *Canadian Pharmacists' Journal: CPJ = Revue des pharmacies du Canada: RPC, 148*(4), 176–179. doi:10.1177/1715163515588106

Bosque, E. (2011). A model of collaboration and efficiency between neonatal nurse practitioner and neonatologist: Application of collaboration theory. *Advances in Neonatal Care, 11*, 108–113. https://doi.org/10.1097/anc.0b013e318213263d

Busari, J., Moll, F., & Duits, A. (2017). Understanding the impact of interprofessional collaboration on the quality of care: A case report from a small scale resource limited health care environment. *Journal of Multidisciplinary Healthcare, 10*, 227–234. http://doi.org/10.2147/JMDH.S140042

Canadian Interprofessional Health Collaborative. (2010). *A national interprofessional competency framework*. https://phabc.org/wp-content/uploads/2015/07/CIHC-National-Interprofessional-Competency-Framework.pdf

Carter, M., Owen-Williams, E., & Della, P. (2015). Meeting Australia's emerging primary care needs by nurse practitioners. *Journal for Nurse Practitioners, 11*(6), 647–652. http://doi.org/10.1016/j.nurpra.2015.02.0

Centers for Medicare and Medicaid Services. (2019). *Medicare claims processing manual: Physician/nonphysician practitioners*. http://www.cms.gov/Regulations-and-Guidance/Guidance/Manuals/Downloads/clm104c12.pdf

Clausen., C., Strohschein, F. J., Farems, S., Bateman, D., Posel, N., & Fleiszer, D. M. (2012). Developing an interprofessional care plan for an older adult women with breast cancer: From multiple voices to a shared vision. *Oncology Nursing, 16*, E18–E25. http://doi.org/10.1188/12.CJON.E18-E25

Conflict Resolution Network. (2020). *12 skills summary: Conflict resolution skills* https://www.crnhq.org/12-skill-summary/

Covey, S. R. (1989). *The seven habits of highly effective people*. Simon & Schuster.

Creamer, A. M., & Austin, W. (2017). Canadian nurse practitioner core competencies identified: An opportunity to build mental health and illness skills knowledge. *Journal for Nurse Practitioners, 13*(5), e231–e236. https://doi.org/10.1016/j.nurpra.2016.12.017

Deming, W. E. (1982). *Quality, productivity and competitive position*. Massachusetts Institute of Technology.

Desborough, J. L. (2012). How nurse practitioners implement their roles. *Australian Health Review, 36*(1), 22–26.

Dillon, D., & Gary, F. (2017). Full practice authority for nurse practitioners. *Nursing Administration Quarterly, 41*(1), 86–93. https://doi.org/10.1097/NAQ.0000000000000210

Dumez, A. G. (2011). There is need for broader and more effective cooperation among the health service professions. *American Journal of Pharmaceutical Education, 75*, 99. http://doi.org/10.5688/ajpe75599

Emich, C. (2018). Conceptualizing collaboration in nursing. *Nursing Forum, 53*(4), 567–573. https://doi.org/10.1111/nuf.12287

Frank, J., Snell, L., & Sherbino, J. (2015). CanMEDS 2015 Physician Competency Framework. http://canmeds.royalcollege.ca/uploads/en/framework/CanMEDS%202015%20Framework_EN_Reduced.pdf

Friedman, T. L. (2005). *The world is flat: A brief history of the 21st century*. Farrar, Straus and Giroux.

Ghaffari, F., Dehghan-Nayeri, N., & Shali, M. (2015). Nurses' experiences of humour in clinical settings. *Medical Journal of the Islamic Republic of Iran, 29*, 182.

Global Confederation for Interprofessional Education & Collaborative Practice. (2020). *Interprofessional global*. https://interprofessional.global

Goldsberry, J. W. (2018). Advanced practice nurses leading the way: Interprofessional collaboration. *Nurse Education Today, 65*, 1–3. https://doi.org/10.1016/j.nedt.2018.02.024

Green, B., & Johnson, C. (2015). Interprofessional collaboration in research, education, and clinical practice: Working together for a better future. *Journal of Chiropractic Education, 29*(1), 1–10. https://doi.org/10.7899/JCE-14-36

Gucciardi, E., Espin, S., Morganti, A., & Dorato, L. (2016). Exploring interprofessional collaboration during the integration of diabetes teams into primary care. *BMC Family Practice, 17*(12), 1–14. https://doi.org/10.1186/s12875-016-0407-1

Haney, T. S., Sharp, P. B., Nesbitt, C., & Poston, R. D. (2017). Innovative intraprofessional clinical training for clinical nurse specialists and nurse practitioner students. *Journal of Nursing Education, 56*(12). https://doi.org/10.3928/01484834-20171120-09.748-451.

Health Sciences Institute. (2022). The main causes of poor health and avoidable costs are behavioral not medical. https://health-sciences.org

Institute of Medicine. (2000). *To err is human: Building a safer health system*. National Academy Press.

Institute of Medicine. (2010). *The future of nursing: Leading change, advancing health*. http://nationalacademies.org/HMD/Reports/2010/The-Future-of-Nursing-Leading-Change-Advancing-Health.aspx

Interprofessional Education Collaborative. (2011). Core competencies of interprofessional collaborative practice. www.aacn.nche.edu/education/pdf/IPECreport.pdf

Interprofessional Education Collaborative. (2016). *Core competencies for interprofessional collaborative practice: 2016 update.* https://hsc.unm.edu/ipe/resources/ipec-2016-core-competencies.pdf

Interprofessional Education Collaborative. (2020). *Vision and mission.* https://www.ipecollaborative.org/vision-mission.html

Janotha, B., Tamari, K., & Evangelidis-Sakellson, V. (2018). Dental and nurse practitioner student attitudes about collaboration before and after interprofessional clinical experiences. *Journal of Dental Education, 83*(6), 638–644. http://doi.org/10.21815/JDE.019.073

Karam, M., Brault, I., Van Durme, T., & Macq, J. (2017). Comparing interprofessional and interorganizational collaboration in healthcare: A systematic review of the qualitative research. *International Journal of Nursing Studies, 79*, 70–83.

King, T. L. (2020). The effectiveness of midwifery care in the world health organization year of the nurse and midwife. Reducing the cesarean birth rate. *Journal of Midwifery & Women's Health, 65*(1), 7–9. http://doi.org/10.1111/jmwh.13089

Lencioni, P. (2005). *Overcoming the five dysfunctions of a team: A field guide for leaders, managers, and facilitators.* Jossey-Bass.

Longo, J., & Smith, M. (2011). A prescription for disruptions in care: Community building among nurses to address horizontal violence. *Advances in Nursing Science, 34*, 345–356. http://doi.org/10.1097/ANS.0b013e3182300e3e

Mahler, C., Gutmann, T., Karstens, S., & Joos, S. (2014). Terminology for interprofessional collaboration: Definition and current practice. *GMS Zeitschrift fur medizinische Ausbildung, 31*(4). doi:10.3205/zma000932

Maier, C. B., & Aiken, L. H. (2016). Expanding clinical roles for nurses to realign the global health workforce with population needs: A commentary. *Israel Journal of Health Policy Research, 5*(21). http://doi.org/10.1186/s13854-16-0079-2

Manojlovich, M., Kerr, M., Davies, B., Squires, J., Mallick, R., & Rodger, G. L. (2014). Achieving a climate for patient safety by focusing on relationships. *International Journal of Quality in Health Care, 26*(6), 579–584. http://doi.org/10.1093/intqhc/mzu068

McNamara, S., Lepage, K., & Boileau, J. (2011). Bridge the gap: Interprofessional collaboration between nurse practitioner and clinical nurse specialist. *Clinical Nurse Specialist, 25*(1), 33–40. http://doi.org/10.1097/NUR.0b0e13e31820214d

Monahan, L., Sparbel, K., Heinschel, J., Rugen, K. W., & Rosenberger, K. (2018). Medical and pharmacy students shadowing advanced practice nurses to develop interprofessional competencies. *Applied Nursing Research, 39*, 103–108. http://doi.org/10.1016/j.apnr.2017.11.012

Murray-Davis, B., Marshall, M., & Gordon, F. (2011). What do midwives think about interprofessional working and learning? *Midwifery, 27*(3), 376–381. http://doi.org/10.1016/j.midw.2011.03.011

National Academies of Sciences, Engineering and Medicine. (2021). *The future of nursing 2020-2030: Charting a path to achieve health equity.* The National Academies Press.

National Committee for Quality Assurance [NCQA]. (2019). *Benefits of NCQA patient-centered medical home recognition.* https://www.ncqaorg/wp-content-uploands/2019/09/20190926_PCMH_Evidence_Report.pdf

National Council of State Boards of Nursing. (2016). *Nurse Licensure Compact Forum.* https://www.ncsbn.org/9331.htm

National Institute of Health. (2020). *The common fund.* https://commonfund.nih.gov/hcscollaboratory/fundedresearch

National Organization of Nurse Practitioner Faculties. (2017). *Common advanced practice registered nurse doctoral-level competencies.* https://cdn.ymaws.com/www.nonpf.org/resource/resmgr/competencies/common-aprn-doctoral-compete.pdf

Newhouse, R. P., Stanik-Hunt, J., White, K. M., Johantgen, M., Bass, E. B., Zangaro, G., & Weiner, J. P. (2011). Advanced practice nurse outcomes 1990-2008: A systematic review. *Nursing Economics, 29*, 230e–250.

Nir, N., & Halperin, E. (2018). Effects of humor on intergroup communication in intractable conflicts: Using humor in an intergroup appeal facilitates stronger agreement between groups and a greater willingness to compromise. *Political Psychology, 40*(3), 467–485. https://doi.prg10.1111.pops.12535

Norful, A. A., deJacq, K., Carlino, R., & Poghosyn, L. (2018). Nurse practitioner-physician comanagement: A theoretical model to alleviate primary care strain. *Annals of Family Medicine, 16*, 250–256. http://doi.org/10.1370/afm.2230

Nursing and Midwifery Board of Australia. (2014). Nurse practitioner standards for practice. http://www.nursingmidwiferyboard.gov.au/Search.aspx?q=Competency+Standards+for+the+Nursing+Practitioner

Parker, R., Forrest, L., Ward, N., McCracken, J., Cox, D., & Derrett, J. (2013). How acceptable are primary health care nurse practitioners to Australian consumers? *Collegian, 20*(1), 35–41. http://doi.org/10.1016/j.colegn.2012.03.001

Petri, L. (2010). Concept analysis of interdisciplinary collaboration. *Nursing Forum, 45*(2), 73–82. http://doi.org/10.1111/j.1744-6198.2010.00167.x

Pohl, J. M., Hanson, C. M., Newland, J. A., & Croenwett, L. (2010). Unleashing nurse practitioners' potential to deliver primary care and lead teams. *Health Affairs, 29*, 900–905. http://doi.org/10.1377/hlthaff.2010.0374

Rafferty, A. M., Ball, J., & Aiken, L. H. (2001). Are teamwork and professional autonomy compatible and do they result in improved hospital care? *Quality in Health Care, 10*(Suppl 2), ii32–ii37. http://doi.org/10.1136/qhc.0100032

Reuben, D. B., Levy-Storms, L., Yee, M. N., Lee, M., Cole, K., Waite, M., Nichols, L., & Frank, J. C. (2004). Disciplinary split: A threat to geriatrics interdisciplinary team training. *Journal of the American Geriatrics Society, 52*, 1000–1006. http://doi.org/10.1111/j.1532-5415.2004.52272.x

Rice, K., Zwarenstein, M., Conn, L. G., Kenaszchuk, C., Russell, A., & Reeves, S. (2010). An intervention to improve interprofessional collaboration and communications: A comparative qualitative study. *Journal of Interprofessional Care, 24*, 350–361. http://doi.org/10.3109/13561820903550713

Rider, E. (2002). Twelve strategies for effective communication and collaboration in medical teams. *British Medical Journal Career Focus, 325*, S45.

Safriet, B. J. (1992). Health care dollars and regulatory sense: The role of advanced practice nursing. *Yale Journal on Regulation, 9*,

417–487. https://digitalcommons.law.yale.edu/cgi/viewcontent.cgi?article=1223&context=yjreg

Safriet, B. J. (2002). Closing the gap between "can" and "may" in health care providers' scopes of practice: A primer for policymakers. *Yale Journal on Regulation, 19*, 301–334. https://digitalcommons.law.yale.edu/cgi/viewcontent.cgi?article=5418&context=fss_papers

Selleck, C., Fifolt, M., Burkart, H., Frank, J. S., Curry, W. A., & Hites, L. S. (2017). Providing primary care using an interprofessional collaborative practice model: What clinicians have learned. *Journal of Professional Nursing, 33*(6), 410–416. http://doi.org/10.1016/j.profnurs.2016.11.004

Souter, V., Nethery, E., Kopas, M., Wurz, H., Sitcove, K., & Caughey, A. B. (2019). Comparison of midwifery and obstetric care in low-risk hospital births. *Obstetrics and Gynecology, 134*(5), 1056–1065. http://doi.org/10.1097/AOG.0000000000003352

Sullivan, T. J. (1998). *Collaboration: A health care imperative*. McGraw-Hill Health Professionals Division.

Tamayo, M., Besoain-Saldana, A., Aquirre, M., & Leiva, J. (2017). Teamwork: Relevance and interdependence of interprofessional education. *Revista Saude Publica, 51*, 1–10. http://doi.org/10.1590/S1518-8787.2017051006816

The Joint Commission. (2021). Accreditation and certification. https://www.jointcommission.org

US Department of Health and Human Services. (2011). *Patient Protection and Affordable Care Act*. http://www.healthcare.gov/law/full/index.html

US Preventive Services Task Force. (2020). About the USPSTF. https://www.uspreventiveservicestaskforce.org/uspstf/about-uspstf

Wilson, S. (2013). Collaborative leadership: It's good to talk. *British Journal of Healthcare Management, 19*(7), 335–337. http://doi.org/10.12968/bjhc.2013.19.7.335

World Health Organization. (2010). Framework for action on interprofessional education & collaborative practice. http://whqlibdoc.who.int/hq/2010/WHO_HRH_HPN_10.3_eng.pdf

Young, H., Siegel, E. O., McCormick, W. C., Fulmer, T., Harootyan, L. K., & Dorr, D. A. (2012). Interdisciplinary collaboration in geriatrics: Advancing health for older adults. *Nursing Outlook, 59*, 243–251. http://doi.org/10.1016/j.outlook.2011.05.006

11

ETHICAL PRACTICE

LUCIA D. WOCIAL ■ ELLEN M. ROBINSON

"Clinicians must make a commitment to undertake the work involved to educate themselves if they are to develop their ethical expertise."

~ Ann B. Hamric

CHAPTER CONTENTS

FOUNDATIONS OF ETHICAL PRACTICE 342
- Personal and Professional Values 344
- Moral Distress 345
- Clear Communication 345
- Interprofessional Collaboration 346

OVERVIEW OF ETHICAL APPROACHES TO RESOLVING ETHICAL CONFLICTS 346
- Principle-Based Approach 346
- Casuistry Approach 347
- Narrative Ethics 348
- Care-Based Ethics 348

PROFESSIONAL CODES AND GUIDELINES 348
- Professional Boundaries 350

GOALS OF CARE: A CLINICAL-ETHICAL FRAMEWORK TO ENHANCE APRN PRACTICE 350
- Prognosis 350
- Values, Beliefs, and Preferences 352

ETHICAL COMPETENCY OF APRNS 354
- Knowledge Development 355
- Skill Acquisition 355
- Ethical Decision-Making Frameworks 356
- Addressing Ethical Conflict 357
- Creating Ethical Environments 357
- Preventive Ethics 359

ETHICAL ISSUES AFFECTING APRN PRACTICE 361
- Primary Care Issues 361
- Acute and Chronic Care Issues 361
- End-of-Life Complexities 362
- Conscientious Objection 365

SOCIETAL ISSUES, 366
- Promoting Social Justice 366
- Access to Resources 368
- Genomics 369
- COVID-19 Pandemic 369
- Gun Violence 370
- Participation in Research 370

LEGAL ISSUES 370

NAVIGATING BARRIERS TO ETHICAL PRACTICE AND STRATEGIES TO OVERCOME THEM 371
- Barriers Internal to the APRN 371
- Interprofessional Barriers 372
- Patient–Provider Barriers 372
- Organizational and Environmental Barriers 373

APRN WELL-BEING 373

CONCLUSION 376

KEY SUMMARY POINTS 377

Nurses at all levels of clinical practice, in all areas of health care, routinely encounter ethical challenges, yet how they resolve the situations varies significantly. The relationship centeredness of nursing creates a distinct ethical position for nurses. As the complexity of issues intensifies, the role of the advanced practice registered nurse (APRN) becomes particularly important in the identification, deliberation, and resolution of complicated and difficult moral problems. The American Association of Colleges of Nursing (AACN), in its vision for the future of nursing, identifies competence in ethics as a thread that runs through the spheres of practice beginning at the entry level of practice and building in complexity as nurses advance through masters and doctoral level education (AACN, 2019, 2021). Although all nurses are moral agents, APRNs are expected to be more than leaders in recognizing and resolving moral problems. They act as role models, creating ethical practice environments and promoting social justice in the larger healthcare system. This chapter explores the distinctive ethical competency of advanced practice nursing, the process of developing and evaluating this competency, barriers to ethical practice that APRNs can expect to confront, and potential strategies for overcoming those barriers.

FOUNDATIONS OF ETHICAL PRACTICE

Perhaps one of the biggest challenges for APRNs in attaining competence and sustaining ethical practice is the path taken to become an APRN. Some individuals will pursue APRN education after years of clinical practice and others will begin practice as an APRN with no experience in nursing or health care. Box 11.1 provides definitions for some foundational concepts in ethics. As a profession, we expect nurses to demonstrate everyday ethical comportment and to integrate a strong moral competence into every aspect of nursing practice (Milliken, 2017).

This requires at the very least cultivating one's *moral sensitivity*, which is an individual's capacity, acquired through experience, to sense the moral significance of a situation (Lützén et al., 2006). This necessitates a capacity to distinguish between feelings, facts, and values and reflect on these with the ability to articulate what is good, recognizing that defining what is good can be fraught with pitfalls if one has not engaged in rigorous self-reflection of personal values and potential biases (Feister, 2015).

Evidence suggests that when people face ethical decisions, they engage in mental processes outside their conscious awareness (may rely on intuition) and their decisions may be affected by their emotional state (Guzak, 2015). APRNs are not immune to the strong

BOX 11.1

Ethical Definitions and Terms for APRNs

- Ethical dilemma: Situations in which obligations require that individuals adopt each of two or more alternative but ethically acceptable incompatible actions, such that the individual cannot perform all required actions
- Principle of respect for autonomy: The duty to respect others' personal liberty and individual values, beliefs, and choices
- Principle of nonmaleficence: The duty not to inflict harm or evil
- Principle of beneficence: The duty to do good and prevent or remove harm
- Principle of formal justice: The fair equitable and appropriate treatment in light of what is owed to persons
    - *Distributive justice* refers to the fair, equitable, and appropriate distribution of benefits and burdens determined by societal norms.
    - *Material justice* deals with those characteristics that can be used to identify substantive properties that can be used to determine how to distribute goods and services.
- Rule of veracity: The duty to tell the truth and not to deceive others
- Rule of fidelity: The duty to honor commitments
- Rule of confidentiality: The duty not to disclose information shared in an intimate and trusted manner
- Rule of privacy: The duty to respect limited access to a person

Adapted from Beauchamp, T. L., & Childress, J. F. (2019). *Principles of biomedical ethics* (8th ed.). Oxford University Press.

The authors acknowledge Ann B. Hamric and Sarah A. Delgado for their work on previous editions of this chapter.

emotions evoked by ethically challenging, often tragic situations. Therefore a goal for the APRN, and all clinicians, is to identify the emotion within the situation and its circumstances, while also identifying one's own emotional response to it. The ability to separate the two is necessary to assess and intervene, even if the intervention is simply "bearing witness" alongside the patient, family, and clinical staff.

A rigorous practice of self-reflection to cultivate sensitivity to one's own emotion and hidden biases is essential for APRNs. Honest self-reflection can help minimize the risk of an emotional response to an ethically challenging situation, which in turn helps preserve the self and foster strong moral agency. The *Code of Ethics for Nurses* includes a provision calling attention to the duties nurses owe to themselves, including preservation of wholeness of character and integrity (American Nurses Association [ANA], 2015). This attention to the self enables nurses to hold themselves and others accountable even and especially in emotionally charged situations.

One often overlooked element of ethical practice is a deep understanding of dignity and the role it plays in fostering positive relationships. While each of us desires to be treated with dignity, we have an innate talent for lashing out when we feel our dignity is violated. Our default is to attack, which contributes to a cycle of psychological warfare against others, effectively destroying relationships and poisoning the environment (Hicks, 2011). When we learn to embrace the essential elements of dignity (Table 11.1), we can overcome our autopilot and promote healthy human relationships, which are essential for an ethical environment. Exemplar 11.1 is a brief but powerful example of how an APRN demonstrates how to honor dignity through everyday ethical comportment.

Because the APRN will apply theories, principles, rules, and moral concepts in actual encounters with patients, it is imperative to consider each specific context separately. Simulation has been shown to be an effective environment for students to learn and practice skills necessary to navigate complex environments

TABLE 11.1

Ten Essential Elements of Dignity

Element	Description
Acceptance of identity	Approach people as neither inferior nor superior to you; give others the freedom to express their authentic selves without fear of being negatively judged; interact without prejudice or bias, accepting how race, religion, gender, class, sexual orientation, age, disability, and so on are at the core of their identities; assume they have integrity.
Recognition	Validate others for their talents, hard work, thoughtfulness, and help; be generous with praise; give credit to others for their contributions, ideas, and experience.
Acknowledgment	Give people your full attention by listening, hearing, validating, and responding to their concerns and what they have been through.
Inclusion	Make others feel that they belong at all levels of relationship (family, community, organization, nation).
Safety	Put people at ease on two levels: physically, where they feel free of bodily harm, and psychologically, where they feel free of concern about being shamed or humiliated and feel free to speak without fear of retribution.
Fairness	Treat people justly, with equality, and in an evenhanded way according to agreed-upon laws and rules.
Independence	Empower people to act on their own behalf so that they feel in control of their lives and experience a sense of hope and possibility.
Understanding	Believe that what others think matters; give them the chance to explain their perspectives and express their points of view; actively listen in order to understand them.
Benefit of the doubt	Treat people as trustworthy; start with the premise that others have good motives and are acting with integrity.
Accountability	Take responsibility for your actions; if you have violated the dignity of another, apologize; make a commitment to change hurtful behaviors.

Adapted from *Dignity: Its Essential Role in Resolving Conflict*, by D. Hicks, 2011, Yale University Press. 33-97.

EXEMPLAR 11.1
CLINICAL SITUATION DEMONSTRATING EVERYDAY ETHICAL COMPORTMENT: HONORING DIGNITY[a]

Lori is a clinical nurse specialist who is eager to promote evidence-based practice changes. Armed with the latest research demonstrating the effectiveness of simple interventions to reduce urinary catheter-related infections, she encounters Kathy, a busy direct care nurse. Following (Hicks, 2011) essential elements of dignity (see Table 11.1), Lori approaches Kathy as a colleague, not one who has superior knowledge. Lori knows that Kathy has not attended her in-service program outlining the new protocol, and, rather than mention that, Lori acknowledges the heavy patient assignment Kathy is managing and complements her on her organization. When Kathy mentions that there is an order for a routine culture of the urinary catheter, Lori takes the opportunity to explain key points from the new protocol. Lori cheerfully offers to contact the physician, giving him the benefit of the doubt that he did not realize there was a new nurse-led protocol to guide appropriate removal of urinary catheters and check cultures only when a patient is symptomatic. Despite Lori's best efforts, Kathy feels that Lori has not been responsive to the workload she faces and lashes out at Lori, suggesting she is pushing this new protocol simply because it will save money. Lori does not respond to Kathy's heated comments. She instead helps Kathy focus on the primary goal of reducing the risk of infection for the patient. Lori offers to help Kathy remove the catheter and makes several suggestions to ensure that the patient has assistance to void, including returning in an hour to help Kathy monitor the patient to make sure he has assistance to void.

[a]Thanks to Lori Alesia, MN, RN, CNS, for her assistance with this exemplar.

involving ethical conflict (Calleja et al., 2020). Graduate curricula for APRNs need to go beyond traditional ethical issues to encompass a vast array of issues APRNs will face that have ethical complexity: building trust in the provider–patient relationship, professionalism and patient advocacy, resource allocation decisions, and individual versus population-based responsibilities, to name a few. As technology changes and new dilemmas confront practitioners, the APRN must be prepared to anticipate conditions that erode an ethical environment; for example, introduction of new electronic health records (EHRs) and potential violations of confidentiality because of the ease of access, use of artificial intelligence in EHRs, and the risk of using technology to replace the human connection (Ho, 2017; Stokes & Palmer, 2020; Yuste et al., 2017). Though there is no consensus definition for ethical competency in nursing (Lechasseur et al., 2018) because ethics is ever present in all aspects of nursing care, at a bare minimum, APRNs have an obligation to develop their ethical awareness and learn to apply ethical knowledge in their clinical practice (Milliken, 2018).

In this chapter, the terms *ethics* and *morality* or *morals* are used interchangeably (see Beauchamp & Childress, 2019, for a discussion of the distinctions between these terms). A problem becomes an ethical or moral problem when one's core values or fundamental obligations are in conflict. An *ethical* or *moral dilemma* occurs when obligations require or appear to require that a person adopt two (or more) alternative actions but the person cannot carry out all of the required alternatives. The agent experiences tension because of the moral obligations resulting from the dilemma of differing and opposing demands (Beauchamp & Childress, 2019). In some moral dilemmas, the agent must choose between equally morally unacceptable alternatives. For example, based on her evaluation, a family nurse practitioner (FNP) may suspect that a patient is a victim of domestic violence, although the patient denies it. The FNP is faced with two equally troubling options: connect the patient with existing social services, possibly straining the family and jeopardizing the FNP–patient relationship, or avoid intervention and miss an opportunity to potentially interrupt the cycle of violence. Honoring the FNP's desire to prevent harm (the principle of nonmaleficence) justifies social service referral, whereas respect for the patient's autonomy justifies the opposite course of action.

Personal and Professional Values

An individual's interpretations and positions on issues reflect their underlying value system. An intentional exploration of personal values generates more consistent choices and behaviors; it can also assist APRNs to articulate the boundaries of their personal and professional values.

Personal exploration and reflection upon one's own values and biases enhance APRN practice and promote self-care. Self-exploration provides greater insight into how one's values and bias may impact one's assessment of, interactions with, and recommendations to patients and families. APRNs encounter situations in their practice every day that evoke high emotion: cases with great sadness, family and personal dysfunction, and, at times, violence, to name a few. It is only human for the APRN to experience emotion in such situations, yet the APRN who can be cognizant of their own emotional response as it presents to them has less chance of enmeshing their emotional response in the preexisting high emotion of the case. In this way, the APRN is better equipped to respond to the situation, having harnessed their own emotional response. This takes a conscious, intentional reflective practice whose investment pays off for the good of the patient and for the APRN's ability to sustain involvement in these challenging situations. When given the opportunity to reflect on their own values, nurses reported enhanced skill in ethical discernment (Robinson et al., 2014). Reflection should include an exploration of the complex interplay between cultural values and ethical decision making and the potential for implicit bias on the part of the practitioner (Hall et al., 2015). When patient and family decisions contradict the dominant cultural norm of medical practice, healthcare providers may inadvertently resort to coercive or paternalistic measures to influence patients' choices to be more consistent with the provider's values. APRNs' and other healthcare providers' recommendations for particular treatments may be unduly influenced by their own cultural values. For example, a patient from a Southeast Asian culture may show respect to authority figures by obeying the APRN's treatment suggestions, even if they disagree with the plan. The APRN must be intentional when inviting the patient to ask questions and provide reassurance that disagreements are not signs of disrespect.

By the same token, claims made in the name of religious and cultural beliefs are not absolute. For example, spiritual or cultural claims grounded in an identifiable and established community are more defensible than those that are idiosyncratic to the person making the claim (Lazenby et al., 2014). For example, it is a social norm to recognize long-standing communities of faith (e.g., Catholicism, Islam, Judaism) and thus it may be challenging to accept someone who follows a charismatic leader who is unencumbered by a traditional faith tradition. Although it is critical for caregivers to respond with respectful dialogue, support, and compassionate care, patient and family demands must be considered in relation to other claims that also have ethical weight—the professional integrity of providers, legal considerations, economic realities, and issues of distributive justice. APRNs must maintain a sense of integrity, which is vital for fostering curiosity and respect for people of other cultures (Hemberg & Vilander, 2017).

Moral Distress

Jameton (1984) was the first to describe *moral distress*: the feeling that one believes that they know the ethically appropriate action but feel constrained from carrying out that action because of institutional obstacles (e.g., lack of time or supervisory support, physician power, institutional policies, legal constraints). Scholars now understand that moral distress is a complex construct, and there is considerable debate over an exact definition (Fourie, 2015). Even so, the phenomenon of moral distress has received increasing national and international attention in nursing and medical literature. There is growing recognition that failing to address moral distress may have negative consequences for clinicians and patients.

Moral distress occurs when conscientious persons are practicing in challenging contexts and is not due to moral weakness of the person experiencing it (Garros et al., 2015). Studies have reported that moral distress is significantly related to unit-level ethical climate and to healthcare professionals' decisions to leave clinical practice (Austin et al., 2017; Lamiani et al., 2015). By employing honest self-reflection, education, empowerment, and problem solving, APRNs may be able to enhance their moral agency and in turn decrease the incidence of moral uncertainty and intensity of moral distress for themselves and their colleagues.

Clear Communication

The challenge encountered in many ethical dilemmas is the erosion of open and honest communication. The erosion begins when clinicians fail to speak up in crucial situations, which often arise because of long-standing authority gradient challenges. Research suggests that even when patient safety is at risk, fewer than 2 in 10 clinicians will speak up (Maxfield et al., 2010). Other studies suggest that this problem is not unique to the United States (Dadzie & Aziato, 2020; Pattni et al., 2019). Because medical errors are known to contribute to patient deaths in the United States, it is essential that we focus on stopping the silent erosion of communication. APRNs must be willing and able not only to speak up in high-stakes situations but to coach nurses in how to break the silence and create an atmosphere in which open communication is the rule rather than the exception.

Clear communication is an essential prerequisite for informed and responsible decision making. Some ethical disputes reflect inadequate communication rather than a difference in values (Ulrich, 2012). The APRN's communication skills must include the ability to present information in a precise and succinct manner. In patient encounters, disagreements between the patient and a family member or within the family can be rooted in faulty communication, which then leads to ethical conflict. The skill of listening is just as crucial in effective communication as having proficient verbal skills. Listening involves recognizing and appreciating various perspectives and showing respect to individuals with differing ideas. To listen well is to allow others the necessary time to form and present their thoughts and ideas.

Understanding the language used in ethical deliberations (e.g., terms such as *beneficence*, *autonomy*, and *utilitarian justice*) helps the APRN frame the concern in rational terms. This can help those involved to see the components of the ethical problem rather than be mired in their own emotional responses. When ethical dilemmas arise, effective communication is the first key to negotiating and facilitating a resolution. For example, Jameson (2003) found that when certified registered nurse anesthetists (CRNAs) and anesthesiologists focused on the common goal of patient care (shared values) rather than on the conflicting opinions about supervision and autonomous practice, they were able to transcend role-based conflict and promote effective communication.

Interprofessional Collaboration

The second theme encountered is that most ethical dilemmas that occur in the healthcare setting are multidisciplinary in nature. Issues such as refusal of treatment, end-of-life decision making, cost containment, and confidentiality all have interprofessional elements interwoven in the dilemmas, so a successful resolution depends on an interprofessional approach. When people bring different perspectives to a discussion, it can lead to creative and collaborative decision making or to a breakdown in communication and lack of problem solving. Thus an interprofessional theme is necessary in the presentation and resolution of ethical problems.

For example, a clinical nurse specialist (CNS) is facilitating a discharge plan for an older woman who is terminally ill with heart failure. The plan of care, agreed upon by the interprofessional team, patient, and family, is to continue oral medications but discontinue intravenous inotropic support and all other aggressive measures. Just prior to discharge, the social worker laments to the CNS that medical coverage for the patient's care in the skilled nursing facility will be covered by the insurer only if the patient has an intravenous line in place. The patient's daughter wishes to take her mother home and provide care. The attending cardiologist determines that the patient can be discharged to her daughter's home because she no longer requires skilled care; however, the bedside nurse is concerned that the patient's need for physical assistance will overwhelm her daughter and believes that the patient is better off returning to the skilled nursing facility. The CNS engages the patient in a careful conversation about her condition and her preferences. Although each team member shares responsibility to ensure that the plan of care is consistent with the patient's wishes and minimizes the cost burden to the patient, they differ in perspective and approach for how to achieve these goals. Such legitimate but differing perspectives from various team members can lead to ethical conflict.

OVERVIEW OF ETHICAL APPROACHES TO RESOLVING ETHICAL CONFLICTS

Principle-Based Approach

Although different models to resolve ethical conflicts (typically referred to as *ethical decision making*) in health care are extensively discussed in the bioethics literature, the principle-based model is most dominant

(Box 11.2). In cases of conflict, the principles or rules in contention are balanced and interpreted with the contextual elements of the situation. However, the final decision and moral justification for actions are based on principles. In this way, the principles are binding and tolerant of the particularities of specific cases (Beauchamp & Childress, 2019). Both the ANA (2015) and International Council of Nurses (2012), as delineated in their respective codes of ethics, endorse the principle of respect for persons and underscore the profession's commitment to serving individuals, families, and groups or communities. The emphasis on respect for persons implies that it is not only a philosophic value of nursing but also a binding principle within the profession.

Although ethical principles and rules are the cornerstone of most ethical decisions, the principle-based approach has been criticized because it minimizes the value of relationships, which is central to nursing ethics and reduces the resolution of a clinical case simply to balancing principles (Rushton & Penticuff, 2007). Because all of the principles are considered of equal moral weight, this approach has been seen as inadequate to provide guidance for moral action (Strong, 2007). Another significant challenge to the principled approach is a shallow understanding of autonomy. Honoring a person's autonomy does not mean that that person should get whatever they want. Respect for persons (the broader understanding of autonomy) requires a more nuanced understanding of how to balance what a person may want with the responsibility to avoid harm and promote a person's well-being. This is especially important when, for example, APRNs face pressure from patients to prescribe medication they do not need or (worse) may cause them harm. Despite these critiques, bioethical principles remain the most common ethical language used in clinical practice settings.

Casuistry Approach

The second common approach to ethical decision making is the casuistic model (Box 11.2), in which current cases are compared with precedent-setting cases (Beauchamp & Childress, 2019). The strength of this approach is that a dilemma is examined in a context-specific manner and then compared with an analogous earlier case. The fundamental philosophic assumption of this model is that ethics emerges from human moral experiences. Casuists approach dilemmas from

BOX 11.2

Alternative Ethical Approaches

CASUISTRY

- Direct analysis of particular cases
- Uses previous paradigm cases to infer ethical action in a current case
- Analogs in common law and case law
- Values practical knowledge rather than theory (pretheoretical)
- Privileges experience

NARRATIVE ETHICS

- Supplements principles by emphasizing importance of full context
- Gathers views of all parties to provide more complete basis for moral justification
- Story and narrator substitute for ethical justification, which emerges naturally
- Privileges stories

VIRTUE-BASED ETHICS

- Emphasizes the moral agent, not the situation or the action
- Right motives and character reveal more about moral worth than right actions
- Character more important than conformity to rules
- Right motives make for right actions
- Privileges actor's values and motives

FEMINIST ETHICS

- Views women as embodied, fully rational, and having experiences relevant to moral reasoning
- Emphasizes view of the disadvantaged—women and other underrepresented groups
- Emphasizes importance and value of openness to different perspectives
- Concerned with power differentials that create oppression
- Emphasizes importance of attention to the vulnerable and to resulting inequalities
- Privileges power imbalances

CARE-BASED ETHICS

- Emphasizes creating and sustaining responsive connection with others
- Emphasizes importance of context and subjectivity in discerning ethical action
- Sees individuals as interdependent rather than independent; focuses on parties in a relationship
- Privileges relationships

an inductive position and work from the specific case to generalizations, rather than from generalizations to specific cases.

Using a casuistic model for ethical decision making may be problematic. As a moral dilemma arises, the selection of the paradigm case may differ among the decision makers and thus the interpretation of the appropriate course of action will vary. In nursing, there are few paradigm cases of ethical issues on which to construct a decision-making process. Furthermore, other than the reliance on previous cases, casuists have no mechanisms to justify their actions. The possibility that previous cases were reasoned in a faulty or inaccurate manner may not be fully considered or evaluated (Beauchamp & Childress, 2019). Despite these concerns, the case-based moral reasoning used in casuistry appeals to clinicians because it mimics clinical reasoning, in which providers often appeal to earlier similar cases to make clinical judgments. An adaptation of this approach, sometimes referred to as the "four box" approach, has been developed by Jonsen et al. (2015). These authors have advocated clustering patient information according to four key topics—medical indications, patient preferences, quality of life, and contextual features—and then using that information to resolve a dilemma.

Narrative Ethics

Because neither casuistry nor a principled approach has been seen as fully satisfactory, alternatives have emerged (see Box 11.2). Narrative approaches to ethical deliberation have evoked considerable interest (Montello, 2014). Narrative ethics emphasizes the particulars of a case or story as a vehicle for discerning the meaning and values embedded in ethical decision making. Narrative ethics begins with a patient's story and has some similarities with casuistry in its inductive particularistic approach. Though this approach lacks the rigor of other theoretical approaches, there is recognition that careful consideration of patient's stories can enlarge and enrich ethical deliberations. It is likely that a blending of more than one approach offers the fullest opportunity to explore ethical challenges. Because nurses often find deep meaning in their work through learning the stories of their patient's lives, both casuistry and narrative ethical approaches are consistent with nursing practice (Meyer et al., 2020).

Care-Based Ethics

Other approaches, such as virtue-based ethics, feminist ethics, and care-based ethics, provide alternative processes for moral reflection and argument. Historically, nursing ethics was virtue based, with an emphasis on qualities necessary to be a virtuous nurse. In this approach, the moral problem is described in terms of relationships with others; moral reasoning requires empathy and emphasizes responsibilities rather than rights. The response of an individual to a moral dilemma emerges from important relationship considerations. Although this is no longer a dominant theme in nursing literature, it can still be seen (Meyer et al., 2020).

Although every ethical theory has some limitations and problems, an understanding of contemporary approaches to bioethics enables the APRN to appeal to a variety of perspectives in achieving a moral resolution. In the clinical setting, ethical decision making most often reflects a blend of the various approaches rather than the application of a single approach. Although there is some danger in oversimplifying these rich and complex approaches, Exemplar 11.2 shows how they can be reflected in ethical decision making. A more thorough discussion of ethical theory is beyond the scope of this chapter, but the reader is referred to the references cited for more detail.

PROFESSIONAL CODES AND GUIDELINES

The ANA's *Code of Ethics for Nurses* and the ICN (ANA, 2015; ICN, 2012) both highlight general ethical obligations of the professional nurse. They provide broad guidelines that more reflect the profession's conscience than provide specific directions for particular clinical situations. They provide a framework that delineates the nurse's overriding moral obligations to the patient, family, community, and profession. Professional organizations delineate standards of performance that reflect the responsibilities, obligations, duties, and rights of the members. These standards also serve as guidelines for professional behavior and define desired conduct, often specific to contemporary issues. For example, the American Association of Critical-Care Nurses (2008) issued a position statement on moral distress, acknowledging that it negatively affects quality of care and nurses' well-being. The

EXEMPLAR 11.2

CLINICAL SITUATION DEMONSTRATING DIFFERING ETHICAL APPROACHES

To illustrate different ethical approaches, consider the case of a 64-year-old female, M.H., who presented to the emergency department with jaw pain and was admitted to the hospital. Her medical history is significant for stage IV glioblastoma multiforme and multifocal stroke. The neurosurgeon has no more curative therapy options for M.H. She underwent palliative surgery in an attempt to relieve pain and pressure from an abscess. On a previous hospitalization, M.H. completed an advance directive specifying a preference to forego resuscitation if her condition is not curable. Currently M.H. is not able to communicate beyond tracking with her eyes. Her daughter K.J. is concerned that M.H.'s inability to communicate is due to the high level of pain medication she is receiving. The neurosurgeon believes it is a manifestation of her progressing tumor. The daughter expresses doubts about her mother's wishes to be on do-not-resuscitate (DNR) status and has asked the team to lighten up on pain medication so she can communicate more with her mother and escalate support, including intubation if necessary. The team caring for the patient, including a staff nurse, resident, attending physician, chaplain, social worker, and clinical nurse specialist (CNS), apply different ethical theories when they approach this case.

The staff nurse believes that K.J.'s inability to support her mother's advance directive and lack of concern for her mother's suffering render her an inappropriate decision maker. The nurse believes her first obligation is to M.H. alleviating her pain and not to K.J.'s need for closure.

The attending physician adopts a principle-based approach, favoring patient autonomy and respect for persons. Because M.H. should be respected as a person, reducing her pain medication to alleviate her daughter's fears is unethical. He sees no reason to put M.H. on a ventilator and favors institution of comfort measures only.

The resident had a similar case a year ago. The patient's family insisted on aggressive interventions, even though the team thought it was futile and the patient recovered from the acute episode, lived another 3 months, and was able to attend his daughter's wedding. Applying a casuistry-based approach, the resident supports the daughter's request.

The social worker adopts a care-based approach, privileging the relationships within the patient's family. He has worked with this patient and her family on previous hospitalizations. He believes if K.J. has a chance to see that less medication will not change M.H.'s ability to communicate, she will be able to accept the terminal nature of her mother's condition.

The chaplain learns that prior to M.H.'s diagnosis, the daughter's only interactions with the healthcare system were the births of her two children. Her mother has assisted her in the care of her children, making it possible for her to work. Interpreting the case from a feminist viewpoint, she worries that the family's socioeconomic status and the daughter's educational background are creating a bias against K.J.

The CNS's involvement in the case begins when the staff nurse consults her because his appeals to the resident and attending physician have failed to result in what he believes is the right course of action—maintenance of the current medication schedule. The CNS adopts a narrative-based approach and wants to hear all of the contextual features of the case before deciding about the best course of action to address the conflict. She learns about a conversation between K.J. and her mother shortly before M.H. became unresponsive, in which M.H. expressed a desire to plan her grandson's birthday party. K.J. says "I know she wants to be here for my kids," she weeps; "she wouldn't give up without telling me."

RESOLUTION OF THE CASE

The CNS organizes a team meeting. She has discerned that personal biases may be influencing different perspectives of team members. She asks the members to work toward a consistent message that can be given to M.H.'s daughter because the contrasting views are clearly creating confusion. This request brings the team to an agreement that the patient's condition is most likely unrecoverable, and she is dying. The CNS then moves forward to facilitate the establishment of a mutually acceptable plan of care.

In a subsequent family meeting, the team explains the patient's prognosis to the patient's daughter using layperson's terms and simple pictures to clarify the growth of the tumor and its position. After addressing K.J.'s questions, the CNS explains that the team has met separately to consider carefully her request for a change in medication and that the potential harm of such a plan outweighs potential benefits. The CNS ends the meeting with the family by offering them additional time to discuss their options and ask any further questions. After several hours the daughter asks to speak with someone from hospice. The CNS's impact in this case is through influencing the flow of communication, not controlling the discussion.

---

paper then lists the responsibilities of nurses to address moral distress, some resources that can be helpful to them, and the obligations of nurses' employers to offer support and resources to assist with managing moral distress. An additional example is the International Association of Forensic Nurses, which has several position papers (https://www.forensicnurses.org/page/PositionPapers), including the *Adult and Adolescent Sexual Assault Patients in the Emergency Care Setting* (International Association of Forensic Nurses, 2009), which supports the use of emergency contraception for victims of sexual assault. This document provides ethical and clinical rationales for policies that permit dispensing of these medications.

Professional Boundaries

In their professional capacity, APRNs often develop long-term therapeutic relationships with many of their patients. The intimate nature of the relationship, coupled with the compassionate nature of nurses, may make them vulnerable to boundary violations. A violation may be the result of a well-intentioned provider who rationalizes crossing lines for the benefit of the patient (Griffith & Tengnah, 2013; Hanna & Suplee, 2012; Holder & Schenthal, 2007). For example, the APRN forms a close relationship with a terminally ill patient and his spouse. When the patient dies, the APRN feels compelled to offer support to his wife and agrees to go to lunch with her. The death of her patient is the catalyst that causes the APRN to drift across a boundary, profoundly altering the expectations and therapeutic nature of the relationship. All nurses, including APRNs, have an obligation to maintain professional boundaries within a therapeutic relationship and to intervene when they occur (ANA, 2015; Griffith & Tengnah, 2013).

APRN boundary crossings may lead to transgressions and ultimately violations. This is known as *boundary drift* (Holder & Schenthal, 2007). A frequent opportunity for transgression occurs when patients and families express gratitude for a provider's care. Gifts such as boxes of candy or flowers are routine. When the gifts become excessive or have significant financial worth (e.g., expensive tickets to a sporting event), providers are challenged to acknowledge the gratitude and redirect it; for example, by suggesting a charitable donation to the facility. When the transgression is initiated by the provider, regardless of the magnitude, the behavior must be addressed immediately, and the culpable individual must be removed from interaction with the patient. Other members of the healthcare team will need to step in and reestablish therapeutic boundaries (National Council of State Boards of Nursing, 2018).

Although the scope and nature of moral problems in patient care experienced by nurses, and more specifically APRNs, reflect the varied clinical settings in which they practice, we believe being mindful of both professional discipline and interprofessional collaboration sets the stage for effective, high-quality, and ethical care that provides a laser focus on the patient while also preserving interprofessional relationships. To this end, we propose a "goals of care" framework to approach patient cases. The following section describes this clinical–ethical framework as one that serves to prevent and mitigate communication problems, interprofessional conflict, and ethical problems that can negatively affect patient care and clinician experience at all levels. Though we provide this framework within an end-of-life context simply as an example, we believe that the categories of prognosis, values, beliefs, and preferences that support ethically and legally accepted options can be applied in other areas of APRN practice as well.

GOALS OF CARE: A CLINICAL-ETHICAL FRAMEWORK TO ENHANCE APRN PRACTICE

A goals of care model as an organizing framework emphasizes ethical practice in that it is grounded in a patient's values. This framework values interprofessional collaboration and communication in all aspects of patient care, from assessment through intervention and to evaluation for the good of the patient. Developing goals of care requires input from medical and surgical physician and APRN consultants. In addition, clinical nurses and all other health professionals offer important contributions to the formulation of goals of care via their assessment, intervention, and evaluation of patient response to intervention.

Three components constitute a goals of care framework: medical and rehabilitative prognosis; values, beliefs, and preferences of the patient; and options that are ethically and legally permissible (Robinson et al., 2020).

Prognosis

The concept of *medical prognosis* in patient care is primary and integral in addressing goals of care for a patient. Medical prognosis is defined by the Harvard Dictionary of Health Terms (2022) as "a prediction on how a person's disease will progress in the future."

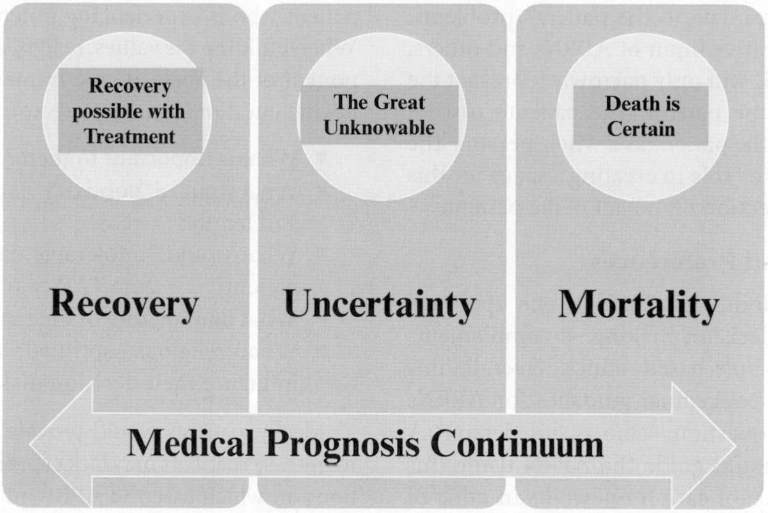

Fig. 11.1 ■ **Medical prognosis: A continuum.** There are situations where medical facts clearly indicate recovery is possible with treatment and when death is certain. Within those two ends lies and area of significant uncertainty that varies with disease complexity and available diagnostic information.

This strict definition falls short. Speaking strictly about the medical prognosis in the absence of rehabilitation potential omits important information that is material to sound healthcare decision making. Medical prognosis can be thought of on a continuum (Fig. 11.1), with clarity at either end: expectation toward clear recovery versus certain death. At either end of the continuum, the collective direction of care in the patient's case is generally evident and health professionals, physicians, and families are all aligned. Unfortunately, prognostication comes with significant uncertainty.

In an age of advanced medical–surgical life-sustaining treatments, pharmacology, cancer treatments, etc., it is more critical than ever to regularly address the question of medical prognosis. Clarity may be elusive and require time and patience as patients respond or fail to respond to interventions. The leadership role of APRNs in these discussions is essential and never to be underestimated. The APRN's blend of medical and nursing expertise lends them clinical credibility in promoting ongoing, open and transparent discussions of prognosis with all members of the team.

An intentional examination of the patient's medical prognosis is the first step in a process of determining goals of care for a patient. The following questions should be considered by APRNs in collaboration with responsible physicians:

- What is medically possible for the patient?
- Can the opinions of medical and surgical consultants be brought to bear on the whole patient?
- What is the rehabilitation potential for the patient?
- Are life-sustaining treatments including pharmacologic therapies effective or likely to be ineffective in restoring the patient to an acceptable functional status and quality of life?

Though the establishment of medical prognosis may theoretically rest within the domain of the responsible physician, given the ever increasing complexity of patients' illnesses, it is imperative that APRNs see their roles as partner to the physician and promote input from medical specialties, highly skilled nurses, and other health professionals, including rehabilitation professionals such as occupational therapists, physical therapists, speech–language therapists, nutrition specialists, social workers, hospice and palliative care consultants, and chaplains to gain a full picture of the patient's response to medical–surgical interventions.

Families of patients often look to the physician and APRN for guidance about whether the patient can get better during a patient's prolonged illness both in the ambulatory and hospital care setting. Considering a patient's projected functional status as an important adjunct to medical prognosis requires the input of rehabilitation and palliative care professionals whose expertise lends critical data to the patient's problems. Without the collaborative input of APRNs and others, the medical prognosis will only narrowly represent the pathophysiology of the patient (the patient's disease process) rather than the patient as a whole person. The APRN often plays a key role in creating a space for this interdisciplinary reflection on behalf of the patient.

Values, Beliefs, and Preferences

An ethic of care (Noddings, 2010) is one approach that guides ethical decision making. It complements the often-used principle-based ethics. Overall, this framework provides conceptual guidance for APRNs to answer a central question: Who is this person? A sense of curiosity should guide the APRN using this framework. In a goals of care framework, an ethic of care is made tangible through consideration of the dimensions of particulars, context, and relationships.

Particulars

Eleven functional health patterns described by M. Gordon (2010; see Box 11.3) illustrate how APRNs focus their curiosity to explore the particulars of the patient who is experiencing potential or actual illness. When building the values, beliefs, and preferences component of the goals of care framework, asking the following questions will help create a profile of the patient:

- What is important to them?
- What would a "good day" look like for the patient and family?
- What would "intolerable days" look like for the patient?
- What does quality of life mean for this patient?
- What religious, spiritual, and cultural beliefs influence their decision making?

Ideally, patients would provide answers; however, in many cases patients may lack capacity to answer the questions, in which case the APRN must turn to surrogates for answers. The preferred surrogate decision maker is one named in writing by the patient or a legally appointed guardian. In the absence of a formally appointed decision maker, many jurisdictions identify a default hierarchy list, typically beginning with family members, who may make decisions on behalf of the patient (Wynn, 2014).

Fig. 11.2 illustrates a creative way providers may get to know patients on a personal level, including those who are limited in their ability to communicate. Information alone on this poster would be an insufficient contribution to the values, beliefs, and preferences component; however, it can provide APRNs and direct care clinicians a sense of the person in their care. For any patient who is not able to communicate, hearing statements from professional caregivers that signify their familiarity with them as person can be a source of comfort.

BOX 11.3

Functional Health Patterns

GORDON'S FUNCTIONAL HEALTH PATTERN ASSESSMENT CATEGORIES

- Health perception–Health management
- Nutritional–Metabolic
- Elimination
- Activity–Exercise
- Sleep–Rest
- Cognitive–Perceptual
- Self-perception–Self-concept
- Role relationship
- Sexuality–Reproductive
- Coping–Stress tolerance
- Value–Belief

Basis for nursing assessment with input from all disciplines to answer the question: Who is this person, living with this disease?

Adapted from Gordon, M. (2010). *Manual of Nursing Diagnoses.* Jones & Bartlett Publishers.

Context

Considering the patient's overall context as a dimension of an ethic of care can yield insight for APRNs as leaders in the healthcare team. Full understanding of the patient is not possible without exploration of context. Turning again to questions:

- What most concerns the patient at this time?
- What led the patient to their current situation?
- How are the patient and their family responding to all of it?

Relationships

Though the principle of autonomy overshadows ethical decision making, particularly in the Western world,

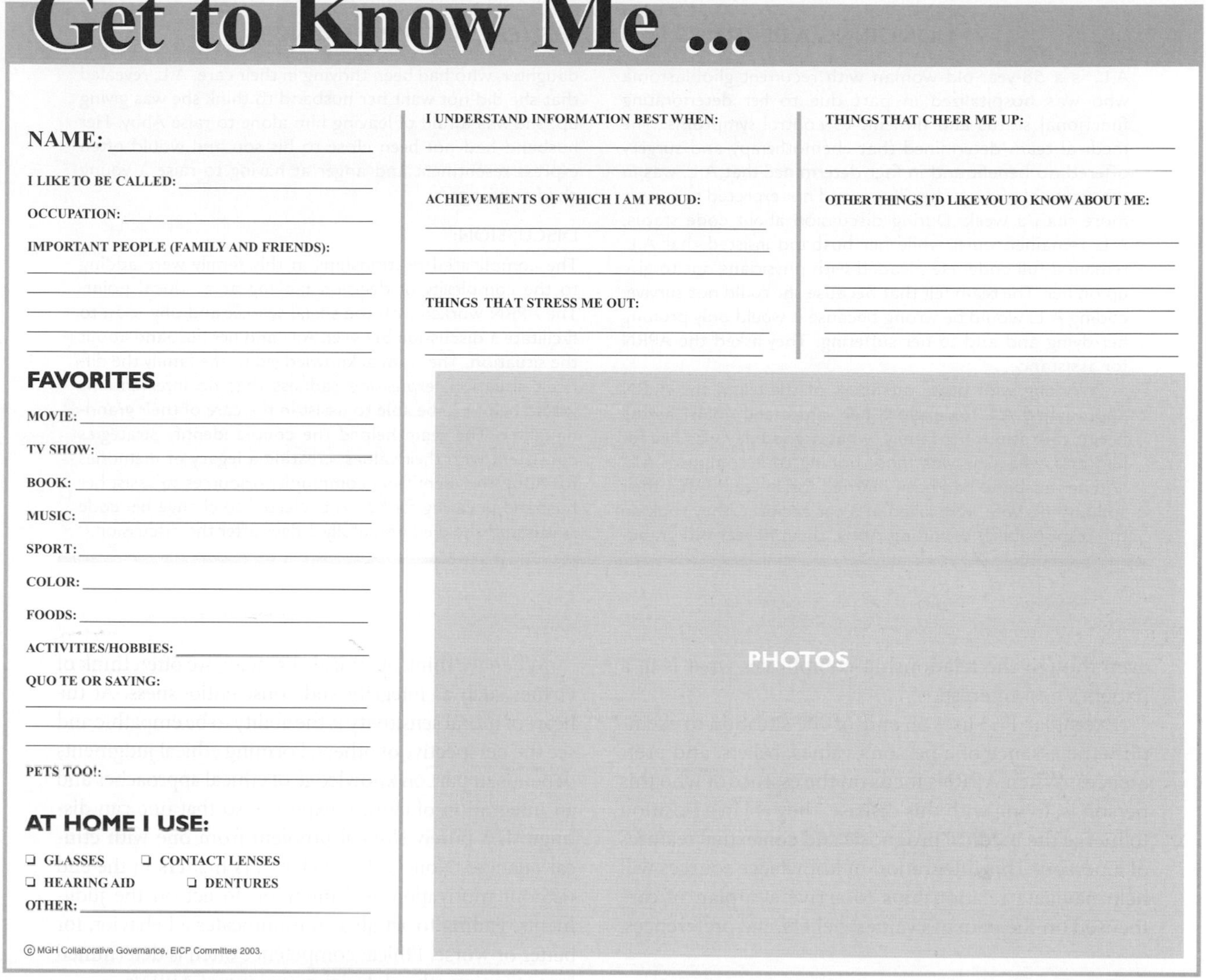
Get to Know Me ...
NAME:
I LIKE TO BE CALLED:
OCCUPATION:
IMPORTANT PEOPLE (FAMILY AND FRIENDS):
FAVORITES
MOVIE:
TV SHOW:
BOOK:
MUSIC:
SPORT:
COLOR:
FOODS:
ACTIVITIES/HOBBIES:
QUO TE OR SAYING:
PETS TOO!:
AT HOME I USE:
❑ GLASSES ❑ CONTACT LENSES
❑ HEARING AID ❑ DENTURES
OTHER:
© MGH Collaborative Governance, EICP Committee 2003.
I UNDERSTAND INFORMATION BEST WHEN:
ACHIEVEMENTS OF WHICH I AM PROUD:
THINGS THAT STRESS ME OUT:
THINGS THAT CHEER ME UP:
OTHER THINGS I'D LIKE YOU TO KNOW ABOUT ME:
PHOTOS

Fig. 11.2 ■ **Poster "Get to know me."** (Used with Permission by Ellen Robinson, PhD, RN, Massachusetts General Hospital)

the reality is that most people, particularly when ill and most especially when facing end of life, look to important relationships in their lives. Being bound in, enriched by, and, at times, injured by relationships contrasts self-determination in isolation with the greater reality of "relational autonomy" (Dove et al., 2017). Even when significant family and friends may be in conflict with the patient, those relationships are important and matter.

APRNs must recognize and navigate both supportive and destructive relationships that may be of importance to the patient and define their network. Recognizing those relationships is the first step to working through dynamics that allow the patient to receive interventions that they need and deserve. As challenging as it may be, attempting to sever a patient's destructive relationships may result in alienating patients from an important person in their network,

EXEMPLAR 11.3

HONORING A PERSON'S VALUES, BELIEFS, AND PREFERENCES

A.L. is a 58-year-old woman with recurrent glioblastoma who was hospitalized in part due to her deteriorating functional status and difficult to control symptoms. The medical team determined that chemotherapy and surgery offered no benefit and in fact determined that A.L. was in the terminal phase of her illness and not expected to survive more than a week. During discussion about code status, A.L. remained quiet while her husband insisted that A.L. remain a full code. He pleaded with physicians not to give up on her. The team felt that because she could not survive, coding A.L. would be wrong because it would only prolong her dying and add to her suffering. They asked the APRN for assistance.

Working with other members of the team, the APRN approached A.L. to explore her values and goals, asking her to talk about her family, what a good day was like for her, and what she was most hoping to accomplish. A.L. and her husband had been married for 35 years. After their son and his wife were killed in a car accident, they took on the responsibility of raising Abby, their 10-year-old granddaughter, who had been thriving in their care. A.L. revealed that she did not want her husband to think she was giving up; she was afraid of leaving him alone to raise Abby. Her husband had not been close to his son and would often express resentment and anger at having to raise a young child at his age.

DISCUSSION:

The complicated relationships in this family were adding to the complexity of decision making at a critical point. The APRN worked with the social worker and physician to facilitate a discussion between A.L. and her husband about the situation. The team acknowledged to the family the difficult situation, expressing sadness that no interventions would help A.L. be able to assist in the care of their granddaughter. The team helped the couple identify strategies consistent with their values, creating a legacy of memories for Abby and identifying community resources to assist her husband in caring for her. A.L. elected to change her code status and she died peacefully 3 days after the discussion.

even though the relationship complicates what is in a patient's best interest.

Exemplar 11.3 uses an end-of-life situation to exemplify the essence of a person's values, beliefs, and preferences. When APRNs focus on the essence of who this person is, living with this disease, they are in a position to merge the medical prognosis and contextual features of a person. This integration of knowledge sources will help navigate relationships to arrive at a plan of care focused on the patient's values, beliefs, and preferences.

ETHICAL COMPETENCY OF APRNS

Others will judge APRN practice as ethical if the APRN demonstrates observable behaviors that adhere to high ethical standards. Ethical practice is not a simple skill demonstration. Ethical behavior depends on adequate functioning on all four interconnected elements: character, sensitivity, judgment, and motivation (Robinson et al., 2014). The APRN must be sensitive to the ethical features of situations, be able to identify the ideal ethical option, be motivated to pursue the ethical course, and have the strength of character to uphold ethical standards and take appropriate action.

When we think of ethical character, we often think of virtues such as integrity and conscientiousness. At the heart of moral sensitivity is the ability to be empathic and see the perspective of others. Forming ethical judgments depends in part on knowledge of ethical approaches and an integration of clinical expertise so that one can distinguish a purely clinical problem from one with ethical nuances. None of these elements matters in the end without motivation and intention to act on the judgments. Failing to act also communicates a behavior, for better or worse. Ethical competence often is determined by evaluating ethical decision making of APRNs.

Clinical practice gives rise to numerous ethical concerns, and APRNs must be able to address these concerns. Ethical involvement follows and evolves from clinical expertise (Benner et al., 2009). Another reason why ethical decision making is a core competency can be seen in the expanded collaborative skills that APRNs develop (see Chapter 10). APRNs practice in a variety of settings and positions but, in most cases, the APRN is part of an interprofessional team of caregivers. The team may be loosely defined and structured, as in a rural setting, or more definitive, as in the acute care setting. The recent reemergence of an interprofessional care model is changing practice for all providers (Brashers et al., 2019). Regardless of the structure of the team, APRNs need the knowledge and skills to avoid power struggles, broker and lead interprofessional communication, and facilitate consensus among team members in ethically difficult situations.

Knowledge Development

The competency of ethical decision making is understood as an evolutionary process in an APRN's development. Novice APRNs should be able to recognize a moral problem and seek clarification and illumination of the concern. Although some beginning graduate students will have had significant exposure to ethical issues in their undergraduate programs, most have not. A 2008 United States survey of nurses and social workers found that only 51% of the nurse respondents had formal ethics education in their undergraduate or graduate education; 23% had no ethics training at all (Grady et al., 2008). APRN students with no ethics education or clinical experience will be at a disadvantage, because graduate education builds on the ethical foundation of professional practice. During graduate school, particular attention should be paid to acquiring deeper knowledge of ethical frameworks and developing moral sensitivity. On this foundation, APRNs will be able to mature in their roles and develop clinical expertise. Achieving that will foster their development as leaders who can build ethical work environments and promote social justice issues central to the identity of the nursing profession.

Exposure to ethical theories, principles, and concepts is not enough. Processes that accommodate and value the unique nature of each ethical problem, incorporating personal values and ethical theories, are gaining influence (Grace et al, 2014). Knowledge development must extend beyond classroom discussions to include discussion of ethical dimensions of clinical practicum experiences. In one study, Laabs (2012) found that APRN graduates, most of whom had completed an ethics course in their graduate curriculum, indicated a fairly high level of confidence in their ability to manage ethical problems, but their overall ethics knowledge was low; this is a compelling commentary on the need for ethics knowledge development in graduate curricula.

Knowledge development is an ongoing process. APRNs will gain core knowledge in graduate education but, as societal issues change and new technologies emerge, new dilemmas and ethical problems arise. The ability to be a leader in creating ethical environments involves a commitment to lifelong learning about ethical issues, of which professional education is just the beginning. It may be continuing education in ethics beyond basic training that has the largest impact on moral action (Grady et al., 2008).

Skill Acquisition

As APRNs acquire core ethical decision-making knowledge, the responsibility to take moral action to address ethical dilemmas becomes more compelling. Action is more successful if the APRN learns to identify situations that are at risk for ethical conflict (Pavlish et al., 2020). When the APRN is proactive in identifying ethical issues and can mount a timely response to an identified ethical conflict, they can change the course in present and future situations. Therefore moral action must be a core APRN skill and should be recognized, fostered, and valued by others. Once an advanced nursing role is assumed, the APRN accepts the responsibility to be a full participant in the resolution of moral dilemmas rather than simply an interested observer or one of many parties in conflict.

When APRNs apply core knowledge of ethical concepts, they begin to develop the practical wisdom of moral reasoning. Mastering the skill of constructively engaging in crucial conversations will enable APRNs to be leaders in resolving conflicts that arise. The success and speed with which the APRN gains these behavioral skills is related to the presence of mentors in the clinical setting and the willingness of the APRN to initiate and stay immersed in ethical discussions.

Institutional resources, such as ethics committees and institutional review boards, provide valuable opportunities for APRNs to participate in the discussion of ethical issues. As a member of an ethics committee, the APRN exchanges ideas with colleagues and gains an understanding of ethical dilemmas from a variety of perspectives. In addition, the APRN is informed of current legislation, regulations, and hospital/clinic policies that have ethical implications. This is an extremely valuable experience that can accelerate the development of ethical decision-making skills. APRNs who have limited access to local resources or mentors who can help them develop the skills of ethical decision making will need to rely on professional organizations and external workshops for guidance in applying knowledge to resolve ethically challenging clinical cases.

Ethical Decision-Making Frameworks

Though there is more than one, Box 11.4 highlights a particular stepwise approach to ethical decision making suggested by Doherty and Purtilo (2016). The reader will note that this framework uses many elements of the various ethical approaches discussed earlier in considering contextual factors, seeking full information on a case, and specifying a step that explicitly appeals to ethical theory. This framework for ethical decision making is intended for all health professionals and therefore is applicable to a wide variety of situations. Models may be helpful; however, there are a number of common mistakes or fallacies that APRNs should avoid when justifying their ethical position. Some examples include giving undue weight to someone in authority, focusing on the characteristics of the people involved in the conflict rather than on their positions, and providing only a basic rationale for their positions (a necessary but not sufficient step) without exploring broader features in the situation (Cooper, 2012).

Problem identification is also a common step in most frameworks. Strong emotional responses to a situation can be the first signal that ethical conflict exists. However, many conflicts that arise in the clinical setting generate powerful emotional responses but may not be ethical in nature. Ethical issues are those that involve some form of controversy about conflicting moral values and/or fundamental duties or obligations. The APRN must distinguish and separate moral dilemmas from other issues, such as administrative concerns, communication problems, and lack of clinical knowledge. For example, a communication problem between a staff nurse and physician may be resolved if an APRN acts as a facilitator, ensuring that each understands the perspective of the other. In this case a framework for ethical decision making may not be needed; the conflict does not result from a difference in values but rather a failure to communicate. As noted, effective and compassionate communication skills undergird this competency.

Although a framework provides structure and suggests a method of examining and studying the ethical

BOX 11.4

Sample APRN Ethical Decision-Making Framework

1. Gather information:
   - Clarify the additional information needed.
   - Categories of information to consider include clinical indications, patient preferences, quality of life, and contextual factors.
   - Caution is advised not to make this step an end in itself.
2. Determine that the problem is an ethical one and identify the type:
   - Locus of authority—conflict involves determining who should make a decision.
   - Ethical dilemma—conflict in which two opposing courses of action are both ethically justifiable but cannot both be satisfied.
   - Moral distress—conflict in which the ethical course of action seems clear but the agent feels unable to carry it out.
3. Use ethical theories or approaches to analyze the problem:
   - A utilitarian approach would focus on the consequences of potential actions.
   - A deontologic approach would focus on the duties of involved parties.
   - Various ethical theories provide additional perspectives (see "Overview of Ethical Approaches" and the references cited).
4. Explore the practical alternatives:
   - Imagination is required to ensure that a wide range of alternatives are identified.
   - Diligence in assessing the feasibility of identified actions is also essential.
5. Complete the action:
   - Once determined, motivation to carry out the ethical action is essential.
   - Not to act at this point is a conscious choice, with consequences.
6. Evaluate the process and outcome:
   - What went well, and why?
   - To what other situations might this experience apply?
   - What do the patient, family, and other providers say about the course of action taken?

Adapted from Doherty, R. F., & Purtilo, R. B. (2016). *Ethical Dimensions in the Health Professions* (6th ed.). Saunders.

issues, the essential component of resolution of ethical dilemmas is moral action. Simply knowing the right course of action does not guarantee that a person has the motivation or courage to act (Rushton & Penticuff, 2007).

Addressing Ethical Conflict

Conflict in any workplace is a daily occurrence. Learning to manage conflict of any kind will make it less likely that individuals will engage in behaviors that are destructive to teams (The Foundation Coalition, n.d.). The challenge in most cases of ethical disputes is to have all involved parties listen to each other's perspectives to understand the basis of the disagreement and work together to create a collaborative solution. In many cases the APRN must serve as a facilitator for the parties in dispute. The objective of successful facilitation in ethical disputes is, whenever possible, to achieve an integrity-preserving solution that is satisfactory to all parties.

Spielman (1993) applied Thomas's five strategies for managing conflict to resolving ethical conflicts, of which collaboration is the preferred approach. Her typology is useful for evaluating ethical conflict resolution. As described in Chapter 10, collaboration is a core competency of advanced practice nursing. Recent attention internationally to interprofessional competencies has also emphasized the importance of collaboration (Brownie et al., 2014; Canadian Interprofessional Health Collaborative, 2010; Interprofessional Education Collaborative [IPEC], 2016). In ethical conflicts, a collaborative approach is the most likely to result in a solution that preserves the integrity of all involved parties. Box 11.5 provides a brief summary of the different approaches to addressing conflict. Exemplar 11.4 provides examples of each of these strategies in a situation that evoked considerable ethical conflict.

BOX 11.5

Highlights of the Different Approaches to Addressing Conflict

1. *Collaboration* works well when members of the team can be assertive and cooperate at a high level but takes a great deal of time and energy.
2. *Compromise* is appropriate when the parties involved are committed to preserving their relationship and each possesses a high moral certainty about their position.
3. *Accommodation* is essential when one party is more committed than the other to preserving the relationship; the committed party defers to the other, with the result that only one perspective directs the outcome. Accommodation is unlikely to promote the integrity of all involved parties and should be used only when time is limited or the issue is trivial.
4. *Coercion* occurs when the more powerful party, who has a strong commitment to a particular position, determines the outcome of the conflict through an aggressive stance.
5. *Avoidance* is the most dangerous of the strategies because the less powerful party does not articulate his or her ethical concerns. Over time, nurses may become so desensitized to ethical conflict, blunting their moral sensitivity.

From Spielman, B. J. (1993). Conflict in medical ethics cases: Seeking patterns of resolution. *Journal of Clinical Ethics, 4*, 212–218.

Some ethically challenging situations retain tension and uneasiness despite ethical practice by the APRN. In true ethical dilemmas, even the best process may still result in a course of action that is not seen positively by all participants. APRNs must be mindful that many issues leave a "moral residue" that continues to trouble participants involved in the conflict (Epstein & Hamric, 2009). Moral residue, initially described by Webster and Bayliss (2000), describes the lingering feelings after a morally problematic situation has passed, a feeling that each of us carries with us from those times in our lives when in the face of moral distress we have seriously compromised ourselves or allowed ourselves to be compromised. This residue, further explicated by Epstein and Hamric (2009), contributes to a crescendo effect, similar to Jameton's coining of the term "reactive distress." (Jameton, 1993, p. 542). Part of the outcome evaluation of actions must address the reality of these lingering feelings and the related tensions that they create.

Creating Ethical Environments

As APRNs become more skilled in the application of ethical knowledge, they are better positioned to help

EXEMPLAR 11.4
STRATEGIES USED IN RESOLVING ETHICAL CONFLICT

An acute care nurse practitioner (ACNP) in an ambulatory clinic provides comprehensive care to patients with narcotics addiction. J.S., a 36-year-old male patient, also has a history of asthma, cigarette smoking, alcohol use, and an anxiety disorder. He arrives at the clinic and is disruptive in the waiting room. He is pacing back and forth and loudly stating that he needs his methadone. In the interval since his last visit, he has wrecked his car and has no easy form of transportation. He has missed multiple days of work and is worried about losing his job.

At this visit, J.S. reports that he has not taken medications for his anxiety because he ran out of pills and had no mechanism for refilling them. He is not carrying an inhaler and is wheezing mildly. He denies any recreational drug use. The ACNP wants to see him for follow-up regarding his asthma and anxiety in 1 week and gives him prescriptions for an anxiolytic and an inhaler.

The following day, J.S. shows up for his methadone. He states that he lost the prescriptions and asks if he could get new ones. The clinic nurse expresses frustration and concern that the patient is "working the system." She claims in exasperation, "He does this all the time!" She feels the patient may be selling his prescriptions and wants to report him to the police. She suggests that the ACNP tell the patient that if he continues to be irresponsible and disrupt the clinic, the clinic will no longer provide treatment.

The social worker, whose ongoing contact with the patient was instrumental in getting him to attend clinic regularly and stay out of trouble, advises the ACNP that there is no evidence of a crime. He states his belief that using coercion will raise the patient's anxiety and likely result in him not following up on treatment for his asthma and will likely not change his disruptive behavior.

The ACNP notes the emotional responses of the interprofessional team members, which signal an ethical conflict. Her initial thought is to provide the new prescriptions and say nothing. This strategy is an example of avoidance. Another avoidance option would be to send the patient to another provider for his medications. For example, a pulmonologist could be consulted for the asthma medication. The ACNP considers but does not select either of these courses of action.

In communicating with the clinic nurse, the ACNP uses accommodation as a strategy for managing ethical conflict. She validates the nurse's concern about the negative impact of the patient's behavior on the other clinic patients and agrees that the behavior is inappropriate and needs to be addressed. The strategy favored by the social worker is also an example of accommodation. He believes that the obligation of the clinic staff is the delivery of patient care and that they should be able to overlook "minor" inconveniences for this patient, who clearly has limited resources. He suggests not providing prescriptions to J.S. again but adopting a policy of calling or faxing all prescriptions for him directly to a pharmacy.

The clinic nurse's strategy is an example of coercion. In coercive strategies, the ethical decision maker resolves the conflict by exerting a controlling influence on another party whose actions or values are fueling the conflict. Suggesting to J.S. that his actions may affect his access to the care he needs exerts power over this patient. The disadvantage of this type of strategy is the powerlessness it imposes.

When J.S. arrives for his follow-up appointment the next week, the ACNP informs him that the staff in the clinic are concerned about his disruptive behavior. She tells the patient, "I do not want you to be in trouble. Being disruptive in clinic is not fair to other patients or the staff who are working to provide care. In addition, losing prescriptions is frustrating and causes others to be suspicious about what happened to the first prescription. I want to work with you to help you stay well." When she invites the patient to help her understand what happened, the patient reveals some important information. J.S. explains that being in the clinic is hard because it makes him more anxious, especially when there are lots of other patients in the waiting room. He accepts his minor wheezing as "normal" and does not see his asthma as a big problem.

The ACNP offers to help J.S. identify strategies to lower his anxiety when he has to wait and offers the suggestion that the clinic fax prescriptions directly to the pharmacy in the future. J.S. agrees to these changes and states he will work harder to be less disruptive in the future.

Another conflict evident in this case is between the clinic nurse and the social worker. Compromise is needed to maintain an effective working relationship because the two provide care to the same patient population. Compromise can be achieved if the two parties focus on a common goal and relinquish control of some elements of the final decision. In this case the ACNP meets with both parties and they identify that their common goal is efficient delivery of quality health care. Through compromise, the clinic nurse recognized the value that the social worker placed on keeping the patient in care and relinquished her desire to coerce the patient to get him to change his behavior. Similarly, the social worker recognized that the nurse wanted to avoid disruptive behavior that upsets other clinic patients. He agreed to relinquish his accommodating approach to the patient's behavior if it negatively affected the clinic's operation in the future.

create and sustain ethical environments. Whether or not ethical problems are productively addressed depends in large part on the ethical health of the work environment. The foundation of an ethical work environment includes respectful, productive interpersonal relationships and skilled communication (American Association of Critical-Care Nurses, 2015). Studies show that poor relationships between physicians and nurses can contribute to moral distress, a sign of ethical conflict (Bruce, Miller & Zimmerman, 2015). Without respect, healthy relationships are doomed and communication is ineffective; not only can this be unethical, it can be harmful (The Joint Commission, 2008).

In one study of nurse practitioners (NPs), the participants' perceptions of the ethical environment were the strongest predictor of ethical conflict in practice; the more ethical the environment, the lower was the ethical conflict (Ulrich et al., 2003). Too often, other nurses and members of the healthcare team remain silent about ethical issues (E. J. Gordon & Hamric, 2006). Once the APRN transforms ethical knowledge into moral action, they will emerge as role models, leading the way in creating ethical work environments in which diverse views are expressed and problems are resolved.

In a classic article, Shannon (1997) noted that the roots of interprofessional conflict in the clinical setting are often based on preconceived stereotypes of the moral viewpoints of other disciplines and perceptions of the moral superiority of one's own discipline. APRNs can help professionals from other disciplines understand the perspectives and socialization of nurses. Teaching and mentoring activities of the mature APRN often focus on other professional colleagues to prepare them to proactively communicate openly with patients about ethical concerns. The APRN is integral to the development and preservation of a collaborative culture that inspires and empowers individuals to respond to moral dilemmas.

An ethically sensitive environment is one in which providers are encouraged to acknowledge when they feel overwhelmed and seek help when they need it (Hamric et al., 2013). The *Code of Ethics for Nurses* (ANA, 2015) has affirmed the importance of nurses contributing to an ethically sensitive healthcare environment, as well as preserving personal integrity. Provision 5 emphasizes that nurses owe the same duty to themselves that they owe to others, including the responsibility to preserve integrity and safety. Only when care providers recognize and attend to their personal needs will they be better able to detect and nurture the needs of others.

Preventive Ethics

An additional important role of the APRN is to extend the concept of ethical decision making beyond problem solving and to move toward a paradigm of preventive ethics. The term *preventive ethics* is derived from the model of preventive medicine. It emphasizes developing effective organizational policies and practices that prevent ethical problems from developing (McCullough, 2005). The ability to predict areas of conflict and develop plans in a proactive rather than reactive manner will avert potentially difficult dilemmas and can lead to more ethically responsive environments (Nelson et al., 2010).

When value conflicts arise, resolution becomes more difficult because one value must be chosen over another. Preventive ethics emphasizes that all important values should be reviewed and examined prior to the conflict so that situations in which values conflict can be anticipated. In other words, the goals of the healthcare team should be articulated as clearly as possible to avoid potential misinterpretations. For example, a CRNA should have an understanding of a terminally ill patient's values regarding aggressive treatment in case a cardiopulmonary arrest occurs during surgery. However, the CRNA's moral and legal obligations should be openly discussed so that the patient and other professionals appreciate and recognize each other's values and moral and legal positions (American Society of Anesthesiologists, 2018). In much the same way, early anticipation of potential complications in patients can lead to proactive discussions of ethical issues and restructuring of the care environment to anticipate and avoid ethical conflict.

By providing knowledge, promoting a positive self-image, and preparing others for participation in decision making, the APRN empowers individuals. APRNs must avoid the trap of trying to fix problems for others. When faced with a dilemma, the APRN is not responsible for identifying the "one right answer." The skill of the APRN is used not to resolve moral dilemmas single-handedly but rather to mentor others to assume a position of moral accountability and

EXEMPLAR 11.5
ADDRESSING STAFF MORAL DISTRESS THROUGH PREVENTIVE ETHICS[a]

Dea, a clinical nurse specialist (CNS) in a neuroscience intensive care unit (ICU), seeks to change the management of patients with traumatic brain injury (TBI). She and other members of the staff have noted that the care of this population is inconsistent, and many staff have a fatalistic attitude about these patients' hope of recovery. She is also aware of research on the use of a new technology, brain tissue oxygen monitoring, that has shown promise in improving outcomes for these patients. As an initial step, she invites an expert in the management of TBI whom she knows to be an inspiring speaker to give a presentation on brain tissue oxygen monitoring. Dea arranges for staff coverage so that all neuroscience ICU registered nurses can attend the presentation and invites staff from other key areas. The speaker describes how the technology is used to prevent progressive injury in patients with TBI. After a successful presentation, Dea then collaborates with the nurse manager and administration to implement brain tissue oxygen monitoring in the neuroscience ICU. She obtains key physician support, provides training sessions, supports the staff when the technology is introduced into patient care, and develops algorithms for acting on the information this technology provides. Dea also creates a Wall of Fame, highlighting all unit patients who have recovered, to help staff celebrate successes in caring for this challenging patient population.

As staff develop expertise with the management of patients with TBI, they notice the improved outcomes in monitored patients promoting early aggressive intervention. Nurses who are expert in the use of the technology develop moral distress because its use varies with attending physicians and depends on patient ICU location. Because the nurses see the better than expected outcomes of monitored patients compared with those who do not receive monitoring, they believe that all appropriate patients should receive this technology. The staff's moral distress heightens after a particularly troubling case of a young patient with a TBI who was never monitored with the new technology and subsequently died.

Using a preventive ethics approach, Dea collaborates with an expert in ethics to coordinate a facilitated discussion about the ethical challenges contributing to the nurses' moral distress. During the discussion, the nurses express the opinion that this new technology has served as the impetus for improving the care of patients with TBI. They feel powerless to help because physicians make the decision about the use of the technology.

During the meeting, the staff identify a number of strategies for decreasing their moral distress. One is directing admission of TBI patients to the neuroscience ICU, recognizing at the same time that patients with thoracic and abdominal trauma as well as TBI would still be admitted to the trauma ICU; in addition, many patients with TBI are first admitted to the trauma ICU while these other problems are ruled out. Better communication between ICU charge nurses was considered as a means to improve nursing input into bed assignment. Another strategy discussed in the meeting was advocacy for patients' needs on the part of the neuroscience nurses with the medical staff. The staff is encouraged to use Dea as a resource when they encounter resistance from their medical colleagues. A final strategy identified at this meeting was to track the outcomes of patients who have received brain tissue oxygen monitoring and thus develop a database to support the value of this tool. Dea agrees to collect the data, review each case, and follow up on quality-of-care issues.

Dea collaborates with physician and nurse colleagues in the trauma ICU, neuroscience ICU, and neurosurgical team. Dea facilitates the development of algorithms for the management of TBI, identifying patients who may benefit from brain tissue oxygen monitoring and facilitating their admission to the neuroscience ICU. These algorithms are incorporated into the trauma manual, a document used by all trauma residents.

Dea coaches the nurses toward effective advocacy and role models collaboration and information sharing in her own communications with residents and attending physicians. Over time, Dea begins to see an increased acceptance of the new technology and of an aggressive approach to managing TBI among the neurosurgery teams.

Two members of the nursing staff, with Dea's encouragement and guidance, developed a poster about their moral distress and steps to address it. The poster was accepted and presented at a national conference (Pracher et al., 2006). The nurses attending the conference to present the poster learned that their situation was not unique; other conference attendees noted similar conflicts in their own units and validated the distress experienced as a result. Two years after the initial education session on this technology, Dea noted that "there is still work to do to optimize the care of these patients." However, because of her proactive response to the staff's distress, champions for this technology now exist on both units, and an environment for effecting positive change has been created.

[a]We gratefully acknowledge Dea Mahanes, MSN, RN, Charlottesville, VA, for sharing this exemplar.

engage in shared decision making. Development and preservation of an ethical environment is the key contribution of the APRN.

Exemplar 11.5 provides an example of preventive ethics in addressing staff moral distress. This case highlights how the ethical decision-making competency of APRNs can lessen the reoccurrence of moral problems. In this situation, Dea's actions went beyond resolving a single case of moral distress and focused on the features of the system that were contributing to the distress of the staff. As this exemplar shows, recurring ethical problems, particularly moral distress, are sometimes a result of the structure of care delivery systems in an institution. Dea's case demonstrates that applying a preventive ethics approach to the system requires perseverance and ongoing identification of new strategies to change complex and interrelated system features.

ETHICAL ISSUES AFFECTING APRN PRACTICE

Primary Care Issues

Situations in which personal values contradict professional responsibilities often confront NPs in a primary care setting. Issues such as abortion, teen pregnancy, patient nonadherence to treatment, vaccination hesitancy, regulations and laws, financial constraints, and delayed implementation of a desired plan of care, whether because of insurance processes or limited availability within a health system, are just some of the ethical challenges for APRNs.

The issues noted by Laabs (2005) likely continue to cause moral dilemmas for APRNs: (1) being required to follow policies and procedures that infringe on personal values, (2) wanting to bend the rules to ensure appropriate patient care, and (3) dealing with patients who have refused appropriate care. Issues leading to NP moral distress included pressure to see an excessive number of patients, clinical decisions being made by others, and a lack of power to effect change (Laabs, 2005). Increasing expectations to care for more patients in less time are routine in all types of healthcare settings as pressures to contain costs escalate. APRNs in rural or ambulatory care settings often have fewer resources to help navigate ethical challenges than their colleagues working in or near academic centers in which ethics committees, ethics consultants, and educational opportunities are more accessible.

Issues of quality of life and symptom management traverse primary and acute healthcare settings. APRNs must confront the various and sometimes conflicting goals of the patient, family, and other healthcare providers regarding the plans for treatment, symptom management, and quality of life. Primary care can result in positive long-term relationships between patients and their care providers. The APRN is often the individual who coordinates the plan of care and thus is faced with clinical and ethical concerns when patients' goals are inconsistent or unrealistic, putting strain on relationships and potentially compromising trusting relationships.

Acute and Chronic Care Issues

Continuity of care and knowing the patient and family are significant issues for APRNs in acute and primary care settings. In outpatient settings, pressures to see more patients in less time can decrease the APRN's opportunity for individualized problem solving for patients and families. However, in time-pressured settings, the emphasis is on efficiency and not on the patient–provider relationship or the provision of holistic care. APRNs struggle in these types of environments to balance the needs of individuals with generalized treatment approaches and productivity targets.

In the acute care setting, APRNs struggle with dilemmas involving pain management, patient capacity to make decisions, end-of-life decision making, advance directives, innovative therapies, and medical errors. Some providers report a variety of morally distressing circumstances: feeling pressured to continue potentially inappropriate treatment, working with colleagues not fully competent, poor team communication, and lack of provider continuity (Hamric et al.,2012; Trautmann et al., 2015).

APRNs often find themselves bridging communication between the medical team and patient or family. In the acute care setting, APRNS are typically responsible for the day-to-day medical management of patients, often establishing a trusting relationship with the patient and family. They are well positioned to learn the patient's values, beliefs, and attitudes that shape decisions. However, they are not ultimately responsible for determining the plan of care, which may place them squarely in the middle between their responsibilities to the medical team and obligations to the patient and can lead to moral distress, particularly when the team's treatment decision carried out by the APRN is incongruent with the APRN's professional judgment or values or patient's wishes.

End-of-Life Complexities

Technological Imperative

The goals of care framework (Robinson et al., 2020) is valuable in that it leads to purposeful and appropriate care at any given time in the patient's trajectory. Advances in life-sustaining medical technology abound, contributing to cures for desperately ill patients with a host of diseases. Cancer treatments can cure and, if not cure, extend patients' lives by years (DeVito et al., 2019). Dialysis as a life-sustaining treatment (LST) is now available in the high-tech environment of the intensive care unit, at dialysis centers in the community, and even on a continuous basis in patients' homes (Daugirdas et al., 2012). Extracorporeal membranous oxygenation (ECMO), once a therapy only for infants, is now available in quaternary care centers for patients with acute cardiac, respiratory, or cardiopulmonary failure who, prior to ECMO, would have died (Roll et al., 2017). This list presents only a snapshot of a multitude of treatment options that can cure disease, palliate symptoms, and, in some cases, prolong the dying process.

When considering whether or not it is ethical to continue LST, the central issue is whether or not the treatment can reasonably advance a patient toward their goals. Within the framework of the right to refuse LST, withholding and withdrawing LSTs are rendered as ethically and legally equivalent. The concept of *time-limited trials* is useful; a treatment can be trialed and, if deemed to be ineffective, can be discontinued (Bruce, Liang et al., 2015). From a qualitative standpoint, clinicians and families may find withdrawing LST, particularly medically supplied nutrition and hydration, to be emotionally challenging. However, ethical and legal equivalence in both withholding and withdrawing life support exists as a steadfast principle in the right to refuse.

When it comes to situations where the advances of medical technology cannot restore a patient to an acceptable quality of life or offer relief regardless of the patient's preferences, providers must focus on end-of-life care. It is critical for the APRN to know what is ethically and legally permissible related to end-of-life care. For example, decision making around LSTs for critically ill patients is fast-moving and has immediate implications for the patient's life or death. The APRN is ethically and professionally bound to participate and write orders that are congruent with acceptable ethical and legal practices, as well as institutional policy. Regardless, concerns about whether or not a plan of care is in a patient's best interest should never be ignored, and APRNs must be prepared to speak up when there is any question about ethical care of patients at the end of life.

In the United States, for example, patients have what is considered a bedrock ethical and legal right to refuse even LST (Cantor, 2001). As medical technology advanced, LSTs became available to stave off death, with the intention of allowing a desperately ill patient to heal and recover. Though lifesaving in many regards, there were also situations where patients would languish on life support, without any hope of recovery. When LST is initiated, it often is unclear which patients will benefit and which patients will be burdened without benefit by the treatment. Often it is the families of patients burdened by technology who request that LST be removed, realizing over time that their loved one is not recovering. Such was one of the major factors leading to case law that accrued to establish the legal right to refuse LST, including artificially provided nutrition and hydration. Box 11.6 highlights some of the precedent setting legal cases that guide ethical decision making around LST in the United States.

Advance Directives

Patients' abilities to state preferences in advance have enhanced and also added to the complexities of end-of-life care. Advance directives come in two broad forms: the appointment of a surrogate decision maker or statements of preference for treatment (often referred to as *living wills*). With the opportunity to identify a legally recognized surrogate decision maker through state laws, persons can name someone to speak on their behalf if a time comes when the person can no longer speak on their own behalf. Even though all 50 states recognize a person's right to appoint a healthcare agent, individual states have specific advance directive forms, underscoring the necessity for APRNs to be knowledgeable about what governs their practice.

When a patient has an advance directive, is unable to speak on their own behalf, and is deemed to lack capacity (Applebaum, 2007), the responsible provider

BOX 11.6

Landmark Legal Cases That Shaped End-of-Life Care: *Sample of Cases That Contributed to Right to Refuse Life Sustaining Treatment*

- Competent patients refusing LST (*Bartling v. Superior Court, California*, 1984)
- Incompetent patients with explicit preferences (*Brophy v. New England Sinai Hospital*, 1986, Massachusetts)
- Incompetent patients without explicit preferences (Matter of Quinlan, 1976, New Jersey; *Cruzan v. Director, Missouri Health Dept.*, 1990)
- Never competent patient (*Superintendent of Belchertown State School v. Saikewicz*, 1977, Massachusetts)

Sources:

Cantor, N. (2001). Twenty-five years after Quinlan: A review of the jurisprudence of death and dying. *Journal of Law, Medicine & Ethics 29*, 182-196.

Emanuel, E. J. (1988). A review of the ethical and legal aspects of terminating medical care. *The American Journal of Medicine, 84*, 291–301.

is required to invoke the advance directive to guide the plan of care. If the advance directive names a surrogate for the patient, that individual is ethically bound to provide the patient's voice, typically through the standard of substituted judgment, which answers the question: What would the patient say if they could participate in this decision making process on behalf of themselves? In the absence of discussions with patients, surrogates will often not be able to accurately predict a patient's preferences or enact the intent of the role in sharing the patient's wishes versus their own wishes for the patient (Nelson et al., 2017). APRNs may be in the position to instruct a healthcare agent in this important obligation. Overall compliance with advance directives is generally only about 33% (Yadev et al., 2017). A patient, of course, can refuse to complete an advance directive. In such cases, it is necessary to turn to a default surrogate decision maker.

In the absence of a patient naming a surrogate decision maker, some states have a rank ordering of default surrogates, based largely on familial relationships (DeMartino et al., 2017). Other states, such as Massachusetts, do not have a rank ordering and seek to identify close family members and domestic partners who seem committed to the patient's care. For patients who have never had capacity (e.g., profound intellectual disability) or who do not yet have capacity (e.g., children), health professionals turn to court-appointed guardians or parents to make healthcare decisions based upon the best interest of the patient. Box 11.7 highlights some of the many resources patients can use to create advance directives. APRNs may be in an excellent position to encourage and work with patients to participate in meaningful conversations about end-of-life preferences and hopefully put those in writing in the form of an advance directive that can be used to guide the establishment of goals of care.

POLST

The POLST (Physician Orders for Life-Sustaining Treatment) approach to end-of-life planning (National POLST, 2022) provides an effective strategy to discuss and document specific patient wishes that extend tangibly from a patient's advance directive when the patient is seriously ill or frail. In states that have adopted the use of POLSTs, patient wishes addressing resuscitation, additional medical interventions, food and fluids, and antibiotics are documented on a form that translates decisions into actionable medical orders. POLST forms are created in collaboration with patients and licensed providers (some states allow APRNs to sign). This means that patients who have completed a POLST may have their preferences honored across settings. In any setting, APRNs may serve as the catalyst for initiating conversations that lead to completion of a POLST, increasing the chances that the care patients receive at the end of life will be consistent with their values and preferences (Hammes et al., 2012).

Medical Aid in Dying

Due to some high-profile cases, Medical Aid in Dying (MAID) has been part of professional discourse for more than 30 years (Quill, 1991). MAID, commonly referred to as physician-assisted suicide (PAS), is a practice that allows terminally ill adults who meet specific criteria to request and receive a prescription for medication that they may choose to self-administer to achieve a peaceful death.

As of early 2021, MAID is in existence in 10 states: Oregon (1994), Washington (2008), Montana

BOX 11.7

Advance Care Planning Resources

Prepare for Your Care www.prepareforyourcare.org This website, developed by geriatricians and other medical professionals, walks people through basic steps in advance care planning and provides prompts and videos to help them get started. Information is available in English and Spanish. https://mydirectives.com/en/how-it-works

Aging With Dignity and **Five Wishes** www.agingwithdignity.org Provides practical information, advice, and legal tools for advance care planning, including the "Five Wishes" Advance Directive. Also offers "Voicing My Choices: A Planning Guide for Adolescents & Young Adults" (in English and Spanish), a tool that helps young people living with a serious illness communicate their preferences to friends, family, and caregivers.

The Center for Practical Bioethics https://www.practicalbioethics.org/resources/advance-care-planning Offers downloadable resources, including the workbook "Caring Conversations," as well as case studies and audio interviews about the importance of advance care planning.

The Conversation Project theconversationproject.org Features *The Conversation Starter Kit*, aimed at helping people overcome barriers to planning and to start talking to family and loved ones. Available in English, Spanish, French, and Mandarin. Theconversationproject.org/starter-kit/intro/

Go Wish game, developed by The Coda Alliance www.codaalliance.org, helps stimulate discussion that would focus in a positive way on values and wishes about end-of-life care. The card game can be an effective tool for elderly people with limited cognition and for people with limited literacy and limited skills in the English language, without seeming too simplistic for those with higher education.

National Hospice and Palliative Care Organization www.nhpco.org The National Hospice and Palliative Care Organization (NHPCO) is the largest nonprofit membership organization representing hospice and palliative care programs and professionals in the United States. Caring Connections (caringinfo.org), a program of the National Hospice and Palliative Care Organization, provides free resources to help people make decisions about end-of-life care before a crisis.

National Institute on Aging Advance Care Planning Tip Sheet https://www.nia.nih.gov/health/publication/advance-care-planning This tip sheet offers advice on advance care planning, including helpful descriptions and definitions of medical situations that may occur and tips for considering decisions around treatment

Online Living Will Registries:

America Living Will Registry: www.alwr.com

US Living Will Registry: www.uslwr.com

MedicAlert Foundation: www.medicalert.org/join/advance-directives.htm

Organ Donation.gov www.Organdonor.gov, run by the US Department of Health and Human Services, offers resources and materials on organ donation.

(2009), Vermont (2013), District of Columbia (2016), Colorado (2016), California (2015), Hawaii (2018), New Jersey (2019), and Maine (2019; https://compassionandchoices.org/end-of-life-planning/learn/understanding-medical-aid-dying/). Oregon was the first state to legalize the practice, setting the model for eligibility criteria and restrictions on the practice to which other states have largely adhered (Oregon Death With Dignity Act Requirements, 2022; Box 11.8). Primary reasons for requesting MAID are generally a fear of loss of autonomy and dignity, inability to participate in activities that make life meaningful, existential suffering, and not being willing to become a burden to others (Oregon Death With Dignity Act, 2016).

Arguments and professional positions against MAID carry ethical weight. Patients are vulnerable, given their illnesses, and therefore it is imperative that health professionals can be trusted to cure when possible and, when

BOX 11.8

Death With Dignity Act Requirements

Under Oregon's Death With Dignity Act (DWDA, 2016), ending one's life in accordance with the law does not constitute suicide. The DWDA specifically prohibits euthanasia, where a physician or other person directly administers a medication to end another's life. To request a prescription for lethal medications, the DWDA requires that a patient must be:

- an adult (18 years of age or older),
- a resident of Oregon,
- capable (defined as able to make and communicate healthcare decisions), and
- diagnosed with a terminal illness that will lead to death within 6 months.

Patients meeting these requirements are eligible to request a prescription for lethal medication from a licensed Oregon physician. To receive a prescription for lethal medication, the following steps must be fulfilled:

- The patient must make two oral requests to his or her physician, separated by at least 15 days.
- The patient must provide a written request to his or her physician, signed in the presence of two witnesses.
- The prescribing physician and a consulting physician must confirm the diagnosis and prognosis.
- The prescribing physician and a consulting physician must determine whether the patient is capable.
- If either physician believes the patient's judgment is impaired by a psychiatric or psychological disorder, the patient must be referred for a psychological examination.
- The prescribing physician must inform the patient of feasible alternatives to DWDA, including comfort care, hospice care, and pain control.
- The prescribing physician must request, but may not require, the patient to notify his or her next of kin of the prescription request.

Physicians must also comply with specific reporting requirements.

The Oregon Revised Statutes specify that action taken in accordance with the DWDA does not constitute suicide, mercy killing, or homicide under the law.

Links to statutes can be found at https://www.oregon.gov/oha/PH/ProviderPartnerResources/Evaluation-Research/DeathwithDignityAct/Pages/index.aspx

not possible, to care well for them until death (Sulmasy & Mueller, 2017). In addition, the tools of palliative care have expanded, with strategies accessible even for health professionals in more remote areas thanks to the Internet and emerging telemedicine technology.

Euthanasia is an intentional act on the part of a health professional to end the life of a patient due to intolerable pain and suffering and is illegal in the United States. As of 2021, it is legal in Belgium, the Netherlands, Colombia, Luxembourg, Canada, Spain, and New Zealand (Rada, 2021). The ethical arguments and laws surrounding MAID and euthanasia can be complicated and are evolving (DePergola, 2018). It is essential that APRNs familiarize themselves with what is legal in their jurisdiction in the event that patients ask about the practice (Hamric et al., 2018).

Conscientious Objection

Resolving situations when an APRN or any healthcare provider refuses to provide a safe, legal medical intervention to preserve their moral integrity requires deep reflection. The tension in such situations is between protecting the healthcare provider without compromising the safety and well-being of persons seeking care. In the end, resolution requires collaboration and compromise. The services often identified with conscientious objection are related to reproductive health and care at the end of life. Except in rare circumstances, the relationship APRNs have with those they serve will be mediated by their employer. We must look to organizations to create policies to mediate this tension. Wicclair (2014) offered four specific criteria to consider in weighing the balance of respecting the integrity of

BOX 11.9

Criteria to Include in Policies Guiding Conscientious Objection

1. Accommodation may not impede a patient's/surrogate's timely access to information, counseling, and referral.
2. Accommodation may not impede a patient's timely access to healthcare services offered within the institution.
3. Accommodation may not impose excessive burdens on colleagues, supervisors, department heads, other administrators, or the institution.
4. Whenever feasible, health professionals requesting accommodation should provide advance notification to department heads or supervisors.

Adapted from Wicclair, M. R. (2014). Managing conscientious objection in healthcare institutions. *HEC Forum, 26*(3), 267–283.

providers with meeting our obligations of justice and beneficence to the patient (see Box 11.9). When it becomes necessary to review a request for accommodation to be excused from providing a service, Wicclair (2014) recommended an approach that encourages the provider to reflect on the depth of their objections to facilitate moral clarity on the part of the provider. Such an approach is consistent with strategies that build moral communities by promoting understanding and may provide an opportunity for the provider to identify a complementary obligation to patients to offset the challenge posed by their objection.

SOCIETAL ISSUES

Florence Nightingale's contribution to nursing went well beyond improved hygiene to fight disease to include a commitment to social change in caring for the homeless or promoting what we think of today as community health nursing (Hegge & Bunkers, 2020). *Nursing's Social Policy Statement* reinforces a broad definition of health that includes addressing social determinants of health such as housing, income, access to healthy food, and education (ANA, 2010). Nurse-led models of care demonstrate how APRNs play a central role in improving the lives of people by emphasizing a broad definition of health that defines the nursing profession (Mason, 2016). This section of the chapter will highlight a few key ethical issues for APRNs that relate to broader social issues.

Promoting Social Justice

APRNs often enlarge their focus of concern, expanding their sphere of involvement beyond their institution into the societal sector. Moving into the arena of social justice is a historic legacy and a moral imperative (Mason, 2016). The nursing literature reflects increasing attention to social justice in the United States and internationally (Perry et al., 2017). Equity is primarily an issue of justice; concerns about access to and distribution of healthcare resources are key justice concerns of APRNs. The clinical expertise and an APRN's cutting-edge understanding of the clinical needs of their patient population provide the platform from which the APRN speaks to social justice issues. APRNs must be prepared to offer expert input when called on by their nurse colleagues working in policy and research roles in support of policy reforms that address social justice issues.

The COVID-19 pandemic forever changed nursing practice. The release of the National Academies of Science, Engineering and Medicine (NASEM) consensus report *The Future of Nursing 2020–2030: Charting a Path to Achieve Health Equity* punctuated a transformative year for nursing (NASEM, 2021). The report provides compelling evidence of the role nurses can play in addressing the health inequities laid bare during the COVID-19 pandemic. APRNs will play a significant role in advancing health equity and addressing social determinants of health. APRNs will be called upon to leverage the profession's ethics, values, and knowledge to build on evidence-informed models, health system policies, and health-related public policies. APRNs will help lead the complex work of integrating the social and health sectors in support of the health and well-being of individuals, families, and communities.

To act at this level requires sophisticated use of all of the core competencies of advanced practice nursing. In particular, advocacy, communication, collaboration (see Chapter 10), and leadership (see Chapter 9) are required. Essential knowledge needed for this element includes an understanding of the concepts of justice, particularly distributive justice (the equitable allocation of scarce resources) and restorative justice (the duty owed to those who have been systematically disadvantaged through no fault of their own). APRNs who move into this type of activity must possess knowledge of the health policy process in general (see Chapter 17) and specific health policies affecting their specialty. Exemplar 11.6 describes one APRN's journey role modeling ethical practice, ultimately promoting social justice. Chapter 17 also provides examples of actions by nurses who have expanded their concerns

EXEMPLAR 11.6

PUTTING IT ALL TOGETHER: DEVELOPMENT OF THE ELEMENTS OF THE ETHICAL DECISION-MAKING COMPETENCY[a]

R.T. is a family nurse practitioner (NP) who is completing a DNP program. Her experience with providing health care to Hispanic migrant farm workers in rural Virginia has given her many opportunities to use her ethical decision-making skills. This exemplar portrays her journey including acting on issues of social justice as she has developed her APRN practice.

One fall evening, R.T. accompanies a team of outreach workers into a migrant farm camp to screen workers for diabetes and heart disease. Three older men approach her with concerns regarding Antonio, one of the new younger workers. They report that he has been losing weight, sweating all the time, and shaking and that he appears ill. They are scared for him and a little frightened that he could be contagious. R.T. encourages the men to have him schedule an appointment with her the following night because she would be staffing a mobile clinic in the community. The men are concerned that Antonio would be unwilling to give his information to anyone because he lacks legal documentation to be in the United States. The men promise that they will encourage Antonio to make an appointment and reassure him that R.T. will not report him to the authorities.

The next night, when Antonio does not show up for an appointment, R.T. walks outside the mobile clinic and luckily sees Antonio. He is easy to identify because he is sweating profusely and his hands are trembling. R.T. asks her community health worker to ask him to join her in the mobile clinic and, to her surprise, he agrees. Antonio looks much older than his reported age of 19. He is frail, anxious-appearing, and sweaty. After taking a history and doing an examination, R.T. suspects that he might have hyperthyroidism. She convinces Antonio to allow her to check some laboratory values.

The laboratory results confirm R.T.'s suspicions. Normally, she could refer a patient with hyperthyroidism to endocrinology for urgent treatment because she is concerned that they could go into a coma or die. Instead, she is faced with many barriers to accessing care for him. He is in this country illegally and uninsured. Although he lives well below the poverty line, he does not qualify for Medicaid. He might qualify for financial assistance but he would be leery of providing any identification or pay stubs. Antonio wants to wait until he returns to Mexico in 6 months to have the issue addressed. He does not want to miss time from work because he thinks he might get fired. In addition, he has transportation and language barriers, which would make it difficult to see a specialist. R.T. struggles to determine whether the principle of beneficence or the principle of respect for autonomy should carry the most weight in her decision making.

Stories such as this are common when working with migrant Hispanic farm workers. Early on R.T. would have thought only about the individual situation. As R.T.'s ethical competency developed, she began to look at the bigger problem: the system. The existing referral system placed most of the burden on patients to obtain appointments with specialists. The referral staff was not allotted the needed time to assist non-English-speaking or illiterate patients, such as Antonio, with obtaining financial assistance at the local academic hospital. R.T. realized that staff and administration for the healthcare center would need to engage in discussions about ethical issues for the culture to change. Antonio's case helped shape a new system. The outreach coordinator now assists migrant farm workers with the financial screening process, interpretation, and transportation. Antonio's case was the first success. Although it took three times as long to get him the care he needed, he finally underwent thyroid ablation and is now a healthy 20-year-old.

As R.T. is developing her practice as a DNP-prepared NP, she is looking for ways to promote social justice within the healthcare system. To have a voice in the larger political arena, R.T. joined the leadership committee of her region's NP organization. She has taken on the role of governmental affairs chairperson. This allows her to be involved in healthcare legislation that affects APRNs and patients. Her hope is that this will become an avenue for addressing the ethical problems associated with caring for undocumented Hispanic migrant farm workers. Though this example is specific to the United States, recent events have made this a global problem. This case demonstrates what is possible for nurses to achieve when caring for vulnerable populations all over the world.

[a]We thank Reagan Thompson Holland, MSN, RN, NP, for her assistance with this exemplar.

about individual patients into working for social justice in the policy arena.

Access to Resources

Issues of access to and distribution of resources create powerful dilemmas for APRNs, many of whom care for underserved populations. Goals of reduced expenditures and increased efficiency, although important, create tension between providers, administrators, and patients.

Costs of the US healthcare system are unsustainably high and growing (Anderson et al., 2019). Improving the efficiency and effectiveness of care delivery at a reduced cost can itself be seen as a moral good, one that requires clinicians to work together with administrators to achieve cost-effective goals. APRNs can bridge clinical and administrative perspectives and collaborate with administrators to help achieve quality patient outcomes at reduced cost to the system, which will indirectly improve access. Removing scope of practice barriers for APRNs may be one way to decrease the cost of care (Emanuel, 2012; Institute of Medicine, 2011).

It may be necessary to question and challenge features in the healthcare system that negatively affect the quality of care delivered. Finally, there is a need to review patient outcomes consistently and the quality of nursing care provided (see Chapters 21 and 23) because these data can be powerful in building the case for quality changes to promote ethically responsive environments.

Issues of social justice and equitable access to resources present formidable challenges in clinical practice. (Milionis's 2013) frank discussion of the consequences of economic hardship on a health system exemplifies a basic challenge; healthcare resources are limited, which means seeking an equitable distribution of the limited resources. Scarcity of resources may be more severe in developing areas of the world, and justice issues of fair and equitable distribution of healthcare services present serious ethical dilemmas for nurses in these regions (Harrowing & Mill, 2010). A report of projects funded by the Robert Wood Johnson Foundation concluded that achieving the objectives of reduced cost and improved quality will require a trusted, widely respected "honest broker" that can convene and maintain the ongoing commitment of health plans, providers, and purchasers (Conrad et al., 2014). APRNs may be in a position to serve as honest brokers.

Allocation conflicts arise in regard to daily decision making; for example, with a CNS guiding the assignment of patients in a staffing shortage or an FNP finding that a specialty consultation for a patient is not available for several months. Whether in community or acute care settings, APRNs must, on a daily basis, balance their obligation to provide holistic, evidence-based care with the necessity to contain costs in an effort to achieve a basic level of fairness in the distribution of healthcare services (Bodenheimer & Grumbach, 2012).

APRNs often bring creativity and a wide range of patient management strategies, which are crucial in caring for large numbers of uninsured and underinsured persons (Garfield et al., 2016). For example, an acute care nurse practitioner (ACNP) managing an underinsured patient with chronic lung disease and heart failure discovers that the patient is unable to pay for all of the medications prescribed and has elected to forego the diuretic and an angiotensin-converting enzyme inhibitor. Because the ACNP knows that angiotensin-converting enzyme inhibitors are associated with reduced morbidity and mortality rates and that diuretics control symptoms and prevent rehospitalization, these changes are discouraged. Instead, the ACNP helps the patient make more suitable choices when altering medications, such as dosing some medications on an every-other-day basis. The ACNP has helped the patient cope with the situation but must face the morally unsettling fact that in the United States, inferior and disturbing shortcuts must be made.

Finally, as nurses in general (NASEM, 2021) and, more specifically, APRNs broaden their perspectives to encompass population health and advocate for sound health policy, both essential competencies of the APRN (AACN, 2019), they will experience the tension between caring for the individual patient and the larger population (DeCamp et al., 2018). Caregivers are increasingly being asked to incorporate population-based cost considerations into individualized clinical decision making (Salvage & White, 2019). Population-based considerations present a challenge to APRNs, many of whom have been educated to focus on the individual rather than consider the broader community in clinical decision making.

Consider this example of how payment issues create ethical tension for an APRN. Knowing a particular patient has a history of diverticulosis and abscess formation, an NP wishes to order a computed tomography scan to evaluate the patient with fever, abdominal tenderness, and abdominal pain. However, the insurance approval process takes a minimum of 24 hours. By sending the patient to the emergency room, the test can be done more quickly, but the patient will also face a long wait and high co-pay if they do not require subsequent hospital admission. Limiting access to computed tomography scans is based on containing costs and avoiding unnecessary testing, which are two laudable goals. In this situation, the lengthy approval process means that the NP must make decisions about the treatment plan without important information. The pressure to alleviate the patient's suffering in a timely manner may tempt the NP to advise the patient to go to the emergency room, which may result in a greater financial burden on the patient and may ultimately prove more expensive to the system. The availability of modern technology forces difficult choices, especially challenging providers to redefine *timely*, *urgent*, and *emergent*, and may cause providers to feel as though they are choosing between what is best for patients and what is best for organizations.

Genomics

Technologic advances, such as the rapidly expanding field of genetics, highlight the need for nurses, particularly APRNs, to have current, up-to-date information to best support patients as they grapple with decisions about using this new technology (Camak, 2016). With all of the advances in precision medicine, we still face enormous ethical challenges in how to apply them to improvements in prevention, diagnosis, and treatment of disease (Quigley, 2015). To counsel patients effectively on the risks and benefits of genetic testing, APRNs need to stay current in this rapidly changing field (Courtwright-Lim & Drago, 2020). A helpful resource for this and other issues is the text by Beery et al. (2018). Genetic testing poses a unique challenge to the informed consent process. Direct-to-consumer marketing with evidence of misinformation through misleading advertisement poses significant problems for consumers and APRNs, who may be asked for advice about whether or not patients should obtain these tests (Fragoulakis et al., 2020; Pandos, 2020).

Because genetic information is crucially linked to the concepts of privacy and confidentiality and the availability of this information is increasing, it is inevitable that APRNs will encounter legal issues and ethical dilemmas related to the use of genetic data. The cost of genomic testing may effectively put this technology out of reach for disadvantaged populations. It will be important for the healthcare system to create a model that will ensure the sustainability of funding for genomic-guided interventions, their adoption and coverage by health insurance, and prioritization of genomic medicine research, development, and innovation, as well as mechanisms to ensure privacy and confidentiality (Fragoulakis et al., 2020).

COVID-19 Pandemic

The arrival of coronavirus (COVID-19), initially in the Wuhan province of China in late 2019, has challenged healthcare systems across the world (Sohrabi et al., 2020). The disease trajectory continues to be complex, and understanding of its pathophysiology and impact remains under study (Yuki et al., 2020; Zhou et al., 2020). The rapid spread of the virus, sheer numbers of infected persons, and societal shutdown strategies have challenged traditional healthcare systems (Barbara, 2020; Feuer & Rashbaum, 2020). Ethical frameworks provide guidance to direct clinicians, disaster teams, and administrators in anticipating ethical issues that this pandemic brings forth, from personal protective equipment to crisis standards of care (Berlinger et al., 2020; Biddison et al., 2019). APRNs will be called upon as clinical leaders in the prevention, mitigation, and contingency crisis management of ethical issues that emerge in this pandemic, which is not expected to end in the immediate future (Morley et al., 2020).

Central to the ethical challenges for APRNs will be the duty to provide care in the context of resource scarcity and the need to consider setting aside best practices to meet the demands of the situation. APRNs will need to balance their clinical expertise, educational training, and respect for evidence-informed practice with shifting standards of care, rapid expansion of scope of practice regulations, rapidly evolving science, and resultant (sometimes conflicting) guidelines for everything from conserving and, when necessary, reusing supplies; substitution of equipment; adapting care delivery models; to reallocation strategies (Benton et al., 2020; Berlinger et al., 2020). As the pandemic drags on, APRNs and others will need to navigate a parallel pandemic: physical, mental, and emotional harms secondary to being a healthcare worker during the pandemic (Chen et al., 2021; Dzau et al., 2020). APRNs will continue to face these situations as future pandemics will undoubtedly occur.

Gun Violence

Gun violence is a public health problem in the United States for which a clear solution has not yet been identified. Though the Second Amendment of the US Constitution proclaims the right to bear arms, doing so with safeguards is a concern for APRNs. According to the Gun Violence Archive, a total of at least 19,223 people lost their lives due to gun violence in 2020—reportedly almost a 25% increase from the prior year (Gun Violence Archive, 2022). This alarming statistic calls attention to gun violence as a public health problem. Data suggest that rather than dangerous people, it is gun access that is more causally linked to death and disability from firearms. Lu and Temple (2019) found that in a study of 663 emerging adults (early 20s), persons with gun access were 18 times more likely to threaten another person with a gun, after controlling for prior gun carrying, mental health treatment, and demographic factors including race and ethnicity. Tying causality to mental illness has obscured the study of etiologies, including dangerous behaviors associated with substance use and domestic violence and widespread access to guns. The exponential rise in the number of mass shootings, defined as a shooting where four or more people are killed with a firearm, underscores the need for APRNs to engage in meaningful dialogue to combat this problem. APRNs have an ethical obligation to inquire and educate patients and families about the presence and safety of firearms in the home, as well as to explore and screen for other risk factors. Community health initiatives, such as the Baltimore Ceasefire 365 Project, where community leaders call for a weekend ceasefire, has demonstrated significant reductions (52%) in firearm violence without a post ceasefire increase (Phalen et al., 2020). This project is community driven by persons who have been affected by gun violence and illustrates how a broad understanding of health beyond the individual to the community can significantly impact individual outcomes.

Participation in Research

APRNs may engage in research as principal investigators, coinvestigators, or data collectors for clinical studies and trials. Ethical issues abound in clinical research, including recruiting and retaining a wide diversity of patients in studies, protecting vulnerable populations from undue risk, and ensuring informed consent, fair access to research, and study subjects' privacy. As APRNs move into quality improvement and research initiatives, they may experience the conflict between the clinician role, in which the focus is on the best interests of an individual patient, and that of the researcher, in which the focus is on ensuring the integrity of the study (Edwards & Chalmers, 2002; Hay-Smith et al., 2016).

LEGAL ISSUES

Over the last 30 years, the complexity of ethical issues in the healthcare environment and the inability to reach agreement among parties has resulted in participants turning to the legal system for resolution. A body of legal precedent has emerged, reflecting changes in society's moral consensus. For example, the culturally and linguistically appropriate services standards mandate that healthcare institutions receiving federal funds provide services that are accessible to patients regardless of their cultural background (US Department of Health and Human Services, Office of Minority Health, 2001). These standards provide legal and regulatory guidance for the ethical obligation to respect all persons, regardless of their cultural background and primary language.

APRNs must use caution and not conflate legal perspectives with ethical practice. In many cases, there is no relevant law to guide decision making. Thoughtful deliberation of the ethical issues rather than searching for a legal answer to avoid litigation offers the best hope of resolution. In addition, looking to the judicial system for guidance in ethical decision making is troubling because the judicial aim is to interpret the law, not to satisfy the ethical concerns of all parties involved. In addition, clinical understanding may be absent from the judicial perspective. Countless examples exist that illustrate how the involvement of the media, especially social media, may further confound the ethical complexity of medical decision making as opinions are confused with facts.

Sometimes the law not only falls short of resolving ethical concerns but contributes to the creation of new dilemmas. Changes in the Medicare hospice benefit under the Patient Protection and Affordable Care Act (2010) offer a clear example. The regulations require a face-to-face assessment by a healthcare provider to recertify hospice eligibility at set intervals after the initial enrollment (Kennedy, 2012). Often, patients with dementia or another slowly progressive disease who enroll in hospice experience an initial period of stability, likely because they have improved symptom management and access to comprehensive services. If this stability extends to the next certification period, the patient may face disenrollment. This situation may cause tension between the APRN's ethical obligation to the patient (advocate for and promote a plan of care consistent with patient values and goals) and being truthful, which would likely result in a lost benefit. Failing to be truthful violates the law, which could have serious legal consequences for the APRN. Society has an ethical obligation to care for patients with potential protracted terminal trajectories such as those with dementia, and a hospice model of care should not be restricted to a 6-month life expectancy (Gillick, 2012). When hospice services become unavailable, the net result may be inadvertently pushing patients toward aggressive treatment, leading to potentially inappropriate treatment because it may be the only support available.

There are also other examples impacting ethical patient care due to regulatory practices such as 30-day mortality statistics for patients undergoing surgeries and procedures. The idea is that should a patient die less than 30 days after a procedure, even if it is considered high risk for such a patient, it creates a mark on the physician's and hospital program's record (Span, 2015).

NAVIGATING BARRIERS TO ETHICAL PRACTICE AND STRATEGIES TO OVERCOME THEM

A number of factors influence how moral issues are addressed and resolved in the clinical setting. Some barriers are easily corrected, but others may require attention at institutional, state, or even national levels. Regardless of type, the APRN must identify and respond to the barriers that inhibit the development of morally responsive practice environments.

Barriers Internal to the APRN

Lack of knowledge about ethics; lack of confidence in one's own ability to name, define, and resolve ethical conflicts; lack of skill in communicating in high-stakes situations; time pressure; and a sense of powerlessness are potent barriers to the APRN achieving competence in ethical decision making. To address these barriers, APRNs need to seek out opportunities for ethics education through schools of nursing and professional organizations. Engaging in periodic values clarification exercises can be helpful for APRNs and all members of the healthcare team who experience conflict. Once personal values are realized, the APRN can more easily anticipate situations in which these conflicts will arise and develop strategies for managing them. For example, an emergency department NP may be faced with providing care for a criminal injured in a gunfight that killed innocent bystanders. The *Code of Ethics for Nurses* (ANA, 2015) emphasizes that all individuals be treated with dignity and respect; however, it can be disturbing and difficult to provide care for an individual who has caused harm to others, particularly if the NP has not examined their own personal views. The process of values clarification is helpful when preparing for this type of situation.

APRNs can empower themselves by role modeling ethical decision making within their team. For example, in the primary care setting, a clinic nurse mentions to the APRN a concern about how a patient situation was handled. In addition to reflective listening and emotional support, the APRN can encourage the nurse to gather all of the necessary information and guide the nurse in an analysis of the ethical elements and consideration of practical solutions. This process demonstrates the process of ethical decision making for the clinic nurse and empowers the APRN in the development of this core competency. Including ethical aspects of a patient's case in interprofessional rounds, scheduling debriefing sessions after a particularly difficult case, reading and discussing ethics articles specific to the specialty patient group in a journal club, and/or using simulation activities in which caregivers role-play different scenarios are additional strategies that APRNs can use to empower themselves and other nurses to examine ethical issues.

Lack of time is often a barrier faced by APRNs seeking to enact this competency. In some cases, the APRN may need to resolve a presenting dilemma in stages, with the most central issue addressed first. The APRN also needs to enlist the aid of administrative and physician colleagues in recognizing the ongoing consequences of lack of time for team deliberations. For example, if a patient is not receiving adequate pain management because the bedside nurse is concerned about hastening death and is unaware of the full treatment plan, the CNS should first focus on relieving the patient's pain. Once the immediate need is addressed, the CNS can help the bedside nurse identify nonpharmacologic interventions to promote comfort and educate the nurse about the dosage and timing of medications to prevent wide fluctuations in pain management. At this point, the administrative leadership should be approached about supporting ongoing staff education. An additional strategy, such as arranging for the nurse to rotate to a hospice unit or attend End-of-Life Nursing Education Consortium training represents a preventive approach to help avert similar dilemmas in the future (Ferrell et al., 2015).

Interprofessional Barriers

Different approaches among healthcare team members can pose a barrier to ethical practice. For example, nurses and physicians often define, perceive, analyze, and reason through ethical problems from distinct and sometimes opposing perspectives (Shannon, 1997). Although the roles are complementary, these differing approaches may create conflict between a nurse and physician, further separating and isolating their perspectives. A physician may be unaware of the nurse's differing opinion or may not recognize this difference as a conflict (Shannon et al., 2002). Similar to an optical illusion, the nurse and physician may look at the same ethically troubling clinical situation but, because of differences in their perspectives, focus on opposing features and arrive at different conclusions about the appropriate course of action (Ponce et al., 2017). In such situations, the APRN first seeks to understand alternative interpretations of the situation and establish respectful and open communication before seeking resolution of ethical problems.

Physicians, nurses, and APRNs need to engage in moral discourse to understand and support the ethical burden that each professional carries (Morley & Shashidhara, 2020). Encouraging examples of interprofessional collaboration include the European Multidisciplinary Research Network on Health and Disability (MURINET) project (Ajovalasit et al., 2012), a joint policy statement on requests for inappropriate treatment (Bosslet et al., 2015), and the National Consensus Project, composed of nursing and medical professional organizations that appointed a team of physicians and nurses to revise the *Clinical Practice Guidelines for Quality Palliative Care* (Ferrell et al., 2018).

A third robust initiative including multiple professions has been the establishment of the IPEC, whose mission is to advance interprofessional education so that students entering the healthcare professions not only seek collaborative relationships with other providers but also view collaboration as the norm and not the exception (IPEC, 2016). An expert panel developed core competencies for interprofessional education; one of the four domains focuses on values and ethics (IPEC, 2016). The emphasis of this domain is developing climates of mutual respect and shared values. Box 11.10 lists the 10 competencies identified. These statements focus on values shared by all healthcare disciplines and can serve as a basis for building collaborative interprofessional teams that emphasize preventive ethics. As noted, collaboration is the key strategy for eliminating interprofessional barriers.

Patient–Provider Barriers

Additional barriers to ethical practice arise from issues in the patient–provider relationship. Regardless of the setting where APRNs practice, developing cultural awareness can enhance relationships with patients and their families. Though there is some evidence that online learning can enhance cultural competence (Lee et al., 2015), issues that result from cultural diversity are difficult to resolve without help from others who are more familiar with the specific cultural practices and beliefs. Occasionally, hospital chaplains, local clergy, or individuals from the patient's culture who may teach in the language department in a local

BOX 11.10

Values and Ethics Competencies[a]

1. Place the interests of patients and populations at the center of interprofessional healthcare delivery.
2. Respect the dignity and privacy of patients while maintaining confidentiality in the delivery of team-based care.
3. Embrace the cultural diversity and individual differences that characterize patients, populations, and the healthcare team.
4. Respect the unique cultures, values, roles and responsibilities, and expertise of other health professions.
5. Work in cooperation with those who receive care, those who provide care, and others who contribute to or support the delivery of prevention and health services.
6. Develop a trusting relationship with patients, families, and other team members.
7. Demonstrate high standards of ethical conduct and quality of care in one's contributions to team-based care.
8. Manage ethical dilemmas specific to interprofessional patient/population-centered care situations.
9. Act with honesty and integrity in relationships with patients, families, and other team members.
10. Maintain competence in one's own profession appropriate to scope of practice.

[a]Competencies as identified by the Interprofessional Education Collaborative.

From Interprofessional Education Collaborative. (2011). *Core competencies for interprofessional collaborative practice: Report of an expert panel.*

university can assist with obtaining an expanded understanding of specific belief systems. Box 11.11 highlights some Internet-based resources to enhance cultural competence.

Another barrier to ethical practice that challenges many APRNs is the issue of patient nonadherence. Patients and families may choose not to be actively involved in their care or resist an APRN's attempts to improve their well-being, which raises clinical and ethical questions. Managing nonadherent patients is ethically troubling because they consume a disproportionate amount of healthcare resources, including the APRN's time, redirecting these resources from patients who are more amenable to the established plan of care. There are no easy solutions to managing the nonadherent patient (Gardner, 2015). Full consideration of this issue is beyond the scope of this chapter (see Chapter 7 for effective strategies for those patients in resistance). APRNs should seek additional support from resources such as social workers or home health nurses to discover the underlying causes and find solutions.

Organizational and Environmental Barriers

Lack of support for nurses who speak up regarding ethical problems in work settings is a potent barrier to ethical practice. Environments in which nurses' concerns are minimized or ignored by physicians, administrators, and even other nurses can lead to moral distress. Recent studies have revealed significant correlations between the level of moral distress and turnover of nurses and physicians (Austin et al., 2017). These findings lend urgency to the need for APRNs to provide leadership in building ethical practice environments. Consideration should be given to organizational ethics programs that focus on building structures and processes to deal with conflicts of roles and expectations (Hamric et al., 2013). APRNs need to develop skills in collaborative conflict resolution and preventive ethics to build ethical practice environments in which moral distress is minimized and the moral integrity of all caregivers is respected and protected.

APRN WELL-BEING

One significant threat to ethical practice is the failure of APRNs to practice self-care. As previously noted from the *Code of Ethics for Nurses* (ANA, 2015), nurses owe the same duty to themselves that they do to their patients. For example, an APRN may receive a referral to see a patient late in the day. They will feel compelled to stay late and meet the patient's needs, even if they already worked well beyond a "normal" day. As a one-time event, this is laudable. When it becomes a pattern, particularly when the APRN is sacrificing personal time or family time, they put themselves at

BOX 11.11

Cultural Competence: Internet-Based Resources to Enhance Cultural Competence: *List provided in part by the Cummings Online Resources (CORE) https://azhin.org/c.php?g=682744&p=4899137*

- **EthnoMed** Information about cultural beliefs related to medical care of recent immigrants. From Harborview Medical Center, University of Washington
- **Cultural Competence Resources for Health Care Providers** Assessment tools and culture- and disease-specific information. From the US Department of Health and Human Services (USDHHS) Health Resources and Services Administration
- **AHRQ: Consider Culture, Customs and Beliefs** The Agency for Healthcare Research and Quality (AHRQ) offers several resources for improving cultural and linguistic competency in delivering health care.
- **National Center for Cultural Competence** Very comprehensive website from Georgetown University devoted to all aspects of cultural competencies across society
- **Office of Minority Health on Cultural Competencies** Developed a comprehensive set of 15 action steps that provide a blueprint for individuals and health and health care organizations to implement culturally and linguistically appropriate services.
- **Culture Clues from the University of Washington** Culture Clues™ are tip sheets for clinicians, designed to increase awareness about concepts and preferences of patients from the diverse cultures served by University of Washington Medical Center.
- **Advancing Effective Communication, Cultural Competence, and Patient- and Family Centered Care for the Lesbian, Gay, Bisexual, and Transgender (LGBT) Community** A new field guide from The Joint Commission
- **National Resource Center** From Drexel University School of Public Health. Website is devoted to providing information and preparing underserved communities to understand and deal with public health crises.
- **Minority Health and Health Equity Archive** The goal of the Archive is to advance the use of new digital technologies to promote transdisciplinary scholarship on race, ethnicity, and disparities research designed to achieve health equity. Through the University of Pittsburgh.
- **Health Disparities Policy Page from the Kaiser Family Foundation**
- **Culture, Language, and Health** US Department of Health and Human Services, Health Resources and Services Administration. Healthy literacy tools and practices to improve individual health and build healthy communities, healthcare providers need to recognize and address the unique culture, language and health literacy of diverse consumers and communities.
- **Culture Vision** An online resource that supports cultural competency in patient care by providing access to information for more than 50 ethnic, cultural, religious, and ability groups
- **A Physician's Practical Guide to Culturally Competent Care** Offers CME/CE credit and equips healthcare professionals with awareness, knowledge, and skills to better treat the increasingly diverse US population they serve.
- **Culture, Language, and Health Literacy** Links to assessment tools, culture/language specific resources, health professions education materials, and more

risk for long-term health consequences. The NASEM has championed clinician wellness as a national priority due in part to an unprecedented rise in burnout and suicide among physicians and nurses (NASEM, 2019). In this consensus study, the authors promote a far-reaching agenda to combat clinical burnout by creating positive work environments. Challenges to self-care will be a constant struggle due to APRNs' multiple competing commitments. Fidelity is an ethical concept that requires persons to be faithful to their commitments and promises. For the APRN, these obligations start with the patient and family but also include physicians and other colleagues, the institution or employer, the larger profession, and oneself. An APRN may face a dilemma if encouraged by a specialist consultant to pursue a costly intervention on behalf

BOX 11.12

Organizations With Electronically Available Ethics Resources

ETHICS POLICY STATEMENTS OR GUIDELINES

- ABCD Caring (Americans for Better Care of the Dying): http://www.abcd-caring.org
- American Academy of Neurology, Practice Guidelines: https://www.aan.com/Guidelines
- American Academy of Pediatrics, Policy Statements: http://www.aap.org/en-us/advocacy-and-policy/Pages/Advocacy-and-Policy.aspx
- American Association of Nurse Anesthesiology: http://www.aana.com
- American College of Medical Genetics: https://www.acmg.net/ACMG/Home/ACMG/Default.aspx?hkey=3f9eaab1-a34c-41f8-a368-3e997ab-cfef4
- American College of Nurse-Midwives: https://www.midwife.org/
- American College of Physicians, Center for Ethics and Professionalism: http://www.acponline.org/ethics
- American College of Surgeons: http://www.facs.org
- American Medical Association, Council on Ethical and Judicial Affairs: https://www.ama-assn.org/about-us/council-ethical-judicial-affairs-ceja
- American Nurses Association, Center for Ethics and Human Rights: http://www.nursingworld.org/MainMenuCategories/EthicsStandards/About
- American Society for Reproductive Medicine: http://www.asrm.org/?vs=1
- American Society of Anesthesiologists, Ethical Guidelines and Statements: http://www.asahq.org/resources/ethics-and-professionalism
- American Society of Law, Medicine and Ethics: http://www.aslme.org
- American Society of Transplantation, Key Position Statements: https://www.myast.org/public-policy/key-position-statements/key-position-statements
- Canadian Resource for Nursing Ethics: http://www.NursingEthics.ca
- Center for Jewish Ethics https://www.reconstructingjudaism.org/connect/center-for-jewish-ethics
- Center for Practical Bioethics: https://www.practicalbioethics.org
- Council for Europe, Committee on Bioethics https://www.coe.int/en/web/bioethics
- Global Network of WHO Collaborating Centers for Bioethics https://www.who.int/ethics/partnerships/global_network/en/
- The Hastings Center: http://www.thehastingscenter.org
- International Care Ethics (ICE) Observatory: https://www.surrey.ac.uk/international-care-ethics-observatory
- International Council of Nurses: http://www.icn.ch
- The National Academies of Sciences, Engineering, and Medicine, Health and Medicine Division: https://www.nationalacademies.org/hmd
- National Catholic Bioethics Center: http://www.ncbcenter.org
- National Hospice and Palliative Care Organization: https://www.nhpco.org
- National Human Genome Research Institute: https://www.genome.gov/
- National Institutes of Health Resources on Bioethics Interest Group: https://oir.nih.gov/sigs/bioethics-interest-group
- Office for Human Research Protections: http://www.hhs.gov/ohrp
- Organ Procurement and Transplantation Network: https://optn.transplant.hrsa.gov
- Presidential Commission for the Study of Bioethical Issues: https://bioethicsarchive.georgetown.edu/pcsbi
- Society for Jewish Ethics: http://societyofjewishethics.org/node/35
- Society of Critical Care Medicine: https://www.sccm.org/Education-Center/Clinical-Resources/Ethics
- United Network for Organ Sharing: http://www.unos.org
- University of Pennsylvania Department of Medical Ethics & Health Policy: http://medicalethicshealthpolicy.med.upenn.edu
- Veterans Administration's National Center for Ethics in Health Care: www.ethics.va.gov

Continued

BOX 11.12

Organizations With Electronically Available Ethics Resources—cont'd

- Yeshiva University Center for Bioethics: https://www.yu.edu/riets/Jewish-Medical-Ethics/programs

ETHICS AND LEGAL SEARCH SITES

- American Bar Association Public Resources: http://www.americanbar.org/portals/public_resources.html
- Bioethics Information Resources, US National Library of Medicine, National Institutes of Health (bioethics online literature search): https://www.nlm.nih.gov/bsd/bioethics.html
- Bioethics Research Library at Georgetown University: https://bioethics.georgetown.edu/
- Legal Information Institute: http://www.law.cornell.edu
- Medical College of Wisconsin, Center for Bioethics and Medical Humanities: http://www.mcw.edu/Center-for-Bioethics-and-Medical-Humanities.htm

of a patient, whereas the APRN's hiring organization has established cost containment as a key objective and does not support use of this intervention (Donagrandi & Eddy, 2000). In this and other situations, APRNs are faced with an ethical dilemma created by multiple commitments and the need to balance obligations to all parties.

The first sign of challenges to ethical practice are feelings of moral distress. The first step in overcoming any barrier to ethical practice is learning how to reflect on and articulate what is causing the moral distress. Mapping the experience of moral distress, especially acknowledging the limits of responsibilities, is one approach that can lead an APRN to critically reflect on what is contributing to moral distress, which makes it possible to see other perspectives and appreciate the ethical complexities in clinical practice (Dudzinski, 2016).

APRNs should identify resources within and outside the institution where they work to assist with the resolution of ethical problems. Internal resources may include chaplains, liaison psychiatrists, patient representatives, social workers, ethics committees and their members, and ethics consultation services. Resources outside the institution include the ANA's Center on Ethics and Human Rights (www.nursingworld.org/ethics), the Veterans Administration's National Center for Ethics in Health Care (www.ethics.va.gov), ethics groups in national specialty organizations, and ethics centers in universities or large healthcare institutions. The recognition of a moral dilemma does not commit the APRN to conducting and managing the process of resolution individually. APRNs should engage appropriate resources to address the identified needs and work toward agreement. Many specialty organizations issue policy statements related to ethical issues or publish guidelines for their members' use in responding to ethical problems. Box 11.12 lists websites that contain valuable ethics resources for clinicians.

CONCLUSION

The changing healthcare environment has placed extraordinary demands on nurses in all care settings. Many forces conflict with nursing's moral imperatives for involvement, connection, and commitment. Professional ethical practice demands that APRNs have knowledge of ethical principles and concepts that are the foundation of our profession and an awareness of the ethical complexities of clinical practice. As a core competency for the APRN, ethical practice reflects the art and science of nursing. The APRN is in a key position to assume a more decisive role in managing the resolution of moral issues and helping create ethically responsive healthcare environments. The identification of patterns in the presentation of moral issues enables the APRN to engage in preventive strategies to improve the ethical climate in patient care environments. Ethical decision-making skills, together with clinical expertise and leadership, empower the APRN to assume leadership roles in public policy processes that promote social justice within the larger healthcare arena. Ethical practice begins during formal education and continues throughout the APRN's career.

KEY SUMMARY POINTS

- APRNs face a variety of ethical challenges typically complicated by problems with communication, the presence of interprofessional conflict, the advances in medical technology, and managing competing commitments and obligations.
- Resolution of ethical challenges for APRNs depends more on thoughtful deliberation than simply following rules or making a choice to avoid litigation.
- APRNs must rigorously and continuously practice self-awareness, becoming exquisitely sensitive to their own hidden biases, which in turn helps develop strong moral agency.

REFERENCES

Ajovalasit, D., Cerniauskaite, M., Aluas, M., Alves, I., Bosisio Fazzi, L., Griffo, G., Leonardi, M., & Pessina, A. (2012). Multidisciplinary research network on health and disability training on the International Classification of Functioning, Disability and Health, Ethics and Human Rights. *American Journal of Physical Medicine and Rehabilitation, 91*(13 Suppl. 1), S168–S172.

American Association of Colleges of Nursing. (2019). AACN's vision for academic nursing. *Journal of Professional Nursing, 35*, 249–259.

American Association of Colleges of Nursing. (2021). *Core competencies for professional nursing education*. American Association of Colleges of Nursing.

American Association of Critical-Care Nurses. (2008). *Position statement: Moral distress*. Author.

American Association of Critical-Care Nurses. (2015). *AACN standards for establishing and sustaining healthy work environments: A journey to excellence* (2nd ed.). http://www.aacn.org/wd/hwe/docs/hwestandards.pdf

American Nurses Association. (2010). *Nursing's social policy statement: The essence of the profession*. Author.

American Nurses Association. (2015). *Code of ethics for nurses, with interpretive statements*. Author.

American Society of Anesthesiologists. (2018). Ethical guidelines for the anesthesia care of patients with do-not-resuscitate orders or other directives that limit treatment. https://www.asahq.org/standards-and-guidelines/ethical-guidelines-for-the-anesthesia-care-of-patients-with-do-not-resuscitate-orders-or-other-directives-that-limit-treatment

Anderson, G. F., Hussey, P., & Petrosyan, V. (2019). It's still the prices, stupid: Why the US spends so much on healthcare, and a tribute to Uwe Reinhart. *Health Affairs, 38*(1), 87–95.

Applebaum, P. S. (2007). Assessment of patient's competence to consent to treatment. *New England Journal of Medicine, 357*, 1834–1840.

Austin, C. L., Saylor, R., & Finley, P. J. (2017). Moral distress in physicians and nurses: Impact on professional quality of life and turnover. *Psychological Trauma: Theory, Research, Practice, and Policy, 9*(4), 399–406. doi:10.1037/tra0000201

Barbara, V. (2020). *Brazil is in Coronavirus free fall*. New York Times. June 8, 2020. https://www.nytimes.com/2020/06/08/opinion/brazil-coronavirus-bolsonaro.html?referringSource=articleShare

Beauchamp, T. L., & Childress, J. F. (2019). *Principles of biomedical ethics* (8th ed.). Oxford University Press.

Beery, T. A., Workman, M. L., & Eggert, J. A. (2018). Genetics and genomics in nursing and health care. FA Davis.

Benner, P., Tanner, C., & Chesla, C. (2009). *Expertise in nursing practice: Caring, clinical judgment, and ethics* (2nd ed.). Springer.

Benton, D. C., Alexander, M., Fotsch, R., & Livanos, N. (2020). Lessons learned and insights gained: A regulatory analysis of the impacts, challenges, and responses to COVID-19. *The Online Journal of Issues in Nursing, 25*(3). doi:10.3912/OJIN.Vol-25No03PPT51

Berlinger, N., Wynia, M., Powell, T., Hester, M., Milliken, A., Fabi, R., Cohn, F., Guidry-Grimes, L. K., Watson, J. C., Bruce, L., Chuang, E. J., Oei, G., Abbott, J., & Jenks, N. P. (2020). *Ethical framework for health care institutions responding to novel coronavirus SARS-CoV-2 (COVID-10): Guidelines for institutional ethics services responding to COVID-19*. The Hastings Center. March 16, 2020. https://www.thehastingscenter.org/ethicalframeworkcovid19/

Biddison, E. L. D., Faden, R., Gwon, H. S., Mareiniss, D. P., Regenberg, A. C., Schoch-Spana, M., Schwartz, J., & Toner, E. S. (2019). Too many patients…A framework to guide statewide allocation of scarce mechanical ventilation during disasters. *CHEST, 155*(4), 848–854.

Bodenheimer, T. S., & Grumbach, K. (2012). *Understanding health policy: A clinical approach* (6th ed.). Lange Medical/McGraw Hill.

Bosslet, G. T., Pope, T. M., Rubenfeld, G. D., Lo, B., Truog, R. D., Rushton, C. H., et al. American Thoracic Society ad hoc Committee on Futile and Potentially Inappropriate Treatment American Thoracic Society American Association for Critical Care. Nurses American College of Chest Physicians European Society for Intensive Care Medicine Society of Critical Care. (2015). An official ATS/AACN/ACCP/ESICM/SCCM policy statement: Responding to requests for potentially inappropriate treatments in intensive care units. *American Journal of Respiratory and Critical Care Medicine, 191*(11), 1318–1330.

Brashers, V., Haizlip, J., & Owen, J. A. (2019). The ASPIRE model: Grounding the IPEC core competencies for interprofessional collaborative practice within a foundational framework. *Journal of Interprofessional Care, 34*(1), 128–132. doi:10.1080/13561820.2019.1624513

Brownie, S., Thomas, J., McAllister, L., & Groves, M. (2014). Australian health reforms: Enhancing interprofessional practice and competency within the health workforce. *Journal of Interprofessional Care, 28*(3), 252–253.

Bruce, C. R., Liang, C., Blumenthal-Barby, J. S., Zimmerman, J., Downey, A., Pham, L., Theriot, L., Delgado, E. D., & White, D.

(2015). Barriers and facilitators to initiating and completing time-limited trials in critical care. *Critical Care Medicine, 43*(12), 2535–2543.

Bruce, C. R., Miller, S. M., & Zimmerman, J. L. (2015). A qualitative study exploring moral distress in the ICU team: The importance of unit functionality and intrateam dynamics. *Critical Care Medicine, 43*(4), 823–831.

Calleja, J. L., Soublette Sánchez, A., & Radedek Soto, P. (2020). Is clinical simulation an effective learning tool in teaching clinical ethics? *Medwave, 20*(02).

Camak, D. J. (2016). Increasing importance of genetics in nursing. *Nurse Education Today, 44*, 86–91.

Canadian Interprofessional Health Collaborative. (2010). A national interprofessional competency framework. www.cihc.ca/files/CIHC_IPCompetencies_Feb1210.pdf

Cantor, N. (2001). Twenty-five years after Quinlan: A review of the jurisprudence of death and dying. *Journal of Law, Medicine & Ethics, 29*, 182–196.

Chen, R., Sun, C., Chen, J. J., Jen, H. J., Kang, X. L., Kao, C. C., & Chou, K. R. (2021). A large-scale survey on trauma, burnout, and posttraumatic growth among nurses during the COVID-19 pandemic. *International Journal of Mental Health Nursing, 30*(1), 102–116.

Conrad, D. A., Grembowski, D., Hernandez, S. E., Lau, B., & Marcus-Smith, M. (2014). Emerging lessons from regional and state innovation in value-based payment reform: Balancing collaboration and disruptive innovation. *Milbank Quarterly, 92*(3), 568–623.

Cooper, R. J. (2012). Making the case for ethical decision making models. *Nurse Prescribing, 10*(12), 607–611.

Courtwright-Lim, A., & Drago, M. (2020). Ethics of genetic testing. *Medicine, 48*(10), 675–679.

Dadzie, G., & Aziato, L. (2020). Perceived interpersonal and institutional challenges to patient advocacy in clinical nursing practice: A qualitative study from Ghana. *International Journal of Health Professions, 7*(1), 45–52.

Daugirdas, J. T., Blake, P. G., & Ing, T. S. (2012). *Handbook of dialysis* (4th ed.). Walters Kluwer-Lippincott, Williams & Williams.

DeCamp, M., Pomerantz, D., Cotts, K., et al. (2018). Ethical issues in the design and implementation of population health programs. *Journal of General Internal Medicine, 33*, 370–375. doi:10.1007/s11606-017-4234-4

DeMartino, E. S., Dudzinski, D. M., Doyle, C. K., Sperry, B. P., Gregory, S. E., Siegler, M., Sulmasy, D. P., Mueller, P. S., & Kramer, D. B. (2017). Who decides when a patient can't? Statutes on alternate decision makers. *New England Journal of Medicine, 376*(15), 1478–1482.

DePergola, P. A. (2018). Euthanasia, assisted-suicide and palliative sedation: A brief clarification and reinforcement of the moral logic. *Online Journal of Health Ethics, 14*(2). doi:10.18785/ojhe.1402.04

DeVito, T., Leavitt, J., & Saleh, N. (2019). Key advances in oncology 2018. *Oncology, 33*(1), 6–8. January 17, 2019. https://www.cancernetwork.com/view/key-advances-oncology-2018

Doherty, R. F., & Purtilo, R. B. (2016). *Ethical dimensions in the health professions* (6th ed.). Elsevier Saunders.

Donagrandi, M. A., & Eddy, M. (2000). Ethics of case management: Implications for advanced practice nursing. *Clinical Nurse Specialist, 14*, 241–249.

Dove, E. S., Kelly, S. E., Lucivero, F., Machirori, M., Dheensa, S., & Prainsack, B. (2017). Beyond individualism: Is there a place for relational autonomy in clinical practice and research? *Clinical Ethics, 12*(3), 150–165.

Dudzinski, D. M. (2016). Navigating moral distress using the moral distress map. *Journal of Medical Ethics, 42*(5), 321–324.

Dzau., V. J., Kirch, D., & Nasca, T. (2020). Preventing a parallel pandemic—a national strategy to protect clinicians' well-being. *New England Journal of Medicine, 383*(6), 513–515.

Edwards, M., & Chalmers, K. (2002). Double agency in clinical research. *Canadian Journal of Nursing Research, 34*, 131–142.

Emanuel, E. J. (1988). A review of the ethical and legal aspects of terminating medical care. *The American Journal of Medicine, 84*, 291–301.

Emanuel, E. J. (2012). Where are the health care cost savings? *JAMA, 307*(1), 39–40. doi:10.1001/jama.2011.1927

Epstein, E. G., & Hamric, A. B. (2009). Moral distress, moral residue, and the crescendo effect. *Journal of Clinical Ethics, 20*(4), 330–342.

Feister, A. (2015). Teaching nonauthoritarian clinical ethics: Using an inventory of bioethical positions. *Hastings Center Report, 45*(2), 20–26.

Ferrell, B., Malloy, P., & Virani, R. (2015). The end of life nursing consortium project. *Annals Palliative Medicine, 4*(2), 61–69.

Ferrell, B. R., Twaddle, M. L., Melnick, A., & Meier, D. E. (2018). National consensus project clinical practice guidelines for quality palliative care guidelines. *Journal of Palliative Medicine, 21*(12), 1684–1689.

Feuer, A., & Rashbaum, W. K. (2020). We ran out of space: Bodies pile up as NY struggles to bury its dead. *New York Times*. April 30, 2020. https://www.nytimes.com/2020/04/30/nyregion/coronavirus-nyc-funeral-home-morgue-bodies.html?referringSource=articleShare

The Foundation Coalition. (n.d.) Understanding conflict and conflict management. http://www.foundationcoalition.org/publications/brochures/conflict.pdf

Fourie, C. (2015). Moral distress and moral conflict in clinical ethics. *Bioethics, 29*(2), 91–97.

Fragoulakis, V., Patrinos, G. P., & Mitropoulou, C. (2020). Economic evaluation of genomic and personalized medicine interventions: Implications in public health. In G. Patrinos (Ed.), *Applied Genomics and Public Health 2020 Jan 1* (pp. 287–304). Academic Press.

Gardner, C. L. (2015). Adherence: a concept analysis. *International Journal of Nursing Knowledge, 26*(2), 96–101.

Garfield, R., Majerol, M., Damico, A., & Foutz, J. (2016). *The uninsured: A primer. Key facts about health insurance and the uninsured in America*. The Henry James Kaiser Family Foundation.

Garros, D., Austin, W., & Carnevale, F. A. (2015). Moral distress in pediatric intensive care. *JAMA Pediatrics, 169*(10), 885–886.

Gillick, M. (2012). How Medicare shapes the way we die. *Journal of Health & Biomedical Law, 8*, 27–55.

Gordon, E. J., & Hamric, A. B. (2006). The courage to stand up: The cultural politics of nurses' access to ethics consultation. *Journal of Clinical Ethics, 17*, 231–254.

Gordon, M. (2010). *Manual of nursing diagnoses*. Jones & Bartlett Publishers.

Grace, P. J., Robinson, E. M., Jurchak, M., Zollfrank, A. A., & Lee, S. M. (2014). Clinical ethics residency for nurses: An education model to decrease moral distress and strengthen nurse retention in acute care. *Journal of Nursing Administration, 44*(12), 640–646.

Grady, C., Danis, M., Soeken, K. L., O'Donnell, P., Taylor, C., Farrar, A., & Ulrich, C. (2008). Does ethics education influence the moral action of practicing nurses and social workers? *American Journal of Bioethics, 8*(4), 4–11.

Griffith, R., & Tengnah, C. (2013). Maintaining professional boundaries: Keep your distance. *British Journal of Community Nursing, 18*(1), 43–46.

Gun Violence Archive. (2022). https://www.gunviolencearchive.org

Guzak, J. R. (2015). Affect in ethical decision making: Mood matters. *Ethics and Behavior, 25*(5), 386–399.

Hall, W. J., Chapman, M. V., Lee, K. M., Merino, Y. M., Thomas, T. W., Payne, K., Eng, E., Day, S. H., & Coyne-Beasley, T. (2015). Implicit racial/ethnic bias among health care professionals and its influence on health care outcomes: A systemic review. *American Journal of Public Health, 105*(12), e60–e76.

Hammes, B. J., Rooney, B. L., Gundrum, J. D., Hickman, S. E., & Hager, N. (2012). The POLST program: A retrospective review of the demographics of use and outcomes in one community where advance directives are prevalent. *Journal of Palliative Medicine, 15*(1), 77–85.

Hamric, A. B., Borchers, C. T., & Epstein, E. G. (2012). Development and testing of an instrument to measure moral distress in healthcare professionals. *AJOB Primary Research, 3*(2), 1–9.

Hamric, A. B., Epstein, E. G., & White, K. R. (2013). Moral distress and the health care organization. In G. Filerman, A. Mills, & P. Schyve (Eds.), *Managerial ethics in healthcare: A new perspective* (pp. 137–158). Health Administration Press.

Hamric, A. B., Schwarz, J., Cohen, L., Mahon, M., & Ayer, C. (2018). Assisted suicide/Aid in dying: What is the nurse's role? A policy dialogue. *American Journal of Nursing, 118*(5), 50–59.

Hanna, A. F., & Suplee, P. D. (2012). Don't cross the line: Respecting professional boundaries. *Nursing2020, 42*(9), 40–47.

Harrowing, J., & Mill, J. (2010). Moral distress among Ugandan nurses providing HIV care: A critical ethnography. *International Journal of Nursing Studies, 47*, 723–731.

Harvard Health Publishing Medical Dictionary of Health Terms. https://www.health.harvard.edu/a-through-c

Hay-Smith, E. J. C., Brown, M., Anderson, L., & Treharne, G. J. (2016). Once a clinician, always a clinician: A systematic review to develop a typology of clinician-researcher dual-role experiences in health research with patient-participants. *BMC Medical Research Methodology, 16*(1), 1–17. 95.

Hegge, M., & Bunkers, S. (2020). Lingering presence: The candle still burns. *Nursing Science Quarterly, 33*(2), 110–114.

Hemberg, J. A., & Vilander, S. (2017). Cultural and communicative competence in the caring relationship with patients from another culture. *Scandinavian Journal of Caring Sciences, 31*(4), 822–829.

Hicks, D. (2011). *Dignity: The essential role it plays in resolving conflict*. Yale University Press.

Ho, A. (2017). Deep ethical learning: Taking the interplay of human and artificial intelligence seriously. *Hastings Center Report, 49*(1), 36–39.

Holder, K. V., & Schenthal, S. J. (2007). Watch your step: Nursing and professional boundaries. *Nursing Management, 38*, 24–29.

Institute of Medicine. (2011). *The future of nursing: Leading change, advancing health*. National Academies Press.

International Association of Forensic Nurses. (2009). The use of emergency contraception post sexual assault. Position paper. http://c.ymcdn.com/sites/www.forensicnurses.org/resource/resmgr/Position_Papers/IAFN_Postion_Statement-Emer.pdf

International Council of Nurses. (2012). *The ICN code of ethics for nurses*. International Council of Nurses.

Interprofessional Education Collaborative. (2011). Core competencies for interprofessional collaborative practice: Report of an expert panel. http://www.aacn.nche.edu/education/pdf/IPECReport.pdf

Interprofessional Education Collaborative. (2016). Core competencies for interprofessional collaborative practice: 2016 update. http://www.aacn.nche.edu/education-resources/IPEC-2016-Updated-Core-Competencies-Report.pdf

Jameson, J. K. (2003). Transcending intractable conflict in health care: An exploratory study of communication and conflict among anesthesia providers. *Journal of Health Communications, 8*, 563–581.

Jameton, A. (1984). *Nursing practice: The ethical issues*. Prentice Hall.

Jameton, A. (1993). Dilemmas of moral distress: Moral responsibility and nursing practice. *AWHONN's Clinical Issues in Perinatalogy and Women's Health Nursing, 4*(1993), 542–551.

The Joint Commission. (2008). Sentinel event alert: Behaviors that undermine a culture of safety. https://www.jointcommission.org/assets/1/18/SEA_40.PDF

Jonsen, A. R., Siegler, M., & Winslade, W. J. (2015). *Clinical ethics: A practical approach to ethical decisions in clinical medicine* (8th ed.). McGraw-Hill.

Kennedy, J. (2012). Demystifying the role of nurse practitioners in hospice: Nurse practitioners as an integral part of the hospice plan of care. *Home Health Care Nurse, 30*, 48–51.

Laabs, C. A. (2005). Moral problems and distress among nurse practitioners in primary care. *Journal of the American Academy of Nurse Practitioners, 17*, 76–84.

Laabs, C. A. (2012). Confidence and knowledge regarding ethics among advanced practice nurses. *Nursing Education Perspectives, 33*, 10–14.

Lamiani, G., Borghi, L., & Argentero, P. (2015). When healthcare professionals cannot do the right thing: A systematic review of moral distress and its correlates. *Journal of Health Psychology, 22*(1), 1–17.

Lazenby, M., McCorkle, R., & Sulmasy, D. P. (2014). *Safe passage: A global spiritual sourcebook for care at the end of life*. Oxford University Press.

Lechasseur, K., Caux, C., Dollé, S., & Legault, A. (2018). Ethical competence: An integrative review. *Nursing Ethics, 25*(6), 694–706.

Lee, A. L., Mader, E. M., & Morley, C. P. (2015). Teaching cross-cultural communication skills online. *Family Medicine, 47*(4), 302–308.

Lu, Y., & Temple, J. R. (2019). Dangerous weapons or dangerous people? The temporal associations between gun violence and mental health. *Preventive Medicine, 121*, 1–6.

Lützén, K., Dahlqvist, V., Eriksson, S., & Norberg, A. (2006). Developing the concept of moral sensitivity in health care practice. *Nursing Ethics, 13*(2), 187–196.

Mason, D. J. (2016). Promoting the health of families and communities: A moral imperative. *Hastings Center Report, 46*, S48–S51.

Maxfield, D., Grenny, J., Lavandero, R., & Groah, L. (2010). The silent treatment: Why safety tools and checklists aren't enough to save lives. https://www.vitalsmarts.com/resource/silent-treatment/

McCullough, L. B. (2005). Practicing preventive ethics—The keys to avoiding ethical conflicts in health care. *The Physician Executive, 31*, 18–21.

Meyer, E. C., Carnevale, F. A., Lillehei, C., & Uveges, M. K. (2020). Widening the ethical lens in critical care settings. *AACN Advanced Critical Care, 31*(2), 210–220.

Milionis, C. (2013). Provision of healthcare in the context of financial crisis: Approaches to the Greek health system and international implications. *Nursing Philosophy, 14*(1), 17–27.

Milliken, A. (2017). Toward everyday ethics: Strategies for shifting perspectives. *AACN Advanced Critical Care, 28*(3), 291–296.

Milliken, A. (2018). Ethical awareness: What it is and why it matters. *The Online Journal of Issues in Nursing, 23*(1). doi:10.3912/OJIN.Vol23No01Man01

Montello, M. (2014). Narrative ethics: The role of stories in bioethics, special report. *Hastings Center Report, 44*(1), S2–S6. doi:10.1002/hast.260

Morley, G., Grady, C., McCarthy, J., & Ulrich, C. M. (2020). COVID-19: Ethical challenges for nurses. *Hastings Center Report, 50*, 1–5.

Morley, G., & Shashidhara, S. (2020). Debriefing as a response to moral distress. *Journal of Clinical Ethics, 31*(3), 283–290.

National Academies of Sciences, Engineering, and Medicine. (2019). *Taking action against clinician burnout: A systems approach to professional well-being*. National Academies Press.

National Academies of Sciences, Engineering, and Medicine. (2021). *The future of nursing 2020–2030: Charting a path to achieve health equity*: The National Academies Press. doi:10.17226/25982

National Council of State Boards of Nursing. (2018). *A nurse's guide to professional boundaries*. Author. www.ncsbn.org

National POLST. (2022). http://www.polst.org

Nelson, J. E., Hanson, L. C., Keller, K. L., Carson, S. S., Cox, C. E., Tulsky, J. A., White, D. B., Chai, E. J., Weiss, S. P., & Danis, M. (2017). The voice of surrogate decision makers: Family responses to prognostic information in chronic critical illness. *American Journal of Respiratory and Critical Care Medicine, 196*(7), 864–872.

Nelson, W. A., Gardent, P. B., Shulman, E., & Splaine, M. E. (2010). Preventing ethics conflicts and improving health care quality through system redesign. *Quality and Safety in Health Care, 19*, 526–530.

Noddings, N. (2010). Complexity in caring and empathy. *Abstracta* Special Issue V, pp. 6–12.

Oregon Death With Dignity Act Data Summary. (2016). https://www.oregon.gov/oha/ph/providerpartnerresources/evaluationresearch/deathwithdignityact/documents/year19.pdf

Oregon Death With Dignity Act Requirements. (2022). https://www.oregon.gov/oha/PH/PROVIDERPARTNERRESOURCES/EVALUATIONRESEARCH/DEATHWITHDIGNITYACT/Documents/requirements.pdf

Pandos, O. C. (2020). DIY genetic tests: A product of fact or fallacy? *Journal of Bioethical Inquiry, 17*(3), 319–324.

Patient Protection and Affordable Care Act, 42 U.S.C. § 18001. (2010).

Pattni, N., Arzola, C., Malavade, A., Varmani, S., Krimus, L., & Friedman, Z. (2019). Challenging authority and speaking up in the operating room environment: A narrative synthesis. *British Journal of Anaesthesia, 122*(2), 233–244.

Pavlish, C. L., Henrikson, J., Brown-Saltzman, K., Robinson, E. M., Shefa Wards, U., Farra, C., Chen, B., & Jakel, P. (2020). A team-based early action protocol to address ethical concerns in the intensive care unit. *American Journal of Critical Care, 29*(1), 49–58.

Perry, D. J., Willis, D. G., Peterson, K. S., & Grace, P. J. (2017). Exercising nursing essential and effective freedom in behalf of social justice: A humanizing model. *Advances in Nursing Science, 40*(3), 244–262.

Phalen, P., Bridgeford, E., Gant, L., Kivisto, A., Ray, B., & Fitzgerald, S. (2020). Baltimore ceasefire 365: Estimated impact of a recurring community-led ceasefire on gun violence. *American Journal of Public Health, 110*(4), 554–559.

Ponce, C. M., Suratt, C. E., & Chen, D. T. (2017). Cases that haunt us: The Rashomon Effect and moral distress on the consult service. *Psychosomatics, 58*(2), 191–196.

Pracher, T., Moss, B., & Mahanes, D. (2006). Moral distress in the care of patients with traumatic brain injury. *Poster presentation at the annual meeting of the American Association of Neuroscience Nurses*, San Diego, CA.

Quigley, P. (2015). Mapping the human genome: Implications for practice. *Nursing2019, 45*(9), 26–34.

Quill, T. E. (1991). Death and Dignity: A case of individualized decision-making. *New England Journal of Medicine, 324*(10), 691–694.

Rada, A. G. (2021). Spain will become the sixth country worldwide to allow euthanasia and assisted suicide. *BMR, 372*(147). doi:10.1136/bmj.n147

Robinson, E. M., Lee, S. M., Zollfrank, A., Jurchak, M., Frost, D., & Grace, P. (2014). Enhancing moral agency: Clinical ethics residency for nurses. *Hastings Center Report, 44*(5), 12–20.

Robinson, E. M., Romain, J. F., & Cremens, M. C. (2020). Ethics and end of life. In R. M. Kacmarek, J. K. Stoller, & A. J. Heuer (Eds.), *Egan's fundamentals of respiratory care* (12th ed.) (pp. 1299–1317). Elsevier Publishing.

Roll, M. A., Kuys, S., Walsh, J. R., Tronstad, O., Ziegenfuss, M. D., & Mullany, D. V. (2017). Long-term survival and health-related quality of life in adults after extra corporeal membrane oxygenation. *Heart, Lung and Circulation, 28*(7), 1090–1098. doi:10.1016/j.hlc.2018.06.1044

Rushton, C. H., & Penticuff, J. H. (2007). A framework for analysis of ethical dilemmas in critical care nursing. *AACN Advanced Critical Care, 18*, 323–328.

Salvage, J., & White, J. (2019). Nursing leadership and health policy: Everybody's business. *International Nursing Review, 66*(2), 147–150.

Shannon, S. E. (1997). The roots of interdisciplinary conflict around ethical issues. *Critical Care Nursing Clinics of North America, 9*, 13–28.

Shannon, S. E., Mitchell, P. H., & Cain, K. C. (2002). Patients, nurses, and physicians have differing views of quality of critical care. *Journal of Nursing Scholarship, 34*, 173–179.

Sohrabi, C., Alsafi, Z., O'Neill, N., Khan, M., Kerwan, A., Al-Jabir, A., Iosifidis, C., & Agha, R. (2020). World Health Organization declares global emergency: A review of the 2019 novel coronavirus (COVID-19). *International Journal of Surgery, 76*, 71–76.

Span, P. (2015). A surgery standard under fire. *The New York Times*. https://www.nytimes.com/2015/03/03/health/a-30-day-surgical-standard-is-under-scrutiny.html

Spielman, B. J. (1993). Conflict in medical ethics cases: Seeking patterns of resolution. *Journal of Clinical Ethics, 4*, 212–218.

Stokes, F., & Palmer, A. (2020). Artificial intelligence and robotics in nursing: Ethics of caring as a guide to divide tasks between AI and humans. *Nursing Philosophy, 21*(4). doi:10.1111/nup.12306

Strong, C. (2007). Specified principlism: What is it and does it really resolve cases better than casuistry? *Journal of Medicine and Philosophy, 25*, 323–341.

Sulmasy, L. S., & Mueller, P. S. (2017). Ethics and the legalization of physician-assisted suicide: An American College of Physicians position paper. *Annals of Internal Medicine, 167*, 576–578.

Trautmann, J., Epstein, E., Rovnyak, V., & Snyder, A. (2015). Relationships among moral distress, level of practice independence, and intent to leave of nurse practitioners in emergency departments: Results from a national survey. *Advanced Emergency Nursing Journal, 37*(2), 134–145.

Ulrich, C. (2012). Nursing ethics in everyday practice. *Sigma Theta Tau International*.

Ulrich, C., Soeken, K., & Miller, N. (2003). Predictors of nurse practitioners' autonomy: Effects of organizational, ethical and market characteristics. *Journal of the American Academy of Nurse Practitioners, 15*, 319–325.

US Department of Health and Human Services Office of Minority Health. (2001). *National standards for culturally and linguistically appropriate services in health care: Final report*. https://minorityhealth.hhs.gov/assets/pdf/checked/finalreport.pdf

Webster, G., and Bayliss, F. (2000). Moral residue. In S. Rubin & L. Zoloth (Eds.), *Margin of error: The Ethics of Mistakes in the Practice of Medicine* (pp. 217–231). University Publishing Group.

Wicclair, M. R. (2014). Managing conscientious objection in health care institutions. *HEC Forum, 26*(3), 267–283. Springer Netherlands.

Wynn, S. (2014). Decisions by surrogates: An overview of surrogate consent laws in the United States. *Bifocal, 36*(1), 10–14. https://www.americanbar.org/groups/law_aging/publications/bifocal/vol_36/issue_1_october2014/default_surrogate_consent_statutes/

Yadev, K. N., Gabler, N. B., Cooney, E., Kent, S., Kim, J., Herbst, N., Mante, A., Halpern, S., & Courtright, K. (2017). Approximately one in three US adults completes any type of advance directive for end of life care. *Health Affairs, 36*(7), 1244–1251.

Yuki, K., Fujiogi, M., & Koutsogiannaki, S. (2020). COVID-19 pathophysiology: A review. *Clinical Immunology, 215*, 1–7.

Yuste, R., & Goering, S. (2017). Four ethical priorities for neurotechnologies and artificial intelligence. *Nature, 551*(7679), 159–163.

Zhou, F., Yu, T., Du, R., Fan, G., Liu, Y., Liu, Z., Xiang, J., Wang, Y., Song, B., Gu, X., Guan, L., Wei, Y., Li, H., Wu, X., Xu, J., Tu, S., Zhang, Y., Chen, H., & Cao, B. (2020). Clinical course and risk factors for mortality of adult inpatients with COVID-19 in Wuhan, China: A retrospective cohort study. *The Lancet, 395*(10229), 1054–1062. doi:10.1016/S0140-6736(20)30566-3

PART III Advanced Practice Roles: The Operational Definitions of Advanced Practice Nursing

12

THE CLINICAL NURSE SPECIALIST

MARY FRAN TRACY ■ SUE SENDELBACH

"If you obey all the rules, you miss all the fun."
~ Katharine Hepburn

CHAPTER CONTENTS

CLINICAL NURSE SPECIALIST PRACTICE: COMPETENCIES WITHIN THE SPHERES OF IMPACT 387
- Direct Clinical Practice 391
- Guidance and Coaching 394
- Evidence-Based Practice 396
- Leadership 398
- Collaboration 401
- Ethical Practice 401

CURRENT MARKETPLACE FORCES AND CONCERNS 402
- Scope of Practice and Delegated Authority 405
- *The Future of Nursing* Reports 405
- Consensus Model for APRN Regulation and Implications for the Clinical Nurse Specialist 406
- Reimbursement for Clinical Nurse Specialist Services 408
- Availability and Standardization of Educational Curricula for Clinical Nurse Specialists 409
- National Certification for Clinical Nurse Specialists 409
- Variability in Individual Clinical Nurse Specialist Practices and Prescriptive Authority 410
- Understanding the Similarities and Differences Between Clinical Nurse Specialists and Nurse Practitioners 410

ROLE IMPLEMENTATION 412
- Evaluation of Practice 412

FUTURE DIRECTIONS 413

CONCLUSION 415

KEY SUMMARY POINTS 415

The clinical nurse specialist (CNS) role was created in response to the increasingly complex nursing care evolving in the early 20th century (Chapter 1). This increasing complexity provided the opportunity for expert nurses to develop specialty knowledge and judgment and to provide expert direct care of patients with increasingly complex conditions. It also allowed for improved outcomes for these populations, particularly in emerging specialty areas such as psychiatry, oncology, and critical care (Chapter 1). Advanced clinical expertise in a specialty population throughout the health continuum in clinical and community settings is the essence, the core value, of the CNS role. Historically, the role has been versatile, evolving, flexing, responding, and adapting to patient populations and healthcare environments. However, the core strength of the CNS in providing complex specialty care while improving the quality of care delivery has remained central to the understanding of this advanced practice registered nurse (APRN) role. The American Nurses Association (ANA) has defined APRNs as nurses who "practice from both expanded and specialized knowledge and skills" (ANA, 2003, p. 9). An expanded knowledge base and skill set refers to the "acquisition of new practice knowledge and skills, including the knowledge and skills that authorize role autonomy within areas of practice that may overlap traditional boundaries of medical practice" (ANA, 2003, p. 9; see Chapter 3). The primary role of the CNS is to continually work toward improving the nursing care of patients and patient outcomes (ANA, 2010; National Association of Clinical Nurse Specialists [NACNS], 2019b), whether at the individual or population level. The purpose of this chapter is to describe the core competencies, current marketplace challenges, and future directions for CNSs.

In its *Statement on Clinical Nurse Specialist Practice and Education*, the NACNS (2019b) defined the CNS as an APRN who directly and indirectly manages the care of complex and vulnerable patients/families, populations, and communities; educates, mentors, and supports nursing and nursing staff; and provides the clinical expertise to facilitate change and innovation in healthcare organizations and systems. CNSs are "uniquely prepared to address healthcare delivery issues at micro, meso, and macro levels" (Tracy et al., 2020, p. 527). NACNS (2019b) describes CNSs as practicing in the three interrelated spheres of impact: patient direct care, nurses and nursing practice, and organizations and systems. As noted earlier in this text, direct care of patients is the primary distinguishing feature of CNS practice (see Chapter 6); CNSs provide this care by carefully considering the individual's environmental context (Tracy et al., 2020).

Interventions in the other two spheres of impact are intended ultimately to affect the care of patients and populations to improve outcomes. Examples of interventions in these two spheres include role modeling effective communication and advancing nursing care through leading staff nurses in evidence-based practice in the nurses and nursing practice sphere and leading quality improvement projects and redesigning the delivery of care in the organizations and systems sphere. In this chapter, the NACNS spheres of impact and the Hamric model (Chapter 3) of competencies are used to illustrate the unique contributions of the role of the CNS and how the CNS role differs from other APRN roles.

A foundation of expert practice and competencies undergirds the CNS role; however, the activities of CNSs are as varied as their individual specialty practices. The diversity of CNS specialties, differences in their individual practices, practice differences seen among CNSs in the same institution, and natural variation of an individual CNS's practice over time have created confusion about what CNSs do. Unlike other APRNs, whose primary role is to deliver direct patient care, the multifaceted CNS delivers direct patient care specifically to complex and vulnerable patients and populations, educates and supports nurses and nursing staff, provides leadership to specialty practice program development, and facilitates change and innovation in healthcare systems (NACNS, 2019b). This variability in CNS practice, even within the same institution, has characterized the role since its creation. The operationalization of the CNS role has remained deliberately broad so that CNSs can respond to rapidly evolving healthcare environments and patient population needs.

A hallmark of the role is the ability of the CNS to adapt to changing needs of patients, nurses, and healthcare systems (Kilpatrick et al., 2016b). For example, a unit- or population-based critical care CNS working with a preponderance of experienced, certified specialty staff may balance their time among direct patient care activities, educating nursing staff, and system-wide improvements. However, if there was an acute increase in staff turnover and the unit had predominantly inexperienced staff, the CNS would likely shift their focus to primarily support, education, and role modeling for the new staff. Conversely, if a preventive cardiology CNS works in an outpatient clinic in the same institution and sees a panel of patients as a provider of expert specialty care, that CNS practice may focus more on direct patient care and less on nursing staff education and system-wide improvements. Several clinical, staff, and system variables must be weighed when planning for CNS positions and implementing the role, including the number, type, and background of nurses and other clinical staff; clinical, educational, or institutional resources; and patient population, acuity, and outcomes.

The versatility of the role is what attracts nurses to become CNSs—the ability to impact patient care on many levels. However, this versatility in CNS practice has continued to challenge understanding of the impact of CNSs on clinical outcomes and healthcare costs. Incorrect utilization of the CNS role by healthcare institutions creates blurring between nursing roles (Sanchez et al., 2019). Cycles of role misunderstanding and variability, regulatory drivers, and fiscal retrenchment in the last 35 years have resulted in cycles of elimination of CNS positions in many parts of the United States to save hospitals money without jeopardizing direct care registered nurse (RN) positions. These cost-cutting measures alternate with cycles of new or re-created CNS positions. The most recent numbers estimate more than 70,000 nurses working as CNSs, with CNS numbers increasing between 2008 and 2018 (Campaign for Action, 2017; National Academies of Sciences, Engineering and Medicine [NASEM], 2021). It is difficult to know the exact number of CNSs in the United States because the Bureau of Labor Statistics currently embeds CNSs within the general RN category when tracking numbers of nurses. However, NP, certified registered nurse anesthetist (CRNA), and certified nurse-midwife (CNM) numbers are identified specifically in an APRN category (US Department of Labor, 2018a, 2018b). This creates an enormous data gap for determining an accurate CNS count, which is needed to ensure adequate CNS numbers to meet the needs of society. CNS clinical practices are shaped by many factors, such as healthcare agency needs, community needs, payer and other regulatory agency mandates, statutory limitations, supervisor requests, and individual CNS interests. Over the past few decades, CNSs have evolved their practices in response to these influential forces.

Clarifying the work and core competencies of all CNSs, regardless of specialty, has been complicated because specialty organizations have historically established varying educational, competency, and practice standards for CNSs (e.g., critical care, oncology, and neuroscience specialties). NACNS was not established until 1995 (see Chapter 1; www.nacns.org). The NACNS itself has acknowledged that advanced practice organizations for the other three APRN roles had a significant head start in defining competencies and influencing health policies related to advanced practice nursing (NACNS, 2004). The NACNS, in collaboration with ANA, the American Association of Colleges of Nursing (AACN), and specialty nursing organizations have worked diligently to define CNS practice, standards, and competencies and to develop CNS curricula (see Chapter 1; NACNS, 2019b). Ongoing work, however, is required to educate colleagues, administrators, and the public about the role of the CNS; delineation of the role from other nursing roles is feasible (Brooks, 2020; Sanchez et al., 2019). With the increasing emphasis on patient outcomes, efficiencies, patient safety, and appropriate use of technology, the CNS is uniquely prepared to address the nation's healthcare needs (Hansen et al., 2019; Storfjell et al., 2017; Tracy et al., 2020). According to the *Consensus Model for APRN Regulation*, a defining factor for all APRNs is that a significant component of the education and practice be focused on direct care of individuals (APRN Joint Dialogue Group, 2008). If CNSs want to be recognized nationally or statewide as APRNs, they must have a component of direct care of individuals in their role. If the focus is primarily on educating nurses or process improvement without direct care of individuals, the clinician is not fully enacting the role of the CNS (Cronenwett, 1995). It is the unique combination of formal specialty expertise, direct care, and evidence-based practice (EBP)/quality improvement (QI) skills that sets CNSs apart from other roles such as the expert staff nurse, nurse manager, or QI specialist (NACNS, 2019b). For the purposes of clinical practice and licensure, accreditation, credentialing, and education, the work and contributions of CNSs as APRNs must be made unambiguously clear.

New opportunities for CNS practice are presented with the continued evolution of the healthcare system (Fels et al., 2015). CNSs have consistently delivered direct and indirect care that improves patient care quality and outcomes, patient safety, and nursing practice and that ensures efficient use of resources, cost efficiency, cost savings, and revenue generation (Coen & Curry, 2016; Hansen et al., 2019; Kilpatrick et al., 2014; Purvis et al., 2018; Spruce & Butler, 2017; see Chapter 21). This is in complete alignment with the public's and health care's interests in improving the overall quality of health care. CNSs' clinical acumen and expertise are not limited to their patients' physiologic and psychological needs. Their clinical expertise permeates the other elements of their multifaceted responsibilities—education, EBP, health policy, organizational and system factors, and political change—and they are highly qualified to lead interprofessional teams in healthcare reform.

CLINICAL NURSE SPECIALIST PRACTICE: COMPETENCIES WITHIN THE SPHERES OF IMPACT

The NACNS's three spheres of impact and Hamric's six competencies (see Chapter 3 and Chapters 6 through 11) will be used to organize and explain CNS practice in this chapter. CNS students are encouraged to familiarize themselves with the *Statement on Clinical Nurse Specialist Practice and Education* (NACNS, 2019b) and with specialty specific standards (e.g., American Association of Critical-Care Nurses, 2014; Emergency Nurses Association, 2011) to supplement the population-based competencies required for licensure. Regardless of setting, specialty, or population, optimization of the CNS role involves application of the six competencies across all three spheres of impact.

Advanced practice competencies are categories of expected proficient performance and include specific knowledge and skill sets. The NACNS, along with other nursing organizations, has endorsed and defined entry-level competencies to be used by graduate programs in the preparation of CNSs (NACNS, 2019b; Table 12.1). According to the NACNS model, CNSs function within three spheres of impact—direct care of patients, nurses and nursing practice, and organizations and systems (NACNS, 2019b; see Chapter 2, Fig. 2.2). The direct care of patients and families is the central competency in Hamric's model (see Chapter 2, Fig. 2.4, 2019) and links every other competency.

The NACNS model also emphasizes the importance of direct care; clinical expertise and direct care are basic to CNS practice. Therefore the direct care of patients sphere encompasses the other two spheres of impact to depict the centrality of the patient care focus (NACNS, 2019b; see Chapter 2, Fig. 2.2). Box 12.1 presents examples of activities in the direct patient care sphere.

CNSs often execute several competencies simultaneously. They can serve as mentors, coaches, educators, guides, and role models for nursing staff and other caregivers while providing patient care or consultation. They demonstrate EBP competencies by working with staff to develop, implement, and

BOX 12.1

Examples of Clinical Nurse Specialist (CNS) Interventions in the Care of Complex and/or Vulnerable Patients

DIRECT CARE AND EVIDENCE-BASED PRACTICE

1. Provide expert, specialized assessment of complex patients.
2. Provide evidence-based treatment and care of illness, symptoms, and responses to illness using advanced concepts related to the nursing process.
3. Provide guidance and coaching to patients and families regarding illness management, health maintenance, and health behavior goals.
4. Monitor and prescribe pharmacologic and nonpharmacologic therapies.
5. Order and interpret laboratory and diagnostic tests.
6. Perform advanced procedures.

COLLABORATION AND ETHICAL PRACTICE

1. Facilitate movement of patients and families through and across healthcare settings.
2. Facilitate healthcare system access.
   a. Provide outcomes management.
   b. Provide discharge planning, providing and/or ensuring ambulatory and community follow-up.
3. Advocate for patient and family.
   a. Promote collaboration between the patient and family and the nurse and interprofessional team.
   b. Provide leadership in interprofessional ethical situations.
   c. Utilize sound ethical principles when partnering with patients and families to determine therapeutic options and plans of care.
   d. Facilitate patient/family and/or healthcare team conferences.
4. Facilitate communication among interprofessional team members.

TABLE 12.1

National Association of Clinical Nurse Specialists Core Competencies

Sphere of Impact	Competency Statement
Patient and direct care sphere	P.1 Uses relationship-building communication to promote health and wellness, healing, self-care, and peaceful end of life.
	P.2 Conducts a comprehensive health assessment in diverse care settings including psychosocial, functional, physical, and environmental factors.
	P.3 Synthesizes assessment findings using advanced knowledge, expertise, critical thinking, and clinical judgment to formulate differential diagnosis.
	P.4 Designs evidence-based, cost-effective interventions, including advanced nursing therapies, to meet the multifaceted needs of complex patients.
	P.5 Implements customized evidence-based advanced nursing interventions, including the provision of direct care.
	P.6 Prescribes medications, therapeutics, diagnostic studies, equipment, and procedures to manage the health issues of patients.
	P.7 Designs and employs educational strategies that consider readiness to learn, individual preferences, and other social determinants of health.
	P.8 Uses advanced communication skills in complex situations and difficult conversations.
	P.9 Provides expert consultation based on a broad range of theories and evidence for patients with complex healthcare needs.
	P.10 Provides education and coaching to patients with complex learning needs and atypical responses.
	P.11 Evaluates impact of nursing interventions on patients' aggregate outcomes using a scientific approach.
	P.12 Leads and facilitates coordinated care and transitions in collaboration with the patient and interprofessional team.
	P.13 Facilitates patient and family understanding of the risks, benefits, and outcomes of proposed healthcare regimens to promote informed shared decision making.
	P.14 Facilitates resolution of ethical conflicts in complex patient situations.
	P.15 Analyzes the ethical impact of scientific advances, including cost and clinical effectiveness, on patient and family values and preferences.
	P.16 Advocates for patients' preferences and rights.
Nurses and nursing practice sphere	N.1 Provides expert specialty consultation to nurses related to complex patient care needs.
	N.2 Promotes interventions that prevent the impact of implicit bias on relationship building and outcomes.
	N.3 Advocates for nurses to practice to the full extent of their role in the delivery of health care.
	N.4 Leads efforts to resolve ethical conflict and moral distress experienced by nurses and nursing staff.
	N.5 Fosters a healthy work environment by exhibiting positive regard, conveying mutual respect, and acknowledging the contributions of others.
	N.6 Employs conflict management and negotiation skills to promote a healthy work environment.
	N.7 Assesses the nursing practice environment and processes for improvement opportunities.
	N.8 Uses evidence-based knowledge as a foundation for nursing practice to achieve optimal nurse-sensitive outcomes.
	N.9 Mentors nurses and nursing staff in using evidence-based practice principles.
	N.10 Leads nurses in the process of planning, implementing, and evaluating change considering intended and unintended consequences.

TABLE 12.1

National Association of Clinical Nurse Specialist Core Competencies—cont'd

Sphere of Impact	Competency Statement
	N.11 Evaluates the outcomes of nursing practice using methods that provide valid data.
	N.12 Facilitates opportunities for nurses, students, and other staff to acquire knowledge and skills that foster professional development.
	N.13 Engages nurses in reflective practice activities that promote self-awareness and invites peer feedback to improve the practice of nursing.
	N.14 Mentors nurses to analyze legislative, regulatory, and fiscal policies that affect nursing practice and patient outcomes.
Organizations/systems sphere	O.1 Cultivates a practice environment in which mutual respect, communication, and collaboration contribute to safe, quality outcomes.
	O.2 Uses leadership, team building, negotiation, collaboration, and conflict resolution to build partnerships within and across systems and/or communities.
	O.3 Consults with healthcare team members to integrate the needs, preferences, and strengths of a population into the healthcare plan to optimize health outcomes and patient experience within a healthcare system.
	O.4 Leads and participates in systematic quality improvement and safety initiatives based on precise problem/etiology identification, gap analysis, and process evaluation.
	O.5 Provides leadership for the interprofessional team in identifying, developing, implementing, and evaluating evidence-based practices and research opportunities.
	O.6 Partners with research-focused, doctoral-prepared (i.e., PhD) colleagues to translate, conduct, and disseminate research that addresses gaps and improves clinical knowledge and practice.
	O.7 Leads and participates in the process of selecting, integrating, managing, and evaluating technology and products to promote safety, quality, efficiency, and optimal health outcomes.
	O.8 Leads and facilitates change in response to organizational and community needs in a dynamic healthcare environment.
	O.9 Evaluates system-level interventions, programs, and outcomes based on the analysis of information from relevant sources.
	O.10 Demonstrates stewardship of human and fiscal resources in decision making.
	O.11 Disseminates CNS practice and fiscal outcomes to internal stakeholders and the public.
	O.12 Promotes nursing's unique contributions to advancing health to stakeholders (e.g., the organization, community, public, and policymakers).
	O.13 Advocates for equitable health care by participating in professional organizations and public policy activities.
	O.14 Advocates for ethical principles in protecting the dignity, uniqueness, and safety of all.

Adapted from *Statement on Clinical Nurse Practice and Education* (3rd ed.), by National Association of Clinical Nurse Specialists, 2019b, p. 26–28.

evaluate EBP changes. They may collaborate in clinical research, which can impact nurses and result in system changes. CNSs provide support to nurses to promote ethical practice and mitigate the moral distress staff nurses may experience in the healthcare environment. Box 12.2 lists examples of CNS interventions in the nurses and nursing practice sphere. CNSs exert influence in the organizations and systems sphere by providing clinical and systems leadership through articulating nursing perspectives and nursing science in healthcare teams, advocating for patients or nurses, or leading quality and cost-effective improvements with technology and care processes. In addition, CNSs must be assertive and diligent in addressing embedded organizational systems and processes that promote and maintain disparities in healthcare

BOX 12.2

Examples of Clinical Nurse Specialist (CNS) Interventions in the Nurses and Nursing Practice Sphere

GUIDANCE AND COACHING

1. Educate nurses and interprofessional staff.
   a. Provide formal classes.
   b. Provide informal, bedside teaching.
   c. Develop skills of experienced staff nurses to perform as consultants on basic nursing care for colleagues so the CNS can focus on consultations for complex and vulnerable patients.
2. Provide role modeling, preceptorship, and mentoring.
3. Ensure professional growth opportunities for both novice and experienced nurses.
4. Disseminate knowledge through publication and conference presentations.

COLLABORATION

1. Collaborate with nurse manager.
   a. Assist with financial planning for units.
   b. Assist in recruiting and retaining staff.
   c. Contribute to formal and informal evaluation of nursing staff.
2. Collaborate with researchers on clinical research projects.

LEADERSHIP

1. Provide unit leadership.
   a. Develop and contribute to staff communication forums.
   b. Assist in conflict resolution among staff.
   c. Inform staff of organizational changes.
2. Evaluate and introduce new technology.

EVIDENCE-BASED PRACTICE (EBP)

1. Role-model use of EBP when developing guidelines, developing new procedures, and evaluating new technology.
2. Educate and mentor nurses and interprofessional staff in the process of evaluating and implementing new evidence.

access and resources. Box 12.3 lists example activities in this sphere.

Throughout all three spheres, CNSs apply the steps of the nursing process (e.g., assessment, planning, implementation, evaluation) at an advanced level. Experienced CNSs understand that activities in each sphere of impact and their advanced practice competencies exert reciprocal influences on each other with synergistic effects. Implementing competencies across the three spheres can result in improvements in clinical outcomes, patient safety, patient/family satisfaction, resource allocation, professional nursing staff knowledge and skills, advancement of clinical nursing practice, healthcare team collaboration, and organizational efficiency (Abela-Dimech et al., 2017; Catania & Tippett, 2015; Frankenfield et al., 2018; Fulton et al., 2016; Zavotsky et al., 2016).

The diversity of activities, the challenge of in-the-moment problem solving that characterizes clinical work, and intermediate- and long-range planning efforts to improve the care of patients attract CNSs to this work. Throughout the history of CNS practice, and despite the changes in health care, reimbursement, and credentialing that have affected advanced practice nursing, CNSs have remained focused on championing excellence in nursing practice and on improving clinical care and the systems in which the care is delivered. This is exemplified by the support of CNSs to attain and maintain Magnet status (Hanson, 2015; Speroni et al., 2020) and achieve specialty accreditation such as Joint Commission disease-specific certification (Frost et al., 2019).

Without sustained engagement in direct care, it would be difficult, if not impossible, to continue to be effective in the other two spheres because the effectiveness of CNSs depends on their clinical credibility and the ability to evaluate practice at the patient interface. However, because CNSs provide leadership in the other two spheres, maintaining their commitment to patient care is often challenged as organizational priorities change. In the following sections, the ways in which CNSs implement the six competencies across three spheres of impact are described.

BOX 12.3

Examples of Clinical Nurse Specialist Interventions in the Organizations and Systems Sphere

1. Assess needs of patients, families, communities, nurses, and organizations.
2. Develop evidence-based protocols, policies/procedures, clinical pathways, and standards of care.
3. Cultivate unit culture that values evidence-based practice.
4. Lead quality improvement efforts.
   a. Identify and prioritize quality improvement issues.
   b. Develop indicators, methods, and metrics to measure patient outcomes.
   c. Perform quality improvement projects.
5. Develop innovative models of care.
6. Develop, implement, and evaluate programs.
7. Form and lead community advisory panels to address healthcare inequities encountered by racially diverse populations in a specialty area of care.
8. Participate on policymaking boards and committees.

Direct Clinical Practice

Specialization was the genesis of the CNS role, but expert clinical practice—and direct patient care—is its heart. The central competency of direct clinical practice is explicitly linked to the patient sphere of impact; the insights and outcomes of providing direct care influence the CNS's work in the other two spheres of nursing practice and systems. It is direct practice that is core to the CNS role; otherwise the CNS can be replaced with experts in project management, policy revision, QI, and nursing education. The direct care expertise at the APRN level adds a unique perspective not provided by others.

Each strategy is highly dependent on the individual CNS and the practice setting; it can fluctuate from year to year in relation to the prevailing healthcare environment. It is easy for the direct care component of the role to be overemphasized or underemphasized because of institutional priorities and competition for CNS expertise. The unique skill set of CNSs may result in them being continually pulled away from direct care to lead projects that are of high priority for the institution. In addition, CNSs are increasingly being asked to function at a system level, rather than a unit or hospital level, leading system EBP/QI initiatives. Conversely, healthcare organizations may require CNSs to solely provide direct patient care for revenue generation, allowing little, if any, time for activities related to advancing nursing practice or quality improvement. The CNS role is optimally enacted when CNSs have the opportunity to use what they learn from direct clinical practice to improve systems of care for individual patients, families, and patient populations, ideally occurring in all three spheres, depending on the issue or priorities.

Providing regular and consistent direct patient care is essential for the CNS in order to:

- Demonstrate one's clinical competency and maintain clinical expertise, thereby role-modeling clinical behaviors, establishing credibility, and maintaining team relationships and collegial trust.
- Identify gaps in the quality, effectiveness, efficiency, and safety of patient care and to apply their expertise in determining root causes of issues (e.g., resources, gaps in workflows, etc.).
- Identify opportunities to address clinical and professional development needs of nursing staff.
- Refine one's clinical expertise and reflective abilities.
- Maintain CNS credentials and certification.

Direct care, or direct clinical practice, refers to CNS activities and responsibilities that occur within the patient–nurse interface (see Chapter 6). Traditionally, CNSs were not proactive in demonstrating the impact of their direct practice such as improved patient outcomes and efficient use of resources. Thus few data were available to justify the role and correlate its expense with the cost avoidance and quality improvement aspects of the role when healthcare institutions were restructuring their operating systems. In today's healthcare environment, it is incumbent on CNSs to measure their direct care impact to demonstrate their value and justify reimbursement, especially in light of the increasing patient frailty and complexity requiring CNS expertise. A CNS is most likely to care directly for a patient whose diagnosis or care is complex, unique, or problematic. Box 12.4 provides examples of patients with these diagnoses. CNS care of these specialty populations has resulted in improved patient outcomes and increased healthcare efficiencies. High-risk patients with complex conditions have consistently shown improved patient outcomes and reduced healthcare costs when CNSs and other APRNs were directly involved with patient care, including assessing, teaching, counseling, and negotiating systems (Chanyeong & Young, 2019).

CNSs are skilled at not only caring for and addressing a patient's physical complexities but also caring for the patient holistically, forming therapeutic relationships and incorporating the environmental context and social determinants of health into the plan of care. This is even more imperative in today's context of inequities in health care and the ability or willingness of some patients to fully participate in a healthcare partnership (NASEM, 2021). The CNS has the ability to evaluate the latest evidence and apply it in unique ways to manage complex cases, taking into account the needs of an ever-expanding diverse population.

Direct care also affords a CNS the opportunity to assess the quality of care for a specific patient population. The astute recognition of patterns can optimize care improvements. For example, a CNS might notice a pattern of frequently missed clinic appointments for a patient with heart failure. Through the therapeutic partnership, the CNS may determine that a lack of clinic parking results in a barrier for this patient to keep appointments. The cause is not one of a nonadherent patient but of a logistical failure that requires immediate resolution for the benefit of all patients with heart failure.

A CNS's clinical practice may occur in different ways. The CNS practice may be continuous, in which they carry a consistent patient caseload, or primarily time-limited or episodic, in which the CNS cares for patients with complex cares or problems as they arise. See Box 12.5 for examples of continuous and episodic CNS practice. Involvement in direct care, whether regular or episodic, enables CNSs to address nursing or

BOX 12.4

Examples of Patients With Complex or Unique Care Requirements

COMPLEX OR MULTIPLE COMORBIDITIES

- A very-low-birth-weight infant
- A frail older person with multiple chronic conditions
- A child requiring an organ transplant
- A young pregnant person with a newly discovered congenital heart defect and cystic fibrosis
- A man diagnosed with bipolar disorder who survived a suicide attempt but who requires prolonged physical rehabilitation

UNIQUE SITUATIONS

- Care of a child with a rigid external distraction device for midface advancement
- Evaluation and implementation of a new intervention, such as teletechnology, to assess the efficacy of preventive interventions for pressure ulcers
- Introduction of an experimental surgical intervention

BOX 12.5

Examples of Clinical Nurse Specialist Continuous and Episodic Patient Care

CONTINUOUS PATIENT CARE

- Providing care for high-risk newborns in a pediatric special care clinic
- Providing support groups and medication management for patients requiring mental health care
- Delivering total patient care to patients in an innovative pulmonary hypertension clinic
- Providing comprehensive care for children with asthma in a hospital-based clinic

EPISODIC PATIENT CARE

- Planning and coordinating a patient's complex hospital discharge
- Stabilizing a patient with complex diabetes and acute renal failure
- Working with a patient and family who are disagreeing about the plan of care in order to facilitate decision making

systems problems that interfere with care and require CNS intervention, such as provide staff education, update clinical policies or procedures based on new evidence, or streamline the process to initiate ethics consults. For each clinical situation, a CNS uses a comprehensive and holistic approach, using advanced knowledge and judgment, and expert skills, including expertise in the technical, humanistic, and organizational aspects of care. In these situations, CNSs are particularly skilled at the use of surveillance, quickly identifying patient and system issue patterns and intervening to avoid further complications. A CNS intervention may be as simple as assisting a patient and family in navigating a hospital's bureaucracy. A CNS knows when it can be appropriate to bend the rules and when and how to bypass organizational or philosophic roadblocks, thus ensuring patient-centered care to achieve optimal outcomes.

If clinical skills—particularly psychomotor ones, such as inserting arterial or central line access or removal of chest tubes—are not used periodically, CNSs can quickly lose skill proficiency. Regular clinical practice helps a CNS maintain and refine the expertise and clinical competence needed to practice as well as teach and develop the skills of other nurses. Direct clinical practice is imperative when a CNS is new to the role in order to establish credibility. It is also instrumental during implementation of new evidence or with organizational change to evaluate the impact of the change on patient care. CNSs must be cognizant of the benefits and costs of ways to implement direct care.

Indirect Practice

Clinical practice can also occur indirectly. For example, a CNS can guide the direct care being performed by a novice staff nurse with the goal to improve the direct care skills and knowledge of the nurse. A CNS can lead nursing rounds, routinely assessing the care of individual patients with staff nurses to ensure best practices are being used, to problem-solve complex issues, and to identify potential or early complications with initiation of appropriate interventions. A CNS may lead and/or collaborate with the healthcare team to develop and implement standards of care, clinical pathways, clinical procedures, and/or QI projects.

Changes and practice improvements are rarely self-sustaining, and CNSs frequently function as champions to continuously support adherence and to promptly identify and resolve any unintended consequences that arise due to the change. This function is imperative if the algorithm, guideline, or change is to be successful and achieve its intended outcome.

Consultation is an expected skill of CNSs and frequently occurs in the indirect care realm. The CNS can provide consultation to others in the care of a complex patient; however, consultation also occurs when the CNS requests advice from another member of the healthcare team yet retains primary responsibility for that patient's care. The CNS often guides nurses to other resources (e.g., other colleagues, community resources, practice guidelines) that enable them to make the most informed decisions on relevant and appropriate information and evidence. It is important that CNSs document the processes and outcomes of consultations to demonstrate the impact of this less visible, indirect care aspect of the role.

The indirect practice of CNSs is also key in evaluating current and new technology. Technologic advances have resulted in significant and accelerated changes in healthcare delivery. While technologic advances have improved access to objective data for clinical decision making (e.g., medication titration based on hemodynamic indices), alternative interventions to manage and treat disease (e.g., closed-loop systems for insulin infusion and glucose management) and devices for remote assessments (e.g., telemonitoring of vital signs and patient status), they create potential for significant challenges in patient care. These advances, coupled with the pressure of cost containment, increased competition, heightened consumer expectations, and capped budgets, create conflicting demands and priorities. CNSs have a unique role in identifying and evaluating technology for these challenges that include increased healthcare costs, appropriate use of technology including ethical perspectives, and anticipation and evaluation of new types of errors that can occur with new technology (Barton & Makic, 2015).

Patient Safety

Patient safety is integral to all aspects of direct and indirect clinical practice, including CNS availability to and support of nurses (Abela-Dimech et al., 2017; Kirk et al., 2015; Makic, 2015; Patton et al., 2017; Purvis et al., 2018; Sorrentino, 2016). The Joint

Commission's National Patient Safety Goals (2022), the Agency for Healthcare Research and Quality's (AHRQ) Patient Safety Network (PSnet, n.d.), teaching strategies from Quality and Safety Education for Nurses (2020), and the Open School at the Institute for Healthcare Improvement (2022) are resources that the CNS can use to keep abreast of patient safety issues. Direct clinical practice empowers a CNS to assume a leadership role in evaluating patient safety, facilitating root cause analyses, and preventing adverse events. A CNS can build an atmosphere of trust in situations in which adverse events are investigated, bring systems and individual patient-level thinking to the discussion, and then facilitate implementation of changes that are needed to prevent recurrence of those adverse events.

Although providing direct care to patients is a core competency, how CNSs provide direct care varies across CNS specialties and practice settings; it is determined by population needs, influenced by the expertise of other nursing personnel, and affected by regulatory designations of CNSs as APRNs and their scopes of practice. When, how, for whom, and with whom direct care is given are fluid and are negotiated and renegotiated with professional nursing staff and organizational leadership based on patients' needs and the knowledge and clinical skill of nursing personnel. It is a balance for the CNS to manage the necessity of direct patient care against competing demands or time pressures of the other valuable role components.

Exemplar 12.1 illustrates how a pediatric CNS uses her professional competencies to provide expert care to a specific patient population. She demonstrates the importance of direct care to execute the other CNS competencies and how the care impacts functioning across the three spheres of impact.

Guidance and Coaching

One of the essential components of the CNS role is that of expert coach. This role of guide or coach is used during teaching and mentoring to facilitate transition from one situation to another or to promote professional and/or personal growth (see Chapter 7). CNSs use formal and informal coaching and guidance strategies with patients and families, nurse, graduate nursing students, and other CNSs and health professionals.

Patients and Families

A CNS's expert guidance and coaching are pivotal in providing or influencing patient and family education and behavior. CNSs may use coaching and teaching skills in educating patients and families with complex situations to complement the care given by other nurses and health professionals. CNSs continually seek better ways to coach patients and families using combinations of cognitive, educational, and behavioral strategies to improve patient education and adherence to interventions. However, a CNS cannot teach every patient and family and so must assess and prioritize whom to teach. For example, a CNS could mentor a case manager or presurgical program educator to provide routine preoperative teaching for cardiac surgical patients. A CNS could then allocate more time to coach high-risk, complex, unusual, or challenging patients, such as a teenage girl with congenital heart defects with a history of an eating disorder who is afraid she will die if she undergoes another cardiac surgery or a patient with multiple comorbidities who neither speaks nor reads English and who will be going home after surgery to housing with no running water. A CNS may coach nurses in how to facilitate difficult conversations with patients and their families by supporting the parents of a newborn who has died, working with a patient and family on end-of-life decisions, or "translating" a physician's technical explanation into lay terms.

As healthcare systems are restructured, there is increasing emphasis on patients' accountability for their own health. This means that in addition to coaching individuals, CNSs are even more likely to be involved in education program planning and interventions aimed at helping groups of patients manage chronic illnesses and associated symptoms. A study of patients with rheumatoid arthritis in the United Kingdom showed that the patients had positive relationships with their CNSs—viewing the CNSs as their main source of information, providing guidance on how to manage their arthritis and providing them reassurance and self-confidence in knowing how to manage their chronic condition (Hardware et al., 2014). Many patients know that they need to be better informed and educated about health risks, preventive self-care, treatment options, and risks and benefits of treatments, but their healthcare behaviors are influenced

EXEMPLAR 12.1

DIRECT CLINICAL PRACTICE AND CORE COMPETENCIES OF THE CLINICAL NURSE SPECIALIST[a]

C.C., a pediatric neurology clinical nurse specialist (CNS), performs preoperative history and physical examinations in the pediatric neurology clinic; orders appropriate radiographs, laboratory tests, and consultations; and obtains cephalometric measurements and photographs for patients undergoing surgery for craniosynostosis. On the day of surgery, C.C. notifies the staff nurses who will be caring for the patient about pertinent findings and specific needs. Postoperatively, C.C. assesses the patient for adequate pain control, dietary needs, vital sign changes, incision status, swelling, and neurologic function. She facilitates discussions about these findings, staff nurses' concerns, parents' concerns, and the plan of care among care team members. She adapts standing orders for each patient in collaboration with the neurosurgeon.

C.C. is frequently consulted by staff nurses, referring physicians, or other advanced practice registered nurses to assess misshapen heads by physical assessment or reviewing radiographs. These consultations provide opportunities to teach healthcare professionals how to recognize the differences between positional plagiocephaly and craniosynostosis, leading to earlier referrals for improved outcomes.

GUIDANCE AND COACHING

The Internet can be an excellent resource for families seeking healthcare information about medical conditions and treatment options. To help families learn more about craniosynostosis, C.C. created a website that describes the various types of craniosynostosis and treatment options, including a new, less invasive technique. As a result, she receives many inquiries from families seeking information about this new technique for their babies. Providing accurate information on the website is critical so that families can make informed decisions about surgery. Much of the preoperative teaching is done by telephone or in the clinic because parents and other family members have many questions.

C.C. has educated nurses about the early recognition of craniosynostosis, surgical options, and positional plagiocephaly through professional journal articles, a book chapter, presentations at national nursing conferences, teaching at the local school of nursing, and in-service education programs for the staff nurses. Mentoring graduate students has provided additional opportunities for role modeling.

EVIDENCE-BASED PRACTICE

Collaboration on research with the pediatric neurosurgeon has yielded data demonstrating that the new surgical technique decreases patients' hospital stays, lowers costs, and improves patient outcomes. When parents noticed a sharp decrease in fussiness in their baby immediately after surgery, C.C. developed a questionnaire to survey parents' perceptions of fussiness and irritability in their baby before and after surgery. Statistically significant decreases in fussiness and irritability were found postoperatively, suggesting that babies with craniosynostosis experience increases in intracranial pressure.

LEADERSHIP

In this unique role, C.C. can provide care throughout the continuum, using clinical pathways to help families navigate the hospital system in an efficient manner. Bringing a baby to an unfamiliar city for surgery by surgeons whom they have never met is a daunting experience for most parents. C.C.'s leadership skills are put to the test coordinating preoperative directed donor blood; arranging lodging at the Ronald McDonald House; scheduling preoperative workups and follow-up appointments with the neurosurgeon, plastic surgeon, ophthalmologist, and anesthesiologist; and coordinating the postoperative molding helmet.

COLLABORATION

Collaboration occurs at many levels. First, C.C. collaborates with the pediatric neurosurgeon to provide for and coordinate optimal patient and family care. She collaborates with the staff nurses who care for the babies with craniosynostosis, providing in-service educational programs about the disorder and conducting rounds with them on the postoperative patients. Collaboration also occurs with other members of the craniofacial team, such as ophthalmologists, genetics counselors, plastic surgeons, and orthotic designers. C.C. confers with referring healthcare providers to provide continuity after the patient leaves the hospital and between follow-up visits.

ETHICAL PRACTICE

Although this new surgical treatment for craniosynostosis results in minimal blood loss, an infant will occasionally present with a low hemoglobin level or experience excessive intraoperative blood loss. Some families refuse blood transfusions for religious reasons, requiring more intensive preoperative preparation to minimize the need for a blood transfusion. Being present for the conversations that the neurosurgeon has with the family who refuses blood transfusions assists in understanding the reasons for refusal and allows the CNS to reinforce the plan of care should the child need blood during or after surgery. A protocol for preoperative erythropoietin injections can be sent to the patient's pediatrician in an attempt to increase the hemoglobin level.

A great deal of preparation is required for a family to bring their baby to the hospital for this type of surgery. The CNS is instrumental in facilitating this process, using the core competencies and spheres of impact.

[a]The authors thank Cathy Cartwright, MSN, RN, PCNS, FAAN, for this exemplar.

by many personal, psychologic, and sociocultural factors. Because patients are not always able or willing to change their lifestyles or to adhere to healthcare recommendations, a CNS must determine which patients or populations will benefit most from the advanced coaching. For example, a patient with a new diagnosis of renal disease who has poor social support living in an economically depressed community will require skillful and advanced coaching by the CNS.

Nurses

A CNS is a role model for nurses, demonstrating the practical integration of theory and EBP into nursing practice. While CNSs coach patients and families, they also play a large role in coaching nurses to improve clinical practice and integrate new knowledge into their practice. A CNS's time may be better utilized by mentoring and coaching staff nurses to provide common patient interventions rather than repeatedly personally providing those same interventions. As a nurse applies the new knowledge and skills taught by a CNS, the CNS can then attend to new or more complex responsibilities. The nurse can become the role model for the skill mastered or the knowledge gained, and so a CNS's influence will continue to impact patient care. For example, a wound, ostomy, and continence CNS can guide and coach nurses to become "skin champions" to assist their peers to use the latest evidence in caring for patients with simple types of wounds. The CNS is then appropriately consulted for complex wounds. Bedside coaching can reinforce EBP and new skills through real-time feedback to the staff RN.

It is important for a discipline to ensure accountability for its own practice. CNSs have demonstrated coaching and leadership to nurses to be accountable for the safety and quality of their practice through development of clinical nurse peer review processes (Semper et al., 2016; Zavotsky et al., 2016). CNSs may also guide and coach RNs in professional development areas, such as advancing their skills in education, publishing, and presenting (Ansryan et al., 2019). The professional development of nurses in clinical practice settings is a key distinguishing feature of the CNS. CNSs' abilities to guide and mentor nurses toward stronger specialty practice can reduce turnover, improve patient safety, and support enhanced patient outcomes (Muller et al., 2010). In addition, in this complex healthcare environment, incidence of burnout and compassion fatigue is rapidly increasing (NASEM, 2019). CNSs can play a significant role in coaching and supporting clinical nurses to increase resiliency, coping, and well-being (Frankenfield et al., 2018). Extending the reach of the CNS through professional RN expertise, development, and well-being can be considered a defining characteristic of the guidance and coaching competency of CNS practice. See Exemplar 12.2 for an example of a CNS supporting well-being in the nursing sphere.

Students

A CNS has a professional responsibility to educate, guide, and coach graduate nursing students and, when the opportunity arises, to be their mentor. In working with graduate nursing students, a CNS models the integration of practical and scientific knowledge into expert clinical practice and demonstrates the level of advanced practice nursing to which a student can aspire. The reward for presenting to or working with graduate students is to extend one's influence more broadly and make advanced practice expertise more widely available. In addition to precepting graduate students in clinical care, the CNS serves as guide and coach for graduate students to implement QI or EBP projects or activities (e.g., performing a literature review, updating a policy, developing a patient education brochure) that also benefit the practice setting.

Evidence-Based Practice

In implementing the EBP competency, CNS involvement in the evaluation and improvement of nursing practice and activities may range from scholarly inquiry to formal scientific investigation. The doctor of nursing practice (DNP) degree adds to the knowledge base of traditional master's programs for CNSs by expanding depth in EBP and quality improvement knowledge and skills (AACN, 2020). DNP-prepared CNSs can implement the science developed by nurse researchers, such as those with a doctor of philosophy (PhD) or doctor of nursing science (DNS) degree (AACN, 2020). Specific EBP competencies, each of which has basic and advanced levels of activity, include interpretation and use of research findings (evidence- or research-based practice) and participation in collaborative research (see Chapter 8).

EXEMPLAR 12.2

CNS COMPETENCIES IN THE NURSES AND NURSING PRACTICE SPHERE OF IMPACT: PYSCH-MENTAL HEALTH APRN PRACTICE TO PROMOTE NURSE WELL-BEING[a]

K.M., a registered nurse in a busy oncology clinic, slumped against the wall outside the breakroom. I walked up to him and gently called his name. Taking a deep breath, he acknowledged me and went into the breakroom to get his lunch. Like a robot, he grabbed his lunch from the refrigerator, carried it to a table, and sat down. He seemed to stare at the table without seeing. The breakroom was empty except for us. Quietly, I sat at the table with him, gently touched his arm, and said, "Tell me, I'm here."

K.M. took a deep breath, and, fighting emotion, he described his morning. Two of his long-standing patients had cancer progression. Both had chosen the option for hospice care. He would not see them again. He stared numbly at the table, his body still. Matching his posture, I was still. We sat quietly for a few moments and he exclaimed, "This is not fair!" He went on to describe his patients, how young they were, their spouses and children. He began to pull his lunch out of his bag with spiky, jarring movements. After there was nothing left to pull from the bag he slumped back into his chair. I asked, "They are both about your age?" He forcefully said, "Yes" and jumped out of the chair and went to retrieve a soda. He opened the can with a loud "pop," sat down, and banged the can onto the table. Some of the pop spilled from the can. I passed napkins to him and asked, "How is L? How is your wife?" He started to cry without sound. He took a deep breath and shared that they had heard that his wife's breast cancer was gone. She had finished treatment and she had no trace of cancer detected. They had just celebrated their daughter's second birthday.

K.M. began to eat. He talked about the crazy balloons, the backyard full of toddlers, and he and his wife with all of their friends. He had grilled hamburgers. His wife's hair was starting to lose that "chemo fuzz" and it was curly and red. He stated with a soft grin, "I always wanted to date a redhead, isn't that what they say?" He looked me in the eyes for the first time in this encounter. We held the gaze, we held the space. After a moment, I nodded slightly and projected acknowledgment, warmth, and caring. He nodded back. "This just sucks. I feel so lucky and guilty at the same time. I get to keep my wife but my patients don't. This is so hard." He talked about his nursing care for these patients. He described the challenges he faced early on with one of them in particular—the anger about the cancer diagnosis and how he supported the patient and his family through that. He shared funny stories that his patients had shared with him. He began to eat his lunch. I walked with him through these stories, through the laughter and the somber moments.

His lunch was done and he needed to get back to his clinic. Efficiently, he tidied the table and threw away his trash. He came back to the table where I had stood. He took a deep breath and looked me in the eye. "Thank you," he said and nodded. I nodded back. He left the room, his posture strong and sure.

[a]The authors wish to thank Amy E. Rettig, DNP, MALM, APRN-BC, CBCN®, for this exemplar.

CNSs have the knowledge, skills, and clinical expertise to use EBP to advance clinical practice and improve patient outcomes. Nurse-sensitive indicators, such as patient falls or hospital-acquired infections, capture nursing's unique contributions to patient outcomes. Assuming responsibility for identifying nursing-sensitive and interprofessional quality indicators and using outcomes data to improve patient care are prime opportunities for a CNS to assess patient care strategies and community systems, analyze interprofessional communication and collaboration, coordinate care, and monitor patient and system progress. Ongoing work is required, however, to develop the science linking nursing, healthcare processes, available measures, and quality outcomes. All CNSs must demonstrate EBP competency and have ongoing accountability for monitoring and improving their practice and the practice of other nurses. CNSs implement this competency in a variety of ways, depending on experience, expertise, circumstances, setting, and resources.

Interpretation and Use of Evidence in Practice

Integration of new evidence and science-based knowledge into practice is essential to ensure optimal outcomes for patients and is increasingly expected by payers, regulators, and the public. For CNSs, the interpretation and use of research and other evidence often begin with a clinical question identified by the CNS or staff with whom he or she works. Knowledge is the basis for practice but, too frequently, routine practice may not be based on sound evidence. The foundation of improved quality of care and patient outcomes is the evaluation of research-based evidence and expert consensus–dependent practice changes to ensure best practice and achieve quality patient care. Inherent in the CNS role is the evaluation of the appropriateness of evidence and the application of its findings to clinical practice. A CNS is the ideal clinician to assess barriers and facilitators to change and to develop, implement, and evaluate EBP. A CNS's involvement in developing policies and procedures, patient and staff educational materials, and care guidelines means that evidence informs clinical practices and standards. See Exemplar 12.3 demonstrating how a CNS was integral in an evidence-based initiative to improve the safety and quality of patient care while demonstrating financial impact to the organization.

A CNS who develops an evidence-based guideline of care for a patient population promotes improved patient outcomes throughout the three spheres of impact. Multiple examples of CNS-led EBP improvements can be found in the literature. CNS contributions to improving patient outcomes by providing evidence-based care include the following: CNS-led initiative to reduce postoperative urinary retention in spinal surgery patients (Hoke & Bradway, 2016), reduction of hospital-acquired pressure ulcers (Fabbruzzo-Cota et al., 2016), reduction of restraint use in postsurgical patients (Kirk et al., 2015), implementing advanced resuscitation to improve mortality in cardiovascular surgery patients (Roberts, 2018), and early extubation in patients after open heart surgery, resulting in decreased length of stay and pulmonary complications (Soltis, 2015; see Chapter 21).

The role of the CNS in making EBP decisions is particularly important in situations where little evidence exists, yet care decisions must be made (e.g., pandemics, care of patients receiving new techniques or devices). CNSs are skilled at evaluating all levels of evidence and determining whether evidence from similar situations or corresponding to basic physiologic functioning can be applied in these new contexts.

Participation in Collaborative Research

Although the number of PhD-prepared CNSs with the training to conduct research is increasing, most CNSs are prepared at the master's or DNP level and can be partners in collaborating on research relevant to practice. Collaborative research between a CNS and researcher increases the likelihood of translating research findings to clinical practice. Researchers provide CNSs with new evidence for patient care practices and the assessment of their impact. The PhD-prepared CNS collaborates with peer CNSs by using advanced research skills to critically appraise research studies, set up research study designs, as well as facilitate contacts with other faculty. They can be the bridge between basic research and patient care. In turn, master's- and DNP-prepared CNSs stimulate researchers to investigate the science that explains their observations of patients and populations.

Typically, novice CNSs are not immediately involved in collaborative research because they are focused on mastering their newly acquired competencies. For experienced CNSs, collaborative research is often a realistic goal. Whether novice or experienced CNSs become involved in research depends on the setting, pregraduate and graduate school experience, resources within the setting, and access to research expertise. Many CNSs find satisfaction with involvement in research as a consultant or coinvestigator. A CNS is the clinical expert, understands clinical issues, has access to patients, and can anticipate clinical and system challenges that may occur throughout the research process. A nurse researcher is a research expert, knows research methodology, and has access to the resources that support research. The CNS is optimally positioned to stimulate a researcher's interest because of their direct clinical association with patients or participant populations. Interprofessional collaborative research offers opportunities for innovative solutions to complex issues, improved collaboration, richness of expertise and perspectives, and more comprehensive care improvements (Tracy & Chlan, 2014). Before participating in a research project, a CNS must determine whether there is readiness and receptiveness in the practice setting and administrative support and whether research activities are a realistic performance goal. Whatever the model, a CNS is a key player in developing and implementing clinically relevant nursing-sensitive and interprofessional quality indicators for measuring patient and system outcomes through EBP, quality improvement, and research.

Leadership

CNSs serve as leaders of interprofessional quality improvement teams because of their unique

EXEMPLAR 12.3
CNS COMPETENCY IN EVIDENCE-BASED PRACTICE[a]

S.J., a critical care CNS, evaluated the current enteral feeding tube insertion and verification practice in the intensive care units (ICUs) at a quaternary care, Magnet-recognized, nonprofit hospital. The evaluation showed the insertion of over 800 feeding tubes a year with placement done at the bedside by the nurse but without the ability to view where the tip of the tube is during placement (blind placement). A radiographic image (x-ray) for these placements needed to be obtained to verify the tube tip location prior to tube use. If tube placement was questioned or the tube was repositioned on an ongoing basis, additional x-rays were required. Enteral tubes that required tip placement in the duodenum or jejunum (advanced placements) were done in the radiology department using fluoroscopy, with additional fluoroscopy procedures for readjustments or replacement. In the evaluation, S.J. identified patient safety events related to blind placement of the tube resulting in additional patient interventions.

S.J. was aware of Food and Drug Administration–approved technology that would allow safe advanced feeding tube placements and guidewire reinsertions to be performed at the bedside with possible reductions in costs. The safety of using this technology to verify the tube tip compared with the current standard of care, x-ray confirmation, would be needed prior to a practice change at S.J.'s facility.

S.J. created a business plan for a quality improvement (QI) initiative to improve the safety of enteral feeding tube insertion and verification practices in the ICUs with a reduced cost of care outcome. Utilizing cost analysis tools, S.J. evaluated the financial impact of the QI initiative. The cost analysis compared current state to future state related to feeding tube equipment cost and cost of care for tube insertion and verification (see Table). New technology training included 1 hour of hands-on didactic for staff with skill competency verification in bedside tube placements with a trained user. A core team of 20 ICU caregivers, including nurses, dietitians, and CNSs, was initially trained. Due to the limited financial impact of training, it was not included in the cost analysis.

COST ANALYSIS TABLE

		Current State (Pre-Technology Implementation)	Future State (Post-Technology With Practice Change)
Tube placement data	Number of tubes placed annually	800	
	% Patients needing final x-ray confirmation	100	30
	% Patients needing multiple (two) x-ray confirmations	30	5
	% Patients requiring fluoroscopic placement	30	5
Cost data*	Variable cost of x-ray	$40.00	$40.00
	Variable cost of fluoroscopy	$250.00	$250.00
	Old feeding tube cost	$10.00	
	New technology feeding tube cost		$30.00
	Cost of new technology (one-time cost)		$15,000.00
Cost calculations	Total cost of feeding tube	$8000.00 (800 × $10.00)	$24,000.00 (800 × $30.00)
	Cost of final x-ray confirmation	$41,600.00 (800 × $40)	$9600.00 (800(30%) × $40)
	Cost of multiple x-ray confirmations	$9600.00 (800(30%) × $40)	$1600.00 (800(5%) × $40)
	Cost of fluoroscopic placement	$60,000.00 (800(30%) × $250)	$10,000 (800(5%) × $250)

Continued

EXEMPLAR 12.3
CNS COMPETENCY IN EVIDENCE-BASED PRACTICE[a]—cont'd

		Current State (Pre-Technology Implementation)	Future State (Post-Technology With Practice Change)
Total cost	Total cost year 1	$119,200.00	$60,200.00
	Total cost subsequent years	$119,200.00	$45,200.00
Cost of care reduction	Cost of care reduction year 1	−$59,000.00	
	Cost of care reduction subsequent years	−$74,000.00	

*Numbers are meant for example only and do not represent actual cost.

A successful pilot of the technology was completed and, along with the business plan, approval gained for implementation. Radiologists and radiology leadership were included in S.J.'s stakeholder group for their expertise and to evaluate potential revenue loss with reduced radiology procedures.

S.J. led revision of policy language to support the use of the new technology for all enteral feeding tube insertions in the ICUs. One year's worth of enteral tube data (n = 599) was captured and evaluated, comparing the tube tip location interpreted by the trained core team to x-ray interpretation, showing 99.6% core team accuracy. These data also showed that insertion of the tube into the trachea and mainstem bronchus occurred in 7.5% of the placements. With the use of the new technology, an inaccurate placement could be immediately identified and the tube repositioned, avoiding patient harm. S.J. utilized these data to show safety and accuracy in tube placement by the core team and gained approval of policy language supporting the change in practice in confirmation of enteral feeding tube placements.

Long-term financial outcomes were captured by tracking variable cost savings through the avoidance of x-rays and fluoroscopy procedures. These figures were included in the CNS scorecard showing a monthly rolling cost savings and are being presented to senior leadership twice a year. Other cost savings were noted, including reduced transport of critically ill patients to radiology for tube placement, reduced x-ray exposure, and reduced physician time in x-ray read and dictation; however, these indirect cost avoidances were difficult to isolate.

To monitor and track the new technology program, S.J. assisted in the development of a dashboard that shows updated data related to the number of feeding tubes inserted, verified, and re-verified using this technology. The dashboard allows for ongoing quality monitoring related to the change in practice.

[a]The authors wish to thank Stacy Jepsen, MS, RN, APRN-CNS, CCRN, for this exemplar.

preparation at the graduate level, using advanced communication and leadership skills to evaluate practice and effect change in complex healthcare delivery systems (AACN, 2021; Lewis & Allen, 2015; NACNS, 2019b). It is because of these very leadership skills that CNSs are often pulled away by administrators to lead other initiatives. Leadership is integral to the role because a CNS has responsibility for clinical innovation and change within the patient care system to improve outcomes and advance nursing science. A CNS has significant formal and informal impact and must be visionary yet realistic.

CNSs have an important role in helping a hospital achieve and maintain Magnet status (Hanson, 2015; Muller et al., 2010; NACNS, 2021; Walker et al., 2009). The nurses and nursing practice sphere of impact of the CNS role is already recognized by many hospitals seeking to obtain or maintain Magnet status and should make this role even more valuable in the future. CNSs lead and mentor nurses to lead projects that meet the Magnet standards. Particular strengths lie in the areas of nursing education, EBP, and process improvement, which are key concerns for attaining Magnet status (Muller et al., 2010).

A CNS is the link between many disciplines and resources and asserts clinical and professional leadership in the practice setting or healthcare system, in healthcare policy and delivery decisions, and in the administration of direct care programs. Using direct practice, EBP, and consultation, the CNS identifies and plans for changes in practice and care delivery; however, it is through the CNS's leadership skills that change is effectively implemented. Clinical and professional leadership competencies are integrated with the other CNS competencies to support an organization's purpose and goals (NACNS, 2019b). Because of the CNS's communication skills and knowledge of diplomacy, a CNS can be a facilitator among staff, administration, and patients during organizational change, problem solving, or conflict resolution. As leaders, CNSs also help the members of one discipline understand the priorities of another discipline and often negotiate agreements that bring diverse perspectives into alignment. This mediation role benefits patients, promotes communication, and creates an environment that fosters collaboration.

Collaboration

CNSs must be skilled at collaboration because the CNS regularly interacts with a variety of people in order to achieve quality improvements and optimal outcomes (see Chapter 10). A CNS collaborates with nurses, physicians, other healthcare providers, and patients and their families, providing an interface among them (Ulit et al., 2020). Depending on the project, the CNS can literally interact with any department in the hospital, depending on the project—for example, supply chain, finance, security, operations, and facilities. The Institute of Medicine (IOM) report *The Future of Nursing: Leading Change, Advancing Health* has recommended that opportunities be expanded for nurses to "lead and diffuse collaborative improvement efforts" (IOM, 2011, p. 11). Many patients have such complex healthcare needs that no one healthcare professional can independently manage them all; this increasing complexity requires more interdependence to adequately manage. A CNS can partner with patients and family members to determine their needs, help them ask questions and assess treatment options, and facilitate timely referrals to other disciplines to ensure a positive outcome. CNSs can integrate the insights of many individuals with different perspectives, with each providing theoretical and applied knowledge. Throughout their interactions with patients and colleagues, CNSs model the communication and collaboration skills that help teams mature and be effective.

Collaboration is an essential competency—the well-earned result of clinical competence, effective communication, mutual trust, the valuing of complementary knowledge and skills, collegiality, and a favorable organizational structure (see Chapter 10). CNSs often identify potential or actual conflicts when collaboration is not working well, and CNS advocacy often prevents or ameliorates adversarial situations and their negative sequelae. A CNS must be skilled in helping team members address and negotiate conflicts to optimize patient care. The outcome of CNS-coordinated collaboration is the empowerment of nurses and recognition of the nurse as a critical member of the healthcare team. This results in team building, synergy, and integrative solutions. Some practice settings and working relationships are more conducive to partnership than others. It has been recommended that nurses be educated with medical and other healthcare professional students and that interprofessional experiences occur throughout their careers (IOM, 2011; Interprofessional Education Collaborative, 2016). Ongoing research has shown that quality care and patient outcomes improve when CNSs collaborate as equals with other healthcare providers (Naylor et al., 2011), and early joint education may facilitate that partnership.

Blurring of boundaries between healthcare professionals can occur as the CNS role develops. Boundaries can overlap between the CNS and staff nurse, between the CNS and physician, or between the CNS and another APRN. It is important that clear communication occur between collaborators to ensure that the blurring of boundaries does not result in either gaps in or duplication of care due to unclear accountability. CNSs must avoid being territorial; this limits their effectiveness, and they are unlikely to develop positive relationships that can help patients and families navigate the healthcare system efficiently. Chapter 10 provides further information on clarity in roles with collaboration, particularly related to direct care of patients.

Ethical Practice

CNSs often identify or consult on ethical issues and facilitate their resolution. In some cases, a CNS is consulted on what staff perceive is a clinical issue but really turns out to be an ethical concern. Being able to recognize, name, and address the moral distress and ethical concerns that are inherent in clinical care is a crucial part of CNS practice. A CNS can significantly influence the acknowledgment and negotiation of moral dilemmas, direction of patient care, access to care, and allocation of resources. CNSs consider numerous factors such as professional and religious codes, cultural values, bioethical principles, and ethical theories when making decisions that may have ethical implications (see Chapter 11).

CNSs have similar responsibilities when applying ethical decision-making skills to patient and organizational issues. They recognize clinicians' experiences of moral distress and articulate moral dilemmas, often serving as advocates for patients, families, and staff. They interpret and mediate patient, family, and team members' views to ensure as complete a discussion of the dilemma as possible. They recognize when there is a need to consult an ethics committee and often initiate that consult. When necessary, CNSs validate nurses' concerns and help nurses present their concerns to other team members, ensuring that the nursing perspective is considered when ethical issues are discussed. When CNSs are excluded from interprofessional ethical decisions, opportunities for effective nursing care are minimized and outcomes, such as timely and appropriate end-of-life care, can be compromised (Wocial, 2019). Because CNSs facilitate optimal care for complex patients who are sicker and more frail, the ethical challenge is to balance the expectations for quality care with the limitations of appropriate care and assist in articulating the moral dilemmas for patients, nursing personnel, and organizations. When CNSs optimize their knowledge and expertise in the ethical competency domain, they can advance beyond resolution of ethical issues on a case-by-case basis to lead a more ethical environment for all patients, families, and healthcare providers in the setting (Wocial, 2019).

CURRENT MARKETPLACE FORCES AND CONCERNS

Patient safety, equity, and quality care continue to be major concerns in healthcare delivery. Reduction of medical errors has garnered and will continue to garner significant attention to ensure the safe provision of care. Skilled application of the six competencies in all three spheres of impact (patient, nurse/nursing practice, systems/organizations) make CNSs well positioned to contribute to address both patient safety and quality care. Role contributions for expert nurses have focused on improving outcomes primarily for populations of patients through implementing EBP and system improvements. CNSs have demonstrated these contributions in decreasing lengths of stay in the hospital, decreasing costs, reducing complications, and increasing patient satisfaction (Kelvin et al., 2016; Newhouse et al., 2011; Spruce & Butler, 2017).

Internationally, the CNS and NP have been identified as the most common APRN roles (Chapter 5). The role of the CNS is expanding internationally for similar reasons, one of which is the need for quality care of increasingly complex patients (Chapter 5). This complexity of patients is seen not only in hospital settings but also in patients' homes, expanding opportunities for CNSs to practice outside the usual boundaries of a hospital, to include transitional care (i.e., transferring care from one healthcare setting to another healthcare setting) and outpatient care (Bryant-Lukosius et al., 2015; Cavanaugh et al., 2021; Cross et al., 2020; Fels et al., 2015; Marshall et al., 2015; NACNS, 2019b; Negley et al., 2016). While the primary setting of CNS practices continues to be the hospital setting, CNSs are employed in a variety of settings such as public health, ambulatory care, private practices, nursing homes, occupational health, and prison systems (NACNS, 2019a). In a systematic review of CNS-led hospital-to-home transitional care compared with usual care, the authors found that the CNS was able to reduce patient mortality in patients with cancer; delay time to and reduce death or rehospitalization, improve patient treatment adherence and patient satisfaction, and decrease costs and length of rehospitalization in patients with heart failure; improve caregiver depression and decrease rehospitalization, rehospitalization length of stay, and costs for elderly patients; and improve infant immunization rates and maternal satisfaction with care and reduce maternal and infant length of hospital stay and costs for high-risk pregnant women and very-low-birth-weight infants (Bryant-Lukosius et al., 2015; see Exemplar 12.4). CNSs in a small rural community hospital in Vermont

EXEMPLAR 12.4

TRANSITIONAL CARE CNSs NAVIGATING PATIENTS ACROSS THE CARE CONTINUUM[a]

In rural Vermont, three hospital-based acute care clinical nurse specialists (CNSs) began to design an integrated care delivery system for their community. Based on the Mary Naylor Transitional Care Model developed at the University of Pennsylvania, the CNS team partnered with primary care providers (PCPs) to identify high-risk, chronically ill patients who are high users of the healthcare system. In this model, expert CNSs navigate patients from the hospital to home, which can include short-term rehabilitation stays and primary and specialty office visits. Gaps in communication and care delivery that negatively impact the patient and family experience are identified. Over 2 years, this team collaborated with community agencies and local/regional resources to improve population health and quality outcomes while decreasing costs. The CNSs created a community care team to support people with addiction and mental illness who frequently use the emergency department. This team devised a community-based wraparound care plan to meet the person's clinical, social, and emotional needs. The team also supported implementation of INTERACT (Interactions to Reduce Acute Care Transfers), recognizing the need to decrease turnaround readmissions from the local nursing homes.

The CNS team was apprehensive to leave the comfort and familiarity of the hospital setting. However, this journey into the realities of healthcare reform has offered the CNSs the challenge of a lifetime. All healthcare providers must strive to understand what happens with patients outside of their time with them. Building a relationship that allows trust to develop also allows patients to feel safe to confide details of what might negatively impact their recovery and wellness.

The following is an example of how CNSs have been architects of integrated care delivery focusing on shared decision making and goal setting to improve the quality of life for many.

CLINICAL EXAMPLE

H.J., a 68-year-old man, has been admitted to the hospital three times in the past 6 weeks with exacerbation of chronic obstructive pulmonary disease (COPD), resulting in treatment with antibiotics and steroids and adjustment of inhaler therapy. Each time, the hospitalist consults with the pulmonologist and the discharge plan includes ongoing care by the specialist. Since the last admission, the CNS (B.R.) has been consulted by the PCP to evaluate why H.J. is unable to be successful when discharged from the hospital. The PCP reports that the patient appears to understand his treatment plan and medications and seems motivated. B.R. visits the patient in the hospital, introducing herself and explaining that she works with his PCP, who knows he is in the hospital. B.R. has access to the PCP record and shares pertinent information with the hospitalist and pulmonologist. She also shares patient information at daily interprofessional rounds. As B.R. assesses the patient, she recognizes that he seems to have difficulty with simple explanations and is not interested in printed material supplied. H.J. is homebound and meets criteria for home care referral but adamantly refuses when it is suggested. B.R. visits the patient daily in the hospital, meets his family, and develops a relationship.

On day 4, when H.J. is being discharged, he reluctantly agrees to let B.R. see him at home: "Just one visit." B.R. visits H.J. the next day and asks to review his discharge information. He hands her a pile of papers that appear untouched. The discharge packet is 20 pages in length, with information about his chronic disease, inhaler use, and all of his medications. B.R. asks to see where he keeps his medications and he shows her a grocery bag filled with pills collected over several years. She asks him for the new medications just ordered and he blushes with embarrassment. "I went to pick them up and couldn't afford to get them. I will just take what I already have here." Over two more home visits, the real story of H.J. comes together. He has minimal financial resources, minimal social support, limited transportation, and few groceries. B.R. starts to make a plan to better meet his needs. She finds out what is important to him, what he is looking forward to, and what he would like to do that he has not been able to do. She provides hope that it may be possible for him to walk down the driveway to his mailbox again, and he may even get to bingo at the senior center.

While B.R. is at his home, she does a targeted physical assessment, checking blood pressure, pulse, and oxygenation (**Direct Care**). He has crackles in the bases less than 24 hours postdischarge because he has not taken his diuretic or used his inhaler since discharge. She asks him to show her how he uses his inhaler and he tries to do it with the cover on, unable to get any of the medication. B.R. takes the cover off and demonstrates the proper technique. She draws a picture to remind him after she leaves and tapes it to his refrigerator. B.R. offers a medication box and demonstrates how to fill it correctly. She recognizes that H.J. has difficulty reading and plans to consult the transitional care pharmacist to design a notebook with pictures of his medications with sun and moon stickers to identify when the medications are to be taken (**Guidance and Coaching**). As she scans H.J.'s apartment, B.R. notices multiple safety hazards. She asks to see his bathroom and identifies the lack of grab bars or safety handles. Little by little, H.J. lets her into his world, sharing what he was ashamed to admit, trusting that she is there to help and not judge.

Continued

EXEMPLAR 12.4
TRANSITIONAL CARE CNSS NAVIGATING PATIENTS ACROSS THE CARE CONTINUUM[a]—cont'd

B.R. asks H.J. if he would allow the transitional care social worker to visit. She explains that the social worker (N.S.) might be able to help him access funds for food, medications, and living expenses (**Collaboration**). N.S. accompanies B.R. the next day to see H.J. N.S. explains potential options and informs H.J. what Medicaid can offer him. H.J. is at first reluctant, but with gentle persistence, N.S. helps him understand the improvement he may see in his life if he is willing to accept some assistance. B.R. and N.S. are able to access a patient fund at the hospital, which allows them to get H.J.'s medications delivered that day.

At the next visit, B.R. brings the transitional care pharmacist to see H.J. He reviews the medication box and continues to help H.J. learn to take his medications safely by explaining the notebook containing pictures of his medications. The pharmacist also examines the grocery bag of pills, identifying them to see whether they are still current medications and whether they are in date. B.R. explains that she will bring the outdated medications to be discarded at the police station. H.J. agrees reluctantly, commenting that they cost a lot of money! B.R. leaves that day feeling satisfied that she has made a difference by collaborating with her team and building a workable plan of care. She hopes that H.J. is on a path to improved health.

One week later, B.R. returns. Again she completes a targeted assessment and is dismayed to find H.J. with shortness of breath, worsening crackles, and a temperature of 101°F. She inquires how long he has been feeling this way and reminds H.J. that he could have called her. He says he did not want to bother her and knew she was coming today. B.R. is disappointed that she did not clearly explain the COPD action plan in a way that H.J. understood. She quickly messages his PCP with an update and gets new orders to help H.J. avoid a repeat hospitalization. She also shares with him that it might be helpful for a home care nurse to see him a few times a week until he feels better (**Collaboration**). She promises she will come with the nurse the first time.

H.J. has an appointment with the pulmonologist the following day. B.R. offers to meet H.J. at the office to help ensure he understands the discussion. She has forwarded a synopsis of her findings to the specialist via phone note prior to the appointment, targeting what he might choose to focus on. B.R. asks whether "high-flow O_2 therapy" may be effective to decrease H.J.'s bouts of pneumonia and shares an article she researched after attending a conference in Chicago (**Evidence-Based Practice**). The pulmonologist seems interested, and B.R. promises to set up a meeting with the vendor to explore this use. B.R. updates the transitional care team at their weekly meeting and presents this case to the team.

Over the past 2 years, the transitional care team has identified gaps in care delivery and, one by one, implemented solutions. This often involves collaboration with other disciplines, multiple community agencies, and Medicaid case workers. Success has come from bringing all partners to the table, brainstorming solutions, and recognizing that "it takes a village" to create integrated care delivery. Presently, competing home care and long-term care agencies sit together at the table strategizing how to work together and finding cost-effective ways to share resources. Medical home case managers and home care nurses who were initially suspicious of the transitional care model negatively impacting their roles now welcome the ability to deploy this resource when they have concerns about a patient at home. PCPs acknowledge the benefit of the model because they have one more tool in their toolboxes to be the eyes and ears across the care continuum. Little by little, the transitional care personnel are functioning as a cohesive team, recognizing what each member brings to the table and creating a symphony out of the chaos that is health care today.

[a]The authors wish to thank Billie Lynn Allard, MS, RN, FAAN, for this exemplar.

led a model change from inpatient practice to a care model where they focused their practices on following patients across the care continuum and into the community setting (Fels et al., 2015). This program resulted in notable decreases in emergency department visits and hospital admissions. Similarly, when comparing outcomes in an outpatient setting, CNSs were able to demonstrate cost-effectiveness as outpatient alternative providers and as complementary care providers (Kilpatrick et al., 2014).

Although CNSs are very clear about their role, one of the concerns facing them is the clarity of the CNS role to others, resulting in role overlap with clinical nurse leaders, nurse educators, and nurse practitioners (Mohr & Coke, 2018). Resolution of this lack of clarity is essential for successful implementation and optimization of the role. Because of the many facets of the CNS role, from expert clinician to direct care provider to systems change agent, it is challenging to articulate the role succinctly. Although the CNS, NP,

CNM, and CRNA are all direct patient care providers, the CNS is a unique APRN role that also focuses on nurses/nursing practice and systems/organizations as foundational to their work (NACNS, 2019b). Ensuring the survival of the role is essential to ensure that all three spheres of impact continue to benefit from the APRN skill set.

Scope of Practice and Delegated Authority

Scope of practice includes those activities a healthcare individual is permitted to perform within their profession. Scope of practice is specific to each state and is established by state regulations. Although the CNS has the education, competence, skills, and expertise to practice, when they move from one state to another state, it is the practice act of the new state that will determine what the CNS can do. Differences in state practice acts have led to a "crazy quilt" of varied and inconsistent licensure laws (Safriet, 2010, p. 453). Adding to the crazy quilt approach is the fact that the organization/facility where the CNS practices can further restrict the practice of a CNS despite the state's scope of practice. This has led to particular issues for the federal Veterans Health Administration. To standardize CNS practice despite state differences, a ruling by the Department of Veterans Affairs (2016) allows CNSs to work to their full practice authority within Veterans Affairs facilities and not within the individual state's scope of practice.

The National Council of State Boards of Nursing (NCSBN) adopted the APRN Compact in 2020 (2022a). Through the APRN Compact, an APRN would hold a multistate license that would allow them to practice in any state that has enacted compact legislation. To date, only one state has enacted legislation to support the APRN Compact (North Dakota), and it can only be implemented when seven states have enacted the legislation (see Chapter 20).

All health professions have an autonomous domain of practice as well as delegated authority within the medical domain (Lyon, 2004). Historically, the medical profession developed a broad, overarching scope of practice that encompassed almost all healthcare activities (Safriet, 2010; see Chapter 1). As a consequence, other health professionals (e.g., nurses, physical therapists, pharmacists) have had to carve their scopes of practice out of the medical scope of practice over time. The ANA's restrictive 1955 definition of nursing (ANA, 1955) reinforced the practice of nursing as having independent functions and being dependent on and delegated to by the profession of medicine. It also prohibited nurses from diagnosing and prescribing pharmacologic and/or durable goods for patients.

This history has contributed to a false dichotomy of what constitutes nursing practice and medical practice. As Chapter 1 has demonstrated, the practice of nursing has evolved over time to take on more responsibility and skills once considered to be the sole domain of medicine. As discoveries about health and illness continue to progress, the knowledge and skills of professional nurses, and other health professionals, will continue to evolve in their own right with their professional practice advancing into traditional boundaries of medicine (Standards for Supervision of Nursing Practice, 1983). As patients have become more complex and understanding of disease more sophisticated, physicians have become more specialized in treating the most complicated or complex patients. Therefore nursing scopes of practice, educational curricula, and competency validation need to stay flexible to evolve over time (Hartigan, 2011).

For CNSs specifically, delegated authority continues to pose an issue as APRNs establish their independent scopes of practice. Consistent with the IOM's *The Future of Nursing* (IOM, 2011), the *Future of Nursing 2020–2030* (NASEM, 2021), and the *Consensus Model for APRN Regulation* (APRN Joint Dialogue Group, 2008), practice restrictions need to be removed so that CNSs can practice to the full extent of their education to meet the needs of more and increasingly complex patients and resolve inequities in care. Inefficiencies in the healthcare system are present and patients do not obtain timely care when physician supervision of APRN practice is required because of either regulations or institutional requirements.

The Future of Nursing Reports

The IOM report *The Future of Nursing: Leading Change, Advancing Health* (IOM, 2011) clearly articulated four key messages and eight recommendations as a blueprint for change in nursing and advanced practice nursing in the United States to meet the health needs of Americans in the era of healthcare reform. The most specific key message for CNSs is supporting all APRNs being able to practice to the full extent of their education and training. Critical to implementation of this key message is removing scope of practice barriers. The NACNS (2012b) formulated a response to address pertinent recommendations from the perspective of CNSs; these recommendations are still relevant today (Table 12.2).

The National Academy of Medicine (formerly the IOM) recently published its report *The Future of Nursing 2020–2030* (NASEM, 2021). While the 2011 IOM report focused on "building the nursing workforce, this [NASEM] report clearly answers the question of to what end" with a focus on achieving health equity (NASEM, 2021, p. xv). The report emphasizes the fact that there are too few RNs and APRNs to address the healthcare needs of the United States, particularly in relation to the aging population, those with mental healthcare needs, primary care, and maternal care (NASEM, 2021). All of these are areas where CNSs can make a significant impact in care. In addition, the report notes that CNSs, as well as NPs, have remained predominantly non-Hispanic White and female and are falling behind changes in racial diversity of the basic RN workforce. This racial diversity gap needs to be aggressively addressed in order to more closely reflect the diversity of the patients for whom CNSs care.

Consensus Model for APRN Regulation and Implications for the Clinical Nurse Specialist

The main purposes of the consensus model are to delineate the scope of practice for APRNs and define the regulation of APRNs in the areas of licensure, accreditation of education programs, certification, and education program requirements (see Chapter 20). This section focuses on the implications of the consensus model as it relates to the CNS role. It is important to note that this regulatory APRN model does not encompass a full conceptual understanding of advanced practice nursing (see Chapter 2). Some of the debates regarding the CNS role in relation to other APRN roles may trace their points of contention to the differences between a regulatory and a conceptual approach to the CNS. Title protection and scopes of practice for CNSs are highly variable from state to state. The consensus model clarifies that the CNS is one of the four APRN roles and that all APRNs have a patient-focused practice and should have the legal authority to perform acts of advanced assessment, diagnosing, prescribing, and ordering. Currently there are some states where CNSs are not under authorization by the board of nursing but under the Department/Board of Health (NCSBN, 2020a). CNSs must incorporate a component of direct care into their practice to reclaim and maintain the regulatory and professional recognition that CNSs are APRNs.

The consensus model requires title protection for CNSs, which would be a step forward for states not having this basic regulatory requirement. A grandfather clause (i.e., recognizing and granting authority to APRNs who graduated from accredited programs and were in practice before the implementation date of the consensus model) is included in the model regulatory language. This grandfather clause is important for CNSs because certification examinations are not available for all population foci (see National Certification for Clinical Nurse Specialists later). Certification of APRNs at the role (e.g., CNM, NP) and population focus (e.g., neonate, women's health) levels is required for all APRNs to be licensed at the advanced practice level. CNS certification in a specialty (e.g., oncology) is voluntary and outside the licensure of APRNs once an individual state fully adopts the consensus model. A summary of the consensus model implementation (scored according to how much of the model is implemented) revealed that to date there are 16 states and two territories that have implemented 100% of the model (NCSBN, 2022b).

At the 2018 NCSBN meeting, it was recognized that the APRN consensus model was 10 years old and there were inconsistencies in both the regulatory interpretation and the implementation of the model in states (NCSBN, 2019). Resolutions were passed that included convening a forum of state board regulators to examine these issues, and a report was delivered to the 2019 NCSBN annual meeting (NCSBN, 2019). Although issues discussed were of more relevance to NPs and CRNAs, the implication of implementing those decisions would impact CNSs; for example, NPs wanting to be called NPs as opposed to APRNs and CRNAs preferring to be called nurse anesthesiologist. Changing the APRN title would minimally have an impact on CNS billing. The final recommendation of

TABLE 12.2

NACNS Strategies for Enacting the Institute of Medicine's (IOM's) *The Future of Nursing* Recommendations Related to the Clinical Nurse Specialist (CNS) Role

IOM Key Message	NACNS Recommendations for Enactment
Nurses should practice to the fullest extent of their education and training.	Amend nurse practice acts to allow CNSs to diagnose and treat health conditions.
	Eliminate requirements for physician "collaborative practice agreements."
	Remove prescribing restrictions or limitations imposed by required physician oversight, collaboration, or signature.
	Amend requirements for hospital participation in the Medicare program to ensure that CNSs are eligible for clinical privileges, admitting privileges, and membership on medical staffs.
	Advocate for all insurers, including but not limited to Medicare, Medicaid, and third-party insurers, to include coverage of CNS services that are within their scope of practice under state law.
	Amend the Medicare and Medicaid programs to authorize CNSs to perform admission assessments, certify patients for home healthcare services, and admit patients to hospitals, hospice, and skilled nursing facilities.
Nurses should achieve higher levels of education and training through an improved education system that promotes seamless academic progression.	Advocate for academic institutions to offer research and practice doctorates that support CNS specialty-focused advanced practice nursing.
	Advocate for CNS-focused courses in doctoral programs.
	Develop bachelor of science in nursing (BSN)–to–doctor of philosophy (PhD) and BSN-to–doctor of nursing practice (DNP) programs for CNSs to streamline the process for preparing research and clinical scholars.
	Recommend options for seamless progression to DNP preparation for CNSs.
Nurses should be full partners, with physicians and other healthcare professionals, in redesigning health care in the United States.	Promote interprofessional education at the graduate level to optimize collaboration skills.
	Support entrepreneurial opportunities for CNSs in the design, implementation, and evaluation of innovative care models.
	Optimize education related to technology and technology evaluation.
	Revise or amend regulatory language to recognize CNSs as primary care providers for patients with chronic health problems related to medical diagnoses such as diabetes, heart failure, and mental health or chronic conditions such as chronic wounds, chronic pain, or impaired mobility.
	Actively engage CNSs in healthcare policy decisions.
	Advocate for organizational support to increase CNSs' responsibility in implementing system improvements.
	Encourage accountable care organizations to include CNS services among all services provided.
	Facilitate the delivery of CNS specialty services in novel healthcare delivery systems.
	Foster the use of CNS leadership skills in the redesign of healthcare delivery across settings.
	Encourage CNSs to design, implement, and evaluate new systems of providing care to specialty populations.
	Advocate for CNS opportunities for continued development of leadership skills (lifelong learning).
	Encourage and mentor CNSs to participate in policy and regulatory bodies.

Continued

TABLE 12.2

NACNS Strategies for Enacting the Institute of Medicine's (IOM's) *The Future of Nursing* Recommendations Related to the Clinical Nurse Specialist (CNS) Role—cont'd

IOM Key Message	NACNS Recommendations for Enactment
Effective workforce planning and policymaking require better data collection and an improved information infrastructure.	Ensure that the criteria for all future survey designs include CNSs. For example, the Workforce Commission and the Health Resources Services Administration may want to develop an APRN survey focusing on the underserved and vulnerable populations. It is critical that CNSs provide the necessary consultation to ensure that CNS-sensitive outcomes are captured within such a survey.
	Include CNSs in the design of all workforce standardized minimum data sets (MDSs), including work by state licensing boards.
	Increase the sample size and fielding of the survey to every other year, facilitating expanding the data collected on APRNs, and release survey results more quickly.
	Include recommendations by CNSs when establishing a monitoring system that uses data from the MDS to measure systematically and project nursing workforce requirements by role, skill mix, region, and demographics.
	Integrate CNSs when coordinating workforce research efforts with the Department of Labor, state and regional educators, employers, and state nursing workforce centers to identify regional healthcare workforce needs and when establishing regional targets and plans for appropriately increasing the supply of health professionals.

Adapted from "Response to the Institute of Medicine's *The Future of Nursing* Report," by National Association of Clinical Nurse Specialists, 2012b, http://nacns.org/advocacy-policy/position-statements/response-to-the-institute-of-medicines-future-of-nursing-report/

the discussion was that the consensus model should not be revised.

Reimbursement for Clinical Nurse Specialist Services

In October 2019 then-President Trump signed an executive order with the goal of enabling providers to spend more time with their patients (Centers for Medicare and Medicaid Services, 2019). It directed the secretary of Health and Human Services (HHS) to re-form the Medicare program to eliminate excessive supervision requirements for the APRN, provide equal pay for equal work of the physician, remove unspecified conditions of participation requirements, and operationalize the CNS practicing to the full extent of their education. If enacted, unspecified supervision requirements, conditions of participation, and licensure requirements that do not allow clinicians to work at the top of their profession could all be eliminated (Hewitt, 2019). In addition, pay disparities could be eliminated; that is, APRNs being reimbursed at 85% of physician reimbursement (Hewitt, 2019).

In a June 2019 report to Congress by MedPAC, a bipartisan advisory group to Congress on issues related to Medicare, it was identified that APRNs and physician assistants were providing an increasing share of medical services (MedPAC, 2019). Recommended changes specific to "incident to" billing was made. Currently, APRNs, including CNSs, can bill under an "incident to" category (see Chapter 19). This allows the APRN to be reimbursed at 100% if the service provided meets certain criteria including the service is billed under the national provider identifier (NPI) of a supervising physician. However, if that same service is provided under the APRNs NPI, only 85% is reimbursed. The committee recommended that Congress eliminate the "incident to" billing and that the secretary of HHS refine Medicare's specialty designation for APRNs. The committee also found that NPs are increasingly providing more specialty care in addition to primary care. This creates an opportunity for CNSs, whose hallmark is specialty care, to explore options for providing care and obtaining reimbursement.

Availability and Standardization of Educational Curricula for Clinical Nurse Specialists

CNSs have graduate education at either the master's or doctoral level. Post-master's certificate programs are also available. Educational programs are currently guided by AACN's master's *Essentials* (AACN, 2011; Mohr & Coke, 2018) or, if at a doctoral level, AACN's DNP *Essentials* (AACN, 2006; Mohr & Coke, 2018) but will be transitioning to conform with the updated AACN *Essentials* (2021). In addition, education for the CNS is also guided by professional competencies developed by NACNS (2019b) that are based on the three spheres of impact.

The AACN has identified that variability exists in CNS programs, including the curriculum, expectations for student performance, and evaluation processes and tools (AACN, 2015). In addition, AACN's revised *Essentials* document (2021) will compel APRN programs to transition to full competency-based curriculum criteria. NACNS has revised the *Statement on Clinical Nurse Specialist Practice and Education* (NACNS, 2019b), the core competencies for CNSs, regardless of specialty and/or level of graduate education (i.e., master's vs. DNP; see Table 12.1), and the evaluation criteria for CNS programs at all levels to help standardize education and practice for the new graduate CNS. The purpose of the program evaluation criteria is to promote standardization of nationally endorsed criteria that are used for development and/or implementation of CNS programs.

Despite efforts to standardize CNS graduate preparation, there continue to be unique challenges for this APRN role (AACN, 2015). These challenges include state-to-state variations in defining and recognizing CNS scope of practice and licensing, sufficient clinical sites and CNS-prepared preceptors to prepare students in all areas across the wellness continuum, and clinical practicum hours and experiences to prepare students for specialty practice in addition to role and population preparation (AACN, 2015). To ensure that the CNS continues to be a recognized advanced practice nursing role, the need is urgent to continue to clarify competencies, standardize CNS curricula, and reach a rational consensus on how to credential CNSs from multiple specialties. Many initiatives are under way that will directly or indirectly affect future CNS preparation, credentialing, and practice. It is necessary to continuously modify or update program curricula with the purpose of preparing CNSs to provide expert care to patients and improve patient outcomes through education and system changes.

Ongoing initiatives are also challenging traditional CNS education. In 2015 the NACNS endorsed the DNP as entry into practice by 2030 (NACNS, 2015). Although DNP programs have rapidly expanded, the majority of CNSs are still prepared at the master's level (Auerbach et al., 2015; NACNS, 2019a). There is also still debate about the consequences of the DNP requirement, some of which may be unintended. Concerns that it may result in fewer students preparing to be CNSs to meet geographic pockets of shortages have been discussed in the literature. The length of the DNP curriculum and inability of some universities to offer doctorates pose a challenge for both academic institutions and students. The separation of the profession's practice and research missions, the acronym's suggestion that a DNP is an NP, and regulatory considerations are additional concerns about the DNP degree requirement (Chase & Pruitt, 2006; Fulton & Lyon, 2005; Meleis & Dracup, 2005).

National Certification for Clinical Nurse Specialists

Certification at the population level for CNSs by examination is available through the American Nurses Credentialing Center (ANCC) and the American Association of Critical-Care Nurses Certification Corporation. Current certifications are limited to adult/gerontological (American Association of Critical-Care Nurses, 2015), pediatric, and neonatal CNSs and adult/gerontology from ANCC (n.d.). The certified CNSs for adult, pediatric, and neonatal critical care are available only for renewal though AACN Certification Corporation. Specialty CNS certifications are also available from specialty organizations such as the Oncology Nursing Certification Corporation (Oncology Nursing Certification Corporation, 2022). However, certification examinations are not available for many CNS specialties, such as cardiovascular, neuroscience, and perinatal nursing; specialty certification examinations do not meet the role and population foci certification as articulated in the NCSBN consensus model regulatory language. If states are going to adopt the consensus model, it is imperative that nationally recognized CNS certification examinations be developed for the role to survive. In 2002 the NCSBN decided to remove alternative mechanisms for granting APRN licensure, such as a portfolio or clinical practice evaluation (Hartigan, 2011). Today, the NACNS encourages states to analyze how the lack of a certification examination for all population foci for CNSs will have an impact on practice within each state before fully implementing the consensus model (NACNS, 2012a).

Variability in Individual Clinical Nurse Specialist Practices and Prescriptive Authority

The evolution of the CNS role has been dynamic. CNSs who pioneered the role were specialists in psychiatry and mental health. The CNS was initially conceptualized as an expert clinician, consultant, educator, and researcher (Hamric & Spross, 1989). Direct care, although central, was not the only focus. Integrating these role manifestations has been difficult but essential to sustain the role's effectiveness, yet differentiating these elements has not been sufficient to describe what CNSs do.

Variability exists in requirements for prescriptive authority for CNSs (Stokowski, 2018). While states' scopes of practice are changing to support CNS prescription of pharmacologic agents, not all CNSs were prepared in their original education curriculum to prescribe, and states have addressed this using various approaches. For example, in 2005, Oregon recognized CNSs as APRNs, including prescriptive authority (Klein, 2012, 2015). A task force was convened by the Oregon Board of Nursing where the final requirement to allow CNSs to prescribe was equivalent to requirements for NP programs (Berlin et al., 2002), and the final Oregon regulation for prescribing included a course in advanced pharmacology and a minimum of 150 hours of supervised pharmacologic management (Klein, 2012).

In Minnesota, CNSs must practice for 2080 hours within the context of a collaborative agreement within a hospital or integrated care setting with a Minnesota-licensed CNP, CNS, or physician who has experience providing care to patients with similar medical problems before they can prescribe independently (Stokowski, 2018). In contrast, in Wisconsin, APRNs with prescriptive authority are defined as advanced practice nurse prescribers (APNPs) and must pass an examination on Wisconsin statutes and rules pertaining to practice of APNPs (Stokowski, 2018). In addition, there are annual educational requirements for the APNP and requirements that include obliging the APNP to carry personal liability malpractice insurance.

The consensus model supports the prescribing of pharmacologic agents by all APRNs (APRN Joint Dialogue Group, 2008). Most current data show that since 2010, CNSs can prescribe independently in 22 states and territories, though some do have qualifiers for independent prescriptive authority (NCSBN, 2020b). Some CNSs want prescriptive authority, whereas others do not, and both sides have been adamant about their positions rather than acknowledging that prescribing is a privilege that an individual CNS can exercise based on their preference and practice. This latter approach is how NPs handled this issue—they want prescriptive authority; whether they will use it or not is up to the individual. Physicians are also the same; most use it, some do not, but all have the authority. The key to moving forward is to publicly support the safety of prescriptive authority for CNSs and discuss the positive contributions to patient outcomes based on that authority. This consistent messaging will help regulators and other professionals outside the CNS community understand the possibilities for the role.

Understanding the Similarities and Differences Between Clinical Nurse Specialists and Nurse Practitioners

The origins of the CNS and NP roles arose from very different needs in health care when the roles were created. In response to a need for nurses with specialized knowledge and training in psychiatric nursing, Peplau (1952) created the first CNS educational program (see Chapter 1). In the 1960s, clinical nurse specialization, specifically in psychiatry and mental health as well as in critical care units, took its modern form as a result of three forces in health care: (1) an increase in specialty-related information, (2) new technologic advances, and (3) a response to public need and interest. In coronary care units, nurses expanded their knowledge and skills by learning how to identify cardiac arrhythmias, administer intravenous medications, and defibrillate patients. These nurses were, in fact, diagnosing and treating patients (Chapter 1). Therefore the origin of the CNS role was born out of a need for specialty practices. Ironically, today many NPs, a role originally developed to help relieve the shortage of physicians in poor and rural areas, are now entering specialty practice because the need for specialists has grown (Martsolf et al., 2020).

In the 1990s, several forces in health care—a downturn in the fiscal health of hospitals; layoffs or repurposing of CNSs into quality managers, case managers, or nurse educator roles; increased emphasis on primary care and rapid growth of NP programs; and the introduction of acute care NPs—led to a sharp decrease in the number of nurses entering CNS programs (see Chapter 1). Confusion about the CNS role and activities persists today despite the NACNS's historical efforts to publicize core competencies and activities (Mohr & Coke, 2018; The National CNS Competency Task Force, 2010).

As noted, the Commission on Collegiate Nursing Education (CCNE) accreditation mandates that all APRN students receive the three Ps (i.e., pathophysiology, physical assessment, pharmacology; AACN, 2006). Knowledge of the pathophysiology, assessment, and treatment of sepsis, for instance, is no different if a clinician is a CNS, an NP, or a physician.

There are differences, however, between the two roles. Significantly, the amount of time spent performing a particular competency or activity is different for each. For example, adult–gerontology acute and critical care CNSs spend time among the three spheres of impact as outlined by the NACNS (Becker et al., 2020; NACNS, 2019b; Saunders, 2015), whereas adult–gerontology acute care NPs spend most of their time in direct care management of patients (Becker et al., 2020; Buerhaus et al., 2015). In a systematic review of global literature, Cooper et al. (2019) examined the similarities and differences between CNSs and NPs. They found that both roles had improved quality of patient care, provided a similar quality of care as physicians, were cost-effective, reduced waiting times and waiting lists for patients, and had an almost equal positive impact. Differences identified were that NPs were more generalist and the CNS was more of a specialist. Mohr and Coke (2018) examined the similarities and differences between the two roles and found that, although the educational preparation is many times seen as similar, in reality they are two distinct roles and the scope of CNSs is distinguishable from that of other APRNs. With the introduction of the DNP degree, core competencies for APRNs who graduate from these programs will have a balance of direct care management education and didactic instruction in education and systems changes to produce a more well-rounded clinician. CNSs receive more instruction about direct care management and NPs receive more instruction about education and EBP evaluation and implementation than prior to introduction of the DNP. Although the two roles are receiving similar education content and have some overlap in skills, it is unclear whether the shift of education content will substantially change their daily practice patterns due to the fundamentally different underpinnings of the two roles.

In 2007, the American Psychiatric Nurses Association (APNA) and the International Society of Psychiatric Mental Health Nurses (ISPN) published a job analysis between the psychiatric–mental health CNS (PMH-CNS) and the psychiatric–mental health NP (PMH-NP) that found there was 90% commonality in the two roles (Rice et al., 2007). However, a subsequent analysis of the items in the job analysis revealed that there was a heavy emphasis on direct care activities that are more typical to the NP role as opposed to items specific to activities in the nurse/nursing personnel or organization/systems spheres of impact, which are typical components of the CNS role (Jones & Minarik, 2012). Weiss and Talley (2009) studied the differences between CNSs and family psychiatric NPs in adolescents and school-aged children and found that CNSs treated more school-aged children and provided more psychotherapy, especially individual therapy and parent–family life therapy. However, the researchers concluded that there were more commonalities than differences and suggested standards be set for both groups.

For PMH APRNs, competency must be attained in the APRN, medical, and psychotherapy domains. PMH-CNSs have a strong history of in-depth psychotherapy training, whereas PMH-NPs have more training in psychopharmacology. Based on the job analysis findings, the APNA and the ISPN endorsed the recommendation that educational programs prepare PMH APRNs as NPs educated across the life span (APNA, 2011).

All PMH APRNs now take the same examination, titled the Psychiatric–Mental Health Nurse Practitioner–Board Certified (PMHNP-BC) certification examination (ANCC, 2017). As the APNA and the ISPN continue to consider implications for CNSs and NPs in psychiatric and mental health, it will be important to continue to incorporate core competencies of the two roles, which include medical, psychiatric, and psychotherapy treatment modalities; educating and supporting interprofessional staff; and facilitating change and innovation in healthcare systems to provide improved access to high-quality mental health care.

ROLE IMPLEMENTATION

Because of the potential for lack of clarity in the CNS role, it is imperative that CNSs entering a new position understand and prepare for optimal entry into the role. In a Canadian study, Kilpatrick et al. (2016b) had CNSs identify both structure and process factors that can facilitate implementation of the role. Organizational structural factors identified by the CNSs included making certain that orientation is planned and structured rather than having an ad hoc approach with each new CNS, ensuring adequate leadership support and stakeholder involvement, and having a structure that facilitates team support. Something as simple as co-location can facilitate development of team cohesion and complementary role functions (Kilpatrick et al., 2016b). The CNSs identified that it was also important that the CNS take personal accountability to obtain certification in a specialty area of practice. Process factors that the CNSs identified that were important to successful role implementation included consistent role titles and expectations, which facilitated both intraprofessional and interprofessional relationship development.

CNSs have different reporting structures in different organizations (e.g., reporting to physicians, directors of nursing, directors of education, chief nursing officers), all of which have advantages and disadvantages. Understanding the reporting structure and corresponding implications is important for any CNS new to a role. CNSs have identified barriers in fully implementing their role (Mayo et al., 2010): multiple job expectations, lack of time, lack of personnel, and lack of secretarial support. These are not unique solely to the CNS role; however, acknowledging the possibility of these when starting a new position informs the CNS and provides leverage to negotiate resources and expectations when accepting a CNS position.

Additional factors affect CNS role implementation, satisfaction, and intent to stay in the role. Kilpatrick and colleagues (2016a) found that activities such as scholarly and professional development improved role satisfaction and indirectly intent to stay. The authors recommended collaboration between managers and CNSs to find a balance between activities, workloads, patient needs, and optimizing CNS satisfaction (Kilpatrick et al., 2016a).

Use of a framework such as the participatory, evidence-based, patient-focused process for advanced practice nursing (APN) role development, implementation, and evaluation PEPPA framework (Kilpatrick et al., 2016a) or the clinical nurse specialist conceptualization, implementation, and evaluation framework (Jokiniemi et al., 2020) is especially important when implementing the nonclinical components of the CNS role, although it will support implementation of all role components. Use of a framework can also help the organization in the aspects of identifying when a new APRN role is needed, defining new roles, and promoting clarity among team members.

Evaluation of Practice

Because the full extent of a CNS's impact and outcomes may not always be readily visible, it is important that CNSs consider how to evaluate, track, and demonstrate their value and outcomes from day 1 in a new role. Although many CNS specialties develop practice setting–specific evaluation tools, a standardized tool should be developed for expected competencies and the assurance of outcome quality. Lunney et al. (2007) designed a tool for graduate students to use for self-evaluation of CNS competency development that could be adapted for practicing CNSs. Portfolios can be used as a tool to evaluate CNS practice by tracking outcomes related to nurse-sensitive indicators, patient satisfaction, and project-related metrics (Fischer-Cartlidge et al., 2019; Hespenheide et al., 2011). Another example that CNSs can use to quantify and describe their contributions to healthcare organization is the CNS cost analysis toolkit (NACNS, 2017).

CNSs may document the components of their clinical practice, including numbers of patients seen, types and frequencies of interventions, and outcomes achieved; educational activities for staff, including one-on-one coaching, in-service programs, orientation, and continuing education; and system initiatives, such as quality improvement activities and interprofessional rounds (AACN, 2006). To evaluate their ability and effectiveness in exercising influence, CNSs may ask nursing and other professional colleagues to comment on their communication and collaboration skills. CNSs may use this information for self-assessment to determine whether the allocation of activities is consistent with personal, professional, and institutional goals; to prepare quarterly reports; or to assemble a portfolio for their annual evaluations. Tracking these data enables CNSs to identify recurring events that may require an intervention at the staff or system level and midcourse corrections if schedule demands require a shift in goals or a realignment of expectations.

In the early days of CNS practice, few studies documented the impact of CNSs on patient and family outcomes. While evidence is mounting, small local EBP projects or small research studies provide limited evidence from which to draw conclusions (see Chapter 21). Some hospitals hire CNSs specifically for their positive impact on patient outcomes. Outcome studies can help CNSs document their activities and effects on patients and families. Example studies have shown the impact of CNS interventions on causes of medication errors (Flanders & Clark, 2010) and, specifically, in regard to revising a policy on labeling medications and solutions on the sterile field in the operating room (Brown-Brumfield & DeLeon, 2010). As these topics suggest, CNSs can identify relevant structure, process, and outcome variables that can be used to assess the CNSs' contributions to quality patient care, including use of clinical practice guidelines and the effect on clinical outcomes.

Evaluation of CNS practice often includes outcomes management (AACN, 2021). One component of outcomes management is the analysis of data regarding care efficiency and cost-effectiveness, the results of which guide systematic and continuous process and performance improvement. CNSs at one institution, for example, were instrumental in developing a hospital-wide process that promoted EBP guidelines through research, patient safety workshops, nursing staff orientation, professionalism, quality of work life, and prevention of falls (Ford et al., 2011).

Practice evaluation must be integrated into one's daily work. Although researchers have begun to identify the interventions used most often by APRNs, there continues to be a need for demonstrating the outcomes of CNS interventions in all settings (see Chapter 21).

FUTURE DIRECTIONS

Three powerful forces converged to influence the practice and regulation of APRNs: the IOM report on *The Future of Nursing* (IOM, 2011), the consensus model for APRN regulation (APRN Joint Dialogue Group, 2008), and healthcare reform. Undoubtedly, additional forces are impacting and will continue to impact CNS practice to address the increasingly complex problems of patient populations and the healthcare system itself (e.g., COVID-19 pandemic, societal and healthcare inequities). There are many exciting opportunities for CNSs to advance their roles and ensure a unique place in the healthcare system. At the same time, the CNS role is threatened by wide variability in philosophy, education, and operationalization that perpetuates role confusion or ambiguity among those in the CNS community, regulators, educators, employers, and the public. To combat the forces that threaten the survival of the role, CNSs must engage in five action areas:

1. **Cohesive Voice**. CNSs need to unify around the NCSBN regulatory affirmation of CNSs as being APRNs, with a significant component of practice in the direct care of individuals and an expanded scope of practice that includes advanced assessment, diagnosing, prescribing, and ordering (NCSBN, 2008). A cohesive voice from the CNS community must advocate for all activities to be legally permissible in state scopes of practice and in individual practices, regardless of individual practices or preferences. Use of common language shared by all APRN groups is essential for identifying shared knowledge, skills, and practices. This reduces the perception of infighting and advances the CNS as an APRN role in collaboration with other APRNs. There is strength in numbers and internal unity.

2. **Demonstrate Value**. CNSs must clearly articulate their contributions to patients, families, and the healthcare system in the three spheres of impact (NACNS, 2019b). By claiming the definition of CNS practice defined at the beginning of the chapter, CNSs can differentiate themselves from other APRNs and still provide direct and indirect care to patients to improve health outcomes in specialty populations.
3. **Strengthen CNS Specialty Practice Within the Three Spheres of Impact**. CNSs must ensure that educational curricula and continuing education programs prepare current and future CNSs with the knowledge and skills to have an expanded practice at the advanced level with specialty populations, educate interprofessional staff, and facilitate change and innovation in healthcare systems. Adherence to the AACN *Essentials* (AACN, 2021) is mandatory for the accreditation of APRN programs and serves as the basis for educational standards, according to the consensus model for APRN regulation (APRN Joint Dialogue Group, 2008). The core competencies developed by the NACNS should serve as a guide to didactic courses and clinical practice, with an additional focus area on disease management (NACNS, 2019b). Preceptors must have CNS students engage in activities in these three spheres of CNS practice to prepare them for a future successful practice. CNSs have a strong history of continuing educational conferences focused on nursing education and systems or process improvement. Continuing education programs for CNSs should increase the course offerings to include care management of specialty populations, including disease and medication management as well as methods for documenting and demonstrating outcomes and value.
4. **Build a Stronger Research Agenda**. CNSs need to be innovative in partnering with others to reform health care. CNS models of population care should be developed and researched, including those that extend beyond the traditional inpatient CNS role. CNSs should collaborate with nurse researchers in conducting and publishing comparative effectiveness studies that test the efficacy of CNS interventions in complex and vulnerable specialty populations, patient outcomes, and innovative new care models. Comparative effectiveness research "is designed to inform health-care decisions by providing evidence on the effectiveness, benefits, and harms of different treatment options. The evidence is generated from research studies that compare drugs, medical devices, tests, surgeries, or ways to deliver health care" (AHRQ, 2012). CNSs continue to need to establish that patient outcomes are improved, safe, and high quality as a direct result of their interventions compared with other practice models. More studies need to be carried out to compare CNS effectiveness in achieving patient outcomes and system-wide improvements, with CNSs managing care as the intervention.
5. **Lead Policy Efforts to Standardize, Credential, and Legitimize CNS Practice**. CNSs need to seek recognition as APRNs statewide, nationally, and internationally through involvement in policymaking and healthcare reform efforts. Local recognition can be obtained by seeking institutional credentialing and privileging and ensuring that institutional job descriptions incorporate the three spheres of impact, with particular attention to the direct care of individuals. CNSs must become involved in passing regulations and legislation using consensus model language and including CNSs as APRNs in state regulations or statutes. CNSs must lobby and advocate for national certification mechanisms that accurately reflect CNS practice. In addition, CNSs need to monitor national changes to regulation in agencies such as the Centers for Medicare & Medicaid Services to ensure that CNSs continue to be recognized as APRNs for purposes of reimbursement.

Development of CNS and APRN roles will continue to expand internationally. The International Council of Nurses (ICN) has established the ICN Nurse Practitioner/Advanced Practice Nursing Network (see Chapter 5). The goal, aims, and objectives of this group are

> *... to become an international resource for nurses practising in nurse practitioner (NP) or advanced nursing practice (ANP) roles, and interested others (e.g., policymakers, educators, regulators, health planners) by:*

1. *Making relevant and timely information about practice, education, role development, research, policy and regulatory developments, and appropriate events widely available;*
2. *Providing a forum for sharing and exchange of knowledge expertise and experience;*
3. *Supporting nurses and countries who are in the process of introducing or developing NP or ANP roles and practice;*
4. *Accessing international resources that are pertinent to this field.*

(ICN, 2021)

CNS titling, education, and regulatory issues continue to be a challenge to establishing the role internationally; however, there are many driving forces that support role creation (see Chapter 5). CNSs should maintain awareness of these international efforts and participate in educational exchanges to standardize and collaborate on continuing to define CNS practice when feasible and learn from each other on how to optimize the role and role utilization.

CONCLUSION

CNSs have a strong and tumultuous history. Over the past 35 years, the departure from direct patient care as being a main focus to working predominantly in the nursing education and systems improvement domains has created confusion within nursing and the public because non-CNSs (e.g., nurse educators, quality improvement managers, clinical nurse leaders) function in a similar capacity. However, CNSs are uniquely educated to provide advanced practice and specialist expertise when working directly with complex and vulnerable patients, educating and supporting nurses and nursing and interprofessional staff, and facilitating change and innovation in healthcare systems that those in other roles in health care cannot.

As healthcare reform continues to gain momentum to improve healthcare system quality, there will be many new opportunities for CNSs. As masters of flexibility and creativity, CNSs must be innovative to meet the needs of patients and healthcare systems. The possibilities are endless if CNSs understand their role, improve understanding of the importance of this role in advanced practice nursing, and maximize the driving forces and minimize the restraining forces related to the role in the healthcare system.

KEY SUMMARY POINTS

- CNSs demonstrate the six competencies of APRN practice across three spheres of impact—patient direct care sphere, nurses and nursing practice sphere, and systems and organizations sphere—regardless of setting or specialty.
- CNSs must be persistent and unified in clearly articulating their unique contributions and role to patients, families, other healthcare professionals, administrators, and the public.
- There need to be continued efforts to ensure standardization of CNS educational curricula and opportunities for certification in specialty practice.
- CNSs need to lead innovative efforts and document improved patient outcomes in the current environment of healthcare reform.

REFERENCES

Abela-Dimech, F., Johnson, K., & Strudwick, G. (2017). Development and pilot implementation of a search protocol to improve patient safety on a psychiatric inpatient unit. *Clinical Nurse Specialist*, *31*(2), 104–114.

Agency for Healthcare Research and Quality. (2012). What is comparative effectiveness research. Retrieved from https://www.ahrq.gov/sites/default/files/wysiwyg/cpi/about/mission/budget/2012/2012opa.pdf

American Association of Colleges of Nursing. (2006). The essentials of doctoral education for advanced nursing practice. Retrieved from http://www.aacn.nche.edu/publications/position/DNPEssentials.pdf

American Association of Colleges of Nursing. (2011). *The essentials of master's education for advanced practice nursing*. American Association of Colleges of Nursing.

American Association of Colleges of Nursing. (2015). White Paper: Re-envisioning the clinical education of advanced practice registered nurses. Retrieved from https://www.pncb.org/sites/default/files/2017 03/APRN Clinical Education.pdf

American Association of Colleges of Nursing. (2020). Fact sheet: The doctor of nursing practice (DNP). Retrieved from https://www.aacnnursing.org/Portals/42/News/Factsheets/DNP-Factsheet.pdf

American Association of Colleges of Nursing. (2021). *The essentials: Core competencies for professional nursing education*. American Association of Colleges of Nursing. https://www.aacnnursing.org/Portals/42/AcademicNursing/pdf/Essentials-2021.pdf

American Association of Critical-Care Nurses. (2014). *AACN scope and standards for acute care clinical nurse specialist practice*. American Association of Critical-Care Nurses.

American Association of Critical-Care Nurses. (2015). *APRN - advanced practice certification*. https://www.aacn.org/~/media/aacn-website/certification/advanced-practice/aprncertification-brochure.pdf?la=en

American Nurses Association. (1955). ANA board approves a definition of nursing practice. *American Journal of Nursing, 5*, 1474.

American Nurses Association. (2003). *Nursing's social policy statement* (2nd ed.). American Nurses Association.

American Nurses Association. (2010). *Nursing's social policy statement* (3rd ed.). American Nurses Association.

American Nurses Credentialing Center. (2017). Psychiatric–mental health nurse practitioner (across the lifespan) certification (PMHNP-BE). Retrieved from https://www.nursingworld.org/our-certifications/psychiatric-mental-health-nurse-practitioner/

American Nurses Credentialing Center (ANCC). (n.d.). Our certifications. https://www.nursingworld.org/our-certifications/

American Psychiatric Nurses Association. (2011). APNA Board of Directors endorses APNA/ISPN Joint Task Force recommendations on the implementation of the "Consensus model for APRN regulation: Licensure, accreditation, certification & education." Retrieved from https://www.apna.org/m/pages.cfm?pageID=4495

Ansryan, L. Z., Marshall, C., Aronow, H. U., Chan, A., & Coleman, B. (2019). Inspiring writing in nursing: A clinical nurse specialist-led program. *Clinical Nurse Specialist, 33*(2), 90–96.

APRN Joint Dialogue Group. (2008). *Consensus Model for APRN regulation: Licensure, accreditation, certification & education*. Retrieved from http://www.aacn.nche.edu/education-resources/APRNReport.pdf

Auerbach, D. I., Martsolf, G., Pearson, M. L., Taylor, E. A., Zaydman, M., Muchow, A. N., et al. (2015). The DNP by 2015: A study of the institutional, political, and professional issues that facilitate or impede establishing a post-baccalaureate doctor of nursing practice program. RAND Corporation. Retrieved from http://www.rand.org/pubs/research_reports/RR730.html

Barton, A. J., & Makic, M. B. F. (2015). Technology and patient safety. *Clinical Nurse Specialist, 29*, 129–130.

Becker, D., Dechant, L., McNamara, L. J., Konick-McMahon, J., Noe, C. A., Thomas, K., & Fabrey, L. J. (2020). Practice analysis: Adult gerontology acute care nurse practitioner and clinical nurse specialist. *American Journal of Critical Care, 29*(2), e19–e30.

Berlin, L. E., Harper, D., Werner, K. E., & Stennett, J. (2002). *Master's-level nurse practitioner educational programs. Findings from the 2000-2001 collaborative curriculum survey*. American Association of the Colleges of Nursing and National Organization of Nurse Practitioner Faculties. Retrieved from https://files.eric.ed.gov/fulltext/ED481680.pdf

Brooks, E. (2020). From shadow to change agent: Revitalization of the clinical nurse specialist role. *Nursing Forum, 55*(2), 297–300.

Brown-Brumfield, D., & DeLeon, A. (2010). Adherence to a medication safety protocol: Current practice for labeling medications and solutions on the sterile field. *AORN Journal, 91*, 610–617.

Bryant-Lukosius, D., Carter, N., Reid, K., Donald, F., Martin-Misener, R., Kilpatrick, K., Harbman, P., Kaasalainen, S., Marshall, D., Charbonneau-Smith, R., & DiCenso, A. (2015). The clinical effectiveness and cost-effectiveness of clinical nurse specialist-led hospital to home transitional care: A systematic review. *Journal of Evaluation in Clinical Practice, 21*(5), 763–781.

Buerhaus, P. I., DesRoches, C. M., Dittus, R., & Donelan, K. (2015). Practice characteristics of primary care nurse practitioners and physicians. *Nursing Outlook, 63*(2), 144–153.

Campaign for Action. (September 4, 2017). Clinical nurse specialists: A force for improving safety, outcomes, and health care delivery. Retrieved from https://campaignforaction.org/clinical-nurse-specialists-a-force-for-improving-safety-outcomes-and-health-care-delivery/

Catania, K., & Tippett, J. E. (2015). Outcomes of clinical nurse specialist role transformation to population-focused model. *Clinical Nurse Specialist, 29*(6), e1–10.

Cavanaugh, K. J., Kronebusch, B. J., Luedke, T. C., & Pike, M. L. (2021). Reflections on ambulatory care nursing and the clinical nurse specialist. *Clinical Nurse Specialist, 35*(1), 31–37.

Chanyeong, K., & Young, K. (2019). Clinical nurse specialist-led implementation of an early discharge protocol after cardiac surgery. *Clinical Nurse Specialist, 33*(4), 184–190.

Chase, S. K., & Pruitt, R. H. (2006). The practice doctorate: Innovation or disruption? *Journal of Nursing Education, 45*, 155–161.

Centers for Medicare and Medicaid Services. (2019). Trump administration strengthens Medicare by reducing provider burden and valuing spent with patients. https://www.cms.gov/newsroom/press-releases/trump-administration-strengthens-medicare-reducing-provider-burden-and-valuing-time-spent-patients

Coen, J., & Curry, K. (2016). Improving heart failure outcomes: The role of the clinical nurse specialist. *Critical Care Nurse Quarterly, 39*(4), 335–344.

Cooper, M. A., McDowell, J., Raeside, L., & ANP-CNS, Group. (2019). The similarities and differences between advanced nurse practitioners and clinical nurse specialists. *British Journal of Nursing, 28*(20), 1308–3013.

Cronenwett, L. R. (1995). Molding the future of advanced practice nursing. *Nursing Outlook, 43*(3), 112–118.

Cross, K. L., Johnson, P., Allard, B. L., & Shuman, C. J. (2020). Clinical nurse specialist perceptions of transitioning into a rural community-based transitional care role. *Journal of Nursing Administration, 50*(9), 456–461.

Department of Veterans Affairs. (2016). Advanced practice registered nurses. 38 C.F.R. pt. 17. RIN 2900–AP44. Full practice authority for advanced practice registered nurses. AGENCY: Department of Veterans Affairs. ACTION: Final rule with comment period. *Federal Register, 81*(240), 90198–90297.

Emergency Nurses Association. (2011). *Competencies for clinical nurse specialists in emergency care*. Emergency Nurses Association.

Fabbruzzo-Cota, C., Frecea, M., Kozell, K., Pere, K., Thompson, T., & Tjan, T. (2016). A clinical nurse specialist–led interprofessional quality improvement project to reduce hospital-acquired pressure ulcers. *Clinical Nurse Specialist, 30*, 110–116.

Fels, J., Allard, B. L., Coppin, K., Hewson, K., & Richardson, B. (2015). Evolving role of the transitional care nurse in a small rural community. *Home Healthcare Now, 33*(4), 215–221.

Fischer-Cartlidge, E., Houlihan, N., & Browne, K. (2019). Building a renowned clinical nurse specialist team: Recruitment, role development and value identification. *Clinical Nurse Specialist, 33*(6), 266–272.

Flanders, S., & Clark, A. P. (2010). Interruptions and medication errors. *Clinical Nurse Specialist, 24*, 281–285.

Ford, P. E. A., Rolfe, S., & Kirkpatrick, H. (2011). A journey to patient-centered care in Ontario, Canada. *Clinical Nurse Specialist, 25*, 198–206.

Frankenfield, R., Thompson, K., Lindsey, A., & Rettig, A. (2018). Caring for staff: The role of psychiatric mental health advanced practice RNs in supporting oncology nurses. *Clinical Journla of Oncology Nursing, 22*(5), 569–572.

Frost, K., Stafos, S., Barbay, K., & Henderson, K. (2019). Achieving disease-specific care Joint Commission certification: The impact of clinical nurse specialist practice. *Clinical Nurse Specialist, 33*(6), 273–278.

Fulton, J. S., & Lyon, B. L. (2005). The need for some sense making: Doctor of nursing practice. *Online Journal of Issues in Nursing, 10*, 1. doi:10.3912/OJIN.Vol10No03Man03

Fulton, J. S., Mayo, A. M., Walker, J. A., & Urden, L. D. (2016). Core practice outcomes for clinical nurse specialists: A revalidation study. *Journal of Professional Nursing, 32*(4), 271–282.

Hamric, A. B., & Spross, J. A. (1989). *The clinical nurse specialist in theory and practice* (2nd ed.). WB Saunders.

Hansen, M. P., Kollauf, C. R., Saunders, M. M., & Santiago-Rotchford, L. (2019). Clinical nurse specialists: Leaders in managing chronic conditions. *Nursing Economics, 37*(2), 103–109.

Hanson, M. D. (2015). Role of the clinical nurse specialist in the journey to Magnet recognition. *AACN Advanced Critical Care, 26*(1), 50–57.

Hardware, B., Johnson, D., Hale, C., Ndosi, M., & Adebajo, A. (2014). Patients and nursing staff views of using the education needs assessment tool in rheumatology clinics: A qualitative study. *Journal of Clinical Nursing, 24*, 1048–1058.

Hartigan, C. (2011). APRN regulation: The licensure-certification interface. *AACN Advanced Critical Care, 22*, 50–65.

Hespenheide, M., Cottingham, T., & Mueller, G. (2011). Portfolio use as a tool to demonstrate professional development in advanced nursing practice. *Clinical Nurse Specialist, 25*, 312–320.

Hewitt, S. (2019). *What does Trump's new executive order mean for nurses?* Capitol Beat from the American Nurses Association. https://anacapitolbeat.org/2019/10/09/what-does-trumps-new-executive-order-mean-for-nurses/

Hoke, N., & Bradway, C. (2016). A CNS-directed initiative to reduce postoperative urinary retention in spinal surgery patients. *American Journal of Nursing, 16*(8), 47–52.

Institute of Medicine. (2011). *The future of nursing: Leading change, advancing health*. The National Academies Press. doi:10.17226/12956

International Council of Nurses. (2021). ICN nurse practitioner/advanced practice nursing network: Aims and objectives. Retrieved from http://international.aanp.org/About/Aims

Interprofessional Education Collaborative. (2016). *Core competencies for interprofessional collaborative practice: 2016 update*. Interprofessional Education Collaborative. https://hsc.unm.edu/ipe/resources/ipec-2016-core-competencies.pdf

Institute for Healthcare Improvement. (2022). Open school. http://www.ihi.org/education/IHIOpenSchool/Pages/defaultbackup2019.aspx

Jokiniemi, K., Korhonen, K., Karkkainen, A., Pekkarinen, T., & Pietila, A. M. (2020). Clinical nurse specialist role implementation, structures, processes and outcomes: Participatory action research. *Journal of Clinical Nursing*, 15–16. doi:10.1111/jocn.15594

Jones, J. S., & Minarik, P. A. (2012). The plight of the psychiatric clinical nurse specialist: The dismantling of the advanced practice nursing archetype. *Clinical Nurse Specialist, 26*, 121–125.

Kelvin, J. F., Thom, B., Benedict, C., Carter, J., Corcoran, S., Dickler, M. N., Goodman, K. A., Margolies, A., Matasar, M. J., Noy, A., & Goldfarb, S. B. (2016). Cancer and fertility program improves patient satisfaction with information received. *Journal of Clinical Oncology, 34*(15), 1780–1786.

Kilpatrick, K., Kaasalainen, S., Donald, F., Reid, K., Carter, N., Bryant-Lukosius, D., Martin-Misener, R., Harbman, P., Marshall, D. A., Charbonneau-Smith, R., & DiCenso, A. (2014). The effectiveness and cost-effectiveness of clinical nurse specialists in outpatient roles: A systematic review. *Journal of Evaluation in Clinical Practice, 20*(6), 1106–1123.

Kilpatrick, K., Tchouaket, E., Carter, N., Bryant-Lukosius, D., & DiCenso, A. (2016a). Relationship between clinical nurse specialist role implementation, satisfaction, and intent to stay. *Clinical Nurse Specialist, 30*(3), 159–166.

Kilpatrick, K., Tchouaket, E., Carter, N., Bryant-Lukosius, D., & DiCenso, A. (2016b). Structural and process factors that influence clinical nurse specialist role implementation. *Clinical Nurse Specialist, 30*, 89–100.

Kirk, A. P., McGlinsey, A., Beckett, A., Rudd, P., & Arbour, R. (2015). Restraint reduction, restraint elimination and best practice: Role of the CNS in patient safety. *Clinical Nurse Specialist, 29*(6), 321–328.

Klein, T. (2012). Implementing autonomous clinical nurse specialist prescriptive authority: A competency-based transition model. *Clinical Nurse Specialist, 26*, 254–262.

Klein, T. (2015). Clinical nurse specialist prescriber characteristics and challenges in Oregon. *Clinical Nurse Specialist, 29*, 156–165.

Lewis, B., & Allen, S. (2015). Leading change: Evidence-based transition. *Clinical Nurse Specialist, 29*(2), e1–e7.

Lunney, M., Gigliotti, E., & McMorrow, M. E. (2007). Tool development for evaluation of clinical nurse specialist competencies in graduate students. *Clinical Nurse Specialist, 21*, 145–151.

Lyon, B. L. (2004). The CNS regulatory quagmire—We need clarity about advanced nursing practice. *Clinical Nurse Specialist, 18*, 9–13.

Makic, M. B. F. (2015). Maximizing smart pump technology to enhance patient safety. *Clinical Nurse Specialist, 29*, 195–197.

Marshall, D. A., Donald, F., Lacny, S., Reid, K., Bryant-Lukosius, D., Carter, N., Charbonneau-Smith, R., Harbman, P., Kaasalainen, S., Kilpatrick, K., & Martin-Misener, R. (2015). Assessing the quality of economic evaluations of clinical nurse specialists and nurse practitioners: A systematic review of cost-effectiveness. *NursingPlus Open, 1*, 11–17.

Martsolf, G. R., Gigli, K. H., Reynolds, B. R., & McCorkle, M. (2020). Misalignment of specialty nurse practitioners and the Consensus Model. *Nurs Outlook, 68*(4), 385–387.

Mayo, A. M., Omery, A., Agocs-Scott, L. M., Khaghani, F., Meckes, P. G., Moti, N., Redeemer, J., Voorhees, M., Gravell, C., & Cuenca, E. (2010). Clinical nurse specialist practice patterns. *Clinical Nurse Specialist, 24*, 60–68.

MedPAC. (2019). Report to the Congress. Medicare and the health care delivery system. https://www.medpac.gov/wp-content/uploads/import_data/scrape_files/docs/default-source/reports/jun19_medpac_reporttocongress_sec.pdf

Meleis, A. I., & Dracup, K. (2005). The case against the DNP: History, timing, substance, and marginalization. *Online Journal of Issues in Nursing, 10*(3), 3. doi:10.3912/OJIN.Vol10No03Man02

Mohr, L. D., & Coke, L. A. (2018). Distinguishing the clinical nurse specialist from other graduate nursing roles. *Clinical Nurse Specialist, 32*(3), 139–151.

Muller, A. C., Hujcs, M., Dubendorf, P., & Harrington, P. T. (2010). Sustaining excellence: Clinical nurse specialist practice and Magnet designation. *Clinical Nurse Specialist, 24*, 252–259.

National Academies of Sciences, Engineering, and Medicine. (2019). *Taking action again clinician burnout: A systems approach to professional well-being*. Retrieved from https://www.nap.edu/catalog/25521/taking-action-against-clinician-burnout-a-systems-approach-to-professional

National Academies of Sciences, Engineering, and Medicine. (2021). *The future of nursing 2020-2030: Charting a path to achieve equity*. The National Academies Press. doi:10.17226/25982. Retrieved from https://nam.edu/publications/the-future-of-nursing-2020-2030/

National Association of Clinical Nurse Specialists. (2004). *Statement on clinical nurse specialist practice and education* (2nd ed.). National Association of Clinical Nurse Specialists.

National Association of Clinical Nurse Specialists. (2012a). National Association of Clinical Nurse Specialists' statement on the APRN Consensus Model implementation. Retrieved from http://nacns.org/advocacy-policy/position-statements/national-association-of-clinical-nurse-specialists-statement-on-the-aprn-consensus-model-implementation/

National Association of Clinical Nurse Specialists. (2012b). Response to the Institute of Medicine's *The Future of Nursing* report. Retrieved from http://nacns.org/advocacy-policy/position-statements/response-to-the-institute-of-medicines-future-of-nursing-report/

National Association of Clinical Nurse Specialists. (2015). Position statement on the Doctor of Nursing Practice. Retrieved from nacns.org/advocacy-policy/position-statements/position-statement-on-the-doctor-of-nursing-practice/

National Association of Clinical Nurse Specialists. (2017). Cost analysis toolkit. A business guide for the clinical nurse specialist. Retrieved from http://nacns.org/professional-resources/toolkits-and-reports/cost-analysis-toolkit/

National Association of Clinical Nurse Specialists. (2019a). Key findings from the 2018 Clinical Nurse Specialists Census. https://nacns.org/wp-content/uploads/2019/10/NACNS-Census-Infographic-FINAL-10.23.19.pdf

National Association of Clinical Nurse Specialists. (2019b). *Statement on clinical nurse specialist practice and education* (3rd ed.). National Association of Clinical Nurse Specialists.

National Association of Clinical Nurse Specialists. (2021). The role of the clinical nurse specialist: Findings from the 2020 census. Retrieved from https://nacns.org/wp-content/uploads/2021/03/NACNS-2020-Census-Infographic-FINAL.pdf

National Council of State Boards of Nursing. (2008). *Consensus model for APRN regulation: Licensure, accreditation, certification, and education (APRN Consensus Work Group and NCSBN APRN Advisory Committee)*. Retrieved from https://www.ncsbn.org/Consensus_Model_for_APRN_Regu ational Association of Clinical Nurse Specialists lation_July_2008.pdf

Naylor, M. D., Aiken, L. H., Kurtzman, E. T., Olds, D. M., & Hirschman, K. B. (2011). The care span: The importance of transitional care in achieving health reform. *Health Affairs (Project Hope), 30*(4), 746–754.

NCSBN. (2019). 2019 NCSBN annual meeting. https://www.ncsbn.org/2019AM_APRN-Consensus.pdf

NCSBN. (2020a). 2019 Advanced practice registered nurse survey. https://www.ncsbn.org/2019APRN.pdf

NCSBN. (2020b). APRN consensus model by state. https://ncsbn.org/APRN_Consensus_Grid_Apr2019.pdf

NCSBN. (2022a). APRN compact. https://www.ncsbn.org/aprn-compact.htm

NCSBN. (2022b). APRN Consensus implementation status. https://www.ncsbn.org/5397.htm

Negley, K. D., Cordes, M. E., Evenson, L. K., & Schad, S. P. (2016). From hospital to ambulatory care: Realigning the practice of clinical nurse specialist. *Clinical Nurse Specialist, 30*(5), 271–276.

Newhouse, R. P., Stanik-Hutt, J., White, K. M., Johantgen, M., Bass, E. B., & Zangaro, G. (2011). Advanced practice nurse outcomes 1990-2008: A systematic review. *Nursing Economic$, 29*, 230–250.

Oncology Nursing Certification Corporation. (2022). Certifications. https://www.oncc.org/certifications/advanced-oncology-certified-clinical-nurse-specialist-aocns

Patton, L. J., Tidwell, J. D., Falder-Saeed, K. L., Young, V. B., Lewis, B. D., & Binder, J. F. (2017). Ensuring safe transfer of pediatric patients: A quality improvement project to standardize handoff communication. *Journal of Pediatric Nursing, 34*, 44–52.

Peplau, H. E. (1952). *Interpersonal relations in nursing: A conceptual frame of reference for psychodynamic nursing*. Putnam.

PSnet. (n.d.). Promoting patient safety. Agency for Healthcare Research and Quality. PSNet: https://psnet.ahrq.gov

Purvis, S., Kaun, A., McKenna, A., Weber Viste, J., & Fedoror, E. (2018). Outcomes of clinical nurse specialist practice in the implementation of video monitoring at an academic medical center. *Clinical Nurse Specialist, 32*(2), 90–96.

Quality and Safety Education for Nurses. (2020). QSEN home. https://qsen.org/

Rice, M. J., Moller, M. D., DePascale, C., & Skinner, L. (2007). APNA and ANCC collaboration: Achieving consensus on future credentialing for advanced practice psychiatric and mental health nursing. *Journal of the American Psychiatric Nurses Association, 13*, 153–159.

Roberts, M. (2018). Advanced rescuscitation guidelines to improve mortality rates among cardiovascular surgery patients. *Journal of Nursing Administration, 48*(6), 296–297.

Safriet, B. J. (2010). Federal options for maximizing the value of advanced practice nurses in providing quality, cost-effective health care. In *The future of nursing: Leading change, advancing health. Institute of Medicine*, 443–476.

Sanchez, K., Winnie, K., & de Haas-Rowland, N. (2019). Establishing the clinical nurse specialist identity by transforming structures, processes and outcomes. *Clinical Nurse Specialist, 33*(3), 117–122.

Saunders, M. M. (2015). Clinical nurse specialists' perceptions of work patterns, outcomes, desires, and emerging trends. *Journal of Nursing Administration, 45*, 212–217.

Semper, J., Halvorson, B., Hersh, M., Torres, C., & Lillington, L. (2016). Clinical nurse specialists guide staff nurses to promote practice accountability through peer review. *Clinical Nurse Specialist, 30*(1), 19–27.

Soltis, L. M. (2015). Role of the clinical nurse specialist in improving patient outcomes after cardiac surgery. *AACN Advanced Critical Care, 26*(1), 35–42.

Sorrentino, P. (2016). Use of failure and effects analysis to improve emergency department handoff processes. *Clinical Nurse Specialist, 30*(1), 28–37.

Speroni, K. G., McLaughlin, M. K., & Friesen, M. A. (2020). Use of evidence-based practice models and research findings in Magnet-designated hospitals across the United States: National survey results. *Worldviews on Evidence-Based Nursing, 17*(2), 98–107.

Spruce, K., & Butler, C. (2017). Enhancing outcomes for outpatient percutaneous coronary interventions. *Clinical Nurse Specialist, 31*(6), 319–328.

Standards for Supervision of Nursing Practice. Sermchief v. Gonzales, 660 S.W.2d 683 (Mo. 1983) (1983). Retrieved from http://biotech.law.lsu.edu/cases/medmal/Sermchief_v_Gonzales.htm

Stokowski, L. (2018). APRN prescribing law: A state-by-state summary. Retrieved from http://www.medscape.com/viewarticle/440315

Storfjell, J. L., Winslow, B. W., & Saunders, J. S. D. (2017). *Catalysts for change: Harnessing the power of nurses to build population health in the 21st century*. Robert Wood Johnson Foundation. Retrieved from https://campaignforaction.org/resource/catalysts-change-harnessing-power-nurses build-population-health-21st-century/

The Joint Commission. (2022). National patient safety goals. www.jointcommission.org/en/standards/national-patient-safety-goals/

The National CNS Competency Task Force. (2010). Clinical nurse specialist core competencies. Executive summary 2006-2008. https://nacns.org/wp-content/uploads/2016/11/CNSCoreCompetenciesBroch.pdf

Tracy, M. F., & Chlan, L. (2014). Interdisciplinary resource teams. *Clinical Nurse Specialist, 28*, 12–14.

Tracy, M. F., Oerther, S., Arslanian-Engoren, C., Girouard, S., Minarik, P., Patrician, P., Vollman, K., Sanders, N., McCausland, M., Antai-Otong, D., & Talsma, A. (2020). Improving the care and health of populations through optimal use of clinical nurse specialists. *Nursing Outlook, 68*(4), 523–527.

Ulit, M. J., Eriksen, M., Warrier, S., Cardenas-Lopez, K., Cenzon, D., Leon, E., & Miller, J. A. (2020). Role of the clinical nurse specialist in supporting a healthy work environment. *AACN Advanced Critical Care, 31*(1), 80–85.

U.S. Department of Labor, Bureau of Labor Statistics. (2018a). *Occupational employment statistics. Occupational Employment and Wages, May 2018*. 29-1141 Registered Nurses. Retrieved from https://www.bls.gov/oes/current/oes291141.htm

U.S. Department of Labor. Bureau of Labor Statistics. (2018b). *Occupational employment statistics*. May 2018 Occupational Profiles. Retrieved from https://www.bls.gov/oes/current/oes_stru.htm#29-0000

Walker, J. A., Urden, L. D., & Moody, R. (2009). The role of the CNS in achieving and maintaining Magnet status. *Journal of Nursing Administration, 39*, 515–523.

Weiss, S., & Talley, S. (2009). A comparison of the practices of psychiatric clinical nurse specialists and nurse practitioners who are certified to provide mental health care for children and adolescents. *Journal of the American Psychiatric Nurses Association, 12*(2), 111–119. doi:10.1177/1078390309333546

Wocial, L. (2019). Ethical decision making. In M. F. Tracy, & E. O'Grady (Eds.), *Hamric and Hanson's advanced practice nursing: An integrated approach* (6th ed.) (pp. 310–343). Elsevier.

Zavotsky, K. E., Ciccarelli, M., Pontieri-Lewis, V., Royal, S., & Russer, E. (2016). Nursing morbidity and mortality: The clinical nurse specialist role in improving patient outcomes. *Clinical Nurse Specialist, 30*(3), 167–171.

13 THE PRIMARY CARE NURSE PRACTITIONER

MARGARET M. FLINTER ■ SUSANNE J. PHILLIPS

"To pay attention, this is our endless and proper work."
~Mary Oliver

CHAPTER CONTENTS

CURRENT AND HISTORICAL PERSPECTIVES ON PRIMARY CARE AND THE NURSE PRACTITIONER ROLE 422
Current Perspectives on Primary Care 422
Historical Perspectives and the First Nurse Practitioners 423
Progress and Change: 1970 to the Present 424
THE PRIMARY CARE NURSE PRACTITIONER 425
Direct Clinical Practice 426
Guidance and Coaching 436
Evidence-Based Practice 437
Leadership 437
Collaboration 438
Ethical Practice 438
Going Forward With Shared Competencies for Primary Care 439
EMERGENCE OF POSTGRADUATE TRAINING IN PRIMARY CARE 439
PRIMARY CARE AND THE FEDERAL GOVERNMENT 441
Health Resources and Services Administration 441
THE PRIMARY CARE SAFETY NET 443
Community Health Centers 443
Nurse-Led Health Centers 444
School-Based Health Centers 446
Veterans Affairs 446
PRACTICE REDESIGN IN PRIMARY CARE 447
Team-Based Primary Care 447
Disruptive Innovations: From Retail Clinic to the New Primary Care Center 447
PRIMARY CARE WORKFORCE AND THE CONTEXT OF PCNP PRACTICE TODAY 448
Primary Care Nurse Practitioner Workforce 448
Where Are PCNPs Practicing Today? 448
TRENDS IN PRIMARY CARE 450
Home Care 450
Burnout: COVID-19 450
CONCLUSION 450
KEY SUMMARY POINTS 451

This chapter highlights the critical and essential position primary care nurse practitioners (PCNPs) now occupy in the US healthcare system and will for generations to come. We address the historical context and evolution of the PCNP in the changing American healthcare system over 6 decades and its current and growing importance to the country. We write as the country and its healthcare system have experienced the seismic shock of the COVID-19 pandemic—the first pandemic experienced in the lifetime of those practicing today and one that has challenged every level of health and society, including healthcare systems. As this edition is prepared, the death toll in the United States exceeds 650,000, with more than 40 million known cases of infection (Centers for Disease Control and Prevention, 2021), numbers that are continuing to rise, even as vaccination efforts drive the rate of death and infection downward. Racial and ethnic minority groups have suffered disproportionate impact, with American Indian or Alaska Native, Black, and Hispanic or Latino persons suffering hospitalization and death at twice the rate of White, non-Hispanic persons (National Center for Immunization and Respiratory Diseases [NCIRD], Division of Viral Diseases, 2020). The United States has simultaneously confronted social tumult in the political and social spheres and the growing recognition of persistent health inequity, from the beginning through end of life. Length of life itself for all people has markedly dropped to the lowest level since 2006, with non-Hispanic Blacks experiencing the greatest decrease in life expectancy (Arias et al., 2021).

Primary care experienced radical disruption as well. Seemingly overnight, practices and practitioners transitioned to remote work and telehealth, supported by accompanying changes in reimbursement policy on an emergency authorization basis. Patients have delayed essential healthcare services such as cancer screening (Bakouny et al., 2021; Shaukat & Church, 2020) out of fear of contagion or facility restrictions, and the need for psychiatric/mental health support and intervention is increasing (Esterwood & Saeed, 2020). We are in a time of significant flux, with the attendant need and opportunity for change, evolution, action, and progress. Advanced practice registered nurses (APRNs) and PCNPs were born of crisis and opportunity. We have demonstrated our ability to both drive and respond to change. We adapt to and create new models of care both alone and in concert with others when the times call for it. That time is now.

Many of the innovations described in past editions of this text are now part of the bedrock of primary care, though not universally and consistently implemented. Primary care practices, particularly within organized health systems such as Veterans Affairs and federally qualified health centers (FQHCs), have largely embraced team-based care and the integration of behavioral health with medical care (Blasi et al., 2018; NCQA, n.d.). The patient-centered medical home recognition model, a designation now earned by 13,000 practices nationwide (NCQA, n.d.), has continued to advance with rigorous focus on patient access, continuity, care coordination, self-management, and population health (Quigley et al., 2020). Veterans Affairs has been a leader in this area with widespread implementation of patient-aligned care teams (R. S. Phillips et al., 2020). Chronic care management is now a covered, billable service for Medicare enrollees, expected to be delivered outside of the face-to-face encounter, by a range of healthcare professionals, for individuals with multiple chronic conditions (Centers for Medicare & Medicaid Services, 2020).

Myrick and Ogburn (2019) report that electronic health records (EHRs) are almost universal in primary care, with more than 85% of physician practices reporting their use, the vast majority of them certified EHRs. It is unlikely that any PCNP entering practice today does so without expertise in using an EHR.

While the value of EHR is acknowledged, the time and clicks required to meet the standards and execute clinical documentation processes have contributed to new stressors and demands on the primary care team and have even led to a new primary care workforce job, the "scribe," and a call for significant investment of effort in optimizing the use of the electronic record to reduce clinician burnout (Shah et al., 2020). All of this has taken place in the context of further advancement of models of population health that focus on the patient as a whole, not incidents of care, and payment systems that are increasingly focused on value-based payment arrangement with both upside and downside financial risk to practices and providers, including PCNPs.

In the first decade of this century (2000–2010), we recall that the key focus of health care was on managing chronic illness, addressing health promotion and prevention, responding to acute and episodic illness, and ensuring that the needs for long-term, rehabilitative, and palliative care were met—all areas of practice engagement for the PCNP. Of course, cost control has always been on the agenda. In safety net settings like community health centers, access to care remained of paramount concern. In the decade preceding the COVID-19 pandemic (2010–2019), these key areas were joined by the escalation of a major threat to premature deaths from what we now often refer to as deaths of despair from substance use disorder, suicide, and violence (Case & Deaton, 2020; Ruhm, 2018), and the COVID-19 pandemic has only exacerbated the phenomenon of deaths of despair (Petterson et al., 2020). The epidemic of death from opioid use disorder and overdose was a call to action for PCNPs to respond to the Comprehensive Addiction and Recovery Act of 2016, (2016) by pursuing the required training to secure US Drug Enforcement Administration (DEA) X waiver registration to provide medication-assisted treatment (MAT) to this highly vulnerable group of patients. Between 2016 and 2019, APRNs, including PCNPs, and physician assistants (PAs) were responsible for a dramatic rise in the number of rural counties with a DEA X waivered provider, and nurse practitioners (NPs) and PAs represented half of that. Notably, broad scope of practice regulations were significantly and positively associated with states that benefited from this increase (Barnett et al., 2019). Yet despite great progress and more than 12,000 NPs now holding a DEA X waiver, this represents only 5% of the 270,000 NPs in the United States (Gardenier et al., 2020). The intersection of the opioid epidemic and the COVID-19 pandemic has forced further innovation in community-based treatment of opioid use disorder (Volkow, 2020). In April 2021, significant changes to increase the number of prescribers and increase access were made to the Controlled Substance Act. These changes eliminated the requirement for the DEA X waiver and associated additional mandatory hours of training for healthcare providers, including NPs, to prescribe MAT with buprenorphine as long as the provider had valid state and DEA licenses and limited treatment to no more than 30 patients on MAT concurrently (A. Knopf, 2021). This change underscores the urgency of the need for primary care providers (PCPs), including PCNPs, to have maximum ability to address our most pressing healthcare needs.

Our models for education, prelicensure training, and postgraduate training have also evolved and innovated in recent years to reflect changing needs, demands for care, and ever-evolving science. Accredited graduate NP education is preparing more graduates and is increasingly held in hybrid and online environments, and the availability of accredited postgraduate residency and fellowship programs has increased significantly in both primary care/community-based organizations and in the specialty/acute care settings (Johnson et al., n.d.). The National Organization of Nurse Practitioner Faculties (NONPF, 2018) has announced a commitment to move all entry-level nurse practitioner education to the doctor of nursing practice (DNP) degree by 2025. Similarly, the march forward for full practice authority has continued, as we will detail in this chapter.

CURRENT AND HISTORICAL PERSPECTIVES ON PRIMARY CARE AND THE NURSE PRACTITIONER ROLE

Current Perspectives on Primary Care

Fig. 13.1 illustrates the foundation that primary care holds globally (left pyramid) and in the US healthcare system (right pyramid) (Macinko et al., 2003). Primary care is recognized as the foundation of strong national healthcare systems (Bitton et al., 2017). Primary care cannot compensate for the myriad of social determinants of health that affect both health and life expectancy, from race to education to income, and the social needs that follow them, such as food and housing insecurity, nor can primary care ignore them (Berwick, 2020). Consistent access to high-quality primary health care is clearly a factor when considering the discrepancy in life expectancy between the United States and other developed countries (Avendano & Kawachi, 2014; Nolte & McKee, 2012; Singh et al., 2017). Primary care providers (PCPs) comprise the frontline of health care, serving patients and communities and addressing most healthcare needs across the life span, in sickness and in health. The late Barbara Starfield identified the key tasks of primary care as (1) first contact with care, (2) longitudinal care, (3) comprehensiveness of care, and (4) coordination of services (Starfield, 1992). *Longitudinal care* refers to a sustained patient–provider relationship over time. In primary care–oriented health systems, there are fewer disparities in health across population subgroups (Starfield, 2008).

Nearly 30 years ago, the Institute of Medicine (IOM) issued a report on primary care, defining it as "the provision of integrated, accessible healthcare services by clinicians who are accountable for addressing a large majority of personal health needs, developing a sustained partnership with patients, and practicing in the context of family and community" (Institute of Medicine [IOM], 1996, p. 36). In 2021 the National Academies of Science, Engineering and Medicine (NASEM) issued a new report on primary care, *Implementing High-Quality Primary Care*, updating their 1996 definition to include terms such as "whole-person equitable health care" delivered by interprofessional teams (NASEM, Committee on Implementing High-Quality Primary Care, 2021). The World Health Organization's (WHO)

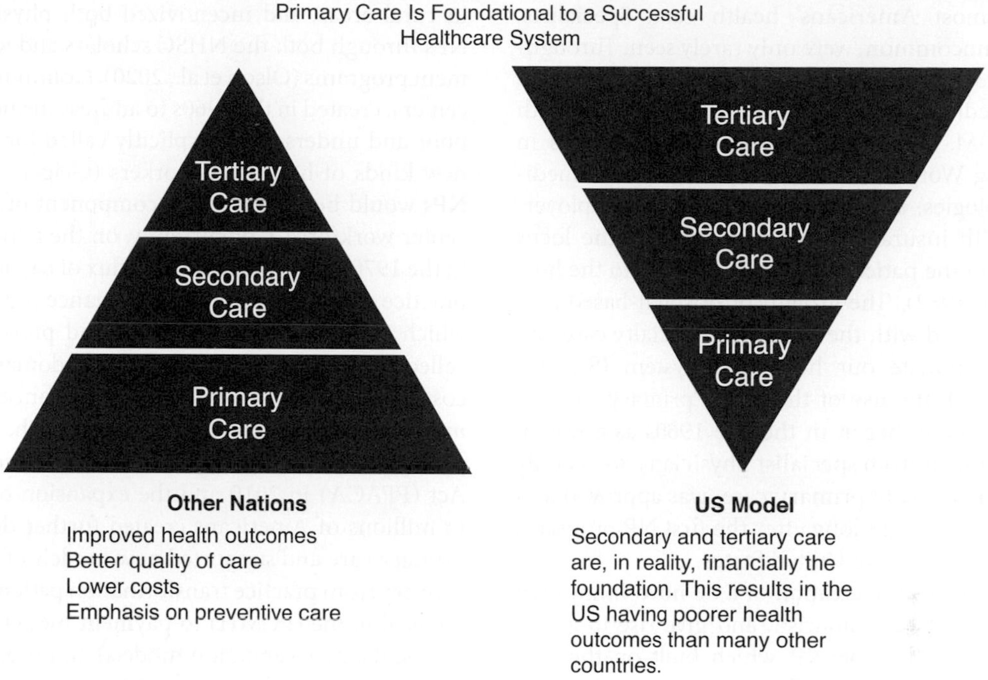

Fig. 13.1 ■ **Models of primary care in other nations and the United States.** (Adapted from "The Contributions of Primary Care Systems to Health Outcomes Within Organization for Economic Cooperation and Development (OECD) Countries, 1970–1998," by J. Macinko, B. Starfield, and L. Shi, 2003, *Health Services Research, 38*, 831–865.)

Commission on Social Determinants of Health (2008) expanded the focus from the delivery of primary care services to addressing the broader issue of the impact of societal and environmental factors on health.

The public health approach builds on *social determinants of health,* defined by the WHO as "the conditions in which people are born, grow, live, work and age, including the health system" (Commission on Social Determinants of Health, 2008, p. 1) and attributes the cause of most health inequities to the distribution of money, power, and resources at the local, national, and global levels. Starfield likely could not have imagined the technological innovations that have made large-scale adoption of telehealth in primary care both possible and imperative since the onset of the COVID-19 pandemic in March 2020.

The centrality of primary care to healthy individuals and healthy, empowered communities has been revisited, restated, and reemphasized (World Health Organization & United Nations Children's Fund [UNICEF], 2018). More specific to the nursing profession, the final recommendation of the NASEM report *Future of Nursing 2020–2030* (NASEM, 2021) calls to make advancing health equity a central focus over the next 10 years. Additional focus on social determinants of health is included in the nine key recommendations that transcend all dimensions of nursing practice.

With this as background, we ask who the PCPs of today and tomorrow are. We answer that PCNPs are increasingly the backbone of the PCP workforce in the United States, growing faster than any other group and demonstrating a commitment to practice in rural and underserved areas and in safety net settings that care for some of the nation's most vulnerable populations (Auerbach et al., 2018).

Historical Perspective and the First Nurse Practitioners

Historians remind us that at one time, all health care was primary care. The United States developed a fixation on specialty care in the last century (Howell, 2010). Before World War II, a generalist physician provided most Americans' health care. Specialists, who were uncommon, were only rarely seen. Throughout the 1930s and 1940s, generalist care expanded to include pediatricians, internists, and public health nurses (IOM, 1996). However, medical advances in care during World War II and rapid growth of medical technologies, along with the advent of employer-based health insurance, combined to shift the locus of care from the patient's home and family to the hospital (Starr, 1982). The growth of hospital-based care was intertwined with the growth of specialty care and came to dominate our healthcare system (Stevens, 1989). Indeed, the use of the term "primary care" in the United States began in the late 1960s as a way of distinguishing it from specialist physician care. Family medicine, essentially primary care, was approved as a specialty in 1969, not long after the first NP programs were established in the United States.

The 1960s saw the creation of a de novo innovation that would take root, flourish, and give rise to a new healthcare provider, the NP, which built on the core tenets of the profession of nursing and reimagined the possibilities for greater service, scope, and impact and specifically in primary care during its early decades. The NP was a new category of health professional, a new role for nursing, and a new kind of PCP. This role was based on a person-centric, holistic approach to the care of individuals and families. Dr. Loretta Ford, public health nurse and educator, and Dr. Henry Silver, a pediatrician, recognized the untapped capability and potential of nurses to expand their primary care practice (Silver et al., 1967). More than 50 years later, one might say that it also inspired and motivated primary care medicine to embrace much of the NP role's focus, with a concerted focus in medical schools and residency programs on social mission and person-centered, holistic, comprehensive primary care (Englander et al., 2013).

Progress and Change: 1970 to the Present

Issues of healthcare access and maldistribution of healthcare resources, along with new federal funding sources, all fueled the continuing development of the NP role and growth in the numbers of nurses pursuing graduate education to become NPs. The legislative creation of the National Health Service Corps (NHSC) in 1972 addressed the problem of maldistribution of healthcare providers in the United States, particularly in rural areas, and incentivized both physicians and NPs through both the NHSC scholars and loan repayment programs (Olson et al., 2020). Community health centers, created in the 1960s to address the needs of the poor and underserved, explicitly called for the use of new kinds of healthcare workers (Geiger, 2005), and NPs would become a major component of the health center workforce. Concurrently, on the national scene in the 1970s, there was a rapid influx of capitated group practice models, or health maintenance organizations, which emphasized primary care and prevention and called for expert providers in those domains. Rising costs in health care saw the creation of concepts such as *managed care* (Bodenheimer & Grumbach, 2016). The passage of the Patient Protection and Affordable Care Act (PPACA) in 2010 and the expansion of coverage to millions of Americans created further demand for primary care and supported new models of healthcare delivery from practice transformation patient-centered medical home (PCMH) to payment models (bundled payments, new capitation models) and organizational models (accountable care organizations), as well as workforce development (Peikes et al., 2020; Redhead & Heisler, 2013). Although a review of each of these is beyond the scope of this chapter, we remind ourselves of the hopes, fears, and aspirations for change that characterized the passage of the PPACA. The implementation of various provisions of the PPACA across states and its ultimate success in reducing the numbers of uninsured, ensured improved access to preventive services at no out-of-pocket cost, making the scourge of denial or exorbitant premium pricing on the basis of preexisting conditions a relic of history (McIntyre & Song, 2019). The third and perhaps final challenge to the constitutionality of the PPACA was based on issues of severability, standing, and constitutionality (Kaplan, 2021). The Supreme Court upheld the constitutionality of the law in a June 17, 2021, opinion (California et al. v. Texas et al., 2021). Now we arrive at a new moment, brought to us by the "twindemics" of COVID-19 and health disparities, and administrative and congressional collaborative leadership is needed that seeks to rectify racial, economic, health and social disparities, and the rapid release of financial resources to accompany sought-after improvements through legislation and appropriations (Health Resources and Services Administration [HRSA], n.d.).

This Is Our Moment

The evidence base for the safety, quality, effectiveness, and patient acceptance of the PCNP has been steadily growing for decades, and we emerge from the COVID-19 pandemic with the public memory of primary care NPs (and all nurses) as a vital, trusted, and vocal profession. The expansion of the NP workforce in primary care and the development of optimal team-based care models were strategies identified by the 2011 IOM document *The Future of Nursing: Leading Change, Advancing Health*. The goal was to ensure that the US healthcare system was adequately prepared to address the aging population, high prevalence of chronic illness, and the demand for primary care (IOM, 2011), but a global pandemic could not have been imagined. The early questions of whether primary care NP practice is "as good as," "as safe as," "as effective as," or accepted by patients have long been put to rest (Lenz et al., 2004; Mundinger et al., 2000) and replaced with calls for research into the contribution of NPs to high-value primary care (Naylor & Kurtzman, 2010).

The attention now is indeed on patient outcomes, the impact of high-value care, and the total commitment to pursuing the elimination of health disparities and inequities. The *Future of Nursing 2020–2030* report (NASEM, 2021) places this charge at the center of focus for the coming decade. In studies of quality of primary care provided by NPs and physicians to vulnerable Medicare beneficiaries, NPs demonstrated improved performance on measures of reduced preventable hospital admissions, readmissions, and inappropriate emergency department utilization (DesRoches et al., 2017); patients cared for by NPs were also more likely to receive chronic disease management and cancer screenings (Buerhaus et al., 2018). Using a more specific focus on primary care management of diabetes, patients cared for exclusively by NPs or by physicians were analyzed on measures of health services utilization, health outcomes, and healthcare costs variables (Lutfiyya et al., 2017). This study demonstrated that patients in the NP-only group showed significantly improved outcomes compared with all–primary care physician provider groups (Lutfiyya et al., 2017). Kurtzman and Barnow (2017) looked at practice patterns and quality of care provided by over 1000 NPs, PAs, and primary care physicians in community health centers over a 4-year period spanning 30 million visits. On seven of nine outcomes studied, no statistically significant differences were detected in NP or PA care compared with MD care, but on the remaining outcomes, visits to NPs were more likely to include recommended smoking cessation counseling and more health education/counseling services than visits to MDs.

Along with the rapid growth of primary care NPs and their importance to the country's health care comes an increased need to identify, examine, and strengthen the practice environment and factors that are associated with professional satisfaction and success. Effective interprofessional teamwork is critical and requires attention to areas such as organizational support, governance, physician–NP relationships, and regulatory and economic issues (Poghosyan et al., 2020).

THE PRIMARY CARE NURSE PRACTITIONER

The PCNP is educated to provide the full spectrum of healthcare services to previously diagnosed and undiagnosed primary care patients and families across the life span, including health promotion, disease prevention, health protection, anticipatory guidance, counseling, disease management, and palliative and end-of-life care (NONPF, 2017). Building on the six APRN competencies described in Chapter 3, the new document *The Essentials: Core Competencies for Professional Nursing Education* (American Association of Colleges of Nursing [AACN], 2021) expands on previous work that identified knowledge, skills, and defined competencies essential to DNP-prepared PCNPs (AACN, 2006). The new *Essentials* are consistent with the recommendations in the new report from NASEM (2021), *The Future of Nursing 2020–2030*.

The *Consensus Model for APRN Regulation: Licensure, Accreditation, Certification, & Education* (APRN Joint Dialogue Group, 2008) states that the role of the certified NP includes diagnosing, treating, and managing patients with acute and chronic illnesses and disease. NP care includes ordering, performing, supervising, and interpreting laboratory, diagnostic, and imaging studies; prescribing medication and durable medical equipment; and making appropriate referrals for patients and families (APRN Joint Dialogue Group, 2008). Further, these role attributes are provided to a specific patient population focus for which the practitioner is specifically educated and licensed (APRN Joint Dialogue Group, 2008; Kleinpell et al., 2012).

The NP community has collaborated to identify competencies for each population focus. Additionally, NPs are now educated and certified in primary care or acute care in the pediatric and adult–gerontology populations, which incorporates the entire spectrum of adults, including young adults and older adults. Population-focused NP competencies with primary care specialization include family/across the life span, pediatric primary care, adult–gerontology primary care, and women's health (NONPF & AACN, 2016; NONPF Population-Focused Competencies Task Force, 2013). These population-focused competencies are guidelines for educational programs preparing NPs with different populations as licensed practitioners and are required for program national accreditation. Foundational to all NP graduates is that they share a generalist nursing foundation, their practice has a base in health promotion, and they have developed advanced assessment and diagnostic reasoning skills. In other words, they have the requisite knowledge, skills, and abilities essential for competent clinical practice, as discussed in Chapter 6 (NONPF & AACN, 2013). Competencies are acquired through mentored patient care experiences while studying a defined curriculum based on role and population focus and occur in clinical settings that support the population focus. Today's curricula prioritize interprofessional learning and collaborative practice.

A discussion of how these PCNP competencies are enacted within the framework of the six APRN core competencies follows. Table 13.1 cross-maps the APRN competencies described in Chapter 3, the new *Essentials* (AACN, 2021), and the NONPF (2017) NP core competencies. In practice, competencies are executed simultaneously to achieve the best outcome. However, for purposes of didactic discussion, specific competencies are discussed separately. Exemplars from primary care practice illustrate the competencies in action and are used throughout discussion of both the APRN competencies and the NP core and specialty competencies.

Although all NPs are educated across the country with the same national standards and competencies and graduate from similar accredited NP programs, scope of NP practice varies widely across the country. While the COVID-19 pandemic brought about positive scope of practice changes in the form of emergency regulations, some states maintained mandatory supervision or collaboration of NP practice (S. Phillips, 2021). S. Phillips (2021) outlined the most up-to-date information on COVID-19 regulatory changes within each state and the status of independent, reduced, and restricted scope of practice as defined by AANP. Overall, states are moving toward independent practice with and without transition to practice periods, a positive sign for access to high-quality, safe, effective health care, yet there is still work to be done to reach independent practice in all states.

The most recent national-level report from the NASEM strongly reiterates previous national calls to remove all barriers to full scope of practice for NPs and registered nurses (NASEM, 2021). At a time of such need for competent, high-quality, safe, and effective NPs, states should look to this newest report to guide legislative and regulatory initiatives to remove scope of practice barriers. Health inequity and disparity will not be solved without it.

Direct Clinical Practice

Direct clinical practice is the central competency of all APRN roles; the delivery of direct care to patients and families is what the PCNP does. In today's hectic care environment, direct clinical practice in primary care includes managing previously diagnosed and undiagnosed increasingly ill and complex patients at a rapid pace and includes growing numbers of aging patients with a range of chronic diseases and multiple comorbidities. It also requires proficiency in addressing behavioral health problems and the socioeconomic challenges that stress so many families, as well as awareness of ongoing, major health problems in our society. Direct clinical practice in primary care builds on patient-centered approaches applied holistically, formation of therapeutic partnerships, expert clinical thinking, use of reflective practice, and use of evidence as a guide to practice yet having the flexibility to integrate diverse, evidence-informed approaches as needed.

One hallmark of the PCNP's direct clinical practice is the breadth and complexity of health issues encountered in a single day in primary care practice, which necessitates triage and constant decision making.

TABLE 13.1

Cross-Mapping of Advanced Practice Registered Nurse (APRN) Competencies, *The Essentials: Core Competencies for Professional Nursing Education*, and National Organization of Nurse Practitioner Faculties (NONPF) 2017 Nurse Practitioner (NP) Core Competencies

APRN Competencies (Chapter 3)	*The Essentials: Core Competencies for Nursing Education*[a]	*NONPF 2017 NP Core Competencies*[b]
Direct Clinical Practice (Chapter 6) Use of a holistic perspective Formation of therapeutic partnerships with patients Expert clinical performance Use of reflective practice Use of evidence as a guide to practice Use of diverse approaches to health and illness management	Domain 1: Knowledge for Nursing Practice Domain 2: Person-Centered Care Domain 3: Population Health Domain 4: Scholarship for the Nursing Discipline Domain 6: Interprofessional Partnerships Domain 8: Informatics and Healthcare Technologies ***Concepts for Nursing Practice*** Clinical Judgment Communication Compassionate Care Diversity, Equity, and Inclusion Ethics Evidence-Based Practice Health Policy Social Determinants of Health Health Policy	***Independent Practice Competencies*** Functions as a licensed independent practitioner. Demonstrates the highest level of accountability for professional practice. Practices independently managing previously diagnosed and undiagnosed patients. Provides the full spectrum of healthcare services to include health promotion, disease prevention, health protection, anticipatory guidance, counseling, disease management, palliative, and end-of-life care. Uses advanced health assessment skills to differentiate between normal, variations of normal, and abnormal findings. Employs screening and diagnostic strategies in the development of diagnoses. Prescribes medications within scope of practice. Manages the health/illness status of patients and families over time. Provides patient-centered care recognizing cultural diversity and the patient or designee as a full partner in decision making. Works to establish a relationship with the patient characterized by mutual respect, empathy, and collaboration. Creates a climate of patient-centered care to include confidentiality, privacy, comfort, emotional support, mutual trust, and respect. Incorporates the patient's cultural and spiritual preferences, values, and beliefs into health care. Preserves the patient's control over decision making by negotiating a mutually acceptable plan of care. Develops strategies to prevent one's own personal biases from interfering with delivery of quality care. Addresses cultural, spiritual, and ethnic influences that potentially create conflict among individuals, families, staff, and caregivers. Educates professional and lay caregivers to provide culturally and spiritually sensitive appropriate care. Collaborates with both professional and other caregivers to achieve optimal care outcomes. Coordinates transitional care services in and across care settings.

Continued

TABLE 13.1

Cross-Mapping of Advanced Practice Registered Nurse (APRN) Competencies, *The Essentials: Core Competencies for Professional Nursing Education*, and National Organization of Nurse Practitioner Faculties (NONPF) 2017 Nurse Practitioner (NP) Core Competencies—cont'd

APRN Competencies (Chapter 3)	*The Essentials: Core Competencies for Nursing Education*[a]	*NONPF 2017 NP Core Competencies*[b]
		Participates in the development, use, and evaluation of professional standards and evidence-based care. ***Scientific Foundation Competencies*** Critically analyzes data and evidence for improving advanced nursing practice. Integrates knowledge from the humanities and sciences within the context of nursing science. Translates research and other forms of knowledge to improve practice processes and outcomes. Develops new practice approaches based on the integration of research, theory, and practice.
Guidance and Coaching (Chapter 7)	Domain 1: Knowledge for Nursing Practice Domain 2: Person-Centered Care **Concepts for Nursing Practice:** Communication Compassionate Care Diversity, Equity, and Inclusion Ethics Evidence-Based Practice Social Determinants of Health	***Independent Practice Competencies (see above)*** ***Technology and Information Literacy Competencies (see below)***
Evidence-Based Practice (Chapter 8)	Domain 2: Person-Centered Care Domain 4: Scholarship for the Nursing Discipline Domain 5: Quality and Safety Domain 6: Interprofessional Partnerships Domain 7: Systems-Based Practice Domain 8: Information and Healthcare Technologies Domain 9: Professionalism **Concepts for Nursing Practice:** Evidence-Based Practice	***Quality Competencies*** Uses best available evidence to continuously improve quality of clinical practice. Evaluates the relationships among access, cost, quality, and safety and their influence on health care. Evaluates how organizational structure, care processes, financing, marketing, and policy decisions impact the quality of health care. Applies skills in peer review to promote a culture of excellence. Anticipates variations in practice and is proactive in implementing interventions to ensure quality.
	Domain 1: Knowledge for Nursing Practice Domain 4: Scholarship for Nursing Practice	***Practice Inquiry Competencies*** Provides leadership in the translation of new knowledge into practice. Generates knowledge from clinical practice to improve practice and patient outcomes. Applies clinical investigative skills to improve health outcomes. Leads practice inquiry, individually or in partnership with others. Disseminates evidence from inquiry to diverse audiences using multiple modalities. Analyzes clinical guidelines for individualized application into practice.

TABLE 13.1

Cross-Mapping of Advanced Practice Registered Nurse (APRN) Competencies, *The Essentials:* Core Competencies for Professional Nursing Education, and National Organization of Nurse Practitioner Faculties (NONPF) 2017 Nurse Practitioner (NP) Core Competencies—cont'd

APRN Competencies (Chapter 3)	*The Essentials: Core Competencies for Nursing Education*[a]	*NONPF 2017 NP Core Competencies*[b]
Leadership (Chapter 9)	Domain 1: Knowledge for Nursing Practice Domain 3: Population Health Domain 6: Interprofessional Partnerships Domain 9: Professionalism Domain 10: Personal, Professional, and Leadership Development **Concepts for Nursing Practice** Communication Evidence-Based Practice Health Policy Social Determinants of Health	***Leadership Competencies*** Assumes complex and advanced leadership roles to initiate and guide change. Provides leadership to foster collaboration with multiple stakeholders (e.g., patients, community, integrated healthcare teams, and policy makers) to improve health care. Demonstrates leadership that uses critical and reflective thinking. Advocates for improved access, quality, and cost-effective health care. Advances practice through the development and implementation of innovations incorporating principles of change. Communicates practice knowledge effectively, both orally and in writing. Participates in professional organizations and activities that influence advanced practice nursing and/or health outcomes of a population focus.
	Domain 2: Person-Centered Care Domain 3: Population Health Domain 7: Systems-Based Practice **Concepts of Nursing Practice** Diversity, Equity and Inclusion Health Policy	***Health Delivery System Competencies*** Applies knowledge of organizational practices and complex systems to improve healthcare delivery. Effects healthcare change using broad-based skills including negotiating, consensus-building, and partnering. Minimizes risk to patients and providers at the individual and systems level. Facilitates the development of healthcare systems that address the needs of culturally diverse populations, providers, and other stakeholders. Evaluates the impact of healthcare delivery on patients, providers, other stakeholders, and the environment. Analyzes organizational structure, functions, and resources to improve the delivery of care. Collaborates in planning for transitions across the continuum of care.
	Domain 2: Person-Centered Care Domain 3: Population Health Domain 4: Scholarship for the Nursing Discipline Domain 5: Quality and Safety Domain 6: Interprofessional Partnerships Domain 7: Systems-Based Care	***Policy Competencies*** Demonstrates an understanding of the interdependence of policy and practice. Advocates for ethical policies that promote access, equity, quality, and cost. Analyzes ethical, legal, and social factors influencing policy development. Contributes in the development of health policy. Analyzes the implications of health policy across disciplines.

Continued

TABLE 13.1

Cross-Mapping of Advanced Practice Registered Nurse (APRN) Competencies, *The Essentials: Core Competencies for Professional Nursing Education*, and National Organization of Nurse Practitioner Faculties (NONPF) 2017 Nurse Practitioner (NP) Core Competencies—cont'd

APRN Competencies (Chapter 3)	*The Essentials: Core Competencies for Nursing Education*[a]	*NONPF 2017 NP Core Competencies*[b]
	Domain 10: Personal, Professional, and Leadership Development **Concepts of Nursing Practice** Diversity, Equity, and Inclusion Health Policy Social Determinants of Health	Evaluates the impact of globalization on healthcare policy development. Advocates for policies for safe and healthy practice environments.
Collaboration (Chapter 10)	Domain 2: Person-Centered Care Domain 3: Population Health Domain 6: Interprofessional Partnerships Domain 7: Systems-Based Practice **Concepts for Nursing Practice** Communication Collaboration Evidence-Based Practice Health Policy	***Independent Practice Competencies (see above)*** ***Scientific Foundation Competencies (see above)*** ***Ethics Competencies (see below)*** ***Leadership Competencies (see below)***
Ethical Practice Decision Making (Chapter 11)	Domain 2: Person-Centered Care Domain 3: Population Health Domain 6: Interprofessional Partnerships Professionalism **Concepts of Nursing Practice** Ethics Compassionate Care Diversity, Equity, and Inclusion	***Ethics Competencies*** Integrates ethical principles in decision making. Evaluates the ethical consequences of decisions. Applies ethically sound solutions to complex issues related to individuals, populations, and systems of care. Integrates appropriate technologies for knowledge management to improve health care.
	Domain 2: Person-Centered Care Domain 6: Interprofessional Partnerships Domain 8: Information and Healthcare Technologies **Concepts of Nursing Practice** Clinical Judgment Communication	***Technology and Information Literacy Competencies*** Translates technical and scientific health information appropriate for various users' needs. Assesses the patient's and caregiver's educational needs to provide effective, personalized health care. Coaches the patient and caregiver for positive behavioral change. Demonstrates information literacy skills in complex decision making. Contributes to the design of clinical information systems that promote safe, quality, and cost-effective care. Uses technology systems that capture data on variables for the evaluation of nursing care.

[a]Source: *The Essentials: Core Competencies for Professional Nursing Education*, by American Association of Colleges of Nursing, 2021, https://www.aacnnursing.org/Portals/42/AcademicNursing/pdf/Essentials-2021.pdf.

[b]Source: "Nurse Practitioner Core Competencies Content: A Delineation of Suggested Content Specific to the NP Core Competencies," by National Organization of Nurse Practitioner Faculties, 2017, https://cdn.ymaws.com/www.nonpf.org/resource/resmgr/competencies/2017_NPCore-Comps_with_Curric.pdf.

The PCNP compares patient data sets with evidence-informed interventions consistent with current standards of care yet tailored to meet the needs of the individual and family in the context of diversity. As with other APRN roles, PCNPs analyze data and evidence critically to improve practice. PCNPs integrate knowledge from the humanities and sciences within the context of nursing science. In particular, the PCNP has a scientific foundation derived from the natural and social sciences that comprises human biology, advanced physiology, genomics, psychology (including behavioral change), epidemiology (for knowledge of population health), and advanced pathophysiology and pharmacotherapeutics. Use of "precision medicine" and genetics is essential in today's practice environment. PCNPs integrate elements of care from nursing and medical models in a collaborative approach to clinical practice that enhances the comprehensiveness and quality of the care rendered. The circle of caring model for PCNPs (Dunphy et al., 2015), for example, integrates a biomedical approach to diagnosis and treatment with a nursing-based, person-centered awareness of patient's responses to health and illness across the life span (see Chapter 2). This model supports PCNPs' understandings of the social determinants of health that exist within the patient's population and environment and how this relates to the patient's health and illness experience. This comprehensive knowledge base enables PCNPs to meet their patients' needs authentically and to hear their voices or "calls for nursing" and respond holistically. PCNPs synthesize concepts from psychology, sociology, biology, and other forms of the human experience within the context of nursing science (Udlis & Jakubis-Konicki, 2016). This care directly affects the health and lives of individuals, families, and whole communities.

Diagnosing and Managing Disease

The PCNP uses advanced health assessment skills to differentiate between normal findings and variations of normal and abnormal findings to manage previously diagnosed as well as undifferentiated or undiagnosed patients. Key skills include using deep questioning and listening, history taking, and use of screening and diagnostic strategies to develop differential diagnoses. This includes obtaining and documenting a relevant health history as well as performing and accurately documenting an appropriate comprehensive or symptom-based physical examination. PCNPs order, perform, and interpret diagnostic tests such as laboratory work and diagnostic studies. Additionally, the PCNP must demonstrate the ability to employ appropriate screening and diagnostic strategies to develop and support diagnoses as well as documenting this using correct diagnostic evaluation and management billing codes. PCNPs are required to manage acute and chronic physical and mental illness independently, including acute exacerbations and injuries, and to minimize the development of complications and promote function and quality of life (NONPF Population-Focused Competencies Task Force, 2013). Disease management may include the ability to perform primary care procedures, which may vary depending on the setting but might include suturing, microscopy, biopsies, Pap smears, joint aspirations and injections, and removal of foreign objects as necessary, to name just a few. PCNPs confirm evidence-informed diagnoses, develop plans of care, prescribe treatments and pharmacotherapeutics, and provide follow-up. Often the plan of care requires coordination of care activities or needed services with multiple professionals.

Health Promotion and Disease Prevention

PCNPs also focus on health promotion, disease prevention, health education, and counseling, guiding patients to make better health and lifestyle choices. PCNPs bring an underlying holistic approach to care, grounded in nursing science and philosophy, an approach that integrates the relationship of the social determinants of health to the overall well-being of the population of patients cared for as well as the individual patient for whom care is provided. The United States continues to lag behind other advanced nations on measures of infant mortality and life expectancy, according to an analysis of more than 300 diseases and injuries in 195 countries and territories (Wong et al., 2016). Drug abuse and diabetes are noted as causing a disproportionate amount of ill health and early death in the United States. PCNPs must be able to respond to the unprecedented level of opioid addiction that has resulted in a fivefold increase in deaths over the past 25 years, an increase from 4000 per year in 1990 to more than 21,300 in 2015 (Wong et al., 2016). Opioid addiction is driving an overall reduction in life expectancy for Americans for the first time in many years (Wong et al., 2016). Alcohol and drug addiction, smoking, and access to guns also pose continuing threats. To combat these health risks, the United States will have to go beyond its reliance on a hospital-centric, drug-centric medical system. According to this study, heart disease remains the leading cause of death (532,000) in the United States, with Alzheimer disease in second place (282,530) and lung cancer ranked third (187,390; Wong et al., 2016).

These statistics reinforce the need for skills and competencies that support patients to achieve and maintain healthy lifestyles, including addressing the community issues of safety, access to healthy food, and opportunities for physical activity. People need providers with strong communication skills, empathy, and an understanding of the environment in which people live. Nursing as a discipline never abandoned its public health roots; community health nursing and population health are integrated in all nursing curriculum and approaches. PCNPs combine "high-tech" and "low-tech" approaches to deal with these population-based health challenges. Specifically, PCNPs must manage and provide a full spectrum of healthcare services that includes health promotion, disease prevention, health protection, anticipatory guidance, counseling, disease management, and palliative and end-of-life care (NONPF & AACN, 2016). Examples of this, building on knowledge about developmental age–related and gender-specific variations, include implementing age-appropriate wellness promotion and disease prevention services; weighing the costs, risks, and benefits to individuals; developing a plan for long-term management of chronic healthcare problems with the individual, family, and healthcare team; and evaluating individuals' and/or caregivers' support systems. It is critical that the PCNP promote safety and risk reduction for vulnerable populations.

Providing Culturally Sensitive, Patient-Centered Care

Care providers who mirror the populations that they care for are more effective; barring that, cultural humility and a commitment to social justice are critical (The Sullivan Commission, 2004; Valentine et al., 2016). PCNPs are educated to provide patients with high-quality, comprehensive, culturally sensitive, and patient-centered care. They use interventions to prevent or reduce risk factors for diverse and vulnerable populations, particularly the young and the frail elderly (NONPF & AACN, 2016). PCNPs counsel and coach as well as educate patients to manage chronic diseases, which are often multiple, and help guide them through difficult decisions related to lifestyles, prioritization, and choices. PCNPs need to be knowledgeable about and integrate behavioral health, in a team-based approach and/or through sensitivity and cultural humility, during their one-to-one encounter with the person/family. They are able to address cultural, spiritual, and ethnic influences that potentially create conflict among individuals, families, staff, and caregivers. They approach persons and families holistically, promote health and hope, and meet persons where they are. Using reflective practice, PCNPs develop strategies to prevent their own biases from interfering with the delivery of quality care. This may involve educating other professionals and lay caregivers to provide culturally and spiritually sensitive, appropriate care. Exemplar 13.1 illustrates how one NP brought culturally competent, patient-centered care to the Community Health Center of New London. These skills are reinforced and expanded upon in *The Future of Nursing 2020–2030* report (NASEM, 2021).

Coordinating Transitional Care Services in and Across Care Settings

Part of the role of the PCNP is to discern gaps in care and barriers to care needing resolution during patient encounters. Coordinated, patient-centered care across settings requires advanced knowledge of the healthcare delivery system as well as an understanding of the payment system. PCNPs apply knowledge of scientific foundations in practice for quality care, they apply skills in technology and information literacy, and they use health information technology (HIT) and enhanced EHRs to provide coordinated care and facilitate better communication among healthcare providers and patients. Even yesterday's nursing care plan has reemerged as a vital tool in the EHR for use by RNs as well as NPs, physicians, social workers, and pharmacists in the coordination of care for our most complex patients—now a billable activity under Medicare. Technology and information literacy competencies also inform NP contributions to the design of clinical

EXEMPLAR 13.1
CULTURALLY SENSITIVE PATIENT-CENTERED CARE AT COMMUNITY HEALTH CENTER OF NEW LONDON[a]

For as long as I can remember, I have always been eager to find ways to better serve my community. This desire stems from the inspiration my parents instilled in me. My father and mother dedicated their lives to serve their communities. My mother, an elementary school teacher, carried hope to every classroom. She believed that every child deserves the opportunity to grow to their best potential, to further enrich their communities. My father, a Peruvian Air Force colonel, exemplified the discipline and tenacity to get things done the right way. He guided many men and women who served our country of Peru.

Since I first started to envision my professional life, I knew I wanted to make important contributions to my community as my parents have. They are my inspiration. Their guidance and example instilled in me early on the importance of family and connection to community and that children who grow in nurturing families and among supportive communities lead healthier lives conducive to fulfilling bright futures. Choosing a career as a family nurse practitioner felt like second nature to me. Family nurse practitioners approach patient care with the understanding that family health and community health underscore the promotion of good individual health. All people deserve an equal opportunity to make the choices that lead to good health. I am on this career path to ensure that they do.

The academic and life preparation to become who I am now is intertwined between two different worlds. The first one was located in Arequipa, Peru, where I was born and raised and was given the building blocks to develop a moral compass that would guide me to lead every human interaction with empathy and compassion. The second location, Burlington, Vermont, is where I moved 2 years after finishing high school. It was here where I learned the "American way of life" and to live independently. Moving to a new country and leaving behind parents, friends, and family was one of the greatest challenges of my life. However, with resilience, perseverance, my family's support, and Adam's (my partner) unconditional love, I excelled academically and graduated with a doctor of nursing practice degree as an NP from the University of Vermont.

After graduating from this prestigious program, I chose the Community Health Center Nurse Practitioner Residency Program as a facilitator to my professional growth. All throughout my collegiate years, and especially during my doctoral degree preparation, I felt supported and inspired by many mentors. They all celebrated my successes but, most important, they offered constructive ideas on how to become my best self. In the residency program, I found myself in a similar environment, where the core belief is to train the next generation of primary care providers and support them to reach full scope of practice. The NP Residency Program deepened my confidence and honed my skills utilizing the evidence-based practice knowledge I acquired through academic study and professional experience. It gave me insights into the ways primary health care is delivered in complex healthcare settings and beyond the four walls of an examination room.

The Community Health Center of New London (CHC) serves a diverse population of patients. It has brought me closer to the Latino community, something I didn't expect after experiencing life in Burlington, Vermont. I knew that one of the requirements to work here was to be bilingual, but I was not prepared to be speaking Spanish on almost every visit. The connections I make with the patients who speak Spanish as their first language go beyond the ability to speak Spanish. I learn about their successes, their struggles, and their different journeys to this country. On most occasions, there is an invisible understanding, a tacit mutual recognition of the sacrifices made to be here, living in the United States, and the support needed to accomplish personal goals while being away from what was once called home. There is a lot to be done to ensure that their voices are heard and to make them

Continued

EXEMPLAR 13.1

CULTURALLY SENSITIVE PATIENT-CENTERED CARE AT COMMUNITY HEALTH CENTER OF NEW LONDON[a]—cont'd

count. That sentiment fuels my desire to empower the Latino community by delivering evidence-based health care to optimize their health, and in the future I long for the day I can influence healthcare policies to promote well-being in this community.

I was also given the opportunity to be part of a strong team at the health center to combat the opioid epidemic, and that filled me with gratitude. Along with gratitude came a big responsibility. It is not easy to care for one of the most disfranchised groups of people in our current society. There is a lot of work to be done, and that sentiment drives my will to work harder. Early in my career at Community Health, during the residency year, my inquisitive spirit drove me to look for opportunities to get involved. On a crisp spring morning, I met with a recovery navigator from Alliance for Living, a nonprofit that services people living with HIV and/or who misuse drugs. Recovery navigators are case managers with lived experience misusing drugs who go in the community looking for people who are ready to enter recovery. We acknowledged that the opioid epidemic takes the lives of many every day and recognized that working together would make us stronger. That was how our New London MAT clinic was born! Alliance for Living partnered with Community Health to have a primary care provider, me, go once a week to their building, to meet people where they are, to offer primary care services and/or initiate medication for addiction treatment.

Joining the residency program and becoming a part of CHC was the best decision I have made for my professional growth. It not only has impacted my clinical expertise but it has enriched my personal growth. When I return home from a busy day at work, I feel that I am on the right path. Working in collaboration with my CHC colleagues and key members of the community at large, I start every day with confidence that I am giving my best effort to positively impact the health of others.

I am honored to be part of the CHC team and I will continue to improve the access to and quality of health care to our nation's most vulnerable populations.

[a]The authors thank Catherine Hirojosa, DNP, NP for this exemplar.

information systems that promote safe, quality, and cost-effective care and enable NPs to use technology systems that capture data variables for evaluating nursing care.

Primary care practice today is a "team sport." For example, the PCNP must demonstrate sensitivity and sound judgment when treating acute and chronic physical and mental health problems and understand when to "hand off" to other members of the team. PCNPs use transition of care theory, handing off care of the patient/family to other team members and reporting information necessary for safe team functioning in the care of patients (NONPF & AACN, 2016).

Primary care practices are developing meaningful systems for the coordination of care needed for populations of patients. This involves the integration of technological solutions for care coordination and microlevel as well as macrolevel approaches. PCNPs effect healthcare change using broad-based skills, including negotiating, consensus building, and collaborating. They work to facilitate the development of healthcare systems that address the needs of culturally diverse populations, providers, and other stakeholders. PCNPs understand that poor communication and lack of patient accountability among multiple providers lead to medical errors, waste, and duplication. PCNPs evaluate the impact of healthcare delivery on patients, providers, other stakeholders, and the environment. Finally, they are competent in analyzing organizational structures, functions, and resources to improve the delivery of care.

Telecare: The Patient Will See You Now

No longer does geographic access limit the healthcare services available. *Telecare,* also known as *telehealth,* is the use of remote healthcare technology to deliver clinical services; specifically, it is the delivery of healthcare services and clinical information using telecommunications technology, including a wide array of clinical services using Internet, wireless, satellite, and telephone media (American Telemedicine Association, n.d.). Whereas HIT is the generation and transmission of digital health data, often through an EHR, telecare is the delivery of an actual clinical service. HIT can facilitate telecare, but it is not a requirement for delivering remote health care. Guided by technical standards and clinical practice guidelines and backed by decades of research and demonstrations, telecare is a safe and cost-effective way to extend the delivery of health care. Exemplar 13.2 describes how a DNP-prepared nurse practitioner and a physician utilize telehealth in their practice.

Currently, telecare in primary care settings is filling a need to improve access to care for anyone, regardless of their location. Some examples of specialty care that is delivered in primary care settings include telestroke, tele-dermatology, and tele-psychiatry, among others, provided to the underserved, especially more remote and rural populations (Henderson et al., 2014). e-Clinics enable PCNPs to deliver primary care to school-based nursing clinics and employee-based health care in workplaces via telecare. Employers benefit by limiting the loss of productivity and by a reduction in healthcare costs; healthier children learn better.

Telecare technologies reduce cost through a variety of means of remote patient monitoring. For example, Pekmezaris et al. (2012) demonstrated cost savings in the care of a population of patients with heart failure. Remote patient monitoring devices enabled PCNPs to intervene when there was a change in health status, thus eliminating the need for costly home care visits, lowered exacerbations of chronic illnesses, and fewer adverse events, hospitalizations, and emergency department visits. Patients with diabetes who were living in rural areas were given a computer tablet through the Mississippi Diabetes Telehealth Network; this

EXEMPLAR 13.2

A VIRTUAL MEDICAL HOME COLLABORATIVE PRACTICE[a]

Sandra Petersen, DNP, and collaborating physician Kim Dunn, MD, PhD, utilize a virtual medical home to create a patient-centered system of "wired" networks built around the virtual medical home model. Telehealth and patient/provider access to a centralized medical record provide a clinically useful pathway for connecting patients, APRNs, physicians, and third parties (home health, hospice, and physical and occupational therapy services) in the community. The model addresses a major problem in the care delivery system in which care is provided in "silos" and patients do not have direct access to their information. Through automating referral and communication processes to improve patient access, the virtual medical home emphasizes the provision of patient-centered care and provides a sustainable approach to health information exchange. Patients are admitted to the primary care practice (medical home) and provide documentation of all providers (and any third parties) that participate in their care. Telehealth allows for Health Insurance Portability and Accountability Act–secure virtual visits and "curbside consults" with specialists (such as neurology, cardiology, and psychiatry) or other providers while the patient is at a primary care visit (whether that is in the office or via telehealth); this allows all providers to be "on the same page" with the plan of care for the patient. Patients are provided with a QR code that can be accessed through their smart phone that allows immediate access to a read-only version of their medical record, including laboratory results, recent medical encounters, imaging, diagnostics, and plan of care. Treating providers can access the record through the QR code and have the opportunity to send a message to the primary care medical home, which is the "hub" for communication, to share treatment information. Patient satisfaction is also queried through the system, which automatically sends a survey to patients after a medical home encounter to ensure that the patient understands the plan of treatment and how to take any medications.

[a]The authors thank Sandra Petersen, DNP, FNP, University of Texas, Tyler for this exemplar.

supported real-time coaching and health education sessions as well as remote monitoring of blood glucose and vital signs and access to specialty care, resulting in better outcomes with cost savings in the primary care context (Henderson et al., 2014).

Use of these virtual modalities, including various remote monitoring devices and sensors—collectively referred to as *telecare*—is exploding. Increasingly, even unstable patients can be at home, managed with the assistance of emerging technologies. Continuous health monitoring for frail elders at home results in timely, quality care and better self-management, keeping patients in their homes longer, more safely, and with better quality of life and decreased costs (Newland et al., 2016). A variant on the hospital-to-home transitional model is equipping assisted living facilities with "smart rooms," complete with smart phones and computer tablets for messaging and sensors to detect injuries, thereby revolutionizing primary care practice (Rantz et al., 2015). PCNPs need to prepare for a more technology-driven practice. Sensor technology has been shown to provide a feeling of connection to the care provider, with the PCNP available by phone or text message or alerts that communicate information about the patient's changing status (Petersen, 2016).

Reflective Practice: A Component of Direct Patient Care

Reflective practice enables nurses to manage the impact of caring for other people on a daily basis. Defined as the process of making sense of events, situations, and actions in the workplace, *reflective practice* is also defined as a process that develops understanding of what it means to be a practitioner and makes the link between theory and practice by means of the practitioner consciously thinking through the experience (Howatson-Jones, 2016). A range of models is available for nurses to use to support reflective practice in clinical practice. Expert clinical thinking and skillful performance are cultivated through repeated evaluation of similar sets of health and illness scenarios and formulating plans of care based on patient expectations, current standards of care, experience, clinical judgment, and current research. Experienced APRNs incorporate this practical wisdom into their decision making, taking actions that they might have been unlikely to take as novice practitioners. Practical wisdom involves knowing what to do and when to do it:

- When is a patient ready to begin home glucose monitoring?
- When is it time to suggest respite or home health care?
- What is the right time to address sexuality issues with a preteen or teenager?
- What is the right time to address an issue directly and when is it time to step back from confronting difficult issues?

Another important strategy for reflective practice is peer review, if done in a supportive collaborative way; this is included in the NONPF (2017) NP core competencies (see Table 13.1). Open, transparent sharing and review of difficult and complex patient situations can lead to important self-reflection.

A new PCNP especially needs time for reflection, conversation, consultation, and collaboration, but all who practice need time for reflection. Time is needed to keep up with the professional literature and learn how to juggle this into an already busy schedule. Technology takes time and is constantly changing. A supportive environment is critical to success. Increasingly, new graduate NPs of all population foci, whether PCNPs or acute care NPs, report a need for additional education and training to manage today's complex care environments (Hart & Bowen, 2016). In Exemplar 13.1, Dr. Hirojosa also reflects on her time spent in an NP residency developing her complex care competencies in a challenging but supportive care environment.

Guidance and Coaching

The competencies of guidance and coaching have been an identified domain of the NP role since its original iteration and description by NONPF in the early 1990s (Lindeke et al., 1997). It is a natural extension of the RN role—a supporter, a facilitator, nonjudgmental in nature, a side-by-side alliance for health or behavioral change, or "getting through" chronic illness, suffering, death, and dying. Many early NPs, all initially in primary care roles, emerged from seasoned RN practice, often as public health or community-based nurses. The relationship between the PCNP and the patient creates a strong foundation for the guidance and coaching competency (see Chapter 7). The PCNP must be skilled at building trust and rapport because the longitudinal nature of primary care relationships can span decades if warmth and trust are established.

Often, an assessment of the chief complaint unearths many issues of which the patient may not be aware. NPs are expert clinical thinkers who understand the need to listen carefully to the patient's story. The skilled practitioner helps the patient sift and sort through issues, establish priorities, and understand the interconnectedness of these priorities, often in a limited time frame. Practical wisdom guides the practitioner to use expert clinical thinking, deep listening, and skillful interviewing, but the plan of care must be patient centered and sometimes coordinated with the healthcare team. PCNPs work to build a plan that is doable and sustainable by the patient and/or her or his family. Patients *must* be at the center of the plan of care for guidance and/or coaching to be effective. As partnerships deepen, the relationship becomes an even more important clinical tool.

Exemplar 13.2 presents a practice in which telecare enhances communication skills of fragile patients and consequently improves the outcomes of care. Today's new PCNPs are entering practice armed with a set of technical competencies unknown to PCNPs just a few years ago. They are trained in complex and sophisticated information management systems via simulation and are increasingly comfortable coaching patients in their use of wearables and home monitoring devices. The PCNP works in teams using actionable clinical dashboards so that data presented may cue the team that more guidance or coaching is needed. Chapter 7, Guidance and Coaching, discusses this in detail.

Evidence-Based Practice

Nursing science foundations have contributed to the discipline of nursing, which is characterized by a "unique perspective, a distinct way of viewing all phenomena, which ultimately defines the limits and nature of its inquiry" (Donaldson & Crowley, 1978, p. 113). According to the AACN *Essentials* (2021), knowledge for nursing practice, person-centered care, and scholarship for nursing discipline guide the practice of all registered nurses. PCNPs will utilize established and evolving disciplinary knowledge and ways of knowing to guide their advanced assessment, diagnostic decision making, and advanced therapeutic interventions.

Evidence-based practice competencies are essential to the PCNP provider role. Doctoral prepared NPs will integrate evidence-based practice theory and translate research and other forms of information to improve practice processes and outcomes. Ultimately, PCNPs are able to develop new practice approaches based on the integration of research, ways of knowing, and practice knowledge.

Clinical practice guidelines ensure that the most current scientific evidence is applied in patient care. Practice patterns, or clinical performance, are evaluated using *process* measures, referring to the types of services delivered by caregivers, as well as *outcome* measures, such as quality indicators, health status, and interventions. The PCNP must participate in measuring outcomes of their practice and make adjustments, because outcomes are heavily influenced by underlying factors such as severity of illness and patient characteristics (King, 2016). Chapters 8, 21, and 23 provide additional information.

Leadership

There are many social forces that shape the future health and professional practice environment for PCNPs. PCNPs assume complex and advanced leadership roles to initiate and guide change. That leadership fosters collaboration with multiple stakeholders (e.g., patients, families, community, integrated healthcare teams, and policymakers) and demonstrates critical and reflective thinking. Given the longitudinal nature of primary care practice, PCNPs are often the long-term member of the team who provides continuity and stability in the care and management of patients over long periods and thus are ideally suited to lead teams. Nurses continue to be identified as the most honest and ethical professionals (Saad, 2020). The PCNP's role as a leader in the community—often via membership on boards of health and education, through active participation in community organizations, and as an influential policymaker—provides evidence of their suitability and ability to *lead* healthcare teams, generating transformational practice change. DNP-prepared NPs are prepared to assess systems and organizations and to evaluate and implement system-level change. PCNPs, particularly doctoral prepared NPs, assume advanced leadership roles to initiate and guide change. The NASEM (2021) cited nursing leadership development as well as leadership in improving healthcare access, quality, and equity as critical to our future as a discipline and profession.

Moreover, PCNPs advocate for improved access, better quality, and cost-effective health care for all populations. They use the development and implementation of innovations that incorporate principles of change to advance practice and promote health at local, national, and global levels. They translate patients' stories. At the local practice level, for example, PCNPs may enact leadership roles when they guide and support staff, triage patients, lead interprofessional teams, coordinate care, and oversee the appropriate use of resources. On a broader level, PCNPs engage in clinical and professional leadership and use effective collaborative skills to assist groups and organizations to envision preferred futures, achieve consensus, and implement change. Where there is need, PCNPs respond.

PCNPs can also demonstrate leadership in advancing practice environments. Bodenheimer and Sinsky (2014) sounded the alarm that the "joy" had gone out of practicing medicine and that a relentless focus on metrics had led to the deterioration of professional practice environments and called for a redesign of the triple aim in health care to a quadruple aim that adds a quadrant for healthcare team well-being (Arnetz et al., 2020). Sometimes called the "missing aim" (Fig. 13.2) or the "forgotten aim," the fourth aim notes that patient outcomes invariably suffer as a result of providers feeling overwhelmed, overworked, and powerless (Chase & Kish, 2015). PCNPs need to lead work to support healthier practice environments that in turn support quality-based outcomes.

Collaboration

Collaboration and leadership are closely linked in the effort to improve healthcare delivery systems. The 1996 IOM definition of primary care implies the use of professional collaboration to deliver integrated and accessible care. Effective collaboration within an interprofessional team context results in more comprehensive, patient-focused care promoting high-quality, cost-effective outcomes both on the local practice level and beyond the walls of the practice into the community (Bodenheimer & Grumbach, 2016). Exemplar 13.3 describes how a family nurse practitioner virtually collaborates and learns from specialists in pain management. Effective collaboration improves institutional performance through processes such as continuous quality improvement, which involves the identification of concrete problems and the formation of interprofessional teams to gather data and propose solutions. Computerized information systems assist all of these components, so technological competencies are essential for the PCNP to be an effective collaborator. Chapter 10 provides additional information on the collaboration competency.

Ethical Practice

Illness can create a range of negative emotions in patients, including anxiety, fear, powerlessness, and vulnerability. In the ever-expanding healthcare system, PCNPs face ethical issues, particularly involving, but not limited to, the allocation of care. How to identify and resolve these ethical issues is an important task for PCNPs. There needs, for example, to be clear separation of financial and clinical decisions. In an era focused on cost containment, the PCNP's accountability to the healthcare system in which they practice may create tension, especially in relation to the use of resources for patient care. PCNPs must always be ethically accountable for their actions, particularly when financial incentives related to resource use are involved (Bodenheimer & Grumbach, 2007). This accountability is aided by increased technology. Despite the familiar pains of adopting new technology and waiting for EHR vendors to "catch up" with practice transformation, technology's impact on primary care has largely been successful.

Additionally, the PCNP will encounter specific patient care concerns that raise ethical issues. Examples include reproductive issues, informed consent, end-of life-issues, conflict of interest on the part of providers, and conflicting healthcare goals among family members, as well as lack of equity, social disparities of health, and in some cases profound suffering.

PCNP practice must embrace thoughtful reflection on the meaning of moral concepts in terms of culture and diversity. Operating with a context-sensitive approach can enable PCNPs to understand and name ethical issues in nursing practice more easily and to integrate ethical principles into their decision making (Lützén, 1997).

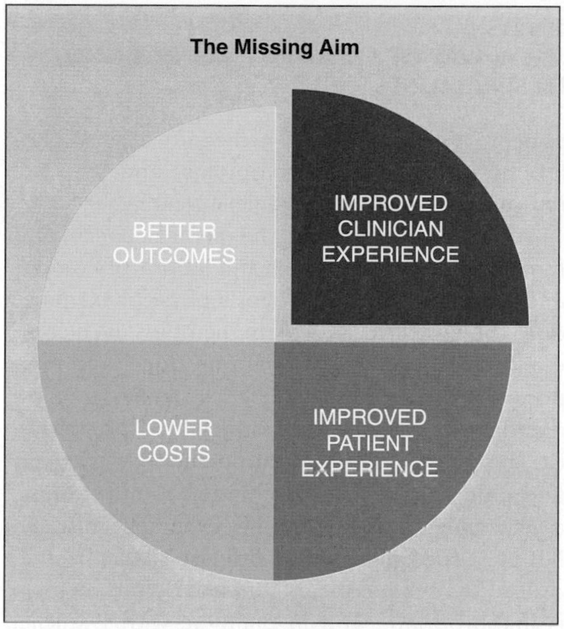

Fig. 13.2 ■ The missing aim: Improved clinician experience. (From "What's Missing From the Triple Aim of Health Care?," by L. Sobal and S. Jaskie, 2016, *Cardiac Interventions Today, 10*[2], 21. http://citoday.com/2016/04/whats-missing-from-the-triple-aim-of-health-care/.)

PCNPs evaluate the ethical consequences of decisions and apply ethically sound solutions to complex issues related to diverse individuals, populations, and systems of care. In today's complex care environments, we must confront moral distress in care providers as they confront the complexity of people's problems and lives. Additional information is found in Chapter 11, Ethical Practice.

Going Forward With Shared Competencies for Primary Care

Englander et al. (2016) identified eight domains of general physician competency from the taxonomy used to map what are called core "entrustable professional activities" for entering medical residency (Box 13.1). This evolved into a list of 58 competencies within eight domains. As can be seen from this list, there is some convergence between these medical domains of competence, the NONPF core NP competencies (Table 13.1), and AACN's 10 domains for nursing competence (Box 13.2). This promising work from medicine, regardless of specialty, provides clear performance outcomes that are expected of all students receiving an MD degree. Medicine, like advanced practice nursing, is shifting from focusing on *time* and predefined curricula to focusing on *competency-based* medical education. These "guidelines" evolved from a grounding in the literature and were vetted through a process that broadly engaged the medical education community, sparked by a desire to improve the quality and safety of the care that new resident physicians provide to patients.

In April 2021, AACN approved a new and updated version of the *Essentials* that incorporates all nursing program levels. *The Essentials: Core Competencies for Professional Nursing Education* (2021) *(Essentials)* provides a newly envisioned educational framework for nurses prepared at the baccalaureate and graduate levels, creating a *competency-based* foundation for nursing education across nursing curricula. The *Essentials* provide clearly defined competencies for professional nursing practice, framed within 10 domains, exemplifying nursing's unique contribution to care in a common language understood across health professions, learners, employers, faculty, and the public (AACN, 2021). The document specifically outlines advanced-level nursing education competencies preparing graduate nurses for practice in an APRN role or an advanced nursing practice specialty. As universities and colleges begin to re-envision their curriculum to incorporate competency-based learning in alignment with the new *Essentials* as well as the NONPF core competencies (2017) and specialty competencies (2013; 2016), competency-based curricula are emerging. This new era will provide a new evidence-based way of educating our PCNPs.

EMERGENCE OF POSTGRADUATE TRAINING IN PRIMARY CARE

Over the past 20 years, studies have documented the experience of new NPs and their interest in a postgraduate, intensive period of clinical training following completion of the academic credential that qualifies for certification as an NP, sometimes referred to as an *NP residency* or *fellowship* (Hart & Bowen, 2016). Since the development of the first models in FQHCs (Flinter, 2012) and the Veterans Affairs (VA; Zapatka et al., 2014), there are currently more than 200 postgraduate NP residency and fellowship programs, with over half focused on primary care (National Nurse Practitioner Residency & Fellowship Training Consortium, n.d.). A

EXEMPLAR 13.3

MOVING KNOWLEDGE, NOT THE PATIENT: A NEW WAY OF LEARNING, CONSULTING, AND WORKING WITH SPECIALISTS

Danielle is a family nurse practitioner (NP) at a rural community health center in Arizona. Like primary care providers across the country, she faces the challenge of caring for patients with chronic pain. She must assess, diagnose, manage, and treat pain in the context of the patient's life and preferences and consider all of the risks and benefits of pharmacologic treatment, especially opioids. But she is not alone in this.

On Thursdays, from noon to 2:00 p.m., Danielle heads to her desk, turns on her computer, and logs into a Zoom videoconference to join Project ECHO-Pain, where for 2 hours she will take a pause from her intensely busy clinical schedule. She will listen to a didactic lecture on an element of pain management, hearing cases presented by primary care colleagues across the country and the advice given to them by a team of pain management experts. This electronic chat includes 30 participants who share their own clinical experiences and lessons learned. She does this with the support of the rural health center leadership, who recognize how challenging this area of practice can be.

Today, Danielle has asked to present a case and get some guidance. She describes a 60-year-old female patient with chronic and generalized pain who first came to her several months ago. Due to back pain and diffuse joint pain, the patient has been treated with opioid medication for 10 years, along with medication for depression. She is obese (body mass index of 42), post-gastric bypass surgery, and disabled from an injury while working. Danielle's assessment was that the opioid regimen was inappropriate, and she referred the patient to a pain management center. The report from the care provider at that pain center was that the patient "threw a scene" in the office when they attempted to reduce her opioids, and they are returning the patient to Danielle's care.

After Danielle presents the medical, social, and family history, medications and laboratory values, and the results of the patient's physical examination, the Project ECHO team members each comment in turn, ask additional questions, and then pose a second round of queries, making recommendations. Unlike a consult with "a" specialist, this is a team consult: an orthopedic surgeon and pain specialist, a psychiatrist, a nutritionist, a pharmacist, a physical medicine specialist, an NP pain specialist, and a Chinese medicine specialist. The team concurs that the opioid regimen is inappropriate, and in dialogue with Danielle, they create an action plan of care that Danielle can implement, incorporating behavioral health, physical medicine, pharmacologic, and nutrition-based approaches.

(Project ECHO is a case-based, distance learning strategy first developed by Dr. Sanjeev Arora at the University of New Mexico as a model to support primary care providers in assuming the responsibility for treating patients with hepatitis C in their practices versus referring them to an academic medical center for treatment with a specialist. The model has been replicated around the United States and the world. Danielle is participating in Project ECHO-Pain, sponsored by the Weitzman Institute, a federally qualified health center–based research and innovation center. For Danielle, participation in Project ECHO is a strategy for ongoing learning in a clinically challenging area, expert feedback on specific cases, and support from a community of primary care providers.)

study of the experience of PCNPs showed the effectiveness of the program in the achievement of competence, confidence, and a sense of mastery by the end of the program (Flinter & Hart, 2017). Similar FQHC-based postgraduate programs have been developed in other FQHCs (Norwick, 2016), in the VA system (Meyer et al., 2015; Rugen et al., 2014), and in private health systems (Bush, 2014; Bush & Lowery, 2016). A 2018 survey of more than 8000 NPs showed that NPs who had done a postgraduate residency or fellowship reported increased

BOX 13.1

Eight Domains of General Physician Competence[a]

1. Patient care
2. Knowledge for practice (medical knowledge for physicians)
3. Practice-based learning and improvement
4. Professionalism
5. Interpersonal and communication skills
6. Systems-based practice
7. Interprofessional collaboration
8. Personal and professional development

[a]Derived from the taxonomy used to map the core entrustable professional activities for entering residency to their critical competencies. From Englander, R., Flynn, T., Call, S., Carraccio, C., Cleary, L., Fulton, T. B., Garrity, M. J., Lieberman, S. A., Lindeman, B., Lypson, M. L., Minter, R., Rosenfield, J., Thomas, J., Wilson, M. C., & Aschenbrener, C. A. (2016). Toward defining the foundation of the MD degree. *Academic Medicine*, 91(10), 1354.

BOX 13.2

Ten Domains for Nursing Competence

1. Knowledge for Nursing Practice
2. Patient-Centered Care
3. Population Health
4. Scholarship for the Nursing Discipline
5. Quality and Safety
6. Interprofessional Partnerships
7. Systems-Based Practice
8. Informatics and Healthcare Technologies
9. Professionalism
10. Personal, Professional, and Leadership Development

From American Association of Colleges of Nursing. (2021). The essentials: Core competencies for professional nursing education. https://www.aacnnursing.org/Portals/42/AcademicNursing/pdf/Essentials-2021.pdf

autonomy, confidence, team collaboration, satisfaction, and intent to stay in practice and, important, were more likely to care for underserved populations (Park et al., 2021). Kesten & El-Banna (2020) studied organizations that sponsored postgraduate training programs for NPs and identified posttraining recruitment and retention of NPs as key positive outcomes. Since 2019, HRSA has funded 36 entities in 24 states to develop or expand postgraduate NP residency training programs with a preference for projects benefitting rural or underserved areas (HRSA, 2020).

PRIMARY CARE AND THE FEDERAL GOVERNMENT

Our educational institutions are charged with the academic preparation of each generation of primary care NPs, but we note that the federal government, in its charge to address the healthcare needs of the country, also plays a vital role in supporting the education and training of primary care NPs and their distribution to underserved communities. The federal government, particularly through the addition of Title VIII to the Public Health Service Act (Congressional Research Service, 2005; Glazer & Alexandre, 2008) strengthened the nation's investment in nursing education and, in particular, advanced practice nursing. The late Dr. Fitzhugh Mullan, speaking in an interview shortly before his death in 2019, opined that the Public Health Service Act was a superb example of federal legislation with funding and a robust response from the nursing community. This legislation built the scaffolding that became the NP and APRN educational structure of the country (Hassmiller, 2020). The goals of the PPACA could not be achieved without also addressing issues of the healthcare workforce, and in Title V, Health Care Workforce, legislates the creation of a workforce commission, securing data for workforce planning, and the education, training, and support of the country's healthcare workforce (Patient Protection and Affordable Care Act, 2010).

Health Resources and Services Administration

Through HRSA, a division of the Department of Health and Human Services, the federal government plays a significant role in supporting systems, organizations, and programs that provide primary care services to vulnerable populations (Fig. 13.3). HRSA works to improve the healthcare workforce distribution throughout the nation, particularly in underserved, rural, and tribal areas, and supports the transformation of healthcare delivery by supporting innovative

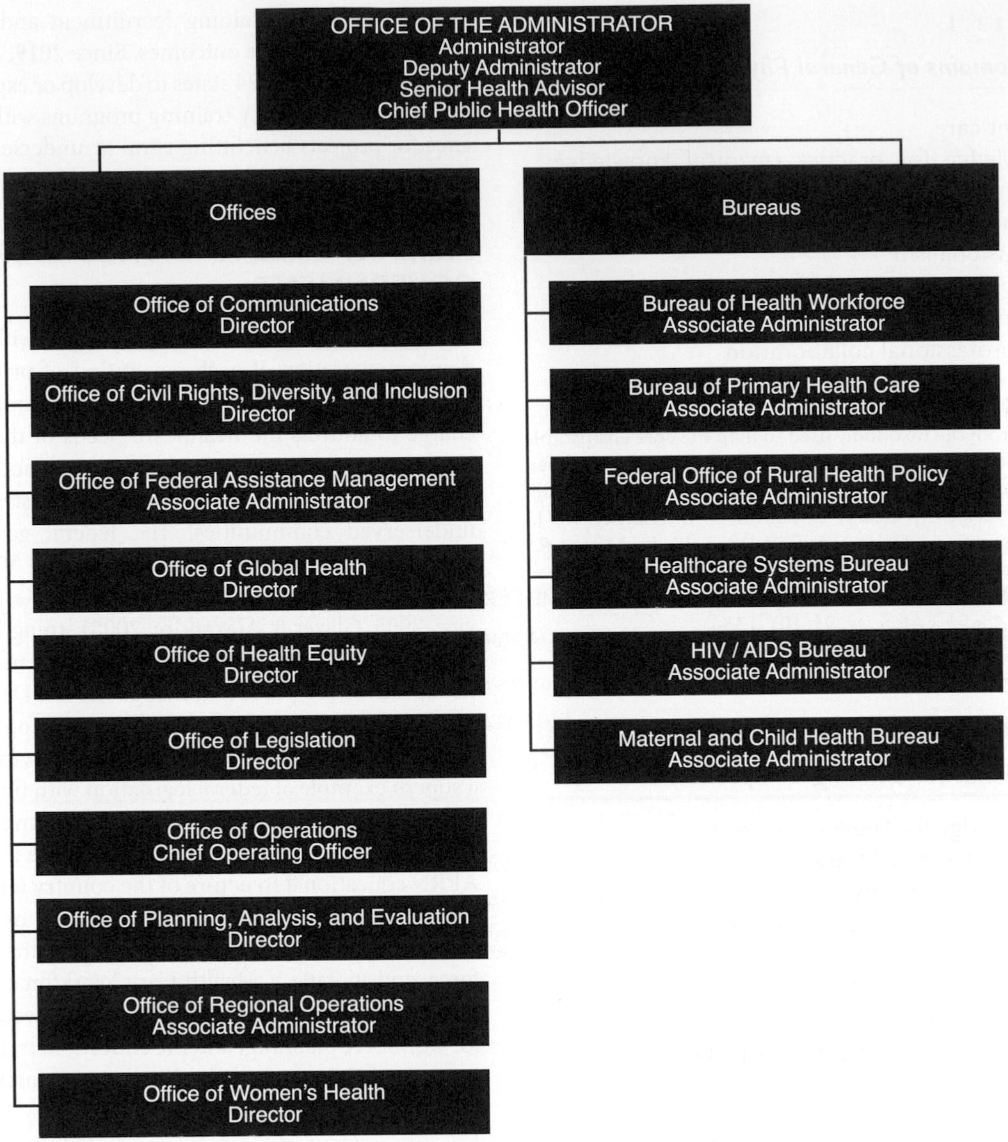

Fig. 13.3 ■ **Health Resources and Services Administration Organization Chart.** (From "HRSA Organization Chart," by Health Resources and Services Administration, 2021a, http://www.hrsa.gov/about/organization/org-chart.html)

models of care. HRSA also plays an important role in educating and training the health professionals who deliver those services. HRSA's Bureau of Health Workforce supports the development and maintenance of an adequate medical, dental, behavioral health, nursing, and public health workforce along with other healthcare workforce–related programs. In addition to collecting data and providing analysis about the healthcare workforce, this bureau offers competitive funding for nursing education programs tailored to areas of greatest need, such as rural health and support for innovations in practice.

One of the most influential pieces of legislation in primary care workforce history in the United States, and a significant milestone in the development of the primary care NPs, was the creation of the NHSC. For a detailed overview of the legislative history and evolution of the NHSC, see Heisler (2018, §4.26.18). Today, NPs are the second largest group of NHSC loan repayment recipients.

The authorizing statute for the NHSC identified shortage areas to fulfill the statutory requirements that direct NHSC personnel to areas of greatest need. Due to limited federal resources, shortage designations help HRSA prioritize and focus resources on the areas of highest need. Generations of NPs, including these authors, have benefited from the financial support of tuition (NHSC scholars) or loan repayment (NHSC loan repayment) and equally from the opportunity to serve through clinical practice in an underserved community, either rural or urban, or with a special population. Similarly, the Nurse Corps helps underserved communities meet their healthcare needs by providing loans and scholarships to nurses and APRNs in rural, urban, and tribal areas. The Bureau of Health Workforce, with the infusion of new federal appropriations as part of the American Rescue Plan (American Rescue Plan Act, 2021), has significantly increased its capacity for Nurse Corps and NHSC awards. These awards are explicit in their focus on creating a workforce that represents underserved communities and populations and is trained in the settings where these populations are cared for (Carthon et al., 2015; Nunez et al., 2021). Underlying most federal support programs for health professional loans and scholarship, as well as many grant-funded programs of interest to primary care NPs, is the concept of *shortages*. These are quantifiable, objective measurements of need that can be scored and ranked in determining priorities and qualifications for resources. Designations include Health Professional Shortage Areas, Medically Underserved Areas/Populations, Exceptional Medically Underserved Populations, and Governor-Designated/Secretary Certified Shortage Areas for Rural Health Clinics (Health Resources and Services Administration, 2021b; Box 13.3).

BOX 13.3

Designation Quick Guide: How the Federal Government Designates Areas for Support

The federal government establishes criteria to designate health professional shortage areas (HPSAs) and to use those designations to provide additional resources such as qualifying for National Health Service Corps clinician awards or funding preference. Health Professional Shortage Areas (HPSAs) identify geographic areas, populations groups, or facilities within the United States that are experiencing a shortage of healthcare professionals. Medically Underserved Areas (MUAs) and Medically Underserved Populations (MUPs) identify geographic areas and populations with a lack of access to primary care services. Exceptional Medically Underserved Populations (Exceptional MUP) identify a specific population subset that does not meet the established criteria to qualify as an MUP but due to unusual circumstance do not have access to primary care services. Governor's Designated Secretary Certified Shortage Areas for Rural Health Clinics are areas that a state governor or designee designates as having a shortage according to the state.

Three scoring criteria are common across all HPSA disciplines:

- Population-to-provider ratio
- Percentage of the population below 100% of the federal poverty level (FPL)
- Travel time to the nearest source of care (NSC) outside the HPSA designation area

The Medically Underserved Area and Medically Underserved Population (MUA/P) score is dependent on the Index of Medical Underservice (IMU) calculated for the area or population proposed for designation.

MUA/P INDICATORS

- Provider per 1000 population ratio
- % Population at 100% of the federal poverty level (FPL)
- % Population age 65 and over
- Infant mortality rate

Health Resources and Services Administration. (2021c). *Medically underserved areas (MUAs) and medically underserved populations (MUA/Ps)*. Bureau of Health Workforce. https://bhw.hrsa.gov/workforce-shortage-areas/shortage-designation#mups

THE PRIMARY CARE SAFETY NET

Community Health Centers

For more than 55 years, providers in community health centers have delivered affordable, accessible, quality, and cost-effective primary health care to patients regardless of their ability to pay. During that time, health centers have become an essential source of comprehensive coordinated primary care encompassing medical, behavioral, and oral health care for America's most vulnerable populations. In 2020, 1395 health centers cared for 29.8 million people (HRSA, n.d.). Community health centers in the United States trace their roots to the work of Drs. Sydney and Emily Kark in South Africa in the 1940s. The Karks developed a new model of population-focused, data-driven, community-oriented health care that engaged local community members in organizing and delivering care (Kark & Kark, 1999), and Dr. Jack Geiger, a US medical student who studied with them, wrote about the model, which ultimately led to the creation of the first US community health centers. Dr. Geiger and fellow activists proposed and secured federal funding that led to the development of the first US health centers in Mound Bayou, Mississippi, and Boston, Massachusetts, as an outgrowth of both the civil rights movement and the War on Poverty (Geiger, 2002, 2005; Lefkowitz, 2005). From early on, health centers were defined by a set of core characteristics: private, independent nonprofit organizations with consumer-controlled boards of directors, sliding scale fees for low-income persons, a comprehensive set of primary care services, and a focus on underserved geographic areas and populations.

The United States has distinct enabling statute, 42 US Code Part D Primary Health Care § 254b-Health Centers, which defines a health center as:

> *... an entity that serves a population that is medically underserved, or a special medically underserved population comprised of migratory and seasonal agricultural workers, the homeless, and residents of public housing by providing, either through the staff and supporting resources of the center or through contracts or cooperative arrangements.*
>
> *(Social Security Act, 2020a)*

FQHCs are community-based health centers that receive funds from the HRSA Health Center Program to provide these primary care services in underserved areas. They must meet a stringent set of requirements, including providing care on a sliding fee scale based on ability to pay, and operate under a governing board that includes patients. The defining statute for federally qualified health centers is Section 1905 (I) (2) (B) of Social Security Act 42 U.S.C. 1396d (Social Security Act, 2020b). Health centers that have not received funding under this authorization may be designated as a FQHC "look alike," which entitles them to some, but not all, of the benefits of being an FQHC. NPs are a vital and growing essential component of the healthcare workforce in FQHCs (10,512 full-time equivalent NPs. vs. 14,082 MDs), and the combined workforce of NPs, PAs, and certified nurse-midwives in FQHCs now outnumber physicians (14,590 vs. 14,082). Health centers now must report annually on their health professions training programs. Health centers make an important contribution to NP training, with 4728 prelicensure NPs and 1808 postgraduate NPs (residencies and fellowships) receiving training in a health center in 2020 (HRSA, 2021d). Health centers were the first healthcare organizations to develop postgraduate primary care NP residency programs and today represent the largest number of primary care–focused postgraduate training programs (Meissen, 2019).

Nurse-Led Health Centers

Originally called nurse-managed health centers, nurse-led health centers are led and staffed by nurses and are typically primary care delivery sites located in the communities they serve, many identifying themselves with the name of that community. They are often located in places traditionally lacking access to care, such as homeless shelters, rural areas, or public housing communities (Sutter-Barrett et al., 2015). Additionally, nurse-led health centers are often associated with academic institutions and provide clinically based educational settings for undergraduate and graduate students across disciplines (Pohl et al., 2011). Exemplar 13.4 describes a medical student's interprofessional training experience in a nurse-led clinic. In Section 5208, the PPACA defined a nurse-managed health center as a "nurse practice arrangement, managed by advanced practice nurses, that provides primary care or wellness services to underserved or vulnerable populations and that is associated with a school, college, university department of nursing, a FQHC, or independent nonprofit health or social services agency" (Patient Protection and Affordable Care Act, 2010). In 2016 there were approximately 153 nurse-led clinics in the United

EXEMPLAR 13.4

INTERPROFESSIONAL, TEAM-BASED EDUCATION IN A NURSE-LED CLINIC[a]

My time at the Florida Atlantic University Christine E. Lynn College of Nursing, Louis and Anne Green Memory and Wellness Center, a nurse-led health center that specializes in the care of patients with memory disorders, fit seamlessly into my interprofessional experience during my third-year medical school rotation. A nurse practitioner (NP) and neuropsychologist evaluate new patients at this center to better characterize their medical concerns and memory impairment. Findings are discussed by an interprofessional team including the NP, social worker, neuropsychologist, and psychotherapist; a therapeutic plan is then developed for the patient and family.

I was able to sit in on a new patient evaluation by Madeline, a primary care advanced practice adult-gerontology NP. A patient, "J," was referred by a transitional program for chronically homeless individuals, where he is a resident. As I listened to the interview that took place, it was apparent that he had some cognitive impairment, which he himself recognized, but it was difficult to determine his reliability as a historian. He had a history of traumatic brain injury from a vehicle–pedestrian accident as well as substance use disorder and an unclear psychiatric history. His perceptions of his relationships and situation gave the impression that he did not realize the severity of his state and did not recognize destructive decisions he had made. He had no contact with his family and could not effectively explain why. As I left, Madeline assured me he would undergo neuropsychological testing to pinpoint his strengths and weaknesses in various cognitive domains. The team would meet to discuss his case and make recommendations.

This rotation allowed me to experience nurse-directed care with heavy involvement from social work and other disciplines. The most striking feature of nurse-led care is an emphasis on continuous communication. Weekly meetings ensure that the team is up to date on patient progress and recommendations. The patients are medically and socially complex and require a cohesive team approach. I think this is the best example of providing care for the individual as a whole that I have observed so far. It was refreshing and eye opening.

[a]The authors thank Ana Duvnjak, Medical Student.

This exemplar was written while the author was a medical student at the Schmidt College of Medicine, Florida Atlantic University, Boca Raton, FL.

States (Hansen-Turton et al., 2016). In these diverse practices, PCNPs provide team-based care in collaboration with other healthcare providers such as nurse-midwives, physicians, dentists, registered nurses (RNs), dietitians, diabetes educators (often nurses), substance abuse counselors, and social workers. In addition, they may collaborate with community sectors such as legal advocates, housing agencies, peer support, community leaders, and churches.

Nurse-led centers typically work with community leaders to advance health equity and expand the definition of health care to address some of the most serious problems facing American society today. These issues include family, adolescent, and neighborhood violence; substance abuse and misuse; environmental aspects of diseases such as asthma and birth defects; and problems such as grief, stress, anxiety, and obesity (Austria, 2015).

An integrative review of characteristics of nurse-led centers' quality and outcomes determined that these centers are consistent with the WHO definition of primary health care that includes the social determinants of health (Holt et al., 2014). Auerbach et al. (2013) posited that nurse-led centers could help mitigate the expected primary care physician shortages. A systematic review of nurse-led clinics studying 15 centers and nearly 4000 respondents documented positive patient satisfaction and positive patient-reported outcomes (Randall et al., 2017). Tine Hansen-Turton et al. (2016), in a comprehensive book on the history, present status, and anticipated future of nurse-led care and nurse-led health clinics, pointed to both the PPACA and the *Future of Nursing 2010–2020* report as major influencers in supporting the continued growth and development of the models of nurse-led clinics.

School-Based Health Centers

Similar to nurse-led FQHCs, school-based health centers (SBHCs) are also innovations that trace their beginning to the 1960s and have become a significant contributor to the healthcare landscape in communities across the United States. While the sponsorship of an individual school-based health center may range from a community health center to a hospital or a school system itself, NPs are the dominant primary care clinical provider. Other models include PAs and, rarely, physicians. SBHC staff often include a behavioral health clinician and oral health provider along with clinical support staff. Multiple studies and systematic reviews have confirmed that SBHCs improve health and advance health equity, particularly for low-income and racial/ethnic minority groups (J. A. Knopf et al., 2016; Lewallen et al., 2015). Most recently, the US Community Preventive Services Task Force noted positive impact on vaccinations, health assessments, oral health, asthma morbidity, access to behavioral health services, and decreased emergency room usage (Arenson et al., 2019; J. A. Knopf et al., 2016; Love, Panchal et al., 2019; Love, Schlitt et al., 2019). A systematic review of studies since 2000 concluded that SBHCs increase access to health services for children, families, and communities and might be well suited to address current challenges affecting youth, including gun violence and adverse childhood experiences, and the health of individuals in American Indian/Alaskan Native communities. The number of SBHCs in the United States doubled between 1999 and 2017, with the majority sponsored by an FQHC (Love, Schlitt et al., 2019). Like all areas of health care, SBHCs were affected by the COVID-19 pandemic due to school closures and disrupted access. Post-pandemic, SBHCs may see significant expansion as the impact of SBHCs in addressing access, health equity, and behavioral health as well as medical concerns is gaining increased recognition and support for expanded investment (Damian & Boyd, 2020).

Veterans Affairs

The VA system is part of the US federal government, separate from Department of Health and Human Services. Its mission is to provide care for the nation's veterans. It is one of the largest employers of NPs, with over 5000 NPs employed in 142 VA medical centers and 800 community-based outpatient clinics (National Center for Veterans Analysis and Statistics, 2018). A comparison study of outcomes of more than 800,000 patients assigned to either MDs or NPs found no significant differences in cost or clinical outcomes between the two groups but did find fewer total hospitalizations and fewer ambulatory care sensitive hospitalizations (Liu et al., 2020). Veterans Affairs has a strong record of innovation. APRNs are widely used in the VA. Innovative programs include the VA's Home-Based Primary Care program for chronically ill individuals; this program has resulted in cost reductions, reduced hospitalizations and emergency room visits by veterans, and fewer disease exacerbations (Edes et al., 2014). In this program, PCNPs function as the PCP and make home visits. Another example of innovation is a Center for Medicare & Medicaid Innovation (CMS Innovation Center) project, currently testing the Home-Based Primary Care approach through the Independence at Home demonstration project. Additionally, the VA system was one of the earliest adopters of EHRs. It also designed the Patient-Aligned Care Teams, which includes physicians, PCNPs, PAs, RNs, licensed practical nurses, medical assistants, and administrative clerks on their clinical teams (Edes et al., 2014). This care team was created specifically to address issues of continuity and access to the PCP as part of the VA's national implementation of the Primary Care Medical Home model (Yano et al., 2014). Patient-Aligned Care Teams became the cornerstone for the way care would be delivered within the VA, and they focused on four key areas: enhanced partnerships between veterans and caregivers, improved access to care, coordinated care among team members, and veteran-centered, team-based care. The VA has been a leader in the development of postgraduate residency training for new PCNPs (Rugen et al., 2014). The team focus has also served as the basis for the development of interprofessional primary care training such as that undertaken at the West Haven, Connecticut, Center for Excellence in Primary Care. Positive outcomes were demonstrated in terms of increased understanding of the role of NPs on the part of internal medicine residents and increased confidence on the part of new NPs relative to their physician counterparts on the team (Meyer et al., 2015). This interprofessional training project was piloted at five different VA settings across the country. Each site has created new understandings of the challenges of fully implementing team-based care (Harada et al., 2019). Alumni of the VA interprofessional postgraduate residency training programs rank the training highly, and 63% of the NPs who completed the program between 2012 and 2018 are actively practicing in primary care (Harada et al., 2019).

On January 13, 2017, NPs along with two other APRN groups, clinical nurse specialists (CNSs) and certified nurse-midwives, were granted full practice authority in the VA system, a landmark decision that overrode state practice authority. In the abstract of their ruling, the VA notes that

> *his rulemaking increases veterans' access to VA health care by expanding the pool of qualified healthcare professionals who are authorized to provide primary health care and other related healthcare services to the full extent of their education, training, and certification, without the clinical supervision of physicians, and it permits VA to use its healthcare resources more effectively and in a manner that is consistent with the role of APRNs in the non-VA healthcare sector, while maintaining the patient centered, safe, high-quality health care that veterans receive from VA.*
>
> ***(US Department of Veterans Affairs, 2016, p. 90199)***

A preliminary evaluation of the impact of the 2017 granting of full practice authority to NPs indicates increased access to timely primary care (Rugs et al., 2021).

PRACTICE REDESIGN IN PRIMARY CARE

Team-Based Primary Care

Whether a practice consists of a single team consisting of one PCP and a medical assistant or a large, multisite organization with both core and extended team members, the evidence base for the advantages of team-based care is well established. Such care improves outcomes, expands access, and contributes to satisfaction (Bodenheimer & Grumbach, 2016; Carter et al., 2009; Coleman et al., 2009; Willard-Grace et al., 2014). The team-based model has been a particular focus in community health centers and Veterans Affairs. As discussed earlier, both were early adopters of the chronic care model for the management of chronic illness, with adaptation for prevention, health promotion, and routine care (Wagner, 2000). The national PCT-LEAP Project (Primary Care Teams, Learning from Effective Ambulatory Care Practices) studied exemplar practices across the country and published a series of articles highlighting the individual and collective impact of individual team members and the team as a whole (Wagner et al., 2017) and leadership attributes of high-performing teams (Crabtree et al., 2020). Additionally, they developed a TEAMS tool to support primary care practices (Jones et al., 2020). Currently, 150 million adults have one or more chronic health conditions, which makes the need for patient self-regulation and family engagement and activation critical in primary care (Bodenheimer & Bauer, 2016).

However, change is difficult. In a discussion paper, the IOM acknowledged openly some of the difficulties, noting, "Health care has not always been ... a team sport" (Mitchell et al., 2012, p. 1). Drawing on data obtained from participants on successful teams, certain personal values were identified as critical to a high-functioning team, including honesty and transparency, discipline, creativity, humility, and curiosity. Pany et al. (2021) studied solo versus team care and the impact on different chronic illnesses and determined that team-based care outperformed solo provider care regardless of team composition (Mitchell et al., 2012; Pany et al., 2021).

Disruptive Innovations: From Retail Clinic to the New Primary Care Center

Convenient Care Clinics

In a classic paper in the *Harvard Business Review* (Christensen et al., 2000), disruptive innovations in health care were described as those that are less expensive, that provide more convenient products and services, and that start by meeting the needs of less-demanding customers. They specifically cited CVS

Minute Clinics, staffed by NPs, as an example of a disruptive innovation in health care, a fundamentally different and new model. Billboards with "You're sick; we're quick" and a smiling healthcare provider—often identified as an NP—indicated that this was new, rich, and valuable setting for NPs to deliver primary care and minor sick care services to those without primary care access—particularly weekends, evenings, and on holidays and just because it was so convenient. Twenty years later, we look back at those years as the start of a sweeping transformation that has made primary health care, urgent care, and even chronic illness management yet another major retail service available at a big box store near you. Questions about quality, over/underutilization, and spending continue, but what is clear is that this has been an area for both innovation and profit in the commercialization of the American healthcare system. While the early models often specifically highlighted NPs as the key and usually solo provider, physicians, PAs, NPs, pharmacists, and, most recently, behavioral health clinicians have all taken their place on the retail clinic team. These clinics report high patient satisfaction with short waiting times and appeal to clientele without insurance or those for whom immediate access is needed and not available (Bachrach et al., 2015). They do not negatively affect preventive care or diabetes management, findings confirmed by Hansen-Turton et al. (2016), who noted improved preventive health in community care clinics over primary care settings. Ashwood and colleagues' 2016 report, showing increased utilization and cost by individuals seeking care in convenient care clinics, sounded a more cautious note. More patients are searching for professional treatment and advice for symptoms they might previously have managed on their own (Ashwood et al., 2016). Increasingly, these clinics are an integral part of a US health system in the throes of massive change. The competitive advantage of data—lots of it—on consumers and their spending, along with predictive analytic data on individuals, neighborhoods, and communities at an unprecedented level, indicates that we will see continued innovation and growth in this space but also an unprecedented engagement of some of the largest corporations in the world in primary care services.

PRIMARY CARE WORKFORCE AND THE CONTEXT OF PCNP PRACTICE TODAY

Primary Care Nurse Practitioner Workforce

Based on a *National Sample Survey of Nurse Practitioners* by HRSA (2012), in 2016 the American Association of Nurse Practitioners (AANP) began assembling a National Nurse Practitioner Database derived from its membership. This sample is dependent on its membership's participation and therefore has limitations, but it is an increasingly important data source nonetheless (Box 13.4, Table 13.2, and Table 13.3; AANP, 2021). The 2021 AANP National Nurse Practitioner Database documents that more than 325,000 NPs are licensed in the United States, with 88.9% of these NPs certified in a primary care specialty. This includes family, pediatric, adult–gerontology, and women's health PCNPs practicing in primary care. The most widely held primary care certification was family NP (FNP), and the average age of practicing NPs is 49 years of age (AANP, 2020, 2021). Diversity of the NP workforce improved from 2018 to 2020; however, there is more work to do, with 79.4% White (down from 87%) and 90% female (down from 93%) in the NP workforce (AANP, 2020).

Most recently published in 2018, the US Health Workforce Chart book (HRSA, 2018) confirmed that the NP workforce is substantially Whiter and older than the working-age population in the United States. As noted, this is a key focus of the *Future of Nursing 2020–2030* report (NASEM, 2021) and its focus on driving toward health equity. A body of research has demonstrated that patient outcomes, including preventive services, patient satisfaction, and ratings of physician's participatory decision-making style, improve in ethnically diverse populations when a healthcare provider cares for a patient who is ethnically and culturally matched (Marrast et al., 2014; Martin et al., 2013).

Where Are PCNPs Practicing Today?

Beyond community health centers, school-based health centers, and Veterans Affairs, where are PCNPs practicing today? At this time, there is no national reporting system based on the NPI (National Provider

BOX 13.4

2020 Facts About Nurse Practitioners

There are more than 325,000 nurse practitioners (NPs) licensed in the United States[a]

- An estimated 30,000 new NPs completed their academic programs in 2018 to 2019[b]
- 99.1% of NPs have graduate degrees[c]
- 88.9% of NPs are certified in an area of primary care[c]
- Nearly three in four NPs are accepting new Medicare patients and 71.7% are accepting new Medicaid patients[c]
- 42.5% of NPs hold hospital privileges; 12.8% have long-term care privileges[c]
- 96.2% of NPs prescribe medications, and those in full-time practice write an average of 21 prescriptions per day[c]
- In 2020, the mean, full-time base salary for an NP was $110,000[c]
- The majority of full-time NPs see three or more patients per hour[c]
- NPs have been in practice an average of 11 years[c]
- The average age of NPs is 49 years[c]

[a]American Association of Nurse Practitioners. (2020). *The state of the nurse practitioner profession 2020.* https://storage.aanp.org/www/documents/no-index/research/2020-NP-Sample-Survey-Report.pdf

[b]American Association of Colleges of Nursing. (2020). *2019-2020 Enrollment and graduations in baccalaureate and graduate programs in nursing.* Washington, DC: AACN.

[c]American Association of Nurse Practitioners. (2021). *NP fact sheet.* https://www.aanp.org/all-about-nps/np-fact-sheet

Identification) number that would provide comprehensive data for all primary care NPs, their community of practice, and characteristics of patients they care for. For now, the best available data are from the AANP periodic survey data on NP practice, geographic distribution and type of practice setting, and compensation. The most recent AANP survey data (2020) acknowledges the potential impact of the COVID-19 pandemic on the healthcare delivery system and health professionals and possible influence on survey participation (Tables 13.2 and 13.3). The simple answer to the question, "Where do PCNPs practice?" remains that they are everywhere. Nearly 30% of respondents cite "family" or "primary care" as their clinical focus. Hospital outpatient clinics, private group practice, and private physician practice, along with private NP practice, rural health clinic, FQHCs and community health centers, and employer/corporate clinics were the top NP work site settings with "family" as the top clinical focus area. Our focus must be on the diversity of our

TABLE 13.2

Distribution: Primary Care Nurse Practitioner Certification

Area of Primary Care Certification	%
Family/life span	69.7
Adult	10.8
Adult/gerontology	7
Pediatrics	3.2
Women's health/gender specific	2.2
Gerontology	1.8

Percentages of PCNPs in each section may reflect those NPs who may be certified in more than one primary care nurse practitioner specialty (i.e., Adult/Gerontology NP may also hold a Pediatrics NP certification as well).

Adapted from *The State of the Nurse Practitioner Profession*, by American Association of Nurse Practitioners, 2020, https://storage.aanp.org/www/documents/no-index/research/2020-NP-Sample-Survey-Report.pdf

TABLE 13.3

Distribution of Primary Care NPs: Top Ambulatory Worksite Settings by Top Clinical Focus Areas

Top NP Practice Settings	%	Top Clinical Focus	%
Hospital outpatient clinic	14.3	Family	12.3
Private group practice	10.4	Family	24.6
Private physician practice	7.8	Family	25.6
Private NP practice	3.8	Family	43.7
Urgent care	4.3	"Urgent care"	91.9
Rural health clinics	3.4	Family	67.8
Federally qualified health centers	3.3	Family	54.6
Community health centers	3.2	Family	48.3
Employer/corporate clinic	2.9	Family	36.7

Adapted from *The State of the Nurse Practitioner Profession*, by American Association of Nurse Practitioners, 2020, https://storage.aanp.org/www/documents/no-index/research/2020-NP-Sample-Survey-Report.pdf.

NP workforce in practice today and the generation that follows, not just on numbers of NPs and where they practice. Poghosyan and Brooks Carthon (2017) pointed to the potential for NPs to reduce health disparities, but an essential element of this must be building a diverse pipeline to the profession.

TRENDS IN PRIMARY CARE

Home Care

Home-based primary care practices are an effective way to meet the needs of frail older adults who find it difficult, if not impossible, to leave home for medical care and may save funds. The PCNP's training and education uniquely prepare them to address whole person aspects of health. After a long legislative battle, President Trump signed the Coronavirus Aid, Relief and Economic Security (CARES) Act (P.L. No. 116-136) in March 2020, which includes a provision in Section 3708 authorizing NPs, CNSs, and PAs as "allowed practitioners" under Medicare and Medicaid. By doing so, this authorized NPs, CNSs, and PAs to certify, recertify, establish, and periodically review the plan of care, as well as perform face-to-face encounters after January 11, 2021 (CMS, 2020).

With improved access to home health services, Medicare and Medicaid beneficiaries will benefit from timely access to PCNPs as they expand their practices in home health (Sapio, 2020). According to Xue et al. (2017), there is a shift toward increasing capacity of the primary care system to serve elderly populations in rural and health professions shortage areas. PCNPs now have the ability through federal authority to improve access for the nation's most vulnerable populations.

Burnout: COVID-19

No discussion of the PCNP would be complete without addressing the issues of burnout and resilience. This was an issue of concern prior to the COVID-19 pandemic; the hundreds of recent articles published on burnout in healthcare professionals reflect that it has been of key concern during the pandemic as well. Perhaps one's lived experience of this pandemic, including one's experience of personal, familial, or community losses and the degree of professional engagement in COVID-related clinical care and practice, will transform us and our practices in ways we cannot yet assess. However, burnout among healthcare providers has been recognized as an issue of concern in health care for years, leading the National Academy of Medicine to launch an initiative to advance research and develop recommendations to improve clinician well-being (NASEM, 2019). Their recommendations call for attention to the practice environment as essential to address burnout. Abraham et al. (2020) conducted a systematic review of predictors and outcomes of burnout among primary care providers inclusive of physicians, NPs, and PAs and identified the primary care practice environment as the most common predictor of PCP burnout, lending support to the importance of improving the primary care practice environment. Goodwin et al. (2021) noted that postgraduate training reduces burnout and turnover among new PCNPs.

A meta-analysis of studies from around the world concluded that a bundled strategy addressing individual, structural, and organizational interventions is required and suggested team-based primary care redesign as one intervention in primary care (Zhang et al., 2020). In 2021 the American Rescue Plan recognized the urgency of increasing reports of burnout among healthcare professionals and charged HRSA with funding initiatives to promote resilience and mental health among the health professions (US Department of Health and Human Services, 2021). The issue and response to health professional burnout and resilience must continue to be a focus of leaders in research, education, and practice not just throughout this pandemic but in the era that will follow.

CONCLUSION

This is an exciting time to be a PCNP for those who seek rigor, challenge, and opportunity to contribute to health and health care. The advent of new payment models (e.g., accountable care organizations), new delivery models (e.g., telehealth/virtual care), new science discoveries (e.g., precision medicine), and new opportunities for education and training (e.g., postgraduate residencies and fellowships) combine with the sheer size and impact of the NP primary care workforce to make primary care NPs essential to any discussion of health and health care in the United States. The question is, what will NPs do with their knowledge, power, and impact? The unconscionable health disparities and equities have not lessened but have worsened during the years in which we have enjoyed rapid growth and acceptance, and the NP workforce falls far short of reflecting the racial and ethnic mix of our country. The promise of access to health care as a basic human right that made forward progress has been challenged, hampered, and stalled in recent years. We have new tools, knowledge, resources, and numbers to exert strong influence on what happens next. The legacy of the first 60 years of PCNPs must be one that is not about us but about the impact we have made on health and health care and building a more just, equal, and healthy society, including taking action to create a more diverse workforce of PCNPs. That is the true path forward for PCNPs.

KEY SUMMARY POINTS

- Historians remind us that all health care was once primary care. The United States developed a fixation on specialty care in the last century, creating an overspecialized tertiary care system with a more fragile primary care system in place.
- PCNPs are fundamental to the nation's safety net for health care; in FQHCs, nurse-led health centers, school-based health centers, and the Veterans Administration; and in caring for the homeless, including veterans.
- PCNPs are well positioned to lead highly innovative practice models such as telecare, to promote aging-in-place innovations and wearable technologies, and to employ big data to move knowledge, not patients.
- As health care evolves in the United States, it is predicted that PCNPs will continue to be a disruptive innovation, delivering care in nontraditional sites and by nontraditional methods.
- PCNPs are uniquely prepared to provide holistic direct care that is patient centered and outcome directed and is based on evidence in the primary care setting.

REFERENCES

Abraham, C. M., Zheng, K., & Poghosyan, L. (2020). Predictors and outcomes of burnout among primary care providers in the United States: A systematic review. *Medical Care Research and Review, 77*(5), 387–401.

American Association of Colleges of Nursing. (2006). *The essentials of doctoral education for advanced nursing practice*. http://www.aacn.nche.edu/publications/position/DNPEssentials.pdf

American Association of Colleges of Nursing. (2021). *The essentials: Core competencies for professional nursing education*. https://www.aacnnursing.org/Portals/42/AcademicNursing/pdf/Essentials-2021.pdf

American Association of Nurse Practitioners. (2020). *The state of the nurse practitioner profession 2020*. https://storage.aanp.org/www/documents/no-index/research/2020-NP-Sample-Survey-Report.pdf

American Association of Nurse Practitioners. (2021). *NP fact sheet*. https://www.aanp.org/all-about-nps/np-fact-sheet

American Rescue Plan Act of 2021, HR1319 §PL117-2. (2021).

American Telemedicine Association. (n.d.). http://www.americantelemed.org/home

APRN Joint Dialogue Group. (2008). *Consensus Model for APRN regulation: Licensure, accreditation, certification & education*. http://www.aacn.nche.edu/education-resources/APRNReport.pdf

Arenson, M., Hudson, P. J., Lee, N., & Lai, B. (2019). The evidence on school-based health centers: A review. *Global Pediatric Health, 6*. *1-10*. https://doi.org/10.1177/2333794X19828745

Arias, E., Tejada-Vera, B., & Ahmad, F. (2021). NVSS statistics rapid release: Provisional life expectancy estimates for January through June, 2020. *Centers for Disease Control and Prevention National Center for Health Statistics National Vital Statistics System*. https://stacks.cdc.gov/view/cdc/100392

Arnetz, B., Goetz, C., Arnetz, J., Sudan, S., vanSchagen, J., Piersma, K., & Reyelts, F. (2020). Enhancing healthcare efficiency to achieve the Quadruple Aim: An exploratory study. *BMC Research Notes, 13*, 362–366.

Ashwood, J. S., Gaynor, M., Setodji, C. M., Reid, R. O., Weber, E., & Mehrotra, A. (2016). Retail clinic visits for low-acuity conditions increase utilization and spending. *Health Affairs, 35*(3), 449–455.

Auerbach, D. I., Chen, P. G., Friedberg, M. W., Reid, R., Lau, C., Buerhaus, P. I., & Mehrotra, A. (2013). Nurse-managed health centers and patient centered medical homes could mitigate expected primary care physician shortage. *Health Affairs, 32*(11), 1933–1941.

Auerbach, D. I., Straiger, D. O., & Buerhaus, P. I. (2018). Growing ranks of advanced practice clinicians-implications for the physician workforce. *The New England Journal of Medicine, 378*(25), 2358–2360.

Austria, J. L. (2015). Urging a practical beginning: Reimbursement reform, nurse-managed health clinics, and complete professional autonomy for primary care nurse practitioners. *DePaul Journal of Health Care Law, 17*, 121–147.

Avendano, M., & Kawachi, I. (2014). Why do Americans have shorter life expectancy and worse health than do people in other high-income countries? *Annual Review of Public Health, 35*, 307–325.

Bachrach, D., Frohlich, J., Garcimonde, A., & Nevitt, K. (2015). *Building a culture of health: The value proposition of retail clinics*: Robert Wood Johnson Foundation. http://www.rwjf.org/content/dam/farm/reports/issue_briefs/2015/rwjf419415

Bakouny, Z., Paciotti, M., Schmidt, A. L., Lipsitz, S. R., Choueiri, T. K., & Trinh, Q. (2021). Cancer screening tests and cancer diagnoses during the COVID-19 pandemic. *JAMA Oncology, 7*(3), 458–460.

Barnett, M. L., Lee, D., & Frank, R. G. (2019). In rural areas, buprenorphine waiver adoption since 2017 driven by nurse practitioners and physician assistants. *Health Affairs, 38*(12), 2048–2056.

Berwick, D. M. (2020). The moral determinants of health. *The Journal of the American Medical Association, 324*(3), 225–226.

Bitton, A., Ratcliffe, H. L., Veillard, J. H., Kress, D. H., Barkley, S., Kimball, M., Secci, F., Wong, E., Basu, L., & Taylor, C. (2017). Primary health care as a foundation for strengthening health systems in low- and middle-income countries. *Journal of General Internal Medicine, 32*(5), 566–571.

Blasi, P. R., Cromp, D., McDonald, S., Hsu, C., Coleman, K., Flinter, M., & Wagner, E. H. (2018). Approaches to behavioral health integration at high performing primary care practices. *The Journal of the American Board of Family Medicine, 31*(5), 691–701.

Bodenheimer, T., & Bauer, L. (2016). Rethinking the primary care workforce: An expanded role for nurses. *New England Journal of Medicine, 375*(11), 1015–1017.

Bodenheimer, T., & Grumbach, K. (2007). *Improving primary care: Strategies and tools for a better practice*. McGraw-Hill.

Bodenheimer, T., & Grumbach, K. (2016). *Understanding health policy: A clinical approach*. Lange/McGraw-Hill.

Bodenheimer, T., & Sinsky, C. (2014). From triple to quadruple aim: Care of the patient requires care of the provider. *Annals of Family Medicine, 12*(6), 573–576.

Buerhaus, P., Perloff, J., Clarke, S., O'Reilly-Jacob, M., Zolotusky, G., & DesRoches, C. M. (2018). Quality of primary care provided to Medicare beneficiaries by nurse practitioners and physicians. *Medical Care, 56*(6), 484–490.

Bush, C. T. (2014). Postgraduate nurse practitioner training: What nurse executives need to know. *The Journal of Nursing Administration, 44*(12), 625–627.

Bush, C. T., & Lowery, B. (2016). Postgraduate nurse practitioner education: Impact on job satisfaction. *The Journal for Nurse Practitioners, 12*(4), 226–234.

California et al. v. Texas et al., 593 U.S. ___ 2021 (2021). https://caselaw.findlaw.com/us-supreme-court/19-840.html

Carter, B. L., Rogers, M., Daly, J., Zheng, S., & James, P. A. (2009). The potency of team-based care interventions for hypertension: A meta-analysis. *Archives of Internal Medicine, 169*(19), 1748–1755.

Carthon, J. M. B., Barnes, H., & Sarik, D. A. (2015). Federal polices influence access to primary care and nurse practitioner workforce. *The Journal for Nurse Practitioners, 11*(5), 526–530.

Case, A., & Deaton, A. (2020). *Deaths of despair and the future of capitalism*. Princeton University Press.

Centers for Disease Control and Prevention. (2021, September 9). *COVID-19 case surveillance public use data*. https://data.cdc.gov/Case-Surveillance/COVID-19-Case-Surveillance-Public-Use-Data/vbim-akqf

Centers for Medicare and Medicaid Services. (2020). CMS manual system: Pub 100-02 Medicare benefit policy. *Transmittal, 10438*. https://www.cms.gov/files/document/r10438bp.pdf

Chase, D., & Kish, L. (2015). 95 theses for a new health ecosystem. *Health Rosetta*. https://medium.com/@healthrosetta/95-theses-for-a-new-health-ecosystem-b32d0cdce2ce

Christensen, C. M., Bohmer, R., & Kenagy, J. (2000). Will disruptive innovations cure health care? *Harvard Business Review, 78*(5), 102–112. 199. https://hbr.org/2000/09/will-disruptive-innovations-cure-health-care

Coleman, K., Austin, B. T., Brach, C., & Wagner, E. H. (2009). Evidence on the chronic care model in the new millennium. *Health Affairs, 28*(1), 75–85. https://doi.org/10.1377/hlthaff.28.1.75

Commission on Social Determinants of Health. (2008). Closing the gap in a generation: Health equity through action on the social determinants of health: Final report of the commission on social determinants of health. *World Health Organization*. https://www.who.int/publications/i/item/WHO-IER-CSDH-08.1

Comprehensive Addiction and Recovery Act of 2016. S.524 §PL 114-198. (2016).

Congressional Research Service. (2005). Nursing Workforce Programs in Title VIII of the Public Health Service Act. *Congressional Research Service*. https://www.everycrsreport.com/files/20050310_RL32805_910d5e128d76f6067cf78119471044661613bba3.pdf

Coronavirus Aid, Relief and Economic Security (CARES) Act. P.L. No. 116-136. (2020). chrome-extension://efaidnbmnnnibpcajpcglclefindmkaj/viewer.html?pdfurl=https%3A%2F%2Fwww.congress.gov%2F116%2Fplaws%2Fpubl136%2FPLAW-116publ136.pdf

Crabtree, B. F., Howard, J., Miller, W. L., Cromp, D., Hsu, C., Coleman, K., Austin, B., Flinter, M., Tuzzio, L., & Wagner, E. H. (2020). Leading innovative practice: Leadership attributes in LEAP practices. *The Milbank Quarterly, 98*(2), 399–445.

Damian, A. J., & Boyd, R. (2020). Advancing the role of school-based health centers in driving health justice. *Journal of School Health, 91*(4), 1–23. https://doi.org/10.1111/josh.12999

DesRoches, C. M., Clarke, S., Perloff, J., O' Reilly-Jacob, M., & Buerhaus, P. (2017). The quality of primary care provided by nurse practitioners to vulnerable Medicare beneficiaries. *Nursing Outlook, 65*(6), 679–688.

Donaldson, S. K., & Crowley, D. M. (1978). The discipline of nursing. *Nursing Outlook, 26*(2), 113–120.

Dunphy, L. M., Winland-Brown, J. E., Porter, B. O., & Thomas, D. J. (2015). *Primary care: The art & science of advanced practice nursing (4th ed.)*. F. A. Davis.

Edes, T., Kinosian, B., Vuckovic, N. H., Nichols, L. O., Becker, M. M., & Hossain, M. (2014). Better access, quality, and cost for clinically complex veterans with home-based primary care. *Journal of the American Geriatrics Society, 62*(10), 1954–1961.

Englander, R., Cameron, T., Ballard, A. J., Dodge, J., Bull, J., & Aschenbrener, C. A. (2013). Toward a common taxonomy of competency domains for the health professions and competencies for physicians. *Academic Medicine: Journal of the Association of American Medical Colleges, 88*, 1088–1094.

Englander, R., Flynn, T., Call, S., Carraccio, C., Cleary, L., Fulton, T. B., Garrity, M. J., Lieberman, S. A., Lindeman, B., Lypson, M. L., Minter, R., Rosenfield, J., Thomas, J., Wilson, M. C., & Aschenbrener, C. A. (2016). Toward defining the foundation of the MD degree: Core entrustable professional activities for entering residency. *Academic Medicine: Journal of the Association of American Medical Colleges, 91*(10), 1352–1358.

Esterwood, E., & Saeed, S. A. (2020). Past epidemics, natural disasters, COVID19, and mental health: Learning from history as we deal with the present and prepare for the future. *Psychiatric Quarterly, 91*(4), 1121–1133.

Flinter, M. (2012). From new nurse practitioner to primary care provider: Bridging the transition through FQHC-based residency training. *The Online Journal of Issues in Nursing, 17*(1), 1–6. https://ojin.nursingworld.org/MainMenuCategories/ANA-Marketplace/ANAPeriodicals/OJIN/TableofContents/Vol-17-2012/No1-Jan-2012/Articles-Previous-Topics/From-New-Nurse-Practitioner-to-Primary-Care-Provider.html

Flinter, M., & Hart, A. M. (2017). Thematic elements of the post-graduate NP residency year and transition to the primary care provider role in a federally qualified health center. *Journal of Nursing Education and Practice, 7*(1), 95–106. http://www.sciedupress.com/journal/index.php/jnep/article/view/9812/6179

Gardenier, D., Moore, D. J., & Patrick, S. R. (2020). Have waivers allowing nurse practitioners to treat opioid use disorder made a difference in the opioid epidemic? *The Journal for Nurse Practitioners, 16*(3), 174–175.

Geiger, H. J. (2002). Community-oriented primary care: A path to community development. *American Journal of Public Health, 92*(11), 1713–1716.

Geiger, H. J. (2005). The first community health centers. *Journal of Ambulatory Care Management, 28*(4), 313–320.

Glazer, G., & Alexandre, C. (2008). Legislative: The nursing shortage: A public health issue for all. *OJIN: The Online Journal of Issues in Nursing, 14*(1), 1–3.

Goodwin, M., Fingerhood, M., Slade, E., & Davidson, P. (2021). Development of an innovative curriculum-to-career transition program for nurse practitioners in primary care. *Nursing Outlook, 69*(3), 425–434.

Hansen-Turton, T., Patric, K. W., & Teske, J. J. (2016). Convenience care and the rise of retail clinics. In R. A. Phillips (Ed.), *America's healthcare transformation: Strategies and innovations* (pp. 197–217). Rutgers University Press.

Harada, N. D., Rajashekara, S., Sansgiry, S., Wirtz Rugen, K., King, S., Gilman, S. C., & Davila, J. A. (2019). Developing interprofessional primary care teams: Alumni evaluation of the department of veterans affairs centers of excellence in primary care education program. *Journal of Medical Education and Curricular Development, 6*, 1–14. https://doi.org/10.1177/2382120519875455

Hart, A. M., & Bowen, A. (2016). New nurse practitioners' perceptions of preparedness for and transition into practice. *The Journal for Nurse Practitioners, 12*(8), 545–552.

Hassmiller, S. B. (2020). Legacies and lessons: A final conversation with Fitzhugh Mullan. *Health Affairs, 39*(2), 334–338. https://doi.org/10.1377/hlthaff.2019.01715

Health Resources and Services Administration. (2012). *The national sample survey of nurse practitioners*. https://bhw.hrsa.gov/data-research/access-data-tools/national-sample-survey-registered-nurse-practitioners

Health Resources and Services Administration. (2018). The US Health Workforce Chartbook: Part I: Clinicians. *US Department of Health and Human Services*. https://bhw.hrsa.gov/sites/default/files/bureau-health-workforce/data-research/hrsa-us-health-workforce-chartbook-part-1-clinicians.pdf

Health Resources and Services Administration. (2020). *Advanced nursing education nurse practitioner residency (ANE-NPR) program award table*. https://bhw.hrsa.gov/funding/advanced-nursing-education-nurse-practitioner-residency-2019-awards

Health Resources and Services Administration. (2021a). *HRSA organization chart*. http://www.hrsa.gov/about/organization/org-chart.html

Health Resources and Services Administration. (2021b). *What is Shortage Designation?* https://bhw.hrsa.gov/workforce-shortage-areas/shortage-designation

Health Resources and Services Administration. (2021c). *Medically underserved areas (MUAs) and medically underserved populations (MUA/Ps)*. https://bhw.hrsa.gov/workforce-shortage-areas/shortage-designation#mups

Health Resources and Services Administration. (2021d). *Health center program uniform data system (UDS) data overview*. https://data.hrsa.gov/tools/data-reporting/program-data

Health Resources and Services Administration. (n.d.). National Health Center Program Uniform Data System (UDS) awardee data. https://data.hrsa.gov/tools/data-reporting/program-data/national#mups

Heisler, E. J. (2018). The National Health Service Corps. *Congressional Research Service*. https://fas.org/sgp/crs/misc/R44970.pdf

Henderson, K., Carlisle, D. T., Smith, M., & King, M. (2014). Nurse practitioners in telehealth: Bridging the gaps in healthcare delivery. *The Journal for Nurse Practitioners, 10*(10), 845–850.

Holt, J., Zabler, B., & Baisch, M. (2014). Evidence-based characteristics of nurse-managed health centers for quality and outcomes. *Nursing Outlook, 62*(6), 428–439.

Howatson-Jones, L. (2016). *Reflective practice in nursing*. Sage.

Howell, J. D. (2010). Reflections on the past and future of primary care. *Health Affairs, 29*(5), 760–765.

Institute of Medicine (IOM). (1996). *Primary care: America's health in a new era*. The National Academies Press.

Institute of Medicine. (2011). *The future of nursing: Leading change, advancing health*. The National Academies Press.

Johnson, L., Jacobs, A., Turley, R., Maphis, S., Coffman, H., George, H. & Wilson, S. (n.d). *Nurse Practitioner Fellowship and Residency Programs*. https://www.graduatenursingedu.org/nurse-practitioner-residency-programs/

Jones, S. M., Parchman, M., McDonald, S., Cromp, D., Austin, B., Flinter, M., Hsu, C., & Wagner, E. (2020). Measuring attributes of team functioning in primary care settings: Development of the TEAMS tool. *Journal of Interprofessional Care, 34*(3), 407–413.

Kaplan, L. (2021). 2020 Supreme Court challenge to the Affordable Care Act and potential implications. *The Nurse Practitioner, 46*(3), 10–11.

Kark, S., & Kark, E. (1999). *Promoting community health: From Pholela to Jerusalem*. University of the Witwatersrand.

Kesten, K. S., & El-Banna, M. M. (2020). Facilitators, barriers, benefits, and funding to implement postgraduate nurse practitioner residency/fellowship programs. *Journal of the American Association of Nurse Practitioners, 33*(8), 611–617. doi:10.1097/JXX.0000000000000412

King, T. (2016). *The medical management of the vulnerable and underserved patient*. McGraw-Hill.

Kleinpell, R., Buchman, T., & Boyle, W. A. (Eds.). (2012). *Integrating nurse practitioners and physician assistants in the ICU: Strategies for optimizing contributions to care*. Society of Critical Care Medicine.

Knopf, A. (2021). HHS exempts bupe prescribers with 30 patients from training. *Alcoholism & Drug Abuse Weekly, 33*(17), 4–5.

Knopf, J. A., Finnie, R. K., Peng, Y., Hahn, R. A., Truman, B. I., Vernon-Smiley, M., Johnson, V. C., Johnson, R. L., Fielding, J. E., & Muntaner, C. (2016). School-based health centers to advance health equity: A community guide systematic review. *American Journal of Preventive Medicine, 51*(1), 114–126.

Kurtzman, E. T., & Barnow, B. S. (2017). A comparison of nurse practitioners, physician assistants, and primary care physicians' patterns of practice and quality of care in health centers. *Medical Care, 55*(6), 615–622.

Lefkowitz, B. (2005). The health center story. *Journal of Ambulatory Care Management, 28*(4), 295–303.

Lenz, E. R., Mundinger, M. O., Kane, R. L., Hopkins, S. C., & Lin, S. X. (2004). Primary care outcomes in patients treated by nurse practitioners or physicians: Two-year follow-up. *Medical Care Research and Review, 61*(3), 332–351.

Lewallen, T. C., Hunt, H., Potts-Datema, W., Zaza, S., & Giles, W. (2015). The whole school, whole community, whole child model: A new approach for improved educational attainment and healthy development for students. *Journal of School Health, 85*(11), 729–739.

Lindeke, L., Canedy, B., & Kay, M. (1997). A comparison of practice domains of clinical nurse specialists and nurse practitioners. *Journal of Professional Nursing, 13*, 281–287.

Liu, C., Hebert, P. L., Douglas, J. H., Neely, E. L., Sulc, C. A., Reddy, A., Sales, A. E., & Wong, E. S. (2020). Outcomes of primary care delivery by nurse practitioners: Utilization, cost, and quality of care. *Health Services Research, 55*(2), 178–189.

Love, H., Panchal, N., Schlitt, J., Behr, C., & Soleimanpour, S. (2019). The use of telehealth in school-based health centers. *Global Pediatric Health, 6*, 1–10. https://doi.org/10.1177/2333794X19884194

Love, H., Schlitt, J., Soleimanpour, S., Panchal, N., & Behr, C. (2019). Twenty years of school-based health care growth and expansion. *Health Affairs, 38*(5), 755–764.

Lutfiyya, M. N., Tomai, L., Frogner, B., Cerra, F., Zismer, D., & Parente, S. (2017). Does primary care diabetes management provided to Medicare patients differ between primary care physicians and nurse practitioners? *Journal of Advanced Nursing, 73*(1), 240–252.

Lützén, K. (1997). Nursing ethics into the next millennium: A context sensitive approach for nursing ethics. *Nursing Ethics, 4*(3), 218–226.

Macinko, J., Starfield, B., & Shi, L. (2003). The contribution of primary care systems to health outcomes within Organization for Economic Cooperation and Development (OECD) countries: 1970-1998. *Health Services Research, 38*, 831–865.

Marrast, L. M., Zallman, L., Woolhandler, S., Bor, D. H., & McCormick, D. (2014). Minority physicians' role in the care of underserved patients: Diversifying the physician workforce may be key in addressing health disparities. *JAMA Internal Medicine, 174*(2), 289–291.

Martin, K. D., Roter, D. L., Beach, M. C., Carson, K. A., & Cooper, L. A. (2013). Physician communication behaviors and trust among black and white patients with hypertension. *Medical Care, 51*(2), 151–157.

McIntyre, A., & Song, Z. (2019). The US Affordable Care Act: Reflections and directions at the close of a decade. *PLoS Med, 16*(2), 1–3. https://doi.org/10.1371/journal.pmed.1002752

Meissen, H. (2019). Nurse practitioner residency and fellowship programs: The controversy still exists. *Journal of the American Association of Nurse Practitioners, 31*(7), 381–383.

Meyer, E. M., Zapatka, S., & Brienza, R. S. (2015). The development of professional identity and the formation of teams in the Veterans Affairs Connecticut healthcare system's center of excellence in primary care education program (CoEPCE). *Academic Medicine: Journal of the Association of American Medical Colleges, 90*(6), 802–809.

Mitchell, P., Wynia, M., Golden, R., McNellis, B., Okun, S., Webb, C. E., Rohrbach, V., & Von Kohorn, I. (2012). *Core principles & values of effective team-based health care*. Institute of Medicine.

Mundinger, M. O., Kane, R. L., Lenz, E. R., Totten, A. M., Tsai, W., Cleary, P. D., Friedewald, W. T., Siu, A. L., & Shelanski, M. L. (2000). Primary care outcomes in patients treated by nurse practitioners or physicians: A randomized trial. *JAMA: The Journal of the American Medical Association, 283*(1), 59–68.

Myrick, K. L., & Ogburn, D. F. (2019, January). Percentage of office-based physicians using any electronic health record (EHR)/electronic medical record (EMR) system and physicians that have a certified EHR/EMR system, by specialty. *National Electronic Health Records Survey* 2017. chrome-extension://efaidnbmnnnibpcajpcglclefindmkaj/viewer.html?pdfurl=https%3A%2F%2Fwww.cdc.gov%2Fnchs%2Fdata%2Fnehrs%2F2017_NEHRS_Web_Table_EHR_Specialty.pdf&clen=366322&chunk=true

National Academies of Sciences, Engineering, and Medicine. (2019). *Taking action against clinician burnout. A systems approach to professional well-being*. The National Academies Press.

National Academies of Sciences, Engineering, and Medicine. (2021). *The future of nursing 2020-2030: Charting a path to achieve health equity*. The National Academies Press.

National Academies of Sciences, Engineering, and Medicine, Committee on Implementing High-Quality Primary Care. (2021). *Implementing high-quality primary care: Rebuilding the foundation of health care*. The National Academies Press.

National Center for Immunization and Respiratory Diseases (NCIRD), Division of Viral Diseases. (2020, December 10). Introduction to COVID-19 racial and ethnic health disparities. *Centers for Disease Control and Prevention*. https://www.cdc.gov/coronavirus/2019-ncov/community/health-equity/racial-ethnic-disparities/index.html

National Center for Veterans Analysis and Statistics. (2018). *VA benefits & health care utilization*. United States Department of Veterans Affairs. https://www.va.gov/vetdata/docs/pocketcards/fy2019q1.pdf

National Nurse Practitioner Residency & Fellowship Training Consortium. (n.d.). *Primary care and psychiatric mental health NP and NP/PA postgraduate residency and fellowship training programs across the country.* https://www.nppostgradtraining.com/wp-content/uploads/2021/06/NNPRFTC_NPProgSheet_0621_R1.pdf

National Organization of Nurse Practitioner Faculties. (2017). *Nurse practitioner core competencies content: A delineation of suggested content specific to the NP core competencies*. http://c.ymcdn.com/sites/www.nonpf.org/resource/resmgr/competencies/2017_NPCoreComps_with_Curric.pdf

National Organization of Nurse Practitioner Faculties. (2018). *The doctor of nursing practice degree: Entry to nurse practitioner practice by 2025.* https://cdn.ymaws.com/www.nonpf.org/resource/resmgr/dnp/v3_05.2018_NONPF_DNP_Stateme.pdf

National Organization of Nurse Practitioner Faculties and American Association of Colleges of Nursing. (2016). *Adult-gerontology acute care and primary care NP competencies.* http://c.ymcdn.com/sites/www.nonpf.org/resource/resmgr/competencies/NP_Adult_Geri_competencies_4.pdf

National Organization of Nurse Practitioner Faculties Population-Focused Competencies Task Force. (2013). *Population-focused nurse practitioner competencies. National Organization of Nurse Practitioner Faculties.* http://c.ymcdn.com/sites/www.nonpf.org/resource/resmgr/Competencies/CompilationPopFocusComps2013.pdf

Naylor, M. D., & Kurtzman, E. T. (2010). The role of nurse practitioners in reinventing primary care. *Health Affairs, 29*(5), 893–899.

NCQA. (n.d.). National committee for quality assurance (NCQA). http://www.ncqa.org/homepage

Newland, P., Wagner, J., Salter, A., Thomas, F., Skubic, M., & Rantz, M. (2016). Exploring the feasibility and acceptability of sensor monitoring of gait and falls in the homes of persons with multiple sclerosis. *Gait and Posture, 49,* 277–282.

Nolte, E., & McKee, C. M. (2012). In amenable mortality—deaths avoidable through health care—progress in the US lags that of three European countries. *Health Affairs, 31*(9), 2114–2122.

Norwick, R. (2016). Family nurse practitioner residency for recruiting and retention. *The Journal for Nurse Practitioners, 12*(5), e231–e233.

Nunez, F. L., Overbeck, M., & Kelly, A. P. (2021). NHSC at 50: New investments for a new workforce. *Journal of Health Care for the Poor and Underserved, 32*(2), xii–xxv.

Olson, D. P., Nunez, F., Overbeck, M., Hotz, J., Billings, A., Frazier, E., Thomsen, K., Kelly, A. P., Diaz, N., & Little, V. (2020). The National Health Service Corps at 50: A legacy of impact in partnership with the association of clinicians for the underserved. *Journal of Health Care for the Poor and Underserved, 31*(2), 542–548.

Pany, M. J., Chen, L., Sheridan, B., & Huckman, R. S. (2021). Provider teams outperform solo providers in managing chronic diseases and could improve the value of care. *Health Affairs, 40*(3), 435–444.

Park, J., Covelli, A. F., & Pittman, P. (2021). Effects of completing a postgraduate residency or fellowship program on primary care nurse practitioners' transition to practice. *Journal of the American Association of Nurse Practitioners, 34*(1), 32–41.

Patient Protection and Affordable Care Act of 2010. 42 U.S.C. §330A-1. (2010).

Peikes, D., Taylor, E. F., O'Malley, A. S., & Rich, E. C (2020). The changing landscape of primary care: Effects of the ACA and other efforts over the past decade. *Health Affairs, 39*(3), 421–428.

Pekmezaris, R., Mitzner, I., Pecinka, K., Nouryan, C., Lesser, M., Siegel, M., Swinderski, J., Moise, G., Yonker Sr., R., & Smolich, K. (2012). The impact of remote patient monitoring (telehealth) upon Medicare beneficiaries with heart failure. *Telemedicine Journal and e-Health, 18*(2), 101–108.

Petersen, S. (2016, January 20). The Virtual Medical Home: New solutions for "connectedness" in healthcare. [Conference Presentation] American Association of Colleges of Nursing Faculty Practice Pre-conference Workshop: Strategies for success in a changing health care system, Naples, FL, United States.

Petterson, S., Westfall, J. M., & Miller, B. F. (2020). Projected deaths of despair during the coronavirus recession. *Well Being Trust.* https://wellbeingtrust.org/wp-content/uploads/2020/05/WBT_Deaths-of-Despair_COVID-19-FINAL-FINAL.pdf

Phillips, R. S., Sullivan, E. E., & Mayo-Smith, M. F. (2020). The patient-centered medical home and the challenge of evaluating complex interventions. *JAMA Network Open, 3*(2), Article e1920827.

Phillips, S. (2021). 33rd annual APRN legislative update: Unprecedented changes to APRN practice authority in unprecedented times. *The Nurse Practitioner, 36*(1), 27–55. https://journals.lww.com/tnpj/Fulltext/2021/01000/33rd_Annual_APRN_Legislative_Update__Unprecedented.6.aspx

Poghosyn, L., & Brooks Carthon, J. (2017). The untapped potential of the nurse practitioner workforce in reducing health disparities. *Policy, Politics, & Nursing Practice, 18*(2), 84–94.

Poghosyan, L., Ghaffari, A., Liu, J., & McHugh, M. (2020). Organizational support for nurse practitioners in primary care and workforce outcomes. *Nursing Research, 69*(4), 280–288.

Pohl, J. M., Tanner, C., Pilon, B., & Benkert, R. (2011). Comparison of nurse managed health centers with federally qualified health centers as safety net providers. *Policy, Politics, & Nursing Practice, 12*(2), 90–99.

Quigley, D. D., Qureshi, N., Al-Masarweh, L., & Hays, R. D. (2020). Practice leaders report targeting several types of changes in care experienced by patients during patient-centered medical home transformation. *Journal of Patient Experience, 7*(6), 1509–1518.

Randall, S., Crawford, T., Currie, J., River, J., & Betihavas, V. (2017). Impact of community based nurse-led clinics on patient outcomes, patient satisfaction, patient access and cost effectiveness: A systematic review. *International Journal of Nursing Studies, 73,* 24–33.

Rantz, M., Lane, K., Phillips, L., Despins, L., Galambos, C., Alexander, G., Kooperman, R., Hicks, L., Skubic, M., & Miller, S. (2015). Enhanced registered nurse care coordination with sensor technology: Impact on length of stay and cost of aging in place technology. *Nursing Outlook, 63*(6), 650–655.

Redhead, C. S., & Heisler, E. J. (2013). Public health, workforce, quality, and related provisions in ACA: Summary and timeline. *Congressional Research Service.* https://fas.org/sgp/crs/misc/R41278.pdf

Rugen, K. W., Watts, S. A., Janson, S. L., Angelo, L. A., Nash, M., Zapatka, S. A., Brienza, B., Gilman, S. C., Bowen, J. L., & Saxe, J. M. (2014). Veteran Affairs centers of excellence in primary care education: Transforming nurse practitioner education. *Nursing Outlook, 62,* 78–88.

Rugs, D., Toyinbo, P., Barrett, B., Melillo, C., Chavez, M., Cowan, L., Jensen, P. K., Engstrom, C., Battaglia, C., & Thorne-Odem, S. (2021). A preliminary evaluation of full practice authority of advance practice registered nurses in the Veterans Health Administration. *Nursing Outlook, 69*(2), 147–158.

Ruhm, C. J. (2018). Deaths of despair or drug problems? *National Bureau of Economic Research.* https://www.nber.org/papers/w24188

Saad, L. (2020). US ethics ratings rise for medical workers and teachers. *Gallup.* https://news.gallup.com/poll/328136/ethics-ratings-rise-medical-workers-teachers.aspx

Sapio, M. (2020, June). AANP forum: CARES Act bolsters access to home health services. *Journal for Nurse Practitioners, 16*(6), A11.

Shah, T., Kitts, A. B., Gold, J. A., Horvath, K., Ommaya, A., Opelka, F., Sato, L., Schwarze, G., Upton, M., & Sandy, L. (2020 August). Electronic health record optimization and clinician well-being: A potential roadmap toward action. *National Academy of Medicine*. https://nam.edu/electronic-health-record-optimization-and-clinician-well-being-a-potential-roadmap-toward-action/

Shaukat, A., & Church, T. (2020). Colorectal cancer screening in the USA in the wake of COVID-19. *The Lancet Gastroenterology & Hepatology, 5*(8), 726–727.

Silver, H. K., Ford, L. C., & Steady, S. G. (1967). A program to increase health care for children: The pediatric nurse practitioner program. *Pediatrics, 39*(5), 756–760.

Singh, G. K., Daus, G. P., Allender, M., Ramey, C. T., Martin, E. K., Perry, C., De Los, Reyes, Andrew, A, & Vedamuthu, I. P. (2017). Social determinants of health in the United States: Addressing major health inequality trends for the nation, 1935-2016. *International Journal of MCH and AIDS, 6*(2), 139–164.

Social Security Act. Title 42 U.S.C. § 254b Health Centers. (2020a). https://www.govregs.com/uscode/42/254b

Social Security Act. Title 42 U.S.C. 1396d § 1905. (2020b). https://www.ssa.gov/OP_Home/ssact/title19/1905.htm

Starfield, B. (1992). *Primary care: Concept, evaluation, and policy*. Oxford Press.

Starfield, B. (2008). Refocusing the system. *New England Journal of Medicine, 359*(20), 2087–2091.

Starr, P. (1982). *The social transformation of American medicine: The rise of a sovereign profession and the making of a vast industry*. Basic Books.

Stevens, R. (1989). *In sickness and in wealth: American hospitals in the twentieth century*. Basic Books.

The Sullivan Commission. (2004). Missing persons: Minorities in the health professions. A report of the Sullivan Commission on Diversity in the Healthcare Workforce. *Sullivan Commission on Diversity in the Healthcare Workforce*. https://www.aacnnursing.org/Portals/42/News/Sullivan-Report.pdf

Sutter-Barrett, R. E., Sutter-Dalrymple, C. J., & Dickman, K. (2015). Bridge care nurse-managed clinics fill the gap in health care. *The Journal for Nurse Practitioners, 11*(2), 262–265.

Udlis, K., & Jakubis-Konicki, A. (2016, November 17-19). NP competencies and progress indicators. Progress indicator report. [Conference Presentation]. In Thomas, A. (Chair), Readiness for practice: Defining progress indicators. Symposium conducted at the meeting of the National Organization of Nurse Practitioner Faculty, Crystal City, VA, United States.

United States Department of Health and Human Services. (2021, July 16). *HHS announces $103 million from American Rescue Plan to strengthen resiliency and address burnout in the health workforce*. https://www.hhs.gov/about/news/2021/07/16/hhs-announces-103-million-arp-funding-to-address-health-workforce-burnout.html

United States Department of Veterans Affairs. (2016). Advanced practice registered nurses: Final rule with comment period. *Federal Register, 81*(240), 90198–90207. https://pubmed.ncbi.nlm.nih.gov/28001018/

Valentine, P., Wynn, J., & McLean, D. (2016). Improving diversity in the health professions. *North Carolina Medical Journal, 77*(2), 137–140.

Volkow, N. D. (2020). Collision of the COVID-19 and addiction epidemics. *Annals of Internal Medicine, 173*(1), 61–62. https://doi.org/10.7326/M20-1212

Wagner, E. H. (2000). The role of patient care teams in chronic disease management. *British Medical Journal, 320*(7234), 569–572.

Wagner, E. H., Flinter, M., Hsu, C., Cromp, D., Austin, B., Etz, R., Crabtree, B., & Ladden, M. (2017). Effective team-based primary care: Observations from innovative practices. *BMC Family Practice, 18*(1), 13–21.

Willard-Grace, R., Hessler, D., Rogers, E., Dube, K., Bodenheimer, T., & Grumbach, K. (2014). Team structure and culture are associated with lower burnout in primary care. *Journal of the American Board of Family Medicine, 27*(2), 229–238.

Wong, H., Naghavi, M., Allen, C., Barber, R. M., Bhutta, Z. A., Carter, A., Casey, D. C., Charlson, F. J., Chen, A. Z., Coates, M. M., Coggeshall, M., Dandona, L, Dicker, D. J., Erskine, E., Ferarri, A. J., Fitzmaurice, C., Foreman, K., Forouzanfar, M. H., Fraser, M. S., …, Murray C.J.L. Global Burden of Disease (GBD) 2015 Mortality and Causes of Death Collaborators. (2016). Global, regional, and national life expectancy, all-cause and cause-specific mortality for 249 causes of death, 1980–2015: A systematic analysis for the Global Burden of Disease Study 2015. *Lancet, 388*, 1459–1544. https://doi.org/10.1016/S0140-6736(16)31012-1

World Health Organization & United Nations Children's Fund (UNICEF). (2018). *A vision for primary health care in the 21st century: Towards universal health coverage and the sustainable development goals*. WHO Press.

Xue, Y., Goodwin, J., Adhikari, D., Raji, M., & Kuo, Y-F. (2017). Trends in primary care provision to Medicare beneficiaries by physicians, nurse practitioners and physician assistants: 2008-2014. *Journal of Primary Care & Community Health, 8*(4), 256–263.

Yano, E. M., Bair, M. J., Carrasquillo, O., Krein, S. L., & Rubenstein, L. V. (2014). Patient Aligned Care Teams: VA's journey to implement patient-centered medical homes. *Journal of General Internal Medicine, 29*(Suppl. 2), S547–S549.

Zapatka, S. A., Conelius, J., Edwards, J., Meyer, E., & Brienza, R. (2014). Pioneering a primary care adult nurse practitioner interprofessional fellowship. *The Journal for Nurse Practitioners, 10*(6), 378–386.

Zhang, X., Song, Y., Jiang, T., Ding, N., & Shi, T. (2020). Interventions to reduce burnout of physicians and nurses: An overview of systematic reviews and meta-analyses. *Medicine, 99*(26), 1–13.

14

THE ACUTE CARE NURSE PRACTITIONER

S. BRIAN WIDMAR ■ KIM STEANSON

"Things do not change, we change."
~ Henry David Thoreau

CHAPTER CONTENTS

EMERGENCE OF THE ACNP ROLE 458

COMPETENCIES OF THE ACNP ROLE 459
- Direct Clinical Practice 461
- Diagnosing and Managing Disease 461
- Promoting and Protecting Health and Preventing Disease 465
- Guidance and Coaching 466
- Evidence-Based Practice 467
- Leadership 467
- Collaboration 468
- Ethical Practice 468

PREPARATION OF ACNPS 469

ACNP SCOPE OF PRACTICE: LEVELS OF INFLUENCE 471
- National Level (Professional Organizations) 472
- State Level (Government) 473
- Institutional Level 473
- Service-Related Level 474
- Individual Level 475

PROFILES OF THE ACNP ROLE AND PRACTICE MODELS 475
- Comparison With Other Advanced Practice Nurse and Physician Assistant Roles 478
- ACNPs and Physician Hospitalists 479
- ACNP Practice Models 479
- Outcome Studies Related to ACNP Practice 479

SPECIALIZATION OPPORTUNITIES WITHIN THE ACNP ROLE 481
- Bone Marrow Transplantation Services 481
- Diagnostic and Interventional Services 481
- Heart Failure Services 482
- Orthopedic Services 482
- Critical Care Teams 482
- Rapid Response Teams 482
- Supportive and Palliative Care 482

CHALLENGES SPECIFIC TO THE ACNP ROLE 483

FUTURE DIRECTIONS 484

CONCLUSION 485

KEY SUMMARY POINTS 485

The acute care nurse practitioner (ACNP) diagnoses and manages disease and promotes the health of individuals with acute, critical, and/or complex chronic health illnesses or injuries who may be physiologically unstable, technologically dependent, and/or highly vulnerable for complications. The ACNP provides care to acutely, critically, and chronically ill patients in any setting where these patients may present (American Association of Colleges of Nursing [AACN], 2012; American Association of Critical-Care Nurses, 2021; National Association of Pediatric Nurse Practitioners, 2011). The ACNP provides comprehensive care in a

The authors would like to acknowledge and thank Marilyn Hravnak, Jane Guttendorf, Ruth M. Kleinpell, and Kathy S. Magdic for their work on previous versions of this chapter.

collaborative model with physicians, staff nurses, and other healthcare providers as well as with patients and their families. The ACNP not only shares common functions and skills with the other nurse practitioner (NP) subspecialties but also applies unique knowledge and skills in caring for very complex and vulnerable patient populations (AACN, 2012; American Association of Critical-Care Nurses, 2021). The *Consensus Model for APRN Regulation* (APRN Joint Dialogue Group, 2008) states that the role of the certified NP includes diagnosing, treating, and managing patients with acute and chronic illnesses and diseases, including the following: ordering, performing, supervising, and interpreting laboratory, diagnostic, and imaging studies; prescribing medication and durable medical equipment; and making appropriate referrals for patients and families. Furthermore, these role attributes are used with a specific patient population for which the practitioner is specifically educated and licensed (APRN Joint Dialogue Group, 2008). For NPs caring for patients within the pediatric or adult–gerontology population focus, the scope of practice is further delineated according to a primary or acute care focus within a population focus (AACN, 2012; National Council of State Boards of Nursing [NCSBN], 2008). Thus NPs can be educated and certified as pediatric acute or primary care and as adult–gerontology acute or primary care. Adult–gerontology acute care incorporates the entire spectrum of adults, including young, middle-aged, and older adults, while pediatric acute care includes care of infants, children, adolescents, and young adults (AACN, 2012; National Association of Pediatric Nurse Practitioners, 2011). Most ACNPs practice in acute and critical care settings that include subacute care (e.g., rehabilitation facilities, long-term care facilities, etc.), emergency care, inpatient units, and intensive care settings. Within these settings, ACNPs may provide care for patients within a wide range of specialties, including but not limited to specialties such as acute and critical care neurology, pulmonology, trauma, transplantation, presurgical and perioperative care, pain management services, rapid response teams, and cardiac surgery (Barocas et al., 2014; Hoyt & Proehl, 2015; Kapu, Wheeler, & Lee, 2014; Kleinpell & Goolsby, 2012; Kleinpell, Avitall et al., 2015). Acute care nurse practitioners also practice in specialty-based practice settings such as specialty clinics, medical rehabilitation, home care, long-term care, medical flight program settings, and telehealth (Alexander-Banys, 2014; Kleinpell & Goolsby, 2012; Rutledge et al., 2014).

In recent years, adult acute care competencies were revised to reflect the evolved focus of acute care of the adult and older adult (i.e., adult–gerontology, AG-ACNP; AACN, 2012). Prior to this revision and titling change, however, adult acute care nurse practitioners who were certified prior to this revision were commonly referred to as ACNPs. These nurse practitioners may retain their title as long as they keep their prior certification active. For ease of discussion, in this chapter, the term *adult–gerontology acute care nurse practitioner* and the abbreviation AG-ACNP will refer to all nurse practitioners certified in adult acute care, and the term *pediatric acute care nurse practitioner* will be abbreviated as AC-PNP. For elements that apply to both roles, the abbreviation ACNP will be used.

Although all ACNPs share specialty role attributes, there may be intrarole variability based on the nature of the care delivery system, characteristics of a particular employment position or location in which they practice (e.g., private practice versus hospital employee, intensive care unit versus hospital unit or ambulatory care facility), and physiologic specialty (e.g., cardiac, pulmonary, orthopedic, oncology). This chapter presents an overview of the ACNP role, including core and role-specific competencies, scope of practice, issues in practice, and future challenges.

EMERGENCE OF THE ACNP ROLE

The role of the ACNP evolved as a result of a number of changes in the delivery of health care, including the need for an advanced practitioner to manage hospitalized patients whose clinical presentations were more complex, changes in the regulations of work hour restrictions for medical residents and fellows, and shortages of intensivist physicians. As early as the 1970s, primary care NPs (family NPs and adult NPs) were recruited to care for adult patients in hospital-based settings, with on-the-job training to provide secondary and tertiary care skills. By the late 1980s, NPs were increasingly used in tertiary care centers, and it became apparent that a new adult NP specialty was emerging. Education was specifically designed to meet the needs of vulnerable adult patients with acute, critical, and complex chronic illness to ensure consistency in the knowledge, training, and quality of care provided by NP graduates in this new specialty. Master's-level graduate AG-ACNP programs began to emerge in the late 1980s, and in 1995, the first national certification examination for AG-ACNPs was administered (AACN, 2012). As of 2020 there were over 28,000 certified (9858 adult ACNPs and 18,259 AG-ACNPs) by the American Nurses Credentialing Center (2020b) and the American Association of Critical-Care Nurses (2020).

Because of these same historical forces, a need for pediatric NPs (CPNP-AC) who are specifically educated to meet the needs of acutely ill children with complex care needs across a variety of settings also emerged (Reuter-Rice et al., 2016). In 2004 the National Association of Pediatric Nurse Associates and Practitioners (NAPNAP) expanded their PNP scope of practice to reflect the acute care role (NAPNAP, 2011). An acute care PNP (CPNP-AC) examination from the Pediatric Nursing Certification Board became available in 2005 and, as of 2020, approximately 3680 pediatric nurse practitioners were certified to practice in acute care (AACN, 2012; Bolick et al., 2012; NAPNAP, 2011; Pediatric Nursing Certification Board [PNCB], 2020a; Reuter-Rice & Bolick, 2012).

Growth within both acute care nurse practitioner roles increases as unique services offered by the ACNP are identified and as constraints in graduate medical resident work hour restrictions drive a growing need for inpatient coverage. In addition, increasing opportunities for third-party billing for inpatient services enhances revenue by use of ACNPs in clinical settings (Garland & Gershengorn, 2013; Kleinpell, Ward et al., 2015; Munro, 2013; Pastores et al., 2011; Ward et al., 2013).

COMPETENCIES OF THE ACNP ROLE

The central and core competencies for the APRN form the foundations of ACNP practice. The central competency for all APRNs is direct clinical practice in concert with the other five core competencies of guidance and coaching, evidence-based practice, leadership, collaboration, and ethical practice. The ways in which ACNPs enact these core competencies are consistent with other APRN specialties. In addition, AG-ACNPs share common entry-level competencies in accordance with the NP core competencies (National Organization of Nurse Practitioner Faculties [NONPF], 2017). Although the ACNP may need to use specialty skills and knowledge in the care of acutely, critically, and complex chronically ill patients, both adult and pediatric ACNPs have the following factors in common with the other NP specialties: (1) a generalist nursing foundation, (2) a health promotion basis to their practice, and (3) the development of diagnostic reasoning skills. ACNPs prepared at the doctor of nursing practice (DNP) level have knowledge and preparation in communication skills, in-depth scientific foundations, analytic skills for evaluating and providing evidence-based practice, advanced knowledge of healthcare delivery systems and population-based care, knowledge of the business aspects of practice, and an emphasis on independent and interprofessional practice (AACN, 2021). The practice focused doctorate prepares graduates for clinical scholarship, including generation of transferrable evidence through innovation of practice changes, the translation of evidence, and the implementation of quality improvement processes to improve health or health care (AACN, 2015).

The *Nurse Practitioner Core Competencies* (NONPF, 2017) outline competencies that are relevant to the practice of all nurse practitioners. In addition, each of the NP specialties has unique competencies that differentiate practice by population focus. AG-ACNP entry-level competencies are illustrated in the *Adult–Gerontology Acute Care Nurse Practitioner Competencies* for entry into practice (NONPF, 2016a) and the *Scope and Standards for Acute Care Nurse Practitioner Practice* for expert practice (see Box 14.1; American Association of Critical-Care Nurses, 2021). Pediatric acute care nurse practitioner competencies are further illustrated in the *Population-Focused Nurse Practitioner Competencies* for pediatric acute care and include the spectrum of care for infants, children, adolescents, and young adults (NONPF, 2013).

The ACNP provides care to patients who are or may be at risk for physiologic instability. These patients may be encountered across the continuum of care settings because the role is not setting specific but is dependent on patient care needs. As a result, the practice of the ACNP can span from outpatient to inpatient settings including hospitals, urgent care, subacute care, and rehabilitation. As scope of practice is largely determined by acuity and patient care needs, due to unique healthcare needs, a patient who is otherwise outside of the traditional definition of "pediatric" age may still be best served by an AC-PNP rather than an AG-ACNP

BOX 14.1

Standards of Clinical Practice and Professional Performance for the Expert Acute Care Nurse Practitioner

STANDARDS OF CLINICAL PRACTICE

Standard 1: Advanced Assessment

The ACNP elicits relevant data and information about patients with acute, critical, and/or complex chronic illnesses or injury.

Standard 2: Differential Diagnosis

The ACNP analyzes and synthesizes the assessment data when determining differential diagnoses for patients with acute, critical, and/or complex chronic illnesses or injury.

Standard 3: Outcomes Identification

The ACNP identifies individualized goals and outcomes for patients with acute, critical, and/or complex chronic illnesses or injury.

Standard 4: Care Planning and Management

The ACNP develops an outcomes-focused plan of care for patients with acute, critical, and/or complex chronic illnesses or injury.

Standard 5: Implementation

The ACNP implements the plan of care for patients with acute, critical, and/or complex chronic illness or injury based on best evidence available.

Standard 6: Evaluation

The ACNP evaluates the patient's progress toward the achievement of goals and outcomes.

STANDARDS OF PROFESSIONAL PERFORMANCE

Standard 1: Professional Practice

The ACNP evaluates their clinical practice in relation to institutional guidelines, professional practice standards, and relevant statutes and regulations.

Standard 2: Education

The ACNP maintains current knowledge according to best available evidence.

Standard 3: Collaboration

The ACNP collaborates with the patient, family, and members of the interprofessional team across the continuum of care.

Standard 4: Ethics

The ACNP integrates ethical considerations into all areas of practice congruent with the ANA Code of Ethics (2015) and patient and family needs.

Standard 5: Advocacy

The ACNP functions as an advocate for patients, families, and the healthcare team.

Standard 6: Systems/Organizational Thinking

The ACNP engages in organizational systems and processes to promote optimal outcomes.

Standard 7: Resource Utilization

The ACNP incorporates best available evidence regarding diagnostic strategies, therapies, and complementary health alternatives to achieve optimal outcomes.

Standard 8: Leadership

The ACNP leads in the profession and the practice setting.

Standard 9: Collegiality

The ACNP promotes respect for colleagues and the interprofessional team.

Standard 10: Quality and Evidence-Based Practice

The ACNP ensures the quality, safety, and effectiveness of care across the continuum of acute care.

Standard 11: Clinical/Practice Inquiry

The ACNP enhances knowledge, attitudes, and skills through participation in research, translation of scientific evidence, and promotion of evidence-based practice.

ACNP, acute care nurse practitioner; ANA, American Nurses Association

Adapted from AACN Scope and Standards for Acute Care Nurse Practitioner Practice, by American Association of Critical-Care Nurses, 2021, p. 12–21.

(PNCB, 2020b). A discussion of how entry-level ACNP competencies are carried out within the framework of the APRN core competencies follows.

Direct Clinical Practice

Direct clinical practice, the central competency of ACNP practice, is the function that consumes the greatest percentage of ACNP practice time. Goals of ACNP care include patient stabilization for acute and life-threatening conditions, minimizing and preventing complications, attending to comorbidities, and promoting physical and psychological well-being. Additional goals include the restoration of maximum age-specific physiologic and psychological health potential or providing for palliative, supportive, and end-of-life care, as well as an evaluation of risk factors in achieving these outcomes (American Association of Critical-Care Nurses, 2021; NONPF, 2013, 2016a). ACNPs achieve these goals through performing cognitive skills such as advanced patient assessment, clinical and diagnostic reasoning, critical thinking, case management, and prescription of therapeutic interventions. Assessing, prioritizing, and intervening in complex, urgent, or emergency situations are key components of ACNP specialty competencies. Expert communication, collaboration, and facilitation of appropriate transitions of care across the patient's care trajectory are core components of the independent practice competency (NONPF, 2013, 2016a).

The central competencies of direct clinical practice as they apply to ACNP specialty practice can be broadly characterized as those related to diagnosing and managing disease and those related to the promotion and protection of health (AACN, 2012; American Association of Critical-Care Nurses, 2021).

Diagnosing and Managing Disease

The varied practice settings of individual ACNPs across the continuum of healthcare delivery services result in associated variance in some of the competencies that they perform (Kapu et al., 2012). Although individual elements of the ACNP role differ depending on these varied practice settings and on the specialty patient populations served, the basic elements necessary to function as a generalist ACNP remain. The top 22 work activities in an ACNP role delineation study performed by the American Nurses Credentialing Center (ANCC, 2020a), arranged by criticality, are listed in Box 14.2. The top 25 diagnoses most frequently managed by acute care nurse practitioners are listed in Table 14.1.

The performance of patient procedures, some of which are invasive, also constitutes a portion of the ACNP's direct clinical practice. Technical procedures commonly performed by ACNPs are listed in Table 14.2. The literature, including ACNP role delineation studies, corroborates ACNP technical skill performance: endotracheal intubation, central line placement, pulmonary artery line placement, needle thoracotomy, chest tube insertion and removal, and cricothyrotomy for the trauma critical care focus; nerve block, joint needle aspiration, diagnostic peritoneal lavage, needle decompression of the chest, lumbar puncture, chest tube insertion, cricothyrotomy and tracheostomy, suturing of lacerations and wounds, and splinting of injuries for the emergency care focus; and endotracheal and nasotracheal intubation (including rapid sequence), chest tube insertion and removal, insertion of central venous and arterial lines, and bronchoscopy for the critical care focus (ANCC, 2020; Dalley et al., 2012; Kleinpell & Goolsby, 2012; Kleinpell et al., 2006; NONPF, 2011). The ACNP procedural role has expanded to include nonvascular radiology procedures such as paracentesis, thoracentesis, and biopsy procedures (Duszak et al., 2015). Practice analysis data specific to the AC-PNP show that the most commonly performed procedures include advanced airway management, vascular access, catheter insertion and removal (arterial and venous), chest tube insertion and removal, defibrillation, lumbar puncture, and suturing (Bolick et al., 2012).

A NONPF publication, *Integrating Adult Acute Care Skills and Procedures Into Nurse Practitioner Curricula* (NONPF, 2011), outlines a number of psychomotor skills and procedures most commonly taught in AG-ACNP education programs, including the following: monitoring intracranial pressure, 12-lead electrocardiogram interpretation, defibrillation and cardioversion, pacemaker interrogation, hemodynamic monitoring, central venous line insertion, arterial puncture or cannulation, interpretation of a chest radiograph, performing thoracentesis for pleural effusions, chest tube insertion and removal, airway management for the non–anesthesia provider

BOX 14.2

Adult–Gerontology Acute Care Nurse Practitioner List of Top Work Activities Arranged by Criticality

1. Maintains patient privacy and confidentiality (including, but not limited to, Health Information Portability and Accountability Act [HIPAA] compliance)
2. Assesses the patient for urgent and emergent conditions
3. Assesses for rapid changes in physiologic and psychological status
4. Differentiates between normal and abnormal findings
5. Prescribes and/or manages nonpharmacologic and pharmacologic treatment (via invasive and noninvasive routes)
6. Formulates differential diagnoses based on synthesized clinical findings
7. Modifies plan of care according to patient's response to treatment
8. Evaluates the safety and efficacy of pharmacologic, behavioral, and other therapeutic interventions
9. Manages rapid pathophysiological changes
10. Prescribes and/or manages intravenous (IV)/intraosseous (IO) medications (including, but not limited to, cardiac medications, pain medications, insulin drips, thrombolytics, chemotherapy, intravenous dyes, radiocontrast agents)
11. Delivers care based on current evidence-based guidelines
12. Conducts a comprehensive or problem-focused history and physical examination
13. Conducts a pharmacologic assessment addressing pharmacogenetic risks, complex medical regimens, drug interactions, and other adverse events; over-the-counter; complementary or alternative medications
14. Orders interventions to minimize risk and promote safety (including, but not limited to, devices to promote mobility and prevent falls, cognitive and sensory enhancements, restraint-free care, monitoring devices, venous thromboembolism, and stress ulcer prophylaxis)
15. Prioritizes differential diagnoses
16. Obtains personal protected health information from collateral sources (including, but not limited to, electronic health records, databases, and other healthcare providers and family members)
17. Establishes therapeutic relationships in acute, urgent, or emergent care situations
18. Interprets diagnostic tests to formulate diagnoses
19. Advocates for the patient's right to self-determination, sense of safety, autonomy, worth, and dignity
20. Prescribes and/or manages blood-based products
21. Determines need for specialty consultation
22. Manages life-threatening conditions

In all, 22 work activities were rated by respondents (N = 343) as highly critical.

From Adult–Gerontology Acute Care Nurse Practitioner Role Delineation Study Executive Summary, by American Nurses Credentialing Center, 2020, https://www.nursingworld.org/~49f2f5/globalassets/certification/certification-specialty-pages/resources/role-delineation-studies/exam-62-agacnp-rds-executive-summary_final_04092020.pdf

in procedural sedation, spirometry and peak flow assessment, paracentesis, local anesthesia application, and cutaneous abscess drainage. The increasing acceptance of invasive procedural skills is within the ACNP scope of practice and is supported by evidence that complication rates are no greater than those of physician providers (Sirleaf et al., 2014) as well as increasing employment of ACNPs in critical care (Kleinpell & Goolsby, 2012) and improved third-party payment for APRN-performed procedures (Squiers et al., 2013).

It must be understood that procedural skill performance is not limited to the task itself but also includes knowledge of the indications, contraindications, complications, and skill in managing complications. When performing a procedural skill to derive

TABLE 14.1
Top 25 Diagnoses Most Frequently Managed by Acute Care Nurse Practitioners

Diagnosis	Percentage Reported
Hypertension	75.9
Heart failure	66.1
Acute upper respiratory illness	60.8
GERD/heartburn	59.8
Abdominal pain	59.6
Arrhythmias	58.4
Anemia	58.3
UTI	57.7
CAD/IHD/angina	57.6
Acute lower respiratory illness	57.3
Hyperlipidemia	56.0
Diabetes	56.0
COPD	51.6
Asthma	50.9
Anxiety	50.1
Back pain or neck pain	45.7
Dizziness/vertigo	44.0
Headache/migraine	41.4
Depression	41.4
Thyroid disease	41.0
Allergic respiratory illness	37.5
Sinusitis	37.1
Obesity	35.5
Dementia	31.7
Insomnia	30.7

CAD, coronary artery disease; *COPD*, chronic obstructive pulmonary disease; *GERD*, gastroesophageal reflux disease; *IHD*, ischemic heart disease; *UTI*, urinary tract infection.

Adapted from "American Association of Nurse Practitioners National Sample Survey: Update on Acute Care Nurse Practitioner Practice," by R. Kleinpell, M. L. Cook, and D. L. Padden, 2018, *Journal of the American Association of Nurse Practitioners, 30*, 140–149.

TABLE 14.2
Procedures Performed as Reported by 962 Acute Care Nurse Practitioners (ACNPs)

Procedures Performed in Hospital	Frequency (%) of Performance of Procedures by ACNPs (No. of Procedures)
High Reported Frequency	
Radiologic studies	79.3 (619)
Vasoactive intravenous drips	67.1 (516)
Resuscitative efforts	67 (516)
Defibrillation	63.4 (512)
Wound care	49.9 (480)
Suture	40.7 (392)
Incisions	40.7 (392)
Ventilation	39.8 (295)
Medium Reported Frequency	
Cardioversion	38.2 (283)
Pacemakers	31.3 (230)
Arterial catheters	25.2 (182)
Central venous catheters	25 (182)
Pulmonary artery catheters	21.7 (157)
Intracardiac catheters	20.3 (165)
Cardiac assistive devices	18.8 (135)
Endotracheal	17.7 (128)
Chest tubes	15.9 (113)
Lower Reported Frequency[a]	
Lumbar puncture	14.4 (103)
Surgical first assist	9.5 (91)
Thoracostomy tubes	7.8 (75)
Cutdowns	5.4 (21)
Bladder aspiration	2.8 (16)

[a]In addition, other procedures that were performed with lower frequencies included bone marrow biopsies (n = 6), removing intraaortic balloon pumps (n = 4), paracentesis (n = 4), joint aspirations (n = 3), and splinting fractures (n = 3).

Adapted from "American Academy of Nurse Practitioners National Nurse Practitioner Sample Survey: Focus on Acute Care," by R. Kleinpell and M. J. Goolsby, 2012, *Journal of the American Academy of Nurse Practitioners, 24*, 694.

physiologic data, such as mean arterial pressure, pulmonary artery pressure, or lumbar cerebrospinal fluid pressure, the ACNP must use this information skillfully for patient diagnosis and management. ACNPs are also compelled to collect their individual practice data related to procedure performance, including number and type of complications, and use these data to document ongoing skill competence to ensure positive patient outcomes and patient safety. The practice of a pediatric ACNP in a cardiothoracic surgical intensive care unit (ICU), which illustrates the integration of technical skills within the context of diagnosis and management of disease, is provided in Exemplar 14.1.

EXEMPLAR 14.1
PEDIATRIC ACUTE CARE NURSE PRACTITIONER (AC-PNP) PRACTICE IN AN INTENSIVE CARE UNIT

The pediatric acute care nurse practitioner (AC-PNP) role in the pediatric cardiac intensive care unit (PCICU) is essential. Emily is part of the care team in the PCICU consisting of attending physicians, a pediatric critical care fellow, and a clinical pharmacist. Emily, an AC-PNP, manages infants and children returning from cardiac surgery through their intensive care stay and transfers the patient to the cardiology floor and to the cardiology service once the patient has met appropriate benchmarks. A cardiology attending also follows the patient through the intensive care period. Other important members of the care team with whom Emily will interact throughout the day include bedside nurses, registered dietitians, and respiratory therapists. Cardiothoracic surgeons and cardiothoracic nurse practitioners work in collaboration with the PCICU team to manage the patient throughout their stay.

Emily's day begins with gathering data on her assigned patients for the day. The night team provides report on the patients, discussing changes in patients' conditions and plans and providing information about the upcoming surgeries for the day. Brief bedside rounds with the cardiac surgeons occur first with Emily presenting a concise picture of the patients' management, progress, and plans for the day. The surgeon and the critical care team discuss next steps in the management plan for the day.

Emily presents her patients during rounds with the critical care team. Family-centered rounds occur with time for parents/caregivers to ask questions and offer suggestions. Information reviewed during rounds includes vital signs, hemodynamic data (central venous pressures, right atrial pressures), ventilator settings, chest radiographs, diagnostic testing, laboratory and culture data, fluid balances, and a complete list of medications and continuous infusions. A comprehensive plan of care is organized based on the physical exam and review of data, along with input from the family and members of the provider and bedside teams. After rounding on each patient, Emily is evaluating the patient issues to be addressed throughout the day. Laboratory and culture data need to be evaluated and acted on, orders need to be written, consultants need to be called, and families need to be updated throughout the day.

Emily initially assesses and evaluates the data for the patient who will be transferred to the cardiology floor that morning. She examines the patient and reviews their data to ensure that the patient's responses to interventions are appropriate. She verifies that the patient has been weaned from vasoactive medications, that their respiratory status is stable, and that they have begun nutritional interventions. Emily calls the cardiology nurse practitioner to provide a comprehensive handoff. She writes a transfer note and transfer orders, ensuring that all patient care issues are addressed prior to transfer. Emily discusses the transfer with the family/caregivers, updating them on the patient's status and answering questions to ensure the smooth transition to the acute care setting.

As Emily finishes the transfer process, the staff assist alert is activated by nursing staff for a patient. Emily runs to the room to find the infant with a heart rate of 50 and apneic. Emily directs the bedside nurse to begin cardiopulmonary resuscitation (CPR) as more team members arrive to assist with the critical situation. The critical care attending arrives and takes the role as leader and Emily steps to the head of the bed to intubate the infant. After successful intubation, the respiratory therapist takes over the ventilation of the infant. After intubation, the infant continues to be pulseless, so the extracorporeal membrane oxygenation (ECMO) and surgical teams are called to the bedside. Emily gives the teams a brief overview of the situation and then places orders for vasoactive infusions, sedation and pain management medications, and chest radiographs; calls the blood bank for blood products; and updates the cardiology team, which has also arrived to provide assistance. An interpreter is called and Emily updates the parents via the interpreter and attends to parent questions and concerns.

Throughout the day, Emily continuously monitors the patient on ECMO along with the three other assigned patients. She provides problem-focused care in response to the changing needs of each of the patients. The bedside nurse contacts Emily for problems such as hypotension, hypertension, bleeding, low oxygen saturations, fever, difficulty with ventilation or ventilator changes, agitation and delirium, inadequate pain management, arrhythmias, electrolyte abnormalities, and problems with lines or catheters. Each incidence of concern will prompt Emily to evaluate the patient, assessing for possible causes, formulating a treatment plan, and circling back to reassess the response to therapy.

Emily consults frequently with the critical care team attending and fellow to maintain open communication with all team members. Some situations are managed independently, but often treatment plans and changes are discussed with the attending and fellow before being implemented. Emily also communicates with consultants from other teams such as cardiology, infectious diseases, nephrology, and general surgery as the need arises.

Emily also participates in admitting patients after surgery. Emily and the critical care team receive handoff from the anesthesiology team including information on the surgery performed, the medications required during and after the surgery, arrhythmias noted during surgery, and

EXEMPLAR 14.1
PEDIATRIC ACUTE CARE NURSE PRACTITIONER (AC-PNP) PRACTICE IN AN INTENSIVE CARE UNIT—cont'd

the findings on the transesophageal echocardiogram performed in the operating room. Emily assesses the patient, noting hemodynamic status, bleeding from chest tubes, ventilator settings, and placement of lines and other drains. She reviews the chart for past medical history and orders medications and initial laboratory studies to be completed. She reviews the overall plan of care with the bedside nurse and the ventilator plan with the respiratory therapist. She updates the parents/family/caregivers and answers their questions and addresses their concerns. Social work and spiritual care services are engaged and provide support to the parents and family. Emily frequently returns to the bedside to assess the patient during the first hours postoperatively to ensure that hemodynamics are within the goals of care. She notes that the patient is hypotensive and orders a bolus of Plasma-Lyte and an increase in the vasoactive medications. She discusses the next options with the critical care attending and fellow if fluid and increasing the medication do not provide appropriate stabilization of the hemodynamics.

Prior to the end of the day, Emily reassesses each of her patients, noting their hemodynamics and fluid status. She makes changes to the plan of care as needed and communicates changes to both the bedside nurse and the critical care attending and fellow. Emily prepares and provides an overview of the plan for the night team.

The PCICU is a challenging and dynamic environment requiring organization and sharp thinking skills. The AC-PNP must be constantly assessing the patients and be alert for subtle changes that require changes to management plans. The family is a critical component of the patient's health and wellness, and communication with the family is imperative for successful patient outcomes.

Emily plays a principal role in the care of the critically ill infants and children in the PCICU. She must communicate with the critical care team, nursing colleagues, consultant teams, and family. She is also a key member of collaborative efforts to ensure pertinent clinical protocols, quality improvement initiatives, and research are ongoing and forward-thinking.

Promoting and Protecting Health and Preventing Disease

In addition to disease diagnosis and management, ACNPs provide services to promote and protect health and prevent disease (AACN, 2012; American Association of Critical-Care Nurses, 2021). Inevitably, some of the methods that ACNPs use to implement health promotion and protection and disease prevention vary from those used by NPs in the primary care specialties, as acute and critical illness warrant prioritization of immediate health needs over chronic health needs. Moreover, in some practice models the episodic nature of the relationship between the ACNP and patient and family is limited to a single acute illness event. However, hospitalization can also provide a critical window of opportunity for AG ACNPs to address health promotion and disease prevention with patients.

ACNPs are skilled in a unique form of health promotion, protection, and disease prevention, recognizing and modifying health risk factors associated with an inpatient stay. The AG-ACNP is qualified to identify the additional health problems for which the acutely, critically, and complex chronically ill are at risk and implement strategies to minimize or prevent that risk. As direct care providers, ACNPs have the ability to activate strategies and systems to implement primary, secondary, or tertiary prevention initiatives related to these unique inpatient risk factors. For example, some risk factors imposed by an inpatient stay are physiologic in nature, such as immobility, decreased nutritional intake, fluid and electrolyte imbalance, altered immunocompetence, impaired self-care ability, existing or developing comorbid disease states, and risks associated with invasive diagnostic and therapeutic interventions. Other risks have a psychological foundation, such as alterations in the patient's physical abilities and their environment, sleep deprivation, communication impairment, alteration of self-image, role reversal, financial challenges, knowledge deficits, and the consequences of medication administration, including but not limited to delirium and depression. Families are also influenced by many of these risks and require ACNP services. ACNPs must often lead difficult conversations with patients and families regarding crisis situations, terminal diagnoses, or deleterious effects of chronic disease. Skillfully navigating conversations regarding goals and expectations of care and care wishes at end of life can be a daunting task for even experienced acute care clinicians (Coates, 2021).

In addition, there are risk factors related to hospitalization itself and the multiplicity of caregivers, including discoordination of care, polypharmacy, system inefficiency and redundancy, miscommunication with families, and miscommunication among caregivers (AACN, 2012; American Association of Critical-Care Nurses, 2021). The ACNP is competent to assess patients for these unique risks and implement interventions to prevent their occurrence or minimize their consequences. As noted in the previous section, 2 of the top 11 critical activities performed by ACNPs are associated with minimizing healthcare-associated risks (i.e., evaluating patients for the safety and efficacy of interventions and ordering interventions to minimize risk; ANCC, 2020). Although these skills are common to all ACNPs, those prepared at the DNP level are equipped to assume leadership roles in developing, implementing, and evaluating evidence-based interventions to address and improve population health and clinical prevention to aggregate patient populations and across care systems (AACN, 2015, 2021).

Innovations in technology have been used to develop advanced methods of care delivery and support frequently used in acute and critical care areas in both diagnosing and managing disease as well as with health promotion and disease prevention. Decision support tools, electronic documentation systems, and electronic medical records are now commonly found in care settings. The nurse practitioner must understand and use technology to appropriately enter, review, appraise, synthesize, translate, and communicate patient health information vital to complex clinical decision making and health coaching (NONPF, 2016a). In addition to decision support in the clinical setting, providers must effectively utilize databases and other forms of technology in order to input, review, and communicate information important to the continuity of care of acute and critically ill patients. ACNPs must navigate information systems successfully in order to coordinate care (NONPF, 2016a). AC-PNPs must also consider the developmental level of both child and family when translating health information (NONPF, 2013).

Guidance and Coaching

Providing expert guidance and coaching of patients, families, and other healthcare providers is a core competency that is also an essential part of ACNP practice. Advancing knowledge of providers through mentorship, coaching, and education delivery is essential to improving care outcomes in both acute care pediatric and adult and older adult populations (NONPF, 2013, 2016a). In the primary care area, the plan of care may be mutually determined and fully implemented between the NP and patient–family dyad. In contrast, the process of assessment and diagnosis, care planning, implementation, and evaluation in the acute care setting, although still centering on the ACNP and patient–family dyad, will likely involve a number of other individuals, including but not limited to physicians, other nurses, respiratory therapists, dietitians, pharmacists, physical and occupational therapists, social workers, and clergy. In this complex setting, the ACNP's ability to plan, interpret, and explain the plan of care while educating others about disease processes is a valued aspect of the ACNP role. Often, critical illness can require many complex treatments, and ACNPs can provide teaching to families, nursing staff, and other members of the healthcare team to facilitate knowledge of indicated care. The core competency of guidance and coaching is played out at the highest levels when ACNPs prepare patients for discharge after serious illness or when they assist and prepare family members to care for loved ones who have undergone catastrophic or debilitating health problems. ACNPs are particularly adept at communicating with families and patients during times of critical stress, when facilitating ethical decision making, or when assisting families in communication with neurologically depressed or deteriorating patients. ACNPs may also follow up with patients after hospital discharge to monitor and treat symptoms, facilitate care transition (Sawatsky et al., 2013), and assess for and mitigate post-ICU syndrome. At times, patients (particularly the poor and uninsured) may not have a consistent primary care provider in the outpatient setting, and the ACNP becomes an important source for health information and promotion and protection interventions during the inpatient encounter. Some patients may be more receptive to health guidance and coaching that occurs in proximity to an acute health event (e.g., diet and exercise information after an acute myocardial infarction). ACNPs also provide coaching for experienced and inexperienced nurses in complex care settings.

Evidence-Based Practice

ACNPs contribute to knowledge development and the application of evidence to practice to improve care delivery through evidence-based care (NONPF, 2013, 2016a). For ACNPs to achieve the competencies to diagnose and manage disease within their specialty patient population, they must demonstrate mastery of advanced pathophysiology and understanding of the pathophysiologic basis of disease, advanced and prioritized health assessment with an understanding of normal physiologic changes of aging and abnormal variations, and the age-related implications of safe and therapeutic pharmacologic and nonpharmacologic interventions (AACN, 2012; American Association of Critical-Care Nurses, 2021; NONPF, 2016a).

ACNPs are expected to effectively evaluate research relevant to their specialty population and identify strategies to disseminate findings as part of an evidence-based practice (NONPF, 2013, 2016a). Evidence-based care competencies are essential to the ACNP provider role, though enactment may vary among ACNP providers. ACNPs work to facilitate individual practice and healthcare system change through clinical inquiry and evidence-based practice initiatives (Kapu & Kleinpell, 2013; Kapu, Kleinpell, & Pilon, 2014; Liego et al., 2014; McCarthy et al., 2013). All ACNPs draw from the literature to deliver evidence-based medical and nursing care and actively participate in evidence-based quality improvement initiatives. ACNPs have been instrumental in both adopting and leading initiatives for implementation of practice standards and guidelines (Fox, 2014) and core measures documentation (Aleshire et al., 2012). Some ACNPs, particularly those prepared at the DNP level, lead interprofessional teams focused on evidence-based practice initiatives (Aleshire et al., 2012). The ACNP may partner with researchers to facilitate conduct of research and in some cases may serve as a clinical member of the research team. ACNPs must be adept in evaluating research findings to assess for their suitability to support clinical practice change (American Association of Critical-Care Nurses, 2021).

In building an evidence-based practice, the ACNP serves as a participant and leader in both the generation of new knowledge and translation of evidence to improve clinical practice and patient outcomes (NONPF, 2013, 2016a). In addition, inherent to the AC-PNP role is ensuring both pediatric assent and consent and obtaining parental consent during the clinical inquiry process (NONPF, 2013).

The ACNP uses the best available evidence to inform clinical practice and applies an understanding of various system-level influences on health care (e.g., access to care, cost, safety, organizational structure, health policy, etc.) and identification of appropriate interventions to address barriers to care and ensure care quality (NONPF, 2016a). The AG-ACNP-level competencies for quality include implementation of evidence-based practice to promote quality and safety and demonstration of continuous improvement within one's own practice (NONPF, 2016a). The AC-PNP must also collaborate with local and state- and national-level child organizations to promote best practices and ensure child safety (NONPF, 2013).

All ACNPs draw from the literature to deliver evidence-based medical and nursing care and actively participate in evidence-based quality improvement initiatives. With the launch of the Value-Based Purchasing Program in 2011, hospitals have been required to improve outcomes and maximize reimbursement for Medicare patients, and the ACNP is a valuable provider in applying evidence-based practices to achieve these goals (Kapu & Kleinpell, 2013; Liego et al., 2014).

Leadership

All ACNPs provide some form of professional, clinical, and systems leadership in their provider role by serving as mentors and role models for staff nurses, taking on selected administrative responsibilities in the healthcare agency, and acting as care facilitators and change agents within the healthcare system. An important competency of the ACNP is to function as a leader in overseeing, coordinating, and directing the delivery of comprehensive clinical services, advocating for the needs of the patient and family within and across the healthcare system (AACN, 2012; NONPF, 2013, 2016a). The AG-ACNP promotes a positive healing environment and demonstrates assertiveness and conflict negotiation skills. Providing leadership in the planning and implementation of system-wide cost containment or cost-effective initiatives is also an aspect of the AG-ACNP role. AG-ACNPs prepared at the DNP level perform these activities at an even higher level of specificity and autonomy.

In addition to each individual ACNP's leadership competencies, some may have leadership responsibilities for groups of ACNPs or other APRNs (as well as physician assistants [PAs] and others). ACNPs may work within teams of advanced practice providers (APPs) and function as the "lead APP," having responsibility for overseeing the practice, performance, productivity, and scheduling of other APPs on the team, using leadership competencies to perform this role. It is also common in large health systems employing large numbers of NPs to have a centralized NP leader serve as a point of contact, liaison, and expert for all matters specific to NP practice (Bahouth et al., 2013).

As a clinical leader, the nurse practitioner must understand healthcare delivery systems and their impact on resource utilization and care delivery. The ACNP must use advanced skills in analysis, critical thinking, communication, and collaboration to navigate processes within the healthcare system and overcome barriers in order to ensure that patients receive safe, high-quality, cost-effective, need-based care, as driven by both acuity and care complexity. Both adult and pediatric ACNPs must be able to evaluate the risks and benefits of advanced therapeutics, as well as collaborate with caregivers and with professionals both within and external to the healthcare system to facilitate the transition to a level of care appropriate for the patient's needs (NONPF, 2016a). In addition, the ACNP must use resources efficiently and identify system barriers to care delivery and coordination (NONPF, 2016a).

Understanding the relationship between policy and practice; advocating for policies that positively impact care access, equity, quality, and cost; and taking an active role in development of policy are key core components of the ACNP role (NONPF, 2013). Nurse practitioners must understand how policy is developed and how it is ultimately influenced by ethical, legal, and social factors (NONPF, 2013). This includes advocating for healthy and safe practice environments, for the full implementation of the AG-ACNP role; developing strategies to mitigate and reduce the impact of bias and prejudices on policies and health systems; and the active participation of the nurse practitioner in the design and implementation of professional standards and guidelines impacting the care of the acute and/or critically ill (NONPF, 2016a). The AC-PNP must understand pediatric and acute care legislation and policy statements and should use policies specific to children to direct patient care.

Collaboration

Collaboration is one of the most frequently practiced core competencies of ACNPs. Collaborative practice in the clinical setting involves working together, with shared responsibilities for clinical decision making for patient care. In the acute care setting, care delivery is always a collaborative effort among interprofessional members of the healthcare team. Therefore the ability to collaborate successfully is one of the critical components of the ACNP role. In a collaborative practice model, the emphasis is on patient outcomes, with professionals responsible for providing the care for which they are best prepared. A collaborative practice model in acute care emphasizes that each patient needs the services of different types of providers simultaneously. The advantage to this model is the ongoing continuity and coordination of care. More recently, there is a focus in healthcare systems to provide patient-centered care or patient and family–centered care, which relies on care being collaborative, holistic, and responsive to patient needs (Sidani et al., 2014). ACNPs are prepared to provide this focus.

Ethical Practice

ACNPs often act as advocates for patients in care dilemmas. Because ACNPs are often involved in planning and implementing end-of-life care, ethical decision-making skills are an essential component of ACNP practice (AACN, 2012; American Association of Critical-Care Nurses, 2021). While considering ethical and legal standards, ACNPs advocate for and facilitate both the patient's and family's right to decision making regarding complex acute, critical, or chronic illness management decisions. Demonstrating respect for autonomy includes allowing the patient to participate in shared decision making and the effective facilitation of difficult conversations regarding goals of care, palliative care options, and advanced care planning influences the perception of care quality by both patients and family (Coates, 2021).

In addition, ACNPs play a key role in interprofessional teams to address ethical issues like patient triage, the utilization of scarce resources, and the impact of treatment decisions upon quality of life (NONPF, 2016a). Mass casualty events or pandemic responses may overwhelm local healthcare systems, exhausting resources and capacity. Hospital surges, or sudden increases in volume or resource demand, create a challenging situation in which the ACNP, as part of an interprofessional team, must implement plans to triage and prioritize patient care needs (Bentley et al., 2019).

PREPARATION OF ACNPS

Education of NPs should be in one of the six population foci outlined in the APRN Consensus Model (APRN Joint Dialogue Group, 2008) and should prepare the student to sit for the certification examination consistent with the appropriate practice population. ACNPs are registered nurses who are prepared at the master's or DNP level of graduate nursing education. All ACNP programs should provide for program requirements as outlined in the *Criteria for Evaluation of Nurse Practitioner Programs* (NONPF, 2016b).

All ACNP programs should build upon *The Essentials: Core Competencies for Professional Nursing Education* (AACN, 2021). This document introduces 10 domains that represent the foundation of professional nursing practice and defines competencies within each domain at both the entry level to professional nursing and the advanced level (AACN, 2021). The ACNP program should then incorporate the graduate core, advanced practice core, NP population, and ACNP specialty competencies into its curricula. DNP curricula combine foundational or core competencies for all DNP program graduates as well as ACNP specialty competencies for the practice doctorate, aligned with the *Practice Doctorate Nurse Practitioner Entry-Level Competencies* (National Panel for NP Practice Doctorate Competencies, 2006).

The ACNP specialty content should focus on the knowledge and skills essential to diagnose and manage the episodic and chronic problems commonly experienced by adult or pediatric patients with acute, critical, and complex chronic illness while performing health promotion and protection and disease prevention activities within the context of the continuum of the healthcare delivery system (AACN, 2012). As illustrated in the conceptual model of care services presented in Table 14.3, ACNPs diagnose and manage not only the acute health problems associated with the patient's chief complaint but also quiescent, stable, and comorbid health conditions. Because ACNPs must be prepared to manage health problems across the full continuum of acute healthcare services, their didactic information and clinical experiences should provide for this broad focus. Similarly, the program should provide didactic and clinical preparation in the NP competencies as delineated in either the *Adult–Gerontology Acute Care Nurse Practitioner Competencies* (NONPF, 2016a) or the *Acute Care Pediatric Population-Focused Nurse Practitioner Competencies* (NONPF, 2013), the *AACN Scope and Standards for Acute Care Nurse Practitioner Practice* (American Association of Critical-Care Nurses, 2021), and the *Nurse Practitioner Core Competencies* (NONPF, 2017).

Teaching skills in screening and prevention specific to acute care practice are also essential. Because ACNP graduates must be competent in critical incident management, clinical simulation and use of standardized patients are helpful strategies to facilitate translating knowledge to practice in ACNP education (Bolick et al., 2012; Hravnak et al., 2007; Pascual et al., 2011). Interprofessional education models can facilitate role definitions and assist ACNP students in integrating into care teams (Corbridge et al., 2013). Technical skills training is also commonly incorporated into ACNP programs. NONPF has published a skills manual to standardize the teaching of clinical skills in ACNP programs (Melander & Settles, 2011).

ACNP education has been actively transitioning to the DNP preparation as entry into practice or as a post-master's program. This expansion in direct practice abilities includes advanced communication (interpersonal and technologic); use of an expanded scientific foundation to provide an evidence basis for practice across settings; advanced participation, collaboration, and leadership within the healthcare delivery system and the business of health care; and a focus on independent practice (NONPF, 2012). An example of the practice skills of an AG-ACNP who has received practice doctorate education is presented in Exemplar 14.2.

TABLE 14.3

Patient Care Problems and Nurse Practitioner Management Interventions Traditionally Associated With Various Health Care Delivery Settings

	HEALTH PROBLEM AND INTERVENTIONS		
Delivery Setting	**Diabetes**	**Hypertension**	**Pneumonia**
Tertiary care management (ICU setting)	Diabetic ketoacidosis management Fluid replacement Electrolyte titration IV insulin	Continuous vasoactive drugs Arterial pressure monitoring Evaluation and management of possible CVA	Mechanical ventilation and artificial airway Pulmonary toilet Culture assessment Sepsis management Continuous monitoring
Secondary care management (inpatient unit)	Diabetic exacerbation management Sliding-scale insulin administration and monitoring Hydration Workup of cause(s)	Hypertensive crisis management Additional antihypertensives Adjunct therapy as needed	IV antibiotics Oxygen therapy Advanced assessment CXR, arterial blood gases, Spo_2
Primary care management (outpatient setting)	Initial Dx or stable management Oral antihyperglycemics or subcutaneous insulin Diet Prevention and assessment of associated complications Foot care Risk factor management	Diet Oral agents Lifestyle changes Prevention and assessment of associated complications Risk factor management	Oral or intramuscular antibiotics

CVA, Cerebrovascular accident; *CXR,* chest x-ray; *Dx,* diagnosis; *ICU,* intensive care unit; *IV,* intravenous; *Spo_2,* peripheral arterial oxygen saturation.

NPs who have been educated in another NP specialty but who are now caring for patients in the population focus specific for adult–gerontology or pediatric acute care and for which additional competencies and skills are required for the quality and safety of practice must ensure that their educational preparation is consistent with this population focus (Kleinpell, Hudspeth et al., 2012). Since neither certification nor licensure grants universal practice rights, it is important that NP practice be substantiated by the appropriate education. Individuals with preparation in another APRN specialty may enroll in an ACNP post-master's or DNP completion program to ensure that they undergo didactic and supervised clinical practica to prepare adequately for caring for this unique and vulnerable patient population (Kleinpell, Hudspeth et al., 2012). Employers are increasingly aligning with requiring ACNP educational preparation as a mandate for practice with adults with complex acute, critical, and chronic health conditions, including the delivery of acute care services, regardless of the geographic practice setting (Kleinpell, Hudspeth et al., 2012), and as consistent with the state boards of nursing (NCSBN, 2008) and the *The Future of Nursing* recommendations (Institute of Medicine [IOM], 2011; National Academies of Science, Engineering and Medicine [NASEM], 2021).

Despite the recent efforts to standardize entry-level competence at the completion of ACNP programs, there is still some variation in the quality of programs and the practice-readiness of graduates. Because of the complexity and vulnerability of the patient population, some healthcare systems have established onboarding programs and postgraduate residencies or fellowships to extend the practice supervision period and transition to practice (Bahouth et al., 2013; Schofield & McComiskey, 2015). This serves to ensure care delivery that is at local standards and mitigate institutional

EXEMPLAR 14.2

ADULT–GERONTOLOGY ACUTE CARE NURSE PRACTITIONER (AG-ACNP) ROLE IMPLEMENTATION FOLLOWING DOCTOR OF NURSING PRACTICE (DNP) PREPARATION

Joyce is a DNP-prepared AG-ACNP currently working in a nephrology practice. The practice consists of one AG-ACNP and five physicians. The practice is organized so that each provider has their own caseload of patients and follows these patients in the office and in the hospital. In addition, Joyce is responsible for one of the outpatient dialysis clinics, where she sees patients three times per week. This particular dialysis clinic is located in a neighborhood consisting mainly of Hispanics and African Americans. Every month, members of the practice meet for breakfast to discuss issues related to patient care and the logistics of the practice. Her usual schedule consists of daily morning rounds on her hospitalized patients followed by afternoon office hours on Tuesdays and Thursdays and outpatient dialysis clinic patients on Mondays, Wednesdays, and Fridays.

To track her patients, Joyce uses an application on her smartphone. As she makes her rounds, she enters the patient data, and at the end of the day she uploads the information into her office computer. Having patient data on a smartphone or tablet allows Joyce to access patient information quickly when, for example, she admits a patient who was seen in the office a week ago but she herself was not in the office.

Recently, Joyce launched a new set of standard admission orders for patients admitted to the hospital with a diagnosis of chronic renal failure. Development of these standard orders resulted from a series of complications that occurred when new medical residents did not order the appropriate laboratory tests or all of the routine medications used to treat renal failure. These complications resulted in increased hospital stays and costs. Joyce searched the literature to provide evidence to support orders that she believed were necessary and then collaborated with the medical staff, nurses, dietitian, pharmacist, and manager of the laboratory to develop this order set. Consensus was reached in 6 months and the orders were approved. Joyce then collaborated with the nursing staff to develop a quality improvement project that looked at whether these orders influenced patient outcomes positively.

In addition to seeing clinical patients, every third month Joyce sits on the credentialing and privileging committee at the hospital. She participates in the review of applicants to ensure that they are qualified to provide competent, safe patient care. Joyce's unique role is to provide peer review on the applications of NPs.

At the dialysis clinic, Joyce is the administrator and patient care provider. Physicians from the practice also provide patient care on a rotating basis and are available for consultation. The staff is composed of registered nurses, nursing assistants, and secretarial support. To maintain optimal patient care, Joyce has implemented policies and evidence-based procedures. A quality improvement committee, led by Joyce, periodically reviews charts for compliance with selected quality indicators. In addition, Joyce coordinates a bimonthly journal club for the clinic's staff as one mechanism to ensure that the staff members are current in their practice. Because of the clinic's location, Joyce sits on the local neighborhood board. Her goal is for the clinic to be a good neighbor. Joyce collaborates with the board members to provide culturally appropriate educational opportunities on topics such as hypertension and diabetes in an effort to reduce the incidence of renal failure in that community.

Joyce serves as adjunct faculty at the local university. She lectures to the AG-ACNP students on renal disease and also serves as a clinical preceptor for AG-ACNP students. In addition, she is a member of the AG-ACNP program's local advisory board, which meets annually. The purpose of this board is to provide consultation to the AG-ACNP faculty on ways to recruit and graduate outstanding students who can meet the needs of the community. At the last meeting, Joyce pointed out that students had poor recall of current guidelines related to the management of diabetes, a leading cause of renal disease. Joyce suggested ways to integrate this information into the curriculum. She pointed out that current guidelines on diabetes management can be found on diabetes professional organization websites and can be accessed through a Smartphone application for easy reference in the clinical area.

liability. Even once they are established in practice, the competence of the care delivered by ACNPs working in entities credentialed by The Joint Commission will need to undergo both focused and ongoing professional practice evaluations, as is required for all licensed and credentialed providers (Hravnak, 2009; Makary et al., 2011).

ACNP SCOPE OF PRACTICE: LEVELS OF INFLUENCE

The scope of ACNP practice is influenced at five levels: national (professional organizations), state (government), local (healthcare institution), service-related, and individual. Like other APRNs, the ACNP's scope of practice is broadly set forth in statements by professional nursing organizations. State regulatory agencies further delineate the scope of practice in statutes such as nurse practice acts or title protection statutes. Because ACNPs frequently provide their services within hospitals, subacute care facilities, nursing homes, and clinics, their scope may be defined further by policies within these institutions, organizations, and healthcare entities and even by the needs of a clinically specialized patient population. Finally, individual ACNPs will further define the scope of their practice based on their own competencies, strengths, and attributes. How ACNP practice is configured at each of these levels is described in the following sections.

National Level (Professional Organizations)

At the national level, the scope of ACNP practice is shaped through established competencies developed and endorsed by leading nurse practitioner organizations and accrediting bodies. Nurse practitioner core competencies are foundational to all nurse practitioners (NONPF, 2017), while population-focused competencies provide additional standards for *entry* into practice as an adult–gerontology acute care nurse practitioner (NONPF, 2016a) or pediatric acute care nurse practitioner (NONPF, 2013). The *AACN Scope and Standards for Acute Care Nurse Practitioner Practice* (American Association of Critical-Care Nurses, 2021) describes standards of clinical practice at the competent level and the standards of professional performance at the advanced ACNP role performance level within both adult–gerontology and pediatric population foci.

The *AACN Scope and Standards for Acute Care Nurse Practitioner Practice* was initially developed jointly by the American Nurses Association and American Association of Critical-Care Nurses in 1995 and later revised by the American Association of Critical-Care Nurses in 2012, 2017, and 2021 to reflect the focus on both adult-gerontology and pediatric acute care nurse practitioner practice (American Association of Critical-Care Nurses, 2021). The population for which the ACNP provides care includes acutely and critically ill patients experiencing episodic illness, stable and/or progressive chronic illness, acute exacerbation of chronic illness, or terminal illness. The ACNP's focus is the provision of curative, rehabilitative, palliative, and maintenance care. Short-term goals include stabilizing the patient for acute and life-threatening conditions, minimizing or preventing complications, attending to comorbidities, and promoting physical and psychological well-being. Long-term goals include restoring the patient's maximum health potential, providing palliative and end-of-life care, and evaluating risk factors in achieving these outcomes. Examples include acute and critical care environments, emergency care, and procedural and interventional settings. This continuum of healthcare services spans the geographic settings of home, ambulatory care, urgent care, long-term acute care, rehabilitative care, and hospice and/or palliative care. The practice environment extends into the mobile environment and virtual locations such as the tele-intensive care unit and areas using telemedicine (American Association of Critical-Care Nurses, 2021). These standards, which are closely aligned with the APRN core competencies, describe a competent level of care and professional performance common to all ACNPs regardless of setting whereby the quality of *expert* ACNP practice can be judged. Some common themes in the standards of ACNP clinical practice and professional performance that distinguish the practice of ACNPs from other NP specialties are the dynamic nature of the patient's health and illness status, vulnerability of the patient population, need for continuous assessment and adjustment of the management plan in the face of rapidly changing patient conditions, and complexity of the required monitoring and therapeutics. Additional themes include the collaborative nature of the practice and interactive relationship between the ACNP and the healthcare system.

Two educational organizations—the AACN and the NONPF—collaborated to define those minimum competencies necessary for safe entry into either adult–gerontology or pediatric ACNP practice (NONPF, 2013, 2016a). Described earlier in this chapter, these population-focused competencies were built upon the generic role competencies for nurse practitioners and, as such, they provide guidance to educational programs preparing ACNPs.

Finally, resources that do not define scope of practice but do specify the knowledge and skills necessary to perform within the specialty scope are the ACNP national certification examinations. APRN specialty certification serves as a primary criterion for APRN practice. In addition, Medicare regulations stipulate completion of a national certification examination as a requirement for ACNPs to obtain reimbursement. ACNP certification examinations are offered by the American Nurses Credentialing Center (ANCC, n.d.) and the American Association of Critical-Care Nurses (2020). Although it is evident that the content of a certification examination should not drive educational standards or curriculum development, the topics and content for the ACNP certification examinations have been validated by role delineation studies and are consistent with the other documents delineating ACNP practice scope (ANCC, 2020). As such, they serve to further articulate the scope of ACNP practice.

State Level (Government)

Each state's government provides the second mechanism whereby the ACNP's professional scope of practice is defined. The nurse practice statute for each state governs nursing practice, which creates a patchwork of rules and regulations to define NP practice (Kleinpell, Hudspeth et al., 2012; NONPF, 2012).

In all states, APRN regulation for practice is based on basic nursing licensure, but many states have additional rules and regulations that delineate specific requirements and define and limit who can use a specific advanced practice nursing title with protection (see Chapter 20). Although at the state level it is relatively easy to define limitations in scope of practice based on the age of the patient population, it is somewhat more difficult to determine scope based on patient acuity and practice setting, which have an impact on population focus (Kleinpell, Hudspeth et al., 2012; NONPF, 2012). Nevertheless, more state boards of nursing are taking a stronger stance to ensure that NP scope of practice at state levels is defined in ways consistent with the APRN *Consensus Model*, particularly in differentiation between primary and acute care (Blackwell & Neff, 2015). This is of particular importance in ensuring that all APRNs are caring for the population for which their education has prepared them. States are bound to do so in order to ensure the public safety of their citizens (Blackwell & Neff, 2015).

Institutional Level

As noted, most ACNPs provide care in healthcare institutions, which may further delineate the institutional ACNP scope of practice by identifying the subpopulation (specialty population) that the ACNP serves and the process and requirements for collaboration with other healthcare providers in the institution (Kleinpell, Hudspeth et al., 2012; Magdic et al., 2005). Further specification of the ACNP's practice scope may be in job descriptions, in hospital policy, or through the institutional credentialing and privileging process.

Employers and hospitals have the right to define a specific healthcare provider's scope of practice within the employment situation. Documentation of initial training and ongoing provider competence in the application of specific skills is needed. This scope of employment may not exceed the scope of practice specified by the state's nurse practice act, but it may curtail the ACNP's scope of practice based on the needs and mission of the employer. The institutional scope of employment may take the form of a job description, hospital policy, or both. In general, the job description should include ACNP performance standards and responsibilities as they relate to patient care, collaborative relationships, professional conduct, and professional development; these institutional performance standards can provide a template for ACNP performance evaluation.

When providing care within a healthcare institution, the ACNP will also undergo the process of provider credentialing and privileging by the institution, whether they are an employee of the hospital or of a hospital-affiliated or private practice plan. For credentialing, the ACNP is required to provide proof of licensure, certification, educational preparation (typically), malpractice insurance, and skill performance (training, numbers of procedures performed, proof of competence). Institutional credentialing is necessary for the ACNP to provide care to patients within the institution, although the ACNP may or may not hold a medical staff appointment (see Chapter 20).

Once an individual is credentialed, a determination is made regarding the clinical privileges that may be granted; this is the process whereby the institution determines which medical procedures may be performed and which conditions may be treated by physician and nonphysician providers (see Chapter 20). Although an appropriately educated provider may be permitted by state statute to perform certain acts or skills, the hospital is not required to grant the provider this privilege. The clinical privileges of the ACNP are based partly on the ACNP's professional license, certification, and inherent scope of practice, as well as documented training, experience, competence, and health status. For example, the ACNP who has received educational preparation for performing invasive diagnostic procedures (e.g., insertion of central line catheters, endotracheal intubation) may request that these privileges be a part of their institutional scope of practice if they can provide proof of training and competency along with documentation that the skill is required for the job. An ACNP may periodically request new privileges based on evolving mastery of skills, further training, and changes in services needed by the patient population and institution. ACNPs must understand that although they may be qualified to perform certain procedures, privileges to perform these acts may not necessarily be granted or renewed (usually on a biannual basis) if the patient population that the ACNP currently serves does not require these skills or if ongoing application and competency in the skill during the renewal period cannot be documented. A number of specific institutional examples of ACNP role development, including discussion of formal orientation programs, are available that further outline considerations for competency assessment, credentialing and privileging considerations, and ongoing professional practice evaluation (Bahouth & Esposito-Herr, 2009; Farley & Lathan, 2011; Foster, 2012; Goldschmidt et al., 2011; Kapu et al., 2012; Kirton et al., 2007; Pascual et al., 2011; Shimabukuro, 2011).

Service-Related Level

ACNP functions are also adjusted according to the needs of the specialty patient population served or the care delivery team (i.e., service) in the organization. This may be inpatient or outpatient based. This service-related scope of practice outlines the clinical functions and tasks that may be administered by the ACNP specific to the service team with which the ACNP works and the needs of the specialty patient population served. Examples of service-related functions for the ACNP include the following:

- An AG-ACNP working with a cardiology service may initiate treatment for myocardial ischemia or infarction.
- An AG-ACNP working in a pulmonary hypertension clinic may see patients on a regular basis to assess response to vasodilator therapy.
- An AC-PNP working with an oncology service may perform bone marrow aspirations or order antibiotics for a suspected opportunistic infection.
- An AC-PNP working on a renal medicine service may write orders for hemodialysis and insert central venous dialysis catheters.
- An AG-ACNP with the cardiovascular surgery service may harvest the vein grafts for coronary artery bypass surgery.
- An AG-ACNP in the medical ICU may intubate and place arterial and central venous catheters.

Therefore service-related scope of practice may vary among ACNPs affiliated with various services or specialties within the same institution and even among those who function under the same generic job description. The service-related scope of practice outlines a more detailed and specific description of the types of activities that the ACNP will perform as a member of the practice.

Though an increasing number of state practice acts no longer require formal or written collaborative agreements, in states in which physician collaboration is a requirement or in cases in which the healthcare organization has collaborative guidelines, the ACNP's institutional and service-related scope of practice and clinical privileges may be determined collaboratively by the physician and ACNP and set forth in a written agreement. This written agreement for collaborative practice then provides the source document on which the hospital makes privileging decisions. Written agreements, often formatted as a checklist, are frequently helpful, because the detail included in a written agreement cannot be spelled out in a job description. The agreement might also specify the level of communication or degree of supervision between the ACNP and physician that is required before the performance of a specific function (Hoffman & Guttendorf, 2017; Kleinpell, Buchman, & Boyle, 2012). For example, an ACNP with novice skills in central line insertion may require direct supervision for a specified period of time or number of successful attempts but, as the ACNP approaches expert status, the level of supervision may be decreased to minimal or none. Eventually, as the ACNP's expertise continues to advance, they may supervise medical trainees or novice ACNPs in these skills. As skills progress, the written agreement, if required, will also need to be modified. In some cases, the written agreement may be used to communicate the ACNP's scope of employment to other members of the healthcare team such as staff nurses and pharmacists.

When negotiating the written agreement, the ACNP must ensure that no function conflicts with the state's nurse practice act or institutional policies. Nevertheless, the agreement should not be a barrier to practice but be written as broadly as reasonable to allow for practicality, flexibility, and optimization of practice within the context of experience and safety.

Individual Level

The final determinant of scope of practice is role individualization by each ACNP. Experience, specialization, interest, motivation, self-esteem, personal ethics, personality traits, and communication style affect the employment opportunities, clinical specialties, skills, practice arrangements, and degree of autonomy that the ACNP will seek out and/or apply in their uniquely personal enactment of the role (Kapu et al., 2012). ACNPs are encouraged to engage in self-reflection and performance appraisal, as well as evaluate their own practice against identified benchmarks, in order to continually assess and improve individual knowledge and skills (AACN, 2012). In addition, ACNPs are encouraged, as they move along the continuum from novice to expert, to be aware of patient care situations that exceed their current skill set and seek advice, assistance, or consultation to ensure patient safety.

PROFILES OF THE ACNP ROLE AND PRACTICE MODELS

Although most ACNPs practice in acute and critical care settings, there are a variety of role implementation models in ever-expanding specialty area practice sites. One ACNP role implementation model focuses on episodic management of patients in a single clinical specialty unit, one model follows a caseload of patients throughout their hospitalization or on providing specialty care such as rapid response team care, and one focuses on managing patients across the entire continuum of acute care services, from hospitalization to home.

The ACNP model focusing on episodic care of patients on a specialty clinical inpatient unit provides the earliest model of ACNP practice (Howie-Esquivel & Fontaine, 2006; Kleinpell & Hravnak, 2005). The ACNP, in collaboration with a physician specialist, might manage the care of a patient admitted to a specialty inpatient unit with an acutely unstable medical or surgical condition. Once the patient is stabilized, the patient is transferred to another clinical unit under the care of another provider. Under this model, ACNPs confine their practice to episodic care at a defined level of acute care, permitting them to develop their skills and knowledge about specific conditions in a delineated setting (see Exemplar 14.1). The limitation of this model is that it does not allow for continuity of care across the continuum.

In a hospital caseload model, the ACNP directly manages a caseload of patients throughout their entire hospitalization, providing individualized ongoing care with continuity to the patient and family. The goal in this model is to facilitate and coordinate a patient's hospital stay to provide high-quality, cost-effective care (Farley & Lathan, 2011; Kapu & Kleinpell, 2013; Kapu et al., 2012; Landsperger et al., 2016). In this model, the ACNP will admit the patient to the hospital, complete the admission history and physical examination, assess the patient's initial clinical status, order and interpret diagnostic and therapeutic tests, perform procedures, evaluate and adjust the plan of care, and prepare the patient for discharge. The ACNP will provide care continuously for patients as they move from high-acuity to lower acuity inpatient care units, facilitate patients' movement through the acute care system, and plan for and implement discharge. Exemplar 14.3 illustrates this model.

In a specialty care model, the ACNP delivers comprehensive specialty care to a group of patients across the entire continuum of care services. For example, an ACNP member of a heart failure care team may oversee patient management during hospitalization, provide postdischarge clinic follow-up, and ultimately manage home-based infusion therapy. The number of ACNPs working in this type of model of care is increasing. Exemplar 14.4 illustrates this model with an AG-ACNP in a pulmonary practice who also bills for her services.

EXEMPLAR 14.3

PEDIATRIC ACUTE CARE NURSE PRACTITIONER (AC-PNP) PRACTICE IN AN INPATIENT SPECIALTY SERVICE

Traci is an acute care pediatric nurse practitioner (AC-PNP) with the pediatric orthopedic team at a large children's hospital. She is the only NP for the inpatient orthopedic team that day, which also consists of a resident physician, an orthopedic fellow, and an attending orthopedic surgeon. The pediatric orthopedic team is responsible for providing care to postoperative and nonoperative orthopedic patients from 7:00 a.m. until 5:00 p.m., when the service is signed out to a pediatric orthopedic fellow for night coverage.

Traci begins the day by printing the pediatric orthopedic patient list from the computer and reviews each patient's chart, noting vital signs, intake and output, laboratory and culture results, surgical drainage amounts, and current medications. She then gathers the day team, receives sign-out from the night fellow, discusses new admissions and surgeries for the day with the oncoming fellow, and assigns patients to herself and the resident physician for the day.

After sign-out is completed, Traci is notified of a child in the emergency department (ED) with fever and leg pain with difficulty walking. Traci goes to the ED to assess the 14-year-old previously healthy boy who presents with a 6-day history of progressively worsening right hip pain with associated fever. He is experiencing significant tenderness over the right hip and is now unable to bear weight and ambulate. His mother is with him and says that they have been treating the pain with acetaminophen and ibuprofen but that the pain is now not well controlled. Traci completes a full history, noting immunization status, family history, and any previous hospitalizations, surgeries, or trauma to the hip. She completes a physical exam and appreciates significant pain with external and internal rotation of the right hip with significant tenderness to the hip. Traci orders initial labs including a complete blood count, C-reactive protein, and blood culture. She discusses the patient presentation and physical exam findings with the orthopedic surgeon. She describes her plan to order a magnetic resonance imaging (MRI) scan of the hip to help further delineate the diagnosis and specific anatomic area of concern. Traci accompanies the surgeon into the patient's room, introduces her to the family, and is available to aid in consenting the patient and family for surgery. Traci communicates with the bedside nurse, the radiology department to coordinate the MRI, and the operating room scheduler to schedule a wash-out of the hip.

Traci returns to her patient list and begins to evaluate her priorities for the remainder of the day. She reviews the charts of the two patients who are being discharged home today. She discusses concerns with the bedside nurses and talks to families and patients about the plan for the day. She identifies specific discharge teaching that is needed for each patient and reaches out to the orthopedic case manager for home care needs. She writes discharge orders and discharge summaries and arranges for postdischarge follow-up appointments with the orthopedic surgeon.

Throughout the day, Traci assigns the new patients to either herself or the resident physician and admits new postoperative patients, ensuring that history and physicals are completed, admission orders and notes are written, and a management plan is discussed with the orthopedic surgeon. Families are updated frequently and patient comfort and progress are assessed continuously during the shift. Traci answers questions from nursing and other collaborative colleagues regarding the patient plan during the day.

At the end of the day, Traci organizes a brief overview of the changes during the day. She updates the surgeon and completes a handoff for the night coverage team.

Diagnostic reasoning and advanced therapeutic interventions, consultation, and referral to other physicians, nurses, and providers are intrinsic components of this role, as described by the ACNP scope of practice (American Association of Critical-Care Nurses, 2021). Although ACNPs might require some variation in skills depending on the care model, strong commonalities exist. As with other APRN roles, all ACNPs are proficient in advanced physical assessment, clinical decision making (diagnostic reasoning), ordering and interpreting laboratory studies and procedures, and collaborating in the development and implementation of a treatment plan that includes prescribing medication. Using diagnostic reasoning, the ACNP diagnoses the origin of a complex medical problem that develops in an acutely or critically ill patient. The skills inherent in effective diagnostic reasoning include the fundamental skills of the ACNP role: history taking, physical examination skills, pattern recognition, ability to analyze and synthesize data, and ability to generate a working diagnosis. A number of factors affect the quality of diagnostic reasoning when applied to the acutely and critically ill, such as multisystem deterioration, hemodynamic instability, depressed level of consciousness, and unavailability of significant others to supply, corroborate, or supplement patient information. All of these factors challenge

EXEMPLAR 14.4

ADULT–GERONTOLOGY ACUTE CARE NURSE PRACTITIONER (AG-ACNP) PRACTICE ACROSS THE CONTINUUM OF HEALTHCARE SERVICES

A community-based pulmonary practice consists of three physicians and Suze, an AG-ACNP. Suze has been with the practice for 4 years. When she was hired, Suze applied for her Medicare national provider identifier (NPI) number, which she then assigned to the practice. This means that when Suze bills for her services, the bill is submitted under her number but payment is made to the practice. Suze's reimbursement rate is at 85% of the physician fee schedule, regardless of whether she bills in the office or in the hospital.

Each member of the practice sees patients in the office and the hospital on a rotating basis. During morning conference, Suze participates with the physicians in reviewing the schedule of that day's office appointments and list of inpatients who need to be followed. Suze sees those patients who have specialized needs relative to learning, treatment adherence, smoking cessation, and caregiver burden or unavailability. Although each one of them has their own daily office schedule of patients, the list of inpatients is divided between Suze and the physician assigned to cover inpatients for the week.

Today, Suze will follow up on 15 inpatients who have specialized needs relative to learning, treatment adherence, smoking examination findings, chest radiograph, and additional diagnostic results. For each of these follow-up visits, she first interviews the patient to confirm and gain additional historical information and then conducts a physical examination. As an example, she sees a 55-year-old man admitted for exacerbation of his chronic obstructive pulmonary disease (COPD) and possible pneumonia. He was treated overnight with broad-spectrum antibiotics, intravenous steroids, oxygen, and a nebulizer and is currently less dyspneic. Suze discusses with the pulmonologist her plan to order a chest computed tomography (CT) scan because this is the patient's third COPD exacerbation in the past 8 weeks. She is concerned that an underlying condition may be causing the exacerbations. In addition, knowing that he is a current cigarette smoker, she adjusts the antibiotic therapy regimen to cover organisms more likely to occur in smokers. She discusses smoking cessation with the patient and they agree to collaborate on developing a smoking cessation strategy at his first office appointment after hospital discharge. Suze and the pulmonologist review the case and treatment plan. He agrees and states that he will also look at the chest radiograph from the office computer but has no need to see the patient that day. Suze writes her progress note and additional orders. At the end of the day, Suze submits her bill for this inpatient under her NPI number to the office manager. Payment will be made to the practice at 85% of the physician fee schedule.

The following day, Suze sees this patient again. She interviews him, performs a physical examination, and reviews the laboratory results and the CT scan. She calls the pulmonologist to tell him that the CT scan is normal. The pulmonologist reviews the CT scan with Suze and visits the patient, asks a few questions related to symptoms, and listens to the patient's lung sounds. He agrees that the chest CT scan is negative; writes a note, which refers to Suze's note and opinion; and documents his history and physical examination findings and interpretation of the CT scan. Because Suze and the pulmonologist have each seen the patient and performed some part of the service, the total work is combined and Suze submits this day's bill as a shared visit under the physician's number. In this case the practice will be paid at 100% of the physician fee schedule. Had the pulmonologist not seen the patient and performed and documented a part of the service, the bill would have been submitted only under Suze's NPI number.

The patient is discharged to home on his routine metered-dose inhalers, a steroid taper, and oral antibiotic. He returns in 2 weeks for a follow-up office appointment scheduled with Suze. Suze interviews the patient, who states that he is feeling much better, and she performs a physical examination. She finds that his lung sounds are much improved. They discuss smoking cessation and the patient agrees to set a stop smoking date. Suze writes a prescription for a drug to help reduce nicotine cravings and also writes refill prescriptions for his inhalers. She documents the events of the visit and later discusses the plan with the pulmonologist. Suze submits the bill under her own NPI number and the practice is reimbursed at 85% of the physician fee schedule.

---

the ACNP's ability to diagnose an acutely or critically ill patient's ever-changing physical condition accurately and expeditiously.

Another inherent portion of the ACNP practice profile is the performance of technical skills, as indicated earlier. Patient needs within a specialty practice ultimately influence the type and level of therapeutic and diagnostic psychomotor skills that an individual ACNP performs (Kapu et al., 2012; Kleinpell & Goolsby, 2012). The ACNP role is one of evidence-based practice, which should be evident in clinical decision making and intervention selection.

As ACNP education increasingly transitions to DNP preparation, emphasis on promoting evidence-based practice for patients with acute, critical, and complex chronic illness and the use of information systems and technology for improving health care, as well as leadership opportunities focused on systems change, quality improvement, and translating research into clinical practice changes, will bring new challenges for the role of ACNPs and the models in which they function.

Comparison With Other Advanced Practice Nurse and Physician Assistant Roles

The ACNP role differs from other APRN roles with regard to the type of patient care problems encountered, acuity of the patient's condition, need for rapid and continuous assessment, planning and intervention, and setting in which the care is delivered. For example, the clinical nurse specialist (CNS) enacts the APRN role through three spheres of impact (e.g., at the patient level in direct care, at the nurse level as with professional development, and at the organizational level, leading system changes to improve patient care). In comparison, the ACNP uses clinical assessment skills to assess complex and acutely ill patients through health history taking, physical and mental status examination, performing procedures, and risk appraisal for complications. Both the ACNP and CNS roles target a patient-centered approach to care for patient populations, but the continuous on-unit presence of the ACNP at the bedside often differentiates the role of the ACNP from the CNS role, while staff education and development and system change responsibilities represent a larger percentage of the CNS's role. Conversely, CNSs do not generally perform many of the procedures and interventions that characterize the ACNP role. Although institutional variations in role implementation for CNSs and ACNPs sometimes lack clear-cut differentiation in role responsibilities, it is acknowledged that the CNS and NP roles are different, with distinct practice foci (Becker et al., 2016).

Table 14.3 can assist readers in conceptualizing where the main focus of ACNP practice falls within the healthcare continuum and where there might be differences or overlap with the primary care NP role. The table presents examples of management strategies for common patient healthcare problems encountered in the traditional geographic primary, secondary, and tertiary healthcare settings. With diabetes care, for example, ACNP practice predominantly involves strategies directed toward management of the patient during an acute exacerbation of the diabetes. Because of the severity of symptoms, the patient must be admitted to the hospital, where they can be continuously monitored and where management strategies may change from hour to hour (tertiary care). During this same hospitalization, the patient may need to have an infected foot ulcer treated with intravenous antibiotics (secondary care). Once the crisis is over, but while the patient is still hospitalized, the ACNP may provide discharge teaching on routine foot care (primary care) as well as diabetic diet and glucose monitoring. At this point, the patient may be referred back to their primary care provider for further follow-up and management.

In comparison, the primary care NP's practice is predominantly directed toward management of the patient's diabetes when it is stable (primary care). This would include ongoing surveillance, guidance and coaching of the patient's self-management of the diabetes, education on diabetes risk factors, and assessment of signs of disease progression and complications. The primary care NP may also assess when the patient's diabetes is not well controlled and requires a continuous glucose monitor or adjustment of insulin or oral hypoglycemic agents (secondary care). At the point when the patient is not responding or becomes acutely ill, the primary care NP will recognize the need for the patient to be referred to a setting in which continuous monitoring and management are provided (tertiary care).

Using these examples helps educators and clinicians understand that there is a natural overlap in some areas of knowledge and practice between acute care and primary care NPs. However, each NP specialty also has its own distinct focus. The knowledge base and practice of the ACNP cannot be limited only to unstable conditions requiring complex technologic diagnostic and management strategies for which the acutely or critically ill patient may be admitted to the hospital; the ACNP also needs to be prepared to manage the range of healthcare problems that accompany the patient. This includes not only the acute illness or exacerbation of chronic illness that requires acute care services but also the patient's comorbidities, which also must be cared for while in the acute care setting. For example, the hospitalized patient with diabetes discussed earlier may also have stable hypertension, stable asthma, osteoarthritis, and an acute episode of mild vaginitis. While the patient is hospitalized, the AG-ACNP must simultaneously attend to these stable comorbid health conditions to maintain their quiescence.

APRNs, including ACNPs, are different from PAs because the PA role is under the jurisdiction of the physician's license. Some overlap exists between the ACNP and PA in terms of the management of disease; however, the ACNP's practice competencies (such as leadership, guidance, and coaching) include nursing's holistic perspective as well as the promotion and protection of health. Whereas PAs are trained in the medical model to focus on providing illness-based care to patients, ACNPs, with their nursing background and practice, bring a wider range of expertise in patient and family education, communication, collaboration, and health promotion and disease prevention for individuals and populations. A growing number of facilities are integrating PA and ACNP practitioners on hospital-based teams to manage care for hospitalized patients (Kleinpell et al., 2019).

ACNPs and Physician Hospitalists

The hospitalist is an internal medicine physician responsible for managing the care of hospitalized patients. The physician hospitalist role is now being incorporated in many academic teaching centers and community settings, and the ACNP has been added as a member of this team (Rosenthal & Guerrasio, 2009). Some ACNPs function as members of the hospitalist team and manage patients independently or in collaboration with the physician hospitalist (Bryant, 2018).

A primary care physician refers the patient to the hospitalist team for management during the acute care admission. The hospitalist team provides care for the patient during hospitalization and refers the patient back to the primary care provider at the time of discharge. The goal of this service is to provide seamless, cost-effective care. This can be an advantage for a primary care physician with busy office hours who may have limited time to make hospital visits and may not be sufficiently familiar with acute care management. The specific role of the ACNP, as a member of the hospitalist team, is similar to the roles previously described, including obtaining an admission history and physical examination, performing daily physical examinations, making rounds with the physician, developing a treatment plan, reviewing laboratory studies and radiographs, and performing procedures. Furthermore, coordinating patient care management when many consultants are involved in decision making is a significant part of the role, as is consultation with the hospice and palliative care team or the case managers to facilitate discharge planning effectively (Cowan et al., 2006). Exemplar 14.5 illustrates the model of an AG-ACNP serving on a hospitalist service.

ACNP Practice Models

As described previously, the ACNP role can be enacted in service-based, unit-based, or specialty-based practice. Each of these roles comprises different practice models for the ACNP. The exemplars in this chapter further provide descriptions of these practice models. Other practice models involve physician/advanced practice provider team-based care, often provided in 24 hours, 7 days a week (24/7) coverage models of care. As more ICU settings adopt a 24/7 model of care, in part to meet workforce demands due to a decrease in resident coverage, the ACNP is now an acknowledged component of such models in the ICU (Garland & Gershengorn, 2013; Ward et al., 2013). The impact of ACNP team-based practice models can be further delineated. Several studies have demonstrated the impact of ACNP team-based models of care provided on a 24/7 basis, validating that ACNP team-based care is similar to care provided by medical teams (Costa et al., 2014; Gershengorn et al., 2012; Landsperger et al., 2016; McCarthy et al., 2013). Differences exist, however, in the specific roles and functions of ACNP practice in different models of care, including differences in provider-to-patient ratios (Kleinpell, Ward et al., 2015).

Outcome Studies Related to ACNP Practice

Measuring practice outcomes is a component of establishing the value of any APRN role (Newhouse et al., 2011). Positive outcomes of ACNP care have been demonstrated in a number of settings, including emergency care (Li et al., 2013), inpatient medical services, geriatric inpatient care, cardiovascular care (Kleinpell,

EXEMPLAR 14.5

ADULT–GERONTOLOGY ACUTE CARE NURSE PRACTITIONER (AG-ACNP) PRACTICE ON A HOSPITALIST TEAM

John is one of three nurse practitioners (NPs) working on a hospitalist team at a community hospital. He is prepared as an AG-ACNP and his colleagues are prepared as adult NPs. They work with a 10-member hospitalist team to provide care to hospitalized patients. The hospitalist service is the primary admitting service for the hospital and provides medical inpatient consultations. John's role consists of managing a group of patients, following up on newly admitted patients, performing a history and physical examination for new admits, discharging patients, and responding to consultation requests. Consultations vary from medical comanagement of surgical patients to the evaluation of acute condition changes and follow-up of diagnostic tests. Condition changes can vary from alterations in vital signs to onset or worsening of symptoms such as nausea, vomiting, shortness of breath, or chest pain, and laboratory results may require further follow-up for possible changes to the treatment plan (e.g., supplemental potassium).

Because he is prepared as an AG-ACNP, John is also called for consultations in the intensive care unit (ICU) or to evaluate patients who might need transfer to the ICU, and he works in collaboration with intensivists to manage acute changes in ICU patients. In addition to serving on the code team, he is a member of the hospital's rapid response team and may be called to further evaluate a patient who has had an acute change in condition anywhere in the hospital.

John will see patients independently but has a hospitalist physician in-house with whom he can further consult for patient care management issues, including generating differential diagnoses, evaluating different treatment options, and discussing care progression in outliers. Often, patients are discussed among the entire team, using the expertise of each member on the hospitalist team.

Other roles of the hospitalist NP include providing patient status updates to family members, explaining the plan of care to clinical nurses, reporting the status of a hospitalized patient to the patient's primary care physician (improving transitions of care communication), planning goals of care for patients being discharged, transferring patients for rehabilitation, ensuring documentation and reporting of core measures (e.g., pneumonia, venous thromboembolism prophylaxis), implementing patient satisfaction activities, planning advance directive care, incorporating integrative and complementary therapies (e.g., acupuncture, healing touch, stress reduction interventions), and coordinating care across the spectrum of consultants who are treating the patient.

Working as a hospitalist AG-ACNP requires John to keep current with requirements for documentation and billing, focused professional practice evaluation (FPPE), and ongoing professional practice evaluation (OPPE). He finds that attending the annual national NP conference and the national hospital medicine conference provides him with essential updates for his practice as well as valuable continuing education. He has negotiated with the hospitalist group to cover travel, registration, hotel costs, and paid time off for these annual conferences. Most recently, John submitted an abstract to present at the national NP conference to speak about the role of the NP on the hospitalist team.

John currently serves on the advanced practice committee for the institution, which reviews the applications for medical staff appointment of advanced practice providers. He also serves on the acute and critical care quality committee, which meets monthly to review quality data such as infection rates and development of acute care protocols.

Although several physician assistants also serve on the hospitalist team, John's role is different in that in addition to managing patient care, he is involved in several performance improvement initiatives. As an APRN, John brings a strong performance and quality improvement perspective to the team, often identifying opportunities to improve care and care delivery, examining possible solutions, and generating consensus among the interprofessional team. One recent initiative targeted the reduction of unplanned readmissions for heart failure patients at risk for rehospitalization within 30 days by initiating a discharge clinic that will be run by the hospitalist NPs. Building on their educational preparation, AG-ACNPs also promote, mentor, and facilitate evidence-based practice by identifying clinical issues, critically examining the literature, and disseminating findings to improve evidence-based practice, minimize variances among providers, and evaluate clinical and administrative outcomes related to practice changes.

As an AG-ACNP on a hospitalist team, John enjoys the flexibility of the role because he is involved in direct patient care management. He also serves in advanced practice consultation roles for committee work for implementing FPPE and OPPE practice standards and for developing NP-run initiatives such as the discharge clinic for heart failure patients. John's role represents a growing opportunity for AG-ACNPs as hospitals develop and expand hospitalist services to assist in the management of hospitalized patients.

Avitall et al., 2015), trauma care (Morris et al., 2012), intensive care (Costa et al., 2014; Farley & Lathan, 2011; Fleming & Carberry, 2011; Gershengorn et al., 2012; Kapu et al., 2012; Landsperger et al., 2016; Shimabukuro, 2011), pediatric intensive care (Gigli et al., 2021), oncology and palliative care (Hutchinson et al., 2014; Kilpatrick et al., 2014), and as rapid response team leaders (Barocas et al., 2014; Kapu, Wheeler et al., 2014). These demonstrated positive outcomes of ACNP care include decreased costs, shorter hospital lengths of stay, decreased rates of hospital readmission, decreased emergency room admissions, decreased use of laboratory tests, lower rates of urinary tract infections and skin breakdown, time savings for house physicians, similar care outcomes compared with physician practices, patient and family satisfaction, and an increased role in discussing patient outcomes with nurses and families.

Although these studies exploring ACNP effectiveness have been conducted in several types of care settings, continued research on the impact of ACNP practice is needed. Over the last decade, the increasing number of studies related to the use and value of ACNPs have focused on outcomes related to care management, continuity of care, safety, patient satisfaction, cost-effectiveness, or the impact of ACNP care on a focused area of care (Jefferson & King, 2018; Kleinpell et al., 2019). Though the added value of ACNP practice is well established, more research would be helpful. ACNPs are practicing in a number of different roles that span the trajectory of acute and critical illness—across the inpatient ICU to the hospitalist team, to the post–acute care area, and on to rehabilitation—and with specialty services such as cardiac arrest, rapid response, and critical care transport teams, among others. Research is needed to delineate the impact of ACNP practice in these broader and less geographically circumscribed areas and across the full spectrum of acute care services, or in more than a single center, to improve generalizability of results. Also, research examining the impact of doctoral preparation would be helpful to support any added benefit to the profession, to patients, and to employers of ACNPs. If ACNPs are to delineate the impact of their care and justify their value, it is imperative that their worth be supported by careful research.

SPECIALIZATION OPPORTUNITIES WITHIN THE ACNP ROLE

As mentioned previously, the ACNP might participate as a member of a specific clinical specialty or consult service practicing in an acute care setting. Some examples of specialty service expansion are highlighted below.

Bone Marrow Transplantation Services

The ACNP working as a member of the bone marrow transplantation service has an autonomous role while functioning as a part of a collaborative practice model; the team may be composed of a resident, fellow, attending physician, and ACNP. The ACNP provides continuity of care for the service by being the only consistent member of the academic healthcare team, in which physicians rotate between clinical and research activities. The ACNP carries a caseload of patients and follows them through their hospital stay until discharge. Role responsibilities include carrying out preliminary daily rounds on each patient, performing physical examinations, interpreting laboratory tests (e.g., electrolytes, radiology studies), performing marrow aspirations, and consulting specialists (e.g., gastroenterology, infectious disease, pulmonary medicine) to assist in patient management. On the basis of the information gathered, the ACNP collaborates with the other provider team members during daily rounds to develop the daily and long-term treatment plan. In addition, the ACNP teaches the house and nursing staff and incorporates health teaching, health promotion, and protection activities into their practice, especially related to risks associated with immunosuppression.

Diagnostic and Interventional Services

In preadmission surgical services, the clinical functions of an ACNP include history taking and physical examinations; performing preprocedure evaluations; providing patient and family education; obtaining and interpreting laboratory, electrocardiographic, and radiologic data; identifying at-risk individuals in need of preadmission discharge planning; initiating contacts with social services; discharge planning; and management recommendations for patients in the surgical holding area. The ACNP consults with the anesthesiologist and surgeon regarding patient health problems that may affect or preclude anesthesia delivery or surgery. ACNPs may provide similar services to patients in the cardiac catheterization suite or the gastrointestinal procedure laboratory. ACNPs may not only support diagnostic and interventional services but may also perform some invasive diagnostic procedures (Duszak et al., 2015).

Heart Failure Services

On the heart failure service in a university medical center, a team of three ACNPs may collaborate with each other and with physician team members to optimize continuity of care for their patients. Each ACNP has a caseload of patients for whom they assume responsibility in the outpatient area. They see each patient in clinic on a regular basis, examine patients, and adjust the treatment plan. They perform follow-up by phone contact on a weekly basis, helping patients assess their symptoms, follow daily weights, discuss dietary changes, and adjust oral medications as needed. Based on information gleaned in follow-up contacts, the ACNP may have the patient come to the outpatient clinic for further clinical assessment and treatment (e.g., a dose of intravenous diuretic, adjustment of continuous inotropic medication infusions). Each ACNP team member provides in-hospital coverage on a weekly rotating basis. When a patient requires admission to the hospital for an acute exacerbation of heart failure, one ACNP, along with the physician, manages the hospitalized patient. They know the patient's problems and treatment plan, can provide continuity, have established a trusting relationship with the patient and care team, and readily facilitate discharge planning and follow-up care.

Orthopedic Services

The ACNP working with patients with orthopedic problems covers a full spectrum of practice settings, including the emergency room, orthopedic clinic, and inpatient orthopedic service. The orthopedic ACNP works closely with the attending physicians, staff nurses, and residents to coordinate care from preadmission testing to discharge. Each ACNP carries a caseload of hospitalized patients and outpatients undergoing short procedures. The role may include perioperative management as first assistant in the operating room.

Critical Care Teams

The ACNP serves as an active member and leader within interprofessional critical care teams. As a critical care expert, the "intensivist" ACNP works closely with attending physician intensivists, critical care staff nurses, residents and fellows, pharmacists, respiratory and physical therapists, and dietitians to provide care to high-acuity patient populations (Kleinpell, Ward et al., 2015; Squiers et al., 2013). Each ACNP on the intensivist team will manage a caseload of patients, including a variety of patient acuities, new admissions, postoperative recoveries, and transfers. The ACNP will perform selected invasive procedures such as central venous line insertion or chest tube insertion. The ACNP may also lead the rapid response team or evaluate and manage unstable patients on step-down units.

Rapid Response Teams

A more recent role for the ACNP may be as team leader or team member of a hospital medical emergency or rapid response team. When hospitalized patients develop sudden physiologic instability outside of critical care areas, a mismatch between patient needs and available supportive resources occurs. Rapid response teams deploy personnel and other resources to meet patient needs in a crisis in any area of the hospital (Aleshire et al., 2012; Barocas et al., 2014; Kapu, Wheeler et al., 2014; Scherr et al., 2012). These teams consist of multidisciplinary members such as ACNPs, physicians, critical care nurses, respiratory therapists, and nursing supervisors. The team might be activated to respond to conditions such as hypotension, acute mental status changes, bleeding, respiratory distress, chest pain, or oliguria. The ACNP may be the team leader, coordinating the assessment, triage, and treatment plan, or they may participate as a team member enacting problem-focused response protocols, placing peripheral or central venous lines, assisting with airway management, and coordinating transfer to another level of care, if necessary (Barocas et al., 2014; Kapu, Wheeler et al., 2014).

Supportive and Palliative Care

The ACNP may serve on inpatient palliative care teams. Working with palliative care attending physicians and consulting services, the ACNP may provide expert consultations, assessing and planning for patient palliative care needs (Coogan et al., 2021). The ACNP helps facilitate discussions of goals of care between the consulting service and the patient and family, in high-risk preoperative situations, or in situations involving the unstable critically ill patient. In addition, the ACNP plays a vital role in palliation or management of symptoms and in entering highly skilled conversations regarding advance care planning with patients and their families. The inpatient palliative care ACNP can also serve as a clinical resource for acute and critical care teams in planning and evaluating palliative care interventions or the deescalation of care, in recommending comfort measures, and by facilitating transition from one level of care to another such as to an inpatient palliative care unit or hospice setting.

CHALLENGES SPECIFIC TO THE ACNP ROLE

The role of the ACNP is continuing to evolve and gain recognition. The increased need for ACNPs to manage patient care directly in an expanding healthcare arena will continue to provide unique practice opportunities. The practice doctorate will provide additional opportunities to expand and increase the emphasis on promoting evidence-based practice and organizational and systems leadership (AACN, 2021; NONPF, 2015). The NASEM report (2021) highlighted the importance of practicing to the full scope of NP practice, and this has direct implications for the ACNP role. Practicing ACNPs continue to report that physicians and hospital administrators are unfamiliar with the full practice role and the differences between the ACNP and primary care NP specialties. Also, some physicians may feel threatened by the role. Misunderstandings about ACNP practice and labeling of the role as a so-called physician extender or midlevel provider have stemmed from the misperception that ACNPs are replacements for house staff and function as resident replacements or hold a practice role "more than a nurse" but "less than a physician." Many of these misperceptions and perceived threats can be addressed through education. ACNPs can use formal and informal opportunities to educate the professional public about the purpose and practice of ACNPs, providing clear and concrete examples of their use and efficacy. To articulate their role, it is extremely important for ACNPs to frame their practice within the nursing paradigm, one that uses the admitting history and physical examination to develop a plan of care that includes the following: recognizing the patient's holistic problems and the medical diagnosis, addressing these nursing and medical problems throughout the hospital stay, using interventions that not only diagnose and manage disease but also promote and protect health, framing the discharge summary so that patients have a continuum of nursing and medical care as they return to the community, and applying all of the ACNP role competencies, not only those related to direct clinical care, to their practice.

Exposure to the comprehensive care that ACNPs provide and the education of the healthcare team about the role will lead to continued role recognition and acceptance. Educating administrators and other healthcare professionals can facilitate acceptance of the role, which will in turn provide an opportunity for independent contracting for ACNP professional services. Awareness of worth in terms of billable revenue and the care that ACNPs can provide is imperative for successful contract negotiations and marketing purposes.

Changing employment trends have also affected ACNP practice. Originally, ACNPs were hired predominantly in tertiary medical center settings. ACNPs now report increased employment with physician practice groups, managed care organizations, accountable care organizations, independent subacute care facilities, and even individual contractual relationships. However, these opportunities also bring the challenges of negotiating legal contracts, multiorganizational credentialing and privileging, group practice, managed care and accountable care organization policies, and reimbursement issues (Kleinpell, Buchman, & Boyle, 2012).

ACNPs need to continue to develop strong collaborative relationships with physicians and others to provide optimal patient care. The DNP-prepared ACNP is well positioned to advocate for advanced interprofessional collaboration for improved health outcomes (AACN, 2021). Working to negotiate a collaborative practice partnership can be a challenge. In working to establish collegial interactions and by sharing successful practice models, ACNPs can promote enhanced collaborative relationships.

FUTURE DIRECTIONS

Forecasts for the need for ACNPs identify that continued role expansion will be needed (Auerbach, 2012) and that the future of ACNP practice will provide a world of opportunity (Aleshire et al., 2012). The ACNP role is also advancing globally (Kleinpell et al., 2014). In alignment with the APRN *Consensus Model*, there is more awareness of the importance of ensuring consistency between NP education, certification, and clinical scope of practice (Kleinpell, Hudspeth et al., 2012). The IOM initiative to ensure that this occurs through fostering adoption of the APRN *Consensus Model* by all boards of nursing is gaining traction, thereby further promoting the ACNP as the appropriate preparation for those caring for acutely and critically ill adults (IOM, 2016). New models of care continue to expand for ACNP practice such as hospitalist team roles as well as 24/7 ICU team-based models of care (Kapu, Kleinpell, & Pilon, 2014). NPs working in hospital inpatient settings are also among the most highly compensated, and this may serve to attract more individuals to this role (American Association of Nurse Practitioners, 2015).

In the future, ACNPs may practice in multiple settings with individually negotiated contracts. Managing episodes of acute illness or exacerbation of chronic illness in home health care, subacute care, and outpatient settings might be directed by the ACNP, as is already the case in some areas. These areas are natural extensions of acute care services and encompass the scope of ACNP practice and the stabilization of acute and complex chronic disease. There are myriad opportunities relative to acute and chronic therapeutic management; for example, the management of renal dialysis or ventilator-dependent patients.

Cost reduction in acute care services will continue. Currently, collaborative teams composed of a physician, resident, and ACNP are popular in many practice settings (Costa et al., 2014; Gershengorn et al., 2012; Landsperger et al., 2016). Some patient populations may be managed by teams composed of several ACNPs with one physician, as in the heart failure service example described previously.

Monitoring outcomes of ACNP practice remains essential. Although a growing number of utilization and outcome-based studies of ACNP practice have been conducted and published, there is still the need to demonstrate the impact of ACNP care in a growing number of specialty practice arenas. The emphasis on continuous quality improvement will continue to mandate the need for ACNPs to become proactive and involved in measuring the impact of their care.

With more ACNPs being educated at the DNP level, there is an increased potential to apply scientific knowledge to clinical practice and establish and uphold evidence-based practice as well as apply research to clinical practice. Information on the impact of the ACNP role at the DNP level is also needed. ACNPs are expected to assume leadership roles in evaluating the scientific literature and applying their findings to change and improve care.

ACNPs must accept the challenge to improve and advance themselves and their profession continually. Strategies for success in the ACNP role include maintaining competency, networking, demonstrating outcomes of practice, and communicating about the role. To provide safe, high-quality, and efficient care, the ACNP must persistently pursue ongoing education and professional development to be knowledgeable about recent advances in health care and be judicious in the application of research findings. ACNPs should not only read the literature but also publish on clinical and role topics. Sharing their clinical expertise and experiences can benefit their peers as those peers seek to develop and enhance their roles. It is important that ACNPs be involved in their NP professional and clinical specialty organizations so that the issues unique to ACNP practice gain recognition by the leaders of national organizations and also to ensure that ACNPs have a voice in the regulatory, legislative, and political decision-making process. Collaboration with public policymakers to influence issues related to the ACNP role or, on a larger scale, health policy issues is also an imperative for all ACNPs (AACN, 2012; American Association of Critical-Care Nurses, 2021; see Chapter 17).

CONCLUSION

The ACNP role provides an opportunity for NPs to have a significant impact on patient outcomes at a dynamic time in the health trajectory of patient populations as well as in the history of healthcare delivery.

As the role continues to evolve, and as healthcare systems respond to market forces and rapidly emerging issues such as global pandemics, opportunities to further develop the ACNP role will arise. Future development of the ACNP role should be based on the need for the role, an understanding of the scope of the role, and role outcomes assessment. Ensuring that ACNPs practice to the full scope of their education and training is in alignment with the recommendations of NASEM (2021). The role of the ACNP is now well established, but because the role continues to evolve, participation in national organizations to refine consensus regarding role components, program curriculum, marketing, and role evaluation is ongoing. ACNP educators and clinicians must work together to ensure that the preparation and practice of ACNPs is safe, effective, and fully represented as the movement of doctoral APRN education evolves. ACNPs also need to thoroughly understand as well as be proponents of the APRN *Consensus Model* (APRN Joint Dialogue Group, 2008) to ensure that licensure and education match the practice setting in order to ensure public safety as well as educate employers in those practice settings where the population focus demands the ACNP as the most appropriate APRN provider. ACNPs must be strong activists in efforts to gain broader recognition of their role within their full scope of practice across acute care settings. In this evolving healthcare arena, ACNP practice is rapidly expanding and holds unlimited potential. Ongoing challenges include ensuring expansion of the ACNP with a focus on advanced practice nursing, rather than as a physician replacement model of care.

KEY SUMMARY POINTS

- The purpose of the ACNP is to diagnose and manage disease and promote the health of patients with acute, critical, and complex chronic health conditions across the continuum of healthcare services.
- Although all ACNPs share specialty role attributes, there may be intrarole variability based on the nature of the care delivery system, characteristics of a particular employment position, location in which they practice, and physiologic specialty.
- For ACNPs to achieve the specialty competencies to diagnose and manage disease in their specialty patient population, they must demonstrate mastery of advanced pathophysiology, completion of a prioritized health history and comprehensive and focused physical examinations, rapid assessment of unstable and complex health problems, implementation of diagnostic strategies and therapeutic interventions to stabilize healthcare problems, technical competence with procedures, modification of the plan of care based on a client's changing condition and response to interventions, and collaboration with other care providers to facilitate positive outcomes.
- Although the ACNP role is the newest NP specialty, there is growing evidence demonstrating that ACNPs deliver care that is safe and cost-effective.

REFERENCES

Aleshire, M. E., Wheeler, K., & Prevost, S. S. (2012). The future of nurse practitioner practice: A world of opportunity. *The Nursing Clinics of North America, 47*, 181–191.

Alexander-Banys, B. (2014). Acute care nurse practitioner managed home monitoring program for patients with complex congenital heart disease: A case study. *Journal of Pediatric Health Care, 28*, 97–100.

American Association of Colleges of Nursing. (2012). *Adult-gerontology acute care nurse practitioner competencies*. Author. https://cdn.ymaws.com/www.nonpf.org/resource/resmgr/competencies/adult geroaccompsfinal2012.pdf

American Association of Colleges of Nursing. (2015). *The Doctor of Nursing Practice: Current issues and clarifying recommendations*. Author. https://www.pncb.org/sites/default/files/2017-02/AACN_DNP_Recommendations.pdf

American Association of Colleges of Nursing. (2021). *The essentials: Core competencies for professional nursing education*. Author. https://www.aacnnursing.org/Portals/42/AcademicNursing/pdf/Essentials-2021.pdf

American Association of Critical-Care Nurses. (2020). Certification exam statistics and cut scores: Exam statistics 2020. Retrieved from http://www.aacn.org/wd/certifications/content/statistical.pcms?menu=certification

American Association of Critical-Care Nurses (2021). In L. Bell, & C. Cain (Eds.), *AACN scope and standards for adult-gerontology and pediatric acute care nurse practitioners*. Author.

American Association of Nurse Practitioners. (2015). *National nurse practitioner compensation survey: An overview*. Author.

American Nurses Association. (2015). *Code of ethics for nurses with interpretive statements*.

American Nurses Credentialing Center (2020a). Adult-gerontology acute care nurse practitioner: Role delineation study executive summary. https://www.nursingworld.org/~49f2f5/globalassets/certification/certification-specialty-pages/resources/role-delineation-studies/exam-62-agacnp-rds-executive-summary_final_04092020.pdf

American Nurses Credentialing Center. (2020b). Certification data. Retrieved from https://www.nursingworld.org/~49930b/global-assets/docs/ancc/ancc-cert-data-website.pdf

American Nurses Credentialing Center. (n.d.). Our certifications. https://www.nursingworld.org/our-certifications/

APRN Joint Dialogue Group. (2008). *Consensus Model for APRN regulation: Licensure, accreditation, certification & education*. http://www.aacn.nche.edu/education-resources/APRNReport.pdf

Auerbach, D. I. (2012). Will the NP workforce grow in the future? New forecasts and implications for healthcare delivery. *Medical Care, 50*, 606–610.

Bahouth, M. N., Ackerman, M., Ellis, E. F., Fuchs, J., McComiskey, C., Stewart, E. S., & Thomson-Smith, C. (2013). Centralized resources for nurse practitioners: Common early experiences among leaders of six large health systems. *Journal of the American Association of Nurse Practitioners, 25*, 203–212.

Bahouth, M. N., & Esposito-Herr, M. (2009). Orientation program for hospital-based nurse practitioners. *AACN Advanced Critical Care, 20*, 82–90.

Barocas, D. A., Kulahalli, C. S., Ehrenfeld, J. M., Kapu, A. N., Penson, D. F., You, C. C., Weavind, L., & Dmochowski, R. (2014). Benchmarking the use of a rapid response team by surgical services at a tertiary care hospital. *Journal of the American College of Surgeons, 218*, 66–72.

Becker, D., Dechan, L. M., McNamara, L. K., Konick-McMahon, J., Noe, C. A., Thomas, K., & Fabrey, L. J. (2016). Practice analysis: Adult-gerontology acute acer nurse practitioner and clinical nurse specialist. *American Journal of Critical Care, 29*, e19–e30.

Bentley, S., Iavicoli, L., Boehm, L., Agriantonis, G., Dilos, B., LaMonica, J., Smith, C., Wong, L., Lopez, T., Galer, A., & Kessle, S. (2019). A simulated mass casualty incident triage exercise: SimWars. *MedEdPORTAL, 15*, 1–9.

Blackwell, C. W., & Neff, D. F. (2015). Certification and education as determinants of nurse practitioner scope of practice: An investigation of the rules and regulations defining NP scope of practice in the United States. *Journal of the American Association of Nurse Practitioners, 27*, 552–557.

Bolick, B. N., Haut, C., Reuter-Rice, K., Leflore, J., McComiskey, C. A., Makhailov, T. A., Cavender, J. D., Creaden, J. A., McLeod, R., & Verger, J. (2012). The acute care pediatric nurse practitioner: Curriculum overview. *Journal of Pediatric Health Care, 26*, 231–237.

Bryant, S. E. (2018). Filling the gaps: Preparing nurse practitioners for hospitalist practice. *Journal of the American Association of Nurse Practitioners, 30*, 4–9.

Coates, J. (2021). The effectiveness of a simulation program to enhance readiness to engage in difficult conversations in clinical practice. *Dimensions of Critical Care Nursing, 40*, 275–279.

Coogan, A. C., Shifrin, M. M., Williams, M. T., Alverio, J., Periyakoil, V. J., & Karlekar, M. B. (2021). Improving medical and nurse practitioner student confidence and clinical skill in advance care plan development: A multidisciplinary mentorship model. *American Journal of Hospice & Palliative Medicine, 39*(2), 184–188. 10499091211017871.

Corbridge, S. J., Tiffen, J., Carlucci, M., & Zar, F. A. (2013). Implementation of an interprofessional education model. *Nurse Educator, 32*, 261–264.

Costa, D. K., Wallace, D. J., Barnato, A. E., & Kahn, J. M. (2014). Nurse practitioner/physician assistant staffing and critical care mortality. *Chest, 146*, 1566–1573.

Cowan, M. J., Shapiro, M., Hays, R. D., Afifi, A., Vazirani, S., Ward, C. R., & Ettner, S. L. (2006). The effect of a multidisciplinary hospitalist/physician and advanced practice nurse collaboration on hospital costs. *Journal of Nursing Administration, 36*, 79–85.

Dalley, C. B., Tola, D. H., & Kesten, K. S. (2012). Providing safe passage: Rapid sequence intubation for advanced practice nursing. *AACN Advanced Critical Care, 23*, 270–283.

Duszak, R., Walls, D. G., Wang, J. M., Hemingway, J., Hughes, D. R., Small, W. C., & Bowen, M. A. (2015). Expanding roles of nurse practitioners and physician assistants as providers of nonvascular invasive radiology procedures. *Journal of the American College of Radiology, 12*, 284–289.

Farley, T. L., & Lathan, G. (2011). Evolution of a critical care nurse practitioner role within a US academic medical center. *ICU Director, 1*, 16–19.

Fleming, E., & Carberry, M. (2011). Steering a course towards advanced nurse practitioner: A critical care perspective. *Nursing in Critical Care, 16*, 67–76.

Foster, S. S. (2012). Core competencies required for the cardiac surgery nurse practitioner. *Journal of the American Academy of Nurse Practitioners, 24*, 472–475.

Fox, K. (2014). The role of the acute care nurse practitioner in the implementation of the Commission on Cancer's Standards on Palliative Care. *Clinical Journal of Oncology Nursing, 18*, 39–44.

Garland, A., & Gershengorn, H. B. (2013). Staffing in ICUs: Physicians and alternative staffing models. *Chest, 143*, 214–221.

Gershengorn, H. B., Johnson, M. P., & Factor, P. (2012). The use of nonphysician providers in adult intensive care units. *American Journal of Respiratory and Critical Care Medicine, 185*, 600–605.

Gigli, K. H., Davis, B. S., Martsolf, G. R., & Kahn, J. M. (2021). Advanced practice provider-inclusive staffing models and patient outcomes in pediatric critical care. *Medical Care, 59*, 597–603.

Goldschmidt, K., Rust, D., Torowicz, D., & Kolb, S. (2011). Onboarding advanced practice nurses: Development of an orientation program in a cardiac center. *Journal of Nursing Administration, 41*, 36–40.

Hoffman, L. A., & Guttendorf, J. (2017). Preparation and evolving role of the acute care nurse practitioner. *Chest, 152*, 1339–1345.

Howie-Esquivel, J., & Fontaine, D. (2006). The evolving role of the acute care nurse practitioner in critical care. *Current Opinion in Critical Care, 12*, 609–613.

Hoyt, S. S., & Proehl, J. A. (2015). Family nurse practitioner or acute care nurse practitioner in the emergency department? *Advanced Emergency Nursing Journal, 37*, 243–246.

Hravnak, M. (2009). Credentialing and privileging for advanced practice nurses. *AACN Advanced Critical Care, 20*, 12–14.

Hravnak, M., Beach, M., & Tuite, P. (2007). Simulator technology as a tool for education in cardiac care. *Journal of Cardiovascular Nursing, 22*, 16–24.

Hutchinson, M., East, L., Stasa, H., & Jackson, D. (2014). Deriving consensus on the characteristics of advanced practice nursing: Meta-summary of more than 2 decades of research. *Nursing Research, 63*, 116–128.

Institute of Medicine. (2011). *The future of nursing: Leading change, advancing health*. National Academies Press.

Institute of Medicine. (2016). *Assessing progress on the Institute of Medicine report: The future of nursing*. National Academies Press.

Jefferson, B. K., & King, J. E. (2018). Impact of the acute care nurse practitioner in reducing the number of unwarranted daily laboratory tests in the intensive care unit. *Journal of the American Association of Nurse Practitioners, 30*, 285–292.

Kapu, A. N., & Kleinpell, R. (2013). Developing nurse practitioner associated metrics for outcomes assessment. *Journal of the American Association of Nurse Practitioners, 25*, 289–296.

Kapu, A. N., Kleinpell, R., & Pilon, B. (2014). Quality and financial impact of adding nurse practitioners to inpatient care teams. *Journal of Nursing Administration, 44*, 87–96.

Kapu, A. N., Thompson-Smith, C., & Jones, P. (2012). NPs in the ICU. *Nurse Practitioner, 37*, 46–52.

Kapu, A. N., Wheeler, A. P., & Lee, B. (2014). Addition of acute care nurse practitioners to medical and surgical rapid response teams: A pilot project. *Critical Care Nurse, 34*, 51–59.

Kilpatrick, K., Kaasalainen, S., Donald, F., Reid, K., Carter, N., Bryant-Lukosius, D., Martin-Misener, R., Harbman, P., Marshall, D. A., Charbonneau-Smith, R., & DiCenso, A. (2014). The effectiveness and cost-effectiveness of clinical nurse specialists in outpatient roles: A systematic review. *Journal of Evaluation in Clinical Practice, 20*, 1106–1123.

Kirton, O. C., Folcik, M. A., Ivy, M. E., Calabrese, R., Dobkin, E., Pepe, J., Mah, J., Keating, K., & Palter, M. (2007). Midlevel practitioner workforce analysis at a university-affiliated teaching hospital. *Archives of Surgery, 162*, 336–341.

Kleinpell, R., Avitall, B., Catrambone, C., Johnson, T., Fogg, L., Moore, S., & Thompson, N. T. (2015). Randomized trial of a discharge planning and telehealth intervention for patients aged 65 and older after coronary artery bypass surgery. *International Journal of Clinical Cardiology, 2*, 1–6.

Kleinpell, R., Buchman, T., & Boyle, W. A. (Eds.). (2012). *Integrating nurse practitioners and physician assistants in the ICU: Strategies for optimizing contributions to care*. Society of Critical Care Medicine.

Kleinpell, R., Cook, M. L., & Padden, D. L. (2018). American Association of Nurse Practitioners national sample survey: Update on acute care nurse practitioner practice. *Journal of the American Association of Nurse Practitioners, 30*, 140–149.

Kleinpell, R., & Goolsby, M. J. (2012). American Academy of Nurse Practitioners National Nurse Practitioner sample survey: Focus on acute care. *Journal of the American Academy of Nurse Practitioners, 24*, 690–694.

Kleinpell, R., Grabenkort, W. R., Kapu, A. N., Constantine, R., & Sicourris, C. (2019). Nurse practitioners and physician assistants in acute and critical care: A concise review of the literature and data 2008-2018. *Critical Care Medicine, 47*, 1442–1449.

Kleinpell, R., & Hravnak, M. (2005). Strategies for success in the acute care nurse practitioner role. *Critical Care Nursing Clinics of North America, 17*, 177–181.

Kleinpell, R., Hravnak, M., Werner, K., & Guzman, A. (2006). Skills taught in acute care NP programs: A national survey. *Nurse Practitioner, 31*, 7–13.

Kleinpell, R., Hudspeth, R., Scordo, K., & Magdic, K. (2012). Defining NP scope of practice and associated regulations: Focus on acute care. *Journal of the American Academy of Nurse Practitioners, 24*, 11–18.

Kleinpell, R., Scanlon, A., Hibbert, D., DeKeyser-Ganz, F., East, L., Fraser, D., Wong, F. K. Y., & Beauchesne, M. (2014). Addressing issues impacting advanced nursing practice worldwide. *Online Journal of Issues in Nursing, 19*(2), 1–12.

Kleinpell, R., Ward, N. S., Kelso, L. A., Mollenkopf, F. P., Jr, & Houghton, D. (2015). Patient to provider ratios for nurse practitioners and physician assistants in the ICU: Results from a national survey. *American Journal of Critical Care, 24*, e16–e21.

Landsperger, J. S., Semler, M. W., Wang, L., Byrne, D. W., & Wheeler, A. P. (2016). Outcomes of nurse practitioner-delivered critical care: A prospective cohort study. *Chest, 149*, 1146–1154.

Li, J., Westbrook, J., Callen, J., Gregiou, A., & Braithwaite, J. (2013). The impact of nurse practitioners on care delivery in the emergency department: A multiple perspectives qualitative study. *BMC Health Services Research, 13*(1), 1–8.

Liego, M., Loomis, J., Van Leuven, K., & Dragoo, S. (2014). Improving outcomes through the proper implementation of acute care nurse practitioners. *Journal of Nursing Administration, 44*, 47–50.

Magdic, K. S., Hravnak, M., & McCartney, S. (2005). Credentialing for nurse practitioners: An update. *AACN Clinical Issues, 16*, 16–22.

Makary, M. A., Wick, E., & Freischlag, J. A. (2011). PPE, OPPE and FPPE: Complying with the new alphabet soup of credentialing. *Archives of Surgery, 146*, 642–644.

McCarthy, C., O'Rourke, N. C., & Madison, J. M. (2013). Integrating advanced practice providers into medical critical care teams. *Chest, 143*, 847–850.

Melander, S., & Settles, J. (2011). Introducing the new NONPF skills manual. *Nurse Practitioner, 36*(11), 14.

Morris, D. S., Reilly, P., Rohrbach, J., Telford, G., Kim, P., & Sims, C. A. (2012). The influence of unit-based nurse practitioners on hospital outcomes and readmission rates for patients with trauma. *The Journal of Trauma and Acute Care Surgery, 73*, 474–478.

Munro, N. (2013). What an acute care nurse practitioner should know about reimbursement. *AACN Advanced Critical Care, 24*, 110–113.

National Academies of Science, Engineering and Medicine. (2021). *The future of nursing 2020-2030: Charting a path to health equity*. The National Academies Press.

National Association of Pediatric Nurse Associates and Practitioners. (2011). NAPNAP position statement on the acute care pediatric nurse practitioner. *Journal of Pediatric Health Care, 25*, e11–e12.

National Council of State Boards of Nursing. (2008). Consensus Model for APRN Regulation: Licensure, accreditation, certification and education. (APRN Consensus Work Group and NCSBN APRN Advisory Committee). https://www.ncsbn.org/Consensus_Model_for_APRN_Regulation_July_2008.pdf

National Organization of Nurse Practitioner Faculties. (2011). *Integrating adult acute care skills and procedures into nurse practitioner curricula*. Author.

National Organization of Nurse Practitioner Faculties. (2012). Statement on acute care and primary care certified nurse practitioner practice. http://c.ymcdn.com/sites/www.nonpf.org/resource/resmgr/imported/acpcstatementfinaljune2012.pdf

National Organization of Nurse Practitioner Faculties. (2013). *Population-focused nurse practitioner competencies.* https://cdn.ymaws.com/www.nonpf.org/resource/resmgr/competencies/population-focusnpcomps2013.pdf

National Organization of Nurse Practitioner Faculties. (2015). The doctorate of nursing practice NP preparation: NONPF perspective. http://c.ymcdn.com/sites/www.nonpf.org/resource/resmgr/DNP/NONPFDNPStatementSept2015.pdf

National Organization of Nurse Practitioner Faculties. (2016a). *Adult-gerontology acute care and primary care NP competencies.* https://cdn.ymaws.com/www.nonpf.org/resource/resmgr/competencies/NP_Adult_Geri_competencies_4.pdf

National Organization of Nurse Practitioner Faculties. (2016b). *Criteria for evaluation of nurse practitioner programs: A report of the National Task Force on Quality Nurse Practitioner Education* (5th ed.). https://cdn.ymaws.com/www.nonpf.org/resource/resmgr/files/2021/20210326_acute_and_primary_c.pdf

National Organization of Nurse Practitioner Faculties. (2017). Nurse practitioner core competencies content. http://c.ymcdn.com/sites/nonpf.site-ym.com/resource/resmgr/competencies/2017_NPCoreComps_with_Curric.pdf?hhSearchTerms=%22Nurse+and+practitioner+and+core+and+competencies+and+content%22

National Panel for NP Practice Doctorate Competencies. (2006). *The practice doctorate nurse practitioner entry-level competencies.* National Organization of Nurse Practitioner Faculties. http://c.ymcdn.com/sites/www.nonpf.org/resource/resmgr/competencies/dnp%20np%20competenciesapril2006.pdf

Newhouse, R. P., Stanik-Hutt, J., White, K. M., Johantgen, M., Bass, E. B., Zangaro, G., Wilson, R. F., Fountain, L., Steinwachs, D. M., Heindel, L., & Weiner, J. P. (2011). Advanced practice nursing outcomes 1990–2008: A systematic review. *Nursing Economic$, 29,* 230–250.

Pascual, J. L., Holena, D. N., Vella, M. A., Palmieri, J., Sicoutris, C., Selvan, B., Fox, A. D., Sarani, B., Sims, C., Williams, N. N., & Schwab, C. W. (2011). Short simulation training improves objective skills in established advanced practitioners managing emergencies in the ward and surgical intensive care. *Journal of Trauma, 71,* 330–338.

Pastores, S. M., O'Connor, M. F., Kleinpell, R. M., Napolitano, L., Ward, N., Bailey, H., & Coopersmith, C. M (2011). The ACGME resident duty-hour new standards: History, changes, and impact on staffing of intensive care units. *Critical Care Medicine, 39,* 2540–2549.

Pediatric Nursing Certification Board [PNCB]. (2020a). 2020 exam statistics. Retrieved from https://www.pncb.org/sites/default/files/resources/PNCB_Exam_Statistics_2020.pdf

Pediatric Nursing Certification Board [PNCB]. (2020b). The PNP-AC role. Retrieved from https://www.pncb.org/cpnp-ac-role

Reuter-Rice, K., & Bolick, B. (2012). *Pediatric acute care: A guide for interprofessional practice.* Jones & Bartlett.

Reuter-Rice, K., Madden, M. A., Gutknecht, S., & Foerster, A. (2016). Acute care pediatric nurse practitioner: The 2014 practice analysis. *Journal of Pediatric Health Care, 30,* 214–251.

Rosenthal, L. D., & Guerrasio, J. (2009). The acute care nurse practitioner as hospitalist: Role description. *AACN Advanced Critical Care, 20,* 133–136.

Rutledge, C. M., Haney, T., Bordelon, M., Renaud, M., & Fowler, C. (2014). Telehealth: Preparing advanced practice nurses to address healthcare needs in rural and underserved populations. *International Journal of Nursing Education Scholarship, 11*(1), 1–9.

Sawatsky, J.-A. V., Christie, S., & Singal, R. K. (2013). Exploring outcomes of a nurse practitioner-managed cardiac surgery follow-up intervention: A randomized trial. *Journal of Advanced Nursing, 69,* 2076–2087.

Scherr, K., Wilson, D. M., Wagner, J., & Haughian, M. (2012). Evaluating a new rapid response team: NP-led versus intensivist-led comparisons. *AACN Advanced Critical Care, 23,* 32–42.

Schofield, D. L., & McComiskey, C. A. (2015). Postgraduate nurse practitioner critical care fellowship: Design, implementation, and outcomes at a tertiary medical center. *The Journal for Nurse Practitioners, 11*(3), e19–e26.

Shimabukuro, D. (2011). Acute care nurse practitioners in an academic multidisciplinary ICU. *ICU Director, 2,* 28–30.

Sidani, S., Collins, L., Harbman, P., MacMillan, K., Reeves, S., Hurlock-Chorostecki, C., Donald, F., Staples, P., & van Soeren, M. (2014). Development of a measure to assess healthcare providers' implementation of patient-centered care. *Worldviews of Evidence Based Nursing, 11,* 248–257.

Sirleaf, M., Jefferson, B., Christmas, A. B., Sing, R. F., Thomason, M. H., & Huhyn, T. T. (2014). Comparison of procedural complications between resident physicians and advanced clinical providers. *The Journal of Trauma and Acute Care Surgery, 77,* 143–147.

Squiers, J., King, J., Wagner, C., Ashby, N., & Parmley, C. L. (2013). ACNP intensivist: A new ICU care delivery model and its supporting educational programs. *Journal of the America Association of Nurse Practitioners, 25,* 119–125.

Ward, N. S., Afessa, B., Kleinpell, R., Tisherman, S., Ries, M., Howell, M., & Kahn, J. Members of Society of Critical Care Medicine Taskforce on ICU Staffing. (2013). Intensivist/patient ratios in closed ICUs: A statement from the Society of Critical Care Medicine Taskforce on ICU Staffing. *Critical Care Medicine, 41,* 638–645.

15

THE CERTIFIED NURSE-MIDWIFE

MELISSA A. SAFTNER ■ MELISSA D. AVERY

"Everything has beauty, but not everyone sees it."

~ Confucius

CHAPTER CONTENTS

MIDWIFE DEFINITIONS 490
- International Definition 490
- US Midwife Definitions 490

HISTORICAL PERSPECTIVE 491

THE NURSE-MIDWIFERY PROFESSION IN THE UNITED STATES TODAY 491
- Recognition of Nurse-Midwifery 491
- Education and Accreditation 492
- Certification and Certification Maintenance 493
- Reentry to Practice 493
- Regulation, Reimbursement, and Credentialing 493
- American College of Nurse-Midwives 496
- Midwifery Internationally 497

IMPLEMENTING ADVANCED PRACTICE NURSING COMPETENCIES 498
- Overview of APRN and Certified Nurse-Midwife Competencies 498
- Direct Clinical Practice 501
- Guidance and Coaching of Patients, Families, and Other Care Providers 502
- Evidence-Based Practice 502
- Leadership 503
- Collaboration 503
- Ethical Practice 505

CURRENT PRACTICE OF NURSE-MIDWIFERY 506
- Scope of Practice 506
- Practice Settings 507
- Certified Nurse-Midwife Practice Summary 508

PROFESSIONAL ISSUES 508
- Image 508
- Work Life 510
- Professional Liability 511
- Diversity 511
- Quality and Safety 514

CONCLUSION 514

KEY SUMMARY POINTS 514

The purpose of this chapter is to describe nurse-midwifery practice in the United States, including a historical perspective and current education, accreditation, and certification of nurse-midwives, along with trends in professional practice. A brief discussion of other models of midwifery in the United States as well as midwifery's place internationally is provided. Although other classifications of midwives in the United States are identified, the focus of the chapter is on certified nurse-midwives (CNMs). CNM competencies, standards and quality metrics, and evidence of outcomes of CNM practice are discussed and numerous interprofessional efforts are emphasized. These partnerships continue to advance excellent clinical care for women.

Nurse-midwifery is approaching 100 years since its initial formal development as a profession in the United States when Mary Breckinridge brought the British model of midwifery, nurse plus midwife, to rural areas of Kentucky in 1925 (Cockerham, 2019).

Nurse-midwifery in the United States has made many contributions that have paved the way for advanced practice registered nurses (APRNs). The American College of Nurse-Midwifery was incorporated in New Mexico in 1955. In 1969 the American College of Nurse-Midwives (ACNM) was formed by the merger of the American College of Nurse-Midwifery and the American Association of Nurse-Midwives. By 1970, the ACNM had developed functions, qualifications, and midwifery standards of practice; within the next several years the ACNM also established criteria for the accreditation of nurse-midwifery education programs and a national certifying examination. Nurse-midwifery activities have been instrumental in securing prescriptive authority and direct reimbursement by insurers for CNMs. These activities have had a favorable direct or indirect impact on all APRNs. Pioneering efforts of CNMs have helped cultivate a clinical and political climate of acceptance, not only for themselves but also for clinical nurse specialists, certified registered nurse anesthetists, and nurse practitioners as highly valued and visible providers of care across all settings.

MIDWIFE DEFINITIONS

Because midwifery and nurse-midwifery in the United States and globally represent different definitions and preparation, it is appropriate to begin by defining the terms internationally and within the US context. The common denominator for all midwives is providing care during pregnancy and birth. The word *midwife* comes from the Old English and means "with woman" (Oxford University Press, n.d.). Although midwifery includes certified midwives (CMs), certified professional midwives (CPMs), and licensed midwives (LMs), this chapter focuses on the profession of nurse-midwifery. Midwives and midwifery practice are distinct from the medical practice of obstetrics and gynecology based on an emphasis on person-centered care and a strong belief that pregnancy and birth, as well as other normal life transitions, are physiologic events that are to be supported as such utilizing medical interventions only as indicated by the person's health status.

International Definition

The International Confederation of Midwives (ICM) defines a midwife as

> *... a person who has successfully completed a midwifery education programme that is based on the ICM Essential Competencies for Basic Midwifery Practice and the framework of the ICM Global Standards for Midwifery Education and is recognized in the country where it is located; who has acquired the requisite qualifications to be registered and/or legally licensed to practice midwifery and use the title "midwife"; and who demonstrates competency in the practice of midwifery.*
>
> *(ICM, 2017)*

Midwifery is a unique profession distinct from nursing and medicine but is combined with nursing in some countries. Midwifery education is recommended to be a minimum 3 years for direct entry (not combined with nursing) and at least 18 months when the midwifery program is completed following basic nursing education (ICM, 2013).

US Midwife Definitions

In the United States, three groups of professionals aim to meet the ICM definition of a midwife. CNMs are educated in the two disciplines of nursing and midwifery and must earn a graduate degree, complete a midwifery education program accredited by the Accreditation Commission for Midwifery Education (ACME), and pass the national certification examination administered by the American Midwifery Certification Board (AMCB) to receive the professional designation CNM (ACNM, 2012a). *Certified midwives* (CMs) are individuals educated in the discipline of midwifery who earn graduate degrees, meet health and science education requirements, and complete an ACME-accredited midwifery education program. They pass the same national certification examination as CNMs to receive the professional designation CM (ACNM, 2012a). The CM direct entry (not combined with nursing) route was developed by ACNM in the mid-1990s in an effort to develop an equivalent midwifery credential (Cockerham, 2019). With the same accreditation requirements and same certification credential as CNMs, the ACNM standards for practice and other ACNM documents such as the *Code of Ethics* also apply to CMs. The regulatory processes are developing; CMs can be licensed in seven states and have prescriptive authority in three (ACNM, 2019b;

Jefferson et al., 2021). An ACNM priority is to make CM practice opportunities and prescriptive authority the same as CNMs in all states. A *certified professional midwife* (CPM) is "a knowledgeable, skilled, and professional independent midwifery practitioner who has met the standards for certification set by the North American Registry of Midwives (NARM)" (NARM, 2021, p.4) and passes the examination administered by NARM. Graduation from an accredited midwifery education program is not required for the NARM examination (NARM, 2020). In addition to CNMs, CMs, and CPMs, there are individuals who use the title direct entry midwife (DEM), lay midwives (also known as *grand midwives*, traditional midwives, traditional birth attendants, empirical midwives, or independent midwives), and licensed midwives (Midwives Alliance of North America, 2016). Some of these practitioners are legally recognized in some states, some have had formal training, and some have had apprenticeship training.

HISTORICAL PERSPECTIVE

Midwifery predates nursing and medicine. Throughout time, and in all cultures, the midwife has played an important and highly respected role in the community. In Biblical times, the midwife assisted a person in labor, helped birth the baby, and provided for aftercare of the mother and infant. Novice midwives acquired knowledge and skill by apprenticing with experienced midwives and through their own observations and experiences.

In colonial times, midwives were an integral part of community life and were highly respected members of society. In the early 1900s a number of developments in the United States considerably diminished that respect and led to a decline in the practice of midwifery. The immigrant population was served by European immigrant midwives, and African American women from the South were cared for by traditional African American midwives. These midwives lacked a national organization, methods of communication, access to the healthcare system, and legal recognition (Cockerham, 2019). During this same time frame, physicians took over the role of birth attendant, obstetrics became a medical specialty, and birth moved into the hospital setting. The medicalization of birth did much to eliminate midwifery and continues to influence and regulate the practice of nurse-midwifery today.

Although midwifery remained part of mainstream health care in many European, Asian, and African countries, US nurse-midwifery was reborn in the 1920s, with growth of nurse-midwifery practice and education in the United States occurring in the 1940s and 1950s. Initial midwifery graduates worked in nursing education and public health because there was a lack of clinical practice opportunities. Like other forms of advanced practice nursing that emerged later, the resurgence of midwifery and the evolution of nurse-midwifery occurred in response to the need for care of underserved persons. By the late 1960s and 1970s, the opportunities for nurse-midwives in clinical practice increased. Demand for nurse-midwifery services for all women grew and the profession responded by opening more education programs and more midwifery practices (Cockerham, 2019; see Chapter 1).

THE NURSE-MIDWIFERY PROFESSION IN THE UNITED STATES TODAY

Recognition of Nurse-Midwifery

In the United States, the Institute of Medicine (IOM) released its report on *The Future of Nursing* (IOM & Committee on the Robert Wood Johnson Foundation Initiative on the Future of Nursing, 2011), the impetus of which was the passage of the Patient Protection and Affordable Care Act (PPACA; see Chapter 17). The report identified CNMs as one of four types of APRNs and called on nurses and midwives to be full partners in redesigning health care in the United States. A report updated in 2015 highlighted progress in obtaining full practice authority for APRNs in the 5 years between the reports and noted that there was still more work to be done (IOM, 2015). Given the need for more work, the National Academy of Medicine (formerly the IOM) convened an expert committee to "examine the lessons learned from the Future of Nursing Campaign for Action as well as the current state of science and technology to inform their assessment of the capacity of the profession to meet the anticipated health and social care demands from 2020 to 2030" (National Academy of Medicine, 2020). This work was completed and published as *The Future of Nursing 2020–2030: Charting a Path to Achieve Health Equity* (National Academies of Sciences, Engineering and Medicine, 2021), informing CNM practice in future policies and clinical practice. The report addresses social determinants of health and health equity, nursing workforce, role of nurses in improving access and quality, educating nurses for the future, disaster preparedness, and nurses leading change.

Nurse-midwives have advocated for enhanced models of care for all people. Shortly after the passing of the PPACA, Childbirth Connection (now known as the National Partnership for Women and Families), a national nonprofit organization dedicated to improving maternity care through consumer engagement and health system transformation, sponsored the Transforming Maternity Care Partnership with participation by CNMs and the ACNM as well as other interdisciplinary professionals. The resulting report, "Blueprint for Action: Steps Toward a High-Quality, High-Value Maternity Care System" (Angood et al., 2010) and follow-up report "Blueprint for Advancing High-Value Maternity Care Through Physiologic Childbearing" (Avery et al., 2018), called for expanding access to midwives and reducing barriers to midwifery practice, among other system-critical focus areas for improvement. The original report led to a partnership with the Centers for Medicare & Medicaid Services (CMS) and the development of the Strong Start initiative. This 4-year initiative aimed to improve maternal and newborn outcomes (CMS, 2020). The initiative found that participants in birth centers and group prenatal care had better outcomes at lower cost relative to other Medicaid participants with similar characteristics (CMS, 2018). These findings, largely midwife led, signal increasing opportunities for CNMs and interprofessional teams as healthcare reform continues in the United States with a goal of achieving the Triple Aim of improved patient experience, improved population outcomes, and reduced costs (Ickovics et al., 2019). These global and domestic initiatives aim to mobilize and intensify worldwide action toward transforming the care that is available to all women and children.

In 2019, the most current year for which data are available, CNMs attended approximately 367,259 births, which constituted 14.3% of vaginal births and 9.8% of all births in the United States (Martin et al., 2021). The majority of midwife-attended births occurred in hospitals, with the other 5% to 6% occurring in freestanding birth centers and at women's homes (MacDorman & Declercq, 2019).

Nurse-midwifery practice is legal in all 50 states, and CNMs have prescriptive authority in 50 states and the District of Columbia (ACNM, 2019b). As with all APRNs, prescriptive authority is regulated by individual states. CNMs are also defined as primary care providers under federal law (ACNM, 2012b).

Education and Accreditation

The ACNM established a national mechanism for the accreditation of nurse-midwifery education programs in 1962 in order to foster a consistent approach to quality education. Because the organization wanted to have its process subject to peer review and recognition, it applied to the US Department of Education for recognition as an accrediting agency. The ACME is the official accrediting body of the ACNM and has been recognized since 1982 by the Department of Education as a programmatic accrediting agency. ACME-accredited programs must receive preaccreditation status before enrolling students and apply for accreditation following graduation of the first class of students. Once the initial accreditation has been granted, the program must be reviewed at least every 10 years (ACNM, 2019a).

Although the American Association of Colleges of Nursing (AACN) recommended the doctor of nursing practice (DNP) as the entry level for clinical practice in 2004, neither the ACNM nor the ACME has endorsed that position. The ACNM supports a graduate degree as basic preparation for midwifery practice consistent with certification requirements, and it does not support the DNP as the entry-level requirement for midwifery education (ACNM, 2015d). Midwifery education has always been more broadly based than nursing. Even at the master's level, degrees may be awarded from schools of nursing, midwifery, public health, or allied health. The ACNM has developed competencies for the practice doctorate in midwifery, recognizing the practice doctorate as one possible option for doctoral preparation for midwives (ACNM, 2011b, 2019c). There currently is no ACNM or AMCB statement about mandatory doctoral preparation, although the ACNM supports and values the attainment of doctoral degrees for CNMs. Lack of a specific degree requirement for graduate preparation for midwifery is the result of a long history of evidence documenting that CNMs provide competent care (ACNM, 2019c).

As of 2021, there are 39 nurse-midwifery graduate programs in the United States accredited or preaccredited by the ACNM's Accreditation Commission for Midwifery Education (ACNM, 2020a). Of these, 36 are located in schools of nursing and three in other graduate programs. Evolving along with other APRN programs, as of 2020, 10 ACME-accredited programs offer master's and DNP options, 18 culminate in a master's degree, and an additional 11 offer the DNP only (ACNM, 2020a). Schools of nursing with DNP midwifery programs also meet the AACN DNP *Essentials* (AACN, 2006). With the approval of the new *Essentials: Core Competencies for Professional Nursing Education* (AACN, 2021), *or Essentials*, DNP programs will be working to align current curricula with the newly published academic standards and competencies.

Certification and Certification Maintenance

A national certification examination for entry into nurse-midwifery practice was instituted in 1971 and serves to protect the public by assuring a common standard for entry into practice. The AMCB credential is required by most states for licensure and by many institutions for credentialing (AMCB, 2018a). Certification is time limited for all CNMs; recertification requires completing three modules provided by the AMCB plus two approved continuing education units or passing the AMCB certification examination (AMCB, 2018b) every 5 years. As of February 2020, there were 12,591 nurse-midwives nationally certified as CNMs by the AMCB, and 116 midwives were certified as CMs (AMCB, 2020).

Reentry to Practice

CNMs may occasionally leave the workforce for a period of time and thus be out of practice. Certification may be maintained during this time by following the AMCB processes described previously. The ACNM has provided guidance to help midwives demonstrate safe, competent practice following a period of time away, which may include didactic learning and precepted clinical practice; a written plan describing the individual identified process is recommended (ACNM, 2016a).

Regulation, Reimbursement, and Credentialing

CNMs are regulated on a state-by-state basis, and there are numerous regulatory and reimbursement barriers at the local, state, and federal levels restricting the full deployment of all APRNs. These barriers are discussed in Chapters 19 and 20. Therefore this section highlights the regulatory, reimbursement, and credentialing considerations that may be distinct to nurse-midwives. CNMs are regulated by boards of nursing in a majority of states and are regulated by boards of medicine, health/public health, and midwifery in others (ACNM, n.d.-g).

The ACNM endorsed the Consensus Model for APRN Regulation (APRN Joint Dialogue Group, 2008) and made additional recommendations specific to midwifery practice (ACNM, 2011a). The first recommendation strongly supports the foundational Consensus Model principle that APRNs are licensed as independent practitioners with no regulatory requirements for collaboration, direction, or supervision. The ACNM has released an official statement about independent nurse-midwifery practice (ACNM, 2017d; Box 15.1). In addition, the ACNM–American College of Obstetricians and Gynecologists (ACOG) document, "Joint Statement of Practice Relations Between Obstetricians and Gynecologists and Certified Nurse-Midwives/Certified Midwives," is a model document that recognizes each group as licensed independent providers who may collaborate based on the needs of their patients (ACOG, 2017; Box 15.2). The ACNM advocates that nursing boards support separate boards of midwifery or boards of nurse-midwifery. Such midwifery boards or subcommittees of other health profession boards led by midwives have been recommended to consistently regulate all midwives in each individual state (Kennedy, Meyers-Ciecko et al., 2018). The ACNM also recommends that the consensus document clarify that a graduate nursing degree is not required to take the AMCB certification examination. This effort supports accredited midwifery programs located in other programs or separate institutions of higher learning (e.g., public health or allied health programs)

BOX 15.1

Independent Midwifery Practice

The following represents the position of the American College of Nurse-Midwives (ACNM):

- Midwifery practice is the independent management of women's health care, focusing particularly on common primary care issues, family planning and gynecologic needs of women, pregnancy, childbirth, the postpartum period, and care of the newborn.
- The practice occurs within a healthcare system that provides for consultation, collaborative management, or referral, as indicated by the health status of the woman or newborn.
- Independent midwifery enables CNMs and CMs to utilize knowledge, skills, judgment, and authority in the provision of primary health services for women while maintaining accountability for the management of health care in accordance with the ACNM Standards for the Practice of Midwifery.

BACKGROUND

Independent practice is not defined by the place of employment, the employee–employer relationship, requirements for a physician's cosignature, or the method of reimbursement for services. Further, *independent* should not be interpreted to mean *alone*, because there are clinical situations when any prudent practitioner would seek the assistance of another qualified practitioner.

Collaboration is the process whereby healthcare professionals jointly manage care. The goal of collaboration is to share authority while providing quality care within each individual's professional scope of practice. Successful collaboration is a way of thinking and relating that requires knowledge, open communication, mutual respect, a commitment to providing quality care, trust, and the ability to share responsibility.

From the American College of Nurse-Midwives. (2017). *Position statement: Independent midwifery practice*.

and institutions with graduate midwifery degrees (ACNM, 2011a, 2015d).

CNMs achieved equitable reimbursement for their services under Medicare in January 2011 and therefore are paid at the same fee schedule rate as physicians for doing the same work. This provision was part of the PPACA (see Chapter 17). Because of this provision, the CNM reimbursement rate increased from 65% of the physician fee schedule to 100% of the Medicare Part B physician fee schedule (ACNM, n.d.-e). CNMs have not yet been included in the wellness examination provision of the PPACA, but the ACNM continues to work to make this change (ACNM, n.d.-e). Medicaid mandates reimbursement for nurse-midwives in all 50 states; all but 15 states reimburse at 100% of the Medicaid physician fee schedule (ACNM, 2019b; A. Kohl, American College of Nurse-Midwives, personal communication, May 2020). Most states also mandate private insurance reimbursement for midwifery services (ACNM, 2019b). The ACNM remains vigilant during ongoing healthcare policymaking and advocates for

> *common-sense policy solutions that ensure women and newborns have guaranteed health coverage and access to a full range of preventative, reproductive and sexual health services under state Medicaid programs and coverage and access to essential health benefits (EHBs), including maternity and newborn care.*
>
> *(ACNM, 2017a, p. 2)*

Multiple authors have called for greater flexibility in state licensing laws (Kennedy, Meyers-Ciecko et al., 2018; Ranchoff & Declercq, 2019; Yang & Kozhimannil, 2015). CNMs and other advanced practice nurses face barriers in state laws and care reimbursement policies that vary widely across the United States. Known barriers to midwifery practice across the United States include various levels of physician supervision, including written practice agreements and restrictions to prescriptive authority preventing midwives and others from practicing their full scope of professional practice. Researchers recently demonstrated that in the United States, higher levels of midwifery integration in states were associated with higher levels of physiologic birth, fewer obstetric interventions, and better neonatal outcomes (Vedam et al., 2018). In addition, more than twice the number of midwives were available to provide midwifery care to women of reproductive

BOX 15.2

Joint Statement of Practice Relations Between Obstetrician-Gynecologists, Certified Nurse-Midwives, and Certified Midwives

The American College of Obstetricians and Gynecologists (ACOG) and the American College of Nurse Midwives (ACNM) affirm our shared goal of safe women's health care in the United States through the promotion of evidence-based models provided by obstetricians–gynecologists (ob-gyns), certified nurse-midwives (CNMs), and certified midwives (CMs). ACOG and ACNM believe health care is most effective when it occurs in a system that facilitates communication across care settings and among clinicians. Ob-gyns and CNMs/CMs are experts in their respective fields of practice and are educated, trained, and licensed independent clinicians who collaborate depending on the needs of their patients.

These clinicians practice to the full extent of their education, training, experience, and licensure and support team-based care. ACOG and ACNM advocate for healthcare policies that ensure access to appropriate levels of care for all women. Quality of care is enhanced by collegial relationships characterized by mutual respect and trust, professional responsibility and accountability, and national uniformity in full practice authority and licensure across all states.

Shortages and maldistribution of maternity care clinicians cause serious public health concerns for women, children, and families. Ob-gyns and CNMs/CMs working together optimize women's health care. ACOG and ACNM recommend increasing the number of ob-gyns and CNMs/CMs, utilizing interprofessional education to promote collaboration and team-based care.

Recognizing the high level of responsibility that ob-gyns and CNMs/CMs assume when providing care to women, ACOG and ACNM affirm their commitment to promote the highest standards for education, national professional certification, and recertification of their respective members and to support evidence-based practice. Accredited education and professional certification preceding licensure are essential to ensure skilled providers at all levels of care across the United States.

ACOG and ACNM recognize the importance of options and preferences of women in their health care. Ob-gyns and CNMs/CMs work in a variety of settings, including private practice, community health facilities, clinics, hospitals, and accredited birth centers. ACOG and ACNM hold different positions on home birth.

Establishing and sustaining viable practices that can provide broad services to women require that ob-gyns and CNM/CMs have access to affordable professional liability insurance coverage, hospital privileges, equivalent reimbursement from private payers and under government programs, and support services including, but not limited to, laboratory, obstetric imaging, and anesthesia. To provide highest quality and seamless care, ob-gyns and CNMs/CMs should have access to a system of care that fosters collaboration among licensed, independent providers.

Adapted from the American College of Obstetricians and Gynecologists. (2018). *Joint Statement of Practice Relations Between Obstetrician-Gynecologists and Certified Nurse-Midwives/Certified Midwives*.

age in states with autonomous practice (Ranchoff & Declercq, 2019). Twenty-six states and the District of Columbia have full practice authority; 14 states require a collaborative agreement for overall practice, 6 states require a collaborative agreement for prescriptive authority, and 4 states require physician supervision as a condition of midwifery practice (ACNM, 2018e). During the COVID-19 pandemic, governors in 22 states implemented emergency waivers temporarily waiving restrictive regulatory requirements for midwifery practice (NCSBN, 2021).

In addition to state regulation, hospitals and health plans have established credentialing requirements for healthcare professionals. These credentialing standards determine who may have hospital admitting privileges, be employed by healthcare systems, and be listed on managed care provider panels. Ideally, health systems would have a mechanism consistent with the profession's standards, recognizing nurse-midwifery as distinct from other healthcare professions, and have processes that guide CNMs in building on entry-level competencies within their scope of practice. Credentialing can be a particularly difficult issue for CNMs, as revealed in a 2011 online survey conducted by the ACNM. A total of 1893 responses were received; 80% of the CNM respondents stated that they did not have full voting privileges within the medical staffs of their local facilities, almost 50% reported that employment by a physician practice or the hospital was a requirement of privileging, and 65% stated that they had privileges to practice but limitations or supervisory restrictions on scope of practice (Bushman, 2014). Medical staff membership is denied in 17 states and allowed in the remaining states (ACNM, n.d.-h). Although CNMs have made significant strides in full participation in the healthcare system, continued work is required to have the authority to practice their full scope in all jurisdictions and health systems.

The federal government, through the CMS, exerts a strong influence over hospitals through its conditions of participation. These are rules with which hospitals are required to comply to maintain eligibility to participate in Medicare and Medicaid programs. In 2012 the CMS issued medical staff participation rules clarifying that hospitals may grant privileges to physicians and nonphysicians and that regardless of whether they were granted medical privileges, practitioners in the institution are required to adhere to the bylaws and regulations of the institution (Cooney & Johnson, 2012). The conditions of participation document urges hospitals to use "nonphysician providers" to help them care for the health of the public and requires that an application for credentialing be reviewed by the medical staff and governing body of the hospital. In all, these regulations send a strong signal about the contributions of CNMs and other APRNs in hospital settings but fall short of requiring that CNMs be credentialed as members of the medical staff (Cooney & Johnson, 2012). Of course, CNMs, like all health professionals, advocate for being referred to by their title rather than as a "non" other professional.

American College of Nurse-Midwives

The National Organization of Public Health Nurses established a section for nurse-midwives in the 1940s. During the reorganization of national nursing organizations, the National Organization of Public Health Nurses was absorbed into the American Nurses Association (ANA) and the National League for Nursing; however, these two organizations did not include a recognizable entity for nurse-midwives. Midwives at the 1954 ANA convention formed the Committee on Organization. This committee approved the definition of a nurse-midwife, but the National League for Nursing and the ANA could not find a place for the nurse-midwives (for various reasons). Subsequently, at their May 1955 meeting, the Committee on Organization voted to form a separate nurse-midwifery organization—the ACNM (Cockerham, 2019).

The growth and development of American nurse-midwifery has been fostered by the ACNM. The ACNM vision is a midwife for every woman and the mission is advancing the practice of midwifery in order to achieve optimal health for women throughout their life spans (ACNM, 2012b). The organization supports members by establishing evidence-based clinical standards, creating liaisons with state and federal agencies and members of congress, providing continuing education, supporting midwifery-relevant research and practice, promoting midwifery globally, and supporting the accreditation of midwifery education programs. In 2020 the ACNM represented 6837 active and student members (C. Neerland, University of Minnesota School of Nursing, personal communication, April 2020), approximately 54% of US CNMs.

The ACNM *Philosophy* (ACNM, 2004; Box 15.3), *Code of Ethics* (ACNM, 2015b; Box 15.4), *Standards for the Practice of Midwifery* (2011c; Table 15.1), and *Core Competencies for Basic Midwifery Practice* (ACNM, 2020b; Box 15.5) are important documents that guide the profession and practitioner. The ACNM is currently promoting a focus on physiologic birth through its national Healthy Birth Initiative, including the creation of the BirthTOOLS tookit for clinical implementation (ACNM, n.d.-d). Midwives are increasingly recognized in the United States for their high-quality care, patient satisfaction, and high-value care—indeed, the parameters of the Triple Aim. This recognition has led

BOX 15.3

Philosophy of the American College of Nurse-Midwives

We, the midwives of the American College of Nurse-Midwives, affirm the power and strength of women and the importance of their health in the well-being of families, communities, and nations. We believe in the basic human rights of all persons, recognizing that women often incur an undue burden of risk when these rights are violated.

We believe that every person has a right to the following:

- Equitable, ethical, accessible quality health care that promotes healing and health
- Health care that respects human dignity, individuality, and diversity among groups
- Complete and accurate information to make informed healthcare decisions
- Self-determination and active participation in healthcare decisions
- Involvement of a woman's designated family members, to the extent desired, in all healthcare experiences

We believe that the best model of health care for a woman and her family:

- Promotes a continuous and compassionate partnership
- Acknowledges a person's life experiences and knowledge
- Includes individualized methods of care and healing guided by the best evidence available
- Involves the therapeutic use of human presence and skillful communication

We honor the normalcy of women's life cycle events. We believe in:

- Watchful waiting and nonintervention in normal processes
- Appropriate use of interventions and technology for current or potential health problems
- Consultation, collaboration, and referral with other members of the healthcare team as needed to provide optimal health care

We affirm that midwifery care incorporates these qualities and that women's healthcare needs are well served through midwifery care.

Finally, we value formal education, lifelong individual learning, and the development and application of research to guide ethical and competent midwifery practice. These beliefs and values provide the foundation for commitment to individual and collective leadership at the community, state, national, and international levels to improve the health of women and their families worldwide.

Adapted from the American College of Nurse-Midwives. (2004). *Philosophy of the American College of Nurse-Midwives.*

to partnerships and recognition from the Alliance for Innovation on Maternal Health, ACOG, and the Association of Women's Health, Obstetric and Neonatal Nurses (AWHONN; ACNM, n.d.-b). Current national legislative objectives include increasing the midwifery workforce, promoting the licensure of CMs in all 50 states, and reimbursement for CNMs who teach learners, including midwifery students, medical students, and residents (ACNM, n.d.-a).

Midwifery Internationally

In 2000 the United Nations set the Millennium Development Goals, increasing the world's attention on women's and children's health. Improvements have been made, and the maternal mortality ratio declined 38% from 2000 to 2017 (World Health Organization, 2019). The new target in the United Nations Sustainable Development Goals, approved in 2015, is to reduce the maternal mortality ratio to below 70 per 100,000 live births by 2030. Midwifery has emerged as a key human resource to help achieve this goal. Internationally, publications such as *The Lancet*'s series on midwifery (Renfrew et al., 2014) and the *State of the World's Midwifery 2014* (United Nations Population Fund, 2014) highlight midwifery as key to continuing to reduce maternal and neonatal mortality. Authors call on the United Nations and world governments to invest in educating and retaining midwives. The

BOX 15.4

American College of Nurse-Midwives: Code of Ethics

CNMs and CMs have three ethical mandates in achieving the mission of midwifery to promote the health and well-being of women and newborns within their families and communities. The first mandate is directed toward the individual women and their families for whom the midwives provide care, the second mandate is to a broader audience for the "public good" for the benefit of all women and their families, and the third mandate is to the profession of midwifery to ensure its integrity and, in turn, its ability to fulfill the mission of midwifery.

Midwives in all aspects of professional relationships will:

- Respect basic human rights and the dignity of all persons.
- Respect their own self-worth, dignity, and professional integrity.

Midwives in all aspects of their professional practice will:

- Develop a partnership with the woman in which each shares relevant information that leads to informed decision-making, consent to an evolving plan of care, and acceptance of responsibility for the outcome of their choices.
- Act without discrimination based on factors such as age, gender, race, ethnicity, religion, lifestyle, sexual orientation, socioeconomic status, disability, or nature of the health problem.
- Provide an environment where privacy is protected and in which all pertinent information is shared without bias, coercion, or deception.
- Maintain confidentiality, except where disclosure is mandated by law.
- Maintain the necessary knowledge, skills, and behaviors needed for competence.
- Protect women, their families, and colleagues from harmful, unethical, and incompetent practices by taking appropriate action that may include reporting as mandated by law.

Midwives as members of a profession will:

- Promote, advocate for, and strive to protect the rights, health, and well-being of women, families, and communities.
- Promote just distribution of resources and equity in access to quality health services.
- Promote and support the education of midwifery students and peers, standards of practice, research, and policies that enhance the health of women, families, and communities.

Adapted from the American College of Nurse-Midwives. (2015). *Code of Ethics*.

World Health Organization in partnership with the United Nations Population Fund released the State of the World's Midwifery 2020 and 2021 in celebration of the year of the nurse and midwife (UNFPA, 2021). In addition to these important reports, the ICM has developed a set of core documents to "strengthen midwifery worldwide in order to provide high-quality, evidence-based health services for women, newborn, and childbearing families" (ICM, 2014a). The ICM documents represent essential competencies for basic midwifery practice, education, regulation, and association strengthening. As a result, midwives from around the world have a common standard against which they can evaluate their profession. Taken together, these reports and ICM documents reflect the urgent need for more and better prepared midwives in developed and developing countries and are a call to action and a blueprint for taking the agenda forward (see Chapter 5).

IMPLEMENTING ADVANCED PRACTICE NURSING COMPETENCIES

Overview of APRN and Certified Nurse-Midwife Competencies

Nurse-midwifery is constantly evolving and has a broader scope of practice now than it did 96 years ago. Nurse-midwifery has six core competencies (see Box 15.5) that are similar to the six identified

TABLE 15.1

Standards for the Practice of Midwifery

Standard I Midwifery care is provided by qualified practitioners.	The midwife: Is certified by the ACNM-designated certifying agent. Shows evidence of continuing competency as required by the ACNM-designated certifying agent. Is in compliance with the legal requirements of the jurisdiction in which the midwifery practice occurs.
Standard II Midwifery care occurs in a safe environment within the context of the family, community, and a system of health care.	The midwife: Demonstrates knowledge of and utilizes federal and state regulations that apply to the practice environment and infection control. Demonstrates a safe mechanism for obtaining medical consultation, collaboration, and referral. Uses community services as needed. Demonstrates knowledge of the medical, psychosocial, economic, cultural, and family factors that affect care. Demonstrates appropriate techniques for emergency management, including arrangements for emergency transportation. Promotes involvement of support persons in the practice setting.
Standard III Midwifery care supports individual rights and self-determination within boundaries of safety.	The midwife: Practices in accord with the *Philosophy* and the *Code of Ethics* of the ACNM. Provides patients with a description of the scope of midwifery services and information regarding the patient's rights and responsibilities. Provides patients with information regarding and/or referral to other providers and services when requested or when care required is not within the midwife's scope of practice. Provides patients with information regarding healthcare decisions and the state of the science regarding these choices to allow for informed decision making.
Standard IV Midwifery care comprises knowledge, skills, and judgments that foster the delivery of safe, satisfying, and culturally competent care.	The midwife: Collects and assesses client care data, develops and implements an individualized plan of management, and evaluates outcome of care. Demonstrates the clinical skills and judgments described. Practices in accord with the ACNM *Standards for the Practice of Midwifery*.
Standard V Midwifery care is based on knowledge, skills, and judgments reflected in written practice guidelines that are used to guide the scope of midwifery care and services provided to patients.	The midwife: Maintains written documentation of the parameters of service for independent and collaborative midwifery management and transfer of care when needed. Has accessible resources to provide evidence-based clinical practice for each specialty area, which may include, but are not limited to, primary health care of women, care of the childbearing family, and newborn care.
Standard VI Midwifery care is documented in a format that is accessible and complete.	The midwife: Uses records that facilitate communication of information to clients, consultants, and institutions. Provides prompt and complete documentation of evaluation, course of management, and outcome of care. Promotes a documentation system that provides for confidentiality and transmissibility of health records. Maintains confidentiality in verbal and written communications.

Continued

TABLE 15.1

Standards for the Practice of Midwifery—cont'd

Standard VII	The midwife:
Midwifery care is evaluated according to an established program for quality management that includes a plan to identify and resolve problems.	Participates in a program of quality management for the evaluation of practice within the setting in which it occurs. Provides for a systematic collection of practice data as part of a program of quality management. Seeks consultation to review problems, including peer review of care. Acts to resolve identified problems.
Standard VIII	The midwife:
Midwifery practice may be expanded beyond the ACNM's core competencies to incorporate new procedures that improve care for women and their families.	Identifies the need for a new procedure, taking into consideration consumer demand, standards for safe practice, and availability of other qualified personnel. Ensures that there are no institutional, state, or federal statues, regulations, or bylaws that would constrain the midwife from incorporation of the procedure into practice. Demonstrates knowledge and competency, including the following: Knowledge of risks, benefits, and patient selection criteria Process for acquisition of required skill Identification and management of complications Process to evaluate outcomes and maintain competency Identifies a mechanism for obtaining medical consultation, collaboration, and referral related to this procedure. Maintains documentation of the process used to achieve the necessary knowledge, skills, and ongoing competency of the expanded or new procedures.

Midwifery practice, as conducted by certified nurse-midwives (CNMs) and certified midwives (CMs), is the independent management of women's health care, focusing particularly on pregnancy, childbirth, the postpartum period, care of the newborn, and the family planning and gynecologic needs of women. The CNM and CM practice within a healthcare system that provides for consultation, collaborative management, or referral, as indicated by the health status of the patient. CNMs and CMs practice in accord with the *Standards for the Practice of Midwifery*, as defined by the American College of Nurse-Midwives (ACNM).
Adapted from *Standards for the Practice of Midwifery*, by American College of Nurse-Midwives, 2011, p. 1–3.

APRN competencies in addition to direct care (see Chapter 3). As with the APRN model in Chapter 3, the direct care role is integral to CNM practice and is well substantiated in both exemplars presented later in this chapter. Consistent with advanced practice nursing, nurse-midwives assume responsibility and accountability for their practice as primary healthcare providers (ACNM, 2018d). Patient-centered assessment and management are hallmarks of all aspects of CNM care. CNMs have, in common with all APRNs, the characteristics of using a holistic, evidence-based perspective. CNMs use research methodologies and ethical decision making to support a caring, low-technology, person-centered approach to childbirth. The ACNM has a well-defined position statement on consultation and collaboration in midwifery practice (ACNM, 2014, 2017b) that has helped inform APRN practice. CNMs have demonstrated leadership in the development of freestanding birth centers, facilities for normal, healthy women who desire a wellness model of pregnancy and birth. It is informative to take a closer look at the competencies related to advocacy and patient education to understand nurse-midwifery practice further. The ACNM-defined competencies in advocacy and patient education parallel the advanced practice core competencies of ethical decision making, guidance, and coaching. CNMs enact the six competencies of advanced practice nursing, as described in the following sections.

BOX 15.5

Core Competencies for Basic Midwifery Practice

The *Core Competencies for Basic Midwifery Practice* include the fundamental knowledge, skills, and behaviors expected of a new practitioner. Accordingly, they serve as guidelines for educators, students, healthcare professionals, consumers, employers, and policy makers.

Major headings and examples/summaries of each include:

HALLMARKS OF MIDWIFERY

Highlights include recognizing developmental and physiologic processes as normal, women as partners in care, cultural humility, health promotion, advocacy for informed choice and evidence-based care.

COMPONENTS OF MIDWIFERY CARE: PROFESSIONAL RESPONSIBILITIES OF MIDWIVES

Includes knowledge of legal basis for practice, engagement in policy related to women's health, international issues in women's health, bioethics, transgender and gender-nonconforming care, collaboration in research, practice according to standards, professional engagement, business knowledge, and supporting the profession through midwifery education.

COMPONENTS OF MIDWIFERY CARE: MIDWIFERY MANAGEMENT PROCESS

Defined process of gathering information, planning care in partnership with individuals, evaluating care, consultation as needed, and adapting care as indicated.

COMPONENTS OF MIDWIFERY CARE: FUNDAMENTALS

Basics underlying care, including anatomy, physiology/pathophysiology, epidemiology, genetics/genomics, phamacotherapeutics, nutrition, and growth and development.

COMPONENTS OF MIDWIFERY CARE

Includes specific competencies in each of the areas of primary, preconception, gynecologic/reproductive/sexual health, antepartum, intrapartum, newborn through the first 28 days of life, and postpartum care.

Adapted from American College of Nurse-Midwives. (2020). *Core competencies for basic midwifery practice*. https://www.midwife.org/acnm/files/acnmlibrarydata/uploadfilename/000000000050/ACNMCoreCompetenciesMar2020_final.pdf

Direct Clinical Practice

CNMs demonstrate a high level of expertise in the assessment, diagnosis, and treatment of sexual and reproductive health life cycle events. They approach these events, such as puberty, pregnancy, birth, and menopause, as physiologic transitions that are best supported by education and midwifery expertise. Nurse-midwives form partnerships with the patients they care for, empowering them to be active participants in their own health care. Nurse-midwives incorporate scientific evidence into clinical practice, are familiar with complementary and alternative therapies, exercise expert clinical thinking and skillful performance, and demonstrate a holistic approach in the care they provide.

The ACNM updated its position statement on CNMs as primary care providers and leaders of maternity care homes in 2012 (ACNM, 2018d). Primary care is included as a core competency for midwifery practice (ACNM, 2020b); it includes the provision of primary health care from the perimenarchal through postmenopausal phases as well as primary care for newborns. This care is provided on a continuous and comprehensive basis by establishing a plan of management with the person. The maternity care home is a concept to address person-centered care before, during, and after pregnancy. It is patterned after the patient-centered medical home (see Chapter 13) and aims to improve neonatal and perinatal health outcomes. Maternity care homes are influencing health outcomes, and the ACNM regards midwives as well positioned to lead patient-centered maternity care teams (ACNM, 2018d). Midwives approach health care holistically and assess the person's environment, relationships, and health status in order to develop a plan of care specific to each person. Nurse-midwives juxtapose nursing knowledge and skills with advanced education in midwifery to enhance outcomes across the life span. DNP-prepared nurse-midwives in particular have additional training and preparation to organize and lead maternity care homes to improve quality and facilitate change in practice delivery in accordance with DNP Essential II (AACN, 2006). With the publication of the newly approved *Essentials* (AACN, 2021), there will be changes to DNP education programs, with the 10 domains of nursing practice outlining a broader scope of responsibility for DNP-prepared midwives.

Guidance and Coaching of Patients, Families, and Other Care Providers

Guidance and coaching are APRN functions that assist patients through life transitions such as illness, childbearing, and bereavement (see Chapter 7). Nurse-midwives offer skillful communication, guidance, and counseling throughout the nurse-midwifery management process (ACNM, 2020b). Client education and engagement in the midwifery model of care are a cornerstone of nurse-midwifery practice (Perriman et al., 2018). For example, when a nurse-midwife counsels a patient regarding antenatal genetic screening, they not only educate the patient about how the test is done but also advise the person as to what the results might indicate, what further testing would then be offered, and what decisions the patient and partner may need to make and offer to provide additional coaching as the process unfolds. In the instance of the first-trimester screen, a combined screen that includes a blood test and ultrasound measurement of the fetal nuchal translucency, the patient would learn that it is a screening test for certain chromosomal conditions, such as Down syndrome, in the fetus. They are informed that it is not diagnostic and that a positive screen means that there is increased risk for the problem, not that the fetus has the problem. A positive result would lead to further decision making on whether to have further testing such as an amniocentesis or high-level ultrasound. The procedures, risks, and benefits of these tests would then be explained. If the person opts for further testing and the results indicate a complication, she would then need to decide whether to continue or terminate the pregnancy. This level of guidance requires time, expertise, skill, and commitment.

As noted in Chapter 7, guidance is an interaction between an expert coach (the nurse-midwife) and the learner (the patient) that enables the learner to develop knowledge and skills within an area of the coach's expertise. An example of this application of knowledge includes health promotion for weight management. Nurse-midwives are trained to understand nutritional needs of women across the life span. Caloric requirements, appropriate food choices, and healthy weight range recommendations are within the scope of care that midwives provide. Nurse-midwives are expected to apply their knowledge to provide guidance through the natural life transitions. In addition to obesity prevention, nurse-midwives apply their knowledge and skills to provide support during pregnancy transitions, childbirth, breastfeeding, grief and loss, parenthood, changes in family constellation, family planning, primary care, and gynecologic/sexual/reproductive health-related issues.

Evidence-Based Practice

Since the early days of the United States, midwives have contributed to knowledge regarding women and infants. Martha Ballard's diary from 1785 to 1812 detailed the care that she gave to women and their families in her rural community. It demonstrated skills, knowledge, outcomes, and political forces that influenced the practice of nurse-midwifery (Ulrich, 1990). The CNM evidence base has grown significantly since Martha Ballard's time. With more nurse-midwives advancing their education in DNP and PhD programs, nurse-midwifery-driven research, theory development, and evidence-based practice projects are enhancing clinical care and patient outcomes.

As an example, Julia Seng has conducted extensive research on posttraumatic stress disorder (PTSD), childhood abuse, and childbirth outcomes (Choi et al., 2017; Seng et al., 2013, 2018). She has extended her research to include a physiologic and biologic focus related to PTSD and trauma that informs care for nurse-midwives and other maternity care providers (Choi & Seng, 2016; Seng et al., 2014, 2018). Seng and colleagues argued that pregnancy is a critical time to interrupt the cycle of intergenerational trauma and violence and advocated for intervention when trauma is identified. Additionally, they noted that women with a past history of violence and trauma may be retraumatized during the birth experience. Holly Powell Kennedy is another example of a CNM researcher who has focused her work on topics important to CNM practice, such as normalizing birth (Avery et al., 2018; Kennedy, 2010), cesarean birth and vaginal birth after cesarean (Dahlen et al., 2016; Shorten et al., 2014, 2015), and extending midwifery care to all women (Kennedy, Kozhimannil & Sakala, 2018; Renfrew et al., 2014). In addition to distinguished individual midwifery researchers, research is incorporated as a core competency of the ACNM foundation documents. Nurse-midwives are charged with infusing scientific evidence into clinical practice to evaluate, apply, interpret, and collaborate in research (ACNM, 2020b).

The ACNM recognizes the importance of building and translating evidence into CNM practice. One mission of the ACNM Division of Research has been to contribute to knowledge about the health of women, infants, and families and advance the practice of midwifery. The Division of Research promotes the development, conduct, dissemination, and translation of midwifery research into practice (ACNM, n.d.-i). Nurse-midwifery has its own journal, the *Journal of Midwifery & Women's Health*, a peer-reviewed, clinically focused publication that publishes research pertinent to pregnancy, gynecologic/sexual/reproductive health, family planning, primary care, and healthcare policies. The ACNM also keeps members up to date via continuing education series and weekly e-newsletters on emerging health crises, such as the COVID-19, Zika, and Ebola viruses, and cooperates with federal agencies and other professional organizations to improve health nationally and internationally.

Leadership

Leadership skills are professional responsibilities that are core competencies for nurse-midwives. DNP-prepared nurse-midwives receive additional education and training related to leadership within organizations and systems. Not only are nurse-midwives knowledgeable regarding national and international issues and trends in women's health and maternal-infant care but they are also expected to be leaders in bringing those issues to the forefront. Nurse-midwives are expected to exercise leadership for the benefit of women, infants, and families; the profession of midwifery; and the ACNM. To this end, the ACNM has state- and federal-level resource centers aimed at advocacy for issues related to women's and children's health as well as for tracking professional and interprofessional issues. Federal advocacy includes participating in the Coalition for Quality Maternity Care, which endorses legislative initiatives and strengthens outreach to the grassroots level. It also includes leadership at the federal level to support women's reproductive rights and access to midwifery care. For example, in 2020, the Health Resources and Services Administration (HRSA) announced the Scholarships for Disadvantaged Students Program funding program (HRSA, 2020). For the first time ever, $2.5 million was earmarked for students attending accredited midwifery education programs. ACNM has lobbied for years to support midwifery education similar to medical training. This funding represents the first time that funding specific to accredited midwifery education programs has been secured during the federal appropriations process. Additionally, the ACNM enhances the ability of CNMs to function as independent practitioners through state-level advocacy (ACNM, 2018a) and supporting full practice authority consistent with the *Consensus Model for APRN Regulation* and the IOM's *The Future of Nursing* report (ACNM, ACME, & AMCB, 2011; IOM, 2011).

Collaboration

Interprofessional collaboration is critical to improving patient and population health outcomes in the complex healthcare environment. Nurse-midwives, particularly those prepared at the doctoral level, have the training and expertise to build interprofessional collaborative teams and facilitate teamwork and often lead these teams to set goals and improve outcomes (AACN, 2006). The ACNM has a series of position statements on collaboration. The 2014 statement focuses on midwifery management as independent, primarily intended for healthy women; however, in the event of complications, collaborative management or referral to a physician may be an appropriate pathway to ensure a patient's well-being (ACNM, 2014). The *Joint Statement of Practice Relations Between Obstetrician-Gynecologists and Certified Nurse-Midwives/Certified Midwives* (ACNM, 2018c; see Box 15.2) includes shared agreement on high standards of education, certification, and accreditation as well as mutual support for ensuring that both professions have access to affordable professional liability insurance coverage, hospital privileges, equivalent reimbursement from private payers, and support services for their work. Interprofessional education to promote team-based care was added to this joint statement; ACNM and ACOG have developed interprofessional modules and learning activities for midwifery students and obstetrics–gynecology residents through a nationally funded project (Avery et al., 2020). There is also agreement that these provider groups have access to a system of care that fosters collaboration among licensed independent providers. The 2018 statement also recognized the need for nurse-midwives and physicians to collaborate but stressed the working relationship, respect for each other's abilities and knowledge, and professional responsibility and accountability. In its position statement *Collaborative Agreement Between Physicians and Certified Nurse-Midwives and Certified Midwives*, the ACNM (2017b) clarified its position regarding collaborative agreements in a continuing attempt to delineate the nature of collaboration between physicians and CNMs. This document notes the limitations of collaborative agreements—they do not guarantee effective communication, may wrongly imply that CNMs need supervision, and also may restrict midwives from exercising their full scope of practice (ACNM, 2017b; Box 15.6).

When a complication occurs, the nurse-midwife can continue to be instrumental in the person's care while benefiting from collaboration with an obstetrician-gynecologist. This involves the nurse-midwife and physician jointly managing the care of a person whose case has become medically, gynecologically, or obstetrically complicated. The collaborating physician and nurse-midwife mutually agree on the scope of care that each will provide. If the physician needs to assume the main role in the person's care, the nurse-midwife will still participate to some degree in the physical care and emotional support and, to a large degree, in counseling, guidance, and teaching. For example, a nurse-midwife caring for a pregnant person identifies that inadequate fetal growth may be an issue. The nurse-midwife then consults with the collaborating physician and, together, they decide on what further testing and care are required under these circumstances. In this case the testing shows inadequate growth; therefore the person will alternate her prenatal visits between the physician and nurse-midwife so that together they can provide frequent fetal surveillance and the best possible outcome for mother and baby. Effective communication is essential in ongoing collaborative management to maintain a healthy working relationship and provide comprehensive care to the individuals under the collaborators' care.

In addition to obstetrician–gynecologists, nurse-midwives collaborate with other providers. During labor, nurse-midwives may collaborate with a doula to provide the laboring person with the best birth experience possible and to meet the goals of her individual birth plan. Doulas are labor support persons who work with pregnant patients and their families to ensure that they are well supported during the labor process. Doulas do not offer medical advice or care. Nurse-midwives collaborate with nurses and maternity unit managers to develop unit policies for the optimal care for the pregnant person and their fetus during the intrapartum and postpartum periods. Nurse-midwives collaborate with other nurse-midwives, labor and delivery nurses, and physician colleagues to develop practice standards and guidelines. These are just a few examples of the myriad ways in which nurse-midwives collaborate in delivering evidence-based care.

Nurse-midwives use consultation in their practice, both as the consultant and as the one seeking consultation. Patients consult with CNMs regarding health care and health promotion. For example, a person may see a nurse-midwife regarding back pain during pregnancy. They want to know what can be done at home to alleviate the discomfort and support a healthy pregnancy. The nurse-midwife may consult with a physical therapist, massage therapist, or other expert in alleviating back pain to get recommendations about activities or exercises that can be safely performed at home to decrease pain. Nurse-midwives often provide consultation in the hospital setting to residents, physicians, and nurses. During a labor and birth, nurses and nurse-midwives may consult each other regarding the interpretation of a fetal monitor tracing. Nurse-midwives serve on hospital quality improvement committees, where they can advocate for evidence-based policies and patient-centered care. Physicians often consult nurse-midwives regarding complementary therapies, breastfeeding, alternative

BOX 15.6

Position Statement: Collaborative Agreement Between Physicians and Certified Nurse-Midwives and Certified Midwives

It is the position of the American College of Nurse Midwives (ACNM) that safe, quality health care can best be provided to women and their infants when policymakers develop laws and regulations that permit certified nurse-midwives (CNMs) and certified midwives (CMs) to provide independent midwifery care within their scopes of practice while fostering consultation, collaborative management, and seamless referral and transfer of care, when indicated. ACNM affirms the following:

- Requirements for a signed collaborative agreement do not guarantee the effective communication between midwives and physicians or other healthcare providers:
  - They do not ensure physician availability when needed.
  - There is no evidence that they increase the safety or quality of patient care.
  - In certain circumstances, such as the aftermath of a natural or declared disaster, such requirements have hampered the ability of CNMs/CMs to provide critically necessary emergency relief services.
- Collaborative agreements signed by individual physicians incorrectly imply that CNMs/CMs need the supervision of those individuals in all situations. Based on this misconception:
  - Professional liability companies have used signed agreements, with their implied requirements for supervision, as the rationale for raising physician premiums, citing increased risk related to such unnecessary supervision.
  - CNMs/CMs may be restricted from exercising their full scope of practice or from receiving hospital credentials, clinical privileges, or third-party reimbursement for services that fall within the scope of their training and licensure.
- Requirements for signed collaborative agreements can create an unfair economic disadvantage for CNMs/CMs:
  - They have been used to limit the number of midwives who can practice collaboratively with any one physician, which effectively bars CNMs and CMs from practice in some cases or restricts the ratio of CNMs and CMs to physicians.
  - They allow potential economic competitors to dictate whether or not midwives can practice in a community.
  - They restrict access to care and choice of provider for women, which is of particular concern in underserved areas.

American College of Nurse-Midwives. (2017). *Position statement: Collaborative agreement between physicians and certified nurse-midwives and certified midwives.*

birthing options such as water birth, or a combination of these therapies.

Nurse-midwives also consult other professionals. There are many situations in which a nurse-midwife may request another's expertise to provide the best care for their patients. For example, a CNM caring for a pregnant person with a low platelet count might consult with the midwife's collaborating physician or a hematologist to decide on the appropriate care and provider for the pregnant person and the fetus. Nurse-midwives frequently consult with lactation consultants to assist with breastfeeding difficulties or with physical therapists to advise on mobility and discomfort problems. Nutritionists, psychologists, chiropractors, acupuncturists, endocrinologists, and cardiologists are other healthcare providers who may be part of the healthcare team of an individual pregnant person.

Ethical Practice

The goal of ethical midwifery practice is to do the right thing for the right reason. Codes of ethics guide moral behavior and are considered part of the criteria that make a practice a profession (J. B. Thompson, 2002). The ACNM *Code of Ethics*, reviewed and approved by the ACNM Board in 2015, has three mandates (ACNM, 2015b; see Box 15.4). The first is directed toward the individual person and their family, the second is for the benefit of all people and their families, and the third is to the profession of midwifery. These mandates are reflected in the *Core Competencies for Basic Midwifery Practice* (see Box 15.5), the *Philosophy* of the ACNM (see Box 15.3), and *Standards for the Practice of Midwifery* (see Table 15.1). The ACNM *Code of Ethics* aligns with the ICM *Code of Ethics*, which overviews the ethics of midwifery relationships, the practice of midwifery, professional responsibilities of midwives, and the advancement of midwifery knowledge and practice (ACNM, 2015b; ICM, 2014b).

Nurse-midwives are faced with ethical decisions in their daily practice, especially in regard to use of interventions; providing competent, evidence-based, client-centered care; informed consent and protecting privacy; and equitable access to health care (Brauer, 2016). Whether and when to use electronic fetal monitoring is an example of a care dilemma. It has become a standard of care to monitor the fetal heart rate during labor by electronic fetal monitoring. Most places of birth (mainly hospitals) have guidelines regarding this practice. Many nurse-midwives provide care in hospital settings with implied and explicit expectations to use routine fetal heart rate monitoring, even though the monitor may be intrusive to the person and not part of the birth plan. However, current evidence does not support routine continuous electronic fetal heart rate monitoring. Instead, intermittent auscultation is supported in healthy pregnancies without risk factors (ACNM, 2015c). Formal informed consent and informal discussions may not be part of the conversation about various options for monitoring the status of the fetus during labor.

Traditional biomedical ethics developed after the atrocities of World War II. Biomedical ethics is a discipline focused on moral philosophy, normative theory, abstract universal principles, and objective problem solving in dilemmas (J. B. Thompson, 2002). The overmedicalization of natural life span transitions in health care has directed the education and practice of nursing and midwifery, and bioethics has guided their codes of ethics. The essence of ethical midwifery practice occurs through human engagement, relationships, and the equilibrium of power within those relationships. Midwives create partnerships with women where the person has autonomy to make informed choices about her health care. This relationship is a collaborative, supportive relationship rather than the patriarchal, provider-dominated interaction that has characterized medical care. In addition, it has been proposed that the ethics of engagement foster ethical midwifery practice by encouraging practitioners to focus on being with women through human engagement (F. E. Thompson, 2003).

Client advocacy is part of the ACNM code of ethics that is central to nurse-midwifery practice. Client education and support of clients' rights and self-determination inform every aspect of nurse-midwifery care. These values have been challenged by the burgeoning growth of medical technology over the past 2 decades and the incursion of managed care in the 1990s. The availability of highly technical interventions for many aspects of childbearing—such as infertility and monitoring pregnancies and birth—conflicts with the traditionally low-technology, low-interventionist approach of nurse-midwives. However, by becoming part of key national movements, such as the Alliance for Innovation on Maternal Health and the US Midwifery Education, Regulation, and Association (US MERA, a group tasked with expanding access to high-quality midwifery care and development of a more cohesive US midwifery presence informed by ICM global standards and competencies), CNMs leverage their ability to ensure that the care they provide is person centered and evidence based. As structures for care delivery continue to evolve from the creation of the PPACA, such as health exchanges and accountable care organizations, it will be crucial for CNMs to be involved in the governance of these entities.

CURRENT PRACTICE OF NURSE-MIDWIFERY

Scope of Practice

Nurse-midwifery practice encompasses a full range of healthcare services for women and others seeking midwifery care, from adolescence to beyond menopause. These services include the independent provision of primary care, gynecologic and family planning services, preconception care, pregnancy care, care during childbirth and the postpartum period, care of the normal newborn during the first 28 days of life, and treatment of male partners for sexually transmitted infections. Midwifery scope of practice also includes care to transgender and gender-nonconforming individuals (ACNM, 2020b) as well as medication-assisted treatment for opioid use disorder (ACNM, 2018b). CNMs provide initial and ongoing comprehensive assessment, diagnosis, and treatment. They conduct physical examinations; prescribe medications, including controlled substances and contraceptive methods; admit, manage, and discharge patients from birth centers or hospitals; order and interpret laboratory and diagnostic tests; and order the use of medical devices. CNMs' care also includes health promotion, disease prevention, and individualized wellness education and counseling. CNMs must demonstrate that they meet the ACNM's *Core Competencies for Basic Midwifery Practice* (ACNM, 2020b) and must practice in accordance with the ACNM's *Standards for the Practice of Midwifery* (ACNM, 2011c). With constant changes in health care, CNMs may need to expand their knowledge and skills beyond those of basic CNM practice. Advanced CNM skills, such as ultrasound or serving as first assistant in surgery, may be incorporated into a CNM's practice as long as the CNM follows the recommendations for acquiring these skills by obtaining formal didactic and clinical training to ensure that the advanced skill is acquired and monitored to ensure patient safety. These steps are outlined in Standard VIII of the ACNM standards for practice (ACNM, 2011c; see Table 15.1).

Practice Settings

CNMs practice in many different settings, including full-scope practice from adolescence though the postmenopausal period and providing care during labor and attending birth. She or he may also choose specific areas of practice—for example, ambulatory care or hospital care—or work exclusively with a population of interest, such as human immunodeficiency virus–positive individuals or young adolescents. Nurse-midwives practice in urban, suburban, and rural areas. Practice settings can include private practice (nurse-midwife-owned or physician-owned), hospitals, freestanding birth centers, clinics, or clients' homes. Nurse-midwifery practice can occur in a group practice, with any combination of physicians, nurse practitioners, physician assistants, or other healthcare providers, or in a solo practice. The nurse-midwife's actual practice depends on the needs of the population and community being served, interest in specific practice models, preferences of those being cared for, and availability of physicians and nurse-midwife colleagues for consultation and collaboration, as well as personal philosophy of the individual midwife.

A nurse-midwife-assisted birth can take place in community settings including client homes and freestanding birth centers, as well as in-hospital birth centers or traditional hospital settings (community, regional, or tertiary). For nurse-midwives and those for whom they provide care, the choice of setting may be a matter of philosophy, comfort, convenience, or degree of medical risk or a combination of these factors. Each setting has unique advantages and disadvantages.

Home births are family and person centered. Risks of iatrogenic and nosocomial infections are minimized. Nonpharmacologic techniques are used for support during labor because analgesia and regional anesthesia are not available in the home setting. After giving birth, the postpartum person can rest or sleep in their own bed, feed their infant at will, and enjoy the attention and support of their family and friends. Cheyney, (Bovbjerg, et al., 2014) documented the outcomes associated with planned home birth among low-risk individuals attended by midwives in the United States. Eighty-six percent of those who gave birth at home were exclusively breastfeeding 6 weeks postpartum. Additionally, the planned home birth group had a cesarean rate of 5.2%, well below the national average of 31.9% (Cheyney et al., 2014). Finally, the rates of intrapartum, early neonatal, and late neonatal mortality were quite low, at 1.3, 0.41, and 0.35 per 1000, respectively. Coordinated access to emergency transfer is critical to safe care and good outcomes, as is an integrated maternity care system with excellent, respectful communication among providers (Cheyney, Everson, & Burcher, 2014; Home Birth Summit, 2016).

The freestanding birth center provides a homelike environment, with selected emergency equipment. Birth centers can be accredited by the Commission for the Accreditation of Birth Centers, which assures compliance with national standards for safety and care. Most birth centers do not use analgesics or narcotics. Local anesthesia may be used for perineal repair. Disadvantages are similar to home birth in that emergency transport to a hospital may be necessary if complications arise during labor, birth, or postpartum. Most families are discharged within 6 to 12 hours of birth. Exemplar 15.1 describes Margaret Dorroh's experience in a freestanding birth center. Exemplar 15.2 describes a collaborative care midwifery practice for Alaska Native and American Indian people.

Current US hospital units for labor and birth tend to be dual-purpose rooms; labor and birth occur in the same room, and most rooms are private. The room may have a rocking chair, pull-out couch, and private bath, with a tub or shower. Although individual and nicely appointed, these rooms are part of the larger medical environment designed to treat illness, with fetal monitoring, operating rooms, anesthesia services, and immediate access to neonatal intensive care. The other support staff available (nurses, physicians) may not hold the same philosophy of birth as a physiologic process as midwives. Even for a person without risk factors, there can be a greater tendency to intervene than to support a normal physiologic birth. Pressure to keep labor moving and a reliance on the use of technology can be palpable on a busy hospital obstetric unit. Traditional hospital labor, delivery, and maternity units are designed to care for many patients at a time, making the units easier for staff to function but not necessarily conducive to the physiologic labor process. These units are well suited for high-risk situations requiring access to higher levels of care and special care nurseries. However, midwife-attended births in the United States primarily occur in hospital environments, where most US births occur. Therefore it is incumbent on midwives to create an atmosphere of normalcy and trust in the midst of a culture of technology. The nurse-midwifery philosophy of the normalcy of pregnancy and birth in most situations is beginning to be embraced more widely by the broader health system.

Certified Nurse-Midwife Practice Summary

Nurse-midwives in the United States have a unique approach to care continuity. Nurse-midwives provide prenatal care for a designated caseload, attend labor and birth (often shared in a group care model), see their patients in the postnatal period, and can then provide primary, or sexual, reproductive, and gynecologic care for individuals seeking midwifery care over their life spans. Not all US or international practice models function using this type of continuity; however, CNMs and their patients have embraced such a model in the United States, similar to the obstetric model of care. Nurse-midwives have many opportunities to influence health care and beyond through direct care, their broad scope of practice, and administrative and other leadership positions and by engaging in legislative and policy work. As the number of doctorally prepared midwives continues to increase, whether through the DNP, PhD, DM (doctor of midwifery), or other related degrees, the scope of influence of midwives on the care system as well as on individual care will continue to increase. Nurse-midwifery care is uniquely person focused, independent, and collaborative. It offers access to high-quality care that is safe, satisfying, and individualized to patients' and their families' needs throughout their lives and during the reproductive years.

PROFESSIONAL ISSUES

Image

The image of the nurse-midwife in the United States varies across communities and healthcare settings. As noted, many practitioners call themselves midwives, although there is no single standard for education, regulation, and practice, which leads to confusion. Some US citizens continue to be unaware of the availability of nurse-midwifery services in the healthcare system and the research documenting their excellent outcomes. However, there is considerable evidence of change (Murphy, 2018). CNM-attended births continue to increase; 9.8% of all US births were attended by CNMs in 2018 (Martin et al., 2021), although this number has plenty of room to increase. *US News & World Report* ranked nurse-midwifery at #82 of the 100 best jobs ("100 Best Jobs: Nurse Midwife Overview," 2020), and job growth of 15.7% is anticipated from 2018 to 2028 according to the US Bureau of Labor Statistics (2020). In addition, improved working relationships and partnerships with obstetrician–gynecologists are exemplified by the 2018 joint statement of practice relationships between the ACNM

EXEMPLAR 15.1

NURSE-MIDWIFERY PRACTICE IN A BIRTH CENTER SETTING[a]

The patient education process begins before a patient is accepted into the practice. Orientation sessions are held to provide prospective patients with information to assist them in determining whether they want to have their baby in a birth center. These sessions, conducted by the certified nurse-midwife (CNM), are designed to provide information and a tour of the facility. Prospective patients can see firsthand the comfort measures (e.g., the whirlpool tub) and equipment to handle normal deliveries and emergencies. Finances are discussed, because the cost of care in the birth center is approximately half of that for obstetric care in a hospital setting with a physician. Many insurers, Medicaid, and Medicare cover birthing center care.

In an autonomous setting such as this, clinical documentation must be meticulous, and an individualized health record ensures that accurate, consistent, and complete information is obtained. Thorough health and family histories are taken, including information about the woman's physical health and her psychological well-being:

- Any recent health concerns, including exposure to infectious agents?
- What type of support system does she have in place?
- What resources might she have that are not currently being called on?
- Was the pregnancy planned or a surprise?
- What are her family circumstances?
- Is there a stable relationship, including past or current history of abuse?
- Are there other children?

It is important to document positive and negative influences that can have an impact on the patient's health and the health of her baby. Once the assessment is complete, risk factors that would prevent us from being able to accept a patient are reviewed; if we cannot accept a patient, we make a referral. If no risk factors are identified, we schedule the patient's first visit.

When patients are accepted into the practice, they are told that they are equal partners in their care. It is the goal of patient education to make this a reality. To be active participants in their care, patients are taught to weigh themselves and do their own urine dipstick tests. They participate in charting the information, thus noting the progress of their pregnancy firsthand. The program of care for pregnant patients at our birth center includes 10 to 15 prenatal visits, childbirth classes, labor and delivery in the birth center, a home visit within 72 hours of birth, and two office follow-up visits for mother and baby, one at 1 week and the other at 6 weeks after birth.

Clinical hours are held daily. The CNMs in the practice share in-office visits, teaching classes, and on-call time. Other responsibilities include administration and facility maintenance. We see pregnant patients, postpartum patients with their babies, and gynecologic patients. The amount of time scheduled for a visit is based on need. A first visit for a pregnant patient is 1 hour long. An established gynecologic patient who is coming for her contraceptive medication requires only a few minutes, long enough to establish that she is having no problems.

When a patient is in active labor or her membranes have ruptured, she calls the CNM on duty. We attribute this largely to the educational process that has taken place. She is met at the birth center and examined. On the rare occasion of false labor or very early labor, we are able to individualize care. If a patient lives far away, we may elect to observe progress for a number of hours. If the woman is sleep deprived, she and her labor may benefit from some sedation. We remain with our patients in the birth center during labor. A registered nurse (RN) is on call for every delivery. If the CNM attending the patient is tiring from having been up for a long labor, or several labors, the RN can be called to come in early to care for the patient while the CNM rests. Sometimes, the RN is not needed until close to time for the birth.

The mother-to-be helps us accommodate her wishes by preparing a birth plan. As her due date nears, one of her tasks (along with packing a bag to bring to the birth center and readying her home for a baby) is to write a birth plan, which will become part of her record. This allows her to tell us who she wants with her during labor, what she imagines labor will be like, what she hopes labor will be like, and what comfort measures would assist her during labor. We use this tool in several ways. We evaluate the effectiveness of our teaching by reading what the woman thinks labor will be like and helping her manage expectations. Mention of fears not previously revealed gives us an opportunity to resolve any emotional factors that could hinder a successful labor. Knowing the person(s) that the patient wants with her during labor informs us about her support system. The people present during labor are an important factor in enhancing the woman's experience of labor.

The list of comfort measures is mainly a reminder to us, although it is a key contribution from the patient. In the midst of labor, a woman may forget that she was looking forward to the whirlpool tub for relaxation and pain relief. A glance at the birth plan helps us try the things that the patient has already identified as being potentially helpful to her. The birth plan helps emphasize to the patient that this is her labor, with its inherent responsibilities and rights. Her dignity and worth as a human being are of highest priority, as are the well-being of mother and baby. We try to nourish the woman's self-esteem and strengths that help in labor, life, and motherhood.

Patients are given ample written material to help with their recall of information covered in classes. (If a patient

Continued

EXEMPLAR 15.1
NURSE-MIDWIFERY PRACTICE IN A BIRTH CENTER SETTING—cont'd

is unable to read, extra time is spent providing information verbally and making sure that the patient understands it.) To help the patient assume responsibility for herself and her labor, she is expected to bring food and beverages with her to the birth center that she would like to have available during labor and certain supplies, such as perineal pads, bed pads, and diapers. Patients take their babies home dressed in their own clothes and wrapped in their own blankets. They take with them an instructional booklet that they were given in the postpartum class. The booklet describes mother and baby care for the first few days in detail. Because mothers and babies are discharged early, often in 4 to 6 hours, it is imperative that the mother be prepared to check the baby's temperature and respirations, check her own uterus, and be able to recognize signs of complications that require attention. These are all enumerated in the instructions, and there is room for notes and questions. Having a reference helps new moms feel more secure. If something needs attention, they can always call the nurse-midwife, but they usually find what they need to know in the booklet. It often confirms what they sensed—that everything was okay or that they need to get in touch with the nurse-midwife. Thus new mothers start out having faith in their own perceptions regarding their infants being reinforced.

Empowering our patients, enhancing their decision-making abilities, reinforcing the mind-body connection, and enhancing family life by helping women find their personal power are goals of CNM care at the birth center. When I think of the enormous effects of empowerment, two new moms come to mind.

M.L.'s case is positive proof of the benefits of teaching new mothers to trust their feelings and make decisions based on them. On the third or fourth day after delivery, M.L.'s baby ceased nursing well. He had been nursing vigorously and now was not. Nursing poorly is one of the signs listed in our booklet that requires professional help. M.L. insisted to her husband that they had to go to the emergency room immediately. They lived a long distance from the birth center and it had been decided earlier that if there should be a problem that seemed serious, she should go to a nearby emergency room rather than try to get to the CNM. Initially, doctors could find nothing wrong, but M.L. insisted they keep looking. As it turned out, the baby had a congenital heart defect that does not show up on a clinical examination until 3 or 4 days after birth. M.L. said she was glad she had been given the information at the birth center; it gave her the confidence to trust her feelings that something was seriously wrong. The baby had heart surgery and is doing well.

A woman with confidence and trust in herself can do almost anything, as shown by the case of S.J. She was 26 years old and came to the birth center soon after it opened, to have her fourth child. S.J. had a high school education and was home with her children, all of whom were younger than 5 years. Her self-esteem was negligible. Her husband came to a few of the prenatal classes but was sullen and unsupportive. S.J. seemed to droop, but she was an excellent mother and was an attentive and fast learner regarding everything to do with childbirth, child rearing, and health in general. Her interest and enthusiasm grew as we reinforced her abilities and strengths. By the time she gave birth to her son, she seemed a different person from the withdrawn, self-effacing young woman we had met 7 months earlier. Two years after this baby's birth, S.J. visited the birth center. "I just wanted to thank you," she said. "Before I came here, I never felt I was any good at anything. You told me I was a good mother, you noticed how well cared for my children were, and you encouraged me to learn all about birth and even let me borrow books and tapes. Well, I learned I was good—at a lot of things! You all showed me that. And I wanted you to know I'm in nursing school now because I want to be able to do what you do—not just take care of people physically, but help people grow."

[a]We wish to acknowledge Margaret W. Dorroh, CNM, for this exemplar.

and the ACOG (ACNM, 2018c). The ACNM moved boldly forward in the 2015–2020 strategic plan in support of members and advancing midwifery and women's health by expanding access to midwifery care to all women (ACNM, 2015a). Consumer outreach, including the Healthy Birth Initiative (ACNM, n.d.-c) and an ACNM-produced promotional video *Midwives in Hospitals: A Great Choice for Childbirth* (https://www.youtube.com/watch?v=15YAObX_lrM)—are evidence of increasing visibility and influence (ACNM, n.d.-j).

Work Life

CNMs provide a full range of primary healthcare services for women and those who seek midwifery care, from adolescence through menopause. There is variety in the way these services can be offered, and CNMs are fortunate to have options from which to choose. Full-scope healthcare services encompass ambulatory and in-hospital care, and midwives in full-scope practice usually work the highest number of hours per week compared with midwives in other practice models. Salaries range from $69,000 to $159,000 (median,

$105,000), according to the 2019 data from the US Bureau of Labor Statistics (2020).

If a practice has several nurse-midwives and the call is shared (e.g., one or two nights of call a week for each midwife), along with 2 to 3 days in the ambulatory clinic setting, the workload can be manageable. To give their best to their patients and stay healthy, nurse-midwives with a heavier on-call schedule need to develop self-care strategies that enable them to balance work with personal responsibilities and relationships (Arbour et al., 2019). Perhaps more important, there is increasing evidence about the relationship between fatigue and medical errors, affecting the call schedule of medical residents and prompting numerous organizations to issue alerts and position papers. Professional midwifery organizations and employers need to be proactive in making recommendations about this aspect of quality and safety. The ACNM published a document with recommendations for sleep and safety for midwives and midwifery students (ACNM, 2017c).

Some nurse-midwives may choose an alternative practice model to enhance their personal interests or maximize work-life balance. They may choose to be a laborist, working specific shifts and providing perinatal services in the hospital, including triage and the management of labor and birth when the provider may be unavailable or for patients who have not enrolled with a provider before labor. An ambulatory-only midwifery position is also an option and gives the advantage of regular hours, although the labor and birth component would not be part of this position. Some midwives teach in midwifery programs and may also follow an academic research trajectory. Others have positions in medical program education, teaching medical students and obstetric and family medicine residents about preventive health care and normal pregnancy and birth. For those who love it, the satisfaction of providing care to people during and following pregnancy, assisting during the physical and mental demands of labor and birth, and seeing the joy of a family greeting their newborn make nurse-midwifery an exciting and personally rewarding career, worth the physical and emotional investment that may be required. It is a privilege to be with families experiencing pregnancy and birth. The opposite kind of experiences, when a stillbirth or a newborn with a major genetic or anatomic abnormality occurs, can be difficult for the midwife and families. Yet even in these difficult situations, there is satisfaction in providing support to families as they cope with complex life situations.

Professional Liability

Midwives need to clarify critical details of professional liability insurance; for example, the specific type of policy, whether the policy is to be from an institutional employer or from an individual (and individual vs. group limits of coverage), whether the employer is self-insured or works with a specific insurance company, whether the employer will pay tail coverage for a claims-made policy, and whether or not the employer provides legal counsel if a claim is made. Nurse-midwifery liability insurance rates are generally higher than those for other APRNs because of the malpractice climate of maternity care (Sakala et al., 2013). Professional organizations and individual nurse-midwives work to stay abreast of legislative and practice changes that may help reframe the current litigious environment in which health care occurs, especially for practitioners of midwifery and obstetrics.

The ACNM, through its state and federal legislative offices, supports tort reform that would cap noneconomic damages, limit the number of years in which a plaintiff can file a healthcare liability action, place reasonable limits on punitive damages, and expand alternative dispute resolution methods. In addition to supporting tort reform, the ACNM has developed a professional liability resource packet that seeks to keep CNMs updated on these issues. The organization also emphasizes quality and safety in practice and risk management strategies that help prevent adverse events from occurring. Finally, it seeks to ensure that midwives have a medical liability insurance option available with a strong underwriter and national coverage endorsed by the professional organization; such an option currently exists (ACNM, n.d.-f).

Diversity

The United States is experiencing a crisis in maternity care. Although the United States spends more money on pregnancy and childbirth than any other high-income country in the world, it is leading its global peers in maternal morbidity and mortality.

EXEMPLAR 15.2

NURSE MIDWIVES PRACTICING IN AN INTRASTATE PRACTICE FOR ALASKA NATIVE AND AMERICAN INDIAN PEOPLE[a]

Women in the Alaska Native healthcare system have many stories about the "old days" in labor and delivery. The facilities at the Anchorage-based Indian Health Service hospital were largely unwelcoming and the experience, not at all consistent with traditional birthing wisdom, often caused emotional distress. Alaska Native people pushed for reforms across the entire system of care, envisioning a customer-centered, relationship-based approach in all clinics and departments. A whole system transformation was made possible when the Native Community compacted with the federal government for ownership of the Alaska Native healthcare delivery system in the late 1990s. Shifting away from the old paradigm of "professionals know best," Alaska Native customer-owners were now in the driver's seat.

With Alaska Native organizations (SCF and the Alaska Native Tribal Health Consortium) heading up the new Alaska Native Medical Center (ANMC), customer-driven changes could be made to all facets of service delivery, including midwifery care. At the time, few models of a collaborative physician/midwifery service existed in a hospital system. Prior to customer-ownership, certified nurse-midwives (CNMs) experienced some autonomy when serving as night-shift providers on the labor and delivery unit, when the physicians were on call from home. Nurse-Midwife Janet Froeschle recalls how they would select "the old hand-cranked metal hospital beds" to offer women options beyond being confined to their backs and in stirrups on the notorious delivery tables. Physician and nurse-midwife practice models on the unit differed starkly. With new operational principles in place, a more collaborative service, with physicians and nurse-midwives working in partnership, could be developed to better fit customer needs.

Obstetrician and gynecologist (ob-gyn) Ben Garnett, who has worked at SCF for over 25 years, recalls the efforts of midwives during this time of whole system transformation. "I watched an ever-growing CNM service begin to not only transform the services available to clients, but to transform the way doctors perceived and practiced obstetrics," said Garnett. "As time passed, a truly collaborative system of care evolved."

This new collaborative care model is in alignment with SCF's Nuka System of Care, which is built on a foundation of long-term relationships; transfer of control to the customer-owner; integration of the mind, body, and spirit; and a commitment to measurement and quality. Customer-owners choose their path to health and wellness, with access to a diverse array of services, including integrative therapies (acupuncture, chiropractic, and massage), traditional healing, lactation, nutritional health, behavioral health, and learning circles (a traditional practice of sharing stories and supporting one another). Sustained for over 2 decades, the Nuka System of Care has helped Alaska Native families and communities achieve better care and better health at lower costs.

Similarly, SCF nurse-midwives work to build trusting, accountable relationships with customer-owners with the goal of honoring each sacred birth experience. They strive to better understand customer-owner family values and the context in which customer-owners live while working to eliminate unnecessary barriers to wellness.

ANMC currently employs 20 CNMs and 16 ob-gyns who provide around-the-clock inpatient care. The nurse-midwives also provide outpatient care in SCF's two locations: the Anchorage Native Primary Care Center and Benteh Nuutah Valley Native Primary Care Center, about 40 miles away. The nurse-midwives based in Anchorage are divided into two teams. One team focuses on care for Anchorage customer-owners and the other serves customers with high-risk pregnancies referred from remote Alaska Native villages for gynecologic and maternity care. Women with high-risk pregnancies are typically transferred to Anchorage from outlying villages at 36 weeks gestation. They are seen by the nurse-midwife with consultation from ob-gyns and maternal–fetal medicine providers as needed. These customers are housed in an all-inclusive facility connected to the ANMC hospital by a sky bridge. The facility offers a cafeteria featuring Alaska Native foods such as seal soup, a fitness center, kitchen area, and phone and Internet access. Customer-owners can be accompanied to Anchorage by a friend or family member to provide support during pregnancy, labor, and birth.

SCF's Nuka System of Care offers nurse-midwives opportunities to practice at the top of their professional scope of practice, while staying true to the core belief that pregnancy and birth are normal physiologic processes. Dedicated to bringing aspects of midwifery care to women with high-risk pregnancies, SCF nurse-midwives participate with their physician consultants in twin and breech vaginal deliveries and manage intrapartum care for women who have experienced preeclampsia, gestational diabetes, and intrahepatic cholestasis of pregnancy. In some cases, physician and midwife collaborative management of very high risk women is appropriate. For example, a laboring customer-owner with severe preeclampsia may require medication to control her blood pressure during labor. In this case the ob-gyn manages the customer-owner's blood pressure and the nurse-midwife manages her labor course, all while working together to deliver holistic, customer-centered care.

The nurse-midwives attend most vaginal births at ANMC. In 2019 CNMs attended 84% of the 1257 vaginal births. The successful collaboration between ob-gyns and

EXEMPLAR 15.2

NURSE MIDWIVES PRACTICING IN AN INTRASTATE PRACTICE FOR ALASKA NATIVE AND AMERICAN INDIAN PEOPLE—cont'd

nurse-midwives has contributed to a cesarean rate consistently below the 2018 national average of 31.9%, as reported by the Centers for Disease Control and Prevention (2020). The primary cesarean rate of women admitted to ANMC's labor and delivery unit in 2019 was 17.8%. The same year, the success rate of vaginal birth after cesarean was 62%.

The presence of nurse-midwives to support normal physiologic labor and birth has advanced a midwifery model of care that includes nursing and physician support and collaboration. The intrapartum care team regularly utilizes midwifery-based practices such as intermittent auscultation for fetal monitoring, oral nutrition in labor, nonpharmacologic pain management (frequent position changes, squatting bar, birthing stool, labor tub), access to a birthing mirror, delayed cord clamping, skin-to-skin contact between mother and baby for the first hour after birth, and encouragement of exclusive breastfeeding. Nitrous oxide and sterile water injections are also available to customer-owners for low-risk labor pain management.

The practice of midwifery at SCF/ANMC has progressed from a model of supervision by ob gyns to a model of strong collaboration and partnership focused on customer-centered care. The nurse-midwives are active in discussions on departmental policies and protocols, participating in quality improvement committees with their physician colleagues and striving to implement evidence-based practice models, a cornerstone of the advanced practice registered nurse (APRN) education.

Within the Nuka System of Care, every customer-owner and employee plays a role in healthcare improvement. In this spirit, the midwifery practice continues to evolve, with new opportunities and long-term goals emerging: supporting the Indigenous birth movement through education and training for Native midwives and doulas (labor support professionals), developing a hospital doula program, constructing a culturally appropriate birth center to support "out-of-hospital" birth practices, and offering water births at ANMC. As APRNs, nurse-midwives are skilled innovators. Within the Alaska Native healthcare system today, nurse-midwives are equipped with the infrastructure and tools needed to help achieve culturally relevant, high-quality midwifery care. In this way, nurse-midwives will continue to play an integral role in achieving the SCF Vision: *A Native Community that enjoys physical, mental, emotional, and spiritual wellness.*

[a]We wish to acknowledge Anjali Madeira, DNP, CNM and Jenni Godbold, DNP, CNM for this exemplar.

The disparity worsens for Black, Indigenous, and People of Color (BIPOC); most deaths are preventable. Greenwood et al. (2020) found that patient outcomes improve when there is racial concordance between the provider and the patient. Yet in the United States, approximately 87% of all midwives certified by AMCB identify as White; only 6% identify as Black, 1% identify as Asian, and 0.58% identify as American Indian/Alaska Native, with the remainder falling into other categories or choosing not to report their demographic data (AMCB, 2019). The profession must recruit and graduate midwives with greater racial diversity to match the patient population.

Given this gap, the midwifery profession is actively working to build a more diverse workforce. In fact, the ACNM 2021–2024 strategic plan lists diversity and inclusivity as the top priority (ACNM, 2020c). As part of this initiative, advocacy will focus on securing more funds for midwifery education programs in order to train a more diverse midwifery workforce (ACNM, 2020c). Furthermore, the ACNM has implemented mandatory diversity, inclusivity, and equity training for any member serving in a volunteer capacity within the organization. The organization continues to develop a plan for ensuring equity within the membership and supporting diverse members to improve maternal child health.

ACNM's targeted efforts to address racism within the institution and create an equitable and just professional organization where all midwives can feel welcome include a reconciliation with the past history of the organization. In March 2021 the ACNM board of directors sent an email to all members to "apologize for the systemic racism that has existed and continued in our organization since it incorporated in 1954" (ACNM, personal communication, March 29, 2021). This email included information about the ACNM Truth and Reconciliation Resolution that "acknowledges the harms caused by its previous actions and establishes a set of resolutions in response." The work to diversify the midwifery workforce and create systems that support BIPOC midwives, patients, and families is ongoing and requires work at the local and national levels.

Quality and Safety

Quality and safety are important topics to nurse-midwives. The ACNM has increased its activity through a position statement, *Creating a Culture of Safety in Midwifery Care* (ACNM, 2016b). This document outlines the principles of evidence-based practice, interprofessional team communication, patient-centered care, and participation in quality management programs. The ACNM is a core member of the Alliance for Innovation on Maternal Health program, a national partnership of organizations dedicated to reducing maternal mortality, improving postpartum care, and providing resources for consistency in providing well-woman care in the United States (ACNM, n.d.-b). The ACNM is also a member of the Council on Patient Safety in Women's Health Care (http://safehealthcareforeverywoman.org), providing information to members of collaborating organizations to provide safe care to every person. Partnership with multiple national women's health professional groups on the development of a safety bundle for postpartum hemorrhage, a common cause of maternal morbidity and mortality, exemplifies this work. The resulting paper was published in several professional journals simultaneously, including the *Journal of Midwifery & Women's Health* (Main et al., 2015). Similarly, the ACNM again partnered with multiple professional organizations in publishing "Transforming Communication and Safety Culture in Intrapartum Care: A Multiorganizational Blueprint" (Lyndon et al., 2015).

Nurse-midwifery has a sustained history of reducing health disparities among disadvantaged groups, starting in rural Eastern Kentucky where, over a 30-year period, low birth weight and maternal mortality rates dropped from levels that were among the highest in the country to those among the lowest. From 1925 to 1958, the maternal mortality rate was 9.1 per 10,000 for the Frontier Nursing Service and 34 per 10,000 for the United States as a whole (Metropolitan Life Insurance Company, 1960). Cochrane Review continues to document that midwife-led care models result in fewer medical interventions, greater maternal satisfaction, and a trend toward lower costs with outcomes at least equivalent to other care models (Sandall et al., 2016).

CONCLUSION

Positive advances in nurse-midwifery and between nurse-midwifery and the broader healthcare system are evident. The ACNM has been extending its reach and is partnering to collaborate broadly with professional nursing, other midwifery groups, medicine (including obstetrics and gynecology), policy, and public health colleagues nationally and internationally. In addition, ACNM is committed to greater racial diversity in the profession and the importance of becoming an anti-racist organization. The need for more midwives has been recognized internationally to continue to reduce maternal and neonatal mortality. In the United States the IOM (2011) report *The Future of Nursing*, the PPACA, increased consumer demand, an improved public image, a growing CNM research evidence base, and strong national quality and educational standards have placed CNMs and other APRNs in a visible leadership role in redesigning the healthcare system for the future. From a midwifery perspective, it is anticipated that a future healthcare system will honor all women and offer support in realizing the satisfaction that comes with a truly person-centered healthcare system.

KEY SUMMARY POINTS

- CNMs are primary care providers who are educated in and practice the two distinct disciplines of nursing and midwifery.
- CNMs are educated in graduate programs accredited by the Accreditation Commission for Midwifery Education and are certified by the American Midwifery Certification Board.
- The midwifery model of care practiced by CNMs includes a strong focus on person-centered care and supporting the normalcy of pregnancy and birth as well as other life transitions.
- Midwifery is recognized internationally as a key resource for improving maternal and newborn health in developed and developing countries.
- CNMs practice and have prescribing authority in all 50 states, practice in all types of healthcare settings, and attend births in hospitals, homes, and freestanding birth centers.
- As the number of CNMs and CNM-attended births continues to grow, nurse-midwives continue

building the required evidence base for practice and are fully engaged in collaborative policy efforts to reform the US healthcare system.

REFERENCES

100 Best jobs: Nurse midwife overview. (2020). *US News & World Report*. https://money.usnews.com/careers/best-jobs/nurse-midwife

American Association of Colleges of Nursing. (2006). *The essentials of doctoral education for advanced nursing practice*. http://www.aacn.nche.edu/dnp/Essentials.pdf

American Association of Colleges of Nursing. (2021). The essentials: Core competencies for professional nursing education. https://www.aacnnursing.org/Portals/42/AcademicNursing/pdf/Essentials-2021.pdf

American College of Nurse-Midwives. (n.d.-a). *ACNM Policy Agenda, 2019-2020*. https://www.midwife.org/acnm-policy-agenda

American College of Nurse-Midwives. (n.d.-b). *Alliance for Innovation on Maternal Health (AIM)*. http://www.midwife.org/Alliance-for-Innovation-on-Maternal-Health-AIM

American College of Nurse-Midwives. (n.d.-c). *American College of Nurse-Midwives Healthy Birth Initiative*. https://www.midwife.org/ACNM-Healthy-Birth-Initiative

American College of Nurse-Midwives. (n.d.-d). *BirthTOOLS*. https://www.birthtools.org/

American College of Nurse-Midwives. (n.d.-e). *Midwives and Medicare after health care reform*. http://www.midwife.org/Midwives-and-Medicare-after-Health-Care-Reform

American College of Nurse-Midwives. (n.d.-f). *Professional liability information*. http://www.midwife.org/Professional-Liability-Information

American College of Nurse-Midwives. (n.d.-g). *State fact sheets*. http://www.midwife.org/acnm/files/ccLibraryFiles/Filename/000000005600/ACNMStateFactSheets8-21-15.pdf

American College of Nurse-Midwives. (n.d.-h). *Understanding state practice environments*. http://www.midwife.org/Understanding-State-Practice-Environments

American College of Nurse-Midwives. (n.d.-i). *Volunteers*. https://www.midwife.org/volunteer.

American College of Nurse-Midwives. (n.d.-j). Video: Midwives in hospitals: A great choice for childbirth. https://www.youtube.com/watch?v=15YAObX_lrM

American College of Nurse-Midwives. (2004). *Philosophy of the American College of Nurse-Midwives*. http://www.midwife.org/index.asp?bid=59&cat=2&button=Search&rec=49

American College of Nurse-Midwives. (2011a). *Midwifery in the US and the consensus model for APRN regulation*. http://www.midwife.org/ACNM/files/ccLibraryFiles/Filename/000000001458/LACE_White_Paper_2011.pdf

American College of Nurse-Midwives. (2011b). *The practice doctorate in midwifery*. http://www.midwife.org/ACNM/files/ACNMLibraryData/UPLOADFILENAME/000000000260/Practice%20Doctorate%20in%20Midwifery%20Sept%202011.pdf

American College of Nurse-Midwives. (2011c). *Standards for the practice of midwifery*. http://www.midwife.org/ACNM/files/ACNMLibraryData/UPLOADFILENAME/000000000051/Standards_for_Practice_of_Midwifery_Sept_2011.pdf

American College of Nurse-Midwives. (2012a). *Definition of midwifery and scope of practice of certified nurse-midwives and certified midwives*. https://www.midwife.org/acnm/files/ccLibraryFiles/Filename/000000007043/Definition-of-Midwifery-and-Scope-of-Practice-of-CNMs-and-CMs-Feb-2012.pdf

American College of Nurse-Midwives. (2012b). *Our mission, vision, and core values*. http://www.midwife.org/Our-Mission-Vision-Core-Values

American College of Nurse-Midwives. (2014). *Position statement: Collaborative management in midwifery practice for medical, gynecologic and obstetric conditions*. http://www.midwife.org/ACNM/files/ACNMLibraryData/UPLOADFILENAME/000000000058/Collaborative-Mgmt-in-Midwifery-Practice-Sept-2014.pdf

American College of Nurse-Midwives. (2015a). *ACNM future focus: ACNM strategic planning 2015-2020*. http://www.midwife.org/ACNM-Future-Focus

American College of Nurse-Midwives. (2015b). *Code of ethics with explanatory statements*. http://www.midwife.org/ACNM/files/ACNMLibraryData/UPLOADFILENAME/000000000293/Code-of-Ethics-w-Explanatory-Statements-June-2015.pdf

American College of Nurse-Midwives. (2015c). Intermittent auscultation for intrapartum fetal heart rate surveillance. *Journal of Midwifery and Women's Health, 60*, 626–632.

American College of Nurse-Midwives. (2015d). *Position statement: Mandatory degree requirements for entry into midwifery practice*. https://www.midwife.org/acnm/files/ACNMLibraryData/UPLOADFILENAME/000000000076/Mandatory-Degree-Requirements-June-2015.pdf

American College of Nurse-Midwives. (2016a). *ACNM re-entry to midwifery practice*. http://www.midwife.org/Re-entry-Guidelines-for-CNMs/CMs

American College of Nurse-Midwives. (2016b). *Position statement: Creating a culture of safety in midwifery care*. http://www.midwife.org/ACNM/files/ACNMLibraryData/UPLOADFILENAME/000000000059/Creating-a-culture-of-safety-in-midwifery-care-MAR2016.pdf

American College of Nurse Midwives. (2017a). *Letter to Senate Majority Leader McConnell and Minority Leader Schumer*. https://www.midwife.org/acnm/files/ccLibraryFiles/Filename/000000006641/ACNM.letter.HELP.SFC.ACA.REFORM.FINAL.pdf

American College of Nurse-Midwives. (2017b). *Position statement: Collaborative agreement between certified nurse-midwives/certified midwives and physicians or other health care providers*. https://www.midwife.org/acnm/files/ACNMLibraryData/UPLOADFILENAME/000000000057/Collaborative-Agreement-PS-FINAL-10-10-17.pdf

American College of Nurse-Midwives. (2017c). *Position statement: Fatigue, sleep deprivation, and safety*. https://www.midwife.org/acnm/files/ACNMLibraryData/UPLOADFILENAME/000000000306/Sleep-Guidelines-04-07-17.pdf

American College of Nurse-Midwives. (2017). *Position statement: Independent midwifery practice*. https://www.midwife.org/acnm/files/ACNMLibraryData/UPLOADFILENAME/000000000073/PS-Independent-Midwifery-Practice-FINAL-Feb-2018.pdf

American College of Nurse-Midwives. (2018a). *2018 annual report.* https://www.midwife.org/acnm/files/cclibraryfiles/filename/000000007568/2018%20Annual%20Report_FINAL.pdf

American College of Nurse-Midwives. (2018b). Medication assisted treatment and certified nurse-midwives. *Policy issue brief.* http://www.midwife.org/acnm/files/cclibraryfiles/filename/000000007450/CNMs%20and%20MAT%20Background%20and%20Issue%20Brief.pdf#:~:text=This%20Act%20expands%20earlier%20legislation,substance%20and%20opioid%20use%20disorder

American College of Nurse-Midwives. (2018c). *Position statement: Joint statement of practice relations between obstetrician/gynecologists and certified nurse-midwives/certified midwives.* https://www.midwife.org/acnm/files/acnmlibrarydata/uploadfilename/000000000224/ACNM-College-Policy-Statement-(June-2018).pdf

American College of Nurse-Midwives. (2018d). *Position statement: Midwives are primary care providers and leaders of maternity care homes.* http://www.midwife.org/ACNM/files/ACNMLibraryData/UPLOADFILENAME/000000000273/Primary%20Care%20Position%20Statement%20June%202012.pdf

American College of Nurse-Midwives. (2018e). *Quick reference: Practice environments for certified nurse-midwives as of June 2018.* https://www.midwife.org/acnm/files/cclibraryfiles/filename/000000007539/practice%20enviro%20map.jpg

American College of Nurse-Midwives. (2019a). *ACME policies and procedures manual for the preaccreditation and accreditation of midwifery education programs.* https://www.midwife.org/acnm/files/cclibraryfiles/filename/000000007635/ACMEPoliciesandProceduresManual(revised%20December%202019).pdf

American College of Nurse-Midwives. (2019b). *Essential facts about midwives.* https://www.midwife.org/acnm/files/cclibraryfiles/filename/000000007531/EssentialFactsAboutMidwives-UPDATED.pdf

American College of Nurse-Midwives. (2019c). *Midwifery education and doctoral preparation.* https://www.midwife.org/acnm/files/acnmlibrarydata/uploadfilename/000000000079/PS%20Midwifery%20Education%20and%20Doctoral%20Preparation%20190927.pdf

American College of Nurse-Midwives. (2020a). *ACME accredited programs.* https://portal.midwife.org/education/accredited-programs

American College of Nurse-Midwives. (2020b). *Core competencies for basic midwifery practice.* https://www.midwife.org/acnm/files/acnmlibrarydata/uploadfilename/000000000050/ACNMCoreCompetenciesMar2020_final.pdf

American College of Nurse-Midwives. (2020c). *Strategic plan 2021–2024.* https://www.midwife.org/acnm/files/cclibraryfiles/filename/000000008086/ACNM%202021-24%20Srategic%20Plan%20Updated%2011.17.2020.pdf

American College of Nurse-Midwives, Accreditation Commission for Midwifery Education and American Midwifery Certification Board. (2011). *Midwifery in the US and the Consensus Model for APRN Regulation.* http://www.midwife.org/acnm/files/ccLibraryFiles/Filename/000000001458/LACE_White_Paper_2011.pdf

American College of Obstetricians and Gynecologists. (2017). Joint statement of practice relations between obstetrician-gynecologists and certified nurse-midwives/certified midwives. *Journal of Obstetrics and Gynecology, 129*, e117–e122.

American Midwifery Certification Board. (2018a). *About American Midwifery Certification Board (AMCB).* https://www.amcbmidwife.org/about-amcb

American Midwifery Certification Board. (2018b). *Certificate maintenance program: Purpose/objective.* https://www.amcbmidwife.org/certificate-maintenance-program/purpose-objectives

American Midwifery Certification Board. (2019). *2019 demographic report.* https://www.amcbmidwife.org/docs/default-source/reports/demographic-report-2019.pdf?sfvrsn=23f30668_2#:~:text=General%20Demographic%20Data&text=Not%20surprisingly%2C%20approximately%2099%25%20of,most%20common%20group%20(6.31%25)

American Midwifery Certification Board. (2020). *Certified nurse-midwives/certified midwives by state.* https://www.amcbmidwife.org/docs/default-source/reports/number-of-cnm-cm-by-state–may-2019.pdf?sfvrsn=4ae04b1e_10

Angood, P. B., Armstrong, E. M., Ashton, D., Burstin, H., Corry, M. P., Delbanco, S. F., Fildes, B., Fox, D. M., Gluck, P. A., Gullo, S. L., Howes, J., Jolivet, R. R., Laube, D. W., Lynne, D., Main, E., Markus, A. R., Mayberry, L., Mitchell, L. V., Ness, D. L., … Salganicoff, A. (2010). Blueprint for action: Steps toward a high-quality, high-value maternity care system. *Women's Health Issues, 20*, S18–S49.

APRN Joint Dialogue Group. (2008). *Consensus model for APRN regulation: Licensure, accreditation, certification and education.* https://www.ncsbn.org/Consensus_Model_Report.pdf

Arbour, M., Tanner, T., Hensley, J., Beardsley, J., Wika, J., & Garvan, C. (2019). Factors that contribute to cxcessive sleepiness in midwives practicing in the US. *Journal of Midwifery and Women's Health, 64*(2), 179–185. doi:10.1111/jmwh.12945

Avery, M. D., Bell, A. D., Bingham, D., Corry, M. P., Delbanco, S. F., Gullo, S. L., Ivory, C. H., Jennings, J. C., Kennedy, H. P., Kozhimannil, K. B., Leeman, L., Lothian, J. A., Miller, H. D., Ogburn, T., Romano, A., Sakala, C., & Shah, N. T. (2018). Blueprint for advancing high-value maternity care through physiologic childbearing. *Journal of Perinatal Education, 27*(3), 130–134.

Avery, M. D., Jennings, J. C., Germano, E., Andrighetti, T., Autry, A. M., Dau, K. Q., Krause, S. A., Montgomery, O. C., Nicholson, T. B., Perry, A., Rauk, P. N., Sankey, H. Z., & Woodland, M. B. (2020). Interprofessional education between midwifery students and obstetrics and gynecology residents: An American College of Nurse-Midwives and American College of Obstetricians and Gynecologists collaboration. *Journal of Midwifery and Women's Health, 65*(2), 257–264.

Brauer, S. (2016). Moral implications of obstetric technologies for pregnancy and motherhood. *Medicine, Health Care, and Philosophy, 19*(1), 45–54.

Bushman, J. (2014). *Letter to Federal Trade Commission on behalf of ACNM.* http://www.midwife.org/acnm/files/ccLibraryFiles/Filename/000000004094/FTCComments-Final.pdf

Centers for Disease Control. (2020). *Births-method of delivery.* https://www.cdc.gov/nchs/fastats/delivery.htm

Centers for Medicare & Medicaid Services. (2018). *Strong start for mothers and newborns: Evaluation of full performance period (2018).* https://innovation.cms.gov/files/reports/strongstart-prenatal-fg-finalevalrpt.pdf

Centers for Medicare & Medicaid Services. (2020). *Strong start for mothers and newborns initiative: General information.* https://innovation.cms.gov/innovation-models/strong-start

Cheyney, M., Bovbjerg, M., Everson, C., Gordon, W., Hannibal, D., & Vedam, S. (2014). Outcomes of care for 16,924 planned home births in the US: The Midwives Alliance of North America Statistics Project, 2004 to 2009. *Journal of Midwifery and Women's Health, 59*(1), 17–27.

Cheyney, M., Everson, C., & Burcher, P. (2014). Homebirth transfers in the US: Narratives of risk, fear, and mutual accommodation. *Qualitative Health Research, 24*(4), 443–456.

Choi, K. R., & Seng, J. S. (2016). Predisposing and precipitating factors for dissociation during labor in a cohort study of posttraumatic stress disorder and childbearing outcomes. *Journal of Midwifery and Women's Health, 61*(1), 68–76.

Choi, K. R., Seng, J. S., Briggs, E. C., Munro-Kramer, M. L., Graham-Bermann, S. A., Lee, R. C., & Ford, J. D. (2017). The dissociative subtype of Posttraumatic Stress Disorder (PTSD) among adolescents: Co-occurring PTSD, depersonalization/derealization, and other sissociation symptoms. *J Am Acad Child Adolesc Psychiatry, 56*(12), 1062–1072.

Cockerham, A. Z. (2019). History of midwifery in the US. In K. Osborne, C. M. Jevitt, T. L. King, & M. C. Brucker (Eds.), *Varney's midwifery* (pp. 3–34): Jones & Bartlett Learning.

Cooney, P., & Johnson, T. (2012). ACNM urges improved access to clinical privileges. *Quickening, 43*(2), 9. Retrieved from http://www.midwife.org/quickening

Dahlen, H. G., Downe, S., Wright, M. L., Kennedy, H. P., & Taylor, J. Y. (2016). Childbirth and consequent atopic disease: Emerging evidence on epigenetic effects based on the hygiene and EPIIC hypotheses. *BMC Pregnancy and Childbirth, 16*(1), 4.

Greenwood, B. N., Hardeman, R. R., Huang, L., & Sojourner, A. (2020). Physician-patient racial concordance and disparities in birthing mortality for newborns. *Proceedings of the National Academy of Sciences of the United States of America, 117*(35), 21194–21200. doi:10.1073/pnas.1913405117

Health Resources & Service Administration. (2020). *Scholarships for disadvantaged students.* https://www.hrsa.gov/grants/find-funding/hrsa-20-006

Home Birth Summit. (2016). *Common ground statements.* http://www.homebirthsummit.org/summits/vision/statements/

Ickovics, J. R., Lewis, J. B., Cunningham, S. D., Thomas, J., & Magriples, U. (2019). Transforming prenatal care: Multidisciplinary team science improves a broad range of maternal child outcomes. *The American Psychologist, 74*(3), 343–355. doi:10.1037/amp0000435

Institute of Medicine. (2015). *Assessing progress on the Institute of Medicine Report The Future of Nursing.* The National Academies Press.

Institute of Medicine (IOM), & Committee on the Robert Wood Johnson Foundation Initiative on the Future of Nursing. (2011). *The future of nursing: Leading change, advancing health.* National Academies Press.

International Confederation of Midwives. (2013). *Global standards for midwifery education* (2010); amended 2013. https://www.internationalmidwives.org/assets/files/general-files/2018/04/icm-standards-guidelines_ammended2013.pdf

International Confederation of Midwives. (2014a). *ICM global standards, competencies and tools.* http://www.internationalmidwives.org/what-we-do/global-standards-competencies-and-tools.html

International Confederation of Midwives. (2014b). *International code of ethics for midwives.* http://internationalmidwives.org/assets/uploads/documents/CoreDocuments/CD2008_001%20V2014%20ENG%20International%20Code%20of%20Ethics%20for%20Midwives.pdf

International Confederation of Midwives. (2017). *ICM international definition of the midwife.* https://www.internationalmidwives.org/assets/files/definitions-files/2018/06/eng-definition_of_the_midwife-2017.pdf

Jefferson, K., Bouchard, M. E., & Summers, L. (2021). The regulation of professional midwifery in the US. *Journal of Nursing Regulation, 11*(4), 26–38. doi:10.1016/S2155-8256(20)30174-5

Kennedy, H. P. (2010). The problem of normal birth. *Journal of Midwifery and Women's Health, 55*, 199–201.

Kennedy, H. P., Kozhimannil, K. B., & Sakala, C. (2018). Using the blueprint for advancing high-value maternity care for transformative change. *Birth Issues in Perinatal Care, 45*(4), 331–335.

Kennedy, H. P., Meyers-Ciecko, J. A., Carr, K. C., Breedlove, G., Bailey, T., Farrell, M. V., Lawlor, M., & Darraugh, I. (2018). US model midwifery legislation and regulation: Development of a consensus document. *Journal of Midwifery and Women's Health, 63*, 652–659.

Lyndon, A., Johnson, C. M., Bingham, D., Napolitano, G. P., Joseph, G., Maxfield, D. G., & O'Keefe, D. G (2015). Transforming communication and safety culture in intrapartum care: A multi-organization blueprint. *Journal of Midwifery and Women's Health, 60*(3), 237–243.

MacDorman, M., & Declercq, E. (2019). Trends and state variations in out-of-hospital births in the US, 2004-2017. *Birth, 46*(2), 279–288. doi:10.1111/birt.12411

Main, E. K., Gofman, D., Scavone, B. M., Low, L. K., Bingham, D., Fontaine, P. L., Gorlin, J. G., Lagrew, D. C., & Levy, B. S. (2015). National partnership for maternal safety consensus bundle on obstetric hemorrhage. *Journal of Midwifery and Women's Health, 60*(4), 458–464.

Martin, J. A., Hamilton, B. E., Osterman, M. J. K., & Driscoll, A. K. (2021). Births: Final data for 2019. *National Vital Statistics Report, 70*(2). doi:10.15620/cdc:100472 National Center for Health Statistics.

Metropolitan Life Insurance Company. (1960). Summary of the tenth thousand confinement records of the Frontier Nursing Service. *Bulletin of the American College of Nurse-Midwifery, 5*(1), 1–9.

Midwives Alliance of North America. (2016). *Types of midwives.* https://mana.org/about-midwives/types-of-midwife

Murphy, C. (2018). Midwives are increasing in popularity. Here's what you need to know. *Healthline Parenthood.* https://www.healthline.com/health/midwives-growing-in-popularity-what-to-know

National Academy of Medicine. (2020). *The future of nursing 2020-2030.* https://nam.edu/publications/the-future-of-nursing-2020-2030/

National Academies of Sciences, Engineering, and Medicine. (2021). *The future of nursing 2020-2030: Charting a path to achieve health equity*. The National Academies Press. doi:10.17226/25982

NCSBN. (2021). *State response to COVID-19 as of April 12, 2021.* https://www.ncsbn.org/State_COVID-19_Response.pdf

North American Registry of Midwives. (2020). *Equivalency applicants.* http://narm.org/equivalency-applicants/

North American Registry of Midwives. (2021). *Candidate information booklet.* http://narm.org/pdffiles/CIB.pdf

Oxford University Press. (n.d.). *Oxford English dictionary.*Retrieved March 16, 2021, from https://www.oed.com/

Perriman, N., Davis, D. L., & Ferguson, S. (2018). What women value in the midwifery continuity of care model: A systematic review with meta-synthesis. *Midwifery, 62*, 220–229.

Ranchoff, B. L., & Declercq, E. R. (2019). The scope of midwifery practice regulations and the availability of the certified nurse-midwifery and certified midwifery workforce, 2012-2016. *Journal of Midwifery and Women's Health, 65*(1), 119–130.

Renfrew, M. J., McFadden, A., Bastos, M. H., Campbell, J., Channon, A. A., Cheung, N. F., Silva, D. R., Downe, S., Kennedy, H. P., Malata, A., McCormick, F., Wick, L., & Declercq, E. (2014). Midwifery and quality care: Findings from a new evidence-informed framework for maternal and newborn care. *Lancet, 384*(9948), 1129–1145.

Sakala, C., Yang, Y. T., & Corry, M. P. (2013). *Maternity care and liability: Pressing problems, substantive solutions.* Childbirth Connection. http://transform.childbirthconnection.org/reports/liability/

Sandall, J., Soltani, H., Gates, S., Shennan, A., & Devane, D. (2016). Midwife-led continuity models versus other models of care for childbearing women. *The Cochrane Database of Systematic Reviews*(4) Art. No.: CD004667.

Seng, J. S., D'Andrea, W., & Ford, J. D (2014). Complex mental health sequelae of psychological trauma among women in prenatal care. *Psychological Trauma, 6*(1), 41–49.

Seng, J. S., Li, Y., Yang, J. J., King, A. P., Low, Kane, L.M., Sperlich, M., Rowe, H., Lee, H., Muzik, M., Ford, J., D., & Liberzon, I. (2018). Gestational and postnatal cortisol profiles of women with posttraumatic stress disorder and the dissociative subtype. *Journal of Obstetrics, Gynecologic, and Neonatal Nurses, 47*(1), 12–22.

Seng, J. S., Sperlich, M., Low, L. K., Ronis, D. L., Muzik, M., & Liberzon, I. (2013). Childhood abuse history, posttraumatic stress disorder, postpartum mental health, and bonding: A prospective cohort study. *Journal of Midwifery and Women's Health, 58*(1), 57–68.

Shorten, A., Fagerlin, A., Illuzzi, J., Kennedy, H. P., Lakehomer, H., Pettker, C. M., Saran, A., Witteman, H., & Whittemore, R. (2015). Developing an Internet-based decision aid for women choosing between vaginal birth after cesarean and planned repeat cesarean. *Journal of Midwifery & Women's Health, 60*(4), 390–400.

Shorten, A., Shorten, B., & Kennedy, H. P. (2014). Complexities of choice after prior cesarean: A narrative analysis. *Birth, 41*(2), 17–84.

Thompson, F. E. (2003). The practice setting: Site of ethical conflict for some mothers and midwives. *Nursing Ethics, 10*, 588–601.

Thompson, J. B. (2002). Moving from codes of ethics to ethical relationships for midwifery practice. *Nursing Ethics, 9*, 522–536.

Ulrich, L. T. (1990). *A midwife's tale: The life of Martha Ballard, based on her diary* (pp. 1785–1812). Knopf/Random House.

UNFPA. (2021). The state of the world's midwifery 2021. unfpa.org/sites/default/files/pub-pdf/21-038-UNFPA-SoWMy2021-Report-ENv4302.pdf

United Nations Population Fund. (2014). *The state of the world's midwifery 2014. A universal pathway. A woman's right to health.* http://www.unfpa.org/sowmy

US Bureau of Labor Statistics. (2020). *Occupational employment statistics: Occupational employment and wages, May 2019: 29-1161 Nurse midwives.* https://www.bls.gov/oes/current/oes291161.htm

Vedam, S., Stoll, K., MacDorman, M., Declercq, E., Cramer, R., Cheyney, M., Fisher, E. B., Yang, Y. T., & Kennedy, H. P. (2018). Mapping integration of midwives across the US: Impact on access, equity, and outcomes. *PLoS ONE, 13*(2), Article e0192523.

World Health Organization. (2019). *Maternal mortality.* https://www.who.int/news-room/fact-sheets/detail/maternal-mortality

Yang, Y. T., & Kozhimannil, K. B. (2015). Making a case to reduce legal impediments to midwifery practice in the US. *Women's Health Issues, 25*, 314–317.

16 THE CERTIFIED REGISTERED NURSE ANESTHETIST

MICHAEL J. KREMER

"Despite everything, no one can dictate who you are to other people."
~ Prince, Musician

CHAPTER CONTENTS

BRIEF HISTORY OF CRNA EDUCATION AND PRACTICE 520
- Education 520
- Certification 520
- Continued Professional Competence 521
- Practice 521
- Role Differentiation Between CRNAs and Anesthesiologists 522

PROFILE OF THE CRNA 523
- Scope and Standards of Practice 524
- Education 524
- Programs of Study 527
- Nurse Anesthesia Educational Funding 529
- Practice Doctorate 530
- Institutional Credentialing 530

ROLE DEVELOPMENT AND MEASURES OF CLINICAL COMPETENCE 531
- Direct Clinical Practice 531
- Guidance and Coaching 534
- Evidence-Based Practice 535
- Leadership 536
- Collaboration 538
- Ethical Practice 541

CURRENT CRNA PRACTICE 542
- Workforce Issues 543
- Access to Care 543
- Reimbursement 544

NURSE ANESTHESIA ORGANIZATIONS 546
- American Association of Nurse Anesthesiology 546
- International Federation of Nurse Anesthetists and International Practice 546

FUTURE DIRECTIONS FOR CRNA PRACTICE 547

CONCLUSION 547

KEY SUMMARY POINTS 548

The author gratefully acknowledges the opportunity to collaborate with Margaret Faut Callahan, PhD, CRNA, FNAP, FAAN, on development of this content for the first six editions of this text.

Nurse anesthesia is the oldest organized advanced practice registered nurse (APRN) specialty (Chapter 1). Standardized postgraduate education, credentialing, and continuing education are all areas pioneered by these APRNs. In 1989 certified registered nurse anesthetists (CRNAs) were the first nurse specialists to receive direct reimbursement for their services. This chapter discusses the professional definitions of nurse anesthesia practice and issues important to this APRN specialty. A profile of current CRNA practice is provided and a model of professional competence for CRNAs is presented. The transition of nurse anesthesia education to the practice doctorate and the associated competencies for CRNAs prepared at the doctoral level will also be reviewed. The American Association of Nurse Anesthesiology (AANA) is described. Finally, challenges and future trends pertinent to the CRNA role are proposed.

The Institute of Medicine (IOM) report on the *Future of Nursing* (IOM, 2011) advocated for nurses and APRNs to practice at the full scope of their education and licensure and assessed progress toward attaining these and other goals in 2015 (Harper, 2016). Like other APRNs, CRNAs have faced physician resistance to a Veterans Administration proposal to expand practice for APRNs to allow them to practice to the full extent of their education and licensure. CRNAs have been part of the movement to transform nursing education and were the first APRN group to require a practice doctorate for entry to practice. As the National Academies of Sciences, Engineering, and Medicine's (NASEM) *Future of Nursing 2020–2030: Charting a Path to Achieve Health Equity* (2021) is rolled out, nurse anesthesia practice will adopt new recommendations where appropriate.

BRIEF HISTORY OF CRNA EDUCATION AND PRACTICE

Nurses have provided anesthesia in the United States since the American Civil War (1861–1865). The first organized program in nurse anesthesia education was offered in 1909. Alumnae from nurse anesthesia programs formed the National Association of Nurse Anesthetists (NANA) in 1931; the organization was renamed the American Association of Nurse Anesthetists (AANA) in 1939. In 2021, AANA re-branded the organization, now known as the American Association of Nurse Anesthesiology (AANA, 2021a). Nurse anesthesia was the first nursing specialty to offer a certification examination (1945) and to have programmatic accreditation (1952), mandatory continuing education (1978), and direct billing under Medicare Part B (1986).

Education

From its inception in 1931, NANA worked to improve and standardize education for nurse anesthetists. In 1933 NANA trustees agreed on minimum standards for schools of anesthesia. By 1937, the NANA Credentials Committee determined that graduation from 1 of 17 approved schools was a requirement for NANA membership. Interprofessional collaboration initiated by NANA to develop a specialty accreditation process began in 1938, when the American Hospital Association and the American Board of Surgery supported its efforts to develop an accreditation mechanism, which was implemented in 1952. The accreditation standards that were developed reflected collaboration between higher education advisors and nurse anesthesia program directors (Horton & Kremer, 2020).

By 1954, there were 106 schools of anesthesia in the United States, 82 of which were fully accredited by AANA. Standardized curricular content was developed by the AANA education director in the form of 13 content modules. In 1955 AANA was recognized by the US Office of Education (OE) as the accrediting body for nurse anesthesia educational programs. The accreditation standards were revised periodically, and AANA held workshops for CRNA educators on topics including the selection of students, transfers between programs, transcripts, course content, teaching, and other issues. By 1970 the AANA criteria for education stipulated an 18-month program of study, with a minimum of 450 clinical cases and at least 300 hours of classroom instruction. A class outline with required content areas and clinical experiences was included with these criteria. The minimum program length was increased to 24 months in 1972 (Horton & Kremer, 2020).

In 1975 the AANA developed autonomous councils to administer the areas of accreditation, certification, recertification, and public interest. The Council on Accreditation of Nurse Anesthesia Educational Programs (COA) was created to be autonomous in decision making and eliminate possible conflicts of interest. COA responsibilities included formulating and adopting accreditation policies and procedures, advising on formulation of educational standards and guidelines, administering the accreditation programs, and investigating complaints submitted against programs. COA mandated a master's degree for entry to practice by 1998, and students entering nurse anesthesia programs on January 1, 2022, and thereafter must be enrolled in a doctoral program (Horton & Kremer, 2020). At this writing, there are 124 accredited nurse anesthesia programs in the United States. The distribution of degrees currently offered by nurse anesthesia programs in the United States is doctor of nursing practice (DNP), 60%; doctor of nurse anesthesia practice (DNAP), 20%; and master's degree, 20% (Council on Accreditation of Nurse Anesthesia Educational Programs [COA], 2021).

Certification

The AANA was responsible for development and administration of the national nurse anesthesia certification examination from 1945 until 1975, when the Council on Certification of Nurse Anesthetists (CCNA) was formed. The CRNA credential came into existence in 1956. AANA members voted to adopt a mandatory continuing education and recertification process in 1978, when the Council on Recertification (COR) of Nurse Anesthetists was formed. In 2007 the CCNA and COR were incorporated as the National Board for Certification and Recertification of Nurse Anesthetists (NBCRNA).

The NBCRNA credentialing process provides assurance to the public, legislators, regulators, and third-party payers that certified individuals have met the qualifications for providing nurse anesthesia services. State licensure provides the legal credential for professional nursing practice, while private voluntary certification demonstrates that successful examinees meet the nurse anesthesia professional practice standards. The CRNA credential is used in many institutional position descriptions. This credential has been recognized through malpractice litigation, through state nurse practice acts, and in state rules and regulations (NBCRNA, 2020a). NBCRNA is accredited by the National Commission for Certifying Agencies (NCCA) and the Accreditation Board for Specialty Nursing Certification (ABSNC) of the American Board of Nursing Specialties (ABNS).

There are 55,700 certified registered nurse anesthetists (CRNAs) in the United States who work in every type of healthcare setting. CRNAs are the sole anesthesia providers in most rural hospitals and are the primary anesthesia providers for members of the US Armed Forces. The initial didactic and clinical education of nurse anesthetists, followed by certification and continued professional competence requirements, demonstrates a commitment to safety and quality in anesthesia care (NBCRNA, 2020a).

NBCRNA determines the eligibility requirements for individuals wishing to take the National Certification Examination (NCE). Those requirements include possession of a current, unrestricted registered professional nursing license, completion of a COA-accredited nurse anesthesia program within the two previous calendar years, and submission of required application documents to the NBCRNA (NBCRNA, 2020d).

The NCE is intended to measure the knowledge, skills, and abilities necessary for entry-level nurse anesthetists. The NCE is a variable-length computerized adaptive test. The examination is for entry into nurse anesthesia practice. Each candidate completes a minimum of 100 test questions, of which 70 items reflect the NCE content outline and 30 questions are random, nongraded pretest questions. The maximum number of questions is 170 items, which include the 30 random, nongraded pretest questions. The national first-time pass rate for the NCE is 84.8%. The content outline for the NCE is in Box 16.1.

Continued Professional Competence

NBCRNA operates a continued professional certification (CPC) program that reflects the professional mandates for maintenance of certification. The CPC program "supports lifelong learning and the strong CRNA credential," protecting continued CRNA practice and meeting the APRN regulatory requirements of every state board of nursing (NBCRNA, 2020b). The CPC program includes four components: Class A and B credits, core modules, and the CPC Assessment. A total of 60 Class A credits are required per 4-year cycle. Class A credits can be earned through participation in approved continuing education courses. There are 40 required Class B credits per 4-year cycle. Class B credits can be earned through a wide range of professional activities; for example, teaching, publishing, and participating in morbidity and mortality conferences. NBCRNA requires completion of four core modules per 4-year cycle. Core modules are specialized Class A credits, focused on recently emerging information and evidence-based knowledge in four core domains of nurse anesthesia practice: airway management, applied clinical pharmacology, human physiology and pathophysiology, and anesthesia equipment and technology. A continued professional certification assessment (CPCA) must be completed every 8 years. The CPCA "is a performance standard assessment" that assesses examinee knowledge in the four core domains of nurse anesthesia practice (NBCRNA, 2020b).

Practice

In addition to 55,700 CRNAs, there are 3114 new students enrolled in US nurse anesthesia programs. CRNAs administer more than 49 million anesthetics to patients annually in the United States and are the primary anesthesia providers in rural areas, enabling

BOX 16.1

National Certification Examination (NCE) Content Outline

Basic sciences (25%)
- Anatomy, physiology, and pathophysiology
- Pharmacology
- Applied chemistry, biochemistry, and physics

Equipment, instrumentation, and technology (15%)
- Anesthetic delivery systems
- Airway equipment
- Monitoring devices
- Imaging

General principles of anesthesia (30%)
- Ethical considerations
- Legal issues
- Safety and wellness
- Preoperative assessment and preparation of patient
- Fluid volume assessment and management
- Positioning
- Utilization and interpretation of data
- Airway management
- Local/regional anesthetics (technique, physiologic alterations, complications)
- Light, moderate, and deep sedation (monitored anesthesia care)
- Pain management
- Pain theory (anatomy, physiology, pathology, psychodynamics)
- Other techniques
- Postanesthesia care/respiratory therapy

Anesthesia for surgical procedures and special populations (30%)
- Surgical and diagnostic anesthesia, including management of complications
- Anesthesia for special populations

Adapted from National Board for Certification and Recertification of Nurse Anesthetists (2020d). *National certification examination content outline.* https://www.nbcrna.com/docs/default-source/publications-documentation/handbooks/nce_hb(1).pdf?sfvrsn=5ed2310c_4

facilities in rural and medically underserved areas to offer obstetric, surgical, pain management, and trauma stabilization services. CRNAs practice in every setting where anesthesia is provided, including traditional hospital operating rooms and obstetric units; critical access hospitals; ambulatory surgical centers; the offices of dentists, podiatrists, ophthalmologists, plastic surgeons, and pain management specialists; and US military, public health services, and Department of Veterans Affairs healthcare facilities. CRNAs are the primary anesthesia providers to US military personnel in all foreign and domestic deployment settings (American Association of Nurse Anesthesiology [AANA], 2019b). CRNAs provide general anesthesia, regional anesthesia (spinal and epidural as well as peripheral nerve blocks), and monitored anesthesia care (local anesthesia with intravenous sedation) to patients across the life span at all acuity levels (AANA, 2019b).

Nurse anesthesia practice involves interactions with patients and their families. Informed consent for anesthesia care includes considering the patient and family cultural values and health beliefs (e.g., socioeconomic status, family structure, health-seeking behaviors, immigration status, country of origin, migration history) and decision-making styles (e.g., familial, individual, delegated, deferential; AANA, 2019a). Decisions related to anesthesia are driven by personal experience and values, healthcare literacy, and information provided by clinicians from surgery and anesthesia during the informed consent process (Feinstein et al., 2018; Gentry et al., 2019; Niyogi & Clarke, 2012). Anesthesia decisions are intertwined with decisions about surgery (Boss et al., 2017; Chan et al., 2019). The decision to have surgery and anesthesia occurs before the anesthesia provider obtains informed consent, which typically occurs shortly before surgery. During this interaction, the patient, or parent/guardian of a minor, is informed about anesthetic options for the planned surgery as well as the associated risks and benefits (Feinstein et al., 2018). It is incumbent on the CRNA to ensure that questions and concerns from the patient and their family members about anesthesia are addressed prior to surgery.

Role Differentiation Between CRNAs and Anesthesiologists

CRNAs provide anesthesia in collaboration with surgeons, dentists, podiatrists, physician anesthesiologists, and other qualified healthcare professionals.

When anesthesia is administered by a nurse anesthetist, it is recognized as the practice of nursing; when administered by a physician anesthesiologist, it is recognized as the practice of medicine. Regardless of whether their educational background is in nursing or medicine, all anesthesia professionals provide anesthesia in a similar manner (AANA, 2019b).

Healthcare systems and facilities have addressed rising costs and flat or declining reimbursement for surgical and diagnostic services, resulting in increased demand for CRNAs, who are paid significantly less than anesthesiologists while providing many of the same services. The mean annual CRNA compensation is $190,247, while the average annual anesthesiologist salary is $436,404. Since outcomes data are positive for CRNAs, this enhances their participation in emerging quality/value-based reimbursement mechanisms (AANA, 2018a, 2020g; Merritt Hawkins, 2019).

CRNAs are responsible for their own professional practice. Surgeons are not legally liable for the actions of CRNAs when they order administration of anesthesia but do not control the course of an anesthetic. Surgeons rely on CRNAs as anesthesia experts who use independent judgment to determine the appropriate type of anesthesia to be administered, including drugs and doses. From a legal perspective, when a surgeon requests that a CRNA administer anesthesia, the surgeon is not liable for the CRNA's actions (AANA, 2020i).

Courts usually apply the same standard of anesthesia care, whether the provider is a CRNA or anesthesiologist. From a legal perspective, *standard of care* refers to what a competent provider in the same field would do in the same situation, with the same resources (Moffett & Moore, 2011). Courts examine the degree of control that surgeons exercise over the anesthesia providers, which typically is minimal, when determining their potential liability for anesthesia outcomes (AANA, 2020i).

PROFILE OF THE CRNA

A shortage of advanced practice providers, including CRNAs, led to a recent study on CRNA job satisfaction and retention (Gilliland, 2022). CRNAs comprise an increasing component of the anesthesia workforce. The average age of CRNAs in 2019 was 48.6 years, and 28% of CRNAs were in practice for 11 to 20 years, indicating a young workforce (Negrusa et al., 2021). In a recent practice survey, the average age at which CRNAs began their careers in nurse anesthesia was 32.7 years old. The gender distribution of CRNAs and nurse anesthesia students was the same in 2019: 41% male and 59% female (NBCRNA, 2020c). Table 16.1 provides information on a breakdown of hours spent providing anesthesia services as well as administrative time and educational activities. Table 16.2 and Table 16.3 provide primary CRNA employment arrangements as well as the distribution of primary positions held by CRNAs.

Over the past 70 years the nurse anesthesia profession has become increasingly diverse. One measure of diversity in nurse anesthesia is the proportion of male CRNAs (41%) versus female CRNAs (59%), which is considerably higher than the overall 12% of registered nurses who are men (Brusie, 2020). Of historic note, the AANA did not permit membership of males or African Americans until 1948 (Horton & Kremer, 2020). Recent AANA member survey data show the following racial/ethnic distribution of CRNAs: White/Caucasian, 88%; Hispanic, 3%; African American, 2%; Asian or Pacific Islander, 3%; other, 4% (AANA, 2018a). The AANA has ongoing efforts to foster

TABLE 16.1

Average CRNA Work Week

Clinical activities: 37.1 hours per week
Administrative activities: 2.8 hours weekly
Educational activities: 3 hours per week
Anesthesia care while on call: 6.3 hours per week

Adapted from *AANA Member Survey Data*, by American Association of Nurse Anesthesiology, 2018a.

TABLE 16.2

Primary CRNA Employment Arrangements

Hospital employee: 41%
Anesthesia group employee: 29%
Independent contractor: 16%
Owner or partner in anesthesia group: 4%
Military, government, or Veterans Administration: 3%
Other employment setting: 0%

Adapted from *AANA Member Survey Data*, by American Association of Nurse Anesthesiology, 2021c.

TABLE 16.3
Distribution of Primary Positions Held by CRNAs

Practice: 92%
Department management/administration: 4%
Education – Administration: 2%

Adapted from *AANA Member Survey Data*, by American Association of Nurse Anesthesiology, 2021c.

diversity, equity, and inclusion in nurse anesthesia. A diversity in nurse anesthesia mentorship program provides prospective nurse anesthesia applicants with guidance on the application process for nurse anesthesia programs and additional information about becoming a CRNA (AANA, 2021b). Diversity, equity, and inclusion efforts in higher education provide an additional impetus for nurse anesthesia programs to admit students from diverse backgrounds. *The Future of Nursing: 2020–2030: Charting a Path to Achieve Health Equity* (NASEM, 2021) calls for nurses, nurse educators, and academic institutions and nursing organizations to prioritize health equity. The AANA has ongoing efforts to foster diversity, equity, and inclusion in the nurse anesthesia profession, including a position statement and a Diversity and Inclusion Committee, along with cultural competency and mentorship resources (AANA, 2021b).

Scope and Standards of Practice

The scope of practice for CRNAs varies depending on institutional credentialing. Although most CRNAs provide general anesthesia and monitored anesthesia care (i.e., local anesthesia, intravenous sedation, and monitoring by an anesthesia provider), regional anesthesia may be performed less frequently by CRNAs compared with general anesthesia due to institutional credentialing and local practice patterns. Placement of invasive monitoring lines and pain management techniques may also be less commonly performed by some nurse anesthetists, also due to institutional credentialing and local practice patterns. Practice restrictions may not always be imposed via the credentialing process; some providers choose not to perform certain types of procedures. The AANA provides guidelines for clinical privileges and other responsibilities of CRNAs, including core privileges that define the scope of clinical procedures that CRNAs are authorized to perform in a healthcare organization based on verification of their education, training, experience, and competence (AANA, 2019d).

The AANA *Scope of Nurse Anesthesia Practice* (2020h) includes five domains: preoperative/preprocedural, intraoperative/intraprocedural, postoperative/postprocedure, pain management, and other services. CRNAs administer anesthesia and anesthesia-related care in four areas: (1) preanesthetic preparation and evaluation; (2) induction, maintenance, and emergence from anesthesia; (3) postanesthesia care; and (4) perianesthetic and clinical support functions. The CRNA scope of practice includes but is not limited to the elements in Box 16.2.

There are 14 components of the *AANA Standards for Nurse Anesthesia Practice* (AANA, 2019a). These standards address topics ranging from ethics to preoperative assessment, implementation, and evaluation of anesthesia care. The standards are described in Box 16.3. The AANA nurse anesthesia scope and standards of practice inform educational and credentialing requirements for CRNAs. These standards reflect a commitment to evidence-based interprofessional practice.

Education

Nurse anesthesia education occurs in diverse settings, including schools or colleges of nursing, allied health, sciences, and medicine. However, the relative value of this diversity has never been quantified in terms of an academic power base or educational credibility. This diversity exists because the nurse anesthesia educational community values various undergraduate degrees for entrance into nurse anesthesia programs and because of the initial difficulty that nurse anesthesia educators met when trying to move certificate nurse anesthesia programs into schools of nursing.

Since 1998, all nurse anesthesia programs have been at the graduate level. As of January 1, 2022, all students entering accredited nurse anesthesia educational programs must be enrolled in a doctoral program (Gerbasi, 2016). However, this requirement for advanced degrees does not dictate the movement of programs into one academic discipline. A reason for this may stem from those programs that in the 1970s established relationships with any academic unit that was

BOX 16.2

AANA Nurse Anesthesia Scope of Practice Domains

1. Preoperative/preprocedural
   a. Provide patient education and counseling.
   b. Perform a comprehensive history and physical examination, assessment, and evaluation.
   c. Conduct a preanesthesia assessment and evaluation.
   d. Develop a comprehensive patient-specific plan for anesthesia, analgesia, multimodal pain management and recovery.
   e. Obtain informed consent for anesthesia and pain management.
   f. Select, order, prescribe, and administer preanesthetic medications, including controlled substances.
2. Intraoperative/intraprocedure
   g. Implement a patient-specific plan of care, which may involve anesthetic techniques, such as general, regional, and local anesthesia; sedation; and multimodal pain management.
   h. Select, order, prescribe, and administer anesthetic medications, including controlled substances, adjuvant drugs, accessory drugs, fluids, and blood products.
   i. Select and insert invasive and noninvasive monitoring modalities (e.g., central venous access, arterial lines, cerebral oximetry, bispectral index monitor, transesophageal echocardiogram [TEE]).
3. Postoperative/postprocedure
   j. Facilitate emergence and recovery from anesthesia.
   k. Select, order, prescribe, and administer postanesthetic medications, including controlled substances.
   l. Conduct postanesthesia evaluation.
   m. Educate the patient related to recovery, regional analgesia, and continued multimodal pain management.
   n. Discharge from the postanesthesia care area or facility.
4. Pain management
   o. Provide comprehensive patient-centered pain management to optimize recovery.
   p. Provide acute pain services, including multimodal pain management and opioid-sparing techniques.
   q. Provide anesthesia and analgesia using regional techniques for obstetric and other acute pain management.
   r. Provide advanced pain management, including acute, chronic, and interventional pain management.
5. Other services
   s. Prescribe medication, including controlled substances (e.g., pain management, medication-assisted treatment, adjuvants to psychotherapy).
   t. Provide emergency, critical care, and resuscitation services.
   u. Perform advanced airway management.
   v. Perform point-of-care testing.
   w. Order, evaluate, and interpret diagnostic laboratory and radiologic studies (e.g., chest x-ray, 12-lead electrocardiogram, TEE).
   x. Use and supervise the use of ultrasound, fluoroscopy, and other technologies for diagnosis and care delivery.
   y. Provide sedation and pain management for palliative care.
   z. Order consults, treatments, or services related to the patient's care (e.g., physical and occupational therapy).

Adapted from American Association of Nurse Anesthesiology. (2020h). *Scope of nurse anesthesia practice*. https://www.aana.com/docs/default-source/practice-aana-com-web-documents-(all)/scope-of-nurse-anesthesia-practice.pdf?sfvrsn=250049b1_6

open to affiliating with a nurse anesthesia program. Programs that pioneered nurse anesthesia education at the graduate level established relationships with those departments in colleges and universities that were willing to take risks with the small numbers of students in nurse anesthesia programs. This diversified model of

BOX 16.3

AANA Standards of Nurse Anesthesia Practice

I. Patient's rights: Respect the patient's autonomy, dignity, and privacy and support the patient's needs and safety.

II. Preanesthesia patient assessment and evaluation: Perform and document or verify documentation of a preanesthesia evaluation of the patient's general health, allergies, medication history, preexisting conditions, anesthesia history, and any relevant diagnostic tests. Perform and document or verify documentation of an anesthesia-focused physical assessment to form the anesthesia plan of care.

III. Plan for anesthesia care: After the patient has had the opportunity to consider anesthesia care options and address his or her concerns, formulate a patient-specific plan for anesthesia care. When indicated, the anesthesia care plan can be formulated with members of the healthcare team and the patient's legal representative.

IV. Informed consent for anesthesia care and related services: Obtain and document or verify documentation that the patient or legal representative has given informed consent for planned anesthesia care or related services in accordance with law, accreditation standards, and institutional policy.

V. Documentation: Communicate anesthesia care data and activities through legible, timely, accurate, and complete documentation in the patient's healthcare record.

VI. Equipment: Adhere to manufacturer's operating instructions and other safety precautions to complete a daily anesthesia equipment check. Verify function of anesthesia equipment prior to each anesthetic. Operate equipment to minimize the risk of fire, explosion, electrical shock, and equipment malfunction.

VII. Anesthesia plan implementation and management: Implement and, if needed, modify the anesthesia plan of care by continuously assessing the patient's response to the anesthetic and surgical or procedural intervention. The CRNA provides anesthesia care until the responsibility is accepted by another anesthesia professional.

VIII. Patient positioning: Collaborate with the surgical or procedure team to position, assess, and monitor proper body alignment. Use protective measures to maintain perfusion and protect pressure points and nerve plexus.

IX. Monitoring, alarms: Monitor, evaluate, and document the patient's physiologic condition as appropriate for the procedure and anesthetic technique. When a physiologic monitoring device is used, variable-pitch and threshold alarms are turned on and audible. Document blood pressure, heart rate, and respiration at least every 5 minutes for all anesthetics.

X. Infection control and prevention: Verify and adhere to infection control policies and procedures as established within the practice setting to minimize the risk of infection to patients, the CRNA, and other healthcare providers.

XI. Transfer of care: Evaluate the patient's status and determine when it is appropriate to transfer the responsibility of care to another qualified healthcare provider. Communicate the patient's condition and essential information for continuity of care.

XII. Quality improvement process: Participate in the ongoing review and evaluation of anesthesia care to assess quality and appropriateness to improve outcomes.

XIII. Wellness: Is physically and mentally able to perform duties of the role.

XIV. A culture of safety: Foster a collaborative and cooperative patient care environment through interdisciplinary engagement, open communication, a culture of safety, and supportive leadership.

Adapted from American Association of Nurse Anesthesiology. (2019a). *AANA standards for nurse anesthesia practice*. https://www.aana.com/docs/default-source/practice-aana-com-web-documents-(all)/standards-for-nurse-anesthesia-practice.pdf?sfvrsn=e00049b1_18 nurse anesthesia education has continued, and many long-established programs would find it strategically and operationally difficult to change their academic affiliations; that is, from allied health to nursing.

Practice doctorates offered in nurse anesthesia programs include the DNP degree and the DNAP degree. Regardless of the degree offered, nurse anesthesia practice doctorates must comport with the COA *Standards for Accreditation of Nurse Anesthesia Programs–Practice Doctorate* (COA, 2019), or revised standards effective for all new CRNA students beginning programs on or after January 1, 2022 (COA, 2022b). These criteria include a minimum program length of 36 months, demonstration of adequate numbers of faculty prepared at the doctoral level, and completion of a final scholarly work (COA, 2019). Current integration of the COA *Standards for Accreditation of Nurse Anesthesia Programs–Practice Doctorate* (2019) and the AACN *Essentials of Doctoral Education* (2006) is depicted in Box 16.4.

In April 2021, AACN updated the *Essentials*, now referred to as *The Essentials: Core Competencies for Professional Nursing Education*. The *Essentials* model contains two levels: AACN essentials for entry-level professional nursing education subcompetencies and AACN essentials for advanced-level nursing education subcompetencies and specialty/role requirements/competencies. There are 10 essential domains for nursing, with associated competencies and subcompetencies for advanced-level nursing education (AACN, 2021). At the time of printing of this book, faculty and academic leadership are working with COA to interpret and implement the new *Essentials* across CRNA programs. For this edition, the author will continue to refer to the AACN *Essentials of Doctoral Education* (2006).

In the mid-1970s, over 170 nurse anesthesia educational programs existed. A rapid decline in the numbers of nurse anesthesia programs occurred in the 1980s, a change that was of great concern to the specialty. The closures were attributed variously to physician pressure, declining support, the inability of hospitals to continue support of small programs, and lack of geographically accessible universities with which a nurse anesthesia program could affiliate (Horton & Kremer, 2020). Despite the decline in the overall numbers of nurse anesthesia programs, many of which were certificate programs with enrollments of less than five students, the level of educational programs changed dramatically. After an initial decline in graduates, the newer graduate programs increased their admissions. To accomplish this, programs had to increase the numbers of clinical training sites. This resulted in a strengthened educational system, deeply entrenched in an academic model.

Colleges and schools of nursing now house more than 60% of nurse anesthesia educational programs in the United States (COA, 2021), reflecting increasing collaboration between all APRN groups on education, legislative, and policy matters. Coalitions of APRNs have effectively worked together on the state and federal levels on professional advocacy issues for many years.

At this writing there are 124 accredited nurse anesthesia programs described on the Council on Accreditation of Nurse Anesthesia Educational Programs CRNA School Search (COA, 2022a). The minimum education and experience required to become a CRNA include:

- A baccalaureate or graduate degree in nursing or another appropriate major.
- An unencumbered license as a registered professional nurse and/or APRN in the United States or its territories and protectorates.
- One year minimum of full-time work experience, or its part-time equivalent, as a registered nurse in a critical care setting within the United States, its territories, or a US military hospital outside of the United States. The average clinical experience of RNs entering nurse anesthesia educational programs is 2.9 years.
- Graduation with a minimum of a master's degree from a nurse anesthesia educational program accredited by the COA.

Programs of Study

The clinical and didactic curriculum requirements for nurse anesthesia educational programs that offer entry practice doctorates are determined by the COA *Standards for Accreditation of Nurse Anesthesia Programs–Practice Doctorate* (2019). The remaining master's-entry nurse anesthesia programs are held to the COA *Standards for Accreditation of Nurse Anesthesia Educational Programs* (COA, 2018). The COA also accredits post-master's doctoral degree and specialty fellowships for practicing CRNAs (COA, 2019).

BOX 16.4

Integration of the AACN Essentials of Doctoral Education for Advanced Nursing Practice *(2006) and the* COA Standards for Accreditation of Nurse Anesthesia Educational Programs–Practice Doctorate *(2019)*[a]

DNP ESSENTIALS AND VALIDATING COMPETENCIES

1. Scientific underpinnings for practice
   a. Uses practice approaches based on scientific findings and theories from relevant disciplines.
2. Organization and systems leadership for quality improvement and systems thinking
   a. Plans cost-effective care.
   b. Applies effective strategies for managing ethical dilemmas.
   c. Uses information technology and quality improvement methods to enhance safety and monitor health outcomes.
   d. Facilitates the development and use of health practices that address the needs of culturally diverse populations, providers, and other stakeholders.
   e. Identifies system factors that contribute to patient and provider risk.
   f. Mitigates risk factors to improve patient and provider quality and safety.
3. Clinical scholarship and analytical methods for evidence-based practice
   a. Participates in practice inquiry.
   b. Evaluates and integrates evidence-based interventions for practice.
   c. Examines patterns of data and outcomes to identify gaps in evidence for practice.
4. Information systems/technology and patient care technology for the improvement and transformation of health care
   a. Uses and evaluates electronic library and Internet resources to guide practice.
   b. Evaluates consumer health information sources for accuracy, timeliness, and appropriateness to client needs.
5. Healthcare policy for advocacy in health care
   a. Identifies practice implications of health policy relevant to clinical situations.
   b. Disseminates relevant policy information to staff, preceptor, and client related to specific health issues.
   c. Practices as a patient advocate.
6. Interprofessional collaboration for improving patient and population health outcomes
   a. Employs effective and respectful verbal, nonverbal, and written communication and collaboration skills with interprofessional team members.
   b. Contributes as an active participant in interprofessional teams in the analysis of practice and organizational issues.
7. Clinical prevention and population health for improving the nation's health
   a. Uses knowledge of economic, environmental, cultural, and psychosocial determinants of health and illness affecting care when developing, implementing, and evaluating health promotion and disease prevention interventions.
8. Advanced nursing practice–CRNA
   a. Incorporates guidance, criticism, and evaluation into clinical practice.
   b. Engages in self-directed learning.
   c. Demonstrates professional behaviors including appearance, reliability, punctuality, accountability, availability, and self-reflection.
   d. Practices within the scope of practice and applicable legal and ethical parameters.
   e. Maintains confidentiality and privacy.
   f. Provides safe perianesthesia care.
   g. Demonstrates knowledge of pharmacology.
   h. Conducts preanesthestic assessment and patient preparation.
   i. Knows principles of physiology and pathophysiology.
   j. Evidences applied knowledge of chemistry and physics and anesthesia principles.
   k. Formulates an appropriate anesthesia care plan.
   l. Shows skill with intraoperative and postoperative care.
   m. Demonstrates skill in management of general anesthesia.
   n. Demonstrates skill with regional anesthesia management.
   o. Demonstrates skill with monitored anesthesia care.

[a]The COA Standards for Accreditation of Nurse Anesthesia Programs - Practice Doctorate (COA, 2022b) and AACN's The Essentials: *Core Competencies for Professional Nursing Education* (AACN, 2021) have been updated. COA accreditation standards, policies and procedures, and guidelines provide guidance for the development of competency crosswalks. Please see https://www.coacrna.org/accreditation/accreditation-standards-policies-and-procedures-and-guidelines/ for updates.

The practice doctorate entry curriculum must meet commonly accepted national standards for similar degrees and the program should entail 3 years of full-time study. The COA curriculum standards apply to programs seeking to award a DNP degree or DNAP degree to graduate students who successfully complete graduation requirements. The curriculum content hours required by the COA with the associated AACN *Essentials* (2006) are intended to prepare graduates for the full scope of nurse anesthesia practice, with didactic content in these areas:

- Advanced physiology/pathophysiology (120 contact hours): Essential I (Scientific Underpinnings for Practice)
- Advanced pharmacology (90 contact hours): Essential I (Scientific Underpinnings for Practice)
- Basic and advanced principles in nurse anesthesia (120 contact hours): Essentials VI and VIII (Interprofessional Collaboration and Advanced Nursing Practice)
- Research (75 contact hours): Essentials III and IV (Clinical Scholarship and Information Systems)
- Advanced health assessment (45 contact hours): Essentials VII, VIII (Clinical Prevention, Population Health and Advanced Practice)
- Other required content areas include human anatomy, chemistry, biochemistry, physics, genetics, acute and chronic pain management, radiology, ultrasound, anesthesia equipment, professional role development, wellness and substance use disorder, informatics, ethical and multicultural health care, leadership and management, health policy, healthcare finance, and integration/clinical correlation: Essentials II, IV, V, VII (Organizational and Systems Leadership, Information Systems, Health Care Policy, Clinical Prevention and Population Health; COA, 2019).

The COA *Standards for Accreditation–Practice Doctorate* (2019) mandate that students complete a minimum of 2000 clinical hours and at least 600 anesthesia cases on patients across the life span at all acuity levels. There are general and specialty case requirements, including obstetrics, pediatrics, neurosurgery, and cardiothoracic surgery. Minimum numbers of anesthetic procedural requirements are also specified, such as airway management techniques, placement of central venous catheters, and regional anesthesia experiences. CRNA students entering on or after January 1, 2022 are required to complete additional cases and experiences (COA, 2022b). Nurse anesthesia programs must verify completion of the required didactic and clinical experiences to demonstrate the eligibility of graduates to take the National Certification Examination offered by the NBCRNA.

COA permits latitude in terms of how programs can implement their curriculum. Some programs may front-load didactic content, with clinical practicum experiences beginning after students have successfully completed the didactic portion of their programs of study. Another curricular model involves the integration of didactic and clinical learning experiences. Regardless of the curricular model employed, nurse anesthesia programs must meet or exceed the COA standards for accreditation to achieve or maintain COA accreditation.

Nurse Anesthesia Educational Funding

The US Health Resources and Services Administration (HRSA) provides competitive funding opportunities that may offset a portion of the educational costs for nurse anesthesia students. The amount of funding available varies from year to year, depending on federal budget allocations. HRSA grant funding that is applicable to nurse anesthesia education includes traineeship funding for advanced nursing education (ANE) and the nurse anesthetist traineeship (NAT; HRSA, 2020).

The NAT program provides support for student registered nurse anesthetists who are enrolled full time in a master's or doctoral nurse anesthesia program. Traineeship funds may be used to offset costs for tuition, books, fees, and reasonable living expenses for students during the period for which the traineeship is provided. During fiscal year 2020, HRSA funded 79 NAT traineeship grants that totaled $2,536,448 (HRSA, 2021). These funds lessen the debt load experienced by nurse anesthesia students. Students are not typically encouraged to work as RNs while enrolled in nurse anesthesia programs, because the rigor of these programs usually entails 60 or more hours per week of committed time. The AANA Division of Federal Government Affairs promotes nurse anesthesia workforce development through legislative advocacy in congress and through representation before the HRSA and its Division of Nursing, which administer the Title VIII NAT program (Kohl, 2022).

The primary funding source for most nurse anesthesia educational programs is tuition. The number of credits required for degree completion and charges per academic credit vary between educational institutions. Some programs may charge a clinical fee in addition to tuition costs.

When demand is high for nurse anesthesia graduates, potential employers may offer sign-on bonuses in exchange for an employment commitment. Some employers may also offer stipends to students during the nurse anesthesia program in exchange for an employment commitment, but this is a less commonly used recruitment strategy. Educational costs may be offset with philanthropic funds in some institutions, but this is less common.

Practice Doctorate

As nurse anesthesia education moved from the hospital-based certificate programs to higher education institutions, the academic units housing nurse anesthesia programs were often in colleges of allied health, medicine, or basic science. Academic affiliations between schools of nursing and nurse anesthesia programs became more common with the COA requirement to implement for master's degree programs by 1998 and practice doctorates by 2022.

The DNAP degree is offered primarily by nonnursing academic units that house nurse anesthesia programs such as health sciences schools. The DNP is typically the exit degree for practice doctorate nurse anesthesia programs in schools of nursing (COA, 2021).

The COA *Standards for Accreditation of Nurse Anesthesia Educational Programs–Practice Doctorate* require that curricula within doctoral programs be designed to award a doctoral degree (DNP or DNAP) to students who complete graduation requirements; waivers to this requirement may be approved by the council (COA, 2019). The primary purpose of the practice-oriented doctoral degree is to prepare nurse anesthetists as practice scholars and requires a minimum of 36 full-time calendar months (COA, 2019). COA requires that a proposed doctoral degree offering be approved by the institutional accreditation agency for the college or university with which the nurse anesthesia program is affiliated (i.e., Higher Learning Commission, Southern Association of Colleges and Schools; COA, 2017).

Nurse anesthesia programs seeking to offer entry or completion doctoral degrees must apply for approval from COA to offer these degrees. For entry into practice doctoral degree applications, programs submit the COA Course Content Map template as part of their COA doctoral program application. The Course Content Map crosswalks how the curriculum complies with the full scope of nurse anesthesia education while linking COA's *Standards for Accreditation of Nurse Anesthesia Programs–Practice Doctorate* competencies (COA, 2017, 2019, 2022b). It additionally ensures that AACN's *The Essentials: Core Competencies for Professional Nursing Education* (2021) competencies and regulatory standards are achieved.

Institutional Credentialing

The terms *credentialing* and *privileging* refer to a two-part process that establishes the qualification of a clinician and their authority to work in a clinical setting. Credentialing involves obtaining and verifying evidence of the qualifications of the healthcare professional to provide care or services. These qualifications or credentials include licensure, education, training, experience, professional and technical competence, or other qualifications. Privileging is the process of granting permission to provide a specific scope of patient care services based on an evaluation of the credentials and performance of a healthcare professional. *Core privileges* refers to the scope of clinical procedures and activities that providers within a specialty area are authorized to perform in a clinical setting based on verification of their education, training, experience, and competence (AANA, 2019c).

The credentialing and privileging process provides an objective mechanism to assess the initial application for privileges based on education, training, experience, legal qualifications, and the individual's competence and ability to render quality care. Renewal of privileges includes review of compliance with licensure and certification requirements, objective measures of clinical performance and outcomes, peer review, risk management findings, and compliance with organization policies. The governing body of an organization approves clinical privileges upon the recommendation of the medical staff (AANA, 2019c).

Clinical privileges for the CRNA should be defined regardless of the contractual employment relationship that exists within the practice setting. CRNAs are responsible for requesting clinical privileges that reflect their educational preparation, clinical experience, and level of professional competence. Evidence of continuing education, which is required for licensure, recertification, and organizational competencies, reflects knowledge of current scientific theories and principles and techniques related to the field of anesthesia and the current practice of the CRNA (AANA, 2019c).

For healthcare organizations that engage in core clinical privileging, the CRNA is granted specialty-specific core clinical privileges consistent with those of other healthcare professionals (e.g., physicians) who are permitted by law and the organization to provide the same patient care services. Individual CRNAs may apply for special privileges related to subspecialty practice. The CRNA scope of practice is dynamic and evolving, and CRNA privileges should reflect the full scope of CRNA practice evidenced by individual credentials and performance (AANA, 2019c).

ROLE DEVELOPMENT AND MEASURES OF CLINICAL COMPETENCE

Nurse anesthesia education focuses on the development of the knowledge, skills, and abilities necessary for qualified applicants to transition from the role of nurse to nurse anesthetist. The didactic and clinical requirements described in the COA *Standards for Accreditation of Nurse Anesthesia Education Programs–Practice Doctorate* (2019, 2022b) provide the necessary structure to facilitate the development of qualified nurse anesthesia graduates. Initial certification and continued professional competence programs overseen by the NBCRNA ensure that graduates possess the necessary knowledge, skills, and abilities for entry into practice and maintenance of certification through an array of lifelong learning activities.

The professional journey of the nurse anesthetist encompasses many facets. Exemplar 16.1 describes how one CRNA functions in practice, as a preceptor and mentor, as a colleague, and as an advocate.

Direct Clinical Practice

Since nurse anesthesia students are experienced critical care nurses, they are accustomed to providing comprehensive holistic nursing services to patients and their families prior to beginning a nurse anesthesia program. Anesthesiology residents complete 1 year of nonanesthesia training before beginning their residency, and anesthesiologist assistants (AAs) are not required to have any clinical background before beginning their educational programs. Therefore nurse anesthesia students typically have more clinical experience caring for high-acuity patients and their families compared with other anesthesia trainees.

Nurse anesthesia practice involves interactions with patients and their families, which often occur in a truncated time period. CRNAs use a nursing model to develop an anesthesia plan of care. CRNAs perform a preoperative assessment, including an examination of the airway anatomy, heart, and lungs. During the preoperative assessment the past medical and surgical histories are elicited, along with information about allergies, medications, and social habits. Laboratory values and the results of diagnostic tests are reviewed. The preoperative assessment informs the anesthetic plan, which is influenced by patient, surgeon, and anesthesia provider preferences, along with the associated risks and benefits of the available anesthetic techniques. The CRNA then implements the anesthetic plan, following the *AANA Standards of Nurse Anesthesia Practice* (AANA, 2019a). CRNAs evaluate the care they provided through monitoring the course of their patient during postanesthesia recovery as well as through involvement with quality improvement processes in their department or practice group.

CRNAs practice according to their expertise, state statutes or regulations, and institutional policy. Unlike AAs, CRNAs can practice without anesthesiologist supervision.

Anesthesia services can facilitate diagnosis, as in the case of the so-called curare test for myasthenia gravis. Anesthesia as a therapeutic modality is seen in the treatment of acute and chronic pain; it is also used in psychiatry for conducting interviews under the influence of ultra-short-acting IV barbiturates and

EXEMPLAR 16.1
A CRNA'S PROFESSIONAL JOURNEY

D.W. has been a CRNA for 6 years. His mother is a clinical nurse specialist. When he was in high school, an online search he performed about nursing education opportunities yielded information about 40 different nursing specialties, including nurse anesthesia. An article he read about CRNAs serving in Afghanistan caught his attention. He liked the responsibility and autonomy that the deployed military CRNAs had in their practice. What was less clear to him was the array of anesthesia practices and varying degrees of CRNA–anesthesiologist collaboration.

D.W. went to nursing school intending to become a CRNA. He completed prerequisite classes at a community college. His mother had a friend who was opening a new diploma-entry nursing program in another state, which he completed, and then he worked in the same area for a year while completing his BSN. He then returned to his hometown in the Midwest and worked as an intensive care unit nurse for 5.5 years in both community and teaching hospitals. A registered nurse at a teaching hospital with a CRNA program told him about an available tuition reimbursement program at that facility, which prompted him to apply to this program, where he was accepted and completed a master's degree. As a student, he found the role differentiation between attending physicians, staff, and trainees frustrating at times.

While D.W. was a student, he attended the AANA Mid-Year Assembly in Washington, DC. This annual meeting provides attendees with current information about federal government affairs that prepares them for lobbying visits on Capitol Hill, as well as valuable networking opportunities. D.W. learned about professional advocacy, billing, and scope of practice at this meeting. He then became active with his state nurse anesthesia association and appreciated being mentored by CRNAs who were both experienced leaders. D.W. became the federal political director for his state, which involved arranging lobbying visits for CRNAs and students attending the Mid-Year Assembly.

Following graduation as a CRNA, D.W. worked at a community hospital where he completed clinical rotations as a student. The practice autonomy at this site was greater than what he experienced at other facilities, and the salary was competitive. After 3 years in this position, he began to feel stagnant in his practice and more jobs became available. He found a CRNA-only practice in a rural area where he worked as a contractor for 9 months and enjoyed the practice. This was followed by other temporary assignments at hospitals in small to midsize cities. During one of those assignments, he worked with the chief medical officer to facilitate development of a more autonomous CRNA practice at that hospital.

D.W. has served as a clinical instructor for nurse anesthesia students in several settings and has taught content including ultrasound-guided peripheral nerve block placement at continuing education conferences. His advice to nurses interested in pursuing nurse anesthesia education is to thoroughly investigate the CRNA role. His impression is that many ICU nurses are motivated to become CRNAs because of the increased CRNA salary but have misconceptions about the CRNA role; that is, that working relationships and scope of practice in critical care and anesthesia are similar. He advocates for all CRNAs to practice at the highest level of their education and training.

for accelerated detoxification of patients with opioid dependency. However, the most common use of anesthesia resources is for the administration of surgical anesthesia. CRNAs select, obtain, or administer the anesthetics, adjuvant drugs, accessory drugs, and fluids necessary to manage the anesthesia, maintain physiologic homeostasis, and correct abnormal responses to anesthesia or surgery (AANA, 2020h). When CRNAs perform these activities, they are legally recognized to be providing anesthesia services on request, not to be prescribing as defined by federal law. Since the advent of legislated prescriptive authority for CRNAs and other APRNs, these providers can prescribe legend and Schedules II through V controlled substances. However, this authority varies from state to state.

Patient monitoring is another key practice area of CRNAs. Nurse anesthetists select, apply, and insert appropriate noninvasive and invasive monitoring modalities for collecting and interpreting physiologic data. These activities are all recognized components of anesthesia services performed by CRNAs on request and are not prescriptive. Criteria for the use of invasive monitors and who places them vary by institution and geographic region. Professional fees associated with the placement of devices such as pulmonary artery catheters at times lead to conflict over which practitioner—anesthetist or surgeon—will place invasive monitors and receive the associated reimbursement.

Nurse anesthesia practice includes airway management, with modalities ranging from ventilation via a face mask to placement of laryngeal mask airways or endotracheal intubation. CRNAs are knowledgeable about mechanical ventilation options and the pharmacologic support needed to maintain mechanical ventilation within and outside of the operating room. In some settings, these APRNs are the sole providers of ventilator management oversight. A combination of technical skills required for airway management using a variety of instruments (e.g., rigid laryngoscope, fiberoptic bronchoscope, video laryngoscope) and knowledge of respiratory anatomy and physiology and pharmacology is important.

Clinicians continue to develop an array of approaches to sedation and analgesia for ventilator-dependent patients. The expertise that CRNAs can provide in the management of ventilator-dependent patients includes reinforcing the need for appropriate sedation and analgesia when critically ill patients are mechanically ventilated, as in the COVID-19 pandemic, when CRNAs provided ventilatory management services in critical care areas (AANA, 2020c). CRNAs can also help patients and families understand the rationale for procedures and treatments related to mechanical ventilation.

Nurse anesthetists manage emergence and recovery from anesthesia by selecting, obtaining, ordering, or administering medications, fluids, or ventilator support to maintain homeostasis, provide relief from pain and anesthesia side effects, and/or prevent or manage complications (AANA, 2020h). These activities also fall within the scope of providing anesthesia services and are not prescriptive in the traditional sense, such as writing a prescription that is filled by a pharmacist. Releasing or discharging patients from a postanesthesia care area can be performed by the CRNA. Providing postanesthesia follow-up evaluation and care related to anesthetic side effects or complications are other CRNA direct care functions.

Regional anesthesia, which includes spinal, epidural, and peripheral nerve blocks, is used by many CRNAs in the management of surgical anesthesia, labor pain, and postoperative pain. CRNAs may be involved with pain management services through the use of epidural and peripheral nerve block analgesic infusions and patient-controlled analgesia, which have greatly contributed to the effective treatment of preventable pain. Nurse anesthetists often have a role in the formulation of protocols and staff education when acute pain treatment regimens are introduced.

Anesthesia services are frequently used in obstetrics to provide analgesia for parturients. Regional anesthesia and applied pharmacology have greatly advanced obstetric anesthesia, which in the past relied on drugs with systemic effects that could cause neonatal depression. Spinal or epidural anesthesia is common for vaginal and cesarean section deliveries, often obviating the need for general anesthesia and its attendant risks. In addition to using regional anesthesia in obstetric and postpartum settings, CRNAs have long worked collaboratively with other clinicians in these areas to manage intrapartum and postpartum pain with various pharmacologic and nonpharmacologic modalities.

Nurse anesthetists respond to emergency situations by providing airway management skills and implementing basic and advanced life support techniques. CRNAs can provide leadership in these settings outside of the operating room, reinforcing the need to apply nationally promulgated standards of anesthesia care. An example of one of these standards of care is the measurement of end-tidal carbon dioxide to rule out esophageal intubation (AANA, 2020h).

Palliative Care

CRNAs possess expert skills in pain and symptom management. Building on experience in acute and critical care nursing, nurse anesthetists have extensive experience with end-of-life care. CRNAs value the close relationship that develops with patients and their families in the critical care environment and may develop close relationships with patients for whom they care during complex surgeries related to serious illness. The knowledge, skills, and experiences of CRNAs have made them uniquely qualified to assist with palliative and end-of-life care (Faut Callahan et al., 2011).

There are tremendous gaps in palliative and end-of-life care resources that have been identified, often in rural areas where CRNAs are the predominant anesthesia care providers. Over the past decade, there have been many efforts to identify gaps and develop strategies to meet the needs of 12 million adults and 400,000 children in the United States who live with serious illnesses (AACN, 2019).

CRNAs have many skills needed to participate in palliative care but do not typically work in these settings. CRNAs' extensive knowledge in pain and symptom management can enhance existing or new palliative care practices. CRNAs, especially those who have recently entered anesthesia practice and have current critical care knowledge and experience with palliative care, may embrace this additional form of patient care because it provides them an opportunity to develop long-term relationships with patients.

Student registered nurse anesthetists have reported an interest in this type of patient care and noted that they are often asked by families about plans of treatment and resources available to them (Faut Callahan et al., 2011). After taking an interdisciplinary palliative care course, student nurse anesthetists demonstrate significant knowledge in all domains of palliative care.

In many rural settings, 100% of anesthesia is delivered by CRNAs. These are the same communities that often do not have palliative and end-of-life services. Recognition of the experience of CRNAs and the knowledge and skills they develop in pain and symptom management may lead to an increase in providers who can assist with the significant gap in palliative care services in the United States.

Specialty Practice Areas

The Council on Accreditation of Nurse Anesthesia Educational Programs accredits five specialty fellowships. Three of these fellowships address specialty competencies in pain management, and the other two fellowships are focused on pediatric anesthesia (COA, 2021). Exemplar 16.2 describes the CRNA's role in pain management. There have been multiple legislative challenges from organized medicine across the United States, seeking to restrict non-physicians from providing pain management services. These initiatives have in some cases limited opportunities for CRNAs to be involved with chronic pain management. AANA member survey data show that 2% of CRNAs are involved in chronic pain management (AANA, 2018a). To date, 105 CRNAs have been certified by the NBCRNA in nonsurgical pain management. This represents 0.1% of all CRNAs (NBCRNA, 2020e).

CRNAs and the Opioid Crisis

In 2016, life expectancy in the United States decreased for the first time in over 20 years. A contributory factor to this decrease in life expectancy included the deaths of 33,000 people who died in 2015 due to opioid misuse. Over 60% of drug-related deaths are opioid related (see Box 16.5). The AANA learning management system has five free courses available for CRNAs with background information on the opioid crisis. Additional information about substance use disorder for patients and providers, management of chronic pain, advocacy comment letters, opioid safety guidelines, and substance use disorder facility policies are available on the AANA website (AANA, 2020f).

The Society for Opioid-Free Anesthesia (SOFA) was founded by CRNAs to foster the use of opioid-free anesthesia, while providing postoperative pain control with strategies such as peripheral nerve blocks and nonopioid analgesics. These measures avoid the side effects of opioids such as respiratory depression, postoperative nausea and vomiting, addiction, and increased length of hospital stay (SOFA, 2021).

Guidance and Coaching

Because surgery and diagnostic procedures are performed primarily on an outpatient or same-day admission basis, CRNAs are challenged to develop a rapport with their patients rapidly and develop a mutually agreed on plan for anesthesia care. Part of the development of the anesthesia plan involves the CRNA coaching the patient and family. The anesthetic options for the involved surgery or procedure need to be thoroughly discussed, along with the associated risks and benefits. This process can involve teaching the patient and family about postoperative analgesic options and coaching patients to avail themselves of the full benefits of the analgesic regimen, whether the treatment for pain entails patient-controlled epidural or IV analgesia.

Patients who undergo outpatient surgery receive coaching from CRNAs about activity, dietary limitations, and use of postoperative analgesics. Patients and their families in these situations also need coaching about when it may be appropriate for them to contact the office of the surgical or anesthesia provider.

Families of infants and children who undergo surgery and anesthesia need to be coached by the CRNA regarding the assessment and management of pain, postoperative nausea, and vomiting. Parameters for advancing activity and diet need to be clearly conveyed to the family or caregiver as part of this coaching process.

EXEMPLAR 16.2

CERTIFIED REGISTERED NURSE ANESTHETIST'S ROLE IN PAIN MANAGEMENT

J.R. has been a practicing certified registered nurse anesthetist (CRNA) for 17 years. The strongest influences in her professional development are "believing in our profession, my knowledge, skills and competencies, while seizing any and all opportunities for professional advancement that crossed my path."

Her interest in nurse anesthesia was stimulated by early exposure to the CRNA role. Her father was an otolaryngologist who practiced in a Midwestern city with a population of 60,000. At the hospital in which he practiced, there were three anesthesiologists and a CRNA on staff. At that time, the surgeons were allowed to post their cases to the surgery schedule and choose the anesthesia provider. Most of the time, J.R.'s father chose the CRNA to provide anesthesia care for his patients. He stated that the CRNA had excellent skills and was wonderful with pediatric patients.

J.R. has practiced as a staff CRNA in a large physician-owned anesthesia group with 11 physicians and 26 CRNAs in the Midwest. She has also been a hospital-employed chief CRNA for an obstetric anesthesia practice involving three network hospitals in another Midwestern city. Most recently, her practice has moved into the realm of interventional pain management for a neurosurgical group. Her time currently is divided among direct patient care (80%), teaching (10%), administration (5%), and professional activities (5%). J.R. acknowledges that working as an employee of a large neurosurgical group in an office-based interventional pain practice is unique. A 2011 American Association of Nurse Anesthesiology (AANA) survey of members showed that 2% of respondents worked in pain management (AANA, 2018a). CRNA involvement in this specialty has been contested in multiple states by other providers.

J.R.'s current practice developed following an initial contact by another advanced practice registered nurse (APRN) who was employed by the neurosurgical group, demonstrating the value of professional networking. J.R. was asked to meet with the group to discuss a practice opportunity. The group was interested in hiring a CRNA to reopen an interventional pain clinic that had been closed for over a year. J.R. was contacted because of her experience with regional anesthesia and her leadership activities in her state nurse anesthesia association. After she met with the physician who championed this effort, she was interested in accepting the challenge. The position "gave me an incredible opportunity for clinical growth and I strongly felt this was a perfect example of how CRNAs are beneficial in an area outside the traditional operating room setting."

A typical day in J.R.'s practice begins with a quick review of her schedule and a safety check of equipment and medications. Her day usually consists of a mixture of diagnostic and therapeutic interventional procedures, such as epidural steroid injections, nerve root blocks, joint blocks, trigger point injections, and lumbar discography.

"In our pain clinic, a patient checks in at the front desk and an escort assesses his or her vital signs and brings the patient to an exam room. A nurse will interview the patient, answer questions, and ensure informed consent." During that time, J.R. "reviews the chart, imaging studies, assessment forms, and the order for treatment." She also interviews the patient prior to the procedure to answer questions or obtain additional information pertinent to the treatment plan before deciding on the type and targeted site of injection.

The patient is taken to the fluoroscopic suite and is prepped and draped under sterile technique. J.R. then performs a diagnostic or therapeutic injection under fluoroscopic guidance. The patient is assessed immediately after the injection and returned to the examination room for 30 minutes for observation. Prior to discharge, the patient is reassessed and information is recorded concerning the type and amount of pain relief provided by the injection. The patient is educated concerning the onset and duration of action of the injected medications and possible complications of the medication and injection and is given discharge and follow-up information.

J.R. describes the greatest challenges in her practice as "initially ... obtaining the necessary knowledge, skills, and competencies to perform the procedures requested by the group that oversees me because there was no other employment situation identical to this practice. Overall, it is dealing with the political environment because there are physicians who feel a CRNA should not be providing pain management care."

J.R.'s story demonstrates the value of professional collaboration, mentoring, networking, and organizational involvement. Her willingness to take risks and improve care elevates the profession.

Evidence-Based Practice

Pioneering Mayo Clinic nurse anesthetist Alice Magaw demonstrated a commitment to evidence-based practice (EBP) more than 100 years ago (Magaw, 1902, 1906). The early adoption of EBP principles by nurse anesthetists contributed to the sustainability of nurse anesthesia despite opposition from organized medicine. "Pioneers are noted for building upon a body of knowledge, establishing a model for continuous improvement, and exemplifying notable methods of

BOX 16.5

Suggested CRNA Strategies to Combat Opioid Misuse

- A thorough preoperative patient assessment, including signs and symptoms of opioid misuse. If there is evidence of opioid misuse, CRNAs are encouraged to consider actions including a frank and nonthreatening discussion with the patient focused on the provider's concern for the patient's well-being. CRNAs may wish to consider referral and expert consultation with pain management, social work, and addiction experts as needed.
- Whether or not CRNAs have prescriptive authority, they need to advocate for responsible prescribing practices through participating in the development of institutional and departmental policies that provide safe, evidence-based guidelines for opioid pain management along with the use of nonopioid analgesics.
- CRNAs are encouraged to participate in continuing education and review of the evolving principles and evidence supporting safe opioid prescribing practices.
- CRNAs can support local, state and federal legislative efforts to mitigate the opioid epidemic, such as making naloxone widely available.

Adapted from Griffis, C., Giron, S., & Darna, J. (2017). The opioid crisis and the certified registered nurse anesthetist: how can we help? *AANA Journal, 85*(4), 19-23. https://www.aana.com/docs/default-source/aana-journal-web-documents-1/guest-editorial-the-opioid-crisis-and-the-certified-registered-nurse-anesthetist-how-can-we-help.pdf?sfvrsn=76ad4ab1_6

research with subsequent documentations of their findings" (Thatcher, 1953, p. 253). Magaw's peer-reviewed data-based publications were described as "a standard for safe, research-based anesthesia delivery. Her publications embodied practice principles that other anesthesia providers would reference in their desires to become more proficient in their own practice …" (Goode, 2015, p. 54).

AANA has a recommended systematic evidence-based research process to analyze and resolve issues pertaining to nurse anesthesia practice. The key components of evidence-based practice identified by AANA include patient preference/values, clinical expertise, and best research evidence. The steps of evidence-based practice as outlined in Chapter 8 and AANA's *Evidence-Based Practice* document (AANA, 2020e) include:

- Ask a clinical question.
- Obtain the best research literature.
- Critically appraise the evidence.
- Integrate the evidence with clinical expertise and patient preferences.
- Evaluate the outcomes of the decision.

Nurse anesthesia has remained a viable specialty because of the commitments of CRNAs to evidence-based practice. The safety and quality of the care provided by CRNAs are enhanced by rigorous and evidence-based education, certification, and continuous professional competence requirements. Evidence-based practice resources for CRNAs are included in Table 16.4.

Leadership

Through application of their clinical acumen and leadership skills, CRNAs promote patient-centered care, which includes:

- Dignity and respect: CRNAs must integrate the patient's point of view and choices when planning anesthesia care. This plan needs to incorporate the knowledge, values, beliefs, and cultural background of patients and their families.
- Information sharing: CRNA practice involves communicating complete, objective information with patients and families in a positive manner.
- Participation: Patients and families need to participate in decision making; that is, discussing anesthesia options with the associated procedures and risks.
- Collaboration: Patients, families, and clinicians should collaborate on all aspects of healthcare delivery (Institute for Patient and Family-Centered Care, 2008).

The CRNA sets the tone in the operating room. As a patient advocate, the CRNA ensures that noise and distractions are kept to a minimum prior to induction of general anesthesia. When anesthetized patients are

TABLE 16.4
Evidence-Based Practice Resources

The Oxford Centre for Evidence-Based Medicine (CEBM) (https://www.cebm.net/)
The Cochrane Collaboration (https://www.cochrane.org/)
The Joanna Briggs Institute (https://jbi.global/)
Evidence-based practice modules and tutorials:
Evidence-Based Behavioral Practice online training modules (https://ebbp.org/)
University of Minnesota online Evidence-Based Practice Interprofessional Tutorial (https://apps.lib.umn.edu/instruction/ebp/story_html5.html)
Guidelines and systematic reviews:
The Agency for Healthcare Research and Quality: Evidence-Based Practice Centers (EBC) (https://www.ahrq.gov/prevention/guidelines/index.html)
Appraisal of Guidelines Research and Evaluation (http://agreecollaboration.org/)
The National Guidelines Clearinghouse (https://www.ahrq.gov/gam/updates/index.html)
PubMed Clinical Queries (https://pubmed.ncbi.nlm.nih.gov/clinical/)

Adapted from *Evidence-Based Practice*, by American Association of Nurse Anesthesiology, 2020e, https://www.aana.com/practice/evidence-based-practice

positioned for surgery, the CRNA ensures that safety straps are applied, pressure points are padded, and patient privacy and dignity are protected. As clinical setting leaders, CRNAs ensure that safety protocols are followed—that is, drugs or solutions to which the patient may be allergic are not administered—and that necessary supplies, including crystalloid and colloid fluid replacement, are readily available. The entire perioperative team completes a time-out, pre- and postprocedural huddle, during which all team members should be empowered to speak. In the case of a life-threatening emergency, such as malignant hyperthermia, anaphylaxis, or bronchospasm, the CRNA exhibits leadership through implementing anesthesia crisis resource management skills, including the use of closed-loop communication, remaining calm, and ensuring that the necessary treatment is provided.

The CRNA graduate's leadership approach must integrate critical and reflective thinking and facilitate collaboration within the profession and among their professional colleagues (COA, 2019, 2022b). COA accreditation standards (2019) also require curricular content on leadership and management, the business of anesthesia/practice management, health policy, and healthcare finance. This didactic content and completion of a scholarly project that often involves use of project management skills provide nurse anesthesia graduates with a solid foundation in leadership knowledge and skills. Exemplar 16.3 demonstrates how a CRNA, over the course of their career, can lead in practice, business and practice management, health policy, and healthcare finance.

AANA continuing education meetings have historically emphasized leadership development. The Fall Leadership Academy provides content for state nurse anesthesia association leaders on effective strategies to manage state government affairs. An engaged State Government Relations Committee is key to addressing proposed statutory or regulatory changes that may adversely impact nurse anesthesia practice. The AANA Mid-Year Assembly, held annually in Washington, DC, provides CRNAs and nurse anesthesia students with current information about federal government affairs that impact nurse anesthesia practice. This content informs advocacy discussions that attendees have with their elected representatives and senators. The annual AANA Assembly of Didactic and Clinical Educators provides participants with current information about curricular and regulatory trends that impact nurse anesthesia education.

CRNAs have held local, state, national, and international leadership roles. These elected and appointed positions have included senior leadership roles in the armed services, higher education, government, and

EXEMPLAR 16.3

A CERTIFIED REGISTERED NURSE ANESTHETIST'S PROFESSIONAL CAREER COMES FULL CIRCLE

C.A. has been a CRNA for 28 years and has practiced in a wide variety of settings as a teacher, practitioner, program administrator, and military officer. She had aunts who were nurses, and nursing was still a common career choice for women when she was growing up. She was a fan of the television show *Julia*, where Diahann Carroll portrayed a nurse and read many of the Cherry Ames student nurse and mystery novels.

Since she had to self-fund her nursing education, C.A. went through a hospital diploma nursing program, which was less costly than the alternatives. She knew about tuition reimbursement through her aunts and planned to obtain her BSN after she became an RN.

As an RN, C.A. worked in two different community hospitals. She obtained intensive care unit experience while completing her BSN degree. In a professional issues class, she learned about nurse anesthesia. She subsequently applied to and was accepted into a nurse anesthesia program that she finished in 1992. C.A. then started taking classes for her DNP degree, working as a teaching assistant and a clinical instructor after graduating from her anesthesia program. Her DNP project was an interprofessional quality improvement initiative for pain assessment and management.

C.A. sought a post-master's DNP because she knew she enjoyed teaching. Her educational costs were reduced through an employer-funded tuition reimbursement plan and federal grant funds obtained by her advisor.

She taught courses that were taken by nurse anesthesia students during their first year in the program. This was satisfying, because at that stage "everything was fresh and new to them." C.A. sought to expand her area of responsibility as a faculty member with designated academic time. She saw this as an opportunity to shape the program and influence curricular content. C.A. later became the assistant program director, which led to reduced clinical time. As technology changed and class sizes increased, the time demands increased. In 2009 C.A. received a national teaching award.

C.A. held elected and appointed positions with her state and national professional organizations because she "felt she owed something to the profession" and wanted to leave it better than she found it. In her association work, she enjoyed lobbying, since this was an opportunity to influence healthcare policy and the future of the profession.

Her interest in the military stemmed from familiarity with an Army Cadet Nurse Program that ceased operation before she was eligible to participate. She liked the idea of serving her country, but the timing never seemed right until she spoke with a recruiter at a state association meeting. C.A. became a commissioned officer in the reserves and was deployed to Kuwait, Afghanistan, Germany, and stateside military hospitals. On her first trip to Afghanistan, the operations tempo was high, with frequent surgeries performed. The professional staff of this forward surgical team included two to three general surgeons, one orthopedic surgeon, and two CRNAs. There were no anesthesiologists. The military team provided humanitarian care to Afghani people with conditions like Ludwig's angina. She received Army Achievement and Commendation medals.

C.A. found that she had to make a concentrated effort to continue her clinical practice over the 20 years she served as a program administrator. It was increasingly challenging to manage the expectations of all stakeholders as a program administrator, along with the teaching and advising requirements associated with larger cohort sizes and a new curriculum. C.A. decided that for the remaining years of her career she wanted to get back to doing what she enjoyed most: patient care. She is currently doing contract clinical anesthesia at different facilities and has enjoyed the transition back to full-time clinical practice.

---

industry. Exemplar 16.4 describes a CRNA's role in leadership and autonomy.

Collaboration

Patient engagement fosters patient-centered care and is central to the provisions of high-quality care (Forbat, 2009). This strategy enhances the relationship between the anesthesia provider, patient, and family through communication, clinical guidance, emotional support, and provision of information. Shared decision making is suited for instances when two or more treatment options—that is, general versus regional anesthesia—are available and both have equivalent clinical outcomes (William, 2009).

Collaboration with CRNAs, patients, and families includes these elements: preoperative education, risk assessment, intervention, patient questions, and shared decision making. This type of communication empowers patients to participate in their care, ask questions, and express feelings and/or concerns. Early patient and family engagement promotes better clinical outcomes by identifying risks, educating

EXEMPLAR 16.4
CERTIFIED REGISTERED NURSE ANESTHETIST ROLE: LEADERSHIP AND AUTONOMY

F.M. has been a certified registered nurse anesthetist (CRNA) for 17 years. His interest in the profession was initiated by a family friend who was a CRNA and who encouraged F.M. to pursue a career as a nurse anesthetist. The factors that have most influenced F.M. in his professional development are his interests in a number of areas, including complex pathophysiology, matching anesthesia techniques to complex patient presentations, pharmacology, and the desire for autonomous practice. F.M. notes, "I get paid to do anesthesia!" This enthusiasm for his specialty is typical of many practicing CRNAs.

F.M. was an active-duty military CRNA and practiced at several military medical centers. As a civilian CRNA, he moved into a group practice based at a rural critical access hospital and other facilities in the Midwest. He spends 90% of his time in direct patient care. Some of that time he oversees a student rotating through his facility because he remains with the student and patient at all times. The balance of F.M.'s time is spent "in the business of anesthesia," related to being part owner of his practice.

A typical day in F.M.'s practice includes meeting in the group's office with colleagues for coffee at 6:00 a.m. Following that, he prepares for anesthetics that he will administer that day. He then meets, interviews, plans, and administers the anesthetic for the first and subsequent cases of the day until the cases are done. If he is on call, he spends the afternoon in the preoperative clinic performing preoperative assessments and interventions for complex patients who will be coming to the operating room in the future.

Some of the unique aspects of F.M.'s practice include autonomy and the use of regional anesthesia techniques. He and his practice partners were early adopters of ultrasound-guided regional block techniques, including interscalene and femoral nerve blocks. He enjoys the challenges of caring for high-acuity patients undergoing complex surgical procedures in a small community hospital.

F.M. describes the greatest challenges in his practice as "autonomy—having to make decisions while caring for very sick and complicated patients with no input from other anesthesia providers [and] the complexity of the patients and the procedures we are performing on them." He also notes that managing a very busy private practice anesthesia group is challenging, "ensuring that we cover all the surgeons and hospitals but at the same time protecting our staff from overwork."

The practice in which F.M. is a partner evolved from a small hospital-employed group of one anesthesiologist and two CRNAs. As the workload grew and more surgeons were added, the group grew larger. "We eventually ended up with three anesthesiologists and six CRNAs. Unfortunately, several members decided to move closer to family. At this point we decided to take advantage of the turmoil and go independent. We formed our own private practice group, a service corporation. We have been functioning like this for the last 9 years."

F.M.'s military background provided knowledge about infrastructure and resources for personal and professional development that carried over into his later career. His CRNA practice partners are all former military CRNAs, and their principal clinical site is a clinical affiliation site for military and civilian nurse anesthesia programs. F.M. has had extensive involvement with his state and national professional organizations and presents to these groups on clinical and nonclinical topics.

patients, and encouraging shared decision making (Becker & Shapiro, 2015).

CRNAs collaborate with peers in the clinical setting, including advanced practice providers (APRNs and physician assistants) in the perioperative setting. Collaboration of this nature may occur in preoperative clinics, and during the intraoperative and postoperative periods, including acute pain management. CRNAs may serve with peers on hospital committees, ranging from quality assurance to APRN-specific committees. CRNAs and other APRNs may belong to organizations that provide advocacy for shared healthcare policy goals, including prescriptive authority full scope of practice and other issues critical to APRNs.

CRNAs provide anesthesia in collaboration with surgeons, dentists, podiatrists, physician anesthesiologists, and other qualified healthcare professionals. Many CRNAs practice collaboratively with anesthesiologists in a care team model. The ratio of CRNAs to anesthesiologists in the care team model is driven by the Centers for Medicare & Medicaid Services (CMS) billing rules (CMS, 2019). There is not uniform agreement in the anesthesia community on the elements of the anesthesia care team. The American Society of Anesthesiologists (ASA) defines anesthesiology as the practice of medicine (ASA, 2019), which is not consistent with historic and legal precedents that also establish anesthesia as the practice of nursing. The ASA's *Statement on the Anesthesia Care Team* (2019) states that all patients deserve the involvement of a physician anesthesiologist in their perioperative care to ensure patient safety and quality of care and describes the physician anesthesiologist as the director of the anesthesia care team. However, research findings published in peer-reviewed journals demonstrate no differences in care when anesthesia is provided by a physician or a CRNA (Dulisse & Cromwell, 2010).

There are four CRNA/physician anesthesiologist anesthesia delivery models commonly used in the United States: CRNA-only, physician anesthesiologist supervision of CRNAs, physician anesthesiologist direction of CRNAs, and physician anesthesiologist–only. Despite the variety of anesthesia delivery models, CRNAs are not required by federal or state laws, except in New Jersey, to be supervised or directed by, or even work with, a physician anesthesiologist (AANA, 2020d).

The distribution of anesthesia providers in the United States does not reflect the ASA mandate for the involvement of a physician anesthesiologist in all anesthetics that are administered. For example, in Illinois, CRNAs are the predominant anesthesia providers in 89% of all counties and the only anesthesia providers in 29% of counties in this state (Illinois Association of Nurse Anesthetists, 2020). Anesthesia providers are not evenly distributed throughout the country, resulting in different populations having disproportionate access to these providers. Compared with anesthesiologists, CRNAs are more likely to be found in counties where populations have lower median incomes, where unemployment, the number of uninsured, and the number of patients using Medicaid are higher. CRNAs provide anesthesia services to these vulnerable populations (Liao et al., 2015).

Collaborative relationships between CRNAs and anesthesiologists are complex, given that these providers are economic competitors. The history of nurse anesthesia in the United States reflects conflicts over control of CRNA education and practice (Horton & Kremer, 2020). However, many CRNAs and anesthesiologists have collegial working relationships. There are CRNA-only anesthesia practices where interprofessional collaboration between CRNAs and surgeons, dentists, and podiatrists is evident. Office-based surgery and forward-deployed military medical units are settings where CRNAs often work without medical direction or supervision by an anesthesiologist.

Federal law requires that CRNAs practice under the supervision of a licensed physician, often a surgeon or anesthesiologist. In 2001 a rule promulgated by CMS allowed states to opt out of the federal requirement for physician supervision of CRNAs (Federal Register, 2001). The rule applies to hospitals and ambulatory surgery centers that meet three criteria. States must:

- Consult with state boards of medicine and nursing about issues related to access to and the quality of anesthesia services in the state.
- Determine that opting out is consistent with state law.
- Determine that opting out is in the best interests of the state's citizens.

The US states and territories that have opted out of the federal physician supervision requirement to date are included in Box 16.6. Additional states do not have

BOX 16.6

Nurse Anesthesia Supervision Opt-Out States and Territories

- Alaska
- Arizona
- Arkansas
- California
- Colorado
- Guam
- Idaho
- Iowa
- Kansas
- Kentucky
- Michigan
- Minnesota
- Montana
- Nebraska
- New Hampshire
- New Mexico
- North Dakota
- Oklahoma
- Oregon
- South Dakota
- Utah (for Critical Access Hospitals and specified rural hospitals)
- Washington
- Wisconsin

Adapted from American Association of Nurse Anesthesiology. (2022b). *Federal supervision rule/opt-out information.* https://www.aana.com/advocacy/state-government-affairs/federal-supervision-rule-opt-out-information supervision requirements in state law and are eligible to opt out should the governors choose to do so. Other states have various laws and regulations that outline the extent to which CRNAs must collaborate with physicians (Merritt Hawkins, 2019).

Findings from a survey of anesthesiologists and CRNAs demonstrated that job stress and dissatisfaction with the work environment were inversely related when collaboration between CRNAs and anesthesiologists was lacking. Other factors that contributed to job stress and dissatisfaction included higher levels of role conflict for CRNAs, unclear work expectations, and limited practice autonomy (Jones & Fitzpatrick, 2009).

Almost half of CRNAs practice in settings where an anesthesiologist concurrently directs up to four CRNAs, which is defined by CMS as *medical direction* and involves seven steps of mandated anesthesiologist participation. Medical supervision is another CMS billing model for anesthesiologist collaboration with CRNAs and does not involve prescribed participation steps for the anesthesiologist and results in less billable revenue per case. One-third of CRNAs practice independently in settings ranging from the military to office-based anesthesia or other clinical settings where medical staff bylaws do not mandate anesthesiologist supervision of CRNAs (Negrusa et al., 2021).

Ethical Practice

CRNAs, like all clinicians, can encounter ethical conflicts in practice. Upholding these ethical principles and accountability in clinical practice, education, and research is critical for CRNAs (Minnesota State University, 2021). CRNAs have an obligation to respect the autonomy of other persons and to not interfere with the decisions of competent adults. For example, a patient with severe chronic obstructive pulmonary disease scheduled for a transurethral resection of the prostate may refuse spinal anesthesia and insist on receiving general anesthesia. The CRNA has the obligation to delineate the risks and benefits of both anesthetic techniques but must respect patient autonomy when formulating the anesthesia care plan.

There is also an obligation to bring about good in all of our actions and to prevent harm. Application of beneficence in clinical practice can be illustrated in a scenario where an anesthetized patient is being placed in the lithotomy position. While the surgical, nursing, and anesthesia teams are all responsible for patient positioning, if the CRNA is the first to notice a positioning error that could result in nerve injury, the CRNA has an ethical obligation to ensure that the patient is correctly positioned. This action helps prevent patient harm in the form of transient or permanent nerve injuries.

As citizens and healthcare providers, CRNAs have an obligation to not harm others; that is, first do no harm. If a CRNA determines that a patient is at risk for pulmonary aspiration of gastric contents and does not implement evidence-based strategies to decrease aspiration risks with consequent patient morbidity or mortality, this violates the principle of nonmaleficence.

We have an obligation to treat all people equally, fairly, and impartially—the principle of justice. Provision of anesthesia care should involve the application of evidence-based practice for each patient, regardless of their ability to pay, and not different standards of care for various patients.

The AANA *Code of Ethics for the CRNA* (2018b) provides guidance for CRNAs for ethical practice in all practice roles. Nurse anesthesia practice may include clinical practice; administrative, educational, or research activities; or a combination of these areas. The AANA *Code of Ethics* contains principles of conduct and professional integrity that guide CRNA decision making and behavior. The primary ethical responsibility of the CRNA is to the patient, as well as to the profession, other healthcare providers, self, and society. "The CRNA acknowledges, understands, and is sensitive to the vulnerability of the patient undergoing anesthesia, pain management, and related care and preserves the patient's trust, confidence and dignity" (AANA, 2018b, p. 1).

Responsibility to the patient is described in the AANA *Code of Ethics* as respect of the CRNA for the patient's moral and legal rights and support of the patient's physical and psychological comfort and well-being. "The CRNA collaborates with the patient and the healthcare team to provide compassionate, holistic, patient-centered anesthesia, pain management and related care" (AANA, 2018b, p. 1).

As licensed independent providers, CRNAs are responsible for their own actions, which is reflected in the *Code of Ethics*.

> *As an independently licensed professional, the CRNA is responsible and accountable for judgments made and actions taken in his or her professional practice. Requests or orders by physicians, other healthcare professionals, or institutions do not relieve the CRNA of responsibility for judgements made or actions taken.*
>
> *(AANA, 2018b, p. 2)*

Responsibility in research is demonstrated by the CRNA protecting the integrity of the research process and the reporting and publication of findings. The CRNA is expected to adhere to the ethical principles of respect for persons, beneficence, and justice relevant to research involving human participants (AANA, 2018b).

Regardless of practice arrangement or setting, CRNAs are expected to maintain ethical business practices in dealing with patients, colleagues, institutions, corporations, and others. The AANA *Code of Ethics* calls for CRNAs to establish and perform contractual obligations consistent with the *Code of Ethics*, professional practice standards, and statutory and regulatory requirements (AANA, 2018b).

The AANA *Code of Ethics* states that CRNAs may endorse products and services only when personally satisfied with the product's or service's safety, effectiveness, and quality. The CRNA may not say that the AANA has endorsed any product or service unless the Board of Directors of the AANA has done so. The CRNA must not endorse any product or service when presenting content for an AANA-approved continuing education activity as this is a prohibited conflict of interest (AANA, 2018b).

CRNAs are expected to collaborate with members of the healthcare professions and others to improve the public health. This includes access to health care and anesthesia, pain management, and related care (AANA, 2018b). Anesthesia care provided by CRNAs to many rural and medically underserved citizens reflects their commitment to this ethical mandate.

CURRENT CRNA PRACTICE

Nurse anesthesia practice includes performing a comprehensive history and physical; conducting a pre-anesthesia evaluation; obtaining informed consent for anesthesia; developing and initiating a patient-specific plan of care; selecting, ordering, prescribing, and administering drugs and controlled substances; and selecting and inserting invasive and noninvasive monitoring modalities. Most CRNAs provide acute pain management services, and some CRNAs administer chronic and interventional pain management therapies. CRNAs may be responsible for critical care and resuscitation services. Anesthesia care can involve ordering diagnostic tests and evaluating the results. CRNAs may request specialty consultation and perform point-of-care testing.

CRNAs plan and initiate anesthetic techniques, including general, regional, and local anesthesia, and intravenous sedation and monitoring. Anesthetic techniques may include the use of ultrasound, fluoroscopy, and other technologies for diagnosis and care delivery and to improve patient safety and comfort. Nurse anesthetists respond to emergency situations using airway management and other skills, facilitate emergence and recovery from anesthesia, and provide postanesthesia care, including medication management. CRNAs conduct postanesthesia evaluation and may be involved with discharging patients from the postanesthesia care area or facility (AANA, 2019c).

CRNAs are interprofessional team members and leaders who practice in these areas: surgical and support services for academic, tertiary, community, ambulatory, office, and critical access, rural facilities; labor and delivery; surgical and nonsurgical pain management; program directors, didactic faculty, and clinical educators; deans; provosts; quantitative and qualitative researchers; and administrators (AANA, 2018a).

Nurse anesthetists administer anesthesia to patients at all acuity levels across the life span, with AANA members reporting caring for patients of varying ages in their clinical practices:

- Neonate, infant 12 months or less: 40%
- Pediatric, more than 12 months to 12 years: 66%
- Adolescent, 13 to 17 years: 89%
- Adult, 18 to 65 years: 99%
- Geriatric, over 65 years: 94% (AANA, 2018a)

Most practicing CRNAs provide general anesthesia and monitored anesthesia care. Depending on the case mix and facility credentialing requirements, CRNAs may also provide regional anesthesia (i.e., spinal, epidural, peripheral nerve blocks) and/or pain management services. CRNAs are also vascular access and airway management experts and are relied on in facilities where they practice to provide these skills (AANA, 2018a).

Mergers and acquisitions of hospitals and healthcare systems are ongoing. These transactions often result in increased market share and improved purchasing power for the involved systems. At the same time, anesthesia practice groups with multistate contracts have emerged. Regardless of whether a CRNA is employed by a hospital (39%), by an anesthesia practice group (35%), or in other practice arrangements, they may be credentialed to provide anesthesia services at multiple clinical sites to maximize their productivity (AANA, 2018a).

The percentage of patients whose health care is publicly funded is rising. Medicare and Medicaid provide lower payment rates than those available through private insurance carriers. As the public payer percentage increases beyond 30% to 40%, some facilities provide financial subsidies to anesthesia groups so that the group can continue to pay its providers market-competitive salaries (Anesthesia Business Consultants, 2019). Findings from a recent study concluded that "direct payments from hospitals are becoming a larger financial consideration for anesthesia groups in California serving nonacademic hospitals and are larger for groups working at hospitals serving publicly insured patients" (O'Connell et al., 2019, p. 534).

Workforce Issues

The US Bureau of Labor Statistics projects job growth for CRNAs to be 26% between 2018 and 2028, while HRSA estimated a 38% increase in the CRNA supply between 2013 and 2015 with a concomitant 16% increase in demand (Bureau of Labor Statistics, n.d.; HRSA, 2016). The AANA member survey data showed that 14% of survey respondents plan to retire from anesthesia practice between 2022 and 2024 (AANA, 2018a).

The Association of American Medical Colleges (AAMC) projected a shortage of up to 122,000 physicians by 2032. This includes shortages of up to 55,000 primary care and 77,000 specialty practice physicians. The specialist shortage is affected by the aging population. Some 10,000 Americans turn 65 each day, and this age cohort utilizes medical services at a higher rate than younger age groups. While seniors represent only 14% of the population, they generate 37.4% of diagnostic tests and treatments and 34% of inpatient procedures, many of which require anesthesia. The US Census Bureau reports that by 2035, senior citizens will outnumber children (Merritt Hawkins, 2019).

Utilization of specialty services, including anesthesia, increased with the economic growth that followed the 2007–2008 recession. There was an increase in ambulatory care sites that influenced utilization of procedures requiring anesthesia. Demand for CRNA services has been driven by the lack of anesthesia providers in rural areas, which are often entirely reliant on CRNAs (Merritt Hawkins, 2019).

There are economic incentives for healthcare systems and facilities to address rising costs and flat or declining reimbursement with increasing use of CRNAs, who are paid considerably less than anesthesiologists while providing many of the same services. Since outcomes data are positive for CRNAs, this enhances their participation in emerging quality/value-based reimbursement (AANA, 2020g; Merritt Hawkins, 2019).

At this writing, the COVID-19 pandemic has had a significant impact on public health and the economy, with 80,440,151 total cases and 986,042 deaths to date in the United States (Centers for Disease Control and Prevention, 2022). Medical group practices of diverse sizes and specialties have felt both direct and indirect impacts of the COVID-19 pandemic. At the height of the COVID-19 pandemic, 97% of practices experienced a negative financial impact directly or indirectly related to COVID-19. On average, practices reported a 55% decrease in revenue and a 60% decrease in patient volume since the beginning of the COVID-19 crisis between January and March 2020. Anesthesia practices reported revenue losses of up to 70%, which led to pay cuts and furloughs (Medical Group Management Association, 2020). In some cases, CRNAs worked in critical care units to maintain their employment (AANA, 2020c). At this writing, elective surgical case volumes in many settings have returned to their pre-COVID-19 levels.

Access to Care

Common staffing models for delivering anesthesia in the United States have been described: services delivered solely by anesthesiologists, services delivered by CRNAs only, and services provided by teams of anesthesiologists and CRNAs. The influence of the opt-out policy enacted by CMS in 2001 was examined through analysis of Medicare claims data. Investigators found that individual facility characteristics and rural/urban considerations played greater roles in the anesthesia service delivery models than did state opt-out status. Allowing CRNAs to provide anesthesia services independently may help alleviate anesthesia provider shortages in rural locations without adversely impacting quality of care and reducing total anesthesia delivery costs (Coomer et al., 2019). Research findings have also demonstrated that opt-out status and less restrictive scope of practice regulations were consistently associated with a greater supply of CRNAs, especially in rural areas. Given the maldistribution of anesthesia providers in the United States (Liao et al., 2015), access to anesthesia services may require addressing issues pertaining to the supply of all anesthesia provider types (Martslof et al., 2019).

While CRNAs are the predominant anesthesia providers in Veterans Administration (VA) hospitals, they lack full practice authority within the VA system, unlike other APRNs who practice in the VA system. The decision to exclude VA CRNAs in the regulatory rule authorizing full practice authority prevents veterans' access to surgical and procedural care requiring anesthesia services, resulting in a delay in care (Wiener, 2017). There are ongoing advocacy efforts to seek full practice authority for the 900 CRNAs who practice in the VA facilities.

Access to health care provided by CRNAs changed as a result of the COVID-19 pandemic. In March 2020, CMS

> *announced an unprecedented array of temporary regulatory waivers and new rules to equip the American healthcare system with maximum flexibility to respond to the pandemic. Waiving the requirements will allow states to optimize their healthcare workforce and enable CRNAs to practice at the top of their license.*
>
> ***(AANA, 2020b)***

States are considering whether to permanently adopt the statutes and rules or allow them to sunset when the declared emergency is over. This is up to each state government.

Reimbursement

Anesthesia billing reflects factors known as *base units*, *time units*, and *modifiers*. Billing services are often incentivized to maximize collections. Box 16.7 defines terms utilized for documenting anesthesia time and Box 16.8 describes general documentation requirements. Additional information on reimbursement can be found in Chapter 19.

Anesthesia Practice Models

There are four anesthesia practice models, including the CRNA-only (modifier code QZ), anesthesiologist-only (modifier code AA), anesthesiologist supervision (more than four concurrent cases; modifier code AD), and anesthesiologist medical direction (one or two to four concurrent cases; modifier codes QX, QY, QK, respectively). Reimbursement by CMS varies by practice model.

According to AANA (2021, December), when the CRNA practices without medical direction, CMS reimburses the CRNA service at 100% of the allowed rate. When the CRNA practices with anesthesiologist supervision, CMS reimburses the CRNA at 50% of the allowed rate. When a CRNA practices under anesthesiologist direction, the CRNA receives 50% of the allowed rate and the anesthesiologist receives 50% of the allowed rate.

Anesthesiologist Billing for Medical Direction vs. Medical Supervision

Medicare pays for medical direction of CRNAs at 50% of the reimbursement for the case. To meet medical direction requirement for two to four concurrent cases, the anesthesiologist must meet the Tax Equity and Financial Reform Act (TEFRA) of Seven Steps rules (Conditions for Payment: Medically Directed Anesthesia Services, 1998). No more than four CRNA cases can be medically directed by an anesthesiologist at one time. An anesthesiologist must document the seven steps, which should be included in the anesthesia record. Two separate claims need to be filed for medically directed anesthesia procedures: one for the anesthesiologist and one for the CRNA. TEFRA steps are included in Box 16.9.

An anesthesiologist may supervise more than four CRNAs concurrently, and billing then occurs at the medically supervised rate. This billing method is

BOX 16.7

Anesthesia Time Definitions

Start time: when the anesthesia provider begins to physically prepare the patient for anesthesia services in the operating room or an equivalent area. This time does not include time spent with the patient during preanesthesia evaluation, as this is bundled into the base unit, which reflects patient acuity. Start time does not include placement of an IV or placing monitors or administration of preanesthesia sedation.

End time is when the anesthesia provider transfers care in the postanesthesia care unit (PACU) to a qualified professional.

Discontinuous time: providers must document the start and end of block or line placement, which occur prior to the primary anesthetic being given; for example:

- 9:00–9:04 AM: IV placement
- 9:05–9:14 AM: discontinuous time
- 9:15–11:15 AM: procedure/surgery

Relief: document start and stop times and the provider who is relieving another provider during the case.

Postoperative pain management: a regional anesthesia block may be billed as a separate service/procedure if placed for postoperative pain management and it is not the primary anesthetic technique.

Other considerations for anesthesia time include:

- Enter exact time, do not round.
- Use one consistent time piece.
- The end time for one case and start time for the next case must be at least 1 minute apart.
- Clearly document names and start/stop times of any relief providers during the case.

Adapted from American Association of Nurse Anesthesiology. (2021, December). *Anesthesia billing basics consideration checklist, version 3.* https://www.aana.com/search?keyword=Anesthesia%20billing%20basics%20considerations%20checklist

seldom used since it does not permit billing for the full reimbursable amount (AANA, 2021, December).

Anesthesia Billing Calculation

Contractual agreements may exist with insurance companies that specify payment of an agreed rate per unit.

BOX 16.8

General Anesthesia Documentation Requirements

- Patient identifiers (name, date of birth, gender)
- Patient diagnosis
- Physical status
- Service date, with anesthesia start, end, and relief times
- Service/procedure performed, which must match the surgeon's operative report
- Type of anesthesia provided
- Patient positioning
- Discontinuous time
- Relief anesthesia provider(s)
- Surgeon request for postoperative pain management and specific information about postoperative pain management provided
- Facility name/OR number
- Provider signature(s)

Adapted from American Association of Nurse Anesthesiology. (2021, December). *Anesthesia billing basics consideration checklist, version 3.* https://www.aana.com/search?keyword=Anesthesia%20billing%20basics%20considerations%20checklist

BOX 16.9

TEFRA (Tax Equity and Financial Reform Act) Steps

1. Performs a preanesthetic examination and evaluation;
2. Prescribes the anesthesia plan;
3. Personally participates in the most demanding procedures in the anesthesia plan, including, if applicable, induction and emergence;
4. Ensures that any procedures in the anesthesia plan that they do not perform are performed by a qualified individual;
5. Monitors the course of anesthesia administration at frequent intervals;
6. Remains physically present and available for immediate diagnosis and treatment of emergencies; and
7. Provides indicated postanesthesia care.

Adapted from Legal Information Institute. (1998). Conditions for Payment: Medically Directed Anesthesia Services, C.F.R. §415.110(a)(1)(iii). https://www.law.cornell.edu/cfr/text/42/415.110

The calculation (Base Units + Time Units + Modifying Units) × Conversion Factor = Billed Amount (AANA, 2021, December) can be adjusted to reflect that negotiated amount. There may be a difference in billed amount and allowed amount.

Anesthesia Claim Modifiers

Box 16.10 describes CRNA, anesthesiologist, and monitored anesthesia care modifiers. Modifiers allow providers to denote additional information related to the procedure code. Every anesthesia claim billed to Medicare must include one of the modifiers. There are a number of variables involved in anesthesia reimbursement. Careful selection of the modifiers, documentation by anesthesia providers, and a competent billing service will maximize revenue for the employer or contractor while avoiding potential exposure to fraudulent billing claims.

BOX 16.10

Anesthesia Care Modifiers

CRNA Modifiers

QX: CRNA service with medical direction by a physician.

QZ: CRNA service without medical direction by a physician.

Anesthesiologist Modifiers

AA: Anesthesia services performed personally by the anesthesiologist.

AD: Medical supervision by a physician; more than four concurrent anesthesia procedures.

QK: Medical direction of two, three, or four concurrent anesthesia procedures involving qualified anesthetists.

QY: Medical direction of one qualified anesthetist by a physician.

GC: Services performed by a resident under the direction of a teaching physician.

Monitored Anesthesia Care

QS: Monitored anesthesia care service. Anesthesia time must be reported.

G8: Monitored anesthesia care for deep complex, complicated, or markedly invasive surgical procedures.

G9: Monitored anesthesia care for patient who has a history of severe cardio-pulmonary condition.

- If the patient loses consciousness or the ability to respond purposefully in any point in the case, the mode is considered general anesthetic.
- The provider of MAC must be qualified to administer anesthesia and be prepared to convert to a general anesthetic if necessary.

Adapted from American Association of Nurse Anesthesiology. (2021, December). *Anesthesia billing basics consideration checklist, version 3*. https://www.aana.com/search?keyword=Anesthesia%20billing%20basics%20considerations%20checklist

NURSE ANESTHESIA ORGANIZATIONS

American Association of Nurse Anesthesiology

The AANA is the professional organization to which over 80% of CRNAs belong. All student registered nurse anesthetists are AANA associate members. The AANA promulgates education and practice standards and guidelines and provides consultative services for members in areas including practice management and research. The AANA Foundation supports the profession by awarding education and research grants to students, faculty, and practicing CRNAs (AANA, 2020a).

The AANA vision is to be the transformative leader driving innovation and patient-centered excellence in anesthesia and health care. AANA's mission is "to advance patient safety and our profession through excellence in practice and service to members" (AANA, 2020a).

The AANA board of directors represents seven geographic regions of the United States. Additional elected positions in AANA are the president, the president-elect, the vice president, and the treasurer. AANA has 18 committees that include staff support and appointed CRNAs. There are opportunities for nurse anesthesia students to serve on some AANA committees, as well on the COA and NBCRNA (AANA, 2020a).

AANA staff members include an executive team comprising four individuals and 15 directors, along with support staff. AANA maintains offices in Park Ridge, Illinois, and Washington, DC.

International Federation of Nurse Anesthetists and International Practice

The International Federation of Nurse Anesthetists (IFNA) was founded in 1989 by 11 countries where nurse anesthetists practiced. IFNA currently has 43 country members (IFNA, 2020). IFNA provides professional advocacy for nurse anesthetists globally while advancing educational standards and the worldwide quality of anesthesia care. IFNA maintains collaborative relationships with institutions worldwide that have a professional interest in nurse anesthesia (IFNA, 2020).

Nurse anesthetists are recognized for their significant contributions to global health care as practitioners, teachers, administrators, researchers, and consultants. IFNA formulates healthcare policies that recognize nurse anesthetists as essential and cost-effective healthcare providers (IFNA, 2020).

IFNA's objectives include:

- Promoting cooperation between nurse anesthetists internationally.
- Developing and promoting educational standards in the field of nurse anesthesia.
- Developing and promoting standards of practice in the field of nurse anesthesia.
- Providing opportunities for continuing education in anesthesia.
- Assisting nurse anesthesia associations in improving the standards of nurse anesthesia and the competence of nurse anesthetists.
- Promoting the recognition of nurse anesthesia.
- Establishing and maintaining effective cooperation between nurse anesthetists, anesthesiologists, and other members of the medical profession, the nursing profession, hospitals, and agencies representing a community of interest in nurse anesthesia (IFNA, 2020).

IFNA has developed Standards of Education, Standards of Practice, and a Code of Ethics for nurse anesthetists. Models of nurse anesthesia program curriculum have been prepared by the IFNA Education Committee. IFNA is an affiliate member of the International Council of Nurses (IFNA, 2020).

FUTURE DIRECTIONS IN CRNA PRACTICE

Negrusa et al. (2021) found that CRNA survey respondents were overall satisfied with their jobs. Factors that increased job satisfaction, which may influence future directions in CRNA practice, included greater autonomy in delivery of anesthesia, utilization of a wide range of clinical skills, and higher levels of compensation. Since supervision ratios in anesthesia are driven by billing requirements, movement from medical direction to medical supervision could increase CRNA job satisfaction. As the number of CRNAs in the anesthesia workforce increases, with a potential concomitant decrease in anesthesiologists, additional reimbursement may become available for CRNAs.

CRNAs seek to augment their clinical skills in areas that are becoming larger components of anesthesia practice; that is, peripheral nerve blocks, advanced airway management, and epidural analgesia. Greater opportunities for nurse anesthesia students to learn and utilize skills in practice will support the market demand for CRNAs who can practice at the full scope of their education and licensure. Facilities and practices that seek to increase CRNA job satisfaction and retention will need to encourage anesthesia care delivery models that do not overly restrict scope of practice and allow CRNAs to fully utilize their education and training (Negrusa et al., 2021).

CONCLUSION

Nurse anesthesia is an established nursing specialty that has withstood significant challenges over its 150-year history. From its inception in 1931, the National Association of Nurse Anesthetists, later the American Association of Nurse Anesthesiology, sought to improve and standardize the education for nurse anesthetists. NANA members were committed to enhancing anesthesia patient safety and quality of care. Nurse anesthesia was the first nursing specialty to offer a certification examination and to have programmatic accreditation, mandatory continuing education, and direct billing under Medicare Part B.

CRNAs in the United States practice in diverse clinical settings, providing anesthesia to patients across the life span at all acuity levels undergoing procedures of varying complexity. Healthcare systems and facilities have addressed rising costs and flat or declining reimbursement for surgical and diagnostic services, resulting in increasing demand for CRNAs, who are paid significantly less annually than anesthesiologists while providing many of the same services. Outcomes data are positive for CRNAs, which enhances their participation in emerging quality/value-based reimbursement mechanisms.

CRNAs practice collaboratively with surgeons, dentists, podiatrists, and anesthesiologists. Staffing ratios when CRNAs work with anesthesiologists are driven by CMS billing requirements. There are CRNA-only practices that provide anesthesia services to hospitals, surgery centers, physician offices, and pain management practices. The AANA scope (2020h) and standards (2019a) of CRNA practice demonstrate the high level of professional responsibility, accountability, and autonomy associated with the CRNA role. Rigorous and evidence-based accreditation, certification, and recertification processes help ensure CRNA workforce competency (AANA, 2022).

The American Association of Nurse Anesthesiology, formerly called the American Association of Nurse Anesthesiology, and state nurse anesthesia associations have repeatedly addressed legal and regulatory challenges to nurse anesthesia practice. Legal and historic precedents have established that when anesthesia is practiced by nurses, it is the practice of nursing; when anesthesia is practiced by a physician, it is the practice of medicine.

While there is some role overlap between critical care nursing and nurse anesthesia, nurse anesthetists function with a high degree of autonomy, with or without medical direction or supervision. This rewarding and challenging specialty offers opportunities in practice, education, research, military service, and industry.

KEY SUMMARY POINTS

- Nurse anesthesia, the earliest nursing specialty, was the first nursing specialty to have standardized educational programs, a certification process, mandatory continuing education, recertification requirements, and the first APRN specialty to adopt a timeline for conversion of educational programs from master's to doctoral entry by January 1, 2022.
- CRNAs are nursing leaders in obtaining third-party reimbursement for professional services and in coping with challenges such as the prospective payment system, managed care, and physician supervision.
- CRNAs work collaboratively with physicians, as do other APRNs, and are capable of providing the full spectrum of anesthesia services.
- Activism at the state and federal legislative and regulatory levels is a recognized CRNA activity. Economics and control of practice continue to be areas of challenge that CRNAs meet proactively, state by state.
- Market demand for CRNAs is high, and additional evidence of the safety, quality, and cost-effectiveness of anesthesia care provided by CRNAs supports the needs of third-party payers, accountable care organizations (ACOs), legislators, and the public for outcome data.
- CRNAs will continue to provide high-quality anesthesia care as practice, education, and reimbursement models evolve to reflect new economic models for the delivery of health care.

REFERENCES

American Association of Colleges of Nursing. (2006). *The essentials of doctoral education for advanced nursing practice*. https://www.aacnnursing.org/DNP/DNP-Essentials

American Association of Colleges of Nursing. (2019). *Palliative care is growing across the US*. https://www.aacnnursing.org/News-Information/News/View/ArticleId/24523/ELNEC-Palliative-Care-is-Growing

American Association of Colleges of Nursing. (2021). *The Essentials: Core competencies for professional nursing education*. https://www.aacnnursing.org/Portals/42/AcademicNursing/pdf/Essentials-2021.pdf

American Association of Nurse Anesthesiology. (2018a). AANA member survey data. *American Association of Nurse Anesthetists*.

American Association of Nurse Anesthesiology. (2018b). *Code of ethics for the CRNA*. https://www.aana.com/docs/default-source/practice-aana-com-web-documents-(all)/code-of-ethics-for-the-crna.pdf?sfvrsn=d70049b1_6

American Association of Nurse Anesthesiology. (2019a). *AANA Standards for Nurse Anesthesia Practice*. https://www.aana.com/docs/default-source/practice-aana-com-web-documents-(all)/standards-for-nurse-anesthesia-practice.pdf?sfvrsn=e00049b1_18

American Association of Nurse Anesthesiology. (2019b). *Certified Registered Nurse Anesthetists Fact Sheet*. https://www.aana.com/membership/become-a-crna/crna-fact-sheet

American Association of Nurse Anesthesiology. (2019c). *Clinical privileges and other responsibilities of certified registered nurse anesthetists*. https://www.aana.com/docs/default-source/practice-aana-com-web-documents-(all)/clinical-privileges-and-other-responsibilities-of-crnas.pdf?sfvrsn=82011b35_2

American Association of Nurse Anesthesiology. (2019d). *Clinical privileges and other responsibilities of CRNAs.* https://www.aana.com/docs/default-source/practice-aana-com-web-documents-(all)/professional-practice-manual/clinical-privileges-and-other-responsibilities-of-crnas.pdf?sfvrsn=82011b35_2

American Association of Nurse Anesthesiology. (2020a). About us. https://www.aana.com/about-us/who-we-are

American Association of Nurse Anesthesiology. (2020b). *CMS suspends CRNA supervision requirements.* https://www.aana.com/news/hot-topics/news-detail/2020/03/31/cms-suspends-supervision-requirements-for-crnas

American Association of Nurse Anesthesiology. (2020c). *CRNAs asked to assume critical care responsibilities during the COVID-19 pandemic.* https://www.aana.com/docs/default-source/practice-aana-com-web-documents-(all)/crnas_asked_to_assume_critical_care_responsibilities_during_the_COVID_19_pandemic.pdf?sfvrsn=ea3630e7_6

American Association of Nurse Anesthesiology. (2020d). *CRNAs: We are the answer.* https://www.aana.com/we-are-the-answer/position-statement

American Association of Nurse Anesthesiology. (2020e). *Evidence-based practice.* https://www.aana.com/practice/evidence-based-practice

American Association of Nurse Anesthesiology. (2020f). *Opioid crisis resources.* https://www.aana.com/practice/clinical-practice-resources/opioid-crisis-resources

American Association of Nurse Anesthesiology. (2020g). *Quality-reimbursement.* https://www.aana.com/advocacy/quality-reimbursement

American Association of Nurse Anesthesiology. (2020h). *Scope of nurse anesthesia practice.* https://www.aana.com/docs/default-source/practice-aana-com-web-documents-(all)/scope-of-nurse-anesthesia-practice.pdf?sfvrsn=250049b1_6

American Association of Nurse Anesthesiology. (2020i). *Surgeon liability.* https://www.aana.com/practice/practice-management/surgeon-liability

American Association of Nurse Anesthesiology. (2021, December). *Anesthesia billing basics consideration checklist, version 3.* https://www.aana.com/search?keyword=Anesthesia%20billing%20basics%20considerations%20checklist

American Association of Nurse Anesthesiology. (2021a). *AANA announces major rebrand and moves forward as the American Association of Nurse Anesthesiology.* https://www.aana.com/news/hot-topics/news-detail/2021/08/14/aana-announces-major-rebrand-and-moves-forward-as-the-american-association-of-nurse-anesthesiology

American Association of Nurse Anesthesiology. (2021b). *AANA diversity and inclusion resources.* https://www.aana.com/about-us/aana-diversity-and-inclusion

American Association of Nurse Anesthesiology. (2021c). *Member survey data.* [PowerPoint slides].

American Association of Nurse Anesthesiology. (2022a). AANA professional practice manual. https://www.aana.com/practice/practice-manual

American Association of Nurse Anesthesiology. (2022b). Federal supervision rule/opt-out information. https://www.aana.com/advocacy/state-government-affairs/federal-supervision-rule-opt-out-information

American Society of Anesthesiologists. (2019). Statement on the anesthesia care team. https://www.asahq.org/standards-and-guidelines/statement-on-the-anesthesia-care-team

Anesthesia Business Consultants. (2019). *The significance of the anesthesia public payer percentage.* https://www.anesthesiallc.com/publications/anesthesia-provider-news-ealerts/1234-the-significance-of-the-anesthesia-public-payer-percentage

Becker, A., & Shapiro, F. (2015). Patient-centered care: Improving patient safety in anesthesia through patient engagement. *ASA Monitor, 75*(5), 10–12. http://monitor.pubs.asahq.org/article.aspx?articleid=2434109

Boss, E. F., Links, A. R., Saxton, R., Cheng, T. L., & Beach, M. C. (2017). Parent experience of care and decision making for children who snore. *JAMA Otolaryngolog—Head & Neck Surgery, 143*(3), 218–225.

Brusie, C. (2020). *Why nursing is a great career choice for men. Nurse.org.* https://nurse.org/articles/Male-Nurses-And-The-Profession/#:~:text=According%20to%20the%20U.S.%20Bureau,in%20the%20U.S.%20are%20men

Bureau of Labor Statistics. (n.d.). Occupational outlook handbook: Nurse anesthetists, nurse midwives, and nurse practitioners. https://www.bls.gov/ooh/healthcare/nurse-anesthetists-nurse-midwives-and-nurse-practitioners.htm

Centers for Disease Control and Prevention. (2022). COVID data tracker. https://covid.cdc.gov/covid-data-tracker/#cases-deaths-testing-trends

Centers for Medicare & Medicaid Services. (2019). Anesthesiologists center. https://www.cms.gov/Center/Provider-Type/Anesthesiologists Center

Chan, K. H., Panoch, J., Carroll, A., Wiehe, S., Downs, S., Cain, M. P., & Frankel, R. (2019). Parental perspectives on decision-making about hypospadias surgery. *Journal of Pediatric Urology, 15*(5). 449.e1–449.e8. https://doi-org.ezproxy.rush.edu/10.1016/j.jpurol.2019.04.017

Coomer, N., Mills, A., Beadles, C., Gillen, E., Chew, R., & Quraishi, J. (2019). Anesthesia staffing models and geographic prevalence post-Medicare CRNA/physician exemption policy. *Nursing Economics, 37*(2), 86–91.

Council on Accreditation of Nurse Anesthesia Educational Programs. (2017). *Guidelines for preparing/reviewing doctoral degree applications.* Council on Accreditation of Nurse Anesthesia Educational Programs.

Council on Accreditation of Nurse Anesthesia Educational Programs. (2018). *Standards for accreditation of nurse anesthesia educational programs.* Council on Accreditation of Nurse Anesthesia Educational Programs.

Council on Accreditation of Nurse Anesthesia Educational Programs. (2019). *Standards for accreditation of nurse anesthesia educational programs – practice doctorate.* Council on Accreditation of Nurse Anesthesia Educational Programs.

Council on Accreditation of Nurse Anesthesia Educational Programs. (2021). *Accredited nurse anesthesia programs in the US.* https://www.coacrna.org/nurse-anesthesia-programs-awarding-masters-and-doctoral-degrees-for-entry-into-practice/

Council on Accreditation of Nurse Anesthesia Educational Programs. (2022a). CRNA school search. https://www.coacrna.org/programs-fellowships/crna-school-search/

Council on Accreditation of Nurse Anesthesia Educational Programs. (2022b). *Standards for Accreditation of Nurse Anesthesia Educational Programs – Practice Doctorate.* https://www.coacrna.org/accreditation/accreditation-standards-policies-and-procedures-and-guidelines/

Dulisse, B., & Cromwell, J. (2010). No harm found when nurse anesthetists work without supervision by physicians. *Health Affairs, 29*(8), 1469–1475.

Faut Callahan, M., Breakwell, S., & Suhayda, R. (2011). Knowledge of palliative and end-of-life care by student registered nurse anesthetists. *AANA J, 79*(4 Suppl), S15–S20.

Federal Register. (2001). *Medicare and Medicaid programs: Hospital conditions of participation: Anesthesia services.* July 4, 2001. https://www.federal-register.gov/documents/2001/07/05/01-16964/medicare-and-medicaid-programs-hospital-conditions-of-participation-anesthesia-services

Feinstein, M. M., Pannunzio, A. E., Lobell, S., & Kodish, E. (2018). Informed consent in pediatric anesthesia: A narrative review. *Anesthesia and Analgesia, 127*(6), 1398–1405. https://doi-org.ezproxy.rush.edu/10.1213/ANE.0000000000003705

Forbat, L. (2009). Engaging patients in healthcare: An empirical study of the role of engagement on attitudes and actions. *Patient Education and Counseling, 74*(1), 84–90.

Gentry, K. R., Arnup, S. J., Disma, N., Dorris, L., de Graaff, J. C., Hunyady, A., Morton, N. S., Withington, D. E., McCann, M. E., Davidson, A. J., Lynn, A. M., & Trial Consortium, GAS. (2019). Enrollment challenges in multicenter, international studies: The example of the GAS trial. *Paediatric Anaesthesia, 29*(1), 51–58.

Gerbasi, F. (2016). *Program directors' update. Issue 71* (pp. 3). Council on Accreditation of Nurse Anesthesia Educational Programs.

Gilliland, J. (2022). *Get ready for a CNS, CRNA, NP and PA labor shortage again in 2022.* https://www.directshifts.com/post/get-ready-for-a-cns-crna-np-and-pa-labor-shortage-again

Goode, V. (2015). Alice Magaw: A model for evidence-based practice. *AANA J, 83*(1), 50–55.

Griffis, C., Giron, S., & Darna, J. (2017). The opioid crisis and the certified registered nurse anesthetist: How can we help? *AANA J, 85*(4), 19–23.

Harper, V. (2016). The Institute of Medicine Report on the future of nursing: Where are we five years later? *Journal of PeriAnesthesia Nursing, 31*(5), 367–369.

Hawkins, M. (2019). *CRNA supply, demand and recruiting trends.* https://www.merritthawkins.com/uploadedFiles/Merritt_Hawkins_CRNA_Whitepaper_2019.pdf

Health Resources and Services Administration. (2016). *Health workforce projects: Certified nurse anesthetists.* https://bhw.hrsa.gov/sites/default/files/bhw/health-workforce-analysis/research/projections/crna-fact-sheet.pdf

Health Resources and Services Administration. (2020). *HRSA health workforce – nursing.* https://bhw.hrsa.gov/grants/nursing

Health Resources and Services Administration. (2021). *FY 2020 nurse anesthetist traineeships (NAT) awards.* https://bhw.hrsa.gov/funding/nurse-anesthetist-traineeships-fy2020-awards

Horton, B., & Kremer, M. (2020). A commitment to quality: Nurse anesthesia accreditation part one: 1930-1982. *AANA Journal, 88*(2), 1–12. https://www.aana.com/docs/default-source/aana-journal-web-documents-1/imagining-in-time-online-content-april-2020.pdf?sfvrsn=ac147c47_6

Illinois Association of Nurse Anesthetists. (2020). *CRNAs improve access to care.* https://www.ilcrna.com/

Institute for Patient and Family-Centered Care. (2008). *Advancing the practice of patient and family-centered care in hospitals.* http://www.ipfcc.org/pdf/getting_started.pdf

Institute of Medicine. (2011). *The future of nursing: Leading change, advancing health.* The National Academies Press. https://www.nap.edu/catalog/12956/the-future-of-nursing-leading-change-advancing-health

International Federation of Nurse Anesthetists. (2020). *About IFNA.* https://ifna.site/about-ifna/

Jones, T., & Fitzpatrick, J. (2009). CRNA-physician collaboration in anesthesia. *AANA Journal, 77*(6), 431–436.

Kohl, R. (2022). AANA federal advocacy hotline. 11, 1-5. American Association of Nurse Anesthesiology.

Legal Information Institute. (1998). Conditions for payment: Medically directed anesthesia services, C.F.R. §415.110(a)(1)(iii). https://www.law.cornell.edu/cfr/text/42/415.110

Liao, C., Quraishi, J., & Jordan, L. (2015). Geographical imbalance of anesthesia providers and its impact on the uninsured and vulnerable populations. *Nursing Economics, 33*(5), 263–270.

Martslof, G., Baird, M., Cohen, C., & Koirala, N. (2019). Relationship between state policy and anesthesia provider supply in rural communities. *Medical Care, 57*(5), 341–347.

Magaw, A. (1902). The administration of anesthetics. *St. Paul Med J, 4*, 11–16.

Magaw, A. (1906). A review of over fourteen thousand surgical anesthesia. *AANA J, 67*(1), 35–38.

Medical Group Management Association. (2020). *COVID-19 financial impact on medical practices.* https://www.mgma.com/getattachment/9b8be0c2-0744-41bf-864f-04007d6adbd2/2004-G09621D-COVID-Financial-Impact-One-Pager-8-5x11-MW-2.pdf.aspx?lang=en-US&ext=.pdf

Minnesota State University. (2021). *Four fundamental ethical principles.* http://web.mnstate.edu/gracyk/courses/phil%20115/Four_Basic_principles.htm

Moffett, P., & Moore, G. (2011). The standard of care: Legal history and definitions: The bad and good news. *Western Journal of Emergency Medicine, 12*(1), 109–112.

National Academies of Sciences, Engineering, and Medicine. (2021). *The future of nursing 2020-2030: Charting a path to achieve health equity.* The National Academies Press. https://doi.org/10.17226/25982

National Board for Certification and Recertification of Nurse Anesthetists. (2020a). About us. https://www.nbcrna.com/about-us,

National Board for Certification and Recertification of Nurse Anesthetists. (2020b). *CPC assessment.* https://www.nbcrna.com/continued-certification/cpc-assessment

National Board for Certification and Recertification of Nurse Anesthetists. (2020c). *Initial certification.* https://www.nbcrna.com/initial-certification

National Board for Certification and Recertification of Nurse Anesthetists. (2020d). *National certification examination content outline.* https://www.nbcrna.com/docs/default-source/publications-documentation/handbooks/nce_hb(1).pdf?sfvrsn=5ed2310c_4

National Board for Certification and Recertification of Nurse Anesthetists. (2020e). Non-surgical pain management. https://www.nbcrna.com/exams/nspm

Negrusa, S., Hogan, P, Jordan, L., Hoyem, R., Cintina, I., Zhou, M., Pereira, A., & Quraishi, J. (2021). Work patterns, socio-demographic characteristics and job satisfaction of the CRNA workforce – Findings from the 2019 AANA survey of CRNAs. *Nursing Outlook, 69*(3), 370–379.

Niyogi, A., & Clarke, S. A. (2012). Elective paediatric surgery: What do parents really want to know. *Scottish Medical Journal, 57*, 65–68. doi:10.1258/smj.2012.012002

O'Connell, C., Dexter, F., Mauler, D., & Sun, E. (2019). Trends in direct hospital payments to anesthesia groups: A retrospective cohort study of nonacademic hospitals in California. *Anesthesiology, 131*(3), 534–542.

Society for Opioid-Free Anesthesia. (2021). *Why should I switch from balanced anesthesia?* https://goopioidfree.com/about-us/

Thatcher, V. (1953). *A history of anesthesia with emphasis on the nurse specialist* (p. 253). JB Lippincott.

Wiener, B. (2017). Six things the VA can do to ensure veterans get the anesthesia care they need. Becker's Hospital Review, October 24, 2017. https://www.beckershospitalreview.com/hospital-physician-relationships/6-things-the-va-can-do-to-ensure-veterans-get-the-anesthesia-care-they-need.html

William, G. (2009). Shared decision-making. *Healthcare Quarterly, 12*(Sp), e186e–e1190.

PART IV Critical Elements in Managing Advanced Practice Nursing Environments

17 MAXIMIZING APRN POWER AND INFLUENCING POLICY

EILEEN T. O'GRADY ■ SUSANNE J. PHILLIPS

"If they don't give you a seat at the table, bring a folding chair."
~ Shirley Chisholm, The United States First Black Woman elected to the House of Representatives (D-NY, 1969–1983)

CHAPTER CONTENTS

POLICY: HISTORIC CORE FUNCTION IN NURSING 555

POLICY: APRNS AND MODERN ROLES 555

POLICY VERSUS POLITICS 556
- Health Policy 556
- Politics 556

UNITED STATES FUNDAMENTALLY DIFFERS FROM THE INTERNATIONAL COMMUNITY 557

KEY POLICY CONCEPTS 559
- Federalism 559
- Incrementalism 559
- Presidential Politics 561
- APRNs, Civic Engagement, and Money 561

POLICY MODELS AND FRAMEWORKS 564
- Longest Model 564
- The Kingdon or Garbage Can Model 564
- Knowledge Transfer Framework 565

CURRENT ADVANCED PRACTICE NURSING POLICY ISSUES 566
- Framing Current Issues: Cost, Quality, Access, and the Value Agenda 566
- Policy Initiatives in Health Reform 570

APRN POLITICAL COMPETENCE IN THE POLICY ARENA 571
- Political Competence 572
- Individual Skills 573
- Moving the APRN Role Forward in Health Policy 582

EMERGING ADVANCED PRACTICE NURSING POLICY ISSUES 584
- APRN Full Practice Authority 584
- APRN Workforce Development 586

CONCLUSION 586

KEY SUMMARY POINTS 586

The purpose of this chapter is to build advanced practice registered nurse (APRN) policy competency. Readers are reminded of nursing's core historical function in policymaking and provided various frameworks to explore the policymaking process and a model for dissemination. Current and emerging APRN policy issues will be emphasized, along with APRN policy leadership skills that comprise the specific attitudes and behaviors necessary to be influential in the policy realm. These skills are highlighted in the exemplars. It is the authors' great hope that students reading this chapter will be moved to expand their roles beyond the clinical and broaden their circle of influence on how health care gets paid for, measured, and delivered.

POLICY: HISTORIC CORE FUNCTION IN NURSING

Florence Nightingale spent much of her career walking the halls of Parliament promoting policy change to improve quality, dignity, and equity, first for the Crimean war soldiers and later for the poor of London. Her 3 years of clinical practice gave her clinical expertise and credibility to assume the role of policymaker. She embraced that role because of her high degree of moral distress and concern about the needless suffering and premature death of her patients (Jameton, 1993; Whitehead et al., 2015). She believed that she knew the right thing to do for the soldiers, and the constraints she faced were significant. Empowered by her clinical practice during the Crimean war, she used data that she had collected systematically to persuade Parliament to make needed military and civic law reforms that promoted health. In 1858 Nightingale became the first woman elected as a member of the Royal Statistical Society, and she later became an honorary member of the American Statistical Association (Gill & Gill, 2005). Her work and prestige were Victorian-era validations of the importance of using evidence to inform policy. Nightingale's activism presaged the APRN as patient advocate and policy shaper. She leveraged statistics and clinical expertise to become an effective advocate for influencing policy. She expected nurses to have a high degree of social interest in the human condition and to be involved in the policymaking process. As Nightingale's work demonstrated, health policy challenges and opportunities can be found in both "big P" policies such as formal laws, rules, and regulations at the local, state, national, and/or international level and in the "small p" policy arena such as nongovernmental organizational guidelines, decisions, and social norms guiding behavior (Brownson et al., 2009).

This historic covenant with the public could be strengthened. APRNs ought to deepen their commitment to and become masterful at critiquing, formulating, and influencing policies that interfere with human dignity, wholeness, and health. Most APRNs in practice today have experienced the effects of polices that lead directly to poor health care. We must substantively weave policy into all APRN roles so that those experiences move APRNs into leadership roles so that they become advocates for change.

POLICY: APRNS AND MODERN ROLES

Powerful APRN clinical experiences, when effectively communicated, serve to deepen policymakers' understanding of health-related issues. APRN practice experiences are poignant stories that enlighten policy issues by providing a human context while bringing nursing's value to the health policy arena. Most APRNs in practice today have experienced the effects of ill-conceived policies that lead to needless suffering, poor resource use, perverse metrics, unmanageable technology intrusions, and poorly coordinated, highly specialized, fragmented health care. This practice experience, coupled with the ability to analyze the policy process, provides a strong foundation to propel APRNs into politically competent action and advocacy.

The *Future of Nursing 2020–2030* report (National Academies of Sciences, Engineering, and Medicine, 2021) has charted a course for nursing to create a culture of health by reducing disparities and to fundamentally improve the health and well-being of the United States. The publication of this report will bring about policy and advocacy opportunities for APRN policy leaders throughout the country to improve health disparities for all, and continuing to ensure that APRNs are at the table when reforms are developed, adopted, and implemented. Increasing numbers of stakeholders are noticing advanced practice nurses and the key role they play in healthcare delivery. During the COVID pandemic of 2020, it was a regular occurrence to see front line APRNs interviewed before huge national audiences on their experience and public health advice during COVID surges. *Reforming America's Healthcare System Through Choice and Competition* (US Department of Health and Human Services, US Department of the Treasury, US Department of Labor, 2018), a report by the US government, recommends allowing all healthcare providers to practice to the "top of their license," utilizing their full skill set. It encourages easy mobility of all healthcare providers across states through interstate compacts. It recognizes that more healthcare competition would ensue if the byzantine patchwork of 50 different state practice acts were streamlined. The risk of anticompetitive harm may be even greater when the regulatory board that imposes restrictions (e.g., in Virginia, nurse practitioners

[NPs], certified nurse-midwives [CNMs], and certified registered nurse anesthetists [CRNAs] are regulated by a joint board of Nursing and Medicine) when one occupation is allowed to control members of another.

POLICY VERSUS POLITICS

Health Policy

All policy involves decisions that affect the daily life of citizens by how resources are allocated. Longest (2016) has defined health policy as "the authoritative decisions pertaining to health or health care, made in the legislative, executive, or judicial branches of government, that are intended to direct or influence the actions, behaviors, or decisions of citizens" (p. 5).

Although there are many definitions of policy and politics, *policy* generally refers to decisions resulting in a law or regulation. It is the responsibility of a multitude of policymakers, whether mayors, county supervisors, government employees, legislators, governors, or presidents, to make health policy. Overall responsibility generally places authority with the legislative branch to craft laws (Box 17.1); the executive branch crafts rules to implement the laws, and the judicial branch interprets conflicts among the spheres of government, citizens, and a public or private entity.

BOX 17.1

How to Find a Legislative Bill and Determine Bipartisan Support

To find a federal bill, go to the Library of Congress website (https://www.congress.gov/) and find the current legislative session.

- Search keywords or enter the bill number.
- Once you get to the bill summary, do an analysis to determine whether the bill has any chance of passing by going to the list of cosponsors.
  - The Library of Congress does not list political affiliation next to the cosponsor's name, which requires looking up each member to find out to which party he or she belongs.
  - Be sure that members of congress from each party are cosponsoring the bill in equivalent numbers. If it is only one party sponsoring the bill, you may conclude that the bill is largely partisan, with small chance of passage.

A politically competent APRN will always look for bipartisan cosponsorship of bills, which indicates the highest chance of actually becoming law. The same method will work for a bill in any state legislature (found on each state's government website).

Politics

Politics refers to power relationships. Politics is the process used to influence those who are making health policy. It introduces nonrational, divisive, and self-interested approaches to policymaking, often along ideological lines. In the United States the core disagreement between the two political parties comes down to what the role of the government should be (if any) in resolving conflicting viewpoints. Any political maneuvering to enhance one's power or status within a group may be described as politics. Politics in a democracy is the nonviolent way of reaching agreement between differing points of view and requires compromise in which neither party gets precisely what it wants. Compromise and deal-making are the only alternatives to coercion or authoritarianism (Crick, 1962). Politics is largely associated with a struggle for ascendancy among groups having different priorities and power relationships. Preferences and interests of stakeholders and political bargaining (favor swapping) are important and extremely influential factors that overlie the policymaking process. The self-interest paradigm suggests that human motives are not any different in political arenas than they are in the private marketplace. This behavioral assumption implies that it is rational for people and organizations to use the power of government to achieve what they cannot accomplish on their own.

Ideally, elected officials seek office to serve the public interest, not their own. However, to be successful in the electoral process, they need electoral support through financial contributions, rendering them beholden to fundraising and funders (Feldstein, 2006). Highly politicized decisions often create outcomes that have little to do with efficient use of scarce resources and what is best for the general public or what is most health-promoting. The intense dependence on fundraising influences decisions that may or may not be based on evidence. This nearly constant financial pressure contributes to the lack of coordination among health policies in the United States, making policy formulation highly complex and exceedingly interesting.

APRNs must engage in the political process to influence public policy and resource allocation decisions within political, economic, and social systems and institutions. APRN political advocacy facilitates civic engagement and collective action, which may be motivated by patient-centered moral or ethical principles or simply to protect what has already been allocated. Advocacy can include many activities undertaken by a person or organization, such as media campaigns, public speaking, commissioning and publishing policy-relevant research or polls, and filing an *amicus curiae* (friend of the court) brief. Lobbying as a political advocacy tool is only effective if a relationship between the advocate and legislator influences or shapes a policy issue. Social media for political advocacy is playing an increasingly significant role in modern politics. Digital advocacy is much more oriented toward gaining political presence, and online and offline activities are highly interconnected (Johansson & Scaramuzzino, 2019). A growing body of research highlights how the Internet and social media offer new platforms for advocacy. For example, the cataclysmic events of 2020 saw the pandemic followed by the murder of George Floyd. These events helped lay the foundation for modern social media activism and a new era of people across the globe leveraging social media to voice support for political or social causes. There is an enlarged capacity for people to speak out against injustices of all kinds. In the United States, more than half of social media users attest to using their accounts for advocacy or activism (Auxier, 2020).

TABLE 17.1

Influencing Health Policy Throughout the Process

Policy Area	Skill	Examples
Formulation	Agenda setting	Defining and documenting problems Developing and evaluating solutions Influencing political circumstances by lobbying or court decisions Educating the public (e.g., writing op-eds)
	Legislation development	Participating in drafting legislation Testifying at hearings Activating the grassroots Forming coalitions
Implementation	Rulemaking	Making formal comments about draft rules Providing input to rulemaking advisory bodies
	Policy operation	Interacting with policy implementers
Modification	Unintended consequences	Creating a case for modification through evaluation and evidence Educating the public about need for change

Adapted from *Health Policymaking in the United States* (6th ed.), by B. Longest, 2016, Health Administration Press.

UNITED STATES FUNDAMENTALLY DIFFERS FROM THE INTERNATIONAL COMMUNITY

The US health system and political process for creating healthcare policy are unique in that the system is decentralized, fragmented, and complex (see Table 17.1). In the United States there is no single entity responsible for healthcare delivery, payment, or policymaking. There are many spheres of policymaking with overlapping authority involving a wide diversity of people, cultures, traditions, and illness patterns. Although the federal government may create broad guidelines, the 50 states, for the most part, have the autonomy to create policies that best serve their citizenry—hence the large patchwork of public, private, local, state, and federal entities. These can be operating as governmental, nonprofit, or for-profit entities, all of which are creating policies and/or delivering care. Moreover, unlike other developed nations, US healthcare policy is highly political and can shift dramatically from one election cycle to another, creating further instability.

The US federal government is also a provider of health services via the Department of Veterans Affairs and the Federal Bureau of Prisons (which has custody of 10% of the 2 million US imprisoned population). The 50 states are responsible for funding health care for their incarcerated population, and 62% of the states contract with for-profit prisons to manage the health of the incarcerated (Szep et al., 2020). This mix of for-profit and government-run correctional facilities and lack of centrality and standards create an uneven health experience for the prison population, who experience poor quality of care, concerning levels of violence, and infectious disease spread behind bars (Andrews, 2017).

In countries such as China, Canada, Great Britain, Switzerland, New Zealand, and the Netherlands, there is a highly centralized health authority for policymaking and a more integrated care delivery system. These nations, with centralized systems of care, can track the impact of their policy decisions more closely and build more tightly controlled surveillance systems to follow epidemics, immunization rates, spending, workforce, and other important markers of a strong healthcare system. Moreover, centralized healthcare systems limit the number of policymakers who need to be influenced, which can be a great advantage. Although there are a smaller number of people to influence, if those policymakers are strongly opposed to issues such as expanded APRN practice, centralization becomes disadvantageous.

The unique US public–private, federal–state, nonprofit, and for-profit arrangements in which most people get their insurance through their employer make it difficult to enact programs that are highly effective in other nations in the United States. Because Americans switch health insurers and healthcare providers as they change jobs, there is no long-term investing or incentive for health delivery businesses to improve the health of the population they serve because of the constant churn. The businesses that provide care are largely focused on short-term thinking and quarterly revenue. For the most part, in the United States, as a person moves from one system or provider to the next, there is no electronic interoperability of their healthcare records. So, for example, if a delivery system was conducting an obesity intervention, they would see a very high "drop-out rate" as patients move, and the delivery system would not be able to reap the benefits of that health intervention. Their public health investment brings no rewards to them as a system in the United States. There are few exceptions, of course, such as Kaiser Permanente, an exemplar of a healthcare delivery system that offers a long-term focus on wellness such as gym memberships, access to wellness coaching, and many more preventive services.

The United States spends nearly twice as much as 10 high-income countries on health care but performs less well on many population health outcomes. A staggering 18% of the US gross domestic product (GDP) goes to health care, with spending in other countries ranging from half of that in Australia to 9.6% to 12% in Switzerland (Papanicolas et al., 2018).

Sadly, but consistently, the US healthcare outcomes are not what would be expected given that the United States spends at least 50% more per capita on health care. Compared with other developed nations, life expectancy in almost all age groups—up to age 75 years—is shorter than that of their counterparts in 16 other wealthy, developed nations (Szmigiera, 2021). The scope of the US health disadvantage is pervasive and involves more than life expectancy; the United States ranks at or near the bottom in both prevalence and mortality for multiple diseases, risk factors, and injuries. Moreover, the national obesity rate in the United States is 42%, a condition that drives coronary heart disease, end-stage renal disease, lower extremity joint replacements, a number of cancers, and metabolic illness such as diabetes (Centers for Disease Control and Prevention [CDC], 2020a). According to the National Research Council and the Institute of Medicine (National Research Council et al., 2013), the US health disadvantage spans many illnesses and injuries compared with peer countries in at least nine areas:

1. Birth outcomes (infant mortality and low birth weight)
2. Injuries and homicides
3. Adolescent pregnancies and sexually transmitted infections
4. HIV/AIDS
5. Drug-related deaths
6. Obesity and diabetes
7. Heart disease
8. Lung disease
9. Disability

Americans are more likely to engage in unhealthy lifestyle behaviors such as heavy caloric intake, drug abuse, and gun ownership. Americans, compared with the international community, tend to live in cites designed for cars, have weak social support, and lack adequate health insurance (Woolf & Aron, 2018).

These findings suggest no support for the oft-repeated claim that US health care is the best in the world. The reason for the US disadvantage has been attributed to four factors: a fragmented health system, poor health behaviors, poor social and economic conditions, and automobile domination of the built environment, minimizing walking as an important physical activity. These challenging problems require a robust public health system (Woolf & Aron, 2018). The APRN is well qualified to lead change in this area.

KEY POLICY CONCEPTS

Federalism

Federalism refers to the allocation of governing responsibility between the states and federal government. The states/provinces and the federal government have a complex relationship governing health policy, which explains a large part of our chaotic and fragmented approach to health care today across the globe. Federalism is a mixed style of government, combining a central government with regional governments (provincial, state, cantonal, or territorial) in a single political system. Its most important feature is a relationship of parity between the two levels of government (Hamilton, et, al., 1788). Federalism is the division of powers between two levels of government of equal status. Its most important distinction is that the states are not subordinate to the federal government. Examples of federalism models include the United States, the European Union, India, Brazil, Mexico, Russia, Germany, Canada, Switzerland, Argentina, and Australia.

It is essential to understand the different responsibilities and authorities of the state and federal governments, because these are highly relevant to most healthcare programs. In the United States, programs such as Medicare (federal) and Medicaid and the State Children's Health Insurance Program (both mixed state and federal) and the effort to create an interoperable health information system are all affected by federalism.

The US Constitution unambiguously gives the federal government absolute power to preempt state laws when it chooses to do so. However, the 50 states are also granted unfettered authority, such as regulation of healthcare professionals and health insurance plans (Bodenheimer & Grumbach, 2012). Ambiguity between state and federal authority allows states to experiment with policy solutions. The "states as learning laboratory" concept has grown out of local health policy problems and enables states to experiment with innovative policy solutions that could not be done on a national level. Moreover, states have local healthcare problems, requiring local, flexible, and humane solutions. Many federal health policy decisions are devolving decision making to the states. Because health care is experienced at the local level, APRNs must be aware of the overlapping state and federal spheres of government and the tension between their authorities.

Internationally, the United Kingdom has a far more centralized health system with components of federalism. The healthcare system across the United Kingdom is a mix, with England, Northern Ireland, Scotland, and Wales each having their own systems of publicly funded health care, funded by and accountable to separate governments and parliaments, together with a smaller private sector. As a result of each country having different policies and priorities, a variety of differences now exist between these systems.

In Canada there is a publicly funded, single payer healthcare system. It consists of 13 provincial and territorial health insurance plans that provide universal healthcare coverage to Canadian citizens. These systems are individually administered by each province with broad guidelines set by the federal government. The provincial governments each set their own budgets, regulate health professionals, and decide on how and when to pay for pharmaceuticals.

Exemplar 17.1 depicts the experience of nurse practitioners (NPs) who practice across the boundaries of the vastly different healthcare systems of two countries, Canada and the United States.

Incrementalism

Although the policymaking process is a continuous interrelated cycle, most efforts to change policy stem from the negative effects of an existing policy. In the United States, we rarely reform, but we frequently modify. This concept of continuous, often modest modification of existing polices is termed *incrementalism*. Major reforms of health policy are seen rarely, usually once in a generation, such as Medicare

EXEMPLAR 17.1
A TALE OF TWO COUNTRIES, TWO NURSE PRACTITIONERS AND TWO HEALTHCARE SYSTEMS

Nancy Brew and Mark Schultz

A husband-and-wife nurse practitioner (NP) team, Nancy (Brew) and Mark (Schultz) (who are now amicably divorced), had been living and practicing in Alaska for over 20 years when they emigrated to British Columbia (BC), Canada. Nancy had worked as a family nurse practitioner (FNP) in Alaska for many years and experienced increasing moral distress[a] (see Chapter 11) from trying to provide equitable and quality care to uninsured and underinsured patients in the expensive, private-payor US healthcare system. Mark was working in an Anchorage intensive care unit and wanted to pursue his graduate degree to become an FNP. They were both drawn to the concept of health care for all, so the idea of working in a country in which everyone had access to health care and no one had to fear bankruptcy or losing their home if medical disaster struck was compelling. Together, they decided to stretch their professional wings and embark on an international practice adventure.

Universal healthcare access to physician and hospital services was established in Canada in the 1960s. The Canadian healthcare system is chiefly administered via provincial and territorial governments. NP-authorizing legislation is now present in all 13 Canadian provinces and territories, and in 2019, 6200 NPs were licensed and practicing in Canada. Similar to NPs in the United States, Canadian NPs are regulated on a province-by-province basis, so there are some variations in scope across the country. The majority of jurisdictions do not require NPs to establish collaborative agreements with a physician or a group of physicians. Many provinces have also given NPs the authority to admit, treat, and discharge patients in a hospital.

Funding in a socialized healthcare system presents unique challenges to moving advanced nursing practice forward. Each regional government determines how to fund advanced practice nurse (APN) practice. In British Columbia (BC), almost all primary care is still provided by small physician group practices in a fee-for-service model in which each patient visit is individually billed to BC's Medical Services Plan. To date, BC NPs have not gained authorization to bill; thus APNs in BC are fiscally unable to open their own practices or freely join existing physician practices, even in the most underserved rural areas. A limited number of salaried positions have been created for BC NPs, but many of these are in specialty areas because the primary care physicians resist APN practice. Hence Mark has worked predominantly in cardiology and orthopedic surgery since becoming an NP, although he was trained in family practice. This is ironic, because the NP role in BC was initially legislated to improve access to primary care. There is a great need for primary care providers in BC, with a significant number of patients unable to find one. NPs could be doing more to address the Canadian primary care shortage, but Canadian health care, as a single-payor, government-run system, lacks a market-based approach to workforce shortages.

Nancy and Mark found it interesting to have worked in health care on both sides of the border while following American healthcare reform debates. The Canadian healthcare system is often held up as a cautionary tale; that is, that the Canadian system was an egregious example of poor care, long waits, and unaccountable, all-empowering bureaucracy that ran health care into the Canadian ground. Although it is true that there can be months' long wait times to see specialists for nonurgent conditions, Nancy and Mark have found that appropriate specialty referrals are given rather freely. Nonurgent computed tomography scans can occur in a week, nonurgent magnetic resonance imaging may take a few months, and the wait times for hip and knee replacements can approach 6 months. The couple found that in Canada, visits are shorter and charting is more concise, but Canadian health care is similarly evidence based and equal in quality. In contrast to in the United States, all Canadian residents and citizens have full access to inpatient and outpatient health care but are likely to pay a monthly affordable premium depending on personal income level. Canadians are responsible for the cost of outpatient prescriptions, which are subsidized to varying degrees by provincial governments.

As they reflect on their years of Canadian practice, while still "locuming" during the summers in the Alaska bush, they have seen firsthand the strengths in each system and how the different healthcare policies play out. In the United States, they see poor care as a result of an individual's inability to pay and cite the example of an uninsured man from a rural fishing village with advanced heart failure. He cannot afford the ferry ride to the clinic and cuts his pills in half or often runs out of them altogether. When he succumbs to cardiac decompensation, he is flown to a regional hospital where he spends several days in the intensive care unit ($40,000), only to return to his village without medication, to repeat the cycle. These costs are ultimately absorbed by the government and healthcare system. Were he in the Canadian system, he would be followed more closely, possibly by a cardiac outreach team; provided with filled prescriptions; and offered a transportation subsidy. However, Canadian NPs have witnessed the moral hazard[b] of unlimited access to health care, in the form of occasionally frivolous visits, such as seeking a bandage for a minor cut or scrape rather than going to the store, or long waits to see a dermatologist for acne that could have been treated in primary care. Both private pay cost barriers and system

EXEMPLAR 17.1
A TALE OF TWO COUNTRIES, TWO NURSE PRACTITIONERS AND TWO HEALTHCARE SYSTEMS—cont'd

overuse issues are policy driven and have enormous impact on the larger economy and lives of individuals.

Although they recognize that the grass is not greener in Canada for APN practice, these two NPs are grateful to live and work in Canada for its all-inclusive healthcare system, provided at a per capita cost that is considerably less than that in the United States. There are times when they wish they could take the best parts of both systems and combine them to decrease the moral distress in the United States and the moral hazard in Canada.

[a]*Moral distress*—when one knows the right thing to do but institutional constraints make it almost impossible to pursue the right course of action (Hamric, 2009; Jameton, 1984).

[b]*Moral hazard*—when a party insulated from risk behaves differently than he or she would behave if he or she were fully exposed to the risk (Jameton, 1984).

and Medicaid in 1965 and the Patient Protection and Affordable Care Act (PPACA) of 2010. Minor changes of existing policies play out slowly over time and are therefore more predictable. Incrementalism promotes stability and stakeholder compromise. A good example of incrementalism is the gradual increase in federal spending for biomedical research from $300 in 1887 to more than $41 billion in 2020, going to the 27 institutes and centers within the National Institutes of Health (Department of Health and Human Services [DHHS], National Institute of Health, 2021). Within that structure, the National Center for Nursing Research was created in 1985 by a congressional override of a presidential veto as a result of the influence of strong nurse leaders. In 1993 the center was elevated to the National Institute for Nursing Research and funded with $50 million; funding levels in 2020 will exceed $140 million (DHHS, 2021). Incrementalism is illustrated in Virginia's 45-year journey on NP scope of practice as told by Dr. Cynthia Fagan in Exemplar 17.2.

Presidential Politics

US presidential politics is playing a larger role in health care in the United States. The presidential candidates frame health issues in ways that greatly influence public perception regarding the severity of health problems and who is responsible for the problem. Presidential candidates are trying to win support for their healthcare priorities and are often unaware of the evidence regarding what is driving cost or disease burden. Even though the United States faces serious health concerns, largely driven by poor health behaviors, and the resulting chronic disease epidemic, there is little political will to address the root cause of these drivers. For example, many of the US agriculture policies subsidize corn, which is used in many processed foods (high-fructose corn syrup). Those processed foods are a large part of the poor American diet, leading to obesity and the long list of health issues that cascade from obesity (Kim et al., 2019).

The very first presidential primary is held in Iowa, a large agriculture state that produces more corn (2.5 billion bushels) than any other state; corn was the most produced crop in 2019 in the United States (US Department of Agriculture, 2019). The economic incentives for Iowa to keep this corn production in place are enormous, thus shutting down any conversation on aligning US farming policy with health policy. Throughout the last two presidential primary and debate processes (2016 and 2020) involving over 30 candidates caucusing in Iowa, not a single candidate addressed America's food system problems and their link to chronic disease and poor health. American presidential politics have become a continuous cycle, making it difficult for candidates to address complex problems that are too big, too difficult to explain, or too unpopular. This exemplifies the impenetrable and complex nature of health policy, which requires considerable political capital to address.

APRNs, Civic Engagement, and Money

Without question, and regardless of one's political affiliation, there is widespread agreement that money has enormous influence on elections, the wealthy have more influence on elections, and candidates who win office promote policies that help their donors. Some of

EXEMPLAR 17.2
A 45-YEAR JOURNEY OF PERSISTENCE FOR VIRGINIA NPS

By Cynthia M. Fagan DNP, RN, FNP-BC

VIRGINIA'S LEGISLATIVE JOURNEY TO NURSE PRACTITIONER AUTONOMOUS PRACTICE LICENSURE

Virginia's journey to expand nurse practitioner (NP) practice authority has been historical for its length and incrementalism. Since the introduction of the NP role in 1973, the regulation of NPs in Virginia has been fraught. From the start, the medical practice act authorized NPs to practice under the supervision of a physician. For decades, NP practice has been regulated by a joint board of medicine and nursing. Over the ensuing years, NPs organized into a grassroots group of six and grew into a statewide, full-service professional advocacy organization, representing over 8000 licensed NPs. The Virginia Council of Nurse Practitioners (VCNP) has been the leading force for professional advancement and NP advocacy for removal of scope of practice barriers to improve access to care.

BABY STEPS

Milestones in Virginia's legislative journey include incremental gains in prescriptive authority with Schedule VI drugs in 1991 following an abandoned first attempt in 1990 where it was discovered that more education of the legislature was necessary. Once Schedule VI drugs were legal to prescribe, the NPs pursued prescriptive authority for Schedule III–V drugs in 2000, the ability to order physical therapy services in 2002, prescriptive authority for Schedule II drugs in 2006, and a mandate for an NP seat on the Board of Nursing in 2008.

NPS DEEMED THREAT TO PUBLIC SAFETY

In 2010, the first attempt at full practice authority (FPA) was undertaken to align Virginia's Nurse Practice Act with modern nursing. The attempt failed to make it out of the subcommittee. This legislation brought out a myriad of medical specialty groups testifying in opposition of NPs' full practice authority, with testimony by the medical society president that "NPs must remain tethered to physicians for public safety and quality of care" without any supporting evidence for this claim. This experience left an indelible mark on NPs present in the room and was instructive for demanding evidence-based data when NP safety and quality were called into question with future legislative endeavors. Legislators also firmly advised NPs to dialogue with organized medicine to work out a compromise before bringing future legislation forward. While this legislative attempt was unsuccessful, it set the stage for future efforts.

LANGUAGE MATTERS ALMOST AS MUCH AS INTEGRITY

Heeding legislators' advice, the NP leadership and the Medical Society Virginia (MSV) embarked on a series of meetings with the intent to craft a consensus bill to move practice authority from physician supervision to a collaborative practice model. While this effort resulted in a 2012 bill for collaborative practice, the final bill language was changed at the 11th hour by the MSV mandating that NPs must collaborate and consult with a physician-led patient care team, language not previously discussed or agreed upon by the NP negotiating team. Another lesson learned was the importance of having control of the bill throughout the process because "words do matter" in legislative language. Passage of this legislation had unintended consequences, causing NPs to pay include for their collaborative agreements with physicians as well as resulting in difficulty securing collaborators. This created numerous barriers to care in rural and underserved areas where existing physician shortages were already a problem.

Sustaining the vision and effort for independent NP practice authority, three separate NP bills were introduced during the 2016 legislative session, with incremental language toward modernizing the Virginia Nurse Practice Act. These bills were either defeated or amended by the MSV to maintain the status quo. For example, in lieu of elimination of the collaborative agreement, one bill was amended to offer an extension of 60 days with a one-time extension (120 days total) for NPs who lose their physician collaborator to avert clinic closure. Another "stall tactic" bill was amended to study telehealth as a vehicle for NP collaborative practice. This legislative session illustrated the continued power gradient and uneven playing field in the legislative arena between medicine and NPs.

BUILD POWERFUL COALITIONS

In 2017, NP legislative efforts for a transition to practice bill were impeded by the hospital association plan to introduce a bill for independent practice autonomy for NPs employed in hospitals and health systems. Fortunately, the hospital association agreed to drop the bill due to NP opposition. This move greatly enlarged the NP stakeholder group to include hospitals and delivery systems that wanted NPs they were employing to practice to the top of their ability and not be hamstrung by outdated state laws.

VICTORY COMES WITH COMPROMISE

After 45 years, in 2018, Virginia finally passed an independent practice bill! Key to this success was presession

EXEMPLAR 17.2
A 45-YEAR JOURNEY OF PERSISTENCE FOR VIRGINIA NPS—cont'd

stakeholder group meetings led by the bill sponsor over 6 months with the single goal of crafting a bill to remove scope of practice barriers. Incumbent physician legislators were invited to participate in these meetings. While dissolution of the Joint Boards of Medicine and Nursing was considered, it was not undertaken as a means of compromise due to posturing from physician legislators that if this was proposed, they would advocate for NP regulation solely under the Board of Medicine. These meetings exposed organized medicine's true intentions to maintain the status quo, which was stated aloud at the conclusion of the meeting period. This, however, set the stage for NPs to craft the bill with a transition to practice period of 1060 hours with either an NP or physician collaborator. It was accepted that the transition hour requirement would be a point of negotiation with organized medicine and would ultimately be lengthier. Organized medicine insisted on a 5-year transition period, which was felt more consistent with the medical education requirement; however, this would make Virginia a significant outlier among all other states with transition hour requirements.

In typical fashion, the MSV orchestrated a substitute bill introduced by a physician legislator for a 5-year transition to practice period for NPs who were licensed and certified in a practice area similar to the collaborating physician's training. This restriction would have precluded all specialty practice NPs from independent practice. The expectation from MSV was that NPs would walk away from the bill; however, NPs used the bill as a vehicle to keep the issue alive and attempt to reduce the practice hour requirement on the senate side. Unfortunately, there was no appetite on the senate side to reduce the practice hour requirement. When presented with the choice of a career-long practice agreement versus independent practice following a 5-year practice period, the NPs accepted the 5-year requirement to increase access to care, which would be especially impactful in rural and underserved areas across the state.

VIRGINIA REMAINS AN OUTLIER AND WE ARE NOT DONE YET

The autonomous practice licensure law for NPs passed the 2018 legislative session and became effective January 7, 2019, through the the Joint Boards of Nursing and Medicine who regulate APNs in Virginia. The new law reforms scope of practice, permitting qualified NPs to be licensed to practice independently. Eligible NPs must meet a 5-year full-time clinical practice experience equivalent and file an attestation from their collaborating physician with the Board of Nursing. Clinical practice experience is delineated as the postgraduate delivery of health care directly to patients, which unfortunately excludes administrative and faculty teaching time. The 5-year full-time equivalent is based on a 36-hour work week and is defined as 1800 hours per year for a total of 9000 hours. Applications require a signature by the patient-care team physician(s) affirming that (1) the physician served as the NP collaborator pursuant to a practice agreement, (2) the physician routinely practiced with a patient population and in a practice area for which the NP is certified and licensed, and (3) the time period practiced with the NP pursuant to the practice agreement.

In the event that circumstances inhibit the NP from obtaining an attestation from the collaborating physician, "other evidence" meeting the qualifications for autonomous practice licensure may be submitted. A one-time administrative fee of $100 per certification category in which the NP is licensed and certified is required. Upon verification that requirements have been met, a new "autonomous practice license" is issued and the NP may practice autonomously.

Since implementation of the new autonomous practice licensure law, nearly 1000 NPs have obtained autonomous licensure. This represents approximately 11% of the 8000 licensed NPs in the state. These numbers are expected to grow with uptake of the new law and development and diffusion of innovative service delivery models.

LESSONS LEARNED

Many lessons have been learned over the decades. A critical first step is to understand the state legislature. Virginia has one of the oldest legislatures in the Western hemisphere and is steeped in tradition. Like other southern states, it is conservative and resists progressive changes, but that is changing as the makeup of the body changes to reflect the population. With conservative decision makers, incremental steps are necessary. The critical element for Virginia's legislative success was finding the right bill patron willing to facilitate stakeholder meetings to fully understand all sides of the issue. Second, it has been imperative to build the professional nursing organizational infrastructure to include paid staff, a dedicated lobbyist, public relations consultants, and an advocacy platform to communicate with members, nonmembers, consumers, and legislators. And, lastly, it is essential to foster long-term relationships with legislators.

TABLE 17.2

Selected APRN and Other Health Professions Organizations' Political Action Committee (PAC) and Lobbying Donations, 2020

Health Professions Organization	2020 PACs	Lobbying FY 2020 Spending
American Association of Nurse Anesthesiology	$926,500 [52% Republican]	$760,000
American College of Nurse-Midwives	$114,809 [28% Republican]	$60,000
American Association of Nurse Practitioners	$478,689 [48% Republican]	$771,764
National Association of Clinical Nurse Specialists	No PAC reported	Less than $5,000 *(last available data 2018)*
American Medical Association	$1,587,859 [43% Republican]	$20,919,000
American Nurses Association	$500,000 [35% Republican]	$1,178,925

Adapted from Center for Responsive Politics, 2021, http://www.opensecrets.org/.

the more effective interest groups do not align with one political party but give equally to both parties so that they can gain access to important decision makers. It is estimated that members of congress spend anywhere from up to two-thirds (and sometimes more) of their time fundraising, especially as an election approaches (Shevlin & Doran, 2016). APRNs have come a long way in supporting candidates. In 2020 there were three nurses elected to congress (Eddie Bernice Johnson [Texas], Lauren Underwood [Illinois; both reelected] and Cori Bush [Missouri; newly elected]) to the House of Representatives. There are no nurses serving in the Senate and no nurses serving as governors at the time of this writing (The Advisory Board, 2020). The easiest form of civic engagement is to vote for or donate to a candidate or political action committee (PAC); next is to work on a campaign, followed by running for office. Table 17.2 outlines health professions' lobbying spending, donations to PACs, and how they distributed those funds across political parties in the United States.

POLICY MODELS AND FRAMEWORKS

Longest Model

Longest (2016) has conceptualized policymaking as an interdependent process. The Longest model defines a policy formulation phase, an implementation phase, and a modification phase (Fig. 17.1). Importantly, this model illustrates the incremental and cyclical nature of policymaking, two of the most important features of the US healthcare policymaking process with which APRNs must be familiar. Essentially, all healthcare policy decisions are subject to modification, because policymaking in the United States involves making decisions that are revisited when circumstances shift. The US system is not designed for big, bold reform. Rather, it considers intended or unintended consequences of existing policy and tweaks changes (Longest, 2016).

Policy Modification

The US system is based on continuous policy modification. Almost every policy creates some form of unintended consequence, which is only learned through implementation of a prior policy. Policies that are appropriate and relevant at one point in time become highly inappropriate as time passes and economic, social, demographic, and commercial circumstances shift. Policy consequences are the reason why stakeholders and policymakers seek to modify policy continually. These policy changes can be driven by stakeholders when a policy negatively affects a group or by members of congress or rule makers when policy does not meet their objective. Understanding the process of policy modification and amendment of earlier polices is a key to mastering political competency.

The Kingdon or Garbage Can Model

Agenda setting is a major component of the Longest policy formulation phase. With so many health policy problems in the United States, why do some problems get attention and others languish at the bottom of the policy agenda for decades? Kingdon (1995)

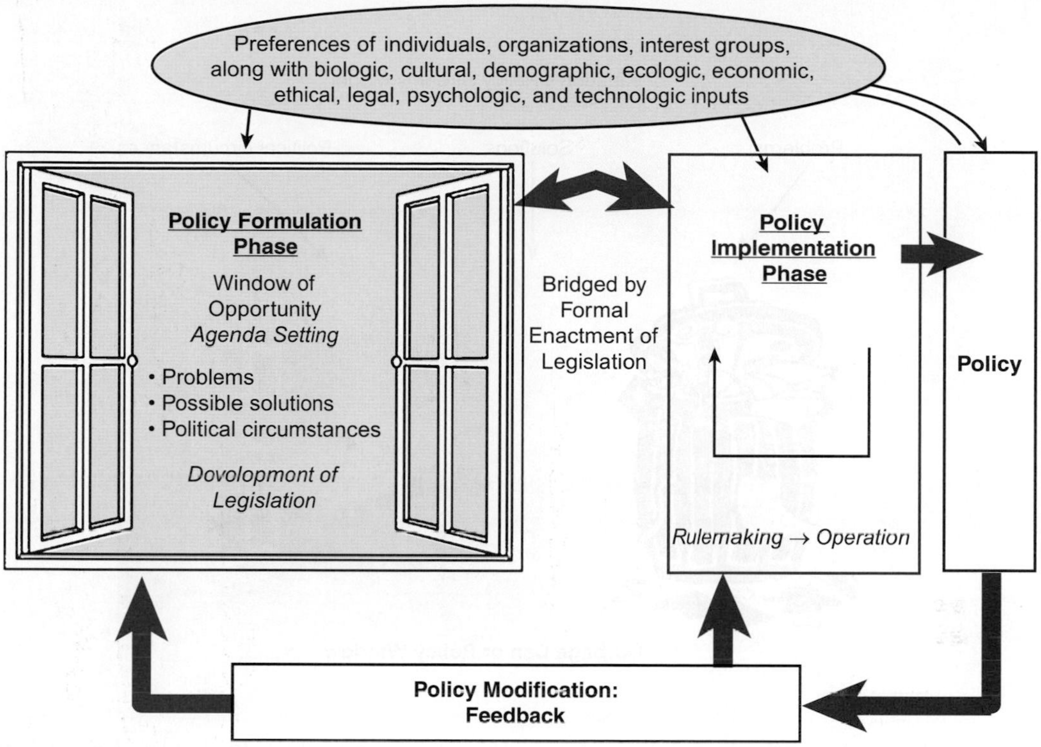

Fig. 17.1 ■ **The Longest model.** (From *Health Policymaking in the United States* [6th ed.], by B. Longest Jr., 2016, Health Administration Press.)

conceptualized an open policy window, with three conditions streaming through the open window at once:

The policy problem must:

1. come to the attention of the policymaker;
2. have a menu of possible policy solutions that have very real potential to solve the issue at hand; and
3. have the right political circumstances.

If all three of these conditions occur simultaneously, the policy window opens and progress can be made on the issue (Fig. 17.2). Conversely, once shut, this policy window (opportunity) may never open again.

Policy Activators

Policy problems come to the attention of policymakers in several ways, including through constituents, litigation, research findings, market forces, fiscal environment, crisis, special interest groups, and the media, singly or collectively. Wakefield (2008) has identified policy dynamics particular to agenda setting (Table 17.3). Additional dynamics have been added, and each dynamic has one or more so-called accelerators that drive the agenda setting or trigger policymakers to take action on an issue. The political circumstances that push problems onto the agenda must have a high degree of public importance and low degree of stakeholder conflict surrounding the policy solution. If there is a great deal of stakeholder disagreement, competing proposals may be put forth, weakening the likelihood that the problem will be addressed. Strong health services research can provide the evidence base to help policymakers specify and therefore accelerate agenda setting (Longest, 2016).

Knowledge Transfer Framework

APRN research must be robust enough and highly relevant to be useful for policymakers. Not all research can or should have an impact. The nature of the political process compels researchers to link their work to

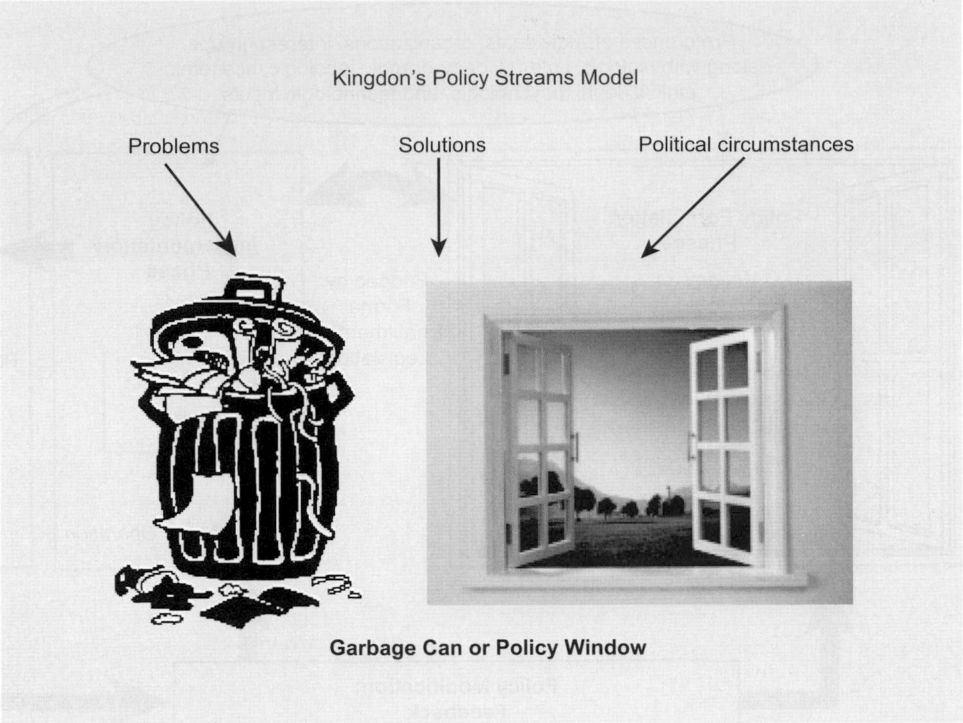

Fig. 17.2 ■ Kingdon's policy streams model. (From *Agendas, Alternatives, and Public Policies* [2nd ed.], by J. Kingdon, 1995, Harper Collins College.)

policy formation. APRNs could more forcefully link their research to policymaking by framing it in a policy context. Gold (2009) has created a framework for researchers to increase the likelihood that their findings will reach some "take-up" of new ideas to be useful and implementable in the policy sphere. It opens a pathway through the unexplored "black box" between health research and its use by policymakers. Such pathways can help stakeholders bridge between the research and the end user by asking five questions (Fig. 17.3). An example of high-quality, nurse practitioner–led research is the well-designed study by Chao et al. (2015) in which they found that chronic stress had a significant direct effect on food cravings and food cravings had a significant direct effect on body mass index. The highly relevant policy link is that interventions aimed at lowering obesity rates must address the underlying emotional and stress landscapes that cause food cravings and not merely focus on food habits. This may well explain why the obesity epidemic is exploding, because current interventions are primarily dietary. Addressing the questions in Fig. 17.3 makes it more likely that the research will be transferred into policy.

CURRENT ADVANCED PRACTICE NURSING POLICY ISSUES

Framing Current Issues: Cost, Quality, Access, and the Value Agenda

The cost–quality–access triad (Fig. 17.4) focuses on the drivers of health policy, across all levels of health care, whether it is at the international, national, state, local, community, institutional, or corporate level. Cost, quality, and access, as health policy drivers, are inherently interdependent; a shift in one inevitably affects the others. Cost, quality, and access issues are not tangential problems to the US healthcare challenges—they are the challenge.

It is important to understand the relationship of quality and cost as it relates to value in health care. Cost containment efforts without attention to access to care or value improvement stifle efforts to reform the

TABLE 17.3

Influence of Policy Dynamics on Agenda Setting

Dynamic	Activator	Examples
Constituents	The constituent can have enormous impact on agenda setting. When members of congress learn from their constituents about deeply moving tragedies that could have been prevented or lessened, the member is moved to introduce legislation.	An automobile accident in a remote area killed three members of a family and seriously injured two. A senator knew the family, which prompted introduction of the Wakefield Act, designed to improve pediatric emergency response in rural areas and honor the family. It became public law, the Wakefield Emergency Medical Services for Children.
Litigation	Court decisions play an increasingly prominent role in setting health policy.	The Supreme Court allows the Newton, CT, parents whose children were gunned down at school to sue the gun manufacturer (Remington Arms Co.) for liability for the violence. This decision could reshape policy on gun violence in the United States.
Research findings	A study in *JAMA Internal Medicine* (Heckert et al., 2019) found that 25% of patients with either type 1 or type 2 diabetes reported underusing insulin because of cost.	A bipartisan bill, The Insulin Price Reduction Act, is introduced in Congress to address the growing public outrage and research findings of insulin underuse due to a cost of $6,000.00 annually for insulin (a 5000% increase over the cost).
Market forces	The pharmaceutical industry greatly expands commercial advertising/marketing of prescribed drugs to consumers. This direct advertising creates higher demands on pharmaceuticals, driving up healthcare costs.	Legislation is introduced to authorize the Food and Drug Administration to restrict direct-to-consumer advertising for prescribed drugs.
Fiscal environment	Very different budget decisions are made when the government is addressing deficit rather than surplus spending.	In 2020, President Trump completely eliminated the Department of Homeland Security's National Biodefense Analysis and Countermeasures Center months before the COVID-19 pandemic hit the United States.
Special interest groups	Well-organized special interest groups with a clear message can have an enormous impact on government action or inaction.	The Newtown, CT, parents whose children were murdered at Sandy Hook Elementary School formed a nonprofit, Sandy Hook Promise, and pushed to get federal legislation introduced for background checks before the purchase of firearms (the measure did not pass). https://www.sandyhookpromise.org/
Crises	Crises can promote rapid response policy changes, usually centered on quality and access.	The startling deadly and rapid coronavirus spread led to scores of wide-ranging bills; for example, mandatory sick leave, partnering with other nations, unemployment benefits, telehealth, and rapid vaccine production, to name a few.
Political ideology	The majority party (Democrat versus Republican) has a large impact on agenda setting. The divide centers on what role the government should play in US society.	Congress has been introducing wildly opposing health policy bills; Republicans want to repeal the Affordable Care Act, whereas Democrats want to improve it. This tension fluctuates depending on the political party in power.
Media	The lay press, reporting on policy issues or crises, often compels policymakers to take action.	Major news outlets report that millions of unencrypted personal healthcare records were stolen or mistakenly made public. Tensions rise between added reporting requirements and privacy. Legislation is introduced on strategies to enforce the Health Insurance Portability and Accountability Act (HIPAA) and mandate encryption.
US president commitment	When the occupant of the White House sets health reform as a major domestic policy agenda versus a focus on deregulation and capitalism as the primary framework, very different outcomes are produced and the power of that office becomes evident.	In March 2010, President Obama signs the historic ACA, after a 2-year debate, town hall meetings across the nation, and multiple national speeches explaining to the public why reform is necessary to help the macroeconomy. It becomes the major initiative of his presidency. President Trump asks the Supreme Court to invalidate the landmark Affordable Care Act.

Adapted from "Agenda Setting: What Rises to a Policymaker's Attention," by E. A. Furlong, in J. A. Milstead and N. M. Short, *Health Policy and Politics: A Nurse's Guide* (6th ed., pp. 17–35), 2019, Jones & Bartlett.

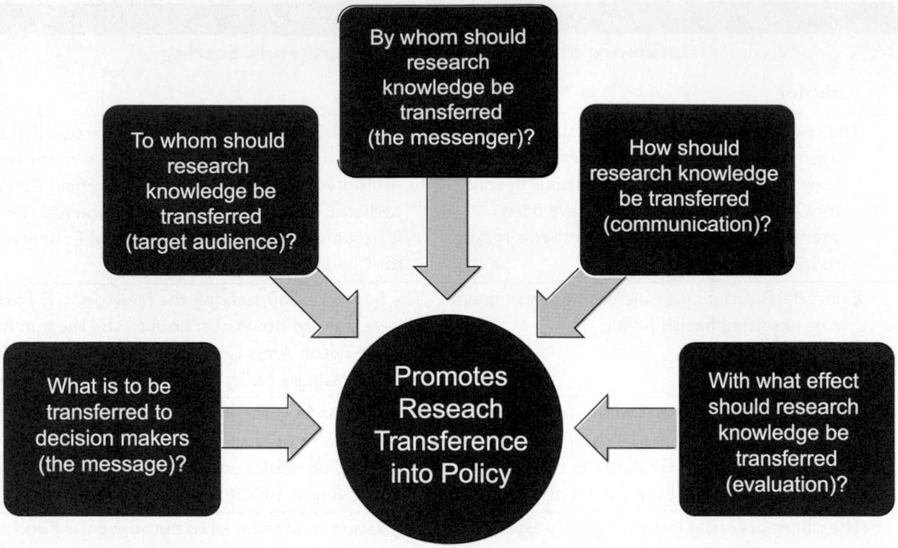

Fig. 17.3 ■ **Pathway to move and accelerate effective research into policy.**

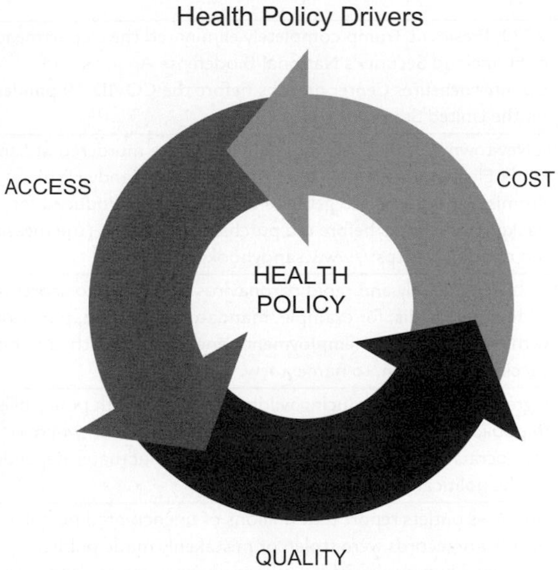

Fig. 17.4 ■ **Cost–quality–access schema.**

healthcare system successfully. The value equation, as described by Porter (2010), is the division of patient outcomes or quality by the total cost care for the condition being treated. The value concept integrates not only quality and cost containment but also safety and patient-centered care as well.

Cost

The PPACA enactment in 2010 stands alongside the passage of Medicaid and Medicare in 1965 as a grand and challenging change in US healthcare policy. This massive bill aimed to improve access, improve quality, and, most important, control the rate of cost increase in health care. In 2019 US health expenditures rose by $1.2 trillion to $3.8 trillion, or $11,597 per capita (Keehan et al., 2020). To put this in perspective, if you take the $1.2 trillion anticipated increase in health costs from 2010 to 2019, you could provide a median family income of about $62,000 for approximately 19.3 million families (Guzman, 2019).

The average annual growth of US health expenditures outpaces the average annual growth of the US GDP. Even with focused efforts to bend the cost curve of health care, increases in health spending are expected to average 5.4% per year until 2028, with the GDP growing only 4.3% per year during the same period (Keehan et al., 2020). By 2028, the health share of the GDP may reach 19.7%. The proportion of the country's GDP expended on health care is of importance to the future of the United States because every dollar spent on health care is a dollar less spent on education, transportation, housing, food, and other essentials. In comparison with the current percentage of GDP, the cost of health care in 1960 was about 6% of the GDP, and in 1980 it was about 9% of GDP (Kaiser Family Foundation, 2011).

Past efforts to control costs included the implementation of health plans in the 1970s, introduction of diagnosis-related groups in the 1980s, and instituting competition in the healthcare market in the 1990s. Efforts in the 2000s were marked by cost control through price regulation and in the 2010s by linking payment to quality (using clinical metrics) and continuing price controls. Even these varied attempts to control costs have had limited impact. Building on these past efforts, the ACA created accountable care organizations (ACOs), integrated systems that bring together hospitals, outpatient clinics, and specialty services to deliver better care coordination and quality of service. ACOs are a vehicle to implement the intent of the ACA by creating integrated systems that can coordinate care better, thus improving quality and managing costs more effectively.

As the ACA continues to evolve, the movement toward value-based care preceded the ACA and has bipartisan support (Muhlestein et al., 2017). Healthcare delivery organizations continue to make great strides in improving care coordination, care delivery, and ultimately value of health care based on ACA principles.

Quality

Attention to quality became a national issue following the Institute of Medicine's (IOM) series of reports, *To Err is Human* (Kohn et al., 2000) and *Crossing the Quality Chasm* (IOM, 2001), focusing on the problems in the healthcare system leading to poor care. In an effort to ensure that cost-saving measures do not impact quality of care, government and private payers, in growing numbers, link quality to reimbursement mechanisms. *Value-based purchasing* is the mechanism by which quality is linked to cost control. As part of value-based purchasing, the Centers for Medicare & Medicaid Services (CMS, 2006) identified 27 "never events" and established a policy whereby hospitals would not be reimbursed for care required when patients experience an event that *should never happen*. "Never events" are referred to as Serious Reportable Events (SREs); the National Quality Forum recognizes 29 SREs. SREs occur not only in hospitals but also in office-based surgery centers, ambulatory practice settings, and long-term care or skilled nursing facilities (National Quality Forum, 2011). APRNs are expected to know SREs and work to ensure that they do not occur. A current compilation of SREs is located at the National Quality Forum (2011) website.

As part of nursing's effort to improve quality of care, the Robert Wood Johnson Foundation initiated the Nursing Alliance for Quality of Care (NAQC) because nursing had no mechanism to bring together stakeholders and there was concern that nursing would not be involved in addressing the critical issues surrounding care (NAQC, 2010). Today, the American Nurses Association manages the NAQC (http://www.naqc.org/), which is composed of nursing organizations and consumer groups. Policymakers recognize the contributions of nurses in advancing consumer centered, high-quality health care. The NAQC was modeled after other alliances that primarily focused on improving the quality of care to report quality measures. In the past decade, several more alliances have emerged that focus on the review and/or development of quality measures. APRNs can obtain information about advancing nursing quality through the work of the NAQC, their professional organizations, and, in general, being aware of the work in quality improvement through organizations such as the Institute for Healthcare Improvement. (See Chapter 19, Chapter 21, Chapter 22, and Chapter 23 for more information on this important topic.)

Access

Access is the ability to obtain needed health care, which is not the same as having health insurance. Many factors hinder a person's ability to access the right health care at the right time. In the United States, health care is considered a privilege and not a right. In order to access health care, one must (1) have health insurance through one's employer, or (2) be insured under a government health insurance program, or (3) be able to purchase health insurance with one's own funds, or (4) be able to pay for services privately, or (5) be able to access the US safety net (federally subsidized care). Once coverage issues are established, there are other barriers to accessing health care. *Timing* is the ability for delivery systems to meet patient appointment needs without long wait times, in the right service setting. *Geography* is the physical location of the health care and the population's ability to access it when needed. This could be public transportation in urban settings or distance in rural settings. *Cultural competency* is when the health care is appropriate to the plurality of the US population and offers methods to overcome language and cultural barriers. The Healthy People 2020 effort has learned that in order for healthcare systems to improve the health of the population they serve in a meaningful way, they must include diverse stakeholders and the public in guiding decision making. Finally, the healthcare providers or teams must have the *capacity to build relationships*. These competencies include excellent communication and emotional intelligence, presence, nonjudgmentalism, and the ability to be empathic, manage conflicts, and know how to collaborate (Johnson et al., 2022).

Healthcare access includes a complex tangle of insurance coverage, financing, affordability, location and welcoming attitude, community building, and provider skills. These are necessary because healthcare access affects a person's overall physical, social, and mental health status and quality of life (Healthy People 2020, 2020).

Policy Initiatives in Health Reform

The ACA and the Health Care and Education Reconciliation Act of 2010, which amended some provisions in the ACA, represent the most far-reaching legislation enacted since the passage of Medicare and Medicaid in 1965. Many requirements in the ACA overlap the issues of cost, quality, and access policy. Now, 10 years later, substantial gains in coverage and access are achieved and new models of care delivery and payment are in place. By 2016, over 20 million previously uninsured individuals held insurance coverage, bringing the number of uninsured to 8.8%, a reduction directly related to ACA provisions (Blumberg et al., 2016). Even with these efforts, according to Sommers (2020), the promise of affordable, comprehensive, person-centered care has been gradual, with expansion in state Medicaid programs increasing from 26 states in 2014 to 37 states in 2020. Yet the nation still faces challenges, with millions of uninsured individuals and issues with affordability (Sommers, 2020). By 2019, under the Trump administration, and before the global pandemic, the uninsured rate rose to 33 million, or 16.8% of the US population (CDC, 2020b). Uninsurance rates in the United States fluctuate with presidential politics. Notwithstanding the difficulties in efforts to implement the ACA, ongoing legal challenges, as well as concerted efforts to repeal or undermine the ACA, this new and complex system continues to evolve and develop. As we move into the next decade, APRN leaders will need to engage in debate, development, and implementation of coverage expansion as well as remedies for reducing underinsurance.

The Value Agenda

The move from fee-for-service to value-based healthcare models is transforming the delivery of healthcare services with emphasis on patient outcomes, not just the number of visits or procedures. An example of a value model is the ACO that links patient outcomes to costs of treatment. An ACO is a system designed to deliver high value by horizontally integrating care across a continuum and includes a primary care provider, specialists, and a hospital. Examples of ACOs include the Geisinger Health System, Kaiser Permanente, and the Mayo Clinic. ACOs are responsible for providing high-quality care to a minimum of 5000 Medicare enrollees while controlling costs. This model shifts the financial risks to the providers rather than the insurers. The savings accrued from reducing costs of care are then given to the providers. Although there have been previous attempts to create coordinated care systems, a new requirement—that ACOs must report quality measures and be highly transparent—is transformational.

According to the American Association of Nurse Practitioners (AANP, 2020), ACOs incentivize team-based care to treat individuals across healthcare settings. Through utilization of shared resources and coordination of care, ACOs are able to meet identified performance standards and quality metrics, thereby lowering the cost of health care. ACOs agree to lower the cost of health care while meeting identified performance standards by sharing resources and coordinating care. NPs are authorized ACO professionals. However, a last-minute change in the Shared Savings section of the ACA for Medicare patients limits its program assignment of patients to those who are being cared for by primary care physicians. Therefore patients who choose an NP as their primary care provider are not counted as beneficiaries and any shared savings are not assigned. Thus, although this does not prevent NPs from joining an ACO, it does prevent their patients from being assigned to a Medicare ACO. Essentially, the structures that are set up to greatly benefit from APRN service lock APRNs out of ACO governance structures, leadership, and cost savings (profit). Progress continues, however, with CMS publishing a final rule in 2019 removing the "one physician visit" requirement in the Medicare Shared Savings Program (MSSP) ACO. The adoption of this provision provides opportunity for beneficiaries to choose an NP ACO professional as their primary care provider (Medicare Shared Savings Program, 2019). It is important for APRNs to be involved in leading, governing, and sharing the ACO savings of these emerging structures. At this time, the AANP and other national APRN organizations continue to push for a policy fix to reinstate assignment of patients of all ACO professionals, including NPs, by adding provider-neutral language.

In April 2016, Medicare bundled payments, in which payment for care is based on a lump sum amount for an episode of care rather than on an individual visit, procedure, or service, began for hip and knee replacements. The bundled payment includes all surgery costs through full recovery for hospitals in 67 geographic areas. In 2014 more than 400,000 Medicare recipients had hip or knee replacements, costing more than $7 billion for just the hospitalization (Delbanco & de Brantes, 2015). Through this new payment model, hospitals benefit financially from high-quality, lower cost service but must repay Medicare if quality and cost targets are not achieved. In addition to efforts to provide better coordination through bundled payments, the ACA specifies development of programs to reduce hospital readmission. Hospitals are required to report on all readmissions in a specific time period, and readmission rates are publicly posted on the Hospital Compare website (https://www.medicare.gov/hospitalcompare/search.html?). Both the bundled payment model and the requirement to reduce admissions are areas in which APRN practice can contribute significant savings and improved outcomes (Newhouse et al., 2011).

In 2010 congress authorized the establishment of an independent Patient-Centered Outcomes Research Institute (PCORI) with a primary goal of funding comparative effectiveness research to identify health interventions that truly make a difference in quality and cost of care to individualized patients. PCORI's research priorities include assessment of prevention, diagnosis, and treatment options; improving healthcare systems; communication and dissemination of research; addressing disparities; and accelerating patient-centered outcomes research and methodological research. The PCORI board of governors represents the broader healthcare community, including patients, providers, payers, manufacturers or developers, quality improvement professionals, and federal and state governments. However, in 2022, board composition continues to be dominated by physician representation, with the minority of members representing a variety of healthcare constituencies; only one PhD-prepared nurse is represented on the board. By the end of 2019, PCORI funded research in 48 states and awarded $2.5 billion funding 1000 projects (PCORI, 2019).

APRN POLITICAL COMPETENCE IN THE POLICY ARENA

The move to doctoral education for APRNs elevates the need for APRN involvement in policy development because effective leadership demands it. Policy competency requires APRNs to incorporate policy strategies continuously among the practice, research, and policy nexus in all practice settings. The American Association of Colleges of Nursing's (AACN) reenvisioned *Essentials* (AACN, 2021) highlights the importance of health policy in nursing education at all levels, threading these concepts across and within multiple newly defined domains of competency (AACN, 2021). It is expected that APRN graduates are prepared to assume a broad leadership role on behalf of the public and nursing profession. The solutions to today's social injustices, politicized delivery systems, perverse financing, and uneven quality in the healthcare system are difficult to both agree upon and implement. Competency in health policy involves goal-directed decision making as a result of an authorized public decision-making process (Keller & Ridenour, 2021). It represents an important aspect of advocacy for patients and for the profession by speaking with a united voice on policy issues that affect nursing practice and health outcomes. APRNs are well positioned and have the clinical credibility to inform, design, and influence policy solutions, but this will happen *only if* they expand their arena of influence beyond the clinical setting (see Exemplar 17.3 on the nation's largest nursing PAC).

EXEMPLAR 17.3
THE ANATOMY OF A SUCCESSFUL POLITICAL ACTION COMMITTEE, FROM ONE OF THE NATION'S STRONGEST[a]

The American Association of Nurse Anesthesiology (AANA) has the largest federal nursing political action committee (PAC) in the nation by far. With donations of over $1.3 million per 2-year election cycle, it is also one of the top federal healthcare PACs in the country. They are very proud of their thoughtful process for governing their PAC and making distributions. The certified registered nurse anesthetist (CRNA)-PAC Mission is *to advance the profession of nurse anesthesia through federal political advocacy*, and they place a strong emphasis on being highly strategic, inclusive, and thoughtful. All operations related to the PAC, including fundraising, research, marketing, communication, and disbursements, stem from strategy and input from the mission, member leadership, and advocacy agenda of the AANA. The PAC is governed by eight CRNAs and one CRNA student. They are assisted by one full-time AANA staff member who regularly works with the PAC committee to serve as liaison and share compliance and political knowledge to make the most informed decisions. There are five key reasons why their PAC is so highly successful.

GRASSROOTS DRIVEN

First, they deploy a highly inclusive process asking grassroots CRNAs for local information about congressional campaigns. Making highly strategic disbursement decisions, they begin with the CRNA community and involve them in identifying key campaigns. Their sole criterion is directed at making disbursements to candidates who will move the CRNA agenda forward. Because the CRNA community is politically diverse, they do not formally endorse candidates. The PAC bases its financial support on the candidate's familiarity with and support of the CRNA profession and ability to influence the overall healthcare agenda in congress. The PAC remains in close contact with individual CRNAs through the process.

EDUCATING POLICYMAKERS

What the PAC disbursements gain for the AANA is access to federal elected officials and other leading policymakers. Policymakers are dealing with a wide breadth of issues and may not know how a policy is being played out in their community. Making PAC donations provides access to policymakers and opportunities for CRNAs to educate them about the benefits of CRNA care and how restricting CRNA practice impacts patients and increases healthcare costs. With the demanding schedule placed on lawmakers, the PAC affords one-on-one opportunities to discuss issues important to CRNAs that are otherwise unattainable.

INSPIRE AND ACCULTURATE CRNA STUDENTS EARLY INTO POLICY ENGAGEMENT

A strong value and part of the culture of the AANA is to involve its student members, which reflects the fact that the AANA has over 90% of all CRNAs as paid members. Nurse anesthesia students learn that their jobs providing anesthesia can be legislated away in an instant, making CRNA students aware of and engaged in policy from the start. The AANA presents policy engagement as having a visible and practical relationship to students' practice and livelihood and encourages early donating to the PAC so that it becomes a pattern as they mature in their careers.

COMMON SINGLE THREAT

Another key aspect of the success of the AANA's CRNA-PAC is that the American Society of Anesthesiologists (ASA) is a very real and outspoken opponent to CRNA practice and has unfortunately tried to block CRNA practice and reimbursement at every turn. While there are decades of peer-reviewed research documenting the safety and efficacy of CRNA practice, the ASA clings to its ideologic agenda that CRNA practice is "unsafe." Moreover, as a physician organization, the ASA has a $3.8 million PAC, nearly double the size of the AANA's CRNA-PAC. A large number of AANA members agree that the ASA opposition is a very real threat to their livelihood. AANA members see PAC contributions as a way to gain access to lawmakers so that they may educate them toward more sound, patient-centered, and evidence-based policymaking.

BIPARTISAN GIVING

Policymakers are carefully vetted, and disbursements target legislators who will carry the CRNA agenda forward. The CRNA-PAC typically gives equally to the Republicans and Democrats with a slight skew toward the party that is in power in the US House of Representatives and the US Senate. This way, the CRNA-PAC is not viewed as being aligned with a single political party, giving members and AANA leadership access to and an information channel with bipartisan legislators and candidates.

[a]Dr. Eileen O'Grady would like to thank Kate Fry of the AANA staff and PAC liaison, who was generous with her time in being interviewed for this exemplar.

Political Competence

Politically competent APRNs serve as content experts with policymakers and their staff. Policymakers have a wide range of knowledge, making it imperative for the APRN to use core nursing skills to determine the policymaker's baseline level of knowledge before launching into information sharing or making suggestions. Often, policymakers in the legislative branch are generalists who have a working knowledge on a broad range of topics such as immigration, transportation, energy, agriculture, and tax policy. However, in the executive branch, where regulations are written, the policymaker will be far more knowledgeable on a narrower range of topics. At the healthcare institution level, the corporate leader is also broad-based, focusing on the institution's profit margin, reputation in the community, and public reporting profile. Serving as a resource to policymakers with evidence-based information and helpful suggestions that are in the public interest is crucial and requires a thoughtful, skillful approach. When serving in this capacity, it is important to avoid a self-serving posture. To influence or participate meaningfully and effectively in policy development, APRNs must be aware of the policymaking process from idea conception to implementation as well as the open windows of political opportunity (see Box 17.1 and Box 17.2). Being effective in policy influence requires having deep knowledge about the problem the policy is intending to solve. Furthermore, intentionally developing and maintaining strong relationships with policymakers and other healthcare interest groups are important APRN activities. This requires asking many questions, building rapport, and seeking to understand where the policymaker is coming from before pushing an APRN or a patient-centered agenda forward. Heeding the US policy process, policymakers seek advisement on highly specific policy modifications rather than major reform recommendations. Elected officials turn over at a far higher rate than civil servants or healthcare executives, who make careers out of formulating and implementing health policy. Because of the longevity of their careers, the strong trustworthy relationships that APRNs make with the policymaker's staff as well as regulatory professionals (see Box 17.3) can yield great results over time.

BOX 17.2

Role of Public Comment

Public laws do not contain specific language about how the policy or program is to be carried out. For health-related issues, the executive branch agency, usually the Department of Health and Human Services, must publish its proposed rules in the daily *Federal Register*, seeking public comment. The public comment opportunity is usually limited to 60 days; however, stakeholder groups can exert an enormous degree of influence in the rulemaking process during this limited period. This public comment stems from two important American principles: (1) that democracy can only work if its citizenry is informed and participates and (2) the federal government does not hold all the expertise but must solicit comment from experts involved in the issue to alert the agency to unforeseen options or consequences (Regulations.gov, 2016). Advanced practice registered nurse (APRN) organizations can powerfully influence rulemaking by submitting evidence-based public comment and by activating the APRN grass roots to launch a public comment campaign. The *Federal Register* will tally the number of responses received and report how many were in favor of or opposed to the proposed rule. Thoughtful, well-crafted public comments submitted by an APRN organization have been directly incorporated into final rules, rendering submission of public comments and the rulemaking process crucially important activities for APRNs.

Individual Skills

Deep Knowledge

Self-Awareness. The value of APRNs is an important idea, but in order for APRNs to communicate that idea effectively, a great degree of maturity, discipline, humility, restraint, and respect for self and others must be practiced. Most careers of any kind are created with small steps; when people are effective, they are elevated into larger and larger spheres of influence. The politically competent APRN develops strong relationships with individuals inside and outside of nursing. The prerequisites for this level of maturity are knowing the self, staying focused on long-range goals, and avoiding being shrill or bringing emotionally charged energy into policy formulation.

For the most part, the APRN must be held in high regard and be knowledgeable, highly competent, and authentic, with solid integrity and a great degree of personal warmth. The APRN must have the trust of others to serve from a universal posture of problem

BOX 17.3

Four Ways to Build and Stay Current With Health Policy Knowledge

1. NEWS FEEDS

The best way to stay informed about current and emerging news is to subscribe to a few news feeds that get pushed to you from reputable, bipartisan policy sources. Glance at the headlines and read only what is of interest. Advanced practice registered nurses (APRNs) must be aware of the larger context of healthcare delivery and develop telescoping skills, in which one hooks smaller institutional policy issues onto what is happening in the larger world. Having knowledge of the larger policy world positions the APRN's capacity to participate more powerfully in institutional policy. Subscribe to three of the following (free) news feeds from the list below:

- The National Academy of Medicine News http://www.nationalacademies.org/hmd/Global/Media%20Room/Updates.aspx
- Commonwealth Fund http://www.commonwealthfund.org/
- Robert Wood Johnson Foundation News Digest http://www.rwjf.org/en.html
- Kaiser Family Foundation http://www.kff.org/
- Rand Corporation https://www.rand.org/
- Agency for Healthcare Research and Quality (AHRQ) https://www.ahrq.gov/news/newsletters/e-newsletter/index.html
- National Academies of Sciences, Engineering, and Medicine. 2021. The future of nursing 2020–2030: Charting a path to achieve health equity. Washington, DC: The National Academies Press. https://doi.org/10.17226/25982. https://nam.edu/publications/the-future-of-nursing-2020-2030/
- Medicare Payment Advisory Commission http://www.medpac.gov/
- Science Daily Health Policy News https://www.sciencedaily.com/news/health_medicine/health_policy/

2. WATCH THE PBS NEWS HOUR

See local listings for your TV station (http://www.pbs.org/newshour/). This hour-long program differs from network news in that there are long conversations with policy experts and the viewpoint is balanced and of the highest quality. It avoids news by sound bite, and there is frequent emphasis on health policy issues. Moreover, listening to the conversations with experts in the field, with a high degree of civility, on topics related to the economy or politics will assist the APRN to become a more informed citizen and raise the level of political competency. This is an easy way to stay informed and experience depth behind the issues.

3. READ/GLANCE AT NEWSPAPERS

Newspaper articles, whether in print or online, have at least one current health policy article. Often, these are found in the business or opinion sections. Read the Sunday opinion pages and the health section of your regional news source.

4. READ ABSTRACTS FROM HEALTH AFFAIRS

Health Affairs is the leading journal of health policy thought and research (http://www.healthaffairs.org/). The peer-reviewed journal explores current health policy issues. Its mission is to serve as a high-level, nonpartisan forum to promote analysis and discussion on improving health and health care and to address such issues as cost, quality, and access. The journal reaches a broad audience that includes government and health industry leaders; healthcare advocates; scholars of health, health care, and health policy; and others concerned with health and healthcare issues in the United States and worldwide. Everybody involved in health policy reads it, so scanning the titles and abstracts is a great way to stay current.

solving and not make decisions solely to elevate the nursing discipline (effective use of power). The locus of responsibility for a politically competent APRN must be far broader than just nursing interests (see Exemplars 17.4 and 17.5 and Box 17.3). There must be a commitment to practical problem solving to increase access to care, lower costs, and/or improve quality of care. This requires the APRN to be careful about

EXEMPLAR 17.4
FROM NURSE PRACTITIONER TO NORTH CAROLINA STATE HOUSE: WHAT PULLED GALE ADCOCK INTO PUBLIC OFFICE

Representative Gale Adcock, NP
North Carolina General Assembly (District 41: Cary, Apex, and Morrisville)
Interviewed by Eileen O'Grady

WHAT SPARKED YOU TO RUN FOR ELECTED OFFICE?

I grew weary trying to influence others to do what I thought they should do. After 27 years working to influence the state house from the outside, I saw over and over how the sausage was made and how bad decisions got made. After 13 years as an elected politician, my main takeaway is this: deal-making is all based on relationships. Relationships drive power in politics, and APNs are great at relationships. Good ideas do not necessarily get off the ground because of *who* had the idea. Bad ideas get made into law based on *who* had the idea. If a politician is not liked by their peers, they have no capacity to convince others to adopt good ideas. This job—being an elected official—requires APN comportment, using nonpolitical language to problem-solve. That includes connecting with constituents effectively. I have to stand up, make my point fast, and not make my opposition wrong or heartless. As nurses, we have the skills to do this.

WHY IS IT IMPORTANT FOR APNS TO BE IN STATE LEGISLATIVE HOUSES?

APNs are in a great position to tell patient stories, bring marginalized voices alive, and put a face on problems and statistics. We understand the cascading impact of not having prenatal care, school nurses, or access to care in rural communities. We are the uncomfortable truth-tellers based on our patient care experiences. When we show up in an elected capacity, for example, the MDs are telling their stories, but the legislation likely will not be provider neutral if we APNs are not there. It's important that we get into elected office to break down the MD dominance mindset. Changing language in legislation to say "healthcare provider" rather than "physician" is a tired fight; in fact, it's exhausting, and we need more of you! I have met doctor of nursing practice (DNP) students who do not regularly vote or know anything about their local candidates. This lack of even the most basic civic engagement is a big disconnect. APNs must become more politically competent by researching candidates who support health care.

The next tier of political competence is to engage with elected officials. Again, this requires relationship building. Meeting with your elected officials to offer your expertise and support *before* you ask them for something is critical in the ever-important stage of relationship building. Use the same skills you would as an APN: establish the relationship with the patient before asking them to manage their chronic illness. We start with small steps and build in bigger asks over time. Do not wait to meet your legislators until you need something. This transfer of nursing skills into the legislative arena is extremely helpful—we can recognize emotional undertones; we can get to the heart of understanding different viewpoints; we can appreciate their home environment. Using nursing skills in the political arena is how we build bipartisanship.

WHAT DO YOU FEEL WAS THE MOST PROFOUND IMPACT YOU HAVE HAD AS AN ELECTED NP?

As a freshman member of the House, I was a primary sponsor of legislation mandating newborn screening for severe combined immunodeficiency disease and it became law! Because of my clinical background, I stepped in for an experienced legislator and lead bill sponsor when he unexpectedly could not testify at committee meetings. The Baby Carlie Nugent Bill was signed into law, and North Carolina was the 34th state to do so. There was bipartisan support, and after the bill signing, the mother of a newborn who died of the disease walked past the governor and hugged me in front of the media.

WHAT HAS SURPRISED YOU ABOUT THE ROLE?

Two things. First, talent, experience, or content expertise are not important for leadership roles. At first, the Speaker of the House did not appoint me to any health committees. It was not obvious. When I went to ask him to be put on the health policy committee, I suggested that my time would not be well spent as a legislator if I couldn't use my clinical and scientific expertise. He agreed to appoint me, and I have served on this committee each term since.

Second, what surprises me still is institutionalized obstruction in policymaking. The legislative body has the mindset of a giant middle school. There are so many shenanigans around bills; they get moved around and stalled only to die a slow death. Rather than being direct and saying, "It's never going to happen," leadership uses indirect means to let good bills and good ideas die. They just never get on a committee calendar and wither away.

HARD PARTS?

The indirect communication. Here in North Carolina, they often don't say it straight.

FUN PARTS?

Everything I do is based on what I've learned as a clinician. Because I'm a nurse sitting in a meeting, I notice when a person's body language does not match their words. I typically say, "I'd appreciate knowing what you think." Or if

Continued

EXEMPLAR 17.4

FROM NURSE PRACTITIONER TO NORTH CAROLINA STATE HOUSE: WHAT PULLED GALE ADCOCK INTO PUBLIC OFFICE—cont'd

one person is dominating, I will say, "We want to hear from those of you in the room that haven't said anything." I try to use silence skillfully when I know a colleague is not speaking their truth.

WHAT ARE THE MOST POLITICALLY COMPETENT ACTIONS YOU HAVE SEEN ADVANCED PRACTICE NURSES ENGAGE IN AS AN ELECTED OFFICIAL?

Establishing relationships early on and building mutual connections by telling stories that are so compelling that legislators remember it every time they see you. Telling stories in such a way that they are remembered years later. Making one specific point in a memorable way can help shift perspective. A powerful, well-told story opens others up, making them less defensive. Tell stories in a way that shows an appreciation for the legislator's context. Nurses must not see this as a linear process. For example, the APRN must be aware of a large Medicaid bill that absorbs everyone's bandwidth or state budget constraints. Always make the gracious assumption that people are trying to do their best and when they *know better*, they do better. So, I recommend that APRNs become as informed as they can be as citizens and guardians of health.

WHAT DO YOU RECOMMEND THEY NOT DO?

NEVER make your message about APRNs and what we deserve. ALWAYS make the focus of your message about patients and what they deserve.

IF YOU COULD SEND ANY TEXT MESSAGE TO EVERYBODY, AS AN ELECTED MEMBER OF A STATE LEGISLATIVE BODY AND A NURSE PRACTITIONER, WHAT WOULD THAT TEXT MESSAGE SAY?

Get involved; get good people in office. "If you're not the lead dog, the view never changes." APRNs must decide to become the lead dog, or nothing will ever change.

EXEMPLAR 17.5

FROM NURSE PRACTITIONER TO EXECUTIVE BRANCH TO LEGISLATIVE BRANCH

Delegate Dawn Adams, DNP
Virginia House of Delegates (68th District, representing Chesterfield Co., Henrico Co., and City of Richmond)
Interviewed by Eileen O'Grady

WHAT SPARKED YOU TO RUN FOR ELECTED OFFICE?

I started in the state's executive branch (Virginia Department of Behavioral Health and Developmental Disabilities). Four years later, I ran for elected office in the legislative branch because I was struck by the lack of clear, productive communication between the two branches of government. I knew how to communicate clearly. As a nurse, I understand that both clear facts and accurate assessment can result in life and death outcomes. I also knew I had the skills to engage in really difficult conversations. As a nurse practitioner, I have had many of these; it is a skill that is honed by years in the profession. We as nurses often change our communication depending on who we are talking to and meet people where they are. I knew I could do a better job communicating between the two branches of government, especially because I had seen up close how ineffective the communication patterns were. I also believed that the only way to truly influence policy was to have a seat at the table discussing and making the decisions that become state law.

WHAT HAS SURPRISED YOU ABOUT THE ROLE?

Lots of things. The true operations I could not have foreseen—maybe I wasn't savvy enough—but I think most people would be truly shocked by how government works. There is a very clear structure. If you are in the majority party, you have unilateral authority—full stop. If you are in the minority party, you have very little say. Expertise does not seem to weigh into leadership decisions regarding committee assignments. Committees are everything during session. Seniority plays an outsized role, and that's why elected politicians want to stay a long time. It may be the last holdout where duration remains more important than quality. But there is an amount of "duration" necessary to make things work. I have had to push hard to be put on health committees. Though I recently completed my third session, this was my first year on any health-related committees. I happen to be the most educated person in health care in the General Assembly, yet when I was serving within the minority party, it was not obvious to put me on health committees.

HARD PARTS?

One of the disheartening parts of politics is seeing that sometimes when there is a choice between policy and politics, politics wins. For example, most people in my party ran on voting for anti-gerrymandering legislation presented

EXEMPLAR 17.5

FROM NURSE PRACTITIONER TO EXECUTIVE BRANCH TO LEGISLATIVE BRANCH—cont'd

in 2019. When my party was in the minority, most voted for this legislation. Because it was legislation that requires a constitutional amendment, it is mandated that the same legislation be voted on 2 years in a row. However, in 2020 the majority party changed and many of the same people who voted for the anti-gerrymandering legislation voted against it, and it got very ugly. So, this is very disappointing, but it is how politics works.

FUN PARTS?

Engaging with people interested in policy! It is really stimulating as a nurse practitioner to be a part of discussing these fascinating ever-changing issues and to have a seat at the table. Every committee meeting I sit on involves intense policy discussions in health care. I love that. I'm never bored shaping a better future.

WHAT ARE THE MOST POLITICALLY COMPETENT ACTIONS YOU HAVE SEEN ADVANCED PRACTICE NURSES ENGAGE IN AS AN ELECTED OFFICIAL?

Just showing up is the most important thing (after voting, of course). Talk to your state representatives, because that is far above what the average citizen does. Share your background and be sure to focus on just one single issue at a time. Describe it as a problem and tell a clinical or real story about it and ask them to support the legislation specific to the issue. I wish that nursing organizations would pick a few issues and stagger their engagement. It would be helpful if the nursing associations coordinated and streamlined their efforts.

We nurses know people and the root causes of their poor health status. APRNs in particular have the experience and the public's trust to explain the impact of food deserts, health disparities, inadequate housing, and the impact the criminal justice system has on vulnerable communities. APRNs are well positioned to work toward decoupling health insurance from employment—it's a model of insurance provision that is in desperate need of an update, because it harms people. We can change minds and bring love and kindness to these persistent problems.

WHAT DO YOU RECOMMEND THEY NOT DO?

Come with a laundry list, especially with issues that are not connected to any active legislation. Nurses who come to the General Assembly and are not strategic about who they see are wasting opportunity. Nurses need to laser focus their energy on their delegate and senator, because they are very concerned about what you think. We should also remember that there are six nurses to every MD in this country, yet MDs are ever present in the General Assembly, showing up and asking for very specific things. Nurses can and must do better to be more present and visible.

It's easy to get through a nursing graduate program and not see how politics is related to you, your job, and your patients because you're busy. You can make excuses about why this is not a priority for you, but this mindset is a mistake. Policy influences every part of your life.

IF YOU COULD SEND ANY TEXT MESSAGE TO EVERYBODY, AS AN ELECTED MEMBER OF A STATE LEGISLATIVE BODY AND A DOCTORALLY PREPARED NURSE PRACTITIONER, WHAT WOULD THAT TEXT MESSAGE SAY?

Where there is opportunity, there is hope, and hope precipitates change. Do not lose faith in the political system. Engage in it.

burning bridges so that there are no individuals or communities of people who want to see the APRN fail.

Content Expertise. Journalists Buresh and Gordon (2006) described three communication challenges that are common across nursing:

1. Not enough nurses are willing to talk about their work.
2. Nurses, media, and health organizations often unwillingly project an inaccurate portrait of nursing as a "virtue" rather than a scientifically based, rigorous, and unique body of knowledge.
3. When nurses do speak about nursing, they often bypass, downplay, or devalue the work of human caring.

These communication challenges capture the central dilemma of modern nursing: that nurses are caring for the sickest or most vulnerable members of society, sometimes without the resources or authority to carry it out. They are unable to fully promote health in the overmedicalized, overspecialized health delivery systems that do not focus on, value, or otherwise profit from early intervention measures that align with nursing core values. Nurses' political competency must be enhanced, and APRNs must fully inhabit the policy realm and move from silence to powerful voice. APRNs ought to be seated at tables of power where government, academic, and corporate decision making occurs. The most pressing healthcare problems in society, especially the chronic disease epidemic, require an intelligence that advanced practice nurses fully own.

Bringing APRN wisdom through a polarity-thinking lens can enhance one's expertise. Many of the most persistent healthcare problems are not really problems to be solved but tensions that need to be leveraged. For example, the problems of cost cutting and improving quality create tensions when one focuses only on one without attention to the other. Polarity thinking helps bring APRN pragmatic wisdom to complex problems. The APRN can identify these polarities and find solutions by connecting interdependent pairs, pointing out that we cannot have one tension without its opposite. Other polarity examples include inhaling versus exhaling, patient care versus self-care, and technology versus human caring. These issues do not go away over time; rather, they are tensions that need to be managed (Wesorick, 2016). APRNs can motivate groups that may be stuck in challenging dilemmas by getting them to move off of "either–or" solutions and move to "both–and" solutions. This may be a more thoughtful and effective way for APRNs to bring their expertise to policy tables.

Seek Out Experts. A great degree of humility is required on the part of the politically active APRN; one effective way to embody humility is to seek out respected individuals with expertise (content experts), including those whose political agenda may be different from one's own. Consulting experts along the way to gain insight and knowledge builds trust because the seeker of expertise does not presume to be an expert in all matters related to health care. The APRN must integrate all sides of an issue (stakeholder analysis) and then decide about how and whether to use that expertise. That means seeking out and engaging experts who may oppose one's policy agenda.

Political Antenna

Policy Process. Content expertise is not the only skill set required to be effective in influencing policy in an interprofessional arena. The APRN must be always mindful of the policy process and carefully measure how one participates in discussions to maximize being heard (political antennae). Developing political antennae can be strengthened by engaging stakeholders who may oppose or support an action that the APRN may want to take. This stakeholder analysis, done privately before issues become public (or before a meeting), is an effective way to learn about all of the issues, especially the opposition viewpoint, so that a creative strategy can be developed to inoculate the opposing ideas with an evidence base or a creative idea. Knowing how others are motivated and what their agenda is places the APRN at an advantage in negotiating a mutually agreeable outcome. By learning others' opinions about contentious issues, the APRN can carefully garner support.

Conduct at Meetings. In terms of public meetings and how APRNs conduct themselves, impromptu remarks should be avoided because they could be used against the person, the nursing profession, or other interests in the future. It is important to continuously gauge the other stakeholders at the meeting; if, for example, a physician has made a point about nursing that the APRN wanted to make, let that external validation stand as a comment that is supportive of nursing, rather than repeating the point. It is important to show restraint in meetings, waiting until an insightful thought comes that forwards the discussion, or to bring more accurate factual data to the conversation, or to help clarify the polarizing issues and areas of agreement in a policy discussion. To be successful, the APRN must keep cool, responding factually and avoiding rhetorical inflammatory comments that might diminish other disciplines (no bashing other provider groups). By participating in meetings with this respectful approach, deep content expertise, and a focus on process, the APRN is well positioned to encourage others to support nursing issues.

Use Power

Contribute to Public Discourse. Another essential responsibility for APRNs is to inform and contribute to the public discourse on important health policy issues, because APRN interests and public interests are not at odds. Gaining public support and influencing public opinion can help get the attention of policymakers or propel issues onto the policy agenda. Submitting a guest essay or op-ed (meaning "opposite the editorial page" in the publication) to major news outlets is a powerful way to do this (Box 17.4). This requires writing that links the health issues to society, uses poignant stories to bring the problem to life, and incorporates evidence to build a strong case about why a policy change is needed. APRNs must use their professional credentials

BOX 17.4

Op-Ed Suggestions

Created by Eileen O'Grady

Op-eds are not formulaic, but some general guidelines may enhance the potential for publication. The term "op-ed" refers to the practice of publishing informed opinions from the public "opposite the editorial pages" which first began in 1921. It was discovered that nothing is more interesting than thought-provoking, well-informed opinions. Advanced practice nurses (APNs) have a unique background and are privileged with the public trust, so we can make our opinions about the public health widely known. Op-eds and letters to the editor are both unsolicited, but letters to the editor are usually shorter and in direct response to a story or article that has previously been published. Op-eds are longer opinion pieces that are usually related to some current event or news story in which the author has an area of expertise. A strong 750-word op-ed piece could include these steps:

1. Begin with the credentials and experience of the author.
2. The policy problem is then hooked to a leading current problem or news story.
3. A specific poignant clinical story is added to describe how the problem affects people.
4. Policy solution(s) are offered backed up by three points of evidence.
5. A "to-be-sure" segment, which anticipates and counters opponents' views
6. An inoculation against those stakeholders who will oppose your ideas.
7. Finally, a conclusion with possible action items for members of the public (e.g., call or write legislator, support a bill).
8. Ask at least five people with strong writing skills to critique the piece prior to submission.

and expertise with a sense of responsibility toward educating the public and not be hesitant to act as advocates based on their knowledge and experience. This could include seeking out media invitations to news programs or starting a podcast to inform the public about the APRN's expertise on major issues of the day.

Serve on Boards. There are numerous opportunities for APRNs to serve on federal, corporate, and health-related advisory boards, which is crucial to integrating APRNs into policymaking. A coalition of nursing stakeholders has created an organization, Nurses on Boards Coalition (http://www.nursesonboardscoalition.org), with the sole purpose of getting nurses on boards in every state, at every level. This is an effort to correct the fact that nurses are underrepresented on policymaking boards, including those of hospitals and health centers. Serving on boards allows APRNs to expand their influence from the front lines to the boardroom and to use that frontline clinical knowledge to inform the boardroom. Often, APRNs are appointed because they have strong working relationships with people who happen to be on boards and are familiar with the APRN as a compelling knowledge source who is effective in groups. A definite set of behaviors is required to serve on national advisory or corporate boards, and a high degree of self-mastery is necessary to be reappointed or invited back (Fig. 17.5).

Use Power Instead of Force. Power accomplishes with ease what force, even with extreme effort, cannot accomplish. On the interpersonal front, it is important for APRNs to avoid using force in advancing their positions in the policy arena. Doing so can diminish one's power. Forcing our power over others is not effective and is harmful when APRNs participate in interprofessional policy or problem-solving meetings. The twin approaches of being judgmental and parochial can quickly compromise effectiveness. *Judgementalism*—criticizing other people or disciplines—distracts from effective problem solving and, in the process, can reflect poorly on the person who judges, greatly diminishing the power to influence. Diminishing others or the work they do can provoke defensiveness and consequently limit the capacity to influence others meaningfully. *Nursing parochialism* occurs when nurses present a narrow, restricted scope or outlook in which only nursing and nursing's interests are offered as solutions. These postures in the policy arena (or any other setting) do not build wide-based support or strong relationships.

Everyone has seen nurses and other leaders who become shrill and consistently present positions that reflect pure self-interest in public arenas, whereby each person in the room knows what the individual will say

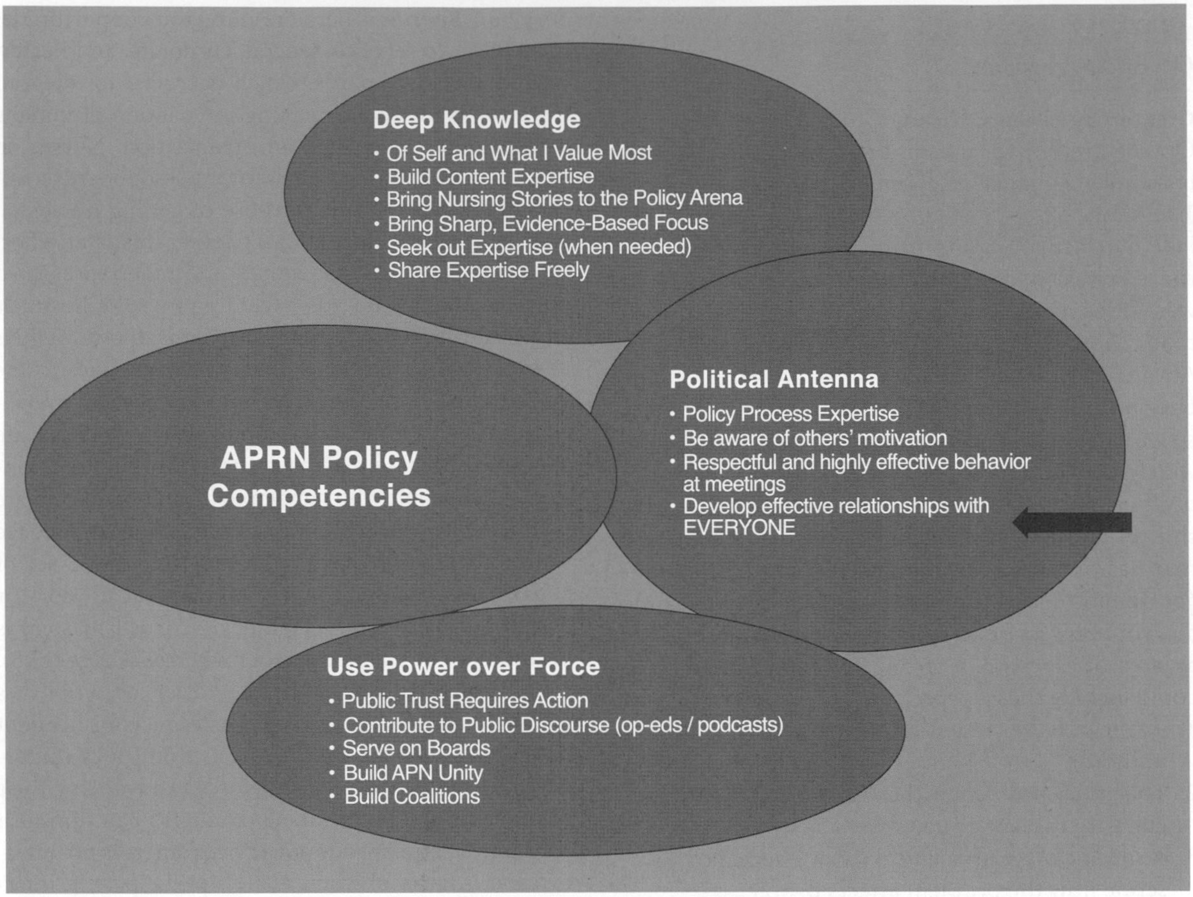
Deep Knowledge
• Of Self and What I Value Most
• Build Content Expertise
• Bring Nursing Stories to the Policy Arena
• Bring Sharp, Evidence-Based Focus
• Seek out Expertise (when needed)
• Share Expertise Freely
APRN Policy Competencies
Political Antenna
• Policy Process Expertise
• Be aware of others' motivation
• Respectful and highly effective behavior at meetings
• Develop effective relationships with EVERYONE
Use Power over Force
• Public Trust Requires Action
• Contribute to Public Discourse (op-eds / podcasts)
• Serve on Boards
• Build APN Unity
• Build Coalitions

Fig. 17.5 ■ Political competence.

before they speak. This is a posture of parochialism that APRNs must work hard to avoid. To be effective in interprofessional and influential arenas and to pursue larger roles, APRNs must build strong relationships founded on trust and respect. In policy-related meetings, APRNs must demonstrate that nurses can solve problems in the healthcare system, not just for nurses' sake. APRNs will inhabit a more powerful stance and become most effective when they bring a broader perspective to all of health care, not just nursing. This may require sharing one's own expertise freely, with a generous spirit, and avoiding the hoarding of information.

The value of APRNs and their potential impact on cost, quality, and access, if fully unleashed, is an enormously powerful solution to some of today's most significant healthcare problems. Power is characterized by humility and truth, which needs no defense or rhetoric; it is self-evident. Force is divisive and exploits people for individual or personal gain (Hawkins, 2002).

Take Action to Create Public Trust. In a study of nursing and power among Canadian nurse practitioners, Quinlan and Robertson (2013) described a form of nonauthoritative power called "communicative power" as the mutual understanding achieved between pairs of individuals by the efforts of a third. It differs from most kinds of informal power in that communicative power is oriented to the collective good, whereas informal power focuses on individual gain. Their study showed that NPs have the greatest amount of communicative power on the healthcare team. This is because they were able to mobilize their holistic practice and bridge the medical and nursing frames of knowledge and thereby were better able to contribute to the knowledge exchange within the teams. It was concluded that NPs have the potential to fully realize their role as knowledge-boundary spanners. The move to doctoral education raises this potential for APRNs even more. Communicative power in the policy arenas could be more fully deployed in light of the public trust. For 19 years in a row, when the public has been asked which professions they trust the most, nurses have ranked at the very top (Saad, 2020) (Table 17.4). This trust creates a social covenant with the public and, by extension, trust in APRNs in the policymaking context. The public trusts nurses to be advocates on their behalf.

Build APRN Unity. There are numerous ways for APRN organizations to exert influence continuously on the policymaking process. Forming coalitions with other APRNs and other nursing, healthcare, and consumer groups strengthens political effectiveness. Although there is a rich diversity of nursing organizations (more than 120 nationally and scores of state and regional organizations), none has a membership base that is more than a fraction of 4 million nurses in the United States. Forming coalitions and strategic plans around policy is necessary to maximize impact. APRN organizational leaders can play a role in defining health policy problems and designing possible solutions. The APRN movement has advanced tremendously, but a greater degree of policy solidarity would significantly strengthen the political effectiveness and power of APRNs. APRNs are characteristically pioneers, blazing new trails that have pushed the role and boundaries of nursing forward. As the total numbers of APRNs and those with doctorates continue to grow exponentially, their political influence will also grow.

Build Coalitions. Longest (2016) has asserted that organizations that form policy communities (build coalitions) can exert enormous influence on the policy process. Policy communities are composed of loosely structured, heterogeneous networks defined by the level of investment that each group has around the issue. There is an enormous difference between defining a health policy problem and reaching concordance

TABLE 17.4

Gallup Poll on Honesty/Ethics in Professions

Nurses Still Rate Highest for Honesty and Ethics **How would you rate the honesty and ethical standards of people in these different fields? Very high, high, average, low, or very low?**	**2020**	**2019**	**2018**	**2017**	**2016**
Nurses	89	85	84	82	84
Engineers	–	66	–	–	65
Physicians	77	65	67	65	65
Pharmacists	–	64	66	62	67
Dentists	52	61	–	–	59
Police officers	–	54	54	56	58
College teachers	–	49	–	–	47
Psychiatrists	–	43	–	–	38
Chiropractors	–	41	–	–	38
Clergy	39	40	37	42	44
Journalists	28	28	33	–	23
Bankers	29	28	27	25	24
Labor union leaders	–	24	21	–	–
Lawyers	21	22	19	18	18
Stockbrokers	–	14	14	–	12
Members of congress	8	12	8	11	8
Car salespeople	8	9	8	10	9

Values are percentages.

Source: "US Ethics Ratings Rise for Medical Workers and Teachers," by L. Saad, 2020, Gallup, https://news.gallup.com/poll/328136/ethics-rating-rise-medical-workers-teacehers.aspx

on policy positions/solutions. Reaching concordance in the development of policy positions is what adds great power to policy communities and is the organizational challenge for APRN groups.

Moving the APRN Role Forward in Health Policy

Communicating Findings

Findings on APRN research must be published in journals outside of nursing to reach a broader policymaking and public audience. Key policymakers and the public must be made more aware of the contributions that APRNs make in reducing healthcare costs and improving access and quality of care. Achieving broader recognition, reducing APRN invisibility, and removing barriers to APRN practice will be contingent on APRNs communicating methodologically sound APRN research with results that are generalizable to the larger delivery system. Moreover, the APRN research agenda could build a portfolio that directly addresses health topics that are important and relevant to a wide swath of public interest. Fig. 17.6 shows an abstract on the policy implications of the rapidly growing nurse practitioner workforce in the United States in the highly regarded journal *Health Affairs*. This journal reaches a wide and highly influential audience. It is read by and used as a reliable knowledge source by health policymakers.

Challenges and Resources in Evidence-Informed Policy Development

As evidence-based clinicians, APRNs may assume that policy is formed by conducting good research, disseminating the findings, and building best practices in a rational, linear process. Another assumption is that once a policy is specified, people will simply implement it. As noted earlier in this chapter, policy in practice is far messier than this. Clearly, evidence needs to influence policy up front. This requires a better relationship between policymakers, researchers, and practitioners and a deeper understanding of each other's priorities and ways of working. The insights from Glasby (2011)

NURSES

By David I. Auerbach, Peter I. Buerhaus, and Douglas O. Staiger

Implications Of The Rapid Growth Of The Nurse Practitioner Workforce In The US

DOI: 10.1377/hlthaff.2019.00686
HEALTH AFFAIRS 39,
NO. 2 (2020): 273–279
©2020 Project HOPE—
The People-to-People Health
Foundation, Inc.

ABSTRACT Concerns about physician shortages have led policy makers in the US public and private sectors to advocate for the greater use of nurse practitioners (NPs). We examined recent changes in demographic, employment, and earnings characteristics of NPs and the implications of those changes. In the period 2010–17 the number of NPs in the US more than doubled from approximately 91,000 to 190,000. This growth occurred in every US region and was driven by the rapid expansion of education programs that attracted nurses in the Millennial generation. Employment was concentrated in hospitals, physician offices, and outpatient care centers, and inflation-adjusted earnings grew by 5.5 percent over this period. The pronounced growth in the number of NPs has reduced the size of the registered nurse (RN) workforce by up to 80,000 nationwide. In the future, hospitals must innovate and test creative ideas to replace RNs who have left their positions to become NPs, and educators must be alert for signs of falling earnings that may signal the excess production of NPs.

David I. Auerbach (davea@alum.mit.edu) is an external adjunct faculty member at the Center for Interdisciplinary Health Workforce Studies, College of Nursing, Montana State University, in Bozeman.

Peter I. Buerhaus is a professor of nursing and director of the Center for Interdisciplinary Health Workforce Studies, both in the College of Nursing, Montana State University.

Douglas O. Staiger is the John Sloan Dickey Third Century Professor in the Social Sciences at Dartmouth College, in Hanover, New Hampshire.

Fig. 17.6 A peer-reviewed abstract in a widely read policy journal on the rapid growth of the nurse practitioner workforce in the United States.

address the challenges of the evidence, policy, and practice interaction (Box 17.5).

Evidence-informed health policy is a growing field that APRNs ought to embrace for deeper knowledge and skill development. See Table 17.5 for a list of professional policy development opportunities for nurses. The World Health Organization (WHO, 2017) sponsors the Evidence-informed Policy Network (EVIPNet), a network established by WHO to promote use of research evidence in policymaking. Through evidence briefs, policy dialogue summaries, rapid synthesis reports, and national clearinghouses, EVIPNet is available to policymakers and researchers to strengthen health systems worldwide. In 2009 BioMed Central Ltd. launched the SUPporting Policy Relevant Reviews and Trials (SUPPORT) project, a series of articles in *Health Research Policy and Systems* that serve as a toolkit for evidence-informed health policymaking (Oxman et al., 2009). Each of the 18 articles in the series presents a proposed tool for use by those involved in finding and using research to inform health policymaking. The series highlights the need for research in policymaking processes, including clarifying problems, framing options, and implementation planning. It instructs on how to assess systematic reviews and other types of evidence to inform policymaking and how to move from evidence to decisions (Oxman et al., 2009). It could serve as an important resource/idea generator for scholarly projects or dissertations.

Building on the work by Oxman et al. (2009), the international organization Health Information for All (HIFA) Working Group on Evidence-Informed Policy and Practice (Pakenham-Walsh, 2016) held a month-long Internet-based discussion representing 16 countries. This group identified five priorities to strengthen evidence-informed policymaking:

1. Build the skills of policymakers
2. Improve the clarity of information for policymakers
3. Engage the public
4. Improve communication and understanding
5. Empower rather than persuade policymakers

The participants emphasized the need to consider tacit forms of knowledge, including experiences, lessons learned, and the voices of patients, as well as the biases of evidence and the manipulation of facts for political purposes. As a first step, researchers must engage stakeholders up front, before the research is designed, to formulate the key questions necessary for making decisions. Finally, the report focuses on the importance of empowerment through evidence, in contrast to persuasion using emotional appeal. These priorities can be directly translated to APRN health policy locally and globally.

The development and evaluation of health policy often take place in organizations referred to as *think tanks*. They can be small, local organizations or large, international, multi-million-dollar organizations such as the Kaiser Family Foundation, the Heritage Foundation, and the Center for American Progress. These organizations seek to shape governmental policy by offering expertise in various areas, including health care (see Exemplar 17.6). Recognizing political bias often held by a think tank is essential when drawing on its work to inform policy. The University of Pennsylvania maintains a list of public policy think

BOX 17.5

Challenges of the Evidence, Policy, and Practice Interaction

1. Evidence is only one voice competing for attention, so researchers need to be committed and passionate.
2. Evidence needs to influence policy early on—not after the policy is formulated or rolled out.
3. Policymakers and researchers need to understand each other's worlds and priorities.
4. Sometimes it may be necessary to gather the best evidence in the time available rather than all of the evidence.
5. Simply "disseminating" more research will not necessarily help embed evidence in practice. Instead, it may be more fruitful to support local leaders to make sense of emerging policy and help create receptive local contexts.

Asking the right question is crucial—asking, "Does this work?" requires a different approach from asking, "If I do this, what might be the implications?"

TABLE 17.5

Selected Health Policy Experiences for Advanced Practice Nurses

Policy Experience, Internship, Fellowship Opportunity	Contact
Academy Health	http://www.academyhealth.org
Nurse in Washington Internship	http://www.nursing-alliance.org/Events/NIWI-Nurse-in-Washington-Internship
National Academy of Social Insurance	https://www.nasi.org/studentopps
Robert Wood Johnson Health Policy Fellowship	http://www.healthpolicyfellows.org/
White House Fellows Program	https://www.whitehouse.gov/participate/fellows
American Association of Nurse Practitioners Health Policy Fellowship	https://www.aanp.org/legislation-regulation/federal-legislation/health-policy-fellowship
Health and Aging Policy Fellowships	http://www.healthandagingpolicy.org/about-the-fellowship/partnerships/
National Academy of Medicine Nurse Scholar-in-Residence	https://www.aannet.org/resources/scholars/nam-scholar-in-residence
American Academy of Nursing Jonas Policy Scholars Program	https://www.aannet.org/resources/scholars/academy-jonas-policy-scholars
The Margaret E. Mahoney Fellowships in Health Policy	https://www.nyam.org/fellows-grants/grants-awards/student-grants/margaret-e-mahoney-fellowships/
American Association of Colleges of Nursing Government Affairs and Policy Internship	https://www.aacnnursing.org/Policy-Advocacy/Get-Involved/Internships
Health Resources and Services Administration (DHHS) Maternal & Child Health Student Internships	https://mchb.hrsa.gov/training/tr_internship-hrsa.asp

tanks according to areas of research, including health. This list includes US and Canadian organizations representing a range of political ideologies (McGann, 2020).

EMERGING ADVANCED PRACTICE NURSING POLICY ISSUES

Nurses in advanced practice face numerous policy challenges in local, state, national, and international arenas. A few of the most important issues facing APRNs in the next decade include continued attainment of full practice authority across APRN roles (see Chapter 20), recognition and reimbursement for services (see Chapter 19), and workforce development.

APRN Full Practice Authority

In 2012, following publication of the 2008 APRN Consensus Model Document, the National Council of State Boards of Nursing (NCSBN) proposed *APRN Model Act and Rules* to assist state legislators, administrators, and stakeholders in developing, enacting, and adopting consistent APRN laws inclusive of all four APRN roles.This model practice act explicitly describes APRN title and scope of practice, licensure requirements, education programs, and defines APRNs as licensed independent practitioners within established professional standards (NCSBN, 2012). The challenge is that achieving this or similar legislation requires that many state licensing laws be relegislated. State licensing laws define the permissible scope of practice for the healthcare professions. The purpose of state health professions laws is to protect the public and to assure consumers that healthcare workers conduct their practices in areas for which they are properly trained. However, according to Martin and Alexander (2019), scope of practice laws too often are unnecessarily restrictive and serve to protect the economic interests of another group. More than 2 decades later, contemporary research continues to reiterate the Pew Health Professions Commission's Task Force on Health Care Workforce Regulation report (1995), which called for

EXEMPLAR 17.6

THINK TANKS TO INFLUENCE POLICY: THE JOURNEY OF DONNA BARRY

By: Donna Barry

While I was directing a Partners In Health project to treat multiple-drug-resistant tuberculosis in Russia, Representative Sherrod Brown from Ohio visited our treatment program in Siberia. That visit and work on that project were my first steps into the world of policy and opened my eyes to the crucial role that advanced practice registered nurses (APRNs) need to take on in policy development.

One of the main points of our project in Russia was to update treatment and show better treatment outcomes using multiple drugs for longer treatment periods and less surgical intervention. The Russia project was part of a bigger policy focus on global treatment policy at the World Health Organization. Senator Brown's visit to the Siberian clinic was to give him on-the-ground stories and experience to shore up his annual defense of increased money for tuberculosis treatment in the State and Foreign Operations budgets in the US House of Representatives and the US Senate.

Eventually I became the first director of policy and advocacy at Partners In Health. During 6 years in that role, I worked alongside several team members and a large coalition, spending our efforts on the following topics, among many others:

- Working on policy related to improving treatment for undernutrition/malnutrition in low-income countries
- Increasing the number of healthcare providers in low-income countries as well as improving their training and retention rates
- Updating outdated US foreign assistance laws and rules that made foreign aid less effective and often more expensive to deliver
- Increasing foreign aid budgets for HIV/AIDS and tuberculosis
- Encouraging the United Nations to consider preventing and treating noncommunicable diseases such as cancer and heart disease as important as preventing and treating infectious diseases

I have since been named the director of the Women's Health and Rights Program at the Center for American Progress (CAP) in Washington, DC. One of the first issues that came up after starting that position was the Supreme Court case on contraceptives and the religious liberty of private corporations (*Hobby Lobby v. Burwell*). There were multiple court cases related to contraception, abortion, the Affordable Care Act, and other key health issues that arose during my time at CAP. Understanding the US court/judicial system was never covered in nursing school or my public health training, but learning how that system works and affects policy is key to comprehending much of US health policy. It is also very important that APRNs understand how laws, regulations, and rules governing health care in our country are made—we APRNs can favorably impact them if we are engaged when they are drafted, reviewed, debated, and implemented.

Change in the domestic and global policy arena is usually incremental and very slow. However, it is critical that nurses, especially APRNs, stay engaged in policy change that affects the fields in which we work, whether that policy is local, state, federal, or global. Our voices and experience are deeply valued by policymakers but also unique and vital for sound policy.

increased regulatory flexibility, as blurred boundaries between professional scopes of practice are recognized with advancement in technology and workforce innovations. The Pew Commission noted that varying objectives and levels of specificity are found in different professions' scopes of practice without rationale and that the system "treats practice acts as rewards for the professions" (p. 6) rather than as rational mechanisms for safe and effective care by competent practitioners. Historically, the Pew report noted the expectation of overlapping scopes of practice among different healthcare professions and emphasized the importance of demonstrated initial and continuing competence as a common thread among healthcare professional practice acts.

Building on this important body of work to reform the existing paradigm, in 2006 Safriet (2011) worked with six professional licensing boards, including the Federation of State Medical Boards and the NCSBN, to achieve consensus on a position paper addressing scope of practice legislation (APRN Joint Dialogue Group, 2008). Notably, the six organizations agreed that the criteria related to who is qualified to perform functions safely without risk of harm to the public are the only justifiable conditions for defining scopes of practice (NCSBN, 2009). Despite these efforts, full practice authority remains a goal for many states. The NCSBN compiles a state-by-state report tracking status of practice and prescribing across all APRN roles accessible to the public and updated regularly

(NCSBN, 2021 August). Provider-neutral language in all rules and regulations would go far in removing artificial barriers to practice that lack an evidence base.

Public Health Crisis

APRNs are familiar with a stepwise legislative approach to full practice authority attainment, but the COVID-19 global pandemic thrust scope of practice limitations into the spotlight in early 2020. Facing an unprecedented number of infected patients, governors across the United States sought to lift scope of practice barriers for APRNs through temporary emergency executive orders and regulatory waivers. To ensure timely access to care during the pandemic, several states enacted permanent legislation authorizing full practice authority for all licensed APRNs (Phillips, 2022), and nearly all states without full practice authority temporarily authorized removal of various regulatory barriers (NCSBN, 2020).

APRN Workforce Development

Data about the US nursing workforce have been critical to formulating rational policies related to APRNs. Inadequacy of census data has been a challenge in defining the benefits of APRNs. The primary source of valid and reliable data has been the U. S. Department of Health and Human Resources, Health Resources and Services Administration's the *National Sample Survey of Nurse Practitioners* (HRSA, 2014). However, this survey does not sample additional APRN roles and has not been updated since 2012. Another data source about NP practice environment is the *National Nurse Practitioner Sample Survey*, which is conducted periodically by the AANP to characterize and review US trends in the NP workforce (AANP, 2019). CRNA and CNM data are of higher quality because each of these advanced nursing practice specialties has a single organization and national certifying body tracking its workforce over time, essentially a census. They are able to analyze their data to answer policy-relevant questions quickly, with a few keystrokes. The National Association of Clinical Nurse Specialists published its first CNS census survey in 2014, and it is conducted every 2 years (National Association of Clinical Nurse Specialists, 2018).

The Bureau of Labor Statistics (2020a) also reports occupational employment statistics for NPs, CRNAs, and CNMs. Occupational employment statistics for the CNS role are included in the registered nurse report (Bureau of Labor Statistics, 2020b). Some data may be available through nursing organizations, current NCSBN national data, and some state nursing workforce centers. The quality of data from these sources is variable.

A policy issue to which APRNs need to continually attend is ensuring that APRN data are identifiable for quality evaluation and outcome assessment. When APRN services are billed "incident-to" the physician services, the value of the APRN work is attributed to the physician (Chapter 19). A model for data collection for APRNs is nurse-managed clinics, which have effective data collecting and reporting systems and are recognized by the National Committee for Quality Assurance as patient-centered medical homes. Having strong, current, reliable APRN workforce data is essential for overcoming invisibility and building political power.

CONCLUSION

APRNs practice in a highly complex, ever-changing environment. The high degree of public trust in nursing points to a social covenant that APRNs have with the public. This covenant is to advocate for sound, clinically informed health policy, which requires engagement in the political process. By the very work they do, APRNs cannot remove themselves from politics, because health care in the United States is inherently political. By framing all healthcare problems in a cost, quality, or access framework, APRNs in any setting or institution (local, state, national, or international) can help others see how policy changes affect patients. Developing political and policy competency is a must to advance the profession.

KEY SUMMARY POINTS

- APRNs must play a larger role in shaping how health care is delivered, because they have a social covenant with the public to serve as patient advocates in the broadest sense. To be able to do this, APRNs must resist the pull of the familiar and overcome invisibility and passivity.

- Policymakers are looking for solutions to escalating costs and continued patient safety problems. Part of the APRN professional role is to assist policymakers in finding practical, evidence-based solutions.
- Membership in professional organizations and coalitions that advance issues critical to APRN practice and the health of the United States is vital to the continued viability of APRNs. The first step to being involved in policy formulation is to be knowledgeable about the policy process and the current and emerging issues relevant to APRNs. To be involved, APRNs need to understand the details related to funding issues, measures of quality, how they reflect APRN practice, and specific programs designed to improve access (Table 17.5).
- An important truth for APRNs and policy is that a single person, with deep understanding of an issue along with highly developed political skills, can make a difference. An individual backed by organizational strength, particularly by coalitions of organizations, can make an even more significant difference.

REFERENCES

The Advisory Board. (November 5, 2020). Meet the 16 doctors, nurses, and other clinicians just elected to Congress. Retrieved from https://www.advisory.com/daily-briefing/2020/11/05/congress-clinicians

American Association of Nurse Practitioners. (2019, January). The State of the Nurse Practitioner Profession, 2018: Results from the National nurse practitioner sample survey. Retrieved from https://www.aanp.org/practice/practice-related-research/research-reports

American Association of Nurse Practitioners. (2020). Federal Issue Briefs: Accountable care organizations (ACOs). Retrieved from https://www.aanp.org/advocacy/federal/federal-issue-briefs/accountable-care-organizations

American Association of Colleges of Nursing (2021). The Essentials: Core competencies for professional nursing education. Retrieved from https://www.aacnnursing.org/Education-Resources/AACN-Essentials

Andrews, J. (2017). The current state of public and private prison healthcare. The Wharton Public Policy Initiative. February 24. Retrieved from https://publicpolicy.wharton.upenn.edu/live/news/1736-the-current-state-of-public-and-private-prison/for-students/blog/news.php

APRN Joint Dialogue Group. (2008). Consensus model for APRN regulation: Licensure, accreditation, certification, and education. http://www.aacn.nche.edu/education-resources/APRNReport.pdf

Auxier, B. (2020). *Activism on social media varies by race and ethnicity, age and political party.* Pew Research Center. Retrieved from https://pewrsr.ch/304HThw

Blumberg, L. J., Garrett, B., & Holahan, J. (2016). Estimating the counterfactual: How many uninsured adults would there be today without the ACA? *Inquiry, 53*, 1–13.

Bodenheimer, T., & Grumbach, K. (2012). *Understanding health policy: A clinical approach* (6th ed.). McGraw-Hill.

Brownson, R. C., Chriqui, J. F., & Stamatakis, K. A. (2009). Understanding evidence-based public health policy. *American Journal of Public Health, 99*(9), 1576–1583.

Bureau of Labor Statistics, US Department of Labor. (2020). *Occupational outlook handbook, nurse anesthetists, nurse midwives, and nurse practitioners.* Retrieved from https://www.bls.gov/ooh/healthcare/nurse-anesthetists-nurse-midwives-and-nurse-practitioners.htm

Bureau of Labor Statistics, US Department of Labor. (2020). *Occupational outlook handbook, registered nurses.* Retrieved from https://www.bls.gov/ooh/healthcare/registered-nurses.htm

Buresh, B., & Gordon, S. (2006). *From silence to voice: What nurses know and must communicate to the public* (2nd ed.). ILR Press.

Centers for Disease Control and Prevention. (2020a). Prevalence of Obesity and Severe Obesity Among Adults: United States, 2017–2018. NCHS Data Brief No. 360, February 2020. Retrieved from https://www.cdc.gov/nchs/products/databriefs/db360.htm

Centers for Disease Control and Prevention, (2020b). Health Insurance Coverage: Estimates from the National Health Interview Survey. May 9, 2019. Retrieved from https://www.cdc.gov/nchs/nhis/healthinsurancecoverage.htm

Centers for Medicare & Medicaid Services. (2006). Eliminating serious, preventable, and costly medical errors—never events. Fact sheet, May 18, 2006. Retrieved from Fact sheets/2006-Fact-sheets-items/2006-05-18.html

Chao, A., Grilo, C. M., White, M. A., & Sinha, R. (2015). Food cravings mediate the relationship between chronic stress and body mass index. *Journal of Health Psychology, 20*(6), 721–729.

Crick, B. (1962). *In defense of politics.* University of Chicago Press.

Delbanco, S., & de Brantes, F. (2015). *The payment reform landscape: Why Medicare's hip and knee replacement payment model may not be the answer for other payers and purchasers.* Health Affairs Blog. Retrieved from http://healthaffairs.org/blog/2015/08/06/the-payment-reform-landscape-why-medicares-hip-and-knee-replacement-payment-model-may-not-be-the-answer-for-other-payers-and-purchasers/

Department of Health and Human Services, National Institute of Health. (2021). Budget. Retrieved from https://www.nih.gov/about-nih/what-we-do/budget

Feldstein, P. (2006). *The politics of health legislation: An economic perspective* (3rd ed.). Health Administration Press.

Furlong, E. A. (2019). Agenda setting: What rises to a policymaker's attention? In J. A. Milstead, & N. M. Short (Eds.), *Health policy and politics: A nurse's guide* (6th ed.) (pp. 17–35). Jones & Bartl

Gill, C., & Gill, G. (2005). Nightingale in Scutari: Her le examined. *Clinical Infectious Diseases: An Officia the Infectious Diseases Society of America, 4*

Glasby, J. (2011, July 1). How evidence, Retrieved from http://www.c how-evidence-policy-and-pr

Gold, M. (2009). Pathways to th policy. *Health Services Research,*

Guzman, G. (2019). New data show income increased in 14 states and 10 of the largest metros. Retrieved from https://www.census.gov/library/stories/2019/09/us-median-household-income-up-in-2018-from-2017.html

Hamilton, A., Madison, J., Jay, J., Chase, S., Hamilton, E. S., & Church, A. S., Jefferson, T., Thomas Jefferson Library Collection, American Imprint Collection, & John Davis Batchelder Collection. (1788). *The federalist: A collection of essays, written in favour of the new Constitution, as agreed upon by the Federal Convention, in two volumes*. https://www.loc.gov/item/09021562/

Hamric, A. B. (2009). Ethical decision-making. In A. B. Hamric, J. A. Spross, & C. M. Hanson (Eds.), *Advanced practice nursing: An integrative approach* (4th ed.) (pp. 315–345). Elsevier Saunders.

Hawkins, D. (2002). *Power vs. force: The hidden determinants of human behavior*. Hay House.

Healthy People. (2020). DHHS, Office of Disease Prevention and Health Promotion, Healthy People 2030 Framework. Retrieved from https://www.healthypeople.gov/2020/About-Healthy-People/Development-Healthy-People-2030/Framework

Health Care and Education Reconciliation Act of 2010, Pub. L. No. 111–152, 124 Stat. 1029. (2010).

Heckert, D., Vijayakumar, P., & Luo, J. (2019). Cost-related insulin underuse among patients with diabetes. *JAMA Intern Med, 179*(1), 112–114. doi:10.1001/jamainternmed.2018.5008

Institute of Medicine. (2001). *Crossing the quality chasm: A new health system for the 21st century*. National Academies Press. Retrieved from http://www.nap.edu/books/0309072808/html

Jameton, A. (1984). *Nursing practice: The ethical issues*. Prentice Hall.

Jameton, A. (1993). Dilemmas of moral distress: Moral responsibility and nursing practice. *AWHONNS Clinical Issues in Perinatal & Women's Health Nursing, 4*(4), 542–551.

Johansson, H., & Scaramuzzino, G. (2019). The logics of digital advocacy: Between acts of political influence and presence. *New Media and Society, 21*(7). doi:10.1177/1461444818822488

Johnson, J., O'Grady, E., & Coetzee, M. (2022). *Intentional therapeutic relationships: Advancing caring in health care*. DesTech Publishing.

Kaiser Family Foundation. (2011, April 12). Snapshots: Health Care Spending in the United States & Selected OECD Countries. Retrieved from http://www.kff.org/health-costs/issue-brief/snapshots-health-care-spending-in-the-united-states-selected-oecd-countries/

Keehan, S. P., Cuckler, G. A., Poisal, J. A., Sisko, A. M., Smith, S. D., Madison, A. J., Rennie, K. E., Fiore, J. A., & Hardesty, J. C. (2020). National health expenditure projections, 2019-28: Expected rebound in prices drives rising spending growth. *Health Affairs (Milwood), 39*, 704–714.

Keller, T., & Ridenour, N. (2021). Ethics. In J. Giddens (Ed.), *Concepts for nursing practice* (pp. 390–398). Elsevier.

Kim, H., Hu, E., & Rebholz, C. (2019). Ultra-processed food intake and mortality in the USA: Results from the Third National Health and Nutrition Examination Survey (NHANES III, 1988–1994). *Public Health Nutrition*, 1–9. 2019 Feb 21.

Kingdon, J. (1995). *Agendas, alternatives, and public policies* (2nd ed.). Harper Collins College.

Kohn, L. T., Corrigan, J. M., & Donaldson, M. S. (Eds.), Committee on Quality of Health Care in America, Institute of Medicine. (2000). To err is human: Building a safer health system. National Academies Press. Retrieved from http://books.nap.edu/books/0309068371/html/index.html

Longest, B. B., Jr. (2016). *Health policymaking in the United States* (6th ed.). Health Administration Press.

Martin, B., & Alexander, M. (2019). The economic burden and practice restrictions associated with collaborative practice agreements: A national survey of advanced practice registered nurses. *Journal of Nursing Regulation*. 9(4), 22–30.

McGann, J. (2020). 2019 Global Go to Think Tank Index Report. https://repository.upenn.edu/think_tanks/17. Retrieved from https://repository.upenn.edu/cgi/viewcontent.cgi?article=1018&context=think_tanks

Medicare Shared Savings Program, 42 C.F.R. § 425.20. (2019). https://ecfr.io/Title-42/Section-425.20

Muhlestein, D., Burton, N., & Winfield, L. (2017). *The changing payment landscape of current CMS payment models foreshadows future plans*. February 3: Health Affairs Blog. Retrieved from https://www.healthaffairs.org/do/10.1377/forefront.20170203.058589/

National Academies of Sciences, Engineering, and Medicine. (2021). *The future of nursing 2020-2030: Charting a path to achieve health equity*. The National Academies Press. doi:10.17226/25982

National Association of Clinical Nurse Specialists. (2018). Key findings from the 2018 clinical nurse specialist census. Retrieved from https://nacns.org/wp-content/uploads/2019/10/NACNS-Census-Infographic-FINAL-10.23.19.pdf

National Council of State Boards of Nursing. (2009). *Changes in healthcare professions' scope of practice: Legislative considerations*. Author.

National Council of State Boards of Nursing. (2012). *NCSBN APRN model act and rules*. Retrieved from https://www.ncsbn.org/2012_APRN_Model_and_Rules.pdf

National Council of State Boards of Nursing. (2020). *State response to COVID-19 (APRNs) as of July 22, 2020*. July. Retrieved from. https://www.ncsbn.org/APRNState_COVID-19_Response_7_22.pdf

National Council of State Boards of Nursing. (2021). *Consensus model implementation status*. August. Retrieved from. https://www.ncsbn.org/5397.htm

National Quality Forum. (2011). *Serious reportable events in healthcare 2011*. Retrieved from http://www.qualityforum.org/Publications/2011/12/Serious_Reportable_Events_in_Healthcare_2011.aspx

National Research Council (US); Institute of Medicine (US) (2013). In S. H. Woolf & L. Aron (Eds.), *US health in international perspective: Shorter lives, poorer health*. National Academies Press (US). Summary. Retrieved from: https://www.ncbi.nlm.nih.gov/books/NBK154469/

Newhouse, R. P., Stanik-Hutt, J., White, K. M., Johantgen, M., Bass, E. B., Zangaro, G., Wilson, R. F., Fountain, L., Steinwachs, D. M., Heindel, L., & Weiner, J. P. (2011). Advanced practice nurse outcomes 1990-2008: A systematic review. *Nursing Economic$, 29*(5), 230–250.

Nursing Alliance for Quality Care. (2010). Strategic policy and advocacy roadmap. Retrieved from http://www.naqc.org/Docs/NewsletterDocs/2010-SPAR.pdf

Oxman, A., Lavis, J., Lewin, S., & Fretheim, A. (2009). December 16. *Health Research Policy and Systems, 7*(Suppl 1), 1–7. Retrieved from https://health-policy-systems.biomedcentral.com/articles/supplements/volume-7-supplement-1

Pakenham-Walsh, N. (2016, April 26). Evidence-informed country-level policymaking 1/3: Selected extracts from discussion. HIFA Working Group on Evidence-Informed Policy and Practice. Retrieved from http://www.hifa.org/sites/default/files/publications_pdf/Evidence%20informed%20country%20level%20policymaking%201.%20Selected%20extracts%20from%20discussion.pdf.

Papanicolas, I., Woskie, L., & Jha, K. (2018). Health care spending in the United States and other high-income countries. *The Journal of the American Medical Association, 319*(10), 1024–1039. doi:10.1001/jama.2018.1150

Patient-Centered Outcomes Research Institute. (2019). *2019 Annual report: Patient-centered outcomes research institute*. Retrieved from https://www.pcori.org/2019-annual-report

Patient Protection and Affordable Care Act, 42 U.S.C. § 18001. (2010).

Pew Health Professions Commission, Task Force on Health Care Workforce Regulation. (1995). *Reforming health care workforce regulation: Policy considerations for the 21st century*. Pew Health Professions Commission.

Phillips, S. J. (2022). 34th annual APRN legislative update. *The Nurse Practitioner, 47*(1), 21–47.

Porter, M. E. (2010). What is value in healthcare? *New England Journal of Medicine, 363*(26), 2477–2481.

Quinlan, E., & Robertson, S. (2013). The communicative power of nurse practitioners in multidisciplinary primary healthcare teams. *Journal of the American Association of Nurse Practitioners, 25*(2), 91–102.

Regulations.gov. (2016). Public comments make a difference. Retrieved from http://www.regulations.gov/docs/FactSheet_Public_Comments_Make_a_Difference.pdf

Saad, L. (2020). *US ethics ratings rise for medical workers and teachers*. Gallup. https://news.gallup.com/poll/328136/ethics-rating-rise-medical-workers-teacehers.aspx

Safriet, B. (2011). Federal options for maximizing the value of advanced practice nurses in providing quality, cost-effective health care. *In Institute of Medicine. The future of nursing: Leading change, advancing health* (pp. 443–476). National Academies Press.

Shevlin, P., & Doran, M. (Producers). (2016, April 24). Dialing for dollars (Season 48, Episode 32) [Television series episode]. *60 Minutes*. CBS News Productions. Retrieved from https://www.cbsnews.com/news/60-minutes-are-members-of-congress-becoming-telemarketers/

Sommers, B. D. (2020). Health insurance coverage: What comes after the ACA? *Health Affairs, 3*(39), 502–508.

Szep, J., Parker, N., So, L., Eisler, P., & Smith, G. (2020). Special report: US jails are outsourcing medical care—and the death toll is rising. Reuters. October 26. Retrieved from https://www.reuters.com/article/us-usa-jails-privatization-special-repor/special-report-u-s-jails-are-outsourcing-medical-care-and-the-death-toll-is-rising-idUSKBN27B1DH

Szmigiera, M. (2021). Life expectancy in industrial and developing countries in 2020. *Stastita*. March 30. Retrieved from https://www.statista.com/statistics/274507/life-expectancy-in-industrial-and-developing-countries/

US Department of Health and Human Services, Health Resources & Services Administration. (2014). *Highlights from the 2012 national sample survey of nurse practitioners*. https://bhw.hrsa.gov.data-research/access-data-tools/national-sample-survey-registered-nurse-practitioners

US Department of Health and Human Services, U.S. Department of the Treasury, U.S. Department of Labor, On Behalf of the President of the United States, Donald Trump. (2018). Reforming America's healthcare system through choice and competition. Retrieved from https://www.hhs.gov/sites/default/files/Reforming-Americas-Healthcare-System-Through-Choice-and-Competition.pdf

US Department of Agriculture. (2019). *Corn is America's largest crop in 2019*. Retrieved from https://www.usda.gov/media/blog/2019/07/29/corn-americas-largest-crop-2019

Wesorick, B. (2016). *Polarity thinking in health care: The missing logic to achieve transformation*. HRD Press.

Wakefield, M. K. (2008). Government response: Legislation. In J. Milstead (Ed.), *Health policy and politics: A nurse's guide* (3rd ed.) (pp. 65–88). Jones & Bartlett.

Whitehead, P. B., Herbertson, R. K., Hamric, A. B., Epstein, E. G., & Fisher, J. M. (2015). Moral distress among healthcare professionals: Report of an institution-wide survey. *Journal of Nursing Scholarship, 47*(2), 117–125.

Woolf, S., & Aron, L. (2018). Failing health of the United States. *BMJ, 360*, k496. doi:10.1136/bmj.k496

World Health Organization. (2017). Evidence-informed policy network (EVIPNet). Retrieved from http://www.euro.who.int/en/data-and-evidence/evidence-informed-policy-making/evidence-informed-policy-network-evipnet

18

MARKETING YOURSELF AS AN APRN: CONTRACTING AND NEGOTIATION

SUSANNE J. PHILLIPS

"Things don't have to change the world to be important."
~ Steve Jobs

CHAPTER CONTENTS

SELF-AWARENESS: FINDING A GOOD FIT 590
CHOOSING BETWEEN ENTREPRENEURSHIP/INTRAPRENEURSHIP 592
Characteristics for Entrepreneurship/Intrapreneurship 593
Entrepreneurial/Intrapreneurial Success 593
Challenges of Innovative Practice 593
MARKETING FOR THE NEW APRN 596
Preparing the New APRN to Market Core Competencies 596
Professional Networking 596
Communication 600
Interview Process 603
NEGOTIATION AND RENEGOTIATION 607
Business and Contractual Arrangements 611
Professional Issues and Practice Arrangements 612
Malpractice Insurance 612
OVERCOMING INVISIBILITY 614
CONCLUSION 614
KEY SUMMARY POINTS 615

The current changes in the healthcare environment for advanced practice registered nurses (APRNs)—brought about by the Institute of Medicine's (IOM's) *The Future of Nursing* report (IOM, 2015; IOM & Committee on the Robert Wood Johnson Foundation Initiative on the Future of Nursing, 2011), the Patient Protection and Affordable Care Act (PPACA, 2010), and the changes in regulation based on the *Consensus Model for APRN Regulation* (APRN Joint Dialogue Group, 2008)—all impact the ways in which APRNs market themselves and negotiate practice contracts. Marketing oneself is an important skill for APRNs to develop in order to become viable members of and achieve stature as principal players in the healthcare arena during these unsettled times.

In marketing themselves successfully, APRNs must integrate clinical expertise, leadership, collaboration, and other APRN competencies and business skills. In addition to understanding reimbursement payment mechanisms, and regulatory and credentialing requirements (discussed in Chapters 19 and 20), all APRNs—new graduates, seasoned professionals, and those striving to develop and maintain independent practices—must understand marketing and negotiation.

This chapter focuses on marketing the role of the APRN both as a new graduate and as an experienced clinician. It includes a discussion on entrepreneurship and intrapreneurship and the need for innovation, marketing, and negotiation skills for all APRNs.

SELF-AWARENESS: FINDING A GOOD FIT

Success in and satisfaction with one's APRN role revolve around the right match between APRNs and the work they do and the ability to be flexible and innovative within the scope of that role. Adaptability to the changing healthcare marketplace is one of the role's greatest strengths. APRNs participate in both clinical and administrative care processes in any practice setting. Examples of indirect processes are the steps taken to market the practice, register a patient, and collect demographics; third-party billing; meeting regulatory, safety, and quality imperatives; and the interaction with medical, pharmaceutical, and office supply vendors. Box 18.1 provides examples of clinical and administrative processes and skills in the APRN role. Both direct and indirect processes are essential to the successful management of any healthcare system, whether it be a small, self-contained APRN or physician practice or a large multiorganizational network.

Over an APRN's career, the balance between direct and indirect process involvement and the size of the system in which these processes occur may vary. At any given time, such shifts in balance and size of the system may require that APRNs adopt an entrepreneurial approach, an intrapreneurial approach, or a mixture of both (Dayhoff & Moore, 2005). An *entrepreneur* plans, organizes, finances, operates, and participates in a new healthcare delivery organization. Entrepreneurs have control over and responsibility for an increased proportion of indirect processes of care in their roles compared with intrapreneurs. Additionally, entrepreneurs assume risk for their project. According to Marques et al. (2019, p. 735), an *intrapreneur* is "one who creates innovation within the healthcare organization through the introduction of a new product, a different service, or simply a new way of doing something." In this case, many of the indirect processes of the care delivery system may be controlled and managed by other employees or departments. The nurse intrapreneur improves, redesigns, or augments an employer's current direct care processes, with a lesser role in day-to-day business administrative functions. Entrepreneurs function within the context of the larger, societal healthcare system. Intrapreneurs function within an institutional healthcare system—a microcosm of the larger arena. Both entrepreneurs and intrapreneurs are risk takers; however, entrepreneurs are likely to take bigger risks and have a higher tolerance for the accompanying uncertainty. Both entrepreneurs and intrapreneurs are individuals who continually search for and are receptive to opportunities and innovation. Innovation comes through the creation of a new process (whether direct, indirect, or both) or through radical changes to an existing process so that it seems "like new."

BOX 18.1

Examples of Clinical and Administrative Advanced Practice Registered Nurse Processes and Skills

CLINICAL PROCESSES AND SKILLS

- Disease management
- Health promotion/disease prevention
- Patient education
- Staff education
- Wound management
- Childbirth education
- Lactation consultation
- Chronic disease consultation
- Prenatal, delivery, and postpartum care
- Adhering to opioid prescribing rules
- Anesthesia
- Patient engagement—group visits
- Minor procedures
- Rapid response policy to emerging public health threats (e.g., COVID-19, Ebola, Zika)

ADMINISTRATIVE PROCESSES AND SKILLS

- Community outreach
- Risk management and assessment
- Reporting mechanisms
- Support staff supervision
- Presentation/teaching/precepting
- Grant writing
- Computer literacy
- Budget development and implementation
- Billing for services
- Research and publishing
- Compliance monitoring related to regulation such as Health Insurance Portability and Accountability Act
- Quality/safety monitoring and reporting

When embarking on program or practice oversight, the APRN needs to understand the balance between direct and indirect processes as well as how much time the APRN wants to devote to each of these. A large portion of time is dedicated to clinical visits and must be financially productive, so there must be a realistic balance between time spent in direct and indirect care. The decision about the proportion of one's role to devote to direct care versus indirect processes is based on the professional and personal values and goals of the APRN and the needs and demands of the practice.

A self-assessment may assist the APRN in clarifying professional and personal values. Types of questions to consider include the following, which are intended to be illustrative only and are not assumed exhaustive:

- ***Philosophic basis for practice.*** What type of nursing practice or approach to care delivery best describes how I perceive my own nursing practice? What do I value most, and how is that value expressed in my practice? Do the options before me favor this model or some other approach? If they favor another approach, how compatible is it with my own beliefs and values? (See Chapter 2.)
- ***Preference for intrapreneurial or entrepreneurial approach.*** Do I thrive on risk taking, like some risk, or prefer situations with a conservative level of risk involved? How is a "loss" or being "unsuccessful" defined? If I like taking risks, how much of a loss can I afford to take—both professionally and personally—if my venture proves to be unsuccessful? (The more risk one is willing to take, the more entrepreneurial one is likely to be.) Do I prefer being a part of a team or being on my own? If I like being on a team, what other team members would I like to be included on this team? How big of a team am I most comfortable with? If I prefer working on my own, how will I interact with my colleagues? (See Chapters 6, 9, and 10.)

CHOOSING BETWEEN ENTREPRENEURSHIP/INTRAPRENEURSHIP

Many nurses seek APRN education with the clear intention of pursuing entrepreneurial or intrapreneurial work. The very first decision an APRN must make is whether to be an employee-intrapreneur, a freelancer, or an entrepreneur. The changing healthcare landscape requires employed APRNs to approach their work with an intrapreneurial spirit. The APRN intrapreneur has the requisite APRN approach that questions the status quo and hunts for innovative solutions that promote health, wellness, and wholeness. Intrapreneurship refers to the APRN who assumes the role to develop new ideas in established organizations, facilitating translation of research, evidence, and evidence-based product evaluation into clinical practice with an acute eye on cost reduction, patient outcomes, and revenue generation (Hewison & Badger, 2006). Intrapreneurship provides the APRN with flexibility to be entrepreneurial within the stability of an employee relationship, while providing transformational leadership in the context of the organization (Hewison & Badger, 2006; Manion, 2001).

The APRN entrepreneur/freelancer is a free agent who often is paid by the hour or project. The APRN freelancer is able to choose the work and the population that is most meaningful to them, who can set their own hours, terms, and conditions. It is possible to have steady work with no overhead, little risk, and a great degree of practice autonomy. Freelancing is a way for APRNs to do the highest quality work with the populations best suited to their skill set. Being successful requires building a strong reputation and cultivating mastery as a clinician. It often requires a contract with the practice or facility and can create an uneven flow of work, and often there are no benefits such as health insurance, malpractice insurance, and paid time off. Nurse entrepreneurs are encouraged to seek professional liability insurance for their business.

The APRN entrepreneur has been described as "an individual who identifies a patient's need and envisions how nursing can respond to that need in an effective way, then formulates and executes a plan to meet that need" (Ieong, 2004, p. 1). In addition to assuming risks of a business, the self-employed entrepreneur is directly accountable to the client or patient (Wilson et al., 2003). Entrepreneurs build a business larger than themselves and earn money when they are not providing services or products themselves. It requires a sharp focus on growth and developing scalable systems.

Characteristics for Entrepreneurship/Intrapreneurship

New APRNs, with prior nursing experience and expertise, may develop interest in entre- or intrapreneurship opportunities following graduation. Doctor of nursing practice (DNP)–prepared APRNs are uniquely positioned to identify innovative opportunities and gaps in service within current healthcare systems when prepared with doctoral competencies. These competencies include business and healthcare delivery, organizational and systems leadership, quality improvement collaboration, healthcare policy, and a unique and acute awareness of patients' unmet needs (American Association of Colleges of Nursing, 2021; Wilson et al., 2012). Likewise, experienced APRNs, motivated by life events, boredom, lack of autonomy, burnout, role constraints, or a general feeling of being stuck in the medical model, may find themselves pursuing these opportunities following years of APRN service. Whether an APRN is a new graduate or a seasoned clinician, advanced practice nurses seek innovative practice settings out of love of nursing and a desire to make a difference. Additionally, strong self-efficacy and influence of mentors and family motivate nurses to pursue an innovative work environment (Shirey, 2007).

APRNs seeking innovative and transformative practice settings envision their individual potential for making a difference in patients' lives and have a desire to stay close to patient care delivery; however, being entrepreneurial or highly innovative within an organization requires tolerating a higher degree of risk taking. These APRNs desire to solve a problem through a unique business or practice venture, providing an alternate and perhaps more flexible professional lifestyle. The bedrock of any entrepreneurial endeavor is for the APRN to have strong clinical competence. This must precede and override all APRN business arrangements regardless of specialty or setting. Characteristics of clinically competent nurse entrepreneurs/intrapreneurs include strong leadership and assertiveness, along with self-confidence and willingness to take risks (Hewison & Badger, 2006; Wilson et al., 2012). Self-discipline, creativity, a need to achieve, and integrity drive their creative vision, providing the necessary motivation to network and market oneself (Hewison & Badger, 2006), and, above all, entrepreneurs are mission driven, placing values above profits (Shirey, 2007).

Entrepreneurial/Intrapreneurial Success

Success is defined individually by attainment of professional goals. Successful APRNs cite a number of reasons for their entrepreneurial achievement: the importance of acquired expertise and skill acquisition through education and consultation, identification of a professional mentor, and assistance from outside experts to provide necessary legal, financial, and business guidance as they embark on their innovative journey (Doerksen, 2010; Shirey, 2007). Exemplar 18.1 provides an example of APRN entrepreneurial success.

Intrapreneurship success is largely dependent on organizational environment and support (Dayhoff & Moore, 2003b). Removal of bureaucratic barriers, multidisciplinary support, access to resources, and organizational flexibility drive success of intrapreneurial initiatives (Dayhoff & Moore, 2003b). The American Association of Colleges of Nursing (AACN), in its original publication *The Essentials of Doctoral Education for Advanced Nursing Practice* (AACN, 2006), emphasized successful entrepreneurship/intrapreneurship through organizational and systems leadership competencies as well as healthcare policy and interprofessional competencies. Attainment of entrepreneurial/intrapreneurial competencies provides nursing expertise in organizational assessment and facilitation of organization-wide changes in practice delivery and prepares APRNs to foster partnerships in social sectors, engaging in policy development and scaling interventions (AACN, 2021). Utilizing political skills, systems thinking, and business analysis, DNP-prepared APRNs are prepared to excel in innovative practice settings. Examples of entrepreneurship and intrapreneurship opportunities across the APRN competencies are provided in Table 18.1.

Challenges of Innovative Practice

Innovative practice arrangements are not without challenges. Historically, factors contributing to difficulty with entrepreneurial and intrapreneurial practice include the APRN's perceived lack of business skills, especially in the areas of healthcare finance, legal and regulatory policies, and business operations (Johnson & Garvin, 2017; Shirey, 2007). Lack of formal educational preparation in traditional APRN master's programs has contributed to this lack of knowledge; however, with the recent move to DNP preparation across

EXEMPLAR 18.1
CLINICAL NURSE SPECIALIST CONSULTANT AND EDUCATION BUSINESS: MAKING THE LEAP

Kathleen Vollman, MSN, RN, CCNS, FCCM, FAAN

Two journeys helped prepare me to launch a successful consultation and education business. The first involved my experience through my master's thesis work of designing, developing, and researching a device that helped position critically ill patients into the prone position (Vollman, 1999; Vollman & Bander, 1996). The clinical and business skills I developed in order to take an idea and bring it to market were completely transferable to intrapreneurial activities while serving as a clinical nurse specialist (CNS) at a large urban medical center and then later when I launched the business full time (Vollman, 2004). While working as a CNS within the hospital, I was able to gather a wealth of knowledge and experience related to leadership, frontline and organizational change in large systems, lean technology, teamwork, and process management, as well as a passion for creating safe work cultures that empower nurses to own their practice. During that time, I also reached out beyond the walls of the organization to share the success of our clinical project work on reducing infections and pressure injuries and improving nurse retention. I wrote abstracts to present at local, regional, and national conferences alone and in partnership with staff nurses. I published articles within my areas of expertise. Through this work, I began to develop an international reputation for speaking and consulting on various pulmonary/critical care, reducing healthcare-acquired injury, and professional nursing topics. This help set the foundation for the development of an independent consultation and education business (Vollman, 2014). Prior to making the official leap to a completely independent business, I straddled the two worlds for 5 years. In 2003 I left my position at the hospital and launched Advancing Nursing, LLC, a company that creates empowered work environments for nurses through the acquisition of greater skills and knowledge to advance the profession of nursing.

In reality, my business parallels the CNS role within a hospital system. If the expectations are unrealistic, the ability of the person to achieve the expected outcomes is limited. Through my CNS journey, I had developed four areas of expertise that serve to guide the scope of the education and consultation product/service:

- Clinical critical care in care of patients with pulmonary disorders and sepsis
- "Back-to-basics" using evidence-based nursing care to prevent patient harm
- Care of the nurse and work environment
- CNS role development and entrepreneurship

In each of these a common thread exists. The goal and the vision for the business are to provide frontline nurses with the necessary knowledge, skills, and resources to enable them to advocate for their patients, the patients' families, and themselves and be fulfilled in their professional work. The next step was to set up the structure (Dayhoff & Moore, 2003a). The structure that best suited Advancing Nursing was a limited liability corporation, a hybrid legal structure that provides the limited liability features of a corporation and the tax efficiencies and operational flexibility of a partnership (Small Business Association, 2016). Once I received the submission document from the state that the business name was official, I set up a separate business checking account at the bank. Minimal capital was required for business start-up, and overhead was very low.

Development of a graphic representation of the business and communication strategies and creating a website were the next steps. Having developed the mission statement made designing the graphic image easier. The image is an inert triangle going from dark to lighter, representing growth as the nurse gains knowledge and skill to increase their personal power to take care of patients and advance the profession of nursing. For a business website, the web address is frequently the business name, but with an already established professional name, it was easy to choose the domain: www.vollman.com.

One of the lessons learned in starting a business is the importance of networking and being comfortable in admitting your limitations. Through networking, I found someone like me but in the tech world who was just starting out and who helped me build the business website. Marketing was done by word of mouth, scientific publications, networking, and ensuring that someone could always connect with me to ask questions, to request a talk or visit, or to comment. As CNSs, we are taught to measure outcomes, and that is true in business as well. I measured both process components and outcomes in a variety of ways, including business growth (new clients), number of referrals, revenue versus expenses, invitations to speak, hits to the website, number of downloads, email follow-through, conference evaluations and posters, and individual clinician and organizational feedback.

One of the largest hurdles I had was determining fee structures for various activities. Determining your worth and asking to be compensated for it is difficult for most nurses, myself included. My colleagues across the country were instrumental in this area because the information is not published anywhere. Through discussion with clinicians who were doing similar work nationally and internationally, I was able to come up with a fee I was comfortable with and that was accepted well by customers. As the business grows, remember to increase your rates based on demand, success of your product/service, and what the market can bear.

EXEMPLAR 18.1

CLINICAL NURSE SPECIALIST CONSULTANT AND EDUCATION BUSINESS: MAKING THE LEAP—cont'd

There were some decisions I made early on. I chose not to be the continuing education provider. I prepare all of the materials necessary but allow the inviting organization to take over all continuing education tasks. I made a conscious decision to work with selected industry partners. Companies that I formed relationships with had products and services that supported the nurse's ability to perform evidence-based care in an effective and efficient manner.

To help maintain life balance, 5 years into the business, I added a 2-day-a-week assistant to help manage invoices, accounting, article retrieval, and some additional activities.

I feel I am one of the most fortunate people in the world, because I am living my dream and sharing my passion of evidence-based practice with other nurses and healthcare practitioners to make an impact in patients' lives. Take the risk of becoming an entrepreneur; you will never regret the journey.

TABLE 18.1

Examples of Entrepreneurship/Intrapreneurship Activities Across the Advanced Practice Registered Nurse (APRN) Competencies

Entrepreneurship Activities	
Direct clinical practice	Nurse-owned primary care clinics, specialty ambulatory practice, birth centers
	Nurse-owned health screening company
	Nurse-owned telehealth company
	Interdisciplinary healthcare business ventures
	APRN-owned healthcare practices
	Interdisciplinary provider–owned healthcare practices
Guidance and coaching	Nurse-owned health promotion/disease prevention company
	Nurse-owned chronic disease management company
	Nurse-owned health coaching company
	Nurse-owned continuing education services
Leadership	Nurse-owned businesses
	Development of new models of reimbursement for nursing care delivery
	APRN executive organizational leadership
	Creating solutions by fostering partnerships in health and social sectors
	Engaging in health policy development

Intrapreneurship Activities	
Direct clinical practice	Development of nurse-triage and telemedicine services
	Development and implementation of group visits
	Nurse-managed chronic disease management clinics
	Transition care
	Development of interdisciplinary care teams
	Facilitation of research results into practice
	CRNA-managed anesthesia provider services
	CNM-managed antepartum services
	Leading interdisciplinary teams to create new models of care
Guidance and coaching	Development and implementation of health coaching programs, quality improvement programs
	Nurse-triage programs
Leadership	Use of informatics to develop and implement new models of care delivery
	Nurse-managed transitional care programs
	Development of nursing care policies
	Nurse-managed palliative care teams
	Development of organizational tele-ICU centers
	Scaling successful interventions
	Engagement in organizational policy development

CNM, Certified nurse-midwife; *CRNA*, certified registered nurse anesthetist; *ICU*, intensive care unit.

APRN roles, business and systems competencies have been addressed in the curriculum.

External forces creating larger systems challenges include organizational strategies that suppress intrapreneurial thinking and lack of APRN identification as a key stakeholder in the development of organizational, local, state, and national health policy. This has created a system of unequal partnership and contribution (Wilson et al., 2012). This particular challenge has led to lack of or limited APRN recognition and reimbursement as an independent profession, a challenge that is particularly difficult when seeking funding for innovative healthcare delivery ideas.

Despite numerous challenges, new and experienced APRNs have risen to the challenge, providing necessary organizational and political leadership. As APRNs enter the world of innovative practice, they will find these opportunities more rewarding with careful attention to collegial working relationships, mentorship, and connectivity from seasoned APRN entrepreneurs and intrapreneurs and active participation in healthcare policy reform.

MARKETING FOR THE NEW APRN

Preparing the New APRN to Market Core Competencies

Graduates of accredited APRN programs are well prepared to market their detailed and often colorful recounting of clinical practicum and procedural portfolios attained during school as well as newly acquired national certification and state licensure. New graduates may find the less-recognized role competencies, such as guidance and coaching, leadership, collaboration, and ethical practice, more difficult to market because many people outside of advanced practice nursing are not familiar with these broad APRN competencies (Spoelstra & Robbins, 2010). As described in Chapter 4, acquisition in each of the core competencies is crucial, with attention to documenting these experiences via a professional portfolio. A guided student self-reflection exercise designed to connect didactic and clinical practicum experiences to APRN role development provides documentation of competency acquisition (Latham & Fahey, 2006). Table 18.2 provides examples of educational activities new APRN graduates may highlight during the interview process with prospective employers or business investors. Marketing the unique skill set of the APRN will enable the applicant to stand out in an interview from other clinicians from different healthcare disciplines. Demonstrating the unique value of APRN care to a practice or organization is essential to a successful job search.

Professional Networking

Professional networking through membership in local, state, and national APRN organizations is of great benefit to APRNs seeking employment or to build a business. Many APRN education programs strongly recommend attendance at a local APRN role-specific meeting for social introduction into the profession, which begins well before graduation. A successful job search incorporates several active strategies and a strong personal organizational approach. Early reflection and identification of clinical strengths, work values and interests, and professional goals, as well as personal areas for growth, are crucial when considering various employment opportunities. As a preliminary step in a job search, it is crucial for each APRN to understand the market for an APRN role within the desired geographic employment area; researching potential employers' opportunities and hiring practices from their websites provides this vital initial information (Vilorio, 2011). In addition to online research of potential employers, a vital search strategy includes personal networking, from which professional relationships are built and which takes time. Networking with faculty, fellow students, and alumni at local, state, and national APRN events, in addition to networking with preceptors and clinicians during clinical rotations, residencies, fellowships, and volunteer opportunities, may lead the novice APRN to their first job as a new graduate or build a client base for the new entrepreneur. Vilorio (2011) reported, "Organizations tend to hire people they know or who are referred to them by someone they trust" (p. 5) and often fill new positions before positions are publicized.

Career centers within APRN academic institutions offer additional assistance with the preparation of cover letters, résumés, and curricula vitae (CVs), as well as interview coaching. Local and regional employment opportunities for APRNs are provided by local and state APRN organizations through webpages, electronic newsletters, and group email. Many of the

TABLE 18.2

Advanced Practice Registered Nurse (APRN) Competencies, Associated Essentials, and Educational Activities to Highlight During an Interview

APRN Core Competency (Chapter 3)	The Essentials: Core Competencies for Nursing Education	Educational Activities to Highlight During the Interview Process
Direct clinical practice (Chapter 6)	Domain 1: Knowledge for Nursing Practice Domain 2: Person-Centered Care Domain 3: Population Health Domain 4: Scholarship for the Nursing Discipline Domain 6: Interprofessional Partnerships Domain 8: Informatics and Healthcare Technologies Concepts for Nursing Practice: Clinical Judgment Communication Compassionate Care Diversity, Equity, & Inclusion Ethics Evidence-Based Practice Health Policy Social Determinants of Health	Population of patients seen during clinical rotations Number of patient encounters by level of complexity Diagnoses managed demonstrating application of evidence-based care Pharmacotherapeutics prescribed Referrals provided Procedures performed Variability of patient care settings appropriate to APRN role preparation including community health centers and settings where vulnerable populations are served Health promotion and disease prevention activities performed specific to APRN role APRN role-specific competencies related to direct clinical practice Entrepreneurship opportunities Approach to diversity, equity, and inclusion in your clinical practice Policy projects you participated in
Guidance and coaching (Chapter 7)	Domain 1: Knowledge for Nursing Practice Domain 2: Person-Centered Care Concepts for Nursing Practice: Communication Compassionate Care Diversity, Equity, and Inclusion Ethics Evidence-based Practice Social Determinants of Health	Anticipatory guidance activities Entrepreneurship/intrapreneurship opportunities Population-specific APRN-led patient education and monitoring programs (obesity management, pain management, diabetes management, family planning, etc.) Development and implementation of tailored patient education materials and programs Team-based care activities Group visit participation Motivational interviewing training and experience Transition care coordination and intervention activities Self-reflection through journal writing
Evidence-based practice (Chapter 8)	Domain 2: Person-Centered Care Domain 4: Scholarship for the Nursing Discipline Domain 5: Quality and Safety Domain 6: Interprofessional Partnerships Domain 7: Systems-Based Practice Domain 8: Information and Healthcare Technologies Domain 9: Professionalism Concepts for Nursing Practice: Evidence-Based Practice	Doctor of nursing practice or Capstone projects Clinical research activities, completed abstracts or proposals, completed literature reviews, projects/posters Evidence-based practice (EBP) presentations given pertinent to APRN role Examples of incorporating EBP in the clinical setting during educational program Practice guideline projects and presentations Projects demonstrating evaluation of clinical guidelines Clinical questions formulated to investigate when in practice

Continued

TABLE 18.2

Advanced Practice Registered Nurse (APRN) Competencies, Associated Essentials, and Educational Activities to Highlight During an Interview—cont'd

APRN Core Competency (Chapter 3)	The Essentials: Core Competencies for Nursing Education	Educational Activities to Highlight During the Interview Process
Leadership (Chapter 9)	Domain 1: Knowledge for Nursing Practice Domain 3: Population Health Domain 5: Quality and Safety Domain 6: Interprofessional Partnerships Domain 9: Professionalism Domain 10: Personal, Professional, and Leadership Development Concepts for Nursing Practice: Communication Evidence-Based Practice Health Policy Social Determinants of Health	Entrepreneurship/intrapreneurship clinical practice experiences Group visit facilitation experience Project planning and management experiences Mentorship of other health professions students Formal and informal networking opportunities Active student membership on curricular or evaluation committees Membership on campus-wide student committees Policy development and implementation Podium and poster presentations Local, state, or national policy fellowships Student leadership roles in professional organizations Development of electronic educational materials/applications Patient advocacy activities Quality improvement and safety activities Scholarly project
Collaboration (Chapter 10)	Domain 2: Person-Centered Care Domain 3: Population Health Domain 5: Quality and Safety Domain 6: Interprofessional Partnerships Domain 7: Systems-Based Practice Concepts for Nursing Practice: Communication Collaboration Evidence-Based Practice Health Policy	Development of legal/regulatory collaboration agreement documents if appropriate for state regulation Interprofessional case-based learning activities Interprofessional patient care clinical experiences Conflict negotiation and resolution workshops and activities Team-leading, team-building, and teamwork experiences Group visit experiences Quality improvement activities Scholarly project if applicable
Ethical practice (Chapter 11)	Domain 2: Person-Centered Care Domain 3: Population Health Domain 5: Quality and Safety Domain 6: Interprofessional Partnerships Domain 9: Professionalism Concepts of Nursing Practice: Ethics Compassionate Care Diversity, Equity, and Inclusion	Demonstration of creating an ethical environment during the practicum experience Case-based ethics simulation activities reflective of the APRN role Reflective evaluation of clinical cases encountered in practicum Obtaining informed consent experiences Reporting of patient concerns to administration Student participation on institutional or academic ethics committees Integration of APRN role-specific code of ethics into APRN role Interprofessional educational experiences focusing on ethical decision making Participation in quality improvement activities during clinical practicum experiences Development of institutional review board protocols for research activities Local, state, and national patient advocacy activities pertaining to safety and patient rights

Source: *The Essentials: Core Competencies for Professional Nursing Education*, by American Association of Colleges of Nursing, 2021, https://www.aacnnursing.org/Portals/42/AcademicNursing/pdf/Essentials-2021.pdf

TABLE 18.3
National Advanced Practice Registered Nurse (APRN) Organizations: Student Information

National Association/Organization	Main Webpage Address	Student Webpage Address
American Association of Nurse Anesthesiology	https://www.aana.com/	https://www.aana.com/about-us/aana-foundation/aana-foundation-student-page
American Association of Nurse Practitioners	https://www.aanp.org/	https://www.aanp.org/student-resources
American College of Nurse-Midwives	http://www.midwife.org/	https://www.midwife.org/Students-and-New-Grads
Gerontological Advanced Practice Nurses Association	https://www.gapna.org/	https://www.gapna.org/just-students
National Association of Clinical Nurse Specialists	http://nacns.org/	All resources may be found on the main webpage
National Association of Pediatric Nurse Practitioners	https://www.napnap.org/	https://www.napnap.org/students
Nurse Practitioners in Women's Health	https://www.npwh.org/	All resources may be found on their main webpage

national APRN organizations offer substantial career assistance to new, recently graduated, and seasoned APRNs. In addition to networking opportunities, these organizations offer national certification preparation resources, mentorship opportunities, scholarship information, online learning, salary surveys, and career resources, including job centers. Some of this information is publicly available, and access to some of this information requires student membership in the organization. Table 18.3 lists national APRN organizational websites pertaining to student and new graduate career resources.

Web-Based Resources

Web-based professional networking sites are available and routinely utilized by APRN recruiters, employers, and potential investors. Approximately 85% of employers report that online profiles influence hiring decisions (University of California, Irvine Career Center, 2016a), and thus APRN students are well advised to review their personal social media to ensure that content such as profiles, images, and communication reflect professional values. All profile pictures should be presentable, and photographs that may not reflect these values should be "untagged" (University of California, Irvine Career Center, 2016a). Preparation of an electronic professional profile, such as a LinkedIn profile, is a great resource for APRN students as well as experienced APRNs. Although business networking sites have numerous similar functions, the advanced job search feature on LinkedIn allows the professional to search by function, geographic area, organizational level, and industry, leveraging employment and entrepreneurial opportunities with online and mobile application capability (Fertig, 2012). With faculty guidance and peer review, students and new entrepreneurs can promote the ideal job they are seeking or business they are marketing while providing a professional profile highlighting unique skills, expertise, experience, and education. A LinkedIn profile allows recruiters, potential employers, and investors looking for specific skills to find a suitable candidate (Fertig, 2012). This activity allows an APRN to build a professional network and provides marketing opportunities in one place that have lasting value. Table 18.4 provides a list of social networking sites for professionals, entrepreneurs, and business owners.

Professional Recruiters

Utilizing a professional recruiter who is well versed in APRN practice is another avenue to ensure a successful job search. APRNs may enlist the services of a recruiter for assistance in finding a position or may be contacted by a recruiter who is searching for qualified candidates. In either case, the recruiter fees are typically paid by the employing agency. Networking through LinkedIn or other professional networking websites will provide an opportunity for recruiters looking for specific APRN qualifications to pull together a pool of prospective employees. An internal recruiter, an external recruiting agency or temporary staffing agency, or an executive "headhunter" may directly contact an

TABLE 18.4

Web-Based Networking Resources for Advanced Practice Registered Nurses

Web-Based Resources	Link
LinkedIn A networking tool to find connections to recommended job candidates, industry experts, and business partners	https://www.linkedin.com/
MedMasters A comprehensive professional networking and career management site for the medical community	http://medmasters.com/
Monster Source for career opportunities nationwide	http://www.monster.com/
For Entrepreneurs	
MakerNURSE "Providing tools, platforms and trainings to make the next generation of health technology"	https://makernurse.com
Johnson & Johnson Innovation Nurses Innovate QuickFire Challenge: Grant Funding	https://jlabs.jnjinnovation.com/quickfire-challenges
National Nurses in Business Association "The Voice of Nurse Entrepreneurship" Business planning & development	https://nursesbusiness.com https://nnbanow.com/category/www-nnba-net/
NP Business Owner NP business blog and podcast	http://NPbusiness.com
National Nurse Practitioner Entrepreneur Network Consulting, credentialing, and revenue cycle management services	https://www.nnpen.org/

APRN. Regardless of the type of recruiter, the employer pays these recruiters typically when and if the recruiter refers the candidate who is hired. Although professional recruiters have an interest in the interviewee's success, they may have a greater interest in the practice for which they are recruiting. After all, the recruiter or recruiting agency is paid based on a percentage of the annual salary of the recruited individual and the number of candidates placed within a practice.

Some of the advantages of enlisting a recruiter for a job search include the fact that these professionals are generally well connected and may have job opportunities that are not published. They typically understand the organizational culture, patient volumes, population, and expectations of the practice or organization and can provide valuable information in preparation to the interviewee. Regardless of whether the APRN seeks the services of a recruiter or a recruiter approaches an APRN for a position, recruiters and recruiting agencies decide which candidates to put forward for interviews, which may result in missed opportunities for those who do not use recruiters. The recruiter may be expected to spend time vetting interviewee qualifications through behavior-based interview questions and clinical-based queries, as well as verification of current certificates, licenses, and privileges, before presenting candidates to a potential employer.

Communication

Expert written and verbal communication skills are vitally important whether conducting a job search or pitching a business proposition or organizational innovation. Business and recruitment experts recommend utilizing a cover letter regardless of the route of communication, including electronic mail; failure to do so may be viewed as unprofessional (Gallo, 2014). The tone of all communication must remain professional at all times (Arndt & Coleman, 2014). Before corresponding with a potential employer, a thorough analysis of the mission and purpose of the organization, including its leadership, must be undertaken (Gallo, 2014). Methods of communicating one's expertise, introduced in a cover letter, may include a professional portfolio comprising multiple documents, such as a résumé or CV.

Cover Letters

Cover letters typically contain detailed information describing why the applicant is qualified for the position, providing an explanation of interest in the specific organization and identification of relevant skills or experiences the applicant possesses. Business experts agree it is important to briefly emphasize personal value to the organization and limit the letter to one page (Gallo, 2014). This is not the format to restate items described in the résumé or CV but rather to highlight relevant experiences. Cover letters are typically sent via electronic mail or uploaded as a document within an electronic application. The literature describes cover letters as referral letters or query letters. *Referral letters* include the individual who referred the applicant to the practice or organization. Referral bonuses may be overlooked if the potential employer is not aware that a referral has been made. *Inquiry (query) letters* typically accompany a résumé and can be sent to organizations or practices that may be hiring but have not advertised a formal job opening. Inquiry letters contain information on why the company is of interest and why the APRN's skills and experience would be assets to the organization. Inquiry letters allow APRNs to expand on their CV by focusing on a few qualifications, using specific examples, and forming a connection between past experience and the position. APRN applicants have to convey why they are motivated to apply for this position and how they will fit in with, and what value they will uniquely bring to, the organization. Box 18.2 provides an example of a cover letter; however, a simple electronic search will yield many excellent examples.

BOX 18.2

Template Cover Letter

May 19, 2021

Name and Address of Company

I am a (university) educated certified registered nurse anesthetist (or recent graduate of a CRNA program at [university]). I am writing in response to the CRNA position recently posted through the California Association of Nurse Anesthetists website. The skills and experience I gained through my clinical education as a CRNA, as well as my experience as a CRNA in a level 1 trauma center in Southern California and as a critical care registered nurse, will enable me to provide both comprehensive and quality anesthesia care to patients at your outpatient surgical center.

I am also an ACLS instructor and have taught this content to a range of intraprofessional specialists. My experience as first an ICU nurse and then a CRNA provided the opportunity to work on or lead interdisciplinary teams. I have become a very effective team member of all healthcare teams that I work on. I believe that interprofessional practice offers the highest quality health care.

Thank you for your time and consideration in review of my qualifications. I look forward to hearing from you.

Signature

Contact information

Adapted from University of California, San Francisco Office of Career & Professional Development. (2021). Advanced practice nurse resumes and cover letters. https://career.ucsf.edu/professional/nursing/cvs-resumes-cover-letters#Advance-Practice-Nurse-Resumes

Professional Portfolio

A professional portfolio is an electronic presentation of an APRN's qualifications and accomplishments. An electronic professional portfolio is often compiled during the APRN program and maintained after graduation, building content as professional opportunities and skills are attained. The portfolio serves to educate prospective employers on the APRN role, scope of practice, and impact on patient outcomes and cost savings, while providing evidence of the individual's professional knowledge, skills, expertise, experience, accomplishments, and scholarly work (Beauvais, 2016). When professionally presented, the portfolio highlights the APRN's potential contribution to the organization, providing a strong base for negotiation (Hespenheide et al., 2011). A portfolio differs from a CV in that a portfolio houses multiple documents, including a résumé or CV, necessary to communicate the APRN's qualifications. Box 18.3 provides a basic list of the documents to be included in a portfolio. An electronic link to the portfolio can be sent to a potential employer prior to the interview.

Résumés and Curricula Vitae

Curriculum vitae (which means "course of life" in Latin) or a résumé, which is often submitted with a cover letter, is usually the first introduction and provides the first impression to a prospective employer.

Described as a marketing document in which the hiring agency is the buyer and the APRN is the product, a *résumé* is a one- to two-page concise introduction of education, experiences, and career-related skills, tailored to a specific job opportunity (Lees, 2013). A résumé typically begins with a short summary of the candidate, including why the candidate is the right person for the job. Experts recommend emphasizing accomplishments over responsibilities as a technique in creating a résumé that stands out. Although various types of résumés exist, a document that concisely combines both the chronology of the APRN's work history and the applicant's unique skills and strengths targeted to the employer is recommended (CAREERwise Education, 2016). Box 18.4 provides a detailed description of the components of a résumé.

A *curriculum vitae* is a document in longer format typically used by those searching for academic, research, or executive leadership positions that require a more comprehensive review of qualifications. Without a page limitation, the CV provides a detailed review of a person's professional accomplishments over a lifetime, listed in reverse chronologic order and added to

BOX 18.3

Components of a Professional Portfolio

- Curriculum vitae and/or résumé
- Biographic sketch or professional introduction
- Professional development and educational activities
- Clinical practice/practicum experience
- Competencies and evaluations
- Pertinent statutes and regulations
- Role-specific professional scope of practice and standards of care
- Collaborative practice agreements (if required)
- Reimbursement guidelines
- Color copies of professional license(s), certifications, diplomas, certificates, awards, Drug Enforcement Agency (DEA) registration, national provider identifier (NPI) registration
- Scholarly work: publications, papers, abstracts, presentations, posters, etc.
- References

BOX 18.4

Components of a Résumé (One Page, Double-Sided Maximum)

- **Contact Information:** Name, degree, license, certifications, email address, phone number with area code (top of page)
- **Summary of Qualifications:** Specific, meaningful description of the type of position desired (optional)
- **Education:** Postsecondary only; name of school, major, degree received, graduation date (or projected), honors. Be sure to put graduation date and month because credentialing committees need it to verify degrees.
- **Experience:** Describe using action verbs. Job title for all paid, volunteer, or internship positions; emphasize duties/responsibilities, skills, abilities, significant/relevant achievements; quantify accomplishments; include job title, employing organization, dates of employment (month, year). Avoid listing nonmedical work experience; avoid complete sentences, abbreviations, or acronyms, and do not begin phrases with "I"; avoid medical abbreviations; do not list unrelated, detailed duties or controversial activities or associations.
- **Licensure and National Certification:** With expiration dates for states in which a license was held (current, inactive, or expired); avoid listing numbers
- **Professional Memberships or Affiliations:** Optional
- **Other Skills:** Bilingual/multilingual (list all languages); proficiency in electronic medical record (EMR) platforms if pertinent; advanced skills: suturing, casting, first assist, etc.
- **References:** "Available upon request"

throughout their career. With components similar to a résumé, the CV adds experiences such as research, teaching, mentoring, professional activities, professional memberships, publications, presentations, honors, and awards. Preparing a comprehensive CV from which a concise résumé can be adapted for individual employment opportunities is advisable. Potential employers or interested clients will indicate whether they require a CV or résumé to be provided with the initial application. Box 18.5 describes the main components of a CV.

Interview Process

There are many types of job interviews and, depending on the practice, group, or organization APRNs choose to work for, they may experience one or more types of interviews during their job search. The interview is an opportunity both for the employer or business to get to know the prospective employee and for the candidate to ask important questions about information unavailable through general job postings and exploration. It is vital that a new APRN be empowered to interview the prospective employer and demonstrates active participation in the process (Kador, 2010). Failure to ask questions during the interview may give the impression that a candidate lacks interest, may not ask questions once hired, or, worse, may accept a position that is a bad fit for the APRN (Warner, 2011). Box 18.6 and Box 18.7 provide examples of questions to be prepared for as well as questions to ask potential employers.

BOX 18.5

Components of a Curriculum Vitae (No Page Limitation)

The information below is provided as a guide. Subsections may be necessary to include all relevant information.

- **Personal Data:** Contact information: name, degree(s) (highest degree in each discipline), license(s), certifications, email address, phone number with area code. Include license numbers/expiration, certification numbers/expiration, and board certification titles and numbers/expiration
- **Education:** Name of schools, major/minor, degree received, graduation date (or projected), honors; may also include title of dissertation or DNP scholarly project title(s), including university and dates attended
- **Professional Experience:** Date, position, institution/city/state. This refers to your professional nursing experience. Prior non-nursing experience is noted only if relevant to the position (i.e., leadership)
- **Academic Experience:** Institutions, dates, academic appointment/positions, leadership and/or program coordination and department chair experience, course numbers and course descriptions of classes taught—specify graduate or undergraduate, guest lectures, mentorship including scholarly project/research project name and dates, school and institutional service responsibilities; additional pedagogical education/training including title/institution/city/state.
- **Grants & Awards:** Refers to management of internal or external funding awards for academic responsibilities of research, training, etc. Include funding amount, source, identification, etc.
- **Scholarly Activities: Research, Scholarship, Publications, Speaking:** Depending on your experience and academic preparation this area may include original research, poster presentations, podium presentations, key-note speaker presentations, peer-reviewed articles and abstracts, journal articles, books, book chapters, editorial board positions, reviewer/contributor activities, continuing education faculty activities, etc. *Notes – organizations may have specific items they would like to see and may have category and page limits; follow all CV instructions if provided. Use APA or other academic formatting method for all scholarly entries; consistency is the key.
- **Professional Activities:** Organization name, role, dates
- **Community Volunteer Work:** Applicable to leadership positions; organization, title, role, dates
- **Awards and Honors:** Date, award, organization

BOX 18.6

Types of Interview Questions and Strategies

- **Open-Ended Questions:** Assess motivation, training, skills, and experiences
  - *Example:* "Why should we hire you?"
  - *Strategy:* Summarize relevant training, experience, and skills in 2 minutes.
- **Behavior-Based Questions:** Based on premise that past behavior is a predictor of future performance; ask for an example of a particular situation you handled or skill you used.
  - *Example:* "Tell me about a time when you disagreed with a professional colleague on a course of treatment and how it got resolved."
  - *Example:* "Tell me about a time when you did or said something that had a negative impact on a customer, peer, or direct report. How did you know the impact was negative?"
  - *Strategy:* Give a SHARE Model response (see Box 18.9).
- **General Questions:** Frequently asked in an interview
  - *Example:* "How do you handle conflict?"
  - *Example:* "Tell me about a situation when you discovered that you were on the wrong course. How did you know? What did you do? What, if anything, did you learn from the experience?"
  - *Strategy:* Give an example demonstrating your approach to handling a situation.
- **Hypothetical Questions:** A vignette common in the practice/organization presented to assess how well you solve problems
  - *Strategy:* Give a SHARE Model response.
- **Clinical Questions:** General or open-ended questions about a particular clinical experience or a vignette aimed at assessing your problem-solving skills
  - *Strategy:* Discuss your thought process, the questions you would ask, investigation/exploration of the situation you would conduct, and how you might present the case to a more experienced clinician.

Adapted from Bielaszka-DuVernay, C. (2008). Hiring for emotional intelligence. *Harvard Management Update*, 13(11), 3–5.; and University of California, San Francisco Office of Career & Professional Development. (2013). Advanced practice nurse job search. https://career.ucsf.edu/sites/g/files/tkssra2771/f/2-APN%20Job%20Search%202016.pdf

Questions related to contracts, salary negotiation, malpractice insurance, on-call responsibility, reimbursement, and billing are discussed later in this chapter.

One-on-one interviews are the most common, in which the candidate is interviewed by one person who represents the employer and who will ask questions of the candidate and, more important, provide an opportunity for the APRN to ask questions about the culture and the company. *Videoconference interviews* may occur initially or may be the only live interview opportunity and are typically initially held with a recruiter or manager of a practice. Some of the advantages to this type of interview include the ability to refer to notes and talking points, and live videoconferencing offers the ability to visualize and interpret body language and facial expressions. Although similar to an in-person interview, unique points to consider include technologic availability and location, including clarifying the time zone for the scheduled interview time. Candidates are notified if this type of interview will be conducted and typically provided instructions on the software installation in advance. Web-based platforms such as Microsoft Teams, Zoom, and Cisco Webex, for example, are easy to install and operate. Candidates should ensure that the software and web camera are installed and tested before the appointment. Candidates should also consider the reliability of their Internet connection and ensure a clean, quiet interview location free of distraction and interruption. Box 18.8 provides important reminders for interviewees.

Committee or panel interviews are common in APRN practice and allow an opportunity for the employer to observe how candidates respond in a team scenario. This type of interview may also be conducted via videoconference technology. A group of providers, administrators, and staff will typically take turns asking questions. Eye contact by the APRN with all panel members is important during this process. In

BOX 18.7

Questions to Ask in an Interview

GENERAL QUESTIONS

- Is this an employee or an independent contractor position?
- Has the organization hired an APRN in this position in the past?
- What would a typical day/week be like for the candidate? Is overtime expected?
- How will the selected candidate's performance be evaluated? Is there a formal process? What constitutes success in this position?
- What is the orientation process at your organization? Are there scaled productivity requirements or transition-to-practice expectations?
- How would you describe the level of autonomy you expect from APRNs in this practice/at this institution?
- What are some changes and challenges you have seen here in the past year, and what are some changes and challenges you forecast in the next year?
- How would you describe the culture and management style of the organization?
- Are there prospects for growth and advancement?
- Is continuing education compensated or reimbursed?
- What are the next steps in the process?

PRACTICE- OR POSITION-SPECIFIC QUESTIONS

- How is productivity measured in this practice setting?
- What electronic medical record program is utilized at this facility? Is there on-site technical assistance following orientation to the program?
- Will the candidate for this position see overflow patients or be expected to develop his/her own panel of patients?
- Is relief provided during extended surgical procedures (CRNA-specific)?
- Does this position have call or after-hours responsibilities?
- What training, support, or mentorship can I expect during the first year with this organization?
- Who will I be assigned to as a supervising or collaborating physician or APRN (if required by state regulation)?
- Will the candidate be employed or paid during the credentialing and privileging process? If so, what responsibilities will the candidate have during that time?
- How long does the credentialing and privileging process take? When would you expect the candidate to begin patient care responsibilities?
- What is the process to implement initiative ideas for improvement?
- What is the reporting structure?
- Will there be staff that report to this APRN?
- How will my services be marketed within the organization?
- What are some of the leadership opportunities for this position?
- Is there ability to infuse evidence into practice? What is the process?
- Ethical dilemmas: how are they named and handled?

NOTE: Questions related to benefits and salaries are typically discussed during the negotiation phase of the job search process.

Adapted from Buppert, C. (2014). 20 Questions to ask a prospective employer. *The Journal for Nurse Practitioners, 10*(1), 62–63; Konop, J. (2014). The 10 questions you should be asking a potential employer. *Huff/Post 50.* http://www.huffingtonpost.com/2014/06/21/interview-questions-to-ask-employer_n_5492147.html; University of California, San Francisco Office of Career & Professional Development. (2011). APN employment interviewing. https://career.ucsf.edu/sites/g/files/tkssra2771/f/PDF/NursingAPNinterviewing.pdf; and Warner, S. (2011). Interview the employer. Advance Healthcare Network. http://nurse-practitioners-and-physician-assistants.advanceweb.com/Features/Articles/Interview-the-Employer.aspx

academic settings, the APRN might be asked to interview with a group during a meal; although less formal, it is still an interview.

Second interviews are common in the healthcare profession. This interview may take place in the unit or office where the candidate would be assigned and

BOX 18.8

Tips for a Successful Interview

- Treat all staff members with respect before, during, and after the interview.
- Speak confidently.
- Be prepared with questions for which you are not able to obtain answers from researching other sources.
- Summarize your relevant skills and restate your interest at the end of the interview.
- Ask about next steps and contact information.
- Alert your references that they may be contacted.
- In-person interviews:
  - Arrive early with your cell phone silenced.
  - Dress in business attire regardless of the setting or culture.
  - Be prepared with copies of your résumé/curriculum vitae.
- Video interviews:
  - Ensure videoconferencing software is downloaded and working prior to interview time; test audio and video prior to interview.
  - Ensure a reliable, hands-free connection.
  - Conduct the interview alone in a quiet place.
  - Utilize a clean, solid background. Avoid background templates with distracting moving features; avoid holding videoconference in bedroom or cluttered spaces.

Adapted from University of California, Irvine Career Center. (2016b). Types of interviews. http://www.career.uci.edu/docs/students/Types-of-Interviews.pdf

can take up a significant portion of the day. A series of interviews with various executives, administrators, and healthcare providers should be anticipated. Second interviews are a further indication that the company is interested in hiring the candidate.

Preparation for the Interview

Interview preparation is essential. An APRN's self-reflection on their strengths, weaknesses, interests, deal breakers, and career goals is good preparation for initial, basic interview questions. An APRN should prepare three to five copies of their résumé or CV, a copy of their transcript and diploma, a reference list, and a professional portfolio with an electronic link (or thumb drive). A notebook with a list of questions is helpful in guiding the question-and-answer period of the interview (University of California, Irvine Career Center, 2017).

The résumé or CV will provide evidence of APRN role-specific direct practice competencies by documenting licensure and certification. In addition to these competencies, healthcare executives and administrators are interested in one's ability to self-regulate, work well in teams, and be an effective communicator. Emotional intelligence—the ability to be aware of one's own feelings, to read accurately the emotions of others—emerges during the interview process and can be confirmed during reference checking. Research suggests that the top 10 skills perceived to be most important to business executives include integrity, communication, courtesy, responsibility, social skills, positive attitude, professionalism, flexibility, teamwork, and work ethic (Robles, 2012). APRNs can exemplify these skills by preparing for interview questions in advance. Interview questions designed to elicit information on the applicant's emotional intelligence include questions about one's self-awareness and self-regulation, the ability to recognize the impact of one's behavior on others, and the ability to learn from mistakes (Bielaszka-DuVernay, 2008). Box 18.6 provides sample questions designed to identify those with high emotional intelligence.

The APRN can be asked behavioral and technical or clinical skills questions during the interview. Technical skills will center on the APRN role and response to common clinical scenarios. Behavior-based questions in an APRN interview will focus on interpersonal and communications skills. According to the University of California, San Francisco's Office of Career and Professional Development (2011) and the University of California, Irvine Career Center (2017), preparing for the interview should include the following at a minimum:

- reflection on situations in which the APRN has experience with conflict resolution (patients and coworkers)
- working with team members, intrapreneurial experience (i.e., developing and implementing innovative solutions and practices)
- leadership abilities

BOX 18.9

SHARE Model®

1. Describe a *specific* **S**ituation.
2. Identify **H**indrances or challenges.
3. Explain the **A**ction taken.
4. Discuss the **R**esults or outcome.
5. **E**valuate or summarize what was learned.

Adapted from Mayo Clinic. (n.d.). Preparing for an interview. http://www.mayoclinic.org/jobs/how-to-apply/preparing-for-interview

- stressful or difficult decision making
- nursing philosophy or approach
- project management skills
- learning curve
- personal motivation

The SHARE Model described in Box 18.9 provides a strategy for answering behavior-based and hypothetical questions. With practice, the APRN candidate can demonstrate and highlight competencies unique to the APRN profession during the interview.

Demonstrating the Value of APRN Care

The core of the nursing profession, the human caring relationship with attention to human experiences and environments (American Nurses Association, 2010), distinguishes APRN care from that of other healthcare providers. Articulating the value of APRN care within the context of a distinct model of care, as described in Chapter 2, is essential when interviewing for a new APRN position. Describing how the APRN will contribute to access, patient satisfaction, improved quality, and enhanced safety within the practice setting will set the APRN apart from other healthcare professions. In addition to the humanistic contribution to patient care, productivity and outcomes are important metrics in demonstrating value to practice. A new graduate's productivity will grow rapidly over the first year, and understanding how a potential employer defines productivity is essential. Value to a healthcare practice or organization is multifaceted and is not strictly a measure of volume but also involves complex payer reimbursement calculations tailored to the healthcare setting (Rhoads et al., 2006). The candidate should ask the interviewer how productivity and value are measured in the organization for the specific APRN role.

The APRN should review, identify, and select a few recent role-specific resources to be included in their portfolio, demonstrating APRN-specific outcomes and emphasizing whole-person, nursing-focused care. There are a number of systematic reviews including research on quality, safety, and cost-effectiveness of APRN care, which the candidate should be prepared to discuss with the interview team (see Chapter 21). Describing how the APRN role provides complementary and value-added resources to the care provided by the healthcare team is essential. Finally, the candidate should avoid delivering a message that the APRN role is "better than" another healthcare provider role. As Newhouse et al. (2011) suggested, APRNs in certain roles have better outcomes in certain areas than providers trained in a separate health discipline, but conveying that an APRN is better than another type of provider is not recommended and may result in a lost job opportunity. Referring to other members of the healthcare team with a great deal of respect is imperative.

NEGOTIATION AND RENEGOTIATION

The process of negotiation begins in the initial interview, although it is rare to ask for specific items, including salary, at this time. A candidate should consider the interview process as a time to gather information about the organization. By the end of the interview process, the APRN should ensure a clear understanding of

- the employment or independent contractor arrangement
- the scope of the job
- the organization, management, and the direct work team
- an idea of the salary and benefits
- opportunities for professional growth
- how this job meets the candidates short- and long-term goals.

(University of California, San Francisco, Office of Career & Professional Development, 2013)

Negotiations may occur informally, initially, with discussion of each party's needs and desires through in-person meetings and/or telephone or email correspondence.

Once a formal written offer is received, the APRN should take an agreed-upon time to consider all aspects of the offer, paying close attention to concerning clauses. Box 18.10 describes concerning elements to consider when negotiating a new agreement or contract. The Office of Career & Professional Development at the University of California, San Francisco (2013) recommends selecting two aspects of the offer to negotiate, starting with the most important aspect first. When negotiating points for the contract, the APRN candidate should provide a brief rationale for the request, explaining their understanding of the current offer and then asking for what they want, avoiding an apologetic tone. A period of "residency" or "transition" is one potential important area for negotiation. As a new clinician or an experienced clinician moving into a new clinical area, it is likely that productivity as defined by the employer will be lower with time built in to orient to the organization and systems. Negotiating ongoing expert clinical mentorship and possibly a reduced workload for a defined period is a reasonable and important request, with evidence suggesting optimal transition to the new role (Davis et al., 1997; Hill & Sawatzky, 2011). Exemplar 18.2 provides case study examples of the importance of mentorship during a new APRN role transition.

In an employment contract, the salary and compensation package typically includes benefits that add value of up to 30% to 40% of the salary (University of California, San Francisco Office of Career & Professional Development, 2013). The methodology for determining pay structure may be an hourly rate, a straight salary, a percentage of net receipts, or a base salary plus percentage (Buppert, 2015; see Chapter 19). Some employers or organizations may base the salary on a pay range developed by the organization commensurate with experience or provide an open offer. APRNs are familiar with hourly and straight salary methods of payment, but they may find their contract written with either payment based on percentage of net receipts or a base salary plus a percentage of net receipts (Buppert, 2015). When salary is based

BOX 18.10

Contract and Negotiation Red Flags

- Negative discussion about the organization or employees during the interview process
- Hesitation or refusal by the employer or organization to provide an employment contract or written agreement
- Lack of reasonable amount of time to review contract or pressure to accept a job offer on the spot
- Financial penalties for leaving the organization or practice
- Lack of mentorship for new APRN
- Lack of APRN recognition on/in marketing materials
- Collaboration/supervision fees
- "Incident-to" billing of services for APRN care
- Lack of understanding of the APRN role
- "Noncompetition (no-compete)" clause: legal and enforceable in some but not all states; a promise not to compete or practice in the APRN role, during or after employment; may include restrictions from practicing within specialty, within a geographic area, within a certain time frame (during and after the employee leaves the business); must be "reasonable," or acceptable by a judge if the clause were questioned in litigation (Buppert, 2008b, 2015).
  - If required and the employment opportunity is necessary or desired, may negotiate something of value in return
- "Termination without cause" clause: allows the employer to terminate the employee any time with 30-day notice (Buppert, 2008b, 2015); defeats the purpose of a contract; no job security
  - Employers are less likely to delete this clause
  - Ensure termination of contract circumstances are clearly stated
- Nonsolicitation provisions: prohibit former employees from soliciting patients or remaining employees when the provider leaves the practice/business
- Supervision requirements in a full practice authority state

EXEMPLAR 18.2
NEW GRADUATE NURSE ANESTHESIA MENTORSHIP

KARYN KARP, MS, CRNA

Newly graduated registered nurse anesthetists (RNAs) are required to meet, and typically exceed, minimum numbers of practice experiences in general and specialty anesthetics for patients of every age group and acuity presenting with multiple combinations of coexisting diseases. However, certified registered nurse anesthetist (CRNA) staffing varies widely among healthcare facilities, ranging from a solo anesthesia practitioner, to operating practitioner (surgeon) supervision, to full medical direction by anesthesiologists.

California has been fortunate to have a long tradition of autonomous practice by nurse anesthetists, who led the nation in 1936 by proving that anesthesia is the practice of nursing as well as the practice of medicine in the Supreme Court of California. Should a new graduate RNA, or only experienced CRNAs, practice in an "independent" setting? A host of factors should be considered carefully before making this decision. Anesthesia services are provided in a range of settings that vary widely, even in healthcare facilities in the same locale. Important questions to ask involve the ability, clinical experience, and confidence of the RNA provider; the type and size of the facility and its staffing, equipment, and resources; and resources available in the immediate area and the community at large. It is critical to consider how many providers make up the anesthesiology department and who will be present and/or available for backup when procedures are scheduled as well as during on-call hours. Patient demographics and surgical service type and caseload are also important, as well as whether the RNA possesses enough experience to administer specialty services competently.

Consider the following real life case examples that occurred over a 3-month period in a designated critical access hospital (CAH) and level IV trauma center offering multiple services, including obstetric and pediatric care. The facility experienced difficulty in attracting qualified, experienced CRNA providers due to its remote location and limited resources. A new graduate RNA was contracted to provide anesthesia services. In the following cases, the senior CRNA was outside the facility on backup call, serving as a mentor to the RNA.

- *Case 1, Obstetric anesthesia consult:* A 39-year-old, gravida 7, para 4, parturient was referred by a family practice physician for an anesthesia consult at 35 weeks' gestation, calculated from estimated delivery date at 40 weeks. The patient was 59.5 inches tall and weighed 432 pounds (196 kg); body mass index (BMI) was 62.9 and met the criteria for super morbid obesity (BMI > 60). Prepregnancy weight was 409 pounds. Examination revealed a Mallampati class II airway (partial view of uvula and soft palate) and inability to palpate lumbar landmarks or iliac crests bilaterally due to a thick fat layer. The patient was prescribed glyburide for type A2 gestational diabetes mellitus, with poor compliance. She received a continuous labor epidural for a prior spontaneous vaginal delivery with documented difficult placement and had a prior cesarean section for arrested fetal descent due to macrosomia with a 12-pound infant. When questioned about anesthetic complications, the patient stated, "The epidural just made me itch." She had complained of terrible, unabated pain during labor and her cesarean section. Should the patient be permitted to have her baby at the CAH hospital?
- *Case 2, General surgery anesthesia consult:* A male patient, age 82, with a history of hypertension, coronary artery disease with anterior myocardial infarction, chronic microcytic anemia, and chronic obstructive pulmonary disease was scheduled for a complex colectomy for colon cancer. The RNA had excellent experiences delivering neuraxial postoperative pain techniques for multiple patients managed in the intensive care units of community hospitals and had placed over 100 arterial lines and 30 central lines. Should the patient receive his surgery at the CAH?
- *Case 3, Pediatric patient, status post-fall:* A male patient, age 6, with no prior medical or surgical history was brought to the emergency department (ED) after a 20-foot fall from a treehouse. Pupils were round, equal, and reactive to light. The patient appeared to respond appropriately to questions but was crying, restless, and inconsolable, complaining of pain where his head was hit. He also had a deep, 6-inch leg wound and would not permit any examination; the ED physician believed it should be sutured. Should the RNA provide sedation or anesthesia so the ED physician can examine and suture the patient's leg wound?

The new graduate RNA considered providing anesthesia for the general surgery and pediatric patients, while the parturient was referred to an alternative facility to deliver her baby. However, after consulting with the senior CRNA, both the general surgery and pediatric patients were referred to a higher level facility for care. The CAH floor nursing staff was not familiar with the epidural management of postoperative pain. If the colectomy patient were to require postoperative ventilation in the two-bed intensive care unit for any reason, it is unknown whether experienced nursing staff would be available to care for the ventilator, an indwelling epidural, or invasive monitoring. The pediatric patient was transferred via Life Flight to a university medical center 60 miles away for a referral to the neurosurgery department.

The parturient surprised everyone by coming into the CAH in active labor dilated to 8 cm. Under the Emergency Medical Treatment and Active Labor Act (EMTALA), the definition of an emergency medical condition includes a pregnant woman having contractions, and transfer of an

Continued

EXEMPLAR 18.2
NEW GRADUATE NURSE ANESTHESIA MENTORSHIP—cont'd

unstable emergency medical condition from another hospital is a violation of the law. The patient requested a labor epidural. After several unsuccessful attempts, the RNA called the backup CRNA; the patient required a 6-inch epidural needle to place the block. A shoulder dystocia and thick meconium were present at delivery. The CRNA and RNA successfully intubated and resuscitated the neonate. The mother experienced a postpartum hemorrhage requiring 14 units of blood products, which exhausted the local blood bank supply.

These cases illustrate the unique challenge of providing independent anesthesia services and the clear advantage appropriate mentorship provides to new graduate RNAs, their patients, and the facilities in which they practice. Strengths and attributes of the RNA provider, the healthcare facility, and its resources, location, and setting all have important consequences for the new graduate and should be considered carefully when selecting an initial practice location.

on a percentage of net receipts, the salary calculation is based on the amount billed for the APRN service, minus the amount received from the payer and the practice expenses for the APRN (Buppert, 2015). The APRN should understand the local salary range for their APRN role prior to asking for flexibility in salary. Highlighting APRN core competencies that may exceed expectations of the role and will immediately add value to the setting is essential when negotiating salary, benefits, and work environment. Some contracts will offer bonuses, and the criteria for calculating bonuses vary greatly. Buppert (2015) described four types of bonus formulas: productivity based, quality based, profit based, and patient satisfaction based. If a bonus is offered in the employment contract, the APRN must be sure that there is a clear understanding of how the bonus will be calculated, realized, and paid. Evidence-based salary negotiation tips offered by Deepak Malhotra, a Harvard Business School professor, include the following (Gallo, 2015):

- Be prepared to answer a potential employer's question regarding salary expectations and to justify your rationale if there is a significant difference.
- Research what other providers are making in similar institutions and be prepared to ask questions that would be helpful in determining a fair salary.
- Once an offer is made, inquire about what went into calculating the figure.
- Avoid making threats; come prepared with collaborative and creative ideas and a rationale for your perceived worth.
- Consider the overall package, including responsibilities, location, flexibility in work hours, opportunities for growth and promotion, support for continued education and mentorship, bonus opportunities, and tuition reimbursement.

When renegotiating a compensation package, the experienced APRN must clearly articulate, with supporting data, their organizational and financial contributions in the past year. The professional portfolio provides a place to document and store data demonstrating excellence in practice, clinical leadership, and personal and professional development (Hespenheide et al., 2011). Data such as patient encounters/visits, individual billing and reimbursement data specific to payer mix, quality metrics, administrative responsibilities, projects, leadership opportunities, patient satisfaction surveys, continuing education, and competency verification can be included for showcase during renegotiation. A wise APRN negotiator will be able to articulate both their financial contribution and expenses (salary, benefits, continuing education, overhead, etc.) to the practice. APRNs should begin collecting these data as soon as they begin their new job so they are prepared for renegotiation during the periodic review.

In a recent randomized, controlled field experiment conducted in Australia, Leibbrandt and List (2015) found that when potential employees were explicitly notified that salary or pay was negotiable, both women and men negotiate equally for a higher wage. In contrast, when salary determination is ambiguous, men are more likely to negotiate for a higher wage and women are more likely to express willingness to work for lower pay. To avoid gender discrepancy in salary negotiations, the APRN should ask whether the salary is negotiable early in the negotiation phase of the interview process.

The entrepreneurial environment is unique with respect to negotiation of fees for work as a consultant. Development of the consultant's contract and fee proposal, including terms and conditions for payment, must be tailored to the scope of work and expected outcomes of the work or project (Stichler, 2002). Experienced entrepreneurial mentors can assist new APRN entrepreneurs in identifying and placing a dollar value on the APRN's unique knowledge, experience, expertise, and skill.

Business and Contractual Arrangements

Depending on the APRN role, new graduates will likely accept their first position as an employee, but in some cases it will be as an independent contractor. The nature of these two business relationships is significantly different with respect to taxation and professional liability. It is essential to have a basic understanding of the business arrangement and the state-specific laws surrounding that arrangement as a new graduate.

Employment Contracts

Employment arrangements may be offered with or without a contract. Employment contracts are recommended and provide a professional platform for negotiation and discussion of issues, offering some protection for the APRN as well as the employer (Buppert, 2015; Hanson & Phillips, 2014). The complexity of an employment contract warrants careful review by an attorney hired by the APRN before it is accepted and signed. Negotiation of the terms of the contract is common and considered a professional imperative. Buppert (2015) described the issues commonly addressed in an employment contract, as shown in Box 18.11.

BOX 18.11

Elements of APRN Employment Contract

- Scope of services: productivity requirements; on-call requirements; hospital/nursing home/satellite responsibilities; administrative responsibilities
- Duration of employment arrangement or contract
- Performance evaluation terms
- Compensation: salary or hourly; bonus or incentive plans (productivity- or quality-based formulas)
- Benefits: health insurance, life/disability insurance, workers compensation, retirement, continuing education expenses, liability insurance, professional dues, license/registration fees, credentialing fees, vacation, holidays, sick time/bereavement, cell phone, mileage, pager
- Malpractice coverage
- Collaboration/supervision requirements (if required by state law)
- Mentorship, consultation, and staff support
- Restriction on outside professional activities
- Termination clause
- Revision and renegotiation provisions
- May specify conflict resolution processes
- Noncompete clause

Adapted from Buppert, C. (2015). *Nurse practitioner's business practice and legal guide* (5th ed.). Jones & Bartlett.

Independent Contractor

Commonly utilized by certified registered nurse anesthetists, certified nurse-midwives, and in some cases certified nurse practitioners, APRNs use this arrangement to contract their services with a business entity and are generally considered to be self-employed (Buppert, 2015; Hanson & Phillips, 2014; Internal Revenue Service, 2015). The US Internal Revenue Service (IRS) has strict regulations pertaining to qualification as an independent contractor, and development and review of the contract by an attorney is advised (Buppert, 2010). To be considered an independent contractor, several business matters are examined, including behavioral and financial control of the services provided and the type of business relationship. The APRN must control how and what services they perform and may be paid a flat fee or, in some professions, may be paid hourly (IRS, 2016). Independent contractors are not considered employees; are responsible for paying their own state and federal taxes; provide their own benefits, uniforms, and equipment (and possibly supplies); and receive an IRS 1099 form compiled by the employing organization at the end of the year (Hanson & Phillips, 2014; IRS, 2015). The rights of the contractor and organization are specified in the contract.

There are advantages and disadvantages to each type of contractual relationship, but professional consensus recommends having a contract agreement in professional business relationships. Careful review of the employee or independent contractor contract by an attorney knowledgeable in APRN practice is essential to ensure that the APRN's interests are taken into account (Buppert, 2008b). Exemplar 18.3 provides real-life examples of contractual language that could have been avoided if the APRN had sought counsel and review of the contract.

Professional Issues and Practice Arrangements

Marketing and negotiation also involve discussion of professional issues such as state practice authority and malpractice insurance requirements. Both issues have legal implications and warrant a unique place in the discussions during negotiation of a potential position. Chapter 20 provides additional details.

APRN laws and regulations vary widely from state to state. New APRNs must be able to articulate statutory and regulatory practice and prescriptive authority, licensure and certification requirements, and controlled substance registration requirements specific for their APRN role. The APRN should not assume that the employer understands nursing scope of practice laws in the state. This knowledge can be highlighted during the interview process, demonstrating leadership in APRN policy—a unique contribution to a future practice or organization. An APRN should provide future employers with sample documents pertaining to the appropriate laws, which can be easily stored in the professional portfolio.

Future employers often have questions surrounding practice laws during the interview process. When appropriate, the APRN should articulate the difference between full practice authority, independent practice (particularly in states where the roles are defined separately), collaborative practice, and supervisory practice. The APRN should be ready to answer questions regarding collaborative and supervisory practice agreement specifications and should ask the interviewer about the physicians or APRNs who will serve in those roles. Regardless of the state's practice authority, an employer may restrict APRN practice or require collaboration or supervision as an organizational policy. This is allowable, and it is a personal decision of the APRN whether or not to work in a more restrictive environment than the state requires. Many states have adopted "transition-to-practice" laws in which a period of oversight is required prior to the APRN enjoying full autonomous practice authority (Phillips, 2016). In states that require transition-to-practice collaboration or supervision, APRNs should discuss this regulatory requirement with potential employers and clarify who will provide the oversight and attestation of this experience once completed. The APRN must interview the person who will be overseeing their practice before a position is accepted.

Malpractice Insurance

Employer-based malpractice insurance coverage is typically provided to APRN employees; however, these policies serve to protect the practice or organization as a whole and, when utilized, the APRN has little or no say in how the claim is resolved (Fetcho, 2013). It is important for the candidate to inquire about the terms of coverage during the interview and negotiation process. Two types of policies exist for malpractice coverage: *claims-made* and *occurrence*. *Occurrence* policies cover the insured for a malpractice claim that occurs during the policy period regardless of when it is reported as long as the policy was in force when the alleged malpractice occurred. *Claims-made* policies cover the insured for a malpractice claim made during an active policy period only if the claim is also made during the active policy period. *Tail coverage* can be purchased and added to a claims-made policy if the insured decides to end the policy. Tail coverage extends the time a claim can be reported as long as the claim occurred while the policy was active. Chapter 19 provides additional detail.

Independent contractors, like employees, are encouraged to purchase individual professional liability insurance. Depending on the business structure of the practice, additional employees or contractors, corporate status, and other variables, the APRN entrepreneur must also consider additional coverage such as premises, worker's compensation, unemployment, disability, and health insurance (Buppert, 2008a). It is essential that APRN entrepreneurs seek legal counsel when setting up a business to determine specific needs.

EXEMPLAR 18.3

DETRIMENTAL CLAUSES IN APRN CONTRACTS THAT SHOULD NOT HAVE BEEN SIGNED

MELANIE BALESTRA, JD, MN, PNP

(http://balestrahealthlaw.com/)

Ms. Balestra's law practice focuses on legal and business issues that affect physicians, physician assistants, nurse practitioners, nurses, and other healthcare providers, as well as representing them before their respective regulatory boards. With a specialization in the legal aspects of starting entrepreneurial practice, Ms. Balestra has assisted over 200 health professionals throughout the United States and has presented numerous workshops on this subject. Ms. Balestra is the only practicing nurse practitioner licensed to practice law before the US Supreme Court and serves as counsel of record for the California Association of Nurse Practitioners. She has supplied the following examples of detrimental clauses in employment contracts that should not have been signed.

COMPUTER LICENSE FEE

"The Employer will guarantee the fee for the computer software license for use of the Employer's electronic medical record. This fee will be forgiven after three years of employment. However, Employee agrees that if termination of this Agreement is at Employee's request, a prorated fee for use of the computer license will be incurred and due upon effective termination date. This fee will be calculated based on total cost of license at time of employment divided by 36 months. If the fee is not paid upon termination of contract, it will be withheld from the final paycheck. The fee repayment in no manner authorizes Employee use of software license after employment ceases with Employer." This clause requires the employee to pay a prorated fee for use of the computer license if the employee leaves the practice early. Use of this license during the provision of professional services is required for creating documentation in the medical record and should be covered by the employer.

MEANINGFUL USE/OTHER INCENTIVES

"Employee expressly understands that the Employer is responsible for providing and maintaining edges that all income fees and incentives obtained by use of software and hardware shall belong to the Employer. This includes government incentives for meaningful use. If Employee elects to terminate employment, incentives will remain with the Employer. Employee expressly agrees to reimburse Employer for incentives paid directly to Employee for incentives earned while employed with Employer." This clause requires the APRN to give all Meaningful Use incentive fees received to the employer. In many group practices, incentive fees are often part of a negotiated bonus rate.

COVENANT NOT TO COMPETE

"Employee covenants to and with Employer that for a period of 12 months after termination of the Contract, whether by expiration of its term or otherwise, the Employee will not, directly or indirectly, engage in providing healthcare to children (including government or private entities, clinics that provide care to children such as pediatric or family practice clinics) within a radius of 25 miles of either campus of ___________." Noncompete clauses are not uncommon. The APRN should seek legal advice on how to negotiate this clause if the employer refuses to remove it.

SALARY

"Salary is $50 per hour based on productivity of seeing 40 patients per 8-hour day. Productivity will be reviewed on a monthly basis and adjusted according." There are a number of issues with this clause, including (but not limited to) a requirement to see five patients per hour or one patient every 12 minutes; lack of specificity when patients do not show up for their appointment or cancel; and quality, safety, and potential malpractice issues.

INDEPENDENT CONTRACTOR

"Contractor cannot work for any other medical practice within a twenty-five mile radius unless approved by Contractee." As an independent contractor, limitations on the APRNs ability to work outside of this contract are constraining and must be considered.

Medical malpractice policies covering a healthcare organization or practice may restrict APRN practice, such as by requiring cosignatory of patient records or physician presence during care delivered by the APRN, and rarely cover expenses related to license discipline or administrative review (Fetcho, 2013). An individual APRN malpractice insurance policy, paid for separately by the APRN, in addition to employer-based coverage, is recommended by Carolyn Buppert (2015), an attorney and APRN. Citing "fracture [in] collegial alliances" (p. 283), Buppert noted that malpractice lawsuits damage the relationship between the APRN employee and the organization. When named in a lawsuit, the organization may blame the APRN, necessitating individual defense (Buppert, 2015). A recent regulatory trend to require APRN liability coverage has passed in some states and is being considered in a majority of the full practice authority legislation (Phillips, 2016). The APRN should ensure that they are versed in the legislation as well as statutory requirements for malpractice coverage in the state where they intend to provide care.

OVERCOMING INVISIBILITY

Novice APRNs or seasoned entrepreneurs must be able to demonstrate their unique value to an organization whether interviewing for their first position or marketing their entrepreneurial/intrapreneurial practice improvement idea. This is important because often the APRN role is invisible to external funding agencies such as insurers, foundations, and governmental bodies. As a result, APRNs' services may also be invisible to potential employers and organizations.

There are a number of situations in which APRNs are invisible. One example is Medicare policy, by which physicians can bill nurse practitioner services "incident-to" in order to receive 100% reimbursement from Medicare. During the interview or negotiation process, the nurse practitioner should emphasize the restrictions placed on the physician when doing this, including mandated physician presence during nurse practitioner-provided patient care and physician-only access for new patients or existing patients with new complaints. Other examples of invisibility include the National Ambulatory Medical Care Survey (https://www.cdc.gov/nchs/ahcd/index.htm), the Center for Studying Health System Change (http://www.hschange.org/), and the Area-Resource File (https://data.hrsa.gov/topics/health-workforce/ahrf). None of these survey studies or databases include APRN distinctions in their data. This is significant because they are used to determine such things as service need, federal funding, and provider shortage areas. Beyond obtaining employment, doctorally-prepared APRNs should strive to be involved in local, state, and national policymaking so that future studies and databases will include such APRN-specific data. This will enable APRNs to demonstrate value, enhance healthcare delivery, and assist in obtaining federal and private funding and reimbursement.

Marketing the APRN's services once established within the organization or practice is an essential step in overcoming invisibility. In addition to including the APRN on organizational signage, the APRN should be prepared to provide a succinct APRN role description, educational background, and skill set for incorporation into print and electronic marketing materials. Skilled in organizational and systems leadership competencies, DNP-prepared APRNs are uniquely qualified to assist in the development of an organizational APRN marketing strategy.

CONCLUSION

Developing skills to market the unique practice and contribution of the APRN role is important to enable APRNs to become viable members of and achieve stature as principal players in the healthcare arena. Evolution of these skills is established in APRN education, and it is important for academic institutions to include such activities for successful acclimation into the professional world. As a new graduate searching for one's first position or a seasoned clinician seeking to redefine one's professional role, reflection and self-assessment of one's philosophic basis for practice and preference for an intrapreneurial or entrepreneurial approach are an important exercise to determine the right professional fit.

Increasingly, educational institutions are preparing APRNs to leverage the innovative call described in the IOM's *The Future of Nursing* report (IOM, 2015; IOM & Committee on the Robert Wood Johnson Foundation Initiative on the Future of Nursing, 2011) and, more recently, *The Future of Nursing 2020–2030: Charting a Path to Achieve Health Equity* (National Academies of Sciences, Engineering, and Medicine, 2021). Doctoral and APRN role-specific competencies addressing concepts of entrepreneurial and intrapreneurial practice have been implemented into APRN education, preparing APRNs to execute innovative ideas with a focus on accessibility and affordability. Although challenging, innovative practice setting opportunities are increasingly sought by new APRN graduates as well as experienced APRNs.

This chapter provides the new APRN with practical information and resources needed for a successful job search. Demonstrating the unique value of APRN care to an organization in an era of invisibility is an essential marketing skill that is practiced and refined during the job search and interview process.

KEY SUMMARY POINTS

- Attention to and reflection on personal professional goals is essential to finding a good career fit as an APRN entrepreneur.
- Despite challenges, APRNs are increasingly prepared for and seeking employee-intrapreneur, entrepreneur, and freelancing career opportunities that provide innovation and flexibility.
- Highlighting and marketing APRN core competencies during the job search process enables the APRN applicant to stand out in an interview.
- Professional networking through professional association membership and utilization of web-based business networking sites increases the success of a job search and supports growth and success of a business.
- Electronic professional portfolios highlight the APRN's potential contribution to an organization, providing a strong base for negotiation.
- Articulating the value of APRN care within the context of a distinct model of care with careful attention to the humanistic contribution to patient care, productivity, and outcomes is essential when interviewing for a new APRN position or when negotiating with investors.
- Negotiation is a two-way street; the APRN applicant should take an agreed-upon time to carefully consider all aspects of the employment offer, including salary compensation, benefits, and time alternatives. Review of contract agreements by an attorney is recommended.

REFERENCES

American Association of Colleges of Nursing. (2006). The essentials of doctoral education for advanced nursing practice. http://www.aacn.nche.edu/dnp/Essentials.pdf

American Association of Colleges of Nursing. (2021). *The essentials: Core competencies for professional nursing education.* https://www.aacnnursing.org/Portals/42/AcademicNursing/pdf/Essentials-2021.pdf

American Nurses Association. (2010). *Nursing's social policy statement* (3rd ed.). Author.

APRN Joint Dialogue Group. (2008). *Consensus model for APRN regulation: Licensure, accreditation, certification & education.* http://www.aacn.nche.edu/education-resources/APRNReport.pdf

Arndt, T., & Coleman, K. (2014). *Backpack to briefcase: Your guide to success* (4th ed.). College Transition Publishing.

Beauvais, A. (2016). Role transition: Strategies for success in the marketplace. In S. M. DeNisco, & A. M. Barker (Eds.), *Advanced practice nursing: Essential knowledge for the profession* (3rd ed.) (pp. 763–784). Jones & Bartlett Learning.

Bielaszka-DuVernay, C. (2008). Hiring for emotional intelligence. *Harvard Management Update, 13*(11), 3–5.

Buppert, C. (2008a). How to start a health care practice. Law office of Carolyn Buppert.

Buppert, C. (2008b). Negotiating terms of employment. Law office of Carolyn Buppert.

Buppert, C. (2010, June 30). How does the IRS define "Independent Contractor"? Medscape. http://www.medscape.com/viewarticle/724060

Buppert, C. (2014). 20 questions to ask a prospective employer. *The Journal for Nurse Practitioners, 10*(1), 62–63.

Buppert, C. (2015). *Nurse practitioner's business practice and legal guide* (5th ed.). Jones & Bartlett.

CAREERwise Education. (2016). Types of resumes. https://www.careerwise.mnscu.edu/jobs/resumecharts.html

Davis, L. L., Little, M. S., & Thornton, W. L. (1997). The art and angst of the mentoring relationship. *Academic Psychiatry, 21*, 61–71.

Dayhoff, N. E., & Moore, P. S. (2003a). Entrepreneurship: Start-up questions. *Clinical Nurse Specialist, 17*, 86–87.

Dayhoff, N. E., & Moore, P. S. (2003b). You don't have to leave your hospital system to be an entrepreneur. *Clinical Nurse Specialist, 17*(1), 22–24.

Dayhoff, N. E., & Moore, P. S. (2005). CNS entrepreneurs: Innovators in patient care. *The Nurse Practitioner, 30*(Suppl. 1), 6–8.

Doerksen, K. (2010). What are the professional development and mentorship needs of advanced practice nurses? *Journal of Professional Nursing, 26*(3), 141–151.

Fertig, A. (2012). 3 ways LinkedIn can help you nab a job. *Huff/Post, 50*. http://www.huffingtonpost.com/2012/12/08/linkedin-tips-how-to-use_n_2257788.html

Fetcho, J. (2013). Supplemental liability coverage now available for employed CRNAs. *AANA News Bulletin, 67*(5), 1, 6–8. http://www.aana.com/insurance/Documents/supplemental-malpractice-insurance-for-crnas.pdf

Gallo, A. (2014). *How to write a cover letter.* February 4: Harvard Business Review. https://hbr.org/2014/02/how-to-write-a-cover-letter/

Gallo, A. (2015). *Setting the record straight on negotiating your salary.* March 9: Harvard Business Review. https://hbr.org/2015/03/setting-the-record-straight-on-negotiating-your-salary

Hanson, C. M., & Phillips, B. C. (2014). Marketing and negotiation. In A. B. Hamric, C. M. Hanson, M. F. Tracy, & E. T. O'Grady (Eds.), *Advanced practice nursing: An integrative approach* (5th ed.) (pp. 538–556). Elsevier Saunders.

Hespenheide, M., Cottingham, T., & Mueller, G. (2011). Portfolio use as a tool to demonstrate professional development in advanced nursing practice. *Clinical Nurse Specialist, 25*(6), 312–320.

Hewison, A., & Badger, F. (2006). Taking the initiative: Nurse intrapreneurs in the NHS. *Nursing Management, 13*(3), 14–19.

Hill, L. A., & Sawatzky, J. V. (2011). Transitioning into the nurse practitioner role through mentorship. *Journal of Professional Nursing, 27*(3), 161–167.

Ieong, S. (2004). Clinical nurse specialist entrepreneurship. *The Internet Journal of Advanced Nursing Practice, 7*(1), 1–5.

Internal Revenue Service. (2015). Independent contractor (self-employed) or employee? https://www.irs.gov/Businesses/Small-Businesses-&-Self-Employed/Independent-Contractor-Self-Employed-or-Employee

Internal Revenue Service. (2016). Financial control. https://www.irs.gov/businesses/small-businesses-self-employed/financial-control

Institute of Medicine. (2015). *Assessing progress on the Institute of Medicine report: The future of nursing*. http://www.nationalacademies.org/hmd/Reports/2015/Assessing-Progress-on-the-IOM-Report-The-Future-of-Nursing.aspx

Institute of Medicine (US), & Committee on the Robert Wood Johnson Foundation Initiative on the Future of Nursing. (2011). *The future of nursing: Leading change, advancing health*. National Academies Press.

Johnson, J. E., & Garvin, W. S. (2017). Advanced practice nurses: Developing a business plan for an independent ambulatory clinical practice. *Nursing Economic$, 35*(3), 126–133. 141.

Kador, J. (2010). Interview the interviewer. http://www.job-interview.net/questionstoask.htm

Konop, J. (2014). The 10 questions you should be asking a potential employer. *Huff/Post, 50*. http://www.huffingtonpost.com/2014/06/21/interview-questions-to-ask-employer_n_5492147.html

Latham, C. L., & Fahey, L. J. (2006). Novice to expert advanced practice nurses role transition: Guided student self-reflection. *Journal of Nursing Education, 45*(1), 46–48.

Lees, J. (2013). *Knock out CV: How to get noticed, get interviewed and get hired*. McGraw Hill Professional.

Leibbrandt, A., & List, J. A. (2015). Do women avoid salary negotiations? *Management Science, 61*(9), 2016–2024.

Manion, J. (2001). Enhancing career marketability through intrapreneurship. *Nursing Administration Quarterly, 25*(2), 5–10.

Marques, C. S., Marques, C. P., Ferreira, J. J., & Ferreira, F. A. (2019). Effects of traits, self-motivation and managerial skills on nursing intrepreneurship. *International Entrepreneurship and Management Journal, 15*, 733–748. https://link.springer.com/content/pdf/10.1007%2Fs11365-018-0520-9.pdf

Mayo Clinic. (n.d.). Preparing for an interview. http://www.mayoclinic.org/jobs/how-to-apply/preparing-for-interview

National Academies of Sciences, Engineering, and Medicine. (2021). *The future of nursing 2020-2030: Charting a path to achieve health equity*. The National Academies Press. doi:10.17226/25982

Newhouse, R., Stanik-Hutt, J., White, K., Johantgen, M., Bass, E., Zangaro, G., Wilson, R. F., Fountain, L., Steinwachs, D. M., Heindel, L., & Weiner, J. P. (2011). Advanced practice nurse outcomes 1990-2008: A systematic review. *Nursing Economic$, 29*(5), 230–250.

Patient Protection and Affordable Care Act, 42 U.S.C. § 18001. (2010).

Phillips, S. (2016). APRN legislative update: Advancements continue for APRN practice. *The Nurse Practitioner, 41*(1), 23–48.

Rhoads, J., Ferguson, L. A., & Langford, C. A. (2006). Measuring nurse practitioner productivity. *Dermatology Nursing, 18*(1), 32–34, 37–38.

Robles, M. M. (2012). Executive perceptions of the top 10 soft skills needed in today's workplace. *Business Communication Quarterly, 75*(4), 453–465.

Shirey, M. R. (2007). An evidence-based understanding of entrepreneurship in nursing. *Clinical Nurse Specialist, 21*(5), 234–240.

Small Business Association. (2016). Starting and managing: Limited liability company. https://www.sba.gov/starting-business/choose-your-business-structure/limited-liability-company

Spoelstra, S. L., & Robbins, L. B. (2010). A qualitative study of role transition from RN to APN. *International Journal of Nursing Education Scholarship, 7*(1), 1–14.

Stichler, J. F. (2002). The nurse as consultant. *Nursing Administration Quarterly, 26*(2), 52–66.

University of California, Irvine Career Center. (2016). *Job Search Guide, 2016*. College Recruitment Media, Inc. http://www.career.uci.edu/docs/students/UCI_Job-Search-Guide2016.pdf

University of California, Irvine Career Center. (2016). *Types of interviews*. http://www.career.uci.edu/docs/students/Types-of-Interviews.pdf

University of California, Irvine Career Center. (2017). *Applying for the job: Interview techniques*. http://www.career.uci.edu/docs/students/Interview-Techniques.pdf

University of California, San Francisco, Office of Career & Professional Development. (2011). APN employment interviewing. https://career.ucsf.edu/sites/career.ucsf.edu/files/PDF/NursingAPNinterviewing.pdf

University of California, San Francisco, Office of Career & Professional Development. (2013). Advanced practice nurse job search. https://career.ucsf.edu/sites/g/files/tkssra2771/f/2-APN%20Job%20Search%202016.pdf

University of California, San Francisco, Office of Career & Professional Development. (2021). *Advanced practice nurse resumes and cover letters*. https://career.ucsf.edu/professional/nursing/cvs-resumes-cover-letters#Advance-Practice-Nurse-Resumes

Vilorio, D. (2011). Focused job seeking: A measure approach to looking for work. *Occupational Health Quarterly, 55*(1), 2–11.

Vollman, K. M. (1999). My search to help patients breathe. *Reflections /Sigma Theta Tau, 25*(2), 16–18.

Vollman, K. M. (2004). Nurse entrepreneurship through inventing: Taking an idea from birth to the market place. *Clinical Nurse Specialist, 8*(2), 68–71.

Vollman, K. M. (2014). Clinical nurse specialist entrepreneurship: A journey from idea to invention, leading to consulting/education business. In J. S. Fulton, B. L. Lyon, & K. Goudreau (Eds.), *Foundations of clinical nurse specialist practice* (2nd ed.) (pp. 403–409). Springer Publishing Company.

Vollman, K. M., & Bander, J. J. (1996). Improved oxygenation utilizing a prone positioner in patients with acute respiratory distress syndrome. *Intensive Care Medicine, 22*, 1105–1111.

Warner, S. (2011). Interview the employer. Advance Healthcare Network. http://nurse-practitioners-and-physician-assistants.advanceweb.com/Features/Articles/Interview-the-Employer.aspx

Wilson, A., Averis, A., & Walsh, K. (2003). The influences on and experiences of becoming nurse entrepreneurs: A Delphi study. *International Journal of Nursing Practice, 9*(4), 236–245.

Wilson, A., Whitaker, N., & Whitford, D. (2012). Rising to the challenge of health care reform with entrepreneurial and intrapreneurial nursing initiatives. *The Online Journal of Issues in Nursing, 17*(2), 5.

19

REIMBURSEMENT AND PAYMENT FOR APRN SERVICES

LYNN RAPSILBER ■ KATHY BALDRIDGE

"Nursing is a progressive art such that to stand still is to go backwards."
~ Florence Nightingale

CHAPTER CONTENTS

HEALTHCARE REFORM HISTORY 618
REIMBURSEMENT MODELS 621
Federally Funded Medical Coverage 621
State-Administered Medical Coverage 622
Third-Party Payers 624
BILLING FOR APRN SERVICES: UNDERSTANDING THE PROCESS 624
The Credentialing Process 625
Provider Panels and Contracts 626
Coding Sets 627
Outpatient Billing 629
Medical Decision Making 630
Inpatient Billing 633
Revenue Cycle Management 635
VALUE-BASED AND FEE-FOR-SERVICE MODELS 636
Resource-Based Relative Value Scale 636
Value-Based Payments 636
REIMBURSEMENT ISSUES AND CHALLENGES 638
Incident-To Billing 638
Liability/Malpractice Insurance 640
Reimbursement Pay Parity 643
BUSINESS DEVELOPMENT 643
Entrepreneurship 643
Business Ownership 644
Additional APRN Compensation Models 644
FUTURE TRENDS 645
CONCLUSION 645
KEY SUMMARY POINTS 645

Health care is fundamentally defined as the organized provision of medical care to individuals or a community. Unfortunately, the term "health care" in today's environment has been relegated to a business term, rather than the provision of medical care (Sawyer, 2018). Throughout the ages, the challenge has been to deliver medical care within a business model that is mutually beneficial for the patient as well as the provider (Teel, 2018). Today, health care looks much different than it did 100 years ago, and 100 years from now, it cannot operate as it does today. Sustainable solutions that are structured, yet flexible, and must be established to improve healthcare infrastructure and thus, patient outcomes (Teel, 2018).

Advanced practice registered nurses (APRNs) are uniquely qualified and positioned in this evolving system to be a sustainable solution to improving access to health care (see Fig. 19.1). APRNs provide a holistic approach to patient care and excel in providing coordinated, comprehensive, and continuous care to

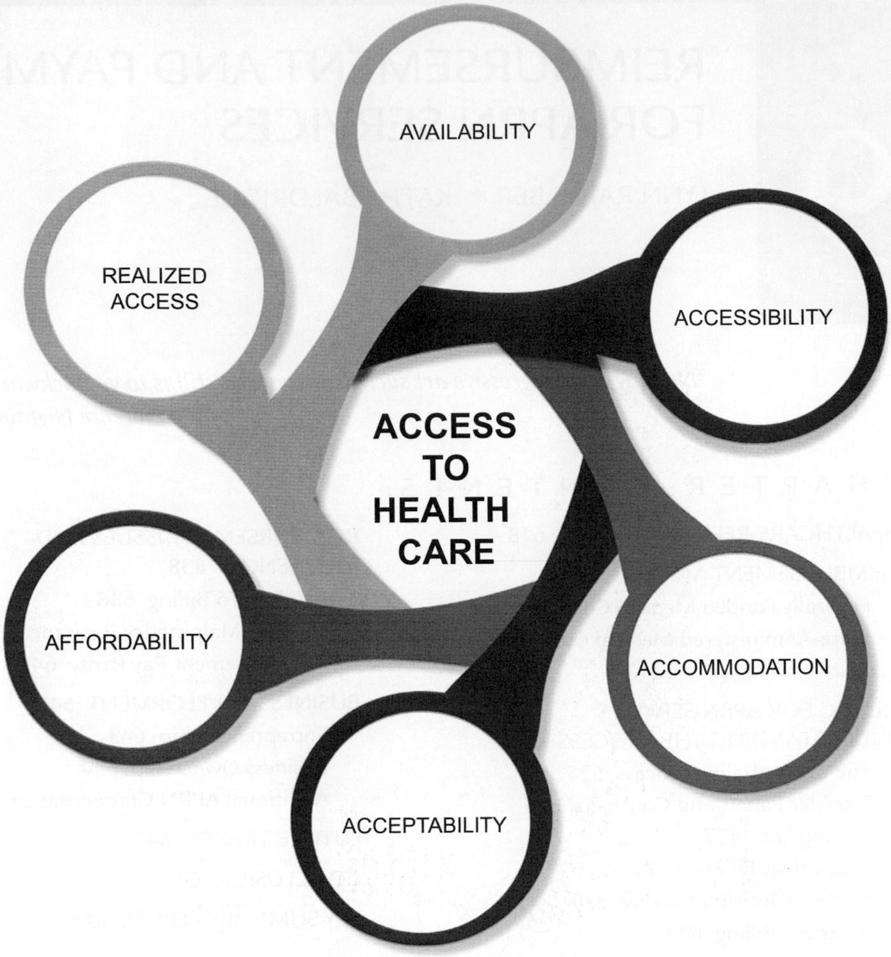

Fig. 19.1 ■ Access to health care components.

patients (Xue et al., 2016). Building upon the strong foundations of the nursing model, APRNs can diagnose patients, prescribe medications, and initiate and manage patient treatments. Yet a distinctive difference from our nursing foundation is the ability to bill for provided services. This makes APRNs "revenue visible," unlike RNs, whose generated revenue is included in facility fees, rendering them "revenue invisible." The role of the APRN is critical to the reformation of healthcare systems, and it is imperative that APRNs understand their value and the value of the services they provide (Safriet, 2011).

HEALTHCARE REFORM HISTORY

To have a visionary view of healthcare reform in the United States, a review of its history is helpful (see Table 19.1). Since the early 1940s, healthcare reform has been the most debated political issue as every newly elected United States president works to increase access, improve quality, and reduce cost. The struggle continues today and is likely to remain on the political agenda for decades to come. Proposed changes to the healthcare system are often highly controversial and heavily debated, leading to bitterness and divisiveness among legislators, healthcare organizations, and the public. Despite partisan politics, there have been some significant changes to health care over the years (Taylor, 2014; Teel, 2018). For example, one of the most notable reforms in history is the Social Security amendment in 1965, which provided health coverage to people 65 years of age and older (Cohen & Ball, 1965). Then in 1985, the Consolidated Omnibus Budget Reconciliation Act (COBRA) made it possible for people to continue their employer-provided insurance coverage after losing their job (Ross & Hayes, 1986). The Omnibus Reconciliation Act, passed in 1989 and 1990, provided for reimbursement of APRNs in rural areas and skilled nursing facilities (Congress.gov, 1989,1990). This was expanded to cover APRNs

TABLE 19.1

US Healthcare Reform Since 1945

Year	Administration	Bill Title	Summary	Outcome
1945–1953	Truman	Universal Health Insurance Coverage	Health insurance for all administered and paid for by the National Health Insurance Board. Heavily opposed by the American Medical Association	Failed to pass
		The Hospital Survey and Construction Act (aka: Hill-Burton Act)	Provided federal grants and loans to build, expand, and modernize hospitals	Passed 1946
1963–1969	L. B. Johnson	Social Security Amendments	Provided healthcare coverage to those 65 years of age and older and to the poor, blind, and disabled	Passed 1965
1969–1974	Nixon	Health Maintenance Organization Act	Laid groundwork for managed care	Passed 1973
1974–1977	Ford	The National Health Planning and Resources Development Act of 1974	Designed to rein in escalating healthcare costs. The goals were to reduce and avoid unnecessary duplication of healthcare facilities and services by mandating certificate of need programs.	Passed 1974 and repealed 1986, but 36 states and the District of Columbia still operate certificate of need programs today.
1981–1989	Reagan	Medicare Catastrophic Coverage Act	Expanded Medicare coverage for outpatient drugs, put a ceiling on out-of-pocket co-pays for hospital and physician services, and modestly expanded payments for long-term care. Program was designed to be funded entirely by Medicare beneficiaries through increased premiums and a surtax on wealthier beneficiaries based on income.	Passed 1988
		Consolidated Omnibus Budget Reconciliation Act	Provides for continuing group health insurance coverage for some employees and their families after a job loss or other qualifying event	Passed 1985
		Omnibus Budget Reconciliation Act	Added nursing home protection rules to Medicare and Medicaid, created no-fault vaccine injury compensation program	Passed 1987

Continued

TABLE 19.1

US Healthcare Reform Since 1945—cont'd

Year	Administration	Bill Title	Summary	Outcome
1989–1993	G. H. W. Bush	Medicare Catastrophic Coverage Act of 1988	Majority of the MCCA repealed due to public outcry and senior revolt at having to pay higher premiums and taxes	Repealed 1989
		Omnibus Budget Reconciliation Act	Changed Medicare's "reasonable charge" method of reimbursing physicians by replacing it with a fee schedule. It also created a new federal agency on research and quality of care. Provided for reimbursement of nurse practitioners in rural health clinics in collaboration with a physician.	Passed 1989
		Omnibus Budget Reconciliation Act	Added cancer screenings to Medicare, required providers to notify patients about advance directives and living wills, expanded Medicaid to all children living below poverty level, required drug companies to provide discounts to Medicaid	Passed 1990
		Omnibus Budget Reconciliation Act	Direct APRN reimbursement by Medicare was available only in rural areas and skilled nursing facilities.	Passed 1990
		Stark Law: Part 1 (Part of the OBRA 1990 Act)	Reduce fraud and abuse to CMS by prohibiting physicians from referring patients for certain designated health services to which they have a financial interest	Passed 1990
		Omnibus Budget Reconciliation Act	Created federal vaccine funding for all children.	Passed 1993
		Stark Law: Part II (Part of the OBRA 1993 Act)	Amended Stark Law Part 1 to extend provisions to Medicaid patients and to DHS except for clinical laboratory services	Passed 1993
1993–2001	Clinton	Welfare Reform Act	Separated Medicaid from welfare	Passed 1996
		Health Insurance Portability and Accountability Act	The Act created federal standards for insurers, health maintenance organizations (HMOs), and employer-provided health plans, including those that self-insure. It also provided for the confidentiality and security of healthcare information and to help the healthcare industry control administrative costs.	Passed 1996
		The Balanced Budget Act	Created the state-federal children's health program called CHIP	Passed 1997
			Medicare expanded reimbursement for clinical nurse specialists (CNS), APRNs, and nurse-midwives to all geographic and clinical settings, allowing direct Medicare reimbursement but at 85% of the physician rate.	Passed 1997

TABLE 19.1
US Healthcare Reform Since 1945—cont'd

Year	Administration	Bill Title	Summary	Outcome
2001–2009	G. H. Bush	Medicare Drug Improvement and Modernization Act of 2003	Noted as one of the largest expansions of Medicare in the program's history, including the establishment of Medicare Part D for prescription drug coverage	Passed 2003
2009–2017	Obama	Patient Protection and Affordable Care Act	Provided for health insurance coverage through private insurers instead, mandated employer health insurance, created state exchanges for insurance, provided federal subsidies for low-income individuals, guaranteed eligibility regardless of preexisting conditions, extended dependent coverage to age 26, and established an individual penalty for no coverage.	Passed 2010
2017–Present	Trump	Tax Cuts and Jobs Act	Repealed the individual mandate that required the payment of a penalty for no health insurance coverage.	Passed 2017

APRN, advanced practice registered nurse; *CHIP*, Children's Health Insurance Program; *CMS*, Centers for Medicaid and Medicare Services; *DHS*, Department of Health and Human Services.
Information from Congress.gov. https://www.congress.gov/search and Taylor, J. W. (2014). A brief history on the road to healthcare reform: From Truman to Obama. Becker's Hospital Review. https://www.beckershospitalreview.com/news-analysis/a-brief-history-on-the-road-to-healthcare-reform-from-truman-to-obama.html

in all geographic areas in 1997 with the Balanced Budget Act but only allowed for reimbursement of 85% of the physician rate (Congress.gov, 1997). Probably the most notable healthcare reform package of the 21st century is the Patient Protection and Affordable Care Act (2010). Consistent throughout history is that no act or reform to health care has been wholly good or bad. They each had components that were beneficial to patients and the healthcare ecosystem. There is no doubt that further reform is on the horizon as policymakers and stakeholders continue efforts to improve the healthcare system in the United States.

REIMBURSEMENT MODELS

Federally Funded Medical Coverage

Having affordable healthcare insurance is critical to improving access to care, and one of the most notable acts of healthcare reform occurred in 1965 when President Lyndon B. Johnson signed into law legislation establishing Medicare and Medicaid services (Taylor, 2014). The Centers for Medicare & Medicaid Services (CMS) is responsible for administering these programs, along with other federal healthcare programs and services. Medicare provides services to people 65 years of age or older, people with certain disabilities, and those with end-stage renal disease. Healthcare services provided by hospital systems, physicians, nursing facilities, and home care providers are covered (CMS, 2018). Medicare is administered by the federal government and consists of Part A, Part B, Part C, and Part D (Table 19.2).

Patients may choose Part A and B services through the original Medicare plan. Part D (i.e., prescription drug benefits) is optional coverage paid for by the patient through a stand-alone plan or through services provided by Part C, also referred to as a Medicare Advantage (MA) Plan, if they reside in the MA service area. Part D coverage is included in some MA Plans. Medicare supplement plans (Medigap) extend coverage to qualified patients who are covered under the original Medicare plan (CMS, 2018).

APRNs who are enrolled as providers in the Medicare program can bill directly for services rendered to its beneficiaries. When billed directly by the APRN, Medicare will reimburse 85% of the allowable physician

TABLE 19.2
Four Parts of Medicare

Part	Entitlement	Coverage
Part A	Hospital insurance	Provides coverage for inpatient hospital services, inpatient skilled nursing facilities, hospice, and some home health services
Part B	Medical insurance	Reimburses for physician services, outpatient care, durable medical equipment, home health services, and a large portion of preventive services
Part C	Medicare Advantage (MA)	Medicare-approved private insurance companies that supply all of Part A and Part B services, as well as some prescription drug coverage and other supplemental benefits
Part D	Prescription drug benefit	Medicare-approved private insurance companies that supply coverage for outpatient prescription drug benefits

TABLE 19.3
Table of Reimbursement

	NP	CRNA	CNM	CNS
Percentage reimbursement of physician rate	85%	Assignment (sign for payment to go directly to the physician) Anesthesia fee schedule	Assignment (sign for payment to go directly to the physician) 80%	85%
Coinsurance		Yes		
Deductible		Yes		
Co-pay		Yes		

CNS, clinical nurse specialist; *CNM*, certified nurse-midwife; *CRNA*, certified registered nurse anesthetist; *NP*, nurse practitioner.

fee schedule (PFS) rate (CMS, 2020b; Table 19.3). The services provided must be within the scope of practice of the APRN as defined by state law.

Services by the APRN may be provided in any setting, and physician cosignature or collaboration is not required unless mandated by state law or the facility. Medicare reimburses for reasonable and necessary services that are not otherwise excluded from the plan. Documentation must reflect the medical necessity of the services rendered and be consistent with the procedure codes. The APRN who is billing Medicare in the inpatient setting will need to adhere to standard rules under Medicare Part A if employed by the hospital or Medicare Part B rules if employed by an outpatient or office practice (CMS, 2020b).

State-Administered Medical Coverage

Medicaid, the nation's public health insurance program, is also administered through CMS (CMS, 2018). As with other areas of healthcare reform, the Medicaid program has evolved over time to meet the changing needs of Americans. The federal government, under Title XIX of the Social Security Act, establishes broad federal statutes, regulations, and policies for the administration of Medicaid (CMS, 2018). Then individual states can decide whether they wish to participate in the Medicaid partnership. If they do participate in the partnership, they are bound to follow the minimum federal guidelines. However, states do have some flexibility to determine covered populations, covered services, healthcare delivery models, and methods for paying providers and hospitals (CMS, 2018). The Medicaid program was designed to be funded through a federal and state partnership to provide health insurance to eligible Americans, with the state receiving matching assistance from the federal government. The Federal Medical Assistance Percentage (FMAP) determines the federal share of the cost of Medicaid in each state. The FMAP is calculated using a formula and is based on state per capita income. The lower a state's per capita income, the higher the state's FMAP, or federal Medicaid matching rate (Rudowitz et al., 2019).

Medicaid is an entitlement program ensuring that any American who meets eligibility criteria is guaranteed coverage and that states are guaranteed federal matching dollars for qualified services provided to Medicaid recipients (CMS, 2018). Mandatory populations, as established by the federal regulations, must be covered by the states in order to receive the federal funding (Rudowitz et al., 2019). The mandatory populations include children through the age of 18 in low-income families, pregnant women with low income, specified parents or caretakers with very low income, most seniors, and people with disabilities who receive cash assistance through the supplemental security income (SSI) program (CMS, 2018). *Low income* is defined as income below 138% of the federal poverty line (FPL). In 2010 Medicaid was expanded through the Patient Protection and Affordable Care Act to include nonelderly, nondisabled adults with income up to 138% of the FPL (Rudowitz et al., 2019). However, nonelderly, nondisabled adults, as well as children, pregnant women, specified parents or caretakers who exceed the FPL, seniors, people with disabilities not receiving SSI and/or low income, and medically needy people (i.e., those whose income exceeds the FPL but have high medical expenses such as nursing home care) are considered "optional" populations that states may choose to cover with Medicaid funds (Rice et al., 2018).

There are certain mandatory services that states are directed to cover under Medicaid. Those services include hospital and provider care, laboratory and x-ray services, home health, and nursing facility services for adults. Early and periodic screening, diagnostic, and treatment (EPSDT) services (e.g., developmental screening, lead toxicity screening, and immunizations) for children under the age of 21 are also required. Most states also cover additional services including dental care, vision services, hearing aids, and personal care services for frail seniors and people with disabilities. Because of the broad federal guidelines and the flexibility afforded to the states, eligibility and benefits may vary by state (Rudowitz et al., 2019).

Medicaid benefits are administered either through a fee-for-service (FFS) model, through managed care plans, or both. In the FFS model, the state determines provider payment rates for delivery of covered services and providers are paid directly from the state (CMS, 2018). The Social Security Administration Act requires that the FFS payment system be consistent with efficiency, economy, and quality of care and is sufficient to provide access that is equivalent to that of the general population (MACPAC, 2022). However, because these rates are often much less than other payers, provider participation in Medicaid programs is low, further decreasing the access to care that this entitlement program was supposed to ensure (Rudowitz et al., 2019).

The majority of states subscribe to a managed care program for the administration and payment of Medicaid services. The culpability of monitoring, measuring, and reporting of outcomes through a managed care program is significantly better than with the FFS model. There are three types of managed care delivery systems through which the state may contract services (Rudowitz et al., 2019).

1. **Comprehensive Risk-Based Managed Care:** Covers a defined set of Medicaid services as negotiated with the state. The state pays the plan a fixed rate per member per month to cover those services. A subsection of the services (e.g., prescription drug coverage) may be provided separately through an FFS or a limited benefit plan.
2. **Primary Care Case Management:** Program enrollees have a designated primary care provider. The provider is paid a monthly case management fee to coordinate and manage the care of the patient. They are also paid on an FFS basis.
3. **Limited Benefit Plans:** Manage specific benefits or provide certain services for a particular subpopulation, such as inpatient mental health or substance abuse inpatient care (CMS, 2018).

Dual Eligibility for Medicare and Medicaid

Some Americans are dual-eligible beneficiaries, meaning that they are qualified for both Medicare and Medicaid coverage. Beneficiaries may be receiving Part A and Part B and getting full Medicaid benefits and/or they may receive assistance with Medicare premiums or cost sharing through the Medicare Savings Program (MSP; CMS, 2018).

Though each State Medicaid Program varies, general rules require that the provider: (1) bill only for covered services; (2) ensure that beneficiaries are eligible for services where they are furnished; (3) ensure that medical records are accurate, legible, signed, and dated; and (4) return any overpayments within 60 days (CMS, 2018).

Third-Party Payers

In addition to the federal payment programs, the APRN needs to be aware of third-party payers. A *third-party payer* is an entity, other than the patient or a healthcare provider, that pays medical claims on behalf of the insured. Examples of third-party payers include government agencies, which include Medicare and Medicaid; insurance companies; and employers. Third-party payers may be public, private, managed care, or preferred provider networks that reimburse fully or partially the cost of healthcare provider services. Examples of healthcare providers include hospitals, physicians, dietitians, pharmacists, and APRNs.

Types of Third-Party Payers

Many types of health insurance options (i.e., third-party payers) are available to patients through either employer-provided plans or commercial plans. Currently, the largest third-party health payer in the United States is UnitedHealth Group (https://www.uhc.com/), which provides networks for care and is a commercial and employer-based insurance company. Third-party payers rarely pay 100% of a patient's bill. The cost of care is split between the insurance carrier and the patient. For example, most plans have a deductible that the patient must pay before the insurance company becomes responsible. Many of today's plans have high deductibles requiring the insured to pay up to $5000 out of pocket before the insurance company starts to cover costs. Some employers share this cost with employees to reduce their out-of-pocket expense. For example, for the employee who has a $3000 deductible, the employer reimburses the first $1500, making the remaining $1500 the employee's responsibility.

Examples of types of third-party payers include (Healthcare.gov, n.d.a):

- Managed care, also called Health Maintenance Organizations or HMOs, empanel healthcare providers to provide services at a lower cost. Patients must choose a permanent provider that is in network. Out-of-network coverage is not available, except in an emergency. If patients go out of network for routine care, they are responsible for 100% of the cost of services provided (Healthcare.gov, n.d.b).
- Preferred Provider Organizations or PPOs provide the insured with a wide choice of preferred providers and broader coverage. These plans cost more than HMOs and are even more expensive if patients go outside the network.
- Health Insurance Exchanges offer patients with no employer-provided insurance or who are self-employed with a marketplace to enroll in affordable health insurance that best meets their needs. Each plan provides core elements of preventative, wellness, ambulatory, obstetrics, mental health, rehabilitation, prescription drugs, emergency, and hospital services.
- High-deductible health plans provide a significant incentive to stay healthy for those who need less-expensive insurance.

Lastly, there is employer-based coverage that is partially or fully funded by the employer. The employer decides what services will be reimbursed and what will not be covered. Escalating costs and the need to control them continue to have significant impact on these businesses. There is concern about the high costs of health care and its impact on small business owners (Buttle et al., 2019).

APRNs must be knowledgeable about all types of coverage in order to plan to bill for their services.

BILLING FOR APRN SERVICES: UNDERSTANDING THE PROCESS

There are many steps APRNs must understand and take before they can see patients, document, code, and bill for services provided. The first step is acquiring knowledge of credentialing, including how to obtain a National Provider Identifier (NPI) number and hospital and insurance credentialing processes. Next is understanding utilization of Current Procedural Terminology (CPT) codes, which is the system used to document "what you do" during the patient encounter. The *International Classification of Diseases* (ICD) code is the "why you are doing" the CPT during the patient encounter (Rapsilber, 2019). Lastly, it is important to understand the nuances to billing appropriately. In total, use of this process results in a revenue stream that keeps a practice, hospital, or organization financially viable.

The Credentialing Process

Obtaining a National Provider Identifier Number

The first step in either hospital or insurance credentialing is to obtain an NPI number (CMS, 2021e). This 10-digit number is a Health Insurance Portability and Accountability Act (HIPAA) Administrative Standard established in 1996 (National Plan and Provider Enumeration System [NPPES], n.d.). The NPI number is a standard, unique number that is a required method of identification for each healthcare provider. Essentially, the individual NPI number functions as a "social security number" in the healthcare arena and is portable regardless of work location. NPIs may also be obtained for organizations such as clinics, practices, and hospitals. The CMS developed the NPPES to assign these unique identifiers. (For more information on obtaining an NPI number, visit https://nppes.cms.hhs.gov/NPPES/Welcome.do.) To apply for an NPI number you will need your Social Security number, date of birth, state nursing license (Certificate of Authority), and practice address(es) and phone and fax numbers. If you are completing the application for an NPI number prior to securing employment, you may use your home address but should update with your practice address as soon as possible (CMS, 2021e).

Hospital Credentialing

Credentialing is the process by which an agency deems a provider qualified to receive privileges to practice (The Joint Commission, 2012). The credentialing process ensures that the provider is competent and meets the necessary requirements to provide services within the organization. Hospital credentialing begins immediately upon hire. The APRN will need to supply information during the credentialing process that includes state licensure, verification of graduation from an approved program, copy of certification, a curriculum vitae, letters of recommendation, malpractice history, additional licensures or certificates (i.e., Controlled Dangerous Substances, Drug Enforcement Agency), educational degree(s), and training/education certificates (McMullen & Howie, 2020). The process may vary by facility, but usually once the application is complete and primary source credentials have been verified, the hospital's credentialing review board will grant or deny the provider privileges to deliver services within their organization. The credentialing process can be daunting and lengthy. To minimize delays and the risk of incomplete applications, it is important to keep well-organized and cataloged essential documentation and licensure information (see Box 19.1). Once privileges have been granted, the APRN will need to maintain ongoing records since recredentialing is required periodically, typically every 1 to 2 years or sooner for changes in information (Patel & Sharma, 2019).

BOX 19.1

Suggested Professional Portfolio Documents

- Education background/copies of degrees earned
- Professional references (at least three)
- Curriculum vitae including employment history
- Malpractice history including past and current policies and any claims information
- Current professional licensure
- Copy of national certification certificate
- Copy of driver's license
- Copy of birth certificate
- Copies of basic life support/advanced cardiac life support
- Collaborative practice agreement/letter of prescriptive authority approval from state board of nursing (if required in your practice state)
- Controlled Drug Substance number
- Drug Enforcement Agency number (if prescribing controlled substances)
- Certificates of procedural training/procedure logs
- Medicare, Medicaid, Council for Affordable Quality Health Care, NPI numbers
- Continuing education log

McMullen, P.C., & Howie, W. O. (2020). Credentialing and privileging: A primer for nurse practitioners. *The Journal for Nurse Practitioners, 16*, 91–95.

Credentialing and privileging are not synonymous. Privileging authorizes the APRN to provide services to patients within a specific scope of practice. APRNs must be cognizant of their scope of practice within the practice state. While the APRN may be credentialed within a specific hospital to perform a procedure, it may not fall within their scope of practice per state regulations. An organization may also further restrict an APRN from performing activities that are within their scope of practice even though the state law allows the APRN authority to perform. Specific patient care services are granted to the provider based on the qualifications verified during credentialing (McMullen & Howie, 2020).

Insurance Credentialing

Reimbursement for services provided is dependent on credentialing with insurance companies. The credentialing process for government agencies (i.e., Medicare, Medicaid) and private payers is very similar to that of hospital credentialing. Again, the purpose is to ensure that APRNs meet the necessary requirements and are appropriately qualified to provide the services for which they will be reimbursed. The required documents for insurance credentialing may vary slightly among payers, but there is basic information that is typical and similar to documentation that is required for hospital credentialing. As with hospital credentialing, it is necessary for the APRN who is billing for services to be intimately familiar with the scope of practice designated by that state's practice act. One of the major criteria for reimbursement listed by the CMS is that APRNs must be practicing within their scope of practice (CMS, 2021c).

Once the APRN has completed the credentialing process with the payer, the payer then determines whether to empanel the APRN as a provider of services to its beneficiaries. A contract between the APRN and the payer is established that determines rates, schedule of benefits, and performance covenants and defines the relationship between the APRN and payer (MedPac, 2019). Once the contract is finalized, the APRN is empaneled as a point of care provider for a panel of subscribers. Unfortunately, there are instances when a third-party payer will deny empanelment to a provider. Not all managed care organizations recognize APRNs as primary care providers. Therefore they will either refuse empanelment or, in states that require supervision or collaboration, will require a collaborating physician to also apply for credentialing (National Credentialing Solutions, n.d.).

In an effort to simplify the credentialing process, the Council for Affordable Quality Healthcare (CAQH; www.caqh.org) Universal Provider Datasource was created. CAQH is a multistakeholder collaboration of more than 120 organizations representing 75% of commercial insurers and Medicare and Medicaid and is designated by the Secretary of the Department of Health and Human Services. This service is provided at no charge and allows providers to create an online profile where professional and practice information can be entered and maintained. The information can then be accessed by payers, hospitals, large provider groups, and health systems with approval from the profile owner/provider. Utilizing the CAQH system greatly reduces the need to duplicate information on credentialing applications. Reattestation that the provider information is current and correct is required at a minimum of every 120 days. The system will notify the provider when it is time to reattest, highlight any missing or expired documents, and provide a log of activity on the provider's account. Accounts can be created on their website (CAQH Solutions, 2021).

Provider Panels and Contracts

The APRN must be credentialed and contracted with a billing entity (i.e., a third-party payer, Medicare or Medicaid) before they can provide patient services. Any missteps in the credentialing process can result in delays in payment. To become a provider, an APRN must apply to provide services for the beneficiaries of a health plan and may not bill for any services until they are credentialed and have a contract. The credentialing process may be completed by the APRN, an office manager, an administrative assistant, or other entity. The APRN should sign the application, including an attestation form, which verifies that the information is correct and true. If the APRN does not see these forms, they should question what insurance companies have credentialed them. It is recommended the APRN review credentialing information by logging on to the CAQH and verifying that the information listed is correct.

Provider contracts detail the specific terms by which the APRN will see patients and be reimbursed.

Contract terms typically include the application process, allowed reimbursement amounts and payment rates, the claim submission process, networks for referrals, and medical necessity. Many of these contracts have embedded legal terminology for amendments and termination clauses (LaPointe, 2018). Unlike federal programs, these contracts are negotiable. Understanding each contract is crucial to avoiding claim denials, acquiring new patients to the practice, and offering comprehensive (and reimbursable) patient services.

Medicare credentialing requires a separate application using the 855i form and cannot be completed through CAQH. This 25-page application is a comprehensive document listing education, training, any legal or disciplinary actions, practice information, billing, and assignment of benefits. An online application process can be found via the Internet-based Provider Enrollment Chain and Ownership System (PECOS) (https://pecos.cms.hhs.gov/providers/index.html). An 855r form reassigns benefits, meaning that you are authorizing the practice to bill and receive payment from Medicare on your behalf for the services you have rendered at the practice location. The APRN will have to notify insurers when they change their practice location or employer. This happens when you go through the credentialing process at the new practice. Notifying insurers ensures that the former practice can no longer bill under your NPI and name (see Fig. 19.2).

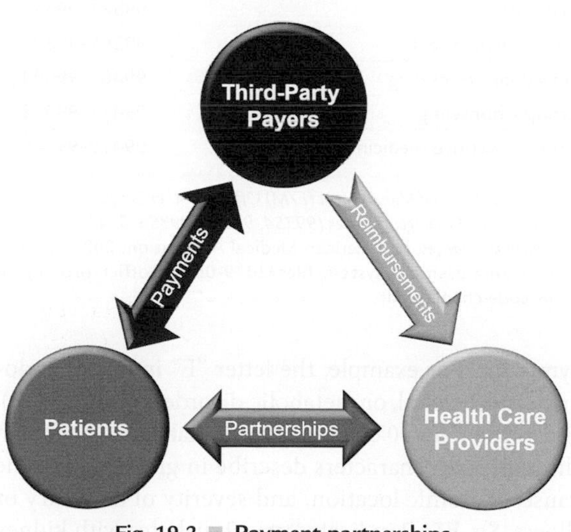

Fig. 19.2 ■ Payment partnerships.

Coding Sets

Once an APRN is credentialed and empaneled, they can bill and be reimbursed for their services. How do APRNs make sure they receive maximum reimbursement without engaging in fraudulent billing practices? The answer to that question is documentation. There are specific documentation requirements allowing providers to communicate with payers the services provided and for which they request reimbursement (CMS, 2021b). There are three main code sets that drive the reimbursement process: CPT codes, ICD classifications, and Healthcare Common Procedure Coding System (HCPCS). When documented in tandem, the CPT and ICD codes communicate a comprehensive picture of the patient and provider encounter. CPT and ICD codes are the most common codes the APRN will encounter. HCPCS codes are used to submit claims to Medicare and comprise two levels:

HCPS Level 1: Encompasses procedures and services provided by physicians, nonphysician providers, and other allied health professionals. These codes are synonymous with CPT codes.

HCPS Level 2: Is a standardized coding system used to identify products, supplies, and services (e.g., ambulance services) and durable medical equipment, prosthetics, orthotics, and supplies (CMS, 2020c).

Current Procedural Terminology Codes

CPT is an expansive list of codes that is developed, maintained, and copyrighted by the American Medical Association (AMA, 2021). These codes are used to describe evaluations, tests, surgeries, and medical procedures performed by a healthcare provider. There are six sections of CPT codes, including evaluation and management (E/M), anesthesiology, surgery, radiology, pathology and laboratory, and medicine. CPT codes are not only central to the billing and reimbursement of services but are also used by various agencies to track prevalence, performance, efficiency, and value of the provision of healthcare services (AMA, 2021). Having a comprehensive understanding of these codes is essential not only for reimbursement but for the value and visibility of APRN services in health care.

The E/M codes are the most commonly utilized CPT codes and define the services of evaluation and management of the patient's health condition during the provider–patient encounter (CMS, 2021b). These codes range from 99202 to 99499 (AMA, 2021) and cover a range of patient encounters in outpatient, inpatient, nursing home, and a variety of other settings. The appropriate CPT codes are selected based on category and subcategory of service (see Table 19.4 for common CPT codes). The E/M codes are utilized by qualified healthcare providers (i.e., physician, APRN) to request reimbursement for their services. Because E/M services are used in high volumes and are linked to reimbursement, it is important to maintain compliance with the current guidelines. Even minor errors can result in major payment issues, and if these errors are recurring, this can result in heightened scrutiny by the payer of the provider's billing and coding practices, sometimes resulting in fraudulent charges.

ICD-10 Coding

The *International Classification of Diseases* (ICD) tenth revision (ICD-10), updated in 2015, is a classification system maintained by the World Health Organization (WHO). ICD-10 coding uses unique alphanumeric codes to catalog specific diagnosis, symptoms, and procedures (WHO, n.d.). In the United States the National Center for Health Statistics and the Centers for Medicare and Medicaid Services (CMS), both federal agencies, are responsible for the use and annual updating of the ICD codes (CMS, 2016). The 2020 update is identified as ICD-10-CM (Clinical Modification; CMS, 2021a). ICD-11 codes were approved by the WHO in 2019 and are set to be released in 2022 once each country's agency has had the opportunity to translate and apply the codes (WHO, 2021).

The ICD tabular list consists of categories, subcategories, and codes (WHO, 2021). Chapters group disease processes together, and within the chapters, the disease processes are further divided into categories and subcategories with assigned codes used as identifiers. All codes have a minimum of three characters, with additional characters added to further specify the disease process, to a maximum of seven characters. The first character is an alpha character that indicates a group of diseases. The second and third characters are numeric, followed by a decimal with one, two, or three more numeric and/or alpha characters after the decimal. The first three characters categorize the disease/

TABLE 19.4
Common CPT Codes

Category/Subcategory	CPT Code(s)
Office or Other Outpatient Services	
New Patient	99201–99205
Established Patient	99211–99215
Hospital Observation Services	
Hospital Observation Care Discharge Services	99217
Initial Observation Care	99218–99220
Hospital Inpatient Services	
Initial Hospital Care	99211–99223
Subsequent Hospital Care	99231–99233
Observation or Inpatient Care Services (including admission and discharge services)	99234–99236
Hospital Discharge Services	99238–99239
Consultation Services	
Office Consultations	99241–99245
Inpatient Consultations	99251–99255
Emergency Department Services	99281–99288
Critical Care Services	
Adult (over 24 months of age)	99291–99292
Pediatric	99293–99294
Neonatal	99295–99296
Continuing Care, Very Low Birth Weight Infant, Low Birth Weight Infant, Normal Weight Newborn	99298–99300
Preventive Medicine Services	
New Patient	99381–99387
Established Patient	99391–99397
Individual Counseling	99401–99404
Group Counseling	99411–99412
Other Preventive Medicine Services	99420–99440

CPT® Evaluation and Management (E/M) Office or Other Outpatient (99202-99215) and Prolonged Services (99354, 99355, 99356, 99417) Code and Guideline Changes, by American Medical Association, 2021, https://www.ama-assn.org/system/files/2019-06/cpt-office-prolonged-svs-code-changes.pdf

symptom. For example, the letter "E" indicates endocrine, nutritional, or metabolic disorders (CMS, 2016); E11 is the ICD-10 code for type 2 diabetes. The fourth through sixth characters describe in greater detail the cause, anatomic location, and severity of an injury or illness. So, E11.2 indicates type 2 diabetes with kidney complications; E11.21 is even more specific indicating type 2 diabetes with diabetic nephropathy. For certain codes, there may be a seventh character used to signify a treatment encounter as initial, subsequent, or sequela (late effect). The longer the number, the more specific the information (CMS, 2016).

Following the ICD coding pattern, you can see how this system serves as a very valuable form of medical communication. Assigning one or more ICD-10 codes to a patient communicates to anyone reading the chart (including billers) the patient's active diagnosis, clinical condition, and plan of care. In addition to medical communication, there are other reasons why designating the most specific and accurate code to the patient encounter is important. These codes, along with CPT codes, guide reimbursement for medical expenses and allow for tracking the incidence and prevalence of diseases, reasons for encounters, factors that influence health status, external causes of disease, and mortality rates (WHO, 2021).

Having the most detailed ICD code possible will help ensure that you are reimbursed appropriately for your service. There are some codes that are considered "unbillable" and are not eligible for reimbursement, such as telephone calls. Reimbursement will be rejected if an invalid code is used. Additionally, reimbursement may be rejected if the ICD code does not align with the CPT code. When CPT codes are out of alignment with ICD codes, it means that the particular service billed would not normally be provided for that diagnosis (e.g., coding the performance of a skin biopsy under a diagnosis code of diabetic nephropathy; CMS, 2016). Codes for signs and symptoms of a disease are appropriate when a related definitive diagnosis has not yet been established. Codes with "not otherwise specified" or "unspecified" terms (e.g., asthma, unspecified) may also result in denied reimbursement.

Regardless of the diagnosis code, there should be sufficient information documented in the medical record to support the clinical knowledge of the patient's health condition. In other words, each healthcare encounter should be coded to the level of clinical information and certainty obtained by the provider, thereby justifying reimbursement for services provided (CMS, 2016, 2020c).

Health statistics globally rely on the accurate assignment of ICD-10 codes to patient charts (WHO, n.d.). The universality of a common language (ICD-10) for diagnosis of diseases and the utilization of electronic health records has made it much easier to (1) store and retrieve health information for analysis and evidence-based decision making; (2) share and compare health information between hospitals, regions, settings, and countries; and (3) compare data in the same location across different time periods. From ICD codes assigned in patient records, morbidity and mortality statistics are tracked and reported. Consider the new (as of April 2020) ICD-10 code U07.0: vaping-related disorders. ICD codes for vaping were not needed 20 years ago, because e-cigarettes, and thus vaping, had not been invented. With the addition of these vaping codes, we will be able to track morbidity and mortality rates related to vaping (WHO, n.d.).

Patient care outcomes, treatment plans, and potential for harm are also dependent on the accuracy and specificity of the ICD code added to the patient record. Once the code is added, it will follow the patient in their medical record across settings. For example, whether the patient has migraine with or without aura will determine whether that patient is prescribed an oral contraceptive at a later visit. Having the most specific and accurate code possible for the patient will assist providers in making clinical decisions and measuring outcomes and care provided to patients. Adding a diagnosis to the chart is more than just random selection. It requires thoughtful prudence to ensure that the patient does not have an inaccurate diagnosis that follows them through the healthcare system (CMS, 2016). Explaining every nuance of intricate billing practice for every setting and situation is beyond the feasible context of this chapter. But it is extremely important that APRNs seek guidance and education on billing and coding relative to their practice setting (LaPointe, 2017). Ultimately, you, as the provider, are legally responsible for assigning the appropriate codes according to the services provided and knowing how your NPI is being utilized.

Outpatient Billing

Evaluation and management (E/M) codes for the outpatient clinical setting are the most frequent codes used by certified nurse practitioners and certified nurse-midwives. In January 2021, the E/M selection of codes in the outpatient setting changed. Revisions made by the AMA were aimed at reducing the administrative burden on documentation and coding, decreasing the need for auditing, decreasing unnecessary documentation, and ensuring that payments are resource based. In the revised version, the complex counting and documentation of elements for history, physical exam, and date were removed. Rather, code selection is determined based on the level of medical decision making or the total time for services performed on the date of the encounter (AMA, 2021). Additionally, the underutilized code 99201 (new patient) has been deleted. While the new guidelines will afford more flexibility, documentation is still important in justifying the choice of E/M code (CMS, 2020b).

In the outpatient clinical setting, the first step in determining the most appropriate code is to identify the patient as a new or established patient. There are two questions to consider when deciding whether a patient is new (99202–99205) or established (99211–99215; CMS, 2020b):

1. Has the patient ever received professional face-to-face services from this provider?
2. Has the patient received professional services at the practice location within the previous 3 years?

Consider these examples:

- If the patient has not received professional services from this provider and/or same specialty in your practice in the previous 3 years, then they are considered a new patient.
- If the patient has received services at the practice but is new to this provider, they are considered an established patient.
- If the patient has received services from this provider but at a different practice, they are considered a new patient.

Once the CPT code is established, the next step is to determine whether to code the visit based on the level of complexity or the total time spent (AMA, 2021).

Medical Decision Making

Determining a code based on medical decision making requires the provider to determine the complexity of establishing a diagnosis and/or selecting a management option. At the time of the encounter, there are three elements to consider in determining the level of medical complexity: (1) the number and complexity of problems addressed (*chronic disease and acute problems*), (2) the amount and/or complexity of data reviewed and analyzed (*including medical records, imaging and laboratory testing*), and (3) the risk of complications, morbidity, and/or mortality of patient management decisions made at the visit, associated with the patient's problem(s) *(any disease which is relevant to the visit can add value)*, the diagnostic procedure(s), and treatment(s). Based on these three elements, the provider will determine whether the complexity of medical decision making is straightforward, low, moderate, or high (AMA, 2021). The E/M code in which the patient encounter meets or exceeds two of the three elements will signal the choice of coding for that visit. As part of the updated guidelines, definitions and examples for criteria within each of the three elements were provided by the AMA (AMA, 2021). (See Table 19.5.)

As stated previously, documentation should accurately reflect the services performed and justify the level of evaluation and management code selected. While documenting specific elements in the history and physical, review of systems, and physical examination is not required, the documentation in each of those areas should be pertinent, relevant, and medically appropriate. The plan of care, CPT codes, and ICD codes should be in alignment and sufficient to be justifiable. Specific rules are described in the evaluation and management services documentation guidelines (CMS, 2020b; see Fig. 19.3).

Time-Based Billing

Establishing the level of visit using time-based billing in the outpatient clinical setting received an update as part of the AMA 2021 guidelines (AMA, 2021). Previously, using time-based billing required that the entirety of the visit be dominated by counseling or coordination of care. That is no longer the case. Determining the level of E/M code may be based solely on time spent; however, there are criteria that must be met. For example, the time must be spent on the date of the face-to-face encounter and may include activities that were non-face-to-face activities (such as reviewing previous diagnostics or hospital records) prior to the visit plus time spent on the face-to-face encounter. It does not include time spent by office staff or time spent on any other calendar day. If services provided extend beyond the maximum total time, a separate

TABLE 19.5

Elements of Medical Decision Making for New/Established Patients

E/M Code New/ Established	99202/99212 Straightforward	99203/99213 Low	99204/99214 Moderate	99205/99215 High
Number and complexity of problems addressed	Minimal ■ One self-limited or minor problem	Low ■ Two or more self-limited or minor problems; or ■ one stable chronic illness; or ■ one acute, uncomplicated illness or injury	Moderate ■ One or more chronic illnesses with exacerbation, progression, or side effects of treatment; or ■ two or more stable chronic illnesses; or ■ one undiagnosed new problem with uncertain prognosis; or ■ one acute illness with systemic symptoms; or ■ one acute complicated injury	High ■ One or more chronic illnesses with severe exacerbation, progression, or side effects of treatment; or ■ one acute or chronic illness or injury that poses a threat to life or bodily function
Amount and/or complexity of data to be reviewed	Minimal or none	Limited (must meet criteria of at least one of two categories)	Moderate (must meet criteria of at least one of three categories)	Extensive (must meet the criteria of at least two of three categories)
	CATEGORY 1: TESTS, DOCUMENTS, OR INDEPENDENT HISTORIAN			
	N/A	*Any combination of two:* ■ Review of prior external note(s) from each unique source ■ Review of the result(s) of each unique source ■ Ordering of each unique test	*Any combination of three:* ■ Review of prior external note(s) from each unique source ■ Review of the result(s) of each unique test ■ Ordering of each unique test ■ Assessment requiring an independent historian(s)	*Any combination of three:* ■ Review of prior external note(s) from each unique source ■ Review of the result(s) of each unique test ■ Ordering of each unique test ■ Assessment requiring an independent historian(s)
	CATEGORY 2: INDEPENDENT INTERPRETATION OF TESTS			
		■ Assessment requiring an independent historian(s) *(See moderate/high for independent interpretation of tests)*	*Independent interpretation of tests* ■ Independent interpretation of a test performed by another physician/other qualified healthcare professional (not separately reported)	*Independent interpretation of tests* ■ Independent interpretation of a test performed by another physician/other qualified healthcare professional (not separately reported)

Continued

TABLE 19.5

Elements of Medical Decision Making for New/Established Patients—cont'd

E/M Code New/ Established	99202/99212 Straightforward	99203/99213 Low	99204/99214 Moderate	99205/99215 High
	CATEGORY 3: DISCUSSION OF MANAGEMENT OR TEST INTERPRETATION			
	N/A	N/A	■ Discussion of management or test interpretation with external physician/other qualified healthcare professional/ appropriate source (not separately reported)	■ Discussion of management or test interpretation with external physician/ other QHP/ appropriate source (not separately reported)
Risk of complications and/or morbidity or mortality of patient management	Minimal risk of morbidity from additional diagnostic testing or treatment	Low risk of morbidity from additional diagnostic testing or treatment	Moderate risk of morbidity from additional diagnostic testing or treatment Examples only: ■ Prescription drug management ■ Decision regarding minor surgery with identified patient or procedure risk factors ■ Decision regarding elective major surgery without identified patient or procedure risk factors ■ Diagnosis or treatment significantly limited by social determinants of health	High risk of morbidity from additional diagnostic testing or treatment Examples only: ■ Drug therapy requiring intensive monitoring for toxicity ■ Decision regarding elective major surgery with identified patient or procedure risk factors ■ Decision regarding emergency major surgery ■ Decision regarding hospitalization ■ Decision not to resuscitate or to deescalate care because of poor prognosis

Billing & Coding in the Outpatient Clinical Setting: A Quick Reference, by K. Baldridge, 2021, Advanced Practice Education Associates.

code can be applied reflecting that additional time was spent. Coding for time in the inpatient setting did not change.

Documentation of time must reflect the services performed and the time spent but does not require itemization of the activities. However, it must be reflective of the services rendered. The new guidelines (AMA, 2021) provide examples of activities that may be included in the non-face-to-face and face-to-face time (See Table 19.6). Example activities of

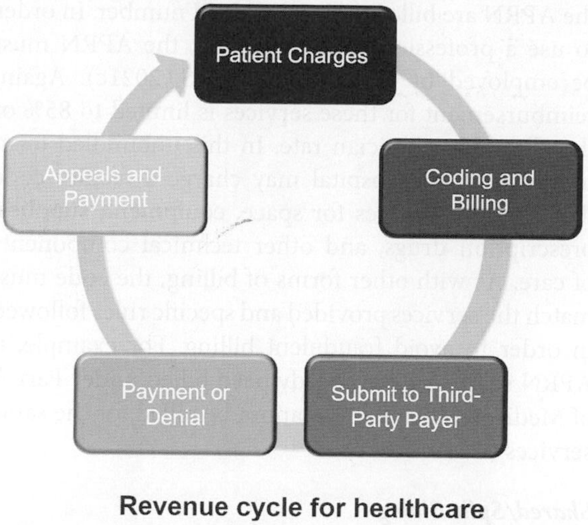

Fig. 19.3 ■ **Revenue cycle for health care.**

non-face-to-face and face-to-face activities include preparing to see the patient (e.g., review of tests); obtaining and/or reviewing a previously obtained history; performing a medically appropriate examination or evaluation; counseling and educating the patient/family/caregiver; ordering medications, tests and/or procedures; referring and communicating with other health care professionals; documenting clinical information in the EHR; independently interpreting results and communicating results to patient/family/caregiver, and care coordination (AMA, 2021).

Modifiers

A modifier is used when additional or more specific information is needed to describe services. Consider a "modifier" in the English language. This helps to explain the who, what, where, when, and how of a story. A CPT modifier provides the same in the medical language and may be used to indicate whether a provider performed multiple procedures, explain why a service was medically necessary, or note the location on the patient where a procedure was performed. Some modifiers do affect reimbursement, whereas others are for information only. CPT modifiers are added to the end of a CPT code with a hyphen. They are always two characters, either numeric or alphanumeric (CMS, 2021d).

Modifier 25 is one of the most commonly used modifiers. When modifier 25 is added, it indicates that two separate but significant services were provided by the same provider on the same day. For example, a patient is seen for follow-up of chronic hypertension but during the same visit, the patient complains of an acute shoulder injury. The APRN determines that a shoulder injection is needed and performs this injection during the same visit. Billing an E/M and the procedure on the same day with a modifier 25 appended to the E/M would be appropriate (CMS, 2021b).

Inpatient Billing

Hospital billing and coding follow the same principles as outpatient billing codes in that the code set allotted

TABLE 19.6
E/M Coding Based on Time for New/Established Patient

E/M Coding Based on Time (Non-Face-to-Face PLUS Face-to-Face)

New Patient	Total Time	Established Patient	Total Time
99201	Deleted code	99211	No encounter with NP. Clinical staff face-to-face time (e.g., nurse visit)
99202	15–29 minutes	99212	10–19 minutes
99203	30–44 minutes	99213	20–29 minutes
99204	45–59 minutes	99214	30–39 minutes
99205	60–74 minutes	99215	40–54 minutes
+G2212	Each additional 15 minutes after 74 minutes[a]	+G2212	Each additional 15 minutes after 54 minutes[a]

[a]+G2212: For both Medicare patients and other non-Medicare patients per payer policy.
Billing & Coding in the Outpatient Clinical Setting: A Quick Reference, by K. Baldridge, 2021, Advanced Practice Education Associates.

drives the documentation required for that patient (CMS, 2020a). In the hospital setting, it is crucial to recognize the differences between billing and coding and how those processes are connected in order to receive payment. Medical coding is the process by which billable information is extracted from the medical record and clinical documentation. Those codes are then used to create insurance claims and bills for patients. There are several distinctions that are specific for hospital and inpatient billing (CMS, 2021c).

Bundled Billing

Bundled payments are an arrangement found in the inpatient setting. With bundled payments, services provided by multiple providers are combined under one episode of care and thus the facility is reimbursed in a single payment. The payment is usually predetermined for a set diagnosis (LaPointe, 2016). For example, if the patient is having a cholecystectomy, the hospital, surgeon, and anesthesia services are bundled and assigned a set fee. If the procedure costs exceed the set reimbursement fee, the hospital, surgeon, and anesthesia services must absorb the remainder of the cost. The purpose of bundled payments is to encourage efficiencies and provider communication in order to provide cost-effective care. Bundling is not without its challenges. For example, the ability to contain costs associated with a procedure is often beyond the control of the providers (e.g., cost of supplies) or the needs of the patient proved to be greater than the preset cost of the procedure. As reimbursement for services moves toward a more value-based model, bundling of healthcare costs is likely to increase. CMS has even taken steps toward bundling payments across facilities; the Comprehensive Care for Joint Replacement model is designed to improve the care coordination between hospitals, skilled nursing facilities, rehabilitation centers, and home health agencies. This bundled reimbursement structure would focus on the episode of care for the patient (i.e., the joint replacement) rather than the individual services required (Gruessner, 2016).

Independent Billing

The independent billing option is another form of coding for inpatient care. It may also be referred to as *unbundling*. In this model, services provided solely by the APRN are billed under their NPI number. In order to use a profession code on billing, the APRN must be employed by the hospital (CMS, 2021c). Again, reimbursement for these services is limited to 85% of the allowable physician rate. In this unbundled form of payment, the hospital may charge a facility code that captures charges for space, equipment, supplies, prescription drugs, and other technical components of care. As with other forms of billing, the code must match the services provided and specific rules followed in order to avoid fraudulent billing. For example, if APRN services have already been billed under Part A of Medicare, then Part B cannot be billed for the same services (CMS, 2021c).

Shared/Split Billing

Shared/split service is another form of billing that may occur. In this form of billing, two providers from the same group may perform a service for the same patient on the same calendar day (CMS, 2021c). If the shared/split billing criteria are met and appropriately documented, then CMS will allow the visit to be combined and reported under a single provider's NPI. Shared/split billing only recognizes E/M services that are provided in emergency departments, outpatient hospital clinics, or inpatient hospitals (excluding critical care services and procedures). Requirements that must be met for this type of billing include:

1. Services are rendered by the attending physician and nurse practitioners, clinical nurse specialists, and certified nurse-midwives.
2. The attending physician and the APRN must be part of the same group practice (e.g., employed by the same cardiology group or contracted to supply services for the same hospitalist group).
3. Services provided should be reasonable and necessary and allowed by the state scope of practice.

In order to induce the correct billing codes, the face-to-face encounter of the physician must be linked to the APRN's face-to-face encounter and documentation. The physician's note must reflect their involvement in the plan of care for the patient. There is no specific length of time required for the face-to-face encounters (CMS, 2021c). Simply agreeing with the APRN's plan and cosignature by the physician do not meet this criterion (Rapsilber, 2019).

Subsequent Hospital Visits

When the provider bills for subsequent hospital visits, the documentation must clearly reflect the need for continued care. Documentation should include at least two of the three key components of the E/M code (i.e., history, physical examination, or medical decision making) and should reflect the patient's status, evolution of medical decision making, and collaboration with other providers and specialists and must support the service provided (Palmetto GBA, 2018). Time-based billing for counseling and/or coordination of care may be billed but must dominate more than 50% of the encounter and follow the same guidelines as time-based billing in the outpatient setting (refer to time-based billing section; CMS, 2021c).

Critical Care Codes

Justification for the use of critical care codes includes medical conditions that impair one or more vital organ systems and/or a high probability that the patient's condition is life-threatening or in imminent threat of deterioration (CMS, 2021c). Critical care services are billed according to time spent caring for the critically ill patient. This is distinctly different from other types of billing. A minimum of 30 minutes, including both direct and indirect patient care time, is required (Dodd & Fan, 2017). Direct patient care is the time spent obtaining the key components of history, physical examination, and medical decision making. Indirect patient care time, including interpreting studies, discussing the case with consultants or admitting teams, retrieving data and reviewing charts, documenting the visit, and performing bundled procedures, should be factored into the critical care time recorded. The provider should be aware of which procedures are bundled in the critical care time and which procedures are billed separately (Dodd & Fan, 2017). It is important to note that critical care time additive may only be billed once per day per patient, does not need to be continuous, and requires direct involvement and documentation by an attending physician (CMS, 2021c).

Revenue Cycle Management

Following the cycle of revenue through the system helps APRNs understand the many steps required to ensure correct billing and proper payment. The patient is in the middle of this process and may incur charges that are not covered by the insurance provider. The APRN is responsible and accountable for what is documented, coded, and billed and must ensure that all services provided during the encounter are captured and that all charges are accounted for and documented correctly (Fig. 19.3).

Walking through the patient visit process can demonstrate the required key components. The registration process is a first critical step to make sure that the patient's demographic and insurance information are correct and current. Insurance coverage can lapse or change from the time an appointment is made to when the patient arrives at the office. Checking and verifying patient insurance information for every patient encounter is important. Accurate information is key to prevent delays in payment.

Co-pays must be collected at the time of service and are never waived as part of the contractual arrangement between the insurance company and the insured. Failure to collect the co-pay is viewed as fraudulent practice.

The APRN performs the necessary history and physical exam and determines the treatment plan, which is documented in the patient's medical record. CPT and ICD codes are selected and submitted for payment. Claims are submitted electronically typically through an electronic claims submission process located within the electronic healthcare record (EHR). Insurance companies typically reimburse the provider directly and, as previously stated, the APRN reassigns the payment to the practice unless the APRN is the practice owner. When the APRN changes employment, payment assignment changes as well. Payment reconciliation ensures that the cycle of reimbursement is complete.

The goal is to submit a "clean claim" for payment the first time. Denials of payment often occur when information is submitted erroneously. Reasons for denials vary and include lack of or incorrect diagnosis code, omission of key patient data requirements such as insurance numbers, omission of a level of service, or the provider is not appropriately credentialed and therefore not allowed to bill for the services. Failure to remediate these claims can adversely affect a practice revenue stream.

Use of electronic medical records (EMRs) is commonplace in the delivery of healthcare services and streamlines the reimbursement process. The APRN should document under their own login and password within the EMR. The EMR will formulate a visit level for billing; however, the APRN should be wary of its accuracy, because any narrative documentation cannot be captured by the EMR and may result in undercoding a visit. Cutting and pasting or copying a previous encounter should be entertained with reservation, because each patient encounter should be unique. Templates can save time documenting in the EMR and can be utilized as prompts to reinforce proper billing for a service. Examples of documentation templates include Medicare Annual Wellness Visit, Review of Systems (ROS) and Physical exam (e.g., well-woman, abdominal pain, back pain). APRNs should avoid cosignature of documents unless it is required by law. A physician cosigning an APRN's documentation does not count as supervision. If the APRN is doing the majority of the work, the APRN should take billing credit as well.

VALUE-BASED AND FEE-FOR-SERVICE MODELS

Reimbursement for healthcare services began as an FFS model where a set fee was reimbursed to a provider for services rendered. This model of payment allows healthcare providers to charge based on individual services (e.g., appointments, treatments, tests ordered, prescriptions given). Services are itemized on billing statements, often making them long and complicated. This model has resulted in many providers taking on more and more patients to gain revenue, placing the emphasis on the quantity of services, rather than the quality of services provided to their patients. This often leads to unnecessary care and increases the cost to deliver health care. The FFS model eventually became unsustainable.

Resource-Based Relative Value Scale

The resource-based relative value scale (RBRVS) is a new method of reimbursement developed to encompass all work required for a provider to render services to a patient. There are three components to this system: (1) provider time and/or work effort, (2) resources of the practice, and (3) provider liability. These are calculated in a formula to determine payment (Hsiao et al., 1988; see Fig. 19.4). A relative value unit (RVU) is a measure of productivity. There are RVUs associated with work effort, practice expense, and malpractice. Work effort includes all provider tasks encompassing the time spent providing the hands-on care to a patient. A geographic practice cost index (GPCI) refers to the cost to deliver care based on location of the care. For example, it is more costly to deliver care in California than in Alabama; therefore payments take these differences into consideration. Practice expense includes the costs to do business, such as office rent, utilities, supplies, technology (e.g., EHR), and employee costs. A conversion factor changes annually based upon factors calculated by CMS. The resulting payment rate can be 100% for a physician, 85% for an APRN, or another payment rate that is negotiated. Even the RBRVS method of reimbursement is flawed. Reimbursement is based upon productivity or how much the provider does for a patient, rather than health outcomes from the provision of quality care. Exemplar 19.1 addresses possible issues with the "gaming" of the RBRVS system.

Value-Based Payments

Value-based payment is poised to replace the current FFS model, with an emphasis on provision of quality care and keeping patients healthy. This system of reimbursement is embraced by the CMS, with a firm commitment to transition to this model as the payment model of the future. The value-based payment model was born from the Medicare Access and CHIP Reauthorization Act (MACRA) of 2015 (CMS, 2019; MACRA, 2015), bipartisan legislation signed into law on April 16, 2015. MACRA created the Quality Payment Program (QPP), which repeals the Sustainable Growth Rate formula and changes the way that Medicare rewards clinicians for value over volume and streamlines multiple quality programs under the new Merit-Based Incentive Payments System (MIPS; CMS, 2017). MIPS is for smaller practices that receive bonus payments based on quality care rendered to Medicare beneficiaries. There is an opportunity to receive bonus payments by taking on more financial risk under alternative payment models (APMs). APMs tend to be typically larger practices or healthcare entities.

The premise of value-based payment is to reward quality care by keeping beneficiaries healthy. APRNs

CONVERTING AN RBRVS TO A DOLLAR AMOUNT

$$(\text{Work RVU} \times \text{Work GPCI}) +$$
$$(\text{Practice Expense RVU} \times \text{Practice Expense GPCI}) +$$
$$(\text{Malpractice RVU} \times \text{Malpractice GPCI}) \times$$
$$\text{Conversion factor} \times \text{Practitioner Payment Rate}$$
$$= \underline{\textit{Allowed Amount}}$$

RVU = relative value unit

GPCI = geographic practice cost indices

Making Sense of the Dollars and Cents Presentation © 2019 L Rapzilber

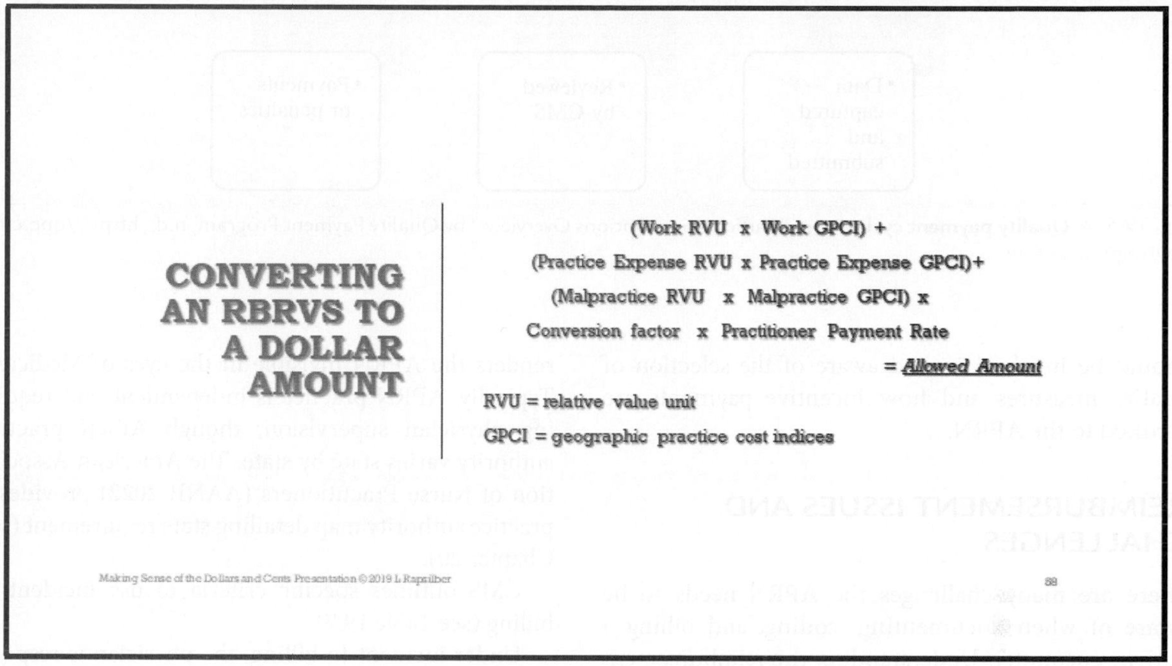

Fig. 19.4 ■ Resource-based relative value scale payment.

EXEMPLAR 19.1
SUSPICION OF FRAUD

Peter is a family nurse practitioner who has a few years of experience practicing in an office setting. During that time, he knew he had to improve his understanding of reimbursement procedures. To that end, he attended classes and worked with his office manager to understand the reports on his productivity. After a year, he moved and joined a practice in a busy metropolitan city. He continued to follow the suggestion of his former office manager who recommended that he keep track of all his services, including ICD-10 and CPT codes. Initially he did not receive any productivity reports from his new officer manager. When he inquired why he was not receiving reports, the response was, "It was not required." This response did not satisfy Peter and he continued to pursue this issue. He spoke with the other NP in the practice but there was no concern for the lack of information. He decided that he would meet with one of the physicians who owned the practice and discuss the lack of productivity reports. The physician's response was similar to the office manager's, and he tried to explain to Peter that he did not need to be concerned about productivity.

The physician assured Peter that he was providing excellent care and improving patient outcomes. Peter remained uncomfortable with this lack of data and was finally able to obtain a report of his activity. To his surprise, the report did not match the data that he was keeping about his billing practices. It seemed that the office was documenting higher levels of care, which was disturbing to Peter.

WHAT SHOULD PETER DO?

The best option for Peter would be to meet with the physician owners of the practice and discuss his concerns. This could have been an unintentional error, which should be easily clarified. However, if this was intentional upgrading of services, this is a fraudulent practice. If there were an investigation of billing practices of this practice, even though Peter did not upgrade the codes, he would be held responsible. This is a very difficult position for an NP to be in, but if there is no clarification or resolution of questionable billing practices, Peter should resign his position and should report these improper practices to CMS.

already provide high-quality care with the focus on disease prevention and health promotion, making this payment model attractive for many practices. Quality measures are selected and reported, and incentive payments are dispersed in a 3-year cycle based on quality benchmark achievements (see Fig. 19.5). APRNs

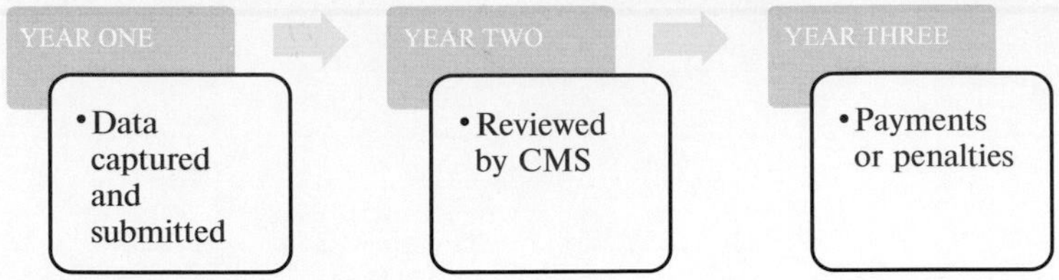

Fig. 19.5 ■ **Quality payment cycle.** From "Participation Options Overview," by Quality Payment Program, n.d., https://qpp.cms.gov/mips/overview

should be involved in and aware of the selection of quality measures and how incentive payments are credited to the APRN.

REIMBURSEMENT ISSUES AND CHALLENGES

There are many challenges the APRN needs to be aware of when documenting, coding, and billing a patient encounter. Understanding the reimbursement process is critical to understanding the financial and legal implications for a practice. Failure to understand these concepts can put the APRN at risk.

APRNS must seek to understand how a practice is billing for their services. This is rarely taught in school and is minimally addressed during job orientation. Sadly, this is the foundation of fiscal responsibility for an APRN to a practice, and lack of knowledge can be detrimental to the patient, APRN, or their practice/employer. Specifically, the APRN should know the difference between the rendering provider and the billing provider, which is important to payers. The rendering provider is the one providing the services to the patient for that encounter. The billing provider is the one authorized to receive payment. Ideally, the rendering and billing provider should be the same provider.

Incident-To Billing

Incident-to billing refers to billing for services or supplies that are incident to the provision of services by or under supervision of a physician. Incident-to billing is only applicable in the outpatient clinical setting (CMS, 2020c). Services that are provided by the APRN are billed under a physician's NPI number, which allows for 100% reimbursement, rather than the 85% allotted for APRN services. Essentially, the incident-to billing renders the APRN invisible in the eyes of Medicare. Typically, APRN practice is independent, not requiring physician supervision, though APRN practice authority varies state by state. The American Association of Nurse Practitioners (AANP, 2022) provides a practice authority map detailing state requirement (see Chapter 20).

CMS outlines specific criteria to use incident-to billing (see Table 19.7).

Under incident-to billing, the physician is responsible to execute the treatment plan upon the initial patient visit. The APRN may see the patient in follow-up care provided that there are no new problems to evaluate. The physician must be in the office at the time of the patient visit, not necessarily seeing the patient but to be available for any questions or render assistance to the APRN (i.e., implied supervision). The physician must have ongoing active care of the patient, meaning that the physician must see the patient in intervals to reassess the treatment plan. Only the physician can implement treatment plan changes under incident-to billing. If the APRN is seeing a new Medicare patient, billing must be under the APRN's NPI.

While incident-to billing results in higher reimbursement, it is not always the best option for the patient or for the practice. If a patient presents to the APRN for follow-up of hypertension but also has a new complaint of sinus congestion, the APRN recognized a new problem, which does not meet incident-to billing. The APRN has a choice: see the patient and consult with the supervising physician to approve a change in the treatment plan (this scenario is not the most efficient business practice) or provide and document the care and submit under the APRN's NPI. The 15% gained when billing incident-to is not likely to cover the time spent by both providers in the care of one patient, creating a revenue loss in this

TABLE 19.7
Incident-To Billing Criteria

Criteria Description	Criteria Fulfilled
Direct supervision by a physician	In the office suite, does not need to see the patient
Physician must perform the initial service	Physician develops the treatment plan
Physician must have active involvement	Physician must see the patient periodically
Patient cannot have new problem	There can be no change to the treatment plan if the APRN sees the patient
APRN must be employed by Physician	Must receive a W-2, leased or independent contractor

"Incident-to Services," by MLN Matters, 2016, Centers for Medicare and Medicaid Services, https://www.cms.gov/outreach-and-education/medicare-learning-network-mln/mlnmattersarticles/downloads/se0441.pdf

EXEMPLAR 19.2
INCIDENT-TO BILLING

Ms. Beatty is a nurse practitioner who sees patients in the office of an internal medicine practice. D.H., a 66-year-old male, covered under Medicare, presents to the office as a new patient for evaluation of increasing shortness of breath. In addition, he has a history significant for hypertension and diabetes. Initially, the office staff schedule D.H. to be seen by Ms. Beatty, but because D.H. is new to the practice and the billing is to be done under the "incident-to" rules, he can only be seen by the physician, Dr. Waters. Dr. Waters does the initial history and physical examination, followed by writing orders for some laboratory and diagnostic testing. He codes the visit as a 99204 (office visit–new patient), submits the bill, and receives 100% reimbursement of the physician fee schedule. He has D.H. schedule a return visit in 2 weeks. Because the plan of care has been established, D.H. is scheduled to be seen by Ms. Beatty. She sees D.H., does a focused history and physical examination, and reviews the results of the tests. Dr. Waters is in the office at the time D.H. is seen. Ms. Beatty codes the visit as a 99213 (office visit–established). The requirements for "incident-to" have been met and the bill is submitted under the physician's number and is reimbursed at 100%. Ms. Beatty schedules the patient to return again in 1 month. During this encounter, Dr. Waters had to leave the office for a meeting. Ms. Beatty does a focused history and physical examination again and codes the visit as a 99213 (office visit–established). Because Dr. Waters is not in the office, the rules for "incident-to" have not been met and the visit must be submitted under Ms. Beatty's number, who is reimbursed at 85% of the physician fee schedule.

A second patient, A.G., is a 73-year-old female who is covered under Medicare and has a history of coronary artery disease presenting to the same internal medicine practice as a new patient due to the fact that her original primary care provider retired. Dr. Waters was busy seeing other patients, so the staff asks whether Ms. Beatty can see the patient. Ms. Beatty agrees, performs a detailed history and physical examination, and bills the visit as a 99204 (office visit–new patient). Even though Dr. Waters is in the office, Ms. Beatty submits the bill under her own number as the rules for "incident-to" billing have not been met (i.e., a physician must see all new patients to establish the plan of care). Reimbursement, in this case, will be at 85%.

scenario. See Exemplar 19.2 for a detailed example of an "incident-to" visit.

Various agencies, including the Medicare Payment Advisory Commission (MedPAC), an independent congressional agency established to advise the United States Congress on issues affecting the Medicare program (MedPac, 2019), and AANP advise that APRNs bill directly for services provided and advocate for the abolishment of incident-to billing (AANP, 2017). It behooves the APRN to identify when this type of billing method is being utilized and question whether there is a suspicion with accuracy since if any of the criteria are not met it can constitute fraudulent billing.

APRNs have a professional obligation to be vigilant in avoiding unethical and fraudulent billing practices. However, the most likely cause of fraudulent billing among APRNs is lack of knowledge (CMS, 2021d). When this occurs, ignorance is not bliss, nor is it a suitable defense in healthcare fraud.

Common activities associated with healthcare fraud include billing for no-show appointments, submitting claims for services at a higher complexity (*upcoding*) or a lower complexity (*downcoding*) than was provided or documented, billing for services not rendered, and inappropriate use of incident-to billing. Regardless of setting, maintaining a proper compliance program, including chart audits and peer reviews, will help reduce the chances of fraudulent billing. However, if documentation does not accurately reflect the level of care provided, the codes will be incorrect (CMS, 2021d).

Any of the examples of fraudulent billing in Box 19.2 can result in financial consequences, loss of revenue, potential audit or worse, exclusion from participation in programs, potential fines, and jail time. It bears repeating: the APRN is responsible for accountable documentation, E/M coding, and billing for each patient encounter.

Liability/Malpractice Insurance

As an APRN, you have increasing responsibilities in patient care and treatment and thus increased risk of malpractice claims. While generating revenue is essential, it is also necessary to ensure that your livelihood is protected against potential malpractice allegations.

A malpractice policy helps to protect you against liability that may occur as a result of rendering—or failure to render—appropriate medical services. A typical malpractice policy will cover the costs of (1) investigating claims, (2) defense of those claims, and (3) legal settlement or court judgment against the insured (up to policy limits). There are a wide variety of settings and specialties, and states vary in their rules and regulations for APRNs; therefore it is important to ensure that you are covered adequately (e.g., different specialties carry higher risks; Flynn, 2017). The cost of malpractice coverage varies according to role,

BOX 19.2

Examples of Fraudulent Billing Practices

- **Overcoding** (Upcoding) results in being reimbursed at a higher rate than the documentation supports. Embellishing the level of history, physical exam, and medical decision making documented is fraudulent. Overvaluing encounters can lead to an audit.
- **Undercoding** (Downcoding) a visit results in undervaluing the services provided, resulting in reduced reimbursement and a loss of revenue to the practice. Some patients may suggest manipulating the codes to reduce an out-of-pocket expense. An example is a patient being seen for diarrhea and a colonoscopy is ordered and the patient asks to be billed as preventative to avoid a co-pay. The patient may have to self-pay for a visit, and to reduce the overall cost, suggests that you bill a 99214 visit as a 99213.
- **Addition of diagnoses** to a claim to enhance reimbursement should only be made when they are relevant to the patient visit. Signs and symptoms should be coded for a patient with right upper quadrant abdominal tenderness, even if suspected acute cholecystitis, until the diagnosis is confirmed. There should be an appropriate level of history, exam, or medical decision making documented and reflective in the level of service billed. Padding the chart with diagnoses in order to enhance reimbursement is unacceptable.
- A service must be medically necessary to be billed. For example, billing an echocardiogram (ECG) when a patient has chest pain is appropriate, but billing for an ECG when a patient is seen for a fractured phalanx does not meet medical necessity. Medical necessity from a Medicare perspective is defined under Title XVIII of the Social Security Act, Section 1862 (a) (1) (a): "No payment may be made under Part A or Part B for expenses incurred for items or services which are not reasonable and necessary for the diagnosis or treatment of illness or injury or to improve the functioning of a malformed body member" (Social Security Act, 2009).
- Coding by time or by medical decision making must be reflected appropriately in the medical documentation and justifiable. For example, billing 1 hour of time for an urgent care visit for acute bacterial rhinosinusitis without additional testing or comorbidities is not likely to be justified.

scope of practice, and even the state where you practice. But whatever the cost of the policy, it is worth it. While malpractice is not a frequent occurrence, just one event can change the life and career of an APRN.

There are various ways in which an APRN may be covered for malpractice. The policy may be (1) owned/paid for by the APRN, (2) owned/paid for by the employer, or (3) owned by the APRN and paid for by the employer (Sweeney et al., 2017). Regardless of how you are covered, there are important questions for an APRN to consider. Are you obtaining coverage as an individual or as a business? If individual, how will you be paid (e.g., 1099 or W-2)? What is your practice setting? Are you working for more than one employer? If the employer is carrying the professional liability insurance, consider these questions. Does the policy name you specifically (owner) or just name "all nurse practitioner employees" that are working for the company? What does the insurance cover? What are its exclusions? What are your obligations if you are named in a suit? Is the policy purchased directly from an insurance company, or are you covered by the employer's self-insurance?

The best scenario is for the individual practitioner to purchase their own malpractice coverage (Pohlman, 2015). This ensures that you will have adequate coverage. Employer-paid policies, while providing you with coverage, are primarily protective of the practice or healthcare institution. The proactive provider will focus on learning the nuances surrounding malpractice insurance. Determining an appropriate amount of coverage based on the unknown of what a claimant may be awarded is nearly impossible in today's world. The typical malpractice policy provides a maximum limit of $1 million per occurrence and $6 million aggregate (maximum combined claims paid). However, quotes for the available limits will be provided based on your professional role, practice state, and practice setting (Nurses Service Organization, 2018; see Table 19.8).

There are many options for additional coverage for issues such as sexual misconduct, information privacy (HIPAA), defense attorneys, defendant expense benefits, personal injury coverage, assault coverage, deposition representation, personal liability coverage and educational and consulting activities (National Service Organization, 2018); determining the best

TABLE 19.8

Steps to Securing Malpractice Coverage

Steps	Considerations
Decide your coverage amounts	Know the minimum coverage requirements for your state. Consider the amount of your assets.
Know factors that influence malpractice rates	The state where you practice Your area of specialty
Know the different medical malpractice plans	Claims made vs. occurrence policies Consider nose and/or tail coverage.
Carefully compare insurance providers	Make sure the company is knowledgeable of APRN practice. Check their rating and financial viability. Check their presence in your state of practice.

coverage at the most affordable price can be confusing. Enlisting the services of an insurance professional may be in your best interest (The Doctors Company, 2018). Finding a broker that is knowledgeable about APRNs and the service they provide is recommended. A broker represents your interests; an insurance agent represents the interest of the insurance company. A well-informed broker can perform a needs assessment and then search for the best policy at the best price. They can also ask about professional discounts (Flynn, 2017). Discounts may be offered if you are new to practice, have not had a recent claim, and/or are willing to complete a risk management course.

There are other terms that you should be familiar with in determining the type of liability insurance that you need. Learning these terms after a malpractice claim is made against you may cost you more than you are able to pay. The two main liability policy types are claims-made and occurrence (Flynn, 2017). Claims-made coverage means that you will be covered for medical liability claims that occur on or after a retroactive date and are reported during the policy period or an extended reporting period (Fig. 19.6).

Extended Reporting Period/Tail Coverage

When the APRN is covered by a claims-made policy and then changes employers or changes liability insurance

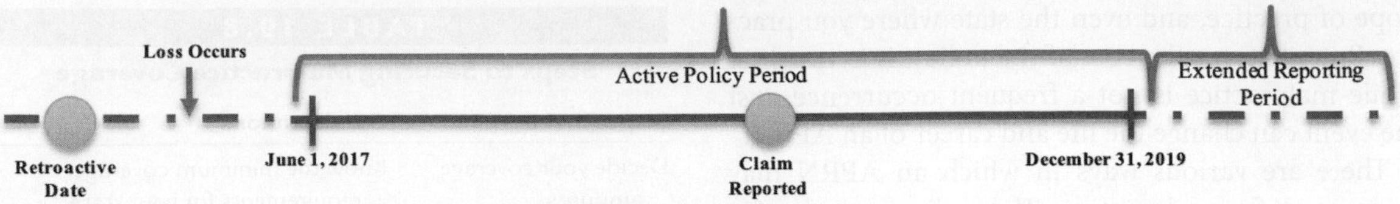

Fig. 19.6 ■ Claims-made policy for malpractice coverage.

companies, a gap period may occur. If a claim is filed after the active policy period has ended, the claim will not be covered. To extend the reporting period of an active policy, the APRN will need to purchase tail coverage. With tail coverage, an event that occurred during the active policy period but is not reported until after the active policy period has ended will then be covered. Preferably the extended reporting period will be unlimited, but this may be limited by the liability carrier to a specific period (e.g., 1 year, 3 years, etc.). A "nose and tail" policy is essentially the same thing as far as coverage goes. It only differs in that a "nose" policy is purchased from the carrier you are joining, whereas a "tail" policy is purchased from the carrier you are leaving (Page, 2020; see Fig. 19.7). Another type of policy is an occurrence policy that covers medical professional liability claims (losses) that occur during a specific coverage period, regardless of when it is reported.

The APRN should also be aware of other liability policies. An umbrella policy is a type of policy that provides additional coverage on top of the primary policy. A vicarious liability policy provides coverage for mistakes made by someone you have contact with, such as an employee of your business. For personal protection, having a "consent to settle" clause in your policy will ensure that a suit cannot be settled without the named insured's written consent (Flynn, 2017).

Mitigating Malpractice Claims

Hopefully APRNs will never need to use their medical liability insurance, but working in a profession that carries increasing responsibility also carries an increased risk of malpractice. Obviously, the best defense is a good offense, so being well versed in key vulnerable areas will help avoid potential litigation. The most common claim against nurse practitioners is failure to diagnose, followed by improper prescribing (especially opioids) and improper treatment/care (Nurses Services Organization, 2021). Other prescribing complaints include failure to explain potential side effects. Patient death is the most common injury, followed by addiction. Claims are made more frequently against adult medical/primary care and family practice, followed by behavioral health and gerontology. The highest average paid indemnities were for neonatal, women's health (obstetrics), and emergency medicine specialties. Physician office practices are the most common practice environments with claims against APRNs, with APRN practice offices and aging service facilities competing for second place (Nurses Service Organization, 2021).

The judicious APRN will actively engage in risk mitigation activities in order to provide safe, cost-effective care and reduce the potential for error. Risk mitigation strategies include (Flynn, 2017):

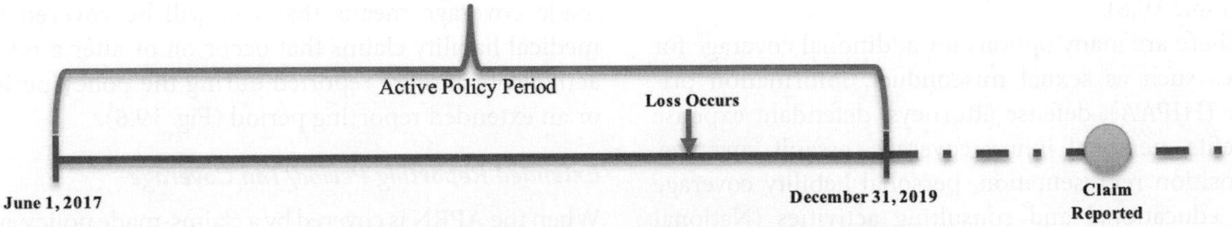

Fig. 19.7 ■ An occurrence policy for malpractice coverage.

- Remaining current in evidenced-based practice guidelines, clinical practice updates, new and revised treatments/medications, and scope of practice.
- Engaging in accurate and clear documentation practices. Make sure your documentation reflects all phases of medical treatment, plan of care, and medication prescribed. Documentation should be timely and objective and include:
  - electronic communication, including diagnostic results
  - nature of proposed treatment, alternatives to treatment, and potential risks and benefits of those treatment options
  - informed consent of prescription medications
  - education of follow-up and signs and symptoms

Documentation is exceptionally important in communicating the patient's medical condition, avoiding fraudulent billing practices, avoiding litigation procedures, and defending your practice if a claim is made. The litigation process is lengthy and grueling. Documentation from 1, 3, 5, or possibly even 10 years prior is what an entire defense will rest on. It is important to document today to tell a story that will be able to be used as a defense in the future (Rosenberg & Page, 2020).

The National Nurse Practitioner Data Bank was established by Congress in 1986 (US Department of Health and Human Services, n.d.). The mission is to improve healthcare quality, protect the public, and reduce healthcare fraud and abuse in the United States by tracking information on medical malpractice payments and adverse actions related to APRNs and other healthcare practitioners and suppliers. State boards of nursing, medical malpractice payers, health plans, hospitals, and other healthcare entities can report and query the data bank (US Department of Health and Human Services, n.d.).

This section cannot be concluded without discussing liability of collaborating physicians in reduced or restricted practice states and tort reform. Whether or not a collaborating physician is included in a malpractice/liability claim is dependent on the facts of the case, involvement of the collaborator in the patient case, and state law. Liability risk is highest when the nurse practitioner is an independent contractor or employed by the physician and lowest when the APRN is engaging in independent practice with a collaborator identified solely to comply with state law (Buppert, 2017).

Reimbursement Pay Parity

Reimbursement and pay parity have been a concern since billing for APRN services became available through the signing of the Balanced Budget Act by President Clinton in 1998. Barbara Safriet, an attorney who is well versed in legislative issues affecting APRN practice, coined the phrase: "Can May Pay" (Safriet, 2002): "Can" we do this based upon our education and training? "May" we do this by our practice authority? "Pay": will we be reimbursed for this? Currently, most APRNs receive 85% reimbursement of the physician rate for Medicare. Private insurers and other third-party payers can set their own contracted rates. The APRN has the potential to negotiate rates with their carriers.

Currently, Oregon is the only state to pass pay parity legislation. In 2016 the Oregon House of Representatives overwhelmingly voted to pass Senate Bill 1503 B (Nurse Practitioners of Oregon, 2016) to continue Oregon's nurse practitioner payment parity law. Oregon's nurse practitioner payment parity law is the first law in the country to require private insurance companies to reimburse primary care and mental health nurse practitioners, physician assistants (PAs), and physicians at the same rates when they perform the same services.

BUSINESS DEVELOPMENT

Entrepreneurship

The *Merriam-Webster dictionary* defines an *entrepreneur* as "one who organizes, manages, and assumes the risk of a business or enterprise" (Merriam-Webster, n.d.). The thought of opening a business is daunting to most APRNs. Changes to health care over the past few years indicate that the nursing model of care is poised to become the healthcare delivery model of the future. APRNS are innovators in health care every day, finding ways to care for patients despite barriers. The APRN who is willing to step out of their comfort zone and deliver care to the full extent of their education and training will find greater fulfillment in caring for patients and reap greater financial rewards for doing so. Education in the nuances of business is key to obtaining the skills necessary for success (see Chapter 18).

Business Ownership

APRNs typically lack training in the business development skills required to start a practice or business. There is also no true accounting of how many APRNs own a practice or business. Many APRNs have the dream and desire to launch a business, but knowing how to operationalize them is the greatest threat to launching a business. Many APRNs express frustration with having to see a predetermined number of patients under the medical model of healthcare delivery in order to meet productivity expectations. The APRN brain is hardwired in the nursing model of holistic, whole-person health care, not disease-specific models. To be successful, the APRN must have the confidence and skill set to pursue business ownership.

There are great opportunities for APRNs to consider practice or business ownership. For example, APRNs can provide direct primary care (e.g., concierge services) to the patient. In this model, the patient pays a set fee and the APRN is available 24/7 to addresses a defined set of primary care needs. A hybrid model occurs when patients pay a fee and the APRN has office hours at a bricks-and-mortar location for care that requires hands-on assessment. Some APRNs are going to patient homes to provide care; for example, with home-based primary care (Home Centered Care Institute, 2022), a house calls practice (Dr. Lawson Nurse Practitioner, 2022), or transitional care management (MLN Network, n.d.), to name a few.

During the recent COVID-19 pandemic, states temporarily removed barriers to APRN care delivery. This has created telehealth practice opportunities that are ripe for APRN ownership (Rutledge et al., 2017). Delivery of services through telehealth works well for rural and underserved areas where access to care is limited. Technological advances allow remote patient monitoring to assess patients, allowing APRNs to provide care where the patients are (Stanik-Hutt et al., 2013). However, telehealth care delivery has limitations of state boundaries for APRNs; APRNs must be licensed in the state where the patient resides. Therefore the APRN must stay abreast of changing rules as the nuances of telehealth are forever in flux. APRNs are cost effective and provide high-quality care with excellent outcomes. The future of healthcare delivery will depend on the ability of APRNs to launch and sustain businesses and practices.

Additional APRN Compensation Models

Beyond reimbursement for services rendered, APRNs should consider other types of compensation. Obviously, the type of environment in which the APRN chooses to work may drive the type of compensation (i.e., business owner vs. employee). Regardless of the environment, APRNs should recognize their value and negotiate the best compensation possible. The APRN needs to be knowledgeable of the community average income within their specialty area and setting.

The easiest and most straightforward method of compensation is an hourly rate. This compensation type may allow flexibility to transfer from one department to another within a facility, without significant change in scheduling and compensation. However, hourly rates do not encourage quality, efficiency, and productivity. Ultimately it may lead to dissension in a practice setting when one provider is less efficient and stays later to complete tasks, thus receiving a higher compensation. This payment model may also be unpredictable for the APRN. When patient volume is low, it will be tempting for the employer to reduce the APRN's hours (ThriveAP, 2019).

Salaried compensation, on the other hand, is predictable and creates a sense of security for the APRN, while also promoting efficiency. However, the salaried provider may feel slighted if providing excellent care to high patient volumes leads to routinely working late. Additional compensation may be expected if there is an increase in responsibilities, patient volumes, and the push to meet quality measures. A salaried compensation structure is not likely to incentivize the APRN to perform to certain metrics or milestones (ThriveAP, 2019).

The combination of a bonus structure with a flat hourly or salaried rate can alleviate some of the disadvantages of a solely hourly or salaried rate. Bonuses can serve as a performance incentive. Bonuses may be tied to patient satisfaction or revenue that is generated. It is important that the APRN clarify exactly how bonuses will be calculated and reported (ThriveAP, 2019).

Productivity-based compensation rewards those providers who generate higher revenue for the practice by seeing higher patient volumes (e.g., RVUs, based on national standards set by CMS). As with the bonus structure, it is important to have a very clear system for calculating payments, and the provider should be familiar with the calculations to ensure accuracy in compensation (ThriveAP, 2019).

Levels-based compensation structures provide for compensation based on specifically outlined expectations by the employer. The employer determines transparent expectations for the provider based on clinical scope, professionalism, and/or experience metrics. This allows the provider to create a path for upward mobility with more than just a "patient-after-patient" cycle.

Competitive compensation packages include more than just salary. Incentives to negotiate include vacation time, malpractice insurance, continuing education allowances, professional leave (e.g., to attend conferences), retirement benefits, disability insurance, allowances for licensure/certifications, professional association membership, long-term care insurance, professional journal allowance, relocation bonus, sign-on bonus, embroidered laboratory coats, and more depending on your setting and needs. When negotiating a contract, determine which points are deal-breakers and which ones are less important. Shoot for the moon and be prepared to negotiate (Dillon & Hoyson, 2014; see Chapter 18).

FUTURE TRENDS

APRNs must have a thorough understanding of the revenue cycle of a practice and the financial role and responsibility they have to a practice. APRNs who make a point of educating themselves about documentation, coding, revenue cycle, and practice payment are invaluable to a practice.

Even if an APRN is not politically savvy, advocacy is a particularly important part of your professional responsibility. Your voice matters! Having a seat at the table when key healthcare decisions are rendered, whether in a practice, in a professional organization, or through legislation, is critical for patients and the APRN profession. Part of your professional responsibility is to belong to your state and national organizations. State organizations focus on day-to-day intricacies of practice authority and regulations within the state, while national organizations address issues at the federal level that affect barriers to care. APRNs must place themselves in positions to influence and effect change within organizations, educate stakeholders about our profession, and change health policy to reduce barriers to practice, patient access to care, and reimbursement and pay parity.

CONCLUSION

Healthcare reform and integration of APRNs into the healthcare system have come a long way since the 1960s, but there is still work to be done. As an integral part of the healthcare system, APRNs should be knowledgeable and competent in healthcare system infrastructures and reimbursement. Creating a revenue stream for the services that APRNs provide is an invaluable asset to all clinical settings. This chapter provided an educational foundation to reimbursement with a succinct and simple introduction to the complex intricacies of the reimbursement process. Understanding these key concepts of the business aspect of providing care, participating in future healthcare reform, and maintaining awareness of regulations at the federal and state level are imperative for the APRN to survive and thrive in the ever-changing healthcare environment.

KEY SUMMARY POINTS

- The APRN must understand how their services are provided and how they are reimbursed.
- The APRN must know the resources used to document, code, and bill for services they render to a patient.
- The APRN is responsible for what they document, code, and bill.
- The APRN must know the nuances of malpractice insurance and what type of coverage they may need.
- The APRN who masters reimbursement will be an asset to any practice or organization.

REFERENCES

American Association of Nurse Practitioners. (2017). AANP comments to CMS innovation center new direction RFI, Nov 2017. https://storage.aanp.org/www/documents/CMMI-Comments.pdf

American Association of Nurse Practitioners. (2022). State practice environment. Retrieved from https://www.aanp.org/advocacy/state/state-practice-environment

American Association of Nurse Practitioners. (2017). Response to CMS regarding CMMI Direction. Retrieved from https://storage.aanp.org/www/documents/CMMI-Comments.pdf

American Medical Association. (2021). CPT® Evaluation and Management (E/M) Office or Other Outpatient (99202-99215) and Prolonged Services (99354, 99355, 99356, 99417) Code and Guideline Changes. pp 1-28. https://www.ama-assn.org/system/files/2019-06/cpt-office-prolonged-svs-code-changes.pdf

Baldridge, K. (2021). Billing & coding in the outpatient clinical setting: A quick reference. Advanced Practice Education Associates.

Buppert, C. (2017). Physicians who work with NPs: What's the liability risk? *Medscape: Legal & Professional Issues for Nurses*. Medscape.com/viewarticle/884585

Buttle, R., Vlietstra Wonnenberg, K., & Simaan, A. (2019). Small-business owners' views on health coverage and costs. The Commonwealth Fund. https://www.commonwealthfund.org/publications/issue-briefs/2019/sep/small-business-owners-views-health-coverage-costs

CAQH Solutions. (2021). ProView Provider User Guide v31. https://proview.caqh.org/Login/Index?ReturnUrl=%2f

Centers for Medicare & Medicaid Services. (2016). ICD-10-CM official guidelines for coding and reporting. *Medicare Learning Network*, 1–115. https://www.cms.gov/Medicare/Coding/ICD10/Downloads/2016-ICD-10-CM-Guidelines.pdf

Centers for Medicare & Medicaid Services Quality Payment Program. (2017). Quality payment program overview. https://qpp.cms.gov/about/qpp-overview

Centers for Medicare & Medicaid Services. (2018). Medicare and Medicaid basics. Medicare Learning Network. pp. 1-23. ICN 006764. https://www.cms.gov/Outreach-and-Education/Medicare-Learning-Network-MLN/MLNProducts/Downloads/ProgramBasicsText-Only.pdf

Centers for Medicare & Medicaid Services. (2019). MACRA. https://www.cms.gov/Medicare/Quality-Initiatives-Patient-Assessment-Instruments/Value-Based-Programs/MACRA-MIPS-and-APMs/MACRA-MIPS-and-APMs#:~:text=The%20Medicare%20Access%20and%20CHIP,clinicians%20for%20value%20over%20volume

Centers for Medicare & Medicaid Services. (2020a, February). Acute inpatient PPS. https://www.cms.gov/Medicare/Medicare-Fee-for-Service-Payment/AcuteInpatientPPS

Centers for Medicare & Medicaid Services. (2020b, April). Advanced practice registered nurses, anesthesiologist assistants, and physician assistants. Medicare Learning Network. pp. 1-17. ICN MLN901623. https://www.cms.gov/Outreach-and-Education/Medicare-Learning-Network-MLN/MLNProducts/Downloads/Medicare-Information-for-APRNs-AAs-PAs-Booklet-ICN-901623.pdf

Centers for Medicare & Medicaid Services. (2020c, September). ICD-10-CM, ICD-10-PCS, CPT, and HCPCS code sets. pp. 1-5. ICN MLN900943. https://www.cms.gov/Outreach-and-Education/Medicare-Learning-Network-MLN/MLNProducts/Downloads/ICD9-10CM-ICD10PCS-CPT-HCPCS-Code-Sets-Educational-Tool-ICN900943.pdf

Centers for Medicare & Medicaid Services. (2021a). 2021 ICD-10-CM. https://www.cms.gov/medicare/icd-10/2021-icd-10-cm

Centers for Medicare & Medicaid Services. (2021b, January). Evaluation and management services guide. Medicare Learning Network. pp. 1-10. ICN 909330. https://www.cms.gov/outreach-and-education/medicare-learning-network-mln/mlnproducts/downloads/eval-mgmt-serv-guide-icn006764.pdf

Centers for Medicare & Medicaid Services. (2021c). Medicare benefit policy manual. Chapter 15, Section 60. https://www.cms.gov/Regulations-and Guidance/Guidance/Manuals/Downloads/bp102c15.pdf

Centers for Medicare & Medicaid Services. (2021d, February). Medicare fraud & abuse: Prevent, detect, report. Medicare Learning Network. pp. 1-27. ICN MLN4649244 https://www.cms.gov/Outreach-and-Education/Medicare-Learning-Network-MLN/MLNProducts/Downloads/Fraud-Abuse-MLN4649244.pdf

Centers for Medicare & Medicaid Services. (2021e). NPI: What you need to know. Medicare Learning Network. pp. 1-6. https://www.cms.gov/Outreach-and-Education/Medicare-Learning-Network-MLN/MLNProducts/Downloads/NPI-What-You-Need-To-Know.pdf

Cohen, W. & Ball, R. (1965). Social Security amendments of 1965: Summary and legislative history. Social Security Administration Bulletin, 1965, pp. 3-21. Retrieved from https://www.ssa.gov/policy/docs/ssb/v28n9/v28n9p3.pdf

Congress.gov. (1989). H.R.2924 - Omnibus Budget Reconciliation Act of 1989. 101st Congress (1989-1990). https://www.congress.gov/bill/101st-congress/house-bill/2924?s=1&r=29

Congress.gov. (1990). H.R.5835 - Omnibus Budget Reconciliation Act of 1990.101st Congress (1989-1990). https://www.congress.gov/bill/101st-congress/house-bill/5835/all-info?r=4&s=2

Congress.gov. (1997). H.R. 2015 – Balanced Budget Act of 1997. 105th Congress (1997-1998). https://www.congress.gov/bill/105th-congress/house-bill/2015

Dillon, D., & Hoyson, P. M. (2014). Beginning employment: A guide for the new nursepractitioner. *The Journal for Nurse Practitioners, 10*(1), 55–59.

The Doctors Company. (2018). Choosing a medical malpractice insurance carrier: A guide for physicians and practices. pp. 1-16. https://www.thedoctors.com/siteassets/pdfs/marketing-order-form-items/choosing-a-medical-malpractice-insurance-carrier-guide2.pdf

Dodd, K., & Fan, T. (2017). ED charting and coding: Critical care time. *Academic Life in Emergency Medicine*. https://www.aliem.com/charting-coding-critical-care-time/

Dr. Lawson Nurse Practitioner. (2022). America's favorite house call nurse practitioner. https://drlawsonnp.com

Flynn, J. (2017). Nurse practitioners and today's professional liability risks. *Minority Nurse*. https://minoritynurse.com/nurse-practitioners-todays-professional-liability-risks/

Gruessner, V. (2016). CMS continues to reform through healthcare bundled payments. *Healthcare Payer Intelligence*. https://healthpayerintelligence.com/news/cms-continues-to-reform-through-healthcare-bundled-payments

HealthCare.gov. (n.d.a). Health insurance plan & network types: HMOs, PPOs, and more. https://www.healthcare.gov/choose-a-plan/plan-types/

HealthCare.gov. (n.d.b). Health maintenance organization. https://www.healthcare.gov/glossary/health-maintenance-organization-hmo/

Home Centered Care Institute. (2022). Advancing home-based primary care. https://www.hccinstitute.org

Hsiao, W. C., Braun, P., Dunn, D., & Becker, E. R. (1988). Resource-based relative values: An overview. *JAMA, 260*(16), 2347–2353.

The Joint Commission. (2012). Ambulatory care program: The who, what, when, and where's of credentialing and privileging. Joint Commission Accreditation PDF Booklet. https://www.jointcommission.org

LaPointe, J. (2016). Understanding the basics of bundled payments in healthcare. Revcycle Intelligence: Practice Management News. https://revcycleintelligence.com/news/understanding-the-basics-of-bundled-payments-in-healthcare

LaPointe, J. (2017). How providers can detect prevent healthcare fraud and abuse. Revcycle Intelligence. https://revcycleintelligence.com/features/how-providers-can-detect-prevent-healthcare-fraud-and-abuse

LaPointe, J. (2018). Key terms, components of payer contracts providers should know. Revcycle Intelligence:Practice Management News. https://revcycleintelligence.com/news/key-terms-components-of-payer-contracts-providers-should-know

MACPAC. (2022). Provider payment and delivery systems. https://www.macpac.gov/medicaid-101/provider-payment-and-delivery-systems/

McMullen, P. C., & Howie, W. O. (2020). Credentialing and privileging: A primer for nurse practitioners. *The Journal for Nurse Practitioners, 16*, 91–95.

Medicare and CHIP Reauthorization Act. (2015). Public Law 114-10 114th Congress. Retrieved on June 15, 2020 from https://www.congress.gov/114/plaws/publ10/PLAW-114publ10.pdf

MedPac. (2019). Improving Medicare's payment policies for advanced practice registered nurses and physician assistants. http://www.medpac.gov/-blog-/the-commission-recommends-aprns-and-pas-bill-medicare-directly-/2019/02/15/improving-medicare's-payment-policies-for-aprns-and-pas

Merriam-Webster. (n.d.). Entrepreneur. *Merriam-Webster.com Dictionary.* Accessed July 29, 2021. https://www.merriam-webster.com/dictionary/entrepreneur

MLN Matters. (2016). Incident-to billing. https://www.cms.gov/outreach-and-education/medicare-learning-network-mln/mlnmattersarticles/downloads/se0441.pdf

MLN Network. (n.d.). Transitional care management services. https://www.cms.gov/outreach-and-education/medicare-learning-network-mln/mlnproducts/downloads/transitional-care-management-services-fact-sheet-icn908628.pdf

National Plan and Provider Enumeration System (NPPES). (n.d.). National plan & provider enumeration system. Centers for Medicare & Medicaid Services. Retrieved from https://nppes.cms.hhs.gov/#1

National Credentialing Solutions. (n.d.). Payor enrollment for nurse practitioners. https://nationalcredentialing.com/?s=payor+enrollment+for+nurse+practitioners (new).

Nurse Practitioners of Oregon. (2016). Legislature votes to make NP payment parity law permanent. Retrieved July 10, 2020 from https://www.nursepractitionersoforegon.org/page/news20160225/Legislature-Votes-to-Make-NP-Payment-Parity-Law-Permanent.htm

Nurses Service Organization. (2018). NSO malpractice insurance for nurse practitioners: Policy features. https://www.nso.com/malpractice-insurance/individuals/nurse-practitioners

Nurses Service Organization. (2021). 10 most surprising things from the nurse's claim report. https://www.nso.com/Learning/Artifacts/Articles/10-most-surprising-things-from-the-nurse-s-claim-report, June 10, 2020.

Page, L. (2020). What you absolutely need to know about tail coverage. Medscape. https://www.medscape.com/viewarticle/924970#vp_4

Palmetto GBA. (2018). Subsequent hospital visit: Coverage and documentation requirements. https://www.palmettogba.com/Palmetto/Providers.nsf/docsCat/JM%20Part%20B~eServices%20Portal~eCBR~Subsequent%20Hospital%20Visit%20(CPT%20Codes%2099231-99233)%20Coverage%20and%20Documentation%20Requirements?open&Expand=1

Patel, R., & Sharma, S. (2019). Credentialing. *Stat Pearls [Internet].* https://www.ncbi.nlm.nih.gov/books/NBK519504/

Patient Protection and Affordable Care Act, 42 U.S.C. § 18001. (2010).

Pohlman, K. (2015). Why you need your own malpractice insurance. *American Nurse Today, 10*(11), 28–30. https://www.myamericannurse.com/wp-content/uploads/2015/11/ant11-Malpractice-1023.pdf

Quality Payment Program. (n.d.). Participation options overview. https://qpp.cms.gov/mips/overview

Rapsilber, L. M. (2019). Reimbursement for nurse practitioner services. In J. G. Stewart Stewart, & S. M. DeNisco (Eds.), *Role development for the nurse practitioner* (pp. 343–366). Jones and Bartlett.

Rice, T., Unruh, L., Ginneken, E., Rosenau, P., & Barnes, A. J. (2018). Universal coverage reforms in the USA: From Obamacare through Trump. *Nursing Outlook, 122*(7), 697–770.

Rosenberg, S. & Page, L. (2020). Malpractice: What to do if you get sued. Medscape. Medscape.com/courses/section/880445

Rudowitz, R., Garfield, R., & Hinton, E. (2019). 10 things to know about Medicaid: Setting the facts straight. Kaiser Family Foundation. https://www.kff.org/medicaid/issue-brief/10-things-to-know-about-medicaid-setting-the-facts-straight/

Rutledge, C. M., Kott, K., Schweickert, P. A., Poston, R., Fowler, C., & Haney, T. S. (2017). Telehealth and eHealth in nurse practitioner training: Current perspectives. *Advances in Medical Education and Practice, 8*, 399–409.

Safriet, B. J. (2002). Closing the gap between can and may in healthcare providers' scopes of practice: A primer for policymakers. *Yale Journal on Regulations.* https://digitalcommons.law.yale.edu/cgi/viewcontent.cgi?article=5418&context=fss_papers

Safriet, B. J. (2011). Federal options for maximizing the value of advanced practice nurses in providing quality, cost-effective health care. In Institute of Medicine (US) Committee on the Robert Wood Johnson Foundation Initiative on the Future of Nursing. National Academies Press. https://www.ncbi.nlm.nih.gov/books/NBK209876/?report=printable

Sawyer, N. T. (2018). In the US "healthcare" is now strictly a business term. *The Western Journal of Emergency Medicine, 19*(3), 494–495.

Social Security Act. (2009). Sec. 2009. [42 U.S.C. 1397h] Retrieved from https://www.ssa.gov/OP_Home/ssact/title20/2009.htm

Stanik-Hutt, J., Newhouse, R. P, White, K. M, Johantgen, M., Bass, E. B., Zangaro, G., Wilson, R., Fountain, L., Steinwachs, D. M., Heindel, L., & Weiner, J. P. (2013). The quality and effectiveness of care provided by nurse practitioners. *The Journal for Nurse Practitioners, 9*(8), 492–500.

Sweeney, C. F., LeMaheiu, A., & Fryer, G. (2017). Nurse practitioner malpractice data: Informing nursing education. *Journal of Professional Nursing, 33*(4), 271–275.

Taylor, J. W. (2014). A brief history on the road to healthcare reform: From Truman to Obama. Becker's Hospital Review. https://www.beckershospitalreview.com/news-analysis/a-brief-history-on-the-road-to-healthcare-reform-from-truman-to-obama.html

Teel, P. (2018). Five top challenges affecting healthcare leaders in the future. Becker's Hospital Review. https://www.beckershospitalreview.com/hospital-management-administration/five-top-challenges-affecting-healthcare-leaders-in-the-future.html

ThriveAP. (2019). Structuring compensation for nurse practitioners: pros and cons. https://thriveap.com/blog/structuring-compensation-nurse-practitioners-pros-cons

US Department of Health and Human Services. (n.d.). National nurse practitioner data bank. https://www.npdb.hrsa.gov/topNavigation/aboutUs.jsp

World Health Organization. (n.d.). ICD-10 version. https://icd.who.int/browse10/2019/en

World Health Organization. (2021). International classification of diseases and related health problems. https://www.who.int/standards/classifications/classification-of-diseases/

Xue, Y., Ye, Z., Brewer, C., & Spetz, J. (2016). Impact of state nurse practitioner scope-of-practice regulation on health care delivery: Systematic review. *Nursing Outlook, 64*(1), 71–85.

20 UNDERSTANDING REGULATORY, LEGAL, AND CREDENTIALING REQUIREMENTS

MAUREEN A. CAHILL ■ MICHELLE BUCK ■ NICOLE LIVANOS

"The surest test of discipline is its absence."
~ Clara Barton

CHAPTER CONTENTS

THE CONSENSUS MODEL FOR APRN REGULATION: LICENSURE, ACCREDITATION, CERTIFICATION, AND EDUCATION 650
- Implementation of Consensus Model Regulation 650
- The Need for Education and Credentialing of APRNs in the US Healthcare System 652

ADVANCED PRACTICE REGISTERED NURSE MASTER'S AND DOCTORAL EDUCATION 652

BENCHMARKS OF ADVANCED PRACTICE NURSING AND EDUCATION 653

ADVANCED PRACTICE REGISTERED NURSE COMPETENCIES 653
- Professional APRN Competencies 653
- APRN Program Oversight and Accreditation 654
- APRN Role and Population Certification 655
- Postgraduate Education 655
- Continued Competency Measured Through Recertification 655
- Mandatory Clinical Education and Clinical Practice Requirements 656

ELEMENTS OF APRN REGULATION AND CREDENTIALING 656

LANGUAGE ASSOCIATED WITH THE CREDENTIALING OF APRNS 657
- Titling of APRNs 657
- State Licensure and Recognition 657
- Institutional Credentialing 658
- Prescriptive Authority 659
- Identifier Numbers 660

SCOPE OF PRACTICE FOR APRNS 661

STANDARDS OF PRACTICE AND STANDARDS OF CARE FOR APRNS 662

ISSUES AFFECTING APRN CREDENTIALING AND REGULATION 662
- Collaborative Practice Arrangements, 662
- Reimbursement 663
- Risk Management, Malpractice, and Negligence 664
- Telehealth, Tele-practice, and Licensure Portability 666

INFLUENCING THE REGULATORY PROCESS 667

CURRENT PRACTICE CLIMATE FOR APRNS 667
- Visioning for Advanced Practice Nursing 667

FUTURE REGULATORY CHALLENGES FACING APRNS 669

CONCLUSION 669

KEY SUMMARY POINTS 670

This chapter delineates the regulatory characteristics and requirements of the four advanced practice nursing roles, certified nurse practitioners (NPs), clinical nurse specialists (CNSs), certified nurse-midwives (CNMs), and certified registered nurse anesthetists (CRNAs). Collectively these roles are described in regulation as advanced practice registered nurses (APRNs). Each role is associated with the direct care of one or more patient populations and, in some cases, a subfocus of acute or primary care. The Consensus Model outlines the elements of common educational preparation and certification requirements, regardless of role, and describes the common requirements of regulation (National Council of State Boards of Nursing [NCSBN], 2008). Regulation of nursing roles exists at the level of the state. Each state must set into law, through legislative act, their requirements for advanced nurse roles. The purpose of this chapter is to help the reader understand the steps required in educational preparation, certification, and maintenance of licensure for the APRN.

Regulation of advanced nursing roles has continued to evolve from the earliest state regulation of an APRN role (Keeling, 2009) to the present day. APRN stakeholders continue efforts each year to align state regulations and rules with those described in the Consensus Model (NCSBN, 2008). All states regulate or coregulate the roles under a board of nursing, a board of health, a board of midwifery, a board of medicine, or a board of professional regulation (NCSBN, 2022c). APRNs need to become familiar with regulations in the states of their practice.

THE CONSENSUS MODEL FOR APRN REGULATION: LICENSURE, ACCREDITATION, CERTIFICATION, AND EDUCATION

Credentialing is used by regulatory boards to ensure that APRNs meet minimum requirements of competency and safety standards in order to protect the public as outlined in each state's nurse practice act (NCSBN, 2020a). Regulatory changes that pertain to APRNs have evolved at different times in different states and with varied elements of what was to be regulated (Kuo et al., 2013). Dialogue began that embraced all credentialing stakeholders and was a major step toward a uniform plan to educate and regulate APRNs.

Describing which advanced roles required regulatory oversight was a first order of business, followed by identifying which populations of patients would be served, such as adult and geriatric, neonatal, pediatric, women's health, mental health, and family health. Educational programs had existed for advanced nursing roles long before such roles were regulated, but the focus of the Consensus Model allowed for common educational pathways, based on role and population, that would provide the basis for preparation and the platform upon which testing (certification) was designed.

Through discussion, brainstorming, and reaching consensus among educators, certifiers, and regulators, the Consensus Model was born (APRN Joint Dialogue Group, 2008; Fig. 20.1). Forty-eight nursing organizations endorsed the work. The vision in creating this Consensus Model was to implement one national regulatory scheme, which could be adopted and carried out at the state level, allowing APRNs to be innovative and meet the needs of patients. State boards of nursing working through the NCSBN agreed to the elements of the Consensus Model as their uniform licensure requirements for the regulation of the four roles. To assist with the implementation of these requirements, NCSBN created model language for bills intended to align state regulation with the elements of the Consensus Model and, thereby, assist state nursing boards in carrying out the new regulations. All states would work toward adoption of this new standard (NCSBN, 2014). A detailed history of this work can be found in The Institute of Medicine's (IOM) report *The Future of Nursing: Leading Change, Advancing Health* (IOM, 2011).

Implementation of Consensus Model Regulation

The Consensus Model has been in existence for more than 10 years. The participating organizations that make up the LACE communication network (licensure, accreditation, certification, and education) have continued to meet regularly to move forward the implementation of the Consensus Model, to keep lines of communication open, maintain transparency, and identify and strategize about important and ongoing issues. The LACE network is a virtual social networking configuration. A platform is in place whereby LACE member organizations pay a membership fee to belong to the working group that sustains the core

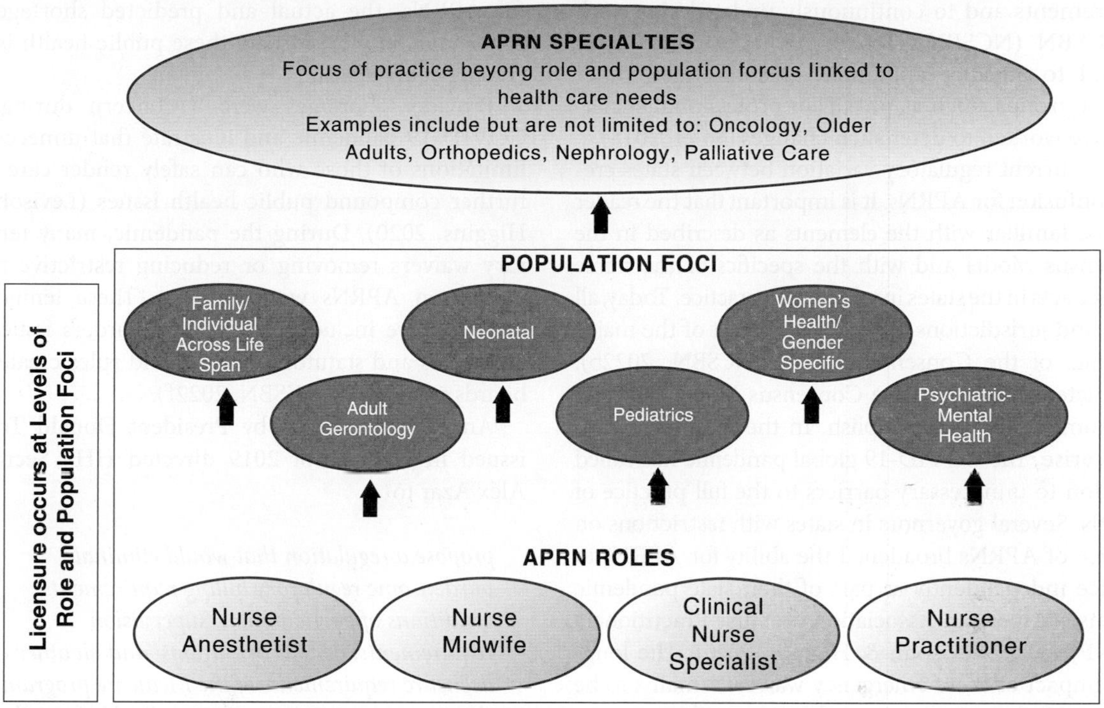

Fig. 20.1 ■ **Advanced practice registered nurse (APRN) regulatory model.** (Adapted from *Consensus Model for APRN Regulation: Licensure, Accreditation, Certification and Education*, by National Council of State Boards of Nursing, 2008, https://www.ncsbn.org/Consensus_Model_for_APRN_Regulation_July_2008.pdf)

TABLE 20.1
APRN Accrediting Bodies

Accrediting Bodies That Oversee APRN Education Programs	Accrediting Bodies That Have Oversight of APRN Certifying Examinations
Commission on Collegiate Nursing Education (CCNE)	American Board of Nursing Specialties (ABNS)
Accreditation Commission for Education in Nursing (ACEN)	National Commission for Certifying Agencies (NCCA), a division of the Institute for Credentialing Excellence (ICE)
Commission for Nursing Education Accreditation (CNEA)	
Council on Accreditation of Nurse Anesthesia Educational Programs (COA)	
Accreditation Commission for Midwifery Education (ACME)	

components of the Consensus Model (LACE Network, 2020).

All four LACE organizational categories (licensure, accreditation, certification, and education) are aimed at meeting any new requirements and assisting with state implementation. There are five programs that have accreditation oversight of APRN education and two accrediting bodies that have oversight of APRN certification programs or examinations (Table 20.1). For questions about current APRN rules and regulations, especially those that pertain to specific state statutes regarding licensing of APRNs, prescriptive authority, and reimbursement, the reader should refer to individual state regulatory bodies for practice requirements and to continuously updated sites such as NCSBN (NCSBN, 2022e). As stakeholders have worked to advance alignment bills in states, other interest groups, such as physician professional societies, have worked to deter such changes (Sofer, 2018).

The current regulatory variation between states creates confusion for APRNs. It is important that the reader become familiar with the elements as described in the Consensus Model and with the specifics of the nurse practice acts in the states in which they practice. Today, all states and jurisdictions have adopted most of the major elements of the Consensus Model (NCSBN, 2022b). Complete transition to the Consensus Model may still take some years to accomplish. In the meantime, new issues arise. The COVID-19 global pandemic has called attention to unnecessary barriers to the full practice of APRNs. Several governors in states with restrictions on practice of APRNs broadened the ability for APRNs to practice independently as part of their state pandemic response (American Association of Nurse Practitioners [AANP], 2020; Levisohn & Higgins, 2020). The long-term impact of these emergency waivers remains to be seen; in the short term, many of the states of emergency have ended and barriers have returned. In early 2021 the governor of Massachusetts made permanent the full practice authority (following a transition to practice period) granted to most APRNs originally through pandemic executive order (An Act Supporting a Resilient Healthcare System That Puts Patients First, 2020)

The Need for Education and Credentialing of APRNs in the US Healthcare System

During the years since 2008, national focus has turned sharply toward healthcare outcomes and costs, following astounding data comparing US health outcomes with those of other high-income countries (Tikkanen & Abrams, 2020). Americans experience some of the worst health outcomes, though the United States spends considerably more on health care than any of the comparison countries (Tikkanen & Abrams, 2020). This trend appeared well before the pandemic and was certainly an issue during it (Hooper et al., 2020). It appears that insurability, access to care (in particular, primary care, mental health services, and maternal/childcare), socioeconomic disparities, and health policy lay at the root of the issue. Despite some physician organizations opposing full practice for APRNs, the actual and predicted shortages of physicians only exacerbate these public health issues (Zhang et al., 2020).

Provider shortages were a concern during the COVID-19 pandemic and illustrate that unnecessary limitations of those who can safely render care only further compound public health issues (Levisohn & Higgins, 2020). During the pandemic, many temporary waivers removing or reducing restrictive regulations on APRNs were adopted. These temporary waivers were included in executive orders issued by governors and statutory changes and rules created by boards of nursing (NCSBN, 2022f).

An executive order by President Donald Trump issued in October of 2019 directed HHS Secretary Alex Azar to

> *propose a regulation that would eliminate burdensome regulatory billing requirements, conditions of participation, supervision requirements, benefit definitions, and all other licensure requirements of the Medicare program that are more stringent than applicable federal or state laws require and that limit professionals from practicing at the top of their profession.*
>
> ***(Whitehouse.gov, 2019)***

President Biden appointed an APRN as acting Surgeon General indicating an understanding of advanced practice nursing roles (De Castella, 2021). It remains to be seen whether the Centers for Medicare & Medicaid Services (CMS) will reduce restrictions on APRNs in Medicare billing and other requirements. The Biden administration has undertaken a review of the previous administrations final orders (Modern Healthcare Policy Tracker, 2021). Expansion of the use of APRNs in health care at all levels requires that nursing ensure the highest levels of education and effective regulation for the advanced nursing roles.

ADVANCED PRACTICE REGISTERED NURSE MASTER'S AND DOCTORAL EDUCATION

The first criterion that any new APRN must meet is successful graduation from an approved, accredited APRN program. Education programs for APRNs must be at the graduate nursing level, resulting in a master's degree in nursing or a doctor of nursing practice (DNP) degree; many programs are transitioning from master's to DNP education (Edwards et al., 2018). The Consensus Model and the NCSBN Nursing Model Act and Model Rules, describing state uniformity in adopting the Consensus Model, do not establish a timeline for the move to doctoral education for APRNs. Currently no state requires a DNP as eligibility for APRN recognition; however, the requirements to meet certification criteria are set by professional organizations and may drive adoption of the DNP degree.

BENCHMARKS OF ADVANCED PRACTICE NURSING AND EDUCATION

Three components of APRN education and practice are related to scope of practice and provide these additional important and currently applied benchmarks: (1) advanced practice nursing core competencies, (2) the APRN role and population, and (2) master's or doctor of nursing practice essentials (American Association of Colleges of Nursing [AACN] 2006, 2011, 2021). These three benchmarks form the foundation on which boards of nursing develop APRN statures and evaluate nursing programs. The Consensus Model delineates six population designations for practice for NPs and CNSs. These populations are adult/gerontology, neonatal, pediatrics, family, psychiatric mental health, and women's health/gender related (Fig. 20.1). In the categories of pediatric and adult/gerontology populations, there was sufficient unique content to create a subfocus of acute care or primary care that is subject to a specific certification category. CNMs have a population that is women's health/gender related and includes care of the newborn as part of maternity-related care. CRNAs are educated to provide anesthesia across the life span. Specialty certification can indicate expertise in a subject area for an APRN, and is encouraged as further role development, when appropriate (NCSBN, 2008). Specialty certification is voluntary and is additive to the education and certification requirements for licensure. The Consensus Model intended that licensure be congruent with the educational preparation and focus of the role and population.

ADVANCED PRACTICE REGISTERED NURSE COMPETENCIES

Nursing program accreditation currently requires that the program be structured based on either *The Essentials of Masters Education in Nursing* (AACN, 2011) or *The Essentials of Doctoral Education for Advanced Nursing Practice* (AACN, 2006), created by the AACN, as previously described. However, the AACN recently released *The Essentials: Core Competencies for Professional Nursing Education* (AACN, 2021), which consolidates the previously separate guidelines into one document for advanced-level nursing education. APRN programs and their accreditors will transition over time to the updated AACN *Essentials*. This document supports scope of practice for APRNs by providing the requirements for graduate core content, the APRN core, and "three Ps." Taken together, the *Essentials*, the common core "three Ps" courses, and the role- and population-specific preparation are an educational blueprint, described in the Consensus Model. Importantly, students must graduate from a program with specific nursing accreditation that aligns with the Consensus Model in order to meet eligibility criteria to sit for certification and to attain licensure or recognition as an APRN. In order to add APRN populations or to change role or role focus, the APRN can complete a postgraduate certification program that has nursing accreditation, as described in the Consensus Model (NCSBN, 2008). It is the incorporation of the most current *Essentials* by APRN programs that adjusts to and encourages the evolution APRN education and influences practice. The new *Essentials* include domains, competencies, subcompetencies, and concepts that build upon the professional practice of nursing from entry to advanced level. They include a competency for compliance with relevant laws, regulations, and policies in practice with subcompetencies that promote the active participation of advanced-level nursing students in advocacy for and participation in regulation and policies impacting nursing practice and healthcare outcomes (AACN, 2021).

Professional APRN Competencies

APRN organizations, such as the National Organization of Nurse Practitioner Faculties (NONPF), the National Association of Clinical Nurse Specialists

(NACNS), the American College of Nurse-Midwives (ACNM), and the American Association of Nurse Anesthesiology (AANA) support each role and population focus with their own set of approved competencies, which are updated to align with the revised *Essentials*. These more specific competencies provide the role and population basis that are used for the certification exams, whether the program prepares the student at the master's or DNP level (Fig. 20.2). See Chapters 12 through 16 for examples of and sources for these competencies. Additionally, the Interprofessional Education Collaborative (IPEC) defined desired core competencies for interprofessional collaborative care, called the ASPIRE model (Brashers, 2020). A review of accreditation requirements related to interprofessional competencies suggested that graduate nursing program requirements were, in large part, representative of interprofessional needs (Zorek & Raehl, 2012). Interprofessional competency assessment and development is ongoing.

APRN Program Oversight and Accreditation

For a master's or DNP nursing program preparing APRNs, credentialing has a somewhat different meaning. Program credentialing includes accreditation for the educational program by one of the four APRN education accrediting organizations. Education programs must also meet state education approval and requirements through each state's department of education or though multistate agreements (US Department of Education, 2016). In many states, the boards of nursing also approve graduate nursing education leading to the APRN roles (NCSBN, 2022c).

The Accreditation Commission for Education in Nursing, the Commission on Collegiate Nursing Education, the Council on Accreditation of Nurse Anesthesia Education Programs (COA), and the Accreditation Commission for Nurse Midwifery Education (Table 20.1) have aligned their standards with the requirements of APRN education as outlined in the

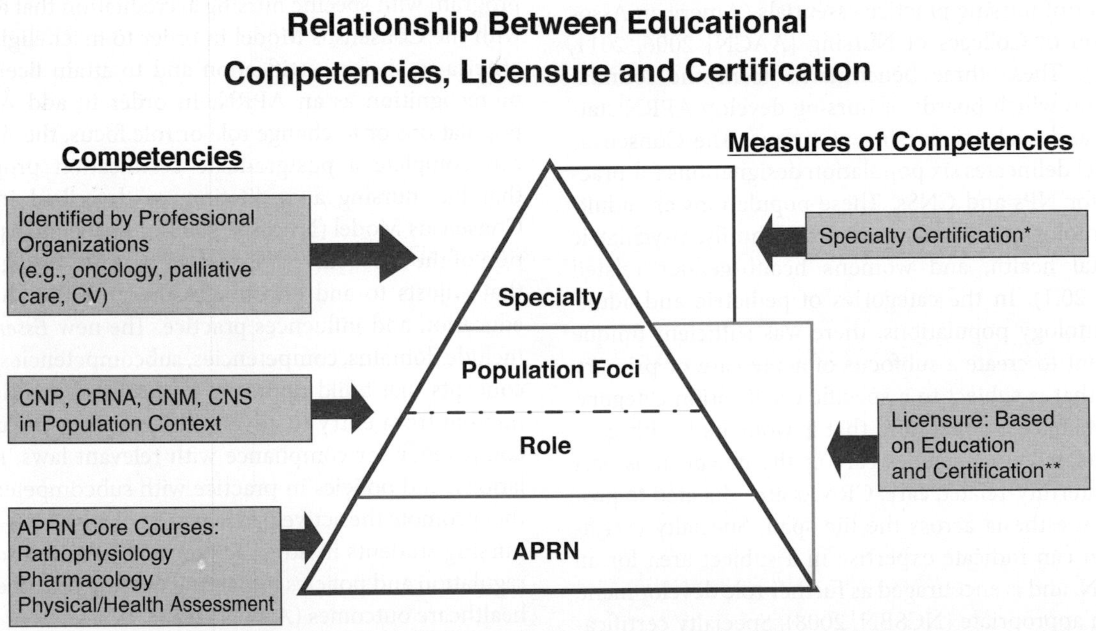

Fig. 20.2 ■ **Relationship between educational competencies, licensure, and certification.** *APRN,* Advanced practice registered nurse; *CNM,* certified nurse-midwife; *CNP,* certified nurse practitioner; *CNS,* clinical nurse specialist; *CRNA,* certified registered nurse anesthetist; *CV,* cardiovascular. *Certification for specialty may include examination, portfolio, peer review, etc. **Certification for licensure will be psychometrically sound and legally defensible examination by an accredited certifying program. (Adapted from *Consensus Model for APRN Regulation: Licensure, Accreditation, Certification and Education,* by National Council of State Boards of Nursing, 2008, https://www.ncsbn.org/Consensus_Model_for_APRN_Regulation_July_2008.pdf)

Consensus Model. The accreditation process provides an overall evaluation of the graduate nursing and APRN curricula and clinical programming.

Preaccreditation review, based on the work of NCSBN and consensus groups, has been adopted by the accreditors. Preaccreditation ensures that all new programs are well developed with appropriate curricula in place prior to student admission. All programs must attain nursing accreditation in order for their graduates to be eligible for certification and licensure.

The multiplicity of populations for the NP and CNS roles necessitates a more complex review structure than that of the CNM or CRNA, who have a single population focus. The NONPF, Pediatric Nursing Certification Board (PNCB), NACNS, and other similar bodies provide curriculum guidelines, program standards, and competencies to assist APRN programs with curriculum planning.

APRN Role and Population Certification

Agencies that offer APRN certification exams such as the American Nurses Credentialing Center and the American Association of Nurse Practitioners Certification Board review APRN educational programs to determine eligibility for APRN graduates to sit for national APRN certification examinations. Advanced practice nursing certification is national in scope, and it is a mandatory requirement for APRNs to obtain and maintain credentialing in most states (NCSBN, 2008, 2022c).

National certification for APRNs is a primary vehicle used by state boards of nursing to ensure a basic measure of competence. Certification examinations for APRNs must be legally defensible and psychometrically sound to be utilized as an element of advanced nursing licensure. Additionally, APRN certification programs must themselves be accredited by the National Commission for Certifying Agencies (Institute for Credentialing Excellence) or by the American Board of Nursing Specialties (ABNS). Certification organizations base content for their exams on role delineation studies that assist in defining the knowledge, skills, and abilities related to that specific role and population (NCSBN, 2012; ANCC, 2020).

CRNAs were credited with the first national certification in 1945, with other APRN specialties following suit, although few standards for certification were in place prior to 1975 (Chapters 1 and 12–16). Certifications exist today for each of the described APRN roles and populations, with the exception of the women's health CNSs, for which competencies are written (NACNS, 2019) but no examination exists. Certification programs rely on a certain number of potential test-takers to offset the expense of creating and maintaining an examination. APRN national certification websites identify the criteria for eligibility, test outlines, and recertification and practice requirements. Certification programs share information on those who hold and maintain certification required for state licensure/recognition with Boards of Nursing. The APRN NurSys database, maintained by NCSBN, houses licensure and certification information for ease of access among state Boards of Nursing and is increasingly utilized across states (NCSBN, 2022e).

Postgraduate Education

Postgraduate APRN programs are offered to students who have already attained a graduate degree in nursing and wish to add an additional population focus. Many individuals who choose to return to school pursue DNP education. The Consensus Model requires that the post-master's education programs obtain formal graduate nursing accreditation. It is important that master's-prepared nurses who aspire to do postgraduate work in order to acquire a new or additional APRN credential attend programs that offer curricula that meet the standards of eligibility for national certification and state licensure.

Continued Competency Measured Through Recertification

Overall, APRNs must fulfill continuing education (CE) and practice requirements to maintain their national certification(s), although requirements differ according to the role. Each APRN certification entity clearly delineates the requirements for recertification. Generally, national certification lasts from 2 to 5 years and requires that the candidate be retested unless established didactic and clinical parameters are met. All APRNs must maintain active certification for licensure eligibility if required in the state where they hold licensure, with the exception of a few states that do not require national certification. In some cases where early exams have been retired, there may not be a testing option left for some who let their credential lapse. For APRNs who are practicing with a retired certification examination, it is important to remain diligent in meeting the requirements for recertification. Retired certification reapproval requirements are available through the certification program's website. If individuals are not maintaining active APRN certification, they should not represent themselves as APRNs.

Mandatory Clinical Education and Clinical Practice Requirements

Continuing education requirements differ based on population focus and may require a prescribed number of clinical practice hours for successful recertification. CE may be a requirement of state licensure renewal, which in some cases may be in addition to those requirements needed for certification renewal. Most APRN roles and specialty areas have specific requirements established by the certifying agency for an adequate number of clinical practice hours between the years of recertification to ensure that APRNs remain clinically current and competent through regular practice. CE should be consistent with role and population, although it may be interprofessional. For example, CRNAs may choose to attend a physician-sponsored anesthesia conference or family NPs may attend a conference with primary care physicians. It is encouraging to note that professional conferences are offering interprofessional speakers and panels. Patient safety organizations such as the Society to Improve Diagnosis in Medicine (SIDM) are focusing their efforts on interprofessional audiences. APRN expert clinicians are serving as conference faculty for medical CE and vice versa. The move to interprofessional offerings has broadened the scope of continuing education resources available.

Ongoing CE hours may be fulfilled in a variety of ways including attending CE courses and workshops, working toward degree requirements, completing journal CE offerings, writing for publication, and completing online offerings, simulations, and webinars. It is important to confirm what type of continuing education is accepted by the certifying body and the APRN's specific state board of nursing.

ELEMENTS OF APRN REGULATION AND CREDENTIALING

As APRNs become more mobile across state and international boundaries, and as communication advances such as telehealth allow for increased interaction, it is important that credentialing and regulatory parameters be well understood. Box 20.1 lists the elements of regulation for APRNs. As noted earlier, credentialing is an umbrella term that refers to the regulatory mechanisms that can be applied to individuals, programs, or organizations. It is the process of collecting and verifying an individual's professional qualifications. Credentialing may occur at a national level by meeting eligibility to sit for a national certification examination. The state verifies graduate or postgraduate education and national certification in the APRN role and population to establish eligibility to confer recognition or licensure. Credentialing can also occur at the level of employment through an institutional process that grants access to the medical staff. Credentialing though this process confirms education and national certification, reviews medical malpractice claims, and describes the standards and duties one is expected to carry out within APRN employment (Buppert, 2019; McMullen & Howie, 2020). This type of credentialing process is increasingly reviewed by regulators and malpractice carriers who seek assurance that APRN practice is congruent with education and certification. While employer credentialing can further limit scope as described in the nurse practice act, it cannot expand it beyond what the state allows in law (Markowitz et al., 2017).

The elements described in Box 20.1 create the standard whereby APRNs are monitored, regulated, and deemed safe or unsafe and whereby APRNs are

BOX 20.1

Elements of Regulation (LACE) for Advanced Practice Registered Nurses

- Licensure
  - Prescriptive authority (see Box 20.3)
- Accreditation of APRN Programs
- Certification (National)
  - Recertification
- Education
  - Master's
  - Post-master's
  - Doctoral

disciplined from state to state. Credentialing changes have occurred, or will occur, as states move toward Consensus-aligned regulations. Titling will require that APRNs legally represent themselves as an APRN, initially, and then by their role (CRNA, CNM, CNP, or CNS). Many states already use these role and population titles, but some do not (Fotsch, 2016). A few states reserve licensure language for the role of the registered nurse and refer to the regulation of advanced practice nursing as an additional certification by the state.

The Consensus Model recommends that boards of nursing provide an APRN license in addition to the Registered Nurse license. A second licensure means that an APRN must meet criteria established by a state board of nursing and is held to the highest level of regulation. Licensure is established in law. Not every state has incorporated a second license in their nurse practice act and may, instead, address the advanced nursing category as a state certification applied by the board of nursing. The issues of titling and second licensure are important to all APRNs and to the public. It validates that each APRN role holds regulatory recognition as both an RN and an APRN, shares a core preparation, and meets uniform regulatory standards intended to offer the highest levels of public protection.

Use of the umbrella term APRN is intended to clarify that advanced practice in nursing is structured on top of the registered nurse foundation and requires an additional approved scope of practice that is additive to and expands on that of the registered nurse. The scope of practice of an APRN, while structured as additional to the registered nurse platform, is unique and is reflected in the requirement of additional regulatory recognition. Licensure remains the highest level of professional regulation in law reflecting the accountability for this evolved and greater nursing scope. Statutes define the title that is legally protected (APRN) and define the minimal requirements of recognition of the four included roles.

LANGUAGE ASSOCIATED WITH THE CREDENTIALING OF APRNS

It is important for APRNs to understand the language and terms used to describe the credentialing process. Credentialing, including education, national certification, and licensure, involves several steps before one has full authority to practice as an APRN. To complicate matters, as previously noted, the credentialing procedures and requirements vary somewhat among states and practice settings. Definitions for the major components of APRN credentialing are presented in Box 20.2.

Titling of APRNs

The issues surrounding the titling and credentialing of APRNs have been difficult since the inception of APRN roles. The preference is to use the title "advanced practice registered nurse" to indicate the uniform preparation and regulation of the four APRN roles (CRNA, CNS, CNM, and CNP). Advanced practice nursing has evolved in differing ways over time, with multiple titles, which confuses policymakers, patients, those within the profession, other healthcare providers, and the public. Currently, not all states recognize all APRN roles for title protection. Several states continue to use titles such as APN or ARNP instead of the widely recognized and accepted APRN (Fotsch, 2016). APRN role and certification programs have aligned title with their credentials, just as they have aligned the Consensus Model educational requirements.

Adding to public confusion about titles is the convention of many large health centers to refer to NPs and physician assistants as advanced practice providers (APPs) as though they are interchangeable roles. However, their preparation, certification, and role orientation are not identical. Another titling quandary is that of a CRNA subgroup who wish to change their title to "nurse anesthesiologist" (Committee for Proper Recognition [CPRC], 2019). While this has become allowable in some settings, it is not a protected title in the vast majority of states. Additionally, it is fiercely opposed by many anesthesiologists (American Medical Association [AMA], 2019). Legal titles are those referenced in the state's nurse practice act.

State Licensure and Recognition

Individual practice acts define the practice of nursing for registered nurses (RNs) throughout the 50 states and territories (NCSBN, 2020a). State laws overseeing APRNs are divided into two forms: (1) statutes or laws as defined by the nurse practice act, which are enacted by the state legislature, and (2) rules and regulations, which are promulgated by state regulatory agencies

BOX 20.2

Advanced Practice Registered Nurse (APRN) Credentialing Definitions

Accreditation: The voluntary process whereby schools of nursing are reviewed by external nursing educational agencies for the purpose of determining the quality of a nursing and/or APRN program.

Certification: A formal process (usually an examination but may be a portfolio) used by a certifying agency to validate, based on predetermined standards, an individual's knowledge, skills, and abilities. Certification provides validation of the APRN's knowledge in a particular role and population or specialty. It is used by most states as one component of second licensure for APRN practice.

Credentialing (institutional level): The process that an individual institution, or health system, uses to permit an APRN to practice in an APRN position within the institution. Generally, APRNs submit particular documentation to an institutional credentialing committee, which reviews and authorizes the APRN's practice.

Credentialing (state level): The requirements that a state uses to assess minimum standards of competency for APRNs to be authorized to practice in an APRN role. The purpose of credentialing is to protect the health and safety of the public. These requirements include an unencumbered registered nurse (RN) license, graduate education transcripts, and national certification in one of six population foci.

Legal authority: The authority assigned to a state or agency with administrative powers to enforce laws, rules, and policies.

Licensure: The process whereby an agency of state government grants authorization to an individual to engage in a given profession. For nursing, licensure is usually based on two criteria—the applicant attaining the essential education and degree of competency necessary to perform a unique scope of practice and passing a national examination. APRNs are licensed first as RNs and second as APRNs.

Regulations: The rules and policies that operationalize the laws and policies that recognize APRNs and credential them for practice in an APRN role and population focus.

under the jurisdiction of the executive branch of state government.

Rules and regulations are created to accompany the nurse practice act and to provide guidance on implementation of the statute. Historically, under the Tenth Amendment of the US Constitution, states have broad authority to regulate activities that affect the health, safety, and welfare of their citizens, including the practice of the healing arts professions within their borders. Licensure stems from this history, grounded in public protection, whereby each state creates standards to ensure basic levels of public safety. In the vast majority of states, boards of nursing have oversight and regulatory authority of APRNs. The CNS role is regulated by boards of nursing in all states that recognize the role. North Carolina, Virginia, and Alabama have joint subcommittees of boards of nursing and boards of medicine regulating CNMs and CNPs. CNMs are also subject to regulation by boards of medicine in New Jersey and Pennsylvania and boards of midwifery in New York, Rhode Island, and North Carolina. Florida requires practice per board of medicine–approved protocols for some APRN roles (NCSBN, 2022c). Some of these regulatory oversights are burdensome and others work under joint committees and toward voluntary collaboration that eases the way for independent practice.

Some states require a temporary permit for a new graduate to practice as an APRN while awaiting national certification results or other requirements, such as a required "gradual" transition to practice or added pharmacology education for prescriptive authority. New graduates should contact their state board of nursing and submit the required application for a temporary APRN permit if the state allows this practice. With the advent of electronic testing, the time lapse between testing and obtaining results for licensure is minimal and markedly reduces the need for a temporary permit. In some states, temporary permits for APRNs no longer exist.

Institutional Credentialing

The need for hospital or outpatient privileges for APRNs varies according to the nurse's practice. For example, CNMs and many rural NPs cannot care for patients properly without the ability to admit patients to the hospital should the need arise. It has not been necessary for CRNAs and some NPs to admit patients to the hospital independently to give comprehensive care, but they may need to see patients in emergency departments. With the advent of hospitalist medicine and the reductions in residency hours, the need for physicians and APRNs with office-based practices to carry hospital privileges is becoming less necessary. The rules for practice as part of the hospital medical staff are even more specific and variable than those for state regulation and are separate from hospital administration; they are bound to the local hospital or medical facility and medical staff of the granting institution. The criteria and guidelines are increasingly considering non-physician providers as part of the medical staff (CMS, 2020a, 2020b). Additionally, medical staff credentialing committees are adding APRN members and facilities are creating APRN advisory committees.

The first step for APRNs seeking hospital privileges is to ask the top-level nurse administrator or APRN leadership how the credentials committee is organized, who makes up the membership, how often it meets, and what support there is for non-physician applicants. Is there a process for APRNs or others to petition for privileges? Nursing administrators are often members of credentials committees, and the APRN should meet with nurse colleagues for advice and support before the application process. A second step is to obtain the application package and begin to collect the necessary documents, which include, for example, licenses and certifications, transcripts, letters of support, and provider numbers. Applicants must confirm that the documentation is completed thoroughly prior to submitting it for review. Support from the collaborating physician, if required, is key. In some cases, a collaborating physician may serve as the sponsor for a nurse colleague, and in other cases they are required to appear before the committee with the APRN. The APRN should review the requested privileges with the collaborating/sponsoring physician at the time the documents are being completed and discuss any details prior to appearing before the credentials committee. Be prepared to strongly represent your qualifications to provide the services requested; do not expect the physician to do this, because it is the responsibility of the APRN. A collaboration describes a two-way relationship that considers input from both parties, whereas sponsorship may simply be the acknowledgment by a member of the medical staff of another provider. A sponsoring physician may only be required to ensure they are available to the APRN as needed and that the APRN meets employment requirements, to the best of their knowledge. It is recommended that the collaborating physicians and APRN have on file an agreement that specifies the elements of their collaboration. The APRN must determine the specific privileges needed to provide care with full scope of practice and top of license. For example, will it be necessary to admit or discharge patients, write orders, perform procedures, visit in-hospital patients, or be available to provide care or consultation to the emergency department? Dialogue among the hospital administration, physician staff, and other stakeholders (e.g., APRN colleagues and other team members) is necessary if admitting privileges will be required for the desired practice role. Alliances with consumers often add support to the application. Some hospitals have specific guidelines and protocols for all providers who are not physicians; others do not.

The Joint Commission requires that APRNs who provide "a medical level of care" be credentialed through the medical staff process. If they do not function at that level of care, they can be credentialed through an "equivalent process" (The Joint Commission, 2016). In today's market, professional "turf issues" are losing ground, and opportunities for hospital privileges are opening the door for new APRN practice.

The Consensus Model stresses that practice should be congruent with APRN education and national certification. Prior to implementation of the Consensus Model, the hiring distinctions of acute and primary care designations and role versus specialty certification were not stressed. Today, alignment with education and certification is vital and, increasingly, facility credentialing and risk management entities are checking such alignment. It is the obligation of the APRN to practice within the privileges granted by each employer as privileges may be more restrictive in scope of practice compared with the nurse practice act. Consider applying for additional privileges during credential renewal.

Prescriptive Authority

In the United States, prescribing by APRNs was an early independent or delegated function. For many states, experience in prescribing by those in APRN roles is now decades old. Evidence suggests safe prescribing within the roles (Jiao et al., 2018).

Credentialing and licensure for prescriptive authority also occur at the state level. Pharmacology education requirements vary among states, although currently most states and all role certification programs require a core advanced pharmacotherapeutics course (a requirement of the Consensus Model) during the graduate APRN education program and some states require yearly CE credits thereafter to maintain prescriptive privilege. Prescriptive authority may be regulated solely by the board of nursing, as it is in several states; jointly by the board of nursing and board of pharmacy, as it is in several others; or by a triad of boards of nursing, medicine, and pharmacy (NCSBN, 2022c). Prescriptive authority may be included in a state's licensure or recognition of APRNs or it may be conferred as a separate license or authority. As prescriptive authority has evolved over the past several years, certain basic requirements have become fairly standard for APRN prescribers (Box 20-3). These requirements vary among states but provide a core regulatory process for prescriptive authority. All states allow for prescribing authority in APRN roles and all have some form of controlled substance prescribing, but variation persists. Concerns regarding opioid abuse and misuse have resulted in additional state regulatory variation within controlled substance prescribing as to the total number of days an opioid may be prescribed and, in some cases, the specific opioids that can be prescribed (NCSBN, 2020b). It is incumbent on the APRN to understand clearly the mechanism of legal prescriptive authority in his or her state and to understand whether ongoing continuing education is required (Maier, 2019).

The reader can check state board of nursing websites to determine the required number of hours of pharmacology needed to qualify and maintain that state's prescribing authority. The Consensus Model clearly outlines requirements for APRN educational programs to comply with pharmacologic content. Pharmacology CE offerings, both classroom and digital, are often interprofessionally focused and are available for the busy clinician (American Society of Addiction Medicine, 2019).

BOX 20.3

Requirements for Advanced Practice Registered Nurse (APRN) Prescribers

- Graduation from an approved master's- or doctoral-level APRN program
- Licensure and recognition as an APRN in good standing
- National certification in an APRN population focus area
- Recent pharmacotherapeutics course of at least 3 credit hours (45 contact hours)
- Evidence of a collaborative practice arrangement (in some states)
- Ongoing continuing education hours in pharmacotherapeutics to maintain prescribing status (in some states)
- State prescribing number (in some states) and national Drug Enforcement Administration number

Identifier Numbers

Drug Enforcement Identifier Number

In some states the licensure or recognition of an APRN is inclusive of prescribing authority. In other states such authority may require an additional registration step. An APRN permitted by their state to prescribe controlled substances must also apply to the US Department of Justice for a unique DEA number. If granted, the approval will indicate which schedules of controlled substances are permitted. The DEA is sending renewal notices by email, so it is imperative that the APRN prescriber keep the DEA apprised of current contact information.

National Provider Identifier Number

In addition to prescriber and DEA registration, APRNs will need to apply for a National Provider Identification (NPI) number (Health Insurance Portability and Accountability Act [HIPAA], 1996). The National Plan and Provider Enumeration System (NPPES) collects identifying information on healthcare providers and assigns each provider a unique number. APRNs should go to the NPPES website for further information or to apply for an NPI number (NPPES, n.d.). Many drugs listed on insurance company formularies are billed via the NPPES system, giving attribution for prescribing to those APRNs who can be identified by their individual number. The NPI number system exists at the level of the practice (NPI type 2) and at the level of the practitioner (NPI type 1). APRNs benefit by attribution of their practice efforts traced correctly to them. The NPI number is used to track billing and can enhance specific attribution of their efforts (CMS, 2020b).

SCOPE OF PRACTICE FOR APRNS

By definition, the term *scope of practice* describes practice limits and sets the parameters within which nurses in the various APRN roles may legally practice. Scope statements define what APRNs may do for and with patients, what they can delegate, and when collaboration with others is required. Scope of practice statements can circumscribe what might actually be beyond the legal limits of an APRN's nursing practice, despite having the education and skills. The scope of practice for each of the four APRN roles differs (see Chapters 12–16). Scope of practice statements are key to the debate about how the US healthcare system uses APRNs as healthcare providers (US Department of Veterans Affairs, Office of Public and Intergovernmental Affairs, 2016). Controversies arise when health professionals' overlapping scopes of practice create interprofessional conflict (Federal Trade Commission [FTC], 2014). For example, CRNAs who administer general anesthesia have a scope of practice markedly different from that of the primary care NP, although both have their roots in basic nursing and have shared a core curriculum in APRN education. In addition, it is important to understand that scope of practice is based on state laws, which impact the state's healthcare delivery.

Revisions to scope of practice statements by APRN role associations and educational programs are informed by collaborative work that reflects current state and national permissions as well as the evolving needs of the roles (Centers for Disease Control and Prevention [CDC], 2018). Accountability becomes crucial as APRNs obtain more authority over their own practices. A scope of practice statement should identify the legal parameters of each APRN role, stating the additional accountabilities beyond those of the RN. These statements then are used by education and certification programs to ensure that the student is educated to those additional accountabilities and tested on them for entry into practice. American society is highly mobile, and practice across state borders is increasingly common. The APRN must be aware of the requirements in every state where his/her patients are physically located at the time care is provided. As professional licensure compacts are adopted, such as the Nurse Licensure Compact for registered nurses and licensed practical nurses and the APRN Compact for APRNs, the APRN must understand multistate practice privileges as they apply to his or her role (NCSBN, 2022a, 2022c, 2022d).

APRNs owe Barbara Safriet, former associate dean at Yale Law School, a debt of gratitude for her vision and clarity in helping APRNs understand and think strategically about scope of practice and regulatory issues. In her landmark 1992 monograph, Safriet (1992) noted that APRNs are unique in that there is a multiprofessional approach to their regulation based on ignorance and on the fallacy that medicine is all-knowing, particularly about advanced practice nursing. As Safriet has implied, restraints on advanced practice nursing result from ignorance about APRNs' abilities, rigid notions about professional roles, and turf protection. She cited reforms in scope of practice laws in Colorado that encouraged solutions to long-time tensions over control of practice between organized medicine and nursing. Colorado's provision defines the term practice authority in terms of ability and thus redirects the regulatory focus from providers' status to the APRN's education and skills (Safriet, 2002, 2010). This example and the imminent move to Consensus Model regulation offer hope that, in the future, policies can be formulated to close the gap between what APRNs are educated and certified to do and what they are allowed to do by scope of practice statutes. Scope of practice is hampered in many states where the APRN practice is carved out of the medical practice act as a medically delegated act that precludes reasonable autonomy for the APRN. Barbara Safriet was inducted as an honorary fellow of the American Association of Nurse Practitioners in 2013, and she was inducted into the American Academy of Nursing in that same year.

It remains important that, although APRNs desire autonomous licensure through the state boards of nursing, the need to work interprofessionally as colleagues and team members is essential to attaining high-quality patient outcomes (Interprofessional Education Collaborative [IPEC], 2016). Changes to American society such as income disparity and rural access to care challenges predict evolving needs for health delivery changes, including borderless care delivery and expansion of non-physician providers of services.

STANDARDS OF PRACTICE AND STANDARDS OF CARE FOR APRNS

Standards of practice for nurses are defined by the profession nationally and help further delineate scope of practice. Standards are overarching authoritative statements that the nursing profession uses to describe the responsibilities for which its members are accountable. As such, they complement and enable the APRN core, population focus, and specialty competencies. APRNs are held to the standards of practice of both the nursing profession and the APRN specialties. At both levels, standards of practice describe the basic competency levels for safe and competent practice (see Chapters 12–16 standards of practice for the CNS, CRNA, CNM, and NP). Professional standards of practice match closely with the core competencies for APRNs outlined in Chapter 3, which undergird advanced practice nursing.

Standards of care differ from standards of practice put forward by the nursing profession. These standards are often termed *practice guidelines.* Practice guidelines provide a foundation for healthcare providers to administer care to patients. Ideally, these guidelines crosscut the health professions' disciplines and provide the framework whereby basic safety and competent care are measured for APRNs. It is therefore logical that APRNs are often held to the same standards used to review the practice of other providers, including that of medicine. Unprofessional competition between provider categories can lead to some casting dispersions on the care of other disciplines. Such contentions must be evaluated against evidence. Clinical guidelines may be used as the standard of care in legal decisions, so it is important for APRNs to be part of the team developing new evidence-based guidelines (Melnyk, 2018).

Standards of care guide what constitutes safe and competent care across the health disciplines, grounded in evidence and evolving in response to the changing healthcare environment. At the federal policy level, the Agency for Healthcare Research and Quality has responsibility for conducting the research needed to evaluate clinical practice guidelines that define a standard of appropriate care. The CDC, professional medical societies, nursing specialty organizations, and other health team member organizations create guidelines for practice, as do many insurers (CDC, 2020; UpToDate, 2022).

ISSUES AFFECTING APRN CREDENTIALING AND REGULATION

The definition of an APRN requires that the four established APRN roles be clinically focused and that the APRN provide direct clinical care to patients (Hamric & Tracy, 2019). From a legal and regulatory perspective, inclusion of the designation of what constitutes an APRN is driven primarily by three factors: (1) the diagnosis and management of patients at an advanced level of nursing expertise, (2) the ability of APRNs to be directly reimbursed, and (3) the degree to which nurses wish to hold prescriptive and hospital admitting privileges. As practice moves across borders and settings, there must be a well-defined and efficacious means for state boards, insurers, prescribing entities, and similar groups to monitor the scope of practice and reimbursement patterns in all settings and sites of service (Center for Connected Health Policy [CCHP], 2021). These groups need clear criteria that can be validated to ensure patient safety and monitor certification and credentialing.

Collaborative Practice Arrangements

In states with regulatory requirements for APRNs to operate under delegated medical authority, a *collaborative practice agreement* may be required. Collaborative agreements provide a written description of the professional relationship between the APRN and a collaborating physician, defining the parameters whereby the APRN may perform delegated medical acts and therefore are, at their core, supervisory. It must be noted that such requirements are without an evidence basis. APRNs have repeatedly demonstrated that they deliver safe and effective care within the scope of their preparation and their role (Kleinpell, 2017).

Collaborative agreements are unnecessary in states that do not require delegated practice. Where such agreements are required, they add costs and restrict access to care without demonstrating a clear benefit to patients. A 2017 study of collaborative requirements conducted by NCSBN concluded that such requirements, in many states, result in excessive costs to APRNs. Those working in rural areas and self-managed clinics were assessed fees for collaborative agreements that fell between $6000 per year to as much as $50,000 per year! The study further found that restrictions beyond fees associated with required collaborations, such as distance restrictions and collaborator turnover, could further restrict APRN's ability to offer care in those areas by as much as 59% (Martin & Alexander, 2019). When utilized, such agreements should be written as broadly as possible to allow for practice variation and evidence-based innovations.

The term *protocol* in relation to advanced practice nursing was common in years past as physician-directed, specific guidance for defined patient problems and treatment approaches. Specific protocols for care are seldom used today because it is difficult to maintain their currency in evolving evidence. It is hoped that collaborative agreements, where required, encourage evidence-based practice and are based on trust and respect between the collaborating APRN and the physician colleague. Collaboration does not need a regulatory mandate; it is a required behavior of all members of the healthcare team to provide the highest level of care (Rosen et al., 2018). Increasingly, required collaborative agreements have been removed from APRN regulatory requirements, but several states have replaced them with a required transition-to-practice period during which an APRN may be required to practice under the supervision of another provider (MD or other APRN) for a specific period of time, after which the APRN can practice independently. The requirements and length of such transition periods are highly variable and lack an evidence basis.

Reimbursement

APRNs should be paid for services rendered for health care whether they work independently or share a joint practice with a physician or are employed in an institution or provider network (see Chapter 19 for detailed discussion). Many private pay insurance standards are based on and modeled after federal Medicare and Medicaid policy.

Federal mandates encourage direct payment to APRNs, but insurance is regulated at the level of the state, and that creates the potential for discriminatory rules and regulations that obscure payment attribution to APRNs for the care they render. From a credentialing standpoint, attention to CMS rules, Medicare and Medicaid provider numbers, Clinical Laboratory Improvement Amendments (CLIAs), and provider requirements is extremely important to ensure that APRNs know how to contract their services at the individual level. APRN credentialing for billing purposes (insurance credentialing) is also done by the insurance companies, who negotiate the bundling of services. It is important for the APRN to be aware of how such negotiations are done and how their work and reimbursement is represented. They should consult an attorney regarding any contract negotiations. It is imperative that APRNs be present at the negotiating table as members of executive management teams who are setting the policies for provider services where the rules of payment are made (see Exemplar 20.1).

In the past, APRNs were reimbursed "incident-to" physicians and at a considerably lower rate. Incident-to billing came into being with the Balanced Budget Act of 1997 through an amendment that allowed NPs to bill Medicare at 85% of the physician fee. The CMS has since clarified this in publications such as the 2022 publication MLN Booklet Advanced Practice Registered Nurses, Anesthesiologist Assistants, & Physician Assistants (CMS, 2022). Today, the attribution of care to the individual practitioner can be tracked and reported with use of the NPI number.

APRNs must have current credentials and regulatory documents organized and available, not only as a novice but over the duration of one's career. It is the responsibility of the APRN to be aware of billing requirements that are consistent with both federal and state requirements. For example, a primary care NP applying for a position would need to meet the criteria listed in Box 20.3. This would include Medicare and Medicaid provider status as well as malpractice history and coverage (see Chapter 19).

EXEMPLAR 20.1

MEETING THE REQUIREMENTS FOR CREDENTIALING AND REGULATION

Laurie is in the final semester of her doctor of nursing practice family nurse practitioner (FNP) program at a state university. She is in the process of negotiating a contract with a provider network of physicians and advanced practice registered nurses (APRNs) in a rural practice. Laurie knows that she must begin the process of acquiring the necessary credentials to be able to practice in her state after she has successfully passed national APRN certification in her population focus area. When she applied to her FNP program, she made sure that the university and graduate program were accredited and in good standing. Now that she is ready to graduate, she must prepare for a new and challenging professional life.

In her seminar class, Laurie received the application to sit for national certification the month after she graduates and has sent the application forward to register the date for her examination. Her next step is to download the advanced practice nursing rules and regulations for her state so that she fully knows the scope of practice she must adhere to. She also obtains the APRN application materials from the state board of nursing. Laurie reviews these documents carefully in order to understand the application process, materials, and fee that she will need to submit to the state licensing board.

Laurie carefully notes that APRNs in her state must show proof that they have completed a 45-contact hour, state-approved graduate nursing course in pharmacotherapeutics. Also, she must complete 6 hours of continuing education in pharmacotherapeutics each year to maintain her status as a prescriber. She makes a note to request the transcript and syllabus for her pharmacotherapeutics course to attach to the application for her APRN license.

Unless she resides in a state with full practice authority, on signing her contract, Laurie will first need to negotiate a written collaborative arrangement with the precepting physician colleague, who will see the patients who are beyond her scope of practice. Second, she needs a Medicaid provider number to see children in the Medicaid program. She will need to apply for her National Provider Identifier and Drug Enforcement Administration numbers. In addition, this healthcare system requires that Laurie apply to the local hospital and nursing home privileging committees so that she can see patients on rounds, do admitting and discharge planning, and follow nursing home patients on a regular basis.

As part of her package, Laurie has negotiated for the employer to pay the premium on her malpractice insurance as an APRN. She also negotiates $3000 per year for continuing education. She needs to call her insurance carrier to discuss the transfer of her student policy to a full malpractice policy to cover her as a certified APRN with the appropriate scope of practice that she will need in her new position. She knows that she wants to purchase an occurrence type of policy. Laurie uses the support of her colleagues and mentors as she works through this important process of preparing her credentials to practice as an APRN (see Box 20.2).

Risk Management, Malpractice, and Negligence

Malpractice suits involving APRNs are rare and increases in numbers of cases correspond to an increasing number of APRN providers. APRNs need to understand clearly what constitutes negligent practice within their scope of practice and grounds for malpractice so they may plan for the safest and most efficient delivery of care. Most malpractice carriers collect and assemble informative trends and guidance documents for their clients and note cases and data that are specific to APRNs, enabling them to be aware of risk issues and behaviors that may be mitigated.

By definition, *negligence* is the failure to act in a professionally, reasonable way as a healthcare clinician. Negligence may lead to malpractice and legal action. The following four factors (the four D's) must be present for a malpractice suit to be valid (Buppert, 2015).

1. A **duty** to care must be owed to the injured party, through direct office or hospital care or through phone or email advice; a patient nurse relationship must be established.
2. The accepted standard of care was breached **(breach of duty)**.
3. The patient must have **damage** or have sustained injury.
4. There must be **direct causation (cause)** demonstrated; that is, the patient has suffered an injury that was caused by the APRN clinician. There may be multiple causative factors based on care by several caregivers over time.

Within the judicial system, care is evaluated by preset criteria in the form of medical and advanced practice standards for appropriate care, as discussed previously. In the case of the APRN, there is blurring between the medical and advanced nursing standards, creating a need for interprofessional standards that hold providers to the same standards as their peers for the same type and level of care. The most common means that a legal standard of care may be established in a specific case is through expert testimony offered by a person who is qualified by education, experience, knowledge, and skill level to judge the actions of the providers in the case. Other mechanisms include review of the professional literature, manufacturer's package inserts, and documented professional standards of care. Additional strategies to prevent malpractice events include establishing a good rapport with patients over time, following an established standard of care to ensure competence, documenting accurately and completely, and taking a course(s) in risk management.

In order to reduce risks of malpractice occurrences, APRNs educated since the publication of the Consensus Model must ensure that their practice is consistent with their education and certification. It is an easy matter for plaintiff attorneys to verify the standards of education and certification for a particular APRN role. Those educated prior to the Consensus Model (before 2008) and whose practice is not congruent with their advanced nursing education should consider advanced certification in their specialty area of practice, if it is available to them. Additionally, to further reduce risks, it is important to maintain a continuing education log and a competency performance record, including a patient profile list and performance review history.

It is important to document thoroughly and accurately and to audit charts frequently for mistakes or omissions that should be appropriately corrected. APRNs must be cognizant, if asked to give advice by phone or to see patients outside their practice setting, of the risk implications of such requests. In such instances, the APRN should treat these events as an office visit with full documentation in the patient record.

APRNs must be knowledgeable about national issues related to timely and accurate patient diagnosis, a major topic in malpractice cases. The use of unnecessary diagnostic tests (laboratory and imaging) contributes to health costs. A national effort is under way to "choose wisely" when selecting appropriate diagnostic tests. The American Board of Internal Medicine [ABIM] Foundation hosts the national "Choosing Wisely®" campaign, which advocates for care that is supported by evidence, not duplicative, free from harm, and truly necessary (ABIM, 2020). The accuracy and timeliness of patient diagnosis have become a national patient safety concern and one that APRNs and nurses at all levels have engaged with physicians to address. Organizations such as the Society to Improve Diagnosis in Medicine introduce practitioners to aggregated data on diagnostic trends and tools that may prove useful for diagnostic accuracy. Evidence-based information about diagnostic processes and tools, including the impact, both good and bad, of electronic medical records systems is increasingly available to APRNs (Society to Improve Diagnosis in Medicine [SIDM], 2020).

Malpractice Insurance

APRNs need a thorough understanding of liability insurance coverage, types of policies, and extent of coverage required. The two most common types of professional liability insurance plans are *claims-made* and *occurrence*. A claims-made insurance policy covers claims made against the APRN only while the policy is in effect. Coverage must be continued indefinitely to ensure coverage for claims filed in the future for actions that occurred in the past. A claims-made policy can be extended by the purchase of additional coverage referred to as a "tail" to cover the APRN during a switch from one carrier to another (American College of Physicians [ACP], 2016). In an occurrence policy, the APRN is covered for alleged acts of negligence that occurred during the time the policy was in effect. An occurrence policy offers coverage even if the policy is cancelled at some future date by honoring coverage for any events that occurred while the policy was in place. The APRN needs a full understanding of the amounts of coverage per incident and how personal legal costs are handled within the policy. The amount of insurance needed is governed by the type of practice in which the APRN is engaged. Roles such as that of CRNAs and CNMs, who are under more risk, are likely to need more coverage. It is important that APRNs carry their own individual liability coverage, even if they are covered by an employer group practice. Employer-based insurance contracts are geared to protect the institution or practice and are not targeted to protect the individual APRN.

Additionally, APRNs have risks associated with provider requirements under HIPAA regulations, which became law in 1996 (HIPAA, 1996). Liability under this law can be aimed at institutional and provider responsibilities. HIPAA requires implementation of statewide, uniform, minimum patient privacy standards. It includes any information that would identify the patient, the patient's problem, the plan of care, and how care is paid for. Institutions must conduct security risk assessments to safeguard private health information. The Office of Civil Rights of the Department of Health and Human Services (DHHS) is charged with enforcing HIPAA requirements, and penalties can be severe (Health and Human Services, Office of Civil Rights [HHS OCR], 2020). If APRNs accept third-party reimbursement or transmit any health information in any form, they are required to comply with HIPAA regulations. In recent years, protected health information has become increasingly at risk from malware and cybercrime. APRNs should be informed of policies and procedures at all sites of care that deter such violation of patient privacy and heed guidance for patient information security.

Telehealth, Tele-practice, and Licensure Portability

Among the most impactful changes to health care in recent years is the shift in care to mobile platforms and care across state and even international borders. The United States and, indeed, the world is on the precipice of a massive shift in health care from the early days of horse and buggy visits to the age of virtual visits, telecare, group care, and remote monitoring. The success of telehealth care is dependent on the providers of care to follow their patients regardless of location. Such change begs change also in the way care providers are regulated, particularly in the area of state licensure. The Nurse Licensure Compact (NLC), applicable to RNs and licensed vocational nurses, allows for a nurse holding a license in a Compact state to practice on that license in other Compact states (NCSBN, 2020a, 2022d). While the NLC is operational, the APRN Compact was adopted in 2020 by the NCSBN Delegate Assembly and will become effective upon seven states enacting the model legislation. The APRN Compact is modeled after the NLC, allowing for an APRN to hold a license in a Compact state with the privilege to practice in other states party to the Compact (see Exemplar 20.2). Physicians have also adopted a state-based portability mechanism through the Federation of State Medical Boards. The Medical Compact license does not eliminate the need to pay multiple state

EXEMPLAR 20.2
INTERSTATE PRACTICE THROUGH LICENSURE PORTABILITY USING THE INTERSTATE COMPACT

Ron Garcia is an advanced practice registered nurse (APRN) clinical nurse specialist who specializes in heart failure. He is a member of a large cardiology team in a multistate health system. Ron leads the heart failure team that includes a pharmacist, a social worker, a physical therapist, home care nurses, and home care aides. Ron's patients are referred to him from cardiologists across this multistate system. His team provides ambulatory and home visits as well as remote monitoring for patients. They have developed a management protocol that has produced remarkable results in improving compliance with home monitoring and reducing readmissions in patients with heart failure. Presently he practices and holds licensure in four states.

Ron is an advocate for interstate licensure. He recognizes that care that is received by his patients can produce benefit or harm. The patients have recourse through their state boards of nursing if they have a complaint with any licensed professional on his teams. This requires that he and his team members hold licenses in each state where their patients receive care. The health system would like to expand care, under his leadership, to the other states. When his state joins the APRN Compact and the Nurse Licensure Compact, both he and the nurses, if they meet qualifications, will be able to practice in any other state that joins those compacts. Ron knows that innovations and breakthroughs in health care are occurring at an amazing rate. Teams like his are discovering socially sensitive care strategies that produce results. His company chooses to expand Ron's team in Compact states preferentially, while they wait for additional states to join the Compacts.

As geography becomes less relevant in care provision, state geographic boundaries will become irrational in a high-value care delivery system. Ron understands that a system of mutual regulatory recognition (licensure portability) through an interstate APRN Compact for APRNs is vitally important. He considers volunteering with the coalition to help with this issue.

licensure fees as the Nurse Compact does, but it does expedite the licensure process across states (Interstate Medical Licensure Compact [IMLC], n.d.).

Regulation for tele-practice by APRNs has been impacted by the need to hold licensure in the state in which the patient receives the care and also by varied regulation between states. The onset of the COVID-19 pandemic compelled states as well as federal agencies to review any restrictions to tele-practice and to expand accessibility to care through teleservice waivers and new sources of funding (Center for Connected Health Policy [CCHP], 2020; Weigel et al., 2020). Clearly, evidence suggests that tele-practice can benefit particular patient groups, and APRNs can and should be part of that care; however, APRNs must be aware of regulations that are inclusive or limiting of their participation. Studies looking at impact and outcomes have thus far indicated that outcomes are comparable and APRNs are able providers of telehealth services (Weiner, 2021). Telehealth is anticipated to continue to expand, and telehealth regulations are certain to change in coming years as a possible solution to access to care issues.

Two million registered nurses have access to the NLC, allowing them to practice across state borders in 39 NLC participating states (NCSBN, 2022c). The APRN Compact has yet to become effective, with variation in regulatory requirements across states complicating its enactment.

Issues that arise are those pertaining to emerging advanced roles such as patient coaches, population health specialists, and informatics specialists, as well as facility practice policies and credentialing. It is advisable to check frequently with state nursing boards for updates and to hold membership in an APRN role organization for additional role-specific information.

INFLUENCING THE REGULATORY PROCESS

Americans are more divided in their political viewpoints than we have seen in many years. Political views are divided by identity with media, economics, geographic location, and progressive versus conservative. Racial disparities have been in evidence in healthcare outcomes and continue to be seen in the COVID-19 pandemic (Jurkowitz et al., 2020). Health care remains a focus of policy attention, both nationally and at the state level. The future of the Affordable Care Act is unclear, and access to care remains a major concern in states. Several strong arguments have been advanced to state regulators to reduce barriers to APRN practice. On both sides of the political divide, APRNs are seen as part of the solution to access to care, yet some representatives of organized medical groups continue to successfully block patient access to APRNs by requiring they remain tethered to physicians in many states.

As major stakeholders in the regulatory environment, it is imperative that APRNs directly influence the process in several ways, including the use of political strategies. At all levels, regulators are eager to find practicing APRNs and advanced practice nursing educators who will take an active role in assisting them to develop and implement sound regulatory policies and procedures. The information explosion has brought the ability to communicate and connect with others at a moment's notice, which makes it easier for APRNs to influence the system directly. Chapters 9 and 17 provide in-depth discussions of skills needed for leadership and political advocacy. Additional ways for novice and expert APRNs to engage actively in any regulatory process that affects their practice are included in Box 20.4.

To accomplish these activities, APRNs need to use research data, a powerful tool for shaping health policy. By actively participating in the regulatory process, APRNs ensure themselves of a strong voice in regulatory and credentialing processes. At the very least, it is incumbent on the practicing APRN to monitor the process carefully through APRN networks and social media to stay informed.

CURRENT PRACTICE CLIMATE FOR APRNS

Visioning for Advanced Practice Nursing

When APRNs seek to change statutes and regulations, it is not because they see themselves as needing to practice in a vacuum of independence apart from the rest of the healthcare team but because they desire to be a valued part of the team. It is a hard fact that APRNs must have authority over their own practices and the decisions they make about patient care. In the

BOX 20.4

Legislative and Regulatory Examples of Engagement

Novice or Experienced APRN	Experienced or Expert APRN
Join and be actively involved in both a statewide and national professional organization.	Seek out a gubernatorial appointment to the board of nursing or advanced practice committee that advises the board of nursing in your state.
Participate in regulatory activities, such as educating lawmakers, providing public comment on APRN issues, writing letters, and being part of an APRN campaign or coalition activities. Join the government relations committee.	Seek membership as the APRN or consumer member of the advisory council for the state medical board or the state board of pharmacy.
Monitor current APRN legislation and legislation that affects patients by subscribing to an electronic legislative resource.	Seek appointment to CMS panels on which Medicare and Medicaid provider issues are decided.
Offer to participate in test-writing committees for national certification examinations as item writers and/or reviewers.	Seek appointment to hospital privileging committees and ensure that privileging materials are appropriate for APRNs.
Respond to offers to review, edit, and provide feedback about circulated draft regulatory policies that directly affect APRN advanced practice nursing education and practice.	Seek appointment on advisory committees and task forces that are advising the NCSBN and other regulatory and credentialing bodies.
	Provide public comment on draft legislation regarding health care and healthcare providers.
	Offer testimony at state and national hearings at which proposed regulatory changes in APRN advanced practice nursing regulation, prescriptive authority, and reimbursement schemes will be discussed.

new *Future of Nursing 2020–2030: Charting a Path to Achieve Health Equity* (National Academies of Science, Engineering and Medicine [NASEM], 2021) report the committee again recommends that nurses be enabled to practice to the full extent of their education and training. The report challenges state and federal entities and all organizations, including employers, to remove barriers, including policy, regulatory, and public and private payment limitations, that prevent nurses from improving access to health care, quality, and value (NASEM, 2021). They must be able to defend their actions within the legal system based on nursing-driven standards and regulation. Only in this way can an APRN move out of the darkness of being a "shadow provider." Issues related to being a shadow provider are best exemplified by "incident-to" billing by NPs using the physician's Medicare number. Advanced practice nursing care is invisible to regulators and insurers with this type of billing procedure. Securing attribution for their unique services in healthcare reimbursement and outcomes will be vital to enabling APRNs to move out of the shadows and into the light.

As care increasingly moves to a team-based model, APRNs are poised to lead teams, when appropriate, and to be valuable team members. Attribution of care to specific team members is an important variable to learn what parts of team-based care contribute to the expected outcomes. This is one example of the challenges APRNs face as they work to clarify state policies. It may be that APRNs will feel comfortable only when their position in the healthcare community is fully secure in all states; this will require focused and coordinated political and legislative work related to credentialing and regulatory issues.

APRNs have already achieved impressive strides over time in the areas of credentialing and regulation of APRNs. The health care provided by APRNs has had far-reaching effects on all members of society. Thus the evolution of advanced practice nursing in the United States is a source of pride to nurses. The IOM's 2011 recommendations were revisited in the 2015 update *Assessing Progress on the Institute of Medicine Report: The Future of Nursing* report, the Josiah Macy Foundation's recommendations, and a White House directive all indicated the need for state-by-state adoption of standardized means to regulate competent practice for a growing number of APRNs (IOM; NASEM, 2016). The progress made in state-by-state adoption of the Consensus Model and uniform licensure requirements have aided in accomplishing the recommendations of these reports.

The Veteran's Health Administration (VHA) implemented full practice authority in specific VHA facilities across the United States for the CNS, NP, and CNM roles, fortunately in time to address the demands of the pandemic. The passage of the Comprehensive Addiction and Recovery Act (CARA) added APRNs to those prescribers who could offer medication-assisted treatment for addiction, also, fortunately, prior to the pandemic (CDC, 2021). The future for APRNs now includes an APRN Compact that will enable practice mobility aligned with the APRN Consensus elements across state borders (NCSBN, 2022a).

Forces within health care, as well as needs within the regulatory and educational climate of advanced practice nursing, have set the stage for an era of progressive change. The pressing healthcare needs in the United States have serious implications for education, practice, and regulation of APRNs. Advancing technologies, enhanced mobility of APRNs across state lines, and diversity among state regulatory mechanisms have brought together APRN leaders and stakeholders to craft a new vision for the future of advanced practice nursing.

FUTURE REGULATORY CHALLENGES FOR APRNS

The current political climate has dismantled parts of the Affordable Care Act, rendering it less effective in addressing the many health outcome challenges we face nationally and at state level (Norris, 2019). While many gains have been realized in Healthy People 2020 objectives, we remain challenged in the areas of access to care, family planning, diabetes care, mental health services, substance abuse services, nutrition, and oral health (U. S. Department of Health and Human Services, 2020). The challenges of the Healthy People 2030 objectives will be to increase the numbers who have access to substance abuse treatment and to reduce disparities in health care so that Americans of every age and condition are able to realize an optimal state of wellness. APRNs when allowed to practice to the full extent of their training can close health outcome gaps. The 2020 pandemic will have changed many things about healthcare delivery, insurance, and public health priorities going forward. APRNs have demonstrated they have a valued place on the teams and can deliver valued care. Perhaps as we move forward to address the many challenges in health for Americans and the disparities in access to care, the unnecessary restrictions that were never based in evidence will be lifted. Many solutions to improved health outcomes may best be addressed in collaborative interdisciplinary care, and APRNs are well on their way to being essential team members.

CONCLUSION

At no time has it been more vital for APRNs to understand and value the important relationships among groups that control the complex processes and systems that regulate practice. New models of health care and varying configurations of how APRNs practice in interprofessional teams have escalated the importance of regulatory considerations. The growth of virtual healthcare delivery makes the picture even more complex. APRNs will need to provide leadership and clear direction to policy makers to ensure the development of broad-based practice standards that will satisfy state statutes and make sense in all areas of advanced practice nursing. The consensus-derived key elements for the preparation and education of the four APRN roles, including the revised *Essentials*, are powerful drivers of the inclusion of APRNs at all levels of US health care. The need for APRNs to move into key roles as healthcare providers in the next decade requires careful vigilance with regard to the LACE components of credentialing and regulation. The ever-changing landscape of America's health system demands vision and a steady hand into the future.

KEY SUMMARY POINTS

- APRNs are increasingly educated, certified, and regulated in alignment with the Consensus Model and uniform license requirements such as those included in the APRN Compact.
- Credentialing procedures and requirements vary from state to state and determine scope of practice. APRNs must strive to achieve a scope of practice in their state that is commensurate with their education and clinical skills.
- Voluntary collaboration among all on healthcare teams is an expectation for patient safety and quality patient care.

REFERENCES

American Association of Colleges of Nursing (AACN). (2006). *The essentials of doctoral education for advanced nursing practice.* www.aacn.nche.edu/education-resources/DNPEssentials.pdf

American Association of Colleges of Nursing (AACN). (2011). *The essentials of master's education in nursing.* https://www.aacnnursing.org/portals/42/publications/mastersessentials11.pdf

American Association of Colleges of Nursing (AACN). (2021). *The essentials: Core competencies for professional nursing education.* https://www.aacnnursing.org/Portals/42/AcademicNursing/pdf/Essentials-2021.pdf

American Association of Nurse Practitioners (AANP). (2020). *Coronavirus disease 2019 (COVID-19) telehealth updates.* https://www.aanp.org/practice/practice-management/technology/telehealth

American Board of Internal Medicine (ABIM). (2020). Choosing Wisely Learning Network. https://www.choosingwisely.org/choosing-wisely-learning-network/

American College of Physicians (ACP). (2016). *Medical malpractice insurance.* https://www.acponline.org/about-acp/about-internal-medicine/career-paths/residency-career-counseling/guidance/medical-malpractice-insurance

American Medical Association. (AMA). *Truth in Advertising, Resolution 228.* https://www.ama-assn.org/, June 2019.

American Society of Addiction Medicine. (2019). AASM and AACN Partner to Increase Critical Addiction Training for Nurse Practitioners. https://www.asam.org/Quality-Science/publications/magazine/article/2019/10/31/asam-and-aacn-partner-to-increase-critical-addiction-training-for-nurse-practitioners

Act Promoting a Resilient Health Care System that Puts Patients First. MA General Law c. 260. (2020). https://malegislature.gov/Laws/SessionLaws/Acts/2020/Chapter260

American Nurses Credentialing Corporation. (2020). *Adult-Gerontology Acute Care Nurse Practitioner Role Delineation Study.* https://www.nursingworld.org/~49f2f5/globalassets/certification/certification-specialty-pages/resources/role-delineation-studies/exam-62-agacnp-rds-executive-summary_final_04092020.pdf

APRN Joint Dialogue Group. (2008). *Consensus model for APRN regulation: Licensure, accreditation, certification & education.* http://www.aacn.nche.edu/education-resources/APRNReport.pdf

Balanced Budget Act of 1997. P. L. 105-33. https://www.congress.gov/bill/105th-congress/house-bill/2015/text?overview=closed

Brashers, V., Haizlip, J., & Owen, J. A. (2020). The ASPIRE Model: Grounding the IPEC core competencies for interprofessional collaborative practice within a foundational framework. *Journal of Interprofessional Care, 34*(1), 128–132.

Buppert, C. (2015). #1 – 4 of 10 things nurse practitioners need to know about the law. *The Journal for Nurse Practitioners, 11*(7), 561–562.

Buppert, C. (2019). *Credentialing the Nurse Practitioner: What NPs and Employers Need to Know.* Medscape.com. June 19, 2019. https://www.medscape.com/viewarticle/914380

Center for Connected Health Policy. (2021). *State telehealth laws and reimbursement policies report.* https://www.cchpca.org/resources/state-telehealth-laws-and-reimbursement-policies-report-fall-2021/https://www.cchpca.org/sites/default/files/2018-10/CCHP_50_State_Report_Fall_2018.pdf

Center for Connected Health Policy (CCHP). (2020). *Telehealth Coverage Policies in the time of Covid.* https://www.cchpca.org/resources/covid-19-telehealth-coverage-policies

Centers for Disease Control and Prevention (CDC). (2018). *From policy to implementation: Practical implications of state law amendments granting nurse practitioner full practice authority.* https://www.cdc.gov/dhdsp/pubs/docs/Nurses_Case_Study-508.pdf

Centers for Disease Control and Prevention (CDC). (2020). Guidelines Library online. https://www.cdc.gov/infectioncontrol/guidelines/index.html

Centers for Disease Control and Prevention (CDC). (2021). Comprehensive Addiction and Recovery Act (CARA) Frequently Asked Questions. https://www.cdc.gov/drugoverdose/drug-free-communities/cara-faq.html

Centers for Medicare & Medicaid Services (CMS). (2020a). *Conditions for coverage (CfCs) and Conditions for Participation (CoPs).* https://www.cms.gov/Regulations-and-Guidance/Legislation/CFCsAndCoPs

Centers for Medicare & Medicaid Services (CMS). (2020b). *Medicare NPI Implementation.* https://www.cms.gov/Regulations-and-Guidance/Administrative-Simplification/NationalProvIdentStand

Centers for Medicare & Medicaid Services (CMS) Medicare Learning Network. (2022, March). *Advanced practice registered nurses, anesthesiologists assistants, and physician assistants.* https://www.cms.gov/Outreach-and-Education/Medicare-Learning-Network-

MLN/MLNProducts/Downloads/Medicare-Information-for-APRNs-AAs-PAs-Booklet-ICN-901623.pdf

The Committee for Proper Recognition of CRNAs (CPRC). (2019). https://www.nurseanesthesiologistinfo.com

De Castella, T. (2021). Delight as Nurse Confirmed as Acting US Surgeon General. *Nursing Times*. https://www.nursingtimes.net/news/leadership-news/delight-as-nurse-confirmed-as-acting-us-surgeon-general-02-02-2021/

Department of Health and Human Services Office for Civil Rights (HHS OCR). (2020). News releases. https://www.hhs.gov/ocr/newsroom/index.html

Edwards, N. E., Coddington, J., Erler, C., & Kirkpatrick, J. (2018). The impact of the role of doctor of nursing practice nurses on healthcare and leadership. *Medical Research Archives, 6*(4) April 2018 issue.

Federal Trade Commission (FTC). (2014). *Policy perspectives: Competition and the regulation of advanced practice nurses*. https://www.ftc.gov/reports/policy-perspectives-competition-regulation-advanced-practice-nurses

Fotsch, R. (2016). What's in a name? Legislative challenges with APRN title change. *Journal of Nursing Regulation, 6*(4), 73–74.

Hamric, A. B., & Tracy, M. F. (2019). A definition of advanced practice nursing. In M. F. Tracy, & E. T. O'Grady (Eds.), *Hamric and Hanson's advanced practice nursing: An integrative approach* (pp. 61–79). Elsevier.

Health Insurance Portability and Accountability Act of 1996, Pub. L. No. 104-191. chrome-extension://efaidnbmnnnibpcajpcglclefindmkaj/viewer.html?pdfurl=https%3A%2F%2Fwww.congress.gov%2F104%2Fplaws%2Fpubl191%2FPLAW-104publ191.pdf

Hooper, M. W., Nápoles, A. M., & Pérez-Stable, E. J. (2020). Covid 19 and Racial/Ethnic Disparities. *Journal of the American Medical Association, 323*(24), 2466–2467. https://doi.org/10.1001/jama.2020.8598

Institute of Medicine (IOM). (2011). *The future of nursing: Leading change, advancing health*. National Academies Press. https://doi.org/10.17226/12956

Institute of Medicine; National Academies of Sciences, Engineering, and Medicine. (2016). *Committee for Assessing Progress on Implementing the Recommendations of the Institute of Medicine Report The Future of Nursing: Leading Change, Advancing Health*. National Academies Press.

Interprofessional Education Collaborative (IPEC). (2016). *Core competencies for interprofessional collaborative practice: 2016 update*. https://www.ipecollaborative.org/ipec-core-competencies

Interstate Medical Licensure Compact (IMLC). (n.d.) https://www.imlcc.org

Jiao, S., Murimi, I. B., Stafford, R. S., Mojtabai, R., & Alexander, G. C. (2018). Quality of prescribing by physicians, nurse practitioners, and physician assistants in the United States. *Pharmacotherapy, 38*(4), 417–427.

The Joint Commission. (2016). *Ambulatory care: The who, what, when, and where's of credentialing and privileging*. https://www.jointcommission.org/-/media/deprecated-unorganized/imported-assets/tjc/system-folders/blogs/ahc_who_what_when_and_where_credentialing_bookletpdf.pdf?db=web&hash=CD838EB80D69FE2FA517285B4F3A0537

Jurkowitz, M., Shearer, E., & Walker, M. (2020). *U.S. media polarization and the 2020 election: A nation divided*. https://www.pewresearch.org/journalism/2020/01/24/u-s-media-polarization-and-the-2020-election-a-nation-divided/

Keeling, A. W. (2009). A brief history of advanced practice nursing in the United States. Chapter 1. In A. B. Hamric, J. A. Spross, & C. M. Hanson (Eds.), *Advanced practice nursing, an integrative approach*. Saunders/Elsevier.

Kleinpell, R. (2017). *Outcome assessment in advanced practice nursing* (4th ed.). Springer Publishing Company.

Kuo, Y. F., Loresto, F. L., Jr., Rounds, L. R., & Goodwin, J. S. (2013). States with the least restrictive regulations experienced the largest increase in patients seen by nurse practitioners. *Health Affairs*, 32(7), 1236–1243. https://doi.org/10.1377/hlthaff.2013.0072

LACE network. (2020). Lace Network login.icohere.com

Levisohn, A., & Higgins, E. (2020). *States address provider shortages to meet the health care demands of the pandemic*. National Academy for State Health Policy. https://nashp.org/states-address-provider-shortages-to-meet-the-health-care-demands-of-the-pandemic/

Maier, S. (2019). *Many nurse practitioners cannot provide medications to treat opioid addiction*. University of San Francisco Research. online. https://www.ucsf.edu/news/2019/04/413856/many-nurse-practitioners-cannot-provide-medications-treat-opioid-addiction

Markowitz, S., Adams, K. E., Lewitt, M., & Dunlop, A. L. (2017). Competitive effects of scope of practice restrictions: Public health or public harm. *Journal of Health Economics, 55*(C), 201–218.

Martin, B., & Alexander, M. (2019). The economic burden and practice restrictions associated with collaborative practice agreements: A national survey of advanced practice registered nurses. *The Journal of Nursing Regulation, 9*(4), P22–P30.

McMullen, P. C., & Howie, W. O. (2020). Credentialing and privileging: A primer for nurse practitioners. *The Journal for Nurse Practitioners, 16*(2), 91–95.

Melnyk, B. (2018). *Why choose evidence-based practice?* American Association of Nurse Practitioners Practice. October 26, 2018. https://www.aanp.org/news-feed/why-choose-evidence-based-practice

Modern Healthcare Policy Tracker. (2021). *Regulation tracker: Biden reviews Trump's final rules*. Modernhealthcare.com Jan 21, 2021. https://www.modernhealthcare.com/policy/regulation-tracker-biden-reviews-trumps-final-rules

National Academies of Sciences, Engineering, and Medicine. (2021). *The Future of Nursing 2020-2030: Charting a Path to Achieve Health Equity*. The National Academies Press. https://doi.org/10.17226/25982

National Association of Clinical Nurse Specialists (NACNS). (2019). *Statement on CNS practice and education* (3rd ed.). https://members.nacns.org/store/viewproduct.aspx?id=19695699

National Council of State Boards of Nursing (NCSBN). (2008). *Consensus model for APRN regulation: Licensure, accreditation, certification and education*. www.ncsbn.org/index.htm

National Council of State Boards of Nursing (NCSBN). (2012). *Requirements for Accrediting Agencies and Criteria for APRN Certification Programs*. https://www.ncsbn.org/12_APRN_Certification_updated.pdf

National Council of State Boards of Nursing (NCSBN). (2014). *Model Act*. https://www.ncsbn.org/3867.htm

National Council of State Boards of Nursing (NCSBN). (2020a). *Nurse Practice Acts*. https://www.ncsbn.org/npa.htm

National Council of State Boards of Nursing (NCSBN). (2020b). *Opioid Toolkit*. https://www.ncsbn.org/opioid-toolkit.htm

National Council of State Boards of Nursing (NCSBN). (2022a). *APRN Compact.com*. https://aprncompact.com/about.htm

National Council of State Boards of Nursing APRN (NCSBN). (2022b). *Consensus Implementation Status*. https://www.ncsbn.org/5397.htm

National Council of State Boards of Nursing (NCSBN). (2022c). *Member Board Profiles*. https://www.ncsbn.org/profiles.htm

National Council of State Boards of Nursing (NCSBN). (2022d). *Nurse Licensure Compact*. https://www.ncsbn.org/nurse-licensure-compact.htm

National Council of State Boards of Nursing (NCSBN). (2022e). Nurse Practice Act Toolkit. *Nurse Practice Act Toolkit*. https://www.ncsbn.org/npa-toolkit.htm

National Council of State Boards of Nursing (NCSBN). (2022f). *State Response to Covid-19 (APRNs)*. https://www.ncsbn.org/APRNState_ COVID-19_Response_4_30.pdf

Norris, L. (2019). *Bottom of Form Understanding Health Insurance Changes for 2020*. Verywellhealth.com

Rosen, M. A., DiazGranados, D., Dietz, A. S., Benishek, L. E., Thompson, D., Pronovost, P. J., & Weaver, S. J. (2018). Teamwork in healthcare: Discoveries enabling safer, high-quality care. *American Psychologist, 73*(4), 433–450. https://doi.org/10.1037%2Famp0000298

Safriet, B. (1992). Health care dollars and regulatory sense: The role of advanced practice nursing. *Yale Journal of Regulation, 9*, 417–487.

Safriet, B. (2002). Closing the gap between can and may in health care providers' scopes of practice: A primer for policymakers. *Yale Journal of Regulation, 19*, 301–334.

Safriet, B. (2010). *Federal options for maximizing the value of advanced practice nurses in providing quality cost effective health care*. www.webNPonline.com

Society to Improve Diagnosis in Medicine SIDM. (2020). Resources for Clinical Teams/SIDM.org https://www.improvediagnosis.org/clinicians/

Sofer, D. (2018). AMA resolution opposes independent practice by APRNs. *American Journal of Nursing, 118*(3), 12.

Tikkanen, R. & Abrams, M. K. (2020). *U.S. health care from a global perspective, 2019: Higher spending, worse outcomes*? The Commonwealth Fund. https://www.commonwealthfund.org/publications/issue-briefs/2020/jan/us-health-care-global-perspective-2019

UpToDate (2022). online: https://www.uptodate.com/home

US Department of Education. (2016). *Education Department Announces Final Rule on State Authorization of Postsecondary Distance Education, Foreign Locations*: ed.gov. https://www2.ed.gov/documents/press-releases/07222016-state-authorization-nprm.pdf

US Department of Health and Human Services. Centers for Disease Control and Prevention. (2020). Healthy people 2020. https://www.cdc.gov/nchs/healthy_people/hp2020.htm

US Department of Veterans Affairs, Office of Public and Intergovernmental Affairs. (2016). *VA Grants Full Practice Authority to Advance Practice Registered Nurses*. https://www.va.gov/opa/pressrel/includes/viewPDF.cfm?id=2793

Weigel, G., Ramaswamy, A., Sobel, L., Salganicoff, A., Cubanski, J., & Freed, M. (2020). *Opportunities and Barriers for Telemedicine in the US During the COVID-19 Emergency and Beyond*. Kaiser Family Foundation. https://www.kff.org/womens-health-policy/issue-brief/opportunities-and-barriers-for-telemedicine-in-the-u-s-during-the-covid-19-emergency-and-beyond/

Weiner, J. P. (2021). In-person and telehealth ambulatory contacts and costs in a large US insured cohort before and during the COVID-19 pandemic. *JAMA Network Open, 4*(3), 1–13. https://jamanetwork.com/journals/jamanetworkopen/fullarticle/2777779

Whitehouse.gov. (2019). *Executive Order on Protecting and Improving Medicare for Our Nation's Seniors*: Whitehouse.gov. https://www.federalregister.gov/documents/2019/10/08/2019-22073/protecting-and-improving-medicare-for-our-nations-seniors

Zhang, X., Lin, D., Pforsich, H., & Lin, V. (2020). Physician workforce in the United States of America: Forecasting nationwide shortages. *Human Resources Health, 18*(1), 8. https://human-resources-health.biomedcentral.com/articles/10.1186/s12960-020-0448-3

Zorek, J., & Raehl, C. (2012). Interprofessional education accreditation standards in the USA: A comparative analysis. *Journal of Interprofessional Care, 27*(2), 123–130. https://pubmed.ncbi.nlm.nih.gov/22950791/

21

APRN OUTCOMES AND PERFORMANCE IMPROVEMENT RESEARCH

PATTI LUDWIG-BEYMER ■ LISA HOPP

"Nature does not hurry, yet everything is accomplished."
~ Lao Tzu

CHAPTER CONTENTS

REVIEW OF TERMS 674
- Why Measure Outcomes? 674
- What Outcome Measures Are Important? 678

CONCEPTUAL MODELS OF CARE DELIVERY IMPACT 680
- Models for Evaluating Outcomes Achieved by APRNs 680
- Outcomes Evaluation Model 680
- Nursing Role Effectiveness Model Adapted for Acute Care Nurse Practitioners 680

EVIDENCE TO DATE 683
- Role Description Studies 683
- Role Perception and Acceptance Studies 684
- Care Delivery Process Studies 684

"PROCESS AS OUTCOME" STUDIES 685

PERFORMANCE (PROCESS) IMPROVEMENT ACTIVITIES 685

OUTCOMES MANAGEMENT ACTIVITIES 686

POPULATION HEALTH ACTIVITIES 686

IMPACT OF APRN PRACTICE 689
- Studies Comparing APRN to Physician and Other Provider Outcomes 689
- Nurse Practitioner Outcomes 695
- Clinical Nurse Specialist Outcomes 695
- Certified Nurse-Midwife Outcomes 696
- Certified Registered Nurse Anesthetist Outcomes 696
- Studies Comparing APRN and Physician Productivity 697
- Relative Work Value of APRNs 697

FUTURE DIRECTIONS FOR USING OUTCOMES IN APRN PRACTICE 698

CONCLUSION 700

KEY SUMMARY POINTS 701

Measuring the impact of advanced practice registered nurse (APRN) practice is an important component in supporting the value of the role with evidence from high-quality research studies. The Patient Protection and Affordable Care Act of 2010 established groundbreaking changes in financial incentives by rewarding better outcomes to improve safety and the quality of care. This value-based purchasing and other quality care initiatives continue to focus on performance monitoring and the development of operational and clinical performance metrics (Centers for Medicare & Medicaid Services [CMS], 2021a).

Several factors have led to the current focus on outcomes of care in health care, including increased emphasis on providing quality care and promoting patient safety, regulatory requirements for healthcare entities to demonstrate care effectiveness, increased health system accountability, the critical need to address health disparities and inequities, and changes

The authors would like to acknowledge Gail Ingersoll, PhD, RN, FANP, FAAN, Ruth Kleinpell, PhD, RN, FAAN, FAANP, FCCM, and Anne W. Alexandrov, PhD, RN, CCRN, ANVP-BC, NVRN-BC, FAAN for their work on previous editions of this chapter.

in the organization, delivery, and financing of health care. APRNs impact patient and system outcomes in many ways, but too often these outcomes remain invisible and are not quantified or attributed to advanced practice nursing (Fulton et al., 2019). Employers, consumers, insurers, and others are calling for APRNs to justify their contribution to health care and to demonstrate the value that they add to the system. The National Academies of Sciences, Engineering and Medicine (NASEM; formerly the Institute of Medicine [IOM]) report *The Future of Nursing* (IOM, 2011) and *Future of Nursing 2020–2030* (NASEM, 2021) highlighted the importance of promoting the ability of APRNs to practice to the full extent of their education and training. When nurses practice at the top of their preparation, they can deliver high-quality, accessible, and equitable care (IOM, 2011; NASEM, 2021). Verifying APRN contributions requires an assessment of the structures, processes, and outcomes associated with APRN performance and the care delivery systems in which they practice. Ultimately, the value proposition of APRN practice requires improved, high-quality economic evaluations using standardized methodological guidelines such as *Guidelines for the Economic Evaluation of Health Technologies: Canada* (Lopatina et al., 2017).

Evaluation of individual APRN impact occurs at multiple levels and contexts, with supporting evidence collected during annual performance reviews, outcomes measurement activities, process improvement analyses, program evaluations, and small- and large-scale clinical, health systems, and outcomes research. At the least, APRNs and/or their supervisors should perform annual individual performance reviews and outcomes measurement, regardless of practice setting, population served, or APRN role and position responsibilities. These assessments will need to consider how APRNs actualize competencies (American Association of Colleges of Nursing [AACN], 2021) and impact outcomes, particularly in underserved populations, who experience disparities in health outcomes (NASEM, 2021).

Outcome evaluation and ongoing performance assessment are essential to the survival and success of advanced practice nursing. The importance of measuring the impact of advanced practice was highlighted repeatedly in the previous *The Essentials of Doctoral Education for Advanced Nursing Practice* (AACN, 2006) and as a key competency for advanced-level nursing education in the recently published *The Essentials: Core Competencies for Professional Nursing Education* (AACN, 2021). Several of the domains and their competencies and subcompetencies of advanced level of nursing education explicitly require knowledge and ability to evaluate APRN practice and decision making (AACN, 2021). A key rationale supporting the development of the doctor of nursing practice degree included industry demand for APRNs capable of gauging baseline clinical outcomes, determining gaps in the use of evidence-based practice (EBP), masterfully leading change that is scientifically sound, and measuring the impact of their interventions.

This chapter focuses on measuring and monitoring the quality of care delivered and the outcomes achieved by APRNs. Performance indicators are discussed at two levels—the aggregate level, at which evidence addresses APRN role impact in one of the four APRN roles, and the individual level, with activities directed at the outcomes of a single APRN's practice. This chapter outlines key terms and describes frameworks for quality and outcomes assessment. Methods supporting comparative effectiveness research led by APRNs are reviewed and strategies for identifying and assessing APRN-sensitive outcome indicators are highlighted. Emphasis is placed on how to use outcomes of APRN practice to showcase impact on the promotion of EBP adoption and health equity (NASEM, 2021).

REVIEW OF TERMS

Numerous interrelated terms are used to define and describe the components of performance appraisal and outcomes assessment. The principal terms used in this chapter are listed alphabetically in Table 21.1.

Why Measure Outcomes?

Measuring outcomes is a required component of health care, based in part on federal and state regulatory agencies, practice guidelines, employers, and consumer groups. Healthcare organizations actively monitor outcomes of care as a means of evaluation, as well as for requirements for accreditation, certification, recognition, and reimbursement. Entities including the CMS, The Joint Commission, the National

TABLE 21.1

Definitions of the Components of Performance Appraisal and Outcomes Assessment

Term	Definition
Benchmark	"An attribute or achievement that serves as a standard for other providers or institutions to emulate. Benchmarks differ from other standard of care goals, in that they derive from empiric data—specifically, performance or outcomes data" (AHRQ, n.d.).
Performance benchmark	An ideal practice standard target that has been achieved by some group or organization known for its quality of services. This process-focused benchmark serves as the gold standard against which others are compared. Some evaluators also use this term to denote achievement of an intermediate outcome (e.g., attainment of desired best practice performance).
Comparative effectiveness research (CER)	"The direct comparison of two or more existing healthcare interventions to determine which interventions work best for which patients and which interventions pose the greatest benefits and harms. The core question of CER is which treatment works best, for whom, under what circumstances" (Patient-Centered Outcomes Research Institute [PCORI], 2021).
Clinical practice guideline	"Statements that include recommendations intended to optimize patient care. They are informed by a systematic review of evidence and an assessment of the benefits and harms of alternative care options." Trustworthiness requires that a knowledgeable, multidisciplinary panel of experts and key stakeholders develop the guideline to consider important patient subgroups and patient preferences. The guideline group uses explicit and transparent processes to minimize bias (Institute of Medicine Committee on Standards for Developing Trustworthy Clinical Practice Guidelines, 2011).
Dashboard	A visual representation of data to enable the review, analysis, and tracking of data trends. The dashboard is like a scorecard because it allows for the visualization of performance and outcome information often in the form of a table or chart (Barnum et al., 2019).
Disease management	An organized process focusing on the patient's disease as the target of interest, with improvements in outcome seen as a result of attention to the attributes or characteristics of the disease. Quality indicators endorsed and adopted by federal and private health plans commonly target adherence to evidence-based processes that are expected to affect disease management.
Effectiveness	Extent to which evidence-based interventions or programs produce desired or intended outcomes in real life. The principle of effectiveness supports the adoption of standardized healthcare processes forming the basis for pay-for-performance core measures because it assumes that widespread use of evidence-based methods should demonstrate reductions in disease and complication incidences and, ultimately, healthcare costs.
Intervention effectiveness	The measurement of results in line with implementation of a specific evidence-based practice. Intervention effectiveness studies are considered *Phase 4 studies* that explore the generalizability of efficacious interventions; specifically, intervention effectiveness studies examine whether results are similar to those produced in *Phase 3* randomized controlled trials that demonstrated initial efficacy of an intervention.
Program effectiveness	Measurement of the results attained through the systematic adoption of evidence-based structures (e.g., systems such as equipment, manpower) and standardized processes.
Efficiency	The effects achieved by some intervention in relation to the effort expended in terms of money, resources, and time.
Evidence-based practice	"The conscientious, explicit, and judicious use of current best evidence in making decisions about the care of individual patients. ... [It] means integrating individual clinical expertise with the best available external clinical evidence from systematic research" (Sackett et al., 1996, p. 71). The shift to pay-for-performance, based on the systematic implementation of evidence-based practice, provides an example of the power of scientifically sound processes and is driving practitioner viability in the healthcare market.
Impact measurement	An analysis of the difference in a targeted outcome measure and growth of practice systems resulting from use of the outcomes management process (Alexandrov et al., 2019). Impact measurement enables advanced practice registered nurses (APRNs) to showcase the effectiveness of programs implemented to improve patient outcomes. Analyzing the impact of an outcomes management process can help identify key aspects of the process that led to changes in an outcome (US Department of Health and Human Services, Administration for Children and Families, 2010).

Continued

TABLE 21.1

Definitions of the Components of Performance Appraisal and Outcomes Assessment—cont'd

Term	Definition
Metric	Also described as a measure or indicator; defines parameters for structure, process, or outcome, depending on its level. For example, a metric for rate-based measures would define population numerators and denominators to ensure that each party using the metric measures the same population (validity) in the same way each time (reliability). The National Quality Forum (NQF) evaluates candidate measures (metrics) against defined criteria and then endorses them; if accepted, the measures are then eligible for pay-for-performance adoption by the Centers for Medicare & Medicaid Services and other third-party payers. These criteria include the following: (1) the importance of studying the measures and publicly reporting findings; (2) the scientific acceptability of measure properties—that they measure validity and reliability; (3) usability, the extent to which payers, providers, and consumers can understand results and use them for healthcare decision making; (4) feasibility, the extent to which the required data are available or could be captured without undue burden; and (5) comparison with related or competing measures to determine how the candidate measure harmonizes or differs from other measures (NQF, 2019).
Outcome	Results produced by inherent characteristics, processes, and/or structures; newly developed processes and/or structures may constitute interventions. Measurement of outcomes will vary according to the intended target. For example, targets may be patients, families, students, other care providers, communities, and in some cases, organizations (if the organization as a whole is the recipient of the intervention). Outcomes may be intended or unintended and reflect positive or untoward results such as complications. Because of this, measurement plans must be cautiously developed to capture all outcomes (positive or negative) that theoretically align with the planned intervention, including the likelihood of no change in pre-intervention status (Alexandrov, 2011; Doran, 2011). Most definitions of outcome have evolved from the original writings of Donabedian (1966, 1980), who defined an outcome as a change in a patient's physiologic health state (i.e., morbidity and mortality; see Chapter 2). This patient-centered understanding of outcomes is particularly relevant to APRNs, whose actions directly or indirectly affect patients and families.
Outcome(s) assessment	An evaluation of the observed results of some action or intervention for recipients of services. Outcome assessments provide the data needed to support or refute the perceived beneficial effect of a clinical decision, care delivery process, or targeted action.
Outcome indicators	Metrics or measures capable of demonstrating actual results produced by the interaction of inherent characteristics, processes, and/or structures. Outcome indicators are derived from systematic determination of all potential results that could occur; these measures should be clearly defined in terms of their measurement properties to ensure validity and reliability, with consideration of their temporal association to the intervention. Today, a variety of well-defined, tested, and endorsed outcome measures are available for use in outcome and disease management programs; however, there are considerably fewer outcome measures available for use compared with process measures. Because the development of sound process and outcome measures requires extensive expertise and testing, APRNs are encouraged to select NQF-endorsed measures to support many of their projects because these are thoroughly vetted and promote meaningful comparisons (NQF, 2017). This approach ensures consistency in the methods used to study and improve phenomena of interest.
Outcome(s) management	The active implementation of processes and/or structures that aim to improve targeted results. According to the classic work of Ellwood (1988), a comprehensive outcomes management program does the following: (1) emphasizes the use of standards to select appropriate interventions; (2) measures a broad array of outcomes, including disease-specific, behavioral, functional, and perception-of-care outcomes; (3) pools outcomes data for groups of like patients in relation to processes of care and patient characteristics; and (4) analyzes and disseminates findings to stakeholders (patients, payers, providers) to inform decision making. The goal is to improve care to aggregate populations.
Outcome(s) measurement	The collection, analysis, and reporting of reliable and valid outcome indicators.
Patient-centered outcomes research	Research that "helps people and their caregivers communicate and make informed healthcare decisions, allowing their voices to be heard in assessing the value of healthcare options" (PCORI, 2013). It assesses both benefits and harms of all types of interventions, is inclusive of individual's preferences, autonomy, and needs and includes a wide variety of settings and diversity of participants. Importantly, it "investigates optimizing outcomes while addressing burden to individuals, availability of services, technology, and personnel, and other stakeholder perspectives" (PCORI, 2013).

TABLE 21.1

Definitions of the Components of Performance Appraisal and Outcomes Assessment—cont'd

Term	Definition
Performance (process and system) improvement	Activities designed to increase the quality of services provided. The focus of attention shifts to the actions taken by the provider and/or new systems that have been developed rather than the outcomes achieved. Although outcomes may be monitored to determine whether the change in process and/or systems produces a desired effect, primary attention is on the interventions (care delivery processes) delivered. Subsumed within performance improvement activities are those associated with quality improvement initiatives, also described by some as *continuous quality improvement* or *total quality management*. Although subtle distinctions are assigned to each of these terms, the focus and the intent are the same—to ensure the delivery of care that is appropriate, safe, competent, and timely and to maximize the potential for favorable patient outcomes. In most cases, the measurement of performance is guided by the use of established indicators of best practice such as national guidelines for care.
Performance evaluation (assessment)	Assessment of individual achievement and the attainment of personal, professional, and organizational goals. Performance assessment activities for APRNs include those associated with evaluating and improving day-to-day interactions with individual patients and healthcare colleagues and those involving the measurement of APRN impact on populations, organizations, and communities.
Process indicator (measure)	A measure of visible behavior or action that a care provider undertakes to deliver care. Process indicators measure the fidelity of targeted interventions and are essential to demonstrating a causal link between new care processes and outcome metrics of interest. When outcome measures are evaluated without process fidelity measurement, it is "assumed" that the targeted process that was changed produced the outcome. But, because this may not be the case, process fidelity has become an important aspect of comparative effectiveness research so that clarity of the intervention's contribution to patient outcomes can be established.
Program evaluation	Assessment of overall programmatic performance, including process fidelity, structural adherence and competency, and the reliable performance of all individual and team contributors to the delivery of health care, in relation to key outcomes of interest. Because APRNs play an integral role in supporting and leading programs, APRN contributions are often evaluated in the context of an overall program.
Proxy indicators	An indirect measure used when a direct measure cannot be obtained or when an accurate indicator has not been identified. An example of a proxy indicator is the collection of self-report data from parents or spouses when patients are unable to respond to questions about perceptions of care or previous health. In the acute care hospital setting, case mix index, patient age, and comorbidity often are used as proxy indicators of risk adjustment for given clinical populations, simply because more direct indicators are not readily accessible. Length of stay has been a commonly measured proxy outcome but there are limitations to its use because many factors can affect length of stay.
Quality of care	A term used to convey overall process utilization and structures of care. Quality of care should be considered a "summary" term because measurement of care quality requires the systematic measurement of processes, structures, and outcomes.
Risk and severity adjustment	A process used to standardize groups according to characteristics that might unduly influence an outcome. An example of severity adjustment would involve leveling a heart failure cohort by controlling for their New York Heart Association Functional Classification at baseline so that patients with severe heart failure can be compared equally against patients with less severe failure; without such an adjustment, baseline severity may affect resource use at discharge, cost of care and length of stay, rehospitalization, functional status, and even mortality. The aim of risk and severity adjustment is to level the field among all patients in a sample so that outcomes associated with interventions may be measured more accurately.
Standards	"A profession's authoritative statements of the actions and behaviors that all registered nurses, regardless of role, population, specialty, and setting, are expected to competently perform" (American Nurses Association, 2021, p. 4). Standards focus on the processes of care delivery and scope of practice, serving as criteria for the establishment of practice-related rules, conditions, and performance requirements.
Structural indicators	Measures of human, technical, and other resources used in care delivery. These structures focus on the characteristics of the setting, system, or care providers and include such elements as numbers and types of providers, provider qualifications, agency policies and procedures, characteristics of patients served, and payment sources.

Quality Forum (NQF), and the Agency for Healthcare Research and Quality (AHRQ), along with individual state-mandated reporting, drive the increased focus on improving outcomes. APRN models of care provide the opportunity to demonstrate impact of care and to improve quality of care outcomes for patients.

What Outcome Measures Are Important?

Many outcomes are important to patients, including perception of the quality of health care, complication rates, return to work after illness/injury, mortality and morbidity rates, and patient/family as well as state and federal costs of care. The *National Patient Safety Goals* of The Joint Commission (2021) continue to evolve as they define specific targets that promote quality and safety outcomes for patients. In the hospital, these include accuracy of patient identification, effectiveness of communication among caregivers, medication safety, avoiding harm with anticoagulant therapy, reducing patient harm related to clinical alarm systems, reducing healthcare-associated infections, identifying patient safety risks, and preventing wrong site, wrong procedure, and wrong person surgery (The Joint Commission, 2021). The NQF has endorsed numerous quality measures for CMS, including provision of venous thromboembolism (VTE) prophylaxis, anticoagulation for atrial fibrillation, patient education for numerous disease states, mortality, early antibiotic administration in sepsis, and smoking cessation counseling; however, most of these indicators are process based, with very few outcome indicators required at this time. Similarly, the AHRQ has developed numerous inpatient quality indicators and patient safety indicators for NQF endorsement and CMS adoption, including prevention of postoperative sepsis, central line–associated bloodstream infection, pressure ulcers, and postoperative respiratory failure among others (AHRQ, 2020).

The Patient Protection and Affordable Care Act's Value-Based Purchasing Program initiative focuses on a hospital's performance on quality measures of clinical process-of-care measures, healthcare-associated infections, claims-based patient safety, and patient experience of care. Under this program, incentive payments are made to hospitals based on quality measure performance and improvement in performance over time; hospitals publicly report these outcomes. Currently, 23 measures are specified under the Hospital Inpatient Quality Reporting program (CMS, 2020). Box 21.1 outlines examples of outcome measures as well as candidate measures for the Hospital Value-Based Purchasing program. Focusing on improving these areas of care has significant implications not only for patient care but also for hospital reimbursement rates. Therefore targeting these identified measures and assessing the impact of APRNs in these areas of care has considerable relevance.

Despite a growing emphasis on outcomes, measuring the outcomes and impact of APRNs is not a consistent part of practice. A survey conducted by the University HealthSystem Consortium (now Vizient), a large national consortium formed from the association of 103 academic medical centers, assessed use of APRNs in 25 organizations (Moote et al., 2011). Productivity was measured using a variety of metrics, including patient encounters, number of procedures, gross charges, collections for professional fees, number of shared visits (Medicare), number of indirect billing visits (Blue Cross), and number of visits billed under the APRN provider number. Very few organizations had defined productivity targets, and despite significant investments in APRN models of care, most organizations reported that they did not measure the financial impact of employing APRNs or had done so in very limited areas. Most organizations (69%) did not track patient outcomes related to APRN care, primarily because of the inability to match patients to providers. A few organizations reported tracking several specific outcomes, often by service, including length of stay (15%), readmission rates (12%), family and patient satisfaction (12%), and specific clinical outcomes such as ventilator days (8%), urinary tract infection rates (4%), ventilator-associated event rates (4%), skin breakdown rates (4%), VTE prophylaxis rates (4%), and catheter-related bloodstream infection rates (4%; Moote et al., 2011). The results of the study identified that even in institutions employing large numbers of APRNs (200 or more), a focused effort at assessing outcomes has not been implemented. This study highlights the current need to reinforce the importance of assessing outcomes of APRNs as an essential component in their utilization and provides a call to action for APRNs to develop initiative and passion for this important work. Without capturing the impact of ARPN care,

BOX 21.1

Examples of Healthcare Outcome Measures by Organization

NATIONAL QUALITY FORUM QUALITY MEASURES EXAMPLES

- Acute otitis externa: percentage of patients age 2 years and older with a diagnosis of acute otitis externa who were not prescribed systemic antimicrobial therapy
- Adult major depressive disorder: percentage of patients age 18 years and older with a diagnosis of major depressive disorder who had a suicide risk assessment completed during the visit in which a new diagnosis or recurrent episode was identified
- Comprehensive diabetes care: percentage of members 18 to 64 years of age with diabetes (type 1 and type 2) whose most recent hemoglobin A1c level is less than 7.0% (controlled)
- Urinary catheter–associated urinary tract infection for patients in the intensive care unit (ICU)
- ICU venous thromboembolism prophylaxis
- Provision of anticoagulation for patients with atrial fibrillation to prevent stroke

AGENCY FOR HEALTHCARE RESEARCH AND QUALITY INDICATOR EXAMPLES

- In-hospital fall with hip fracture rate
- Perioperative pulmonary embolism and deep venous thrombosis rate
- Pressure ulcer rate
- Percentage of ICU patients age 18 and older receiving mechanical ventilation who had an order on the first ventilator day for head-of-bed elevation (30–45 degrees)
- Sepsis: percentage of patients with severe sepsis/septic shock who had two sets of blood cultures collected within 24 hours following severe sepsis/septic shock identification

CENTERS FOR MEDICARE & MEDICAID SERVICES HOSPITAL VALUE-BASED PURCHASING PROGRAM EXAMPLES

- Clinical Processes of Care Measures Examples
  - Influenza immunization
  - Acute myocardial infarction—aspirin prescribed at discharge
  - Heart failure—discharge instructions
  - Healthcare-associated infections—prophylactic antibiotics discontinued within 24 hours after surgery end time
- Hospital-Acquired Condition Measures Examples
  - Surgical site infection for abdominal hysterectomy and colon procedures
  - Methicillin-resistant Staphylococcus aureus bacteremia
  - Central line-associated bloodstream infection
  - *Clostridium difficile* infection
  - Catheter-associated urinary tract infection
- Patient Experience of Care Measures/Person and Community Engagement
  - Communication with nurses
  - Communication with doctors
  - Responsiveness of hospital staff
  - Pain management
  - Communication about medicines
  - Discharge information

THE JOINT COMMISSION NATIONAL PATIENT SAFETY GOALS EXAMPLES

- Improve accuracy of patient identification
- Improve the effectiveness of communication among caregivers
  - Use at least two patient identifiers when providing care, treatment, and services
  - Report critical results of tests and diagnostic procedures on a timely basis
- Improve the safety of using medications
  - Label all medications, containers, and solutions on and off the sterile field in the perioperative areas and other procedural settings
  - Reduce the likelihood of patient harm associated with the use of anticoagulant therapy
  - Maintain and communicate accurate patient medication information
- Reduce patient harm associated with clinical alarm systems
- Reduce the risk of healthcare-associated infections
- Comply with either the current Centers for Disease Control and Prevention hand hygiene guidelines or the current World Health Organization hand hygiene guidelines

contributions to patient care as well as quality of care improvements, patient safety measures, and other salient measures such as family and patient knowledge and satisfaction remain unknown, challenging the overall contribution of APRNs in health care today.

One organization has attempted to improve the ability of advanced practice providers (APRNs and physician assistants [PAs]) to more easily attack the problem of documenting productivity and billing practices to unmask the invisibility of their impact. Brooks and Fulton (2019) tested an algorithm to enable advanced practice providers to more accurately directly bill for their services. Not only did the decision aid significantly improve reimbursement but the APRNs, and PAs, productivity became visible and measurable to administrators and patients.

CONCEPTUAL MODELS OF CARE DELIVERY IMPACT

Because APRNs usually work with other health professionals, their influence on care delivery outcomes can be difficult to assess. They may have a direct effect through their interactions with patients and families and/or they may have an indirect effect through their enhancement of the performance of others. Moreover, many factors can influence APRN practice irrespective of their direct or indirect efforts.

Models for Evaluating Outcomes Achieved by APRNs

Several outcomes measurement and role impact models have been proposed, with most evolving from the original quality-of-care framework proposed by Donabedian (1966, 1980). Donabedian posited that quality is a function of the structural elements of the setting in which care is provided, processes used by care providers, and changes to the recipients of care (i.e., the outcomes; see Chapter 2). Applying these concepts to APRN practice, structural variables relate to the components of a system of care. Process variables pertain to the behavior or actions of the APRN or the activities of an APRN-directed educational or care delivery program. Interactions among structures and processes result in outcomes. Researchers can study Donabedian's elements of structure (attributes of the setting in which care occurs), process (what people do while giving and receiving care), and outcome (describes the effects of care on the health status of patients and populations) or APRNs can use these elements as a model to structure an assessment of their practice. The more complete the model (e.g., the inclusion of all or at least two of the components), the more likely the successful identification of the APRN's impact on care delivery outcome. Two models are described below that rely upon Donabedian's seminal work.

Outcomes Evaluation Model

In 1994, Holzemer designed an outcome evaluation plan using a Donabedian-guided model. Subsequently, others used the three key elements to describe and measure APRN practice (Dwyer et al., 2017; Gardner et al., 2013). A simple organizational approach is to design a table consisting of inputs/context/setting (structure), processes, and outcomes, which are identified along the horizontal axis (Table 21.2).

For the APRN, the patient is any recipient of APRN services (e.g., patients, families). The provider is the person (APRN) or interprofessional group providing the service and potentially could include trained community laypersons who assist with the provision of services. The setting is the local environment in which the services are delivered and includes the resources available to provide care. Table 21.2 illustrates how to use Donabedian's elements to plan APRN outcomes assessment like Holzemer's approach (Holzemer, 1994). Included in the table are potential variables that may facilitate assessment of the APRN's impact. Additional variables would be selected based on specialty service, population specifics, and additional characteristics of the provider, patient, or environment.

Nursing Role Effectiveness Model Adapted for Acute Care Nurse Practitioners

Sidani and Irvine (1999) adapted the nursing role effectiveness model to provide a conceptual approach enabling evaluation of the acute care nurse practitioner (ACNP) role in acute care settings (Fig. 21.1). The model derives from Donabedian's framework, with components focusing on structure (patient, ACNP, and organization), process (ACNP role components, role enactment, and role functions), and outcome (quality and cost outcomes). The model emphasizes

TABLE 21.2

Advanced Practice Registered Nurse Outcomes Planning Grid[a]

	Inputs/Context (Structure)	Processes	Outcomes
Patient	Age Sex Gender Ethnicity Marital status, social supports Educational background Health status (current and past) Previous experience with health system Special needs (e.g., visual, literacy, hearing) Expectations of provider and health system Access to care Insurance coverage	Performance of self-care behaviors Ability Willingness Family involvement in care delivery process Use of alternative or complementary therapies Compliance with evidence-based guideline recommended care for discreet patient diagnoses	***Generic*** Physical health Mental health Symptom control Functional status Perceived well-being Patient perception of the quality of healthcare services Adherence to treatment regimen Knowledge of condition, treatment program, and expected outcomes ***Specific (dependent on patient condition and need; representative examples)*** Serum glucose level Birth weight Reinfarction rate Transplant rejection rate Smoking cessation rate Length of stay Ventilator days Wound closure, wound healing
APRN provider	Educational preparation Specialty focus Years of experience Level of self-esteem Resourcefulness Assertiveness	Expert practice Collaboration Communication patterns Interactions with other care providers and staff Expert guidance and coaching Consultation Clinical and professional leadership Ethical practice Evidence-based practice Case management Care delivery according to practice standards Documentation	Productivity Practice confidence Contributions to science: publications, presentations
Setting	Geographic location (rural, urban, mixed) Type of facility (academic health center, acute care, clinic, industry) Diagnostic equipment Organizational culture and philosophy	Care provider credentialing process Quality improvement process Systems of care Communication patterns Governance process Care provider documentation process	Length of stay Staff turnover rate Cost of services New program development Revenue generated Community satisfaction Provider satisfaction

Continued

TABLE 21.2

Advanced Practice Registered Nurse Outcomes Planning Grid—cont'd

Inputs/Context (Structure)	Processes	Outcomes
Administrative structure	Annual performance review process	Staff satisfaction
State regulations on advanced practice	Provider credentialing process	
Policies and procedures		
Patient mix		
Type of care delivery model		
Availability of other services in vicinity		
Credentialing agency requirements		
State health department regulations		
Annual goals		
Annual budget		

[a]Components are not exhaustive of APRN-related outcomes planning but serve as a guide for planning activities.
Adapted from "The impact of nursing care in Latin America and the Caribbean: A focus on outcomes," by W. L. Holzemer, 1994, *Journal of Advanced Nursing, 20*, 5–12.

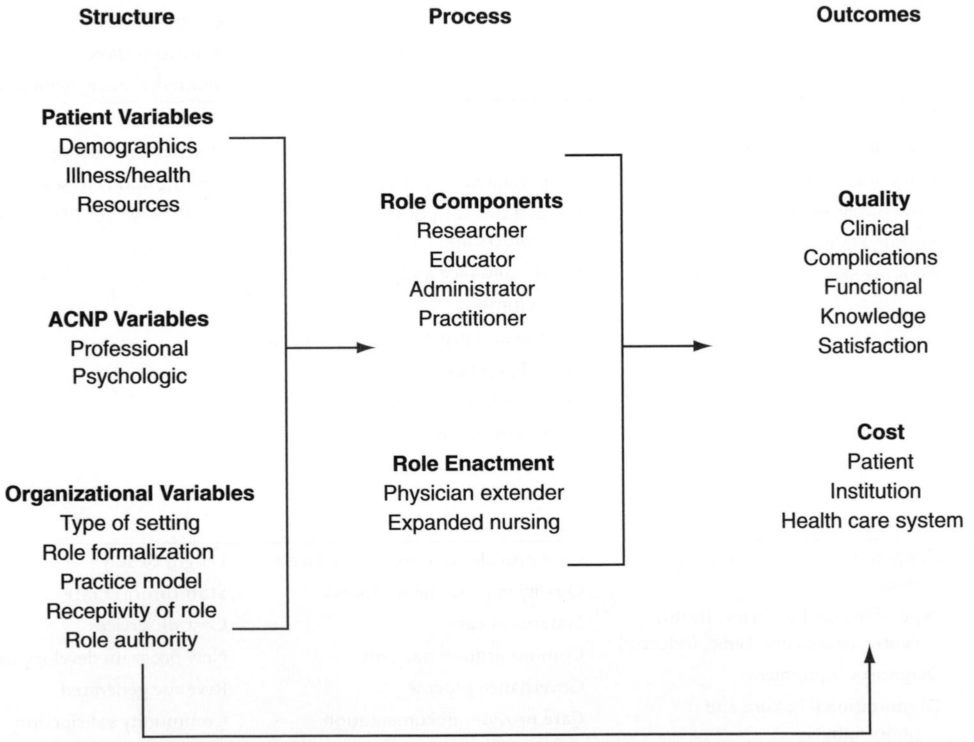

Fig. 21.1 ■ **Nursing role effectiveness model for acute care nurse practitioners.** (From "A conceptual framework for evaluating the nurse practitioner role in acute care settings," by S. Sidani and D. Irvine, 1999, *Journal of Advanced Nursing, 30*, 58–66.)

the interdependence of structure and process on outcomes. Four processes (mechanisms) within the ACNP direct care component are expected to achieve patient and cost outcomes: (1) providing comprehensive care, (2) ensuring continuity of care, (3) coordinating services, and (4) providing care in a timely way (Sidani & Irvine, 1999). Consistent with Donabedian's original writings, when APRNs select practice attributes, they need to realize that the boundaries between structure, process, and outcome may not be distinct and they are interdependent. The ACNP's role functions and how APRNs enact the role within their own practice model will guide how they choose outcome indicators. Practical matters like access to quality tools, data, and their cost will also influence choice of indicators. Doran et al. (2002) tested the utility of the model in registered nursing practice and found that, in general, the results supported the hypothesized relationships. Others have adapted the model for their context including advanced practice in Singapore (MeiLing, 2009), mental health nursing in Portugal (Seabra et al., 2018), and gynecologic oncology in Austria and Switzerland (Kofler et al., 2020). Still others have examined its utility in studies of both general and advanced nursing in specialty populations (Amaral et al., 2014).

EVIDENCE TO DATE

Literature supports that assessment of APRNs' performance and outcomes is critical to their roles. Several systematic reviews highlighted studies that focused on the evaluation of APRN roles and on the outcomes of APRN care (Laurant et al., 2018; Newhouse et al., 2011; Sandall et al., 2016). These studies focused on all four APRN roles, including NP, clinical nurse specialist (CNS), certified registered nurse anesthetist (CRNA), and certified nurse-midwife (CNM); they included two Cochrane Database reviews on the impact of primary care NPs on patient outcomes, processes of care, volume and cost of care (Laurant et al., 2018), NP and other primary care providers versus emergency physicians positioned to care for nonurgent patient problems in emergency rooms (Goncalves-Bradley et al., 2018), and CNM care (Sandall et al., 2016).

Another landmark synthesis focused on research that compared APRN care with that of other providers (e.g., physicians, teams with APRNs) covering published studies between 1990 and 2008. This systematic review identified that APRN care affected outcomes positively (Newhouse et al., 2011). Of 107 studies focused on APRN care in NP, CNS, CNM, and CRNA roles, high-quality evidence supported that APRNs provide effective and high-quality care. The results of the review noted that care provided by NPs and CNMs in collaboration with physicians was similar to, and in some ways better than, care provided by physicians alone, including lower rates of cesarean section deliveries, less epidural use and lower episiotomy rates, and higher breastfeeding rates for CNM patients, as well as more effective blood glucose and serum lipid level control for NP-managed patients. The studies relating to CNS care demonstrated a decrease in length of stay and costs of care and high ratings of satisfaction for hospitalized patients. Studies relating to CRNA care, although few and observational in design, did suggest equivalent complication rates and mortality when comparing care involving CRNAs with care involving only physicians. The largest number of studies related to NP care; these included 37 studies with 14 randomized control trials and 23 observational studies. A high degree of evidence was found for NP care related to improving patient satisfaction, patient self-assessed health status, blood pressure control, duration of mechanical ventilation, and similar rates of emergency department (ED) visits and hospital readmissions in NP and physician comparison groups (Newhouse et al., 2011).

Studies related to the outcomes of APRN care, performance, and impact can be categorized according to whether they focus on role descriptions or practice characteristics, care delivery processes, process (or performance) improvement activities, program evaluation, disease management activities, outcomes management programs, or outcomes research.

Role Description Studies

Role description studies focus on defining and describing role components and job attributes of APRNs. These foundational studies assist in identifying the direct and indirect APRN actions that potentially influence care delivery outcome. As such, they provide information about the structure or process components of Donabedian's model (1966, 1980). Models like the adapted nursing role effectiveness model (Sidani &

Irvine, 1999) illustrate the need to measure and associate role characteristics and behaviors with outcomes and impact on patient care. When studies address the relationship and, indeed, the effect of APRN practice, the evidence can further guide the development of theories about which characteristics of APRN practice or aspects of the APRN role contribute to care delivery outcome. For example, do the APRN's expert coaching or collaboration processes contribute to more favorable outcomes compared with other care providers who may not use these processes?

Role Perception and Acceptance Studies

Studies examining the acceptance of APRNs have been conducted since the various roles were introduced and generally involve surveys of staff nurses, administrators, patients, and other care providers. The contribution of role perception studies to the assessment of APRN impact lies with their potential for clarifying which contextual (structural) factors influence an APRN's ability to perform maximally. If the environment in which an APRN practices does not support the APRN's delivery of services—for instance, if scope of practice is unnecessarily limited—or if colleagues view the APRN's performance as unsatisfactory or unacceptable, outcomes may be affected. These studies identify potential confounding factors that may need to be controlled when measuring APRN effect.

Overall perception of APRN performance has been favorable, with most care providers and patients rating the performance and contribution of APRNs highly (Johantgen et al., 2012; Kahn et al., 2015; Newhouse et al., 2011). Some of the positive regard may be mediated by the patient's perception of enough time spent with the provider (Trentalange et al., 2016). Hardie and Leary (2010) explored patient perceptions of the value of the CNS role within a breast cancer clinic, finding in this small exploratory survey that the CNSs improved respondents' clinic experience.

Care Delivery Process Studies

Studies evaluating care delivery processes often occur in combination with role definition research. The distinction between process and role definition explorations is their attention to what APRNs do as part of their roles. Examples include the delivery of preventive services (Counsell et al., 2007), management of patients in the ED (Lamirel et al., 2012), ordering of antibiotics (Goolsby, 2007), inclusion of physical activity and physical fitness counseling in primary care practices (Buchholz & Purath, 2007), and involvement in performance improvement (Fulton et al., 2019). In these descriptive studies, information is provided about the direct and indirect actions taken by APRNs during the delivery of care. For example, Fulton et al. (2019) suggested that clinical nurse specialists lead system-level nursing practice initiatives to improve care for specialty populations by managing the interactions between people, technology, and organizations. Self-agency, trust, and influence facilitate CNS work. No declarative statements can be made about the relationships between any of these processes and care delivery outcomes, although hypotheses can be generated based on study findings. As a result, these studies are useful as a preliminary step toward outcomes assessment.

In some studies, APRN care delivery processes were compared with those of physicians and other care providers. These studies generally examined NP care and found that they are more likely than physicians and other community health providers to spend more time with patients (Seale et al., 2005), informally manage patient care needs (Sidani et al., 2005, 2006), and discuss treatment options (Seale et al., 2006). In one study, NPs were more likely to provide structural support for the emergency management of closed musculoskeletal injuries, although other interventions were aligned with physician providers (Ball et al., 2007). In another study, physician residents spent significantly more time on coordination of care than NPs (Sidani et al., 2005, 2006). It is interesting to note that despite this difference, patients whom NPs managed reported higher levels of coordination than those overseen by the physician residents.

A scoping review of 78 articles from eight countries (Grant et al., 2017) explored the work of nurse practitioners in primary care settings in developed countries. Practices varied from specific disease processes to managing individual health and well-being through coordination, collaboration, education, counseling, referral for needed services, and advocacy. In addition, APRNs incorporated health promotion activities to improve social determinants of health for vulnerable populations. Prajankett and Markaki (2021) appraised 42 articles to examine the role of APRNs in elderly primary care settings within the United States and Thailand. They found that US APRNs adopted a quality improvement and safety approach, incorporating technology into nursing interventions. In contrast, Thai APRNs empowered individuals through community networks and resources while incorporating care models.

Other studies have demonstrated increased compliance with clinical practice guideline use among NP-led initiatives (Gracias et al., 2008; Smits et al., 2020), a greater focus on population health (Park & Dowling, 2020), integrated person-centered care (Prajankett & Markaki, 2021), and a positive impact on care coordination and patient and family knowledge (Fry, 2011). In a qualitative study describing barriers and facilitators to implementing an APRN-led transitional care intervention for cognitively impaired older adults and their caregivers, Bradway et al. (2012) identified themes that included patients and caregivers having the necessary information and knowledge, care coordination, and caregiver experience. Additional studies are needed to highlight the impact of APRN-led care that is unique to various APRN roles to demonstrate further the distinct features of APRN care that affect patient and healthcare outcomes.

"PROCESS AS OUTCOME" STUDIES

Research studies that measure only processes rather than outcome can elucidate the steps needed to accomplish a certain activity and to compare performances of various providers. Several studies have focused on improving compliance with EBP, demonstrating the benefit of APRN-led initiatives targeting hospitalized patients (Gracias et al., 2008), and improvement in handoff communication for surgical patients (Johnson, 2016). Atkinson et al. (2021) evaluated processes aimed at improving efficiency within a nurse practitioner trauma team. They measured adherence to a standardized rounding process and interruptions via pager. Reigle et al. (2006) conducted a retrospective medical record review of ACNP versus resident performance on patients admitted for cardiac catheterization. They measured two process indicators of provider performance: documentation of education and counseling for risk factors and discharge prescribing practices. The findings demonstrated that ACNPs provided more education and counseling concerning dyslipidemia, exercise, and diabetes, whereas counseling for hypertension and smoking was comparable for both groups. The ACNPs also provided more appropriate medication prescriptions for the management of heart disease.

In a community health center, Park et al. (2020) examined the impact of expanding state scopes of practice for nurse practitioners in 12 states on patient visits to NPs. They used data from 739 community health centers to examine the number of full-time equivalent clinician visits per year. After granting independent practice and prescriptive authority to NPs, there was a statistically significant increase in NP visits and decreases in both physician assistant and primary care physician visits. Additional process as outcome studies are related to specialty care such as urinary incontinence (Albers-Heitner et al., 2012) and osteoporosis management (Greene & Dell, 2010). Differentiating process measures from outcome measures is important. Process measures may be used to evaluate APRN roles and may also have an impact on clinical outcomes.

PERFORMANCE (PROCESS) IMPROVEMENT ACTIVITIES

Performance improvement activities are essential for enhancing patient outcomes, patient experience, and efficient operations. This aspect of outcomes assessment focuses on the value-added complement to medical care provided by APRNs. O'Grady (2008) highlighted the potential to demonstrate APRN importance by evaluating the impact of process improvement initiatives, including the focus on quality of care and patient safety.

Advanced practice nurses are frequently engaged in quality improvement activities. Padula et al. (2021) contend that skilled APRN specialists are needed to evaluate the needs of complex patients, prevent complications, and redesign health systems. Using data from 55 US academic medical centers, they found that adding one board-certified wound care nurse per 1000 hospital beds decreased the pressure ulcer rate by 17.7%. Additionally, nurse anesthetists participated in simulation-based training. As a result, management of hypertensive emergencies, shoulder dystocia, and postpartum hemorrhage improved significantly (Lutgendorf et al., 2017). Internationally, process improvement activities have focused on improving access to health services by implementing a nurse practitioner model within an Australian prison (Wong et al., 2018).

Several studies have discussed specific APRN role components related to performance improvement that affected outcomes. The impact of a home-based APRN intervention for patients with psychiatric illness and human immunodeficiency virus was evaluated in a 4-year randomized controlled trial that studied 238 community residents. Over a 12-month period, those receiving the APRN intervention, which focused on case management and process improvements in the delivery of medical and mental health care, demonstrated improvements in depression and health-related quality of life compared with a control group that received usual care (Hanrahan et al., 2011).

OUTCOMES MANAGEMENT ACTIVITIES

Research suggests some positive results associated with APRN-directed outcomes management programs, many of which incorporate aspects of performance improvement. Multidisciplinary NP-coordinated team visits to medically underserved patients with type 2 diabetes demonstrated improvement in blood glucose and glycated hemoglobin levels and greater patient knowledge and self-efficacy (Jessee & Rutledge, 2012). In a study focusing on APRN care in psychiatry, admission rates to inpatient psychiatric facilities, visits to the ED, referral to rehabilitative services, occupational status, adherence to yearly routine blood tests and medications, and patient satisfaction were found to improve with APRN consultations (Cheng, 2012).

A systematic review of APRN-led interventions for patients with cancer in the ED found the interventions reduced the ED length of stay and improved patient satisfaction without affecting mortality or readmissions (Thamm et al., 2019). A systematic review conducted by Garner et al. (2017) found that nurse-led care for patients with rheumatoid arthritis was as effective and safe as other models of care and was generally superior to other models in terms of patient satisfaction. Patients reported nurse-led care to be superior in terms of education, support, and accessibility. In a study assessing the quality of health care provided at a pediatric nurse–managed clinic, NP care provided to 500 patients was found to improve childhood immunization rates, improve treatment for children with upper respiratory infection, and increase children's access to primary care providers (Coddington et al., 2012).

The Missouri Quality Initiative reviewed the impact of APRNs on the quality measures for 16 participating nursing homes (Rantz et al., 2018). The intervention nursing homes had a full-time APRN embedded in the facility. Their patient quality measure scores were compared from baseline to 36 months to nursing homes in the same counties with similar baseline quality scores, size, and ownership. Composite quality measure scores in intervention homes were significantly better than the comparison group, suggesting that APRNs working full-time in nursing homes can positively influence quality of care. Similarly, Reynolds (2018) found a dramatic decline in 30-day hospital readmissions when patients with systolic heart failure were followed by an APRN who specializes in cardiac care after discharge from the hospital to a skilled nursing facility

Table 21.3 outlines examples of APRN-directed program evaluations. The focus area of the evaluation, target population, and brief study findings are outlined.

POPULATION HEALTH ACTIVITIES

In addition to providing direct care to individual patients, APRNs actively work to improve the health status and health outcomes for groups of people. Examples of APRN actions to address population health with cohorts of patients are discussed elsewhere in this chapter and include a focus on patients with diabetes (Jessee & Rutledge, 2012), heart failure (Craswell et al., 2018), mental health conditions (Alexander & Schnell, 2019; Cheng, 2012), rheumatoid arthritis (Garner et al., 2017), and syncope (Hamdan et al., 2018) and those needing palliative care (Moreton et al., 2020; Walling et al., 2017).

APRNs also focus on population health based on geographic regions. For example, Harrison (2017) found that a fall prevention program provided by a nurse practitioner at community senior centers

TABLE 21.3

Examples of Advanced Practice Registered Nurse (APRN)-Directed Program Evaluations

Study (Year)	Focus of Evaluation	Target Population	Findings
Albers-Heitner et al. (2012)	Urinary incontinence care	Primary care	Improved quality of life; improvement in incontinence severity; more cost-effective care
Anetzberger et al. (2006)	Achievement of program goals—service to at-risk groups and improved outcomes	High-risk older adults	Completed >1600 visits to targeted population; number of referrals doubled; patients highly satisfied with service
Bethea et al. (2019)	Nurse practitioner's (NP) role coordinating care for trauma patients	Elderly trauma patients in level 1 trauma center	Statistically significant decrease in length of stay, hospital charges, and discharge to skilled nursing facility; statistically significant increase in discharge to home
Bissonnette (2011)	APRN-led interprofessional collaborative care model for kidney transplant recipients	Kidney transplant recipients	Improved care for patients with chronic kidney disease awaiting kidney transplantation
Brandon et al. (2009)	Telephone follow-up program for heart failure patients	Primary care patients with heart failure	Reduced rates of rehospitalization and improved patient self-care behaviors
Callahan et al. (2006)	Collaborative care model for Alzheimer disease	Primary care patient	Improved behavioral and psychological symptoms; less caregiver distress
Capezuti et al. (2007)	Consultation and educational services regarding side rail use	Long-term care nursing staff and patients	Reduction in side rail use varied by site; falls significantly reduced for site with reduced use of rails
Cheung et al. (2011)	Certified nurse-midwife–led normal birth unit	Obstetric patients undergoing childbirth	Significant differences in vaginal deliveries, rates of episiotomies and amniotomies (all decreased), and increased postdelivery mobility
Cibulka et al. (2011)	NP-directed oral care program	Low-income pregnant women	Improved oral care, including improved frequency of brushing and flossing teeth, dental checkups, and marked reduction in intake of high-sugar drinks
Collins et al. (2014)	NP-directed care for trauma patients	Trauma patients transferred to step-down unit	Reduction in hospital length of stay and costs of care
Coppa et al. (2018)	Home-based primary care delivered by APRN	Clinically complex patients living at home	Decrease in emergency visits and rehospitalizations
Costa et al. (2014)	NP-directed care for hospitalized patients	Intensive care unit patients	No difference in mortality rates compared with medical resident team
Dickerson et al. (2006)	Support groups	Patients receiving implantable cardioverter-defibrillators	No difference in quality-of-life scores for support group attendees
Greene and Dell (2010)	Disease management program	Patients with osteoporosis	Increased treatment of osteoporosis; decrease in hip fractures
Hamilton and Hawley (2006)	Outpatient management of anemia	Patients with chronic renal disease	Significant improvement in quality of life
Harrison (2017)	Fall prevention program	Community senior centers	Significant improvement in fall risk scores

Continued

TABLE 21.3

Examples of Advanced Practice Registered Nurse (APRN)-Directed Program Evaluations—cont'd

Study (Year)	Focus of Evaluation	Target Population	Findings
Kutzleb and Reiner (2006)	Patient education program	Patients with heart failure	Significant improvement in quality of life
Landsperger et al. (2015)	NP-led team compared with resident-managed patients	Medical intensive care unit	No differences in mortality or hospital length of stay
Lowery et al. (2012)	Disease management model	Patients with chronic heart failure	Significantly fewer congestive heart failure and all-cause admissions at 1-year follow-up, lower mortality at both 1- and 2-year follow-ups
McCorkle et al. (2009)	Postsurgical care for gynecologic cancer	Women who had undergone gynecologic cancer surgery	Improved functional status, less symptom distress, less uncertainty
Moreton et al. (2020)	NP-led palliative care services	Hospital service area in Sydney, Australia	Patients were less likely to die in the hospital and had fewer hospital admissions, and the hospitalization cost per patient were one-half that of those not in the program
Morse et al. (2006)	Assessment of NP-led rapid response team	Hospitalized patients	Significant decrease in in-hospital cardiac arrests, decrease in mortality rates
Patel et al. (2021)	NPs added to provider care team	Hospitalized patients	Care teams with NPs had significantly lower mortality and transfers to higher level of care and significantly higher cost per patient and lengths of stay
Rantz et al. (2018)	Impact of APRNs on quality measure (QM) scores in nursing homes	16 Missouri nursing homes with APRNs compared with similar nursing homes without APRNs	APRN nursing homes had significantly better composite QM scores
Reynolds (2018)	NP interventions for patients with heart failure posthospitalization	Skilled nursing facilities	Decrease in hospital readmissions from 47% to 6%
Rideout (2007)	Care coordination	Hospitalized children with cystic fibrosis	Timeliness of nutrition and social work consultation improved significantly; length of stay declined by 1.35 days
Scherr et al. (2012)	Comparison of NP-led program for rapid response teams compared with physician care	Hospitalized patients	No differences in number of cardiac arrests or mortality rates; nurses reported confidence in knowledge of NP team
Splendore and Grant (2017)	Assessment of NP-led community workshop	Community members	Significant increase in completion rates for advance directives and advance care planning
Stolee et al. (2006)	Role of NP	Long-term care nursing employees	Perception of positive impact; most staff reported improved skill levels
Sung et al. (2011)	NPs as coordinators of acute stroke team	Hospitalized patients with acute stroke onset	Time to computed tomography scan, time to neurology evaluation, and time to initiate thrombolytic therapy significantly improved

TABLE 21.3
Examples of Advanced Practice Registered Nurse (APRN)-Directed Program Evaluations—cont'd

Study (Year)	Focus of Evaluation	Target Population	Findings
Wagner et al., (2007)	Consultation and educational services regarding side rail use	Long-term care patients	Five (median) recommendations per long-term care resident; median cost of intervention per resident was $135
Walling et al. (2017)	Palliative care NP embedded in oncologist practices	Patients seen in oncology clinic with advanced cancer	Patients seen by NP had increased documentation of advance care planning and significantly increased hospice referrals

Abbreviations: APRN, advanced practice registered nurse; NP, nurse practitioner

resulted in a statistically significant improvement in fall risk scores in the elderly population. Pearson (2017) found an increase in patients' knowledge as a result of a nurse practitioner coronary heart disease outreach initiative. Splendore and Grant (2017) found improvement in completion rates for advance directives and advance care planning after providing a nurse practitioner–led community-based program. Impressively, Jakobs and Bigbee (2016) examined the health of populations residing in remote geographic areas of the United States classified as frontier counties. They analyzed data from 308 frontier counties in 14 states, with 858 APRNs residing in those counties. They found a statistically significant lower premature death rate (mortality) and teen birth rate, significantly higher rates of sexually transmitted infections, and no differences in the percentage of low birth rate babies or adult smoking rates in counties with APRNs compared with those without APRNs. Additional geographically focused population health initiatives demonstrated improved outcomes with care delivered by APRNs in nursing homes (Lacny et al., 2016; Rantz et al., 2018; Reynolds, 2018) and prisons (Wong et al., 2018).

IMPACT OF APRN PRACTICE

Several studies have examined the effect of APRN practice on patient and systems outcomes. Table 21.4 organizes these studies by outcome indicator. Studies have investigated care delivery outcomes across providers and among different APRN types. In most cases, physician groups (including physician residents) have been used for comparison. This process is a concern because it implies that physician practice is the gold standard for APRNs and that it encompasses the full range of APRN activity. Physician practice overlaps in some respects and diverges in others. Physician and APRNs approach care differently. For example, Park and Dowling (2020) compared 391 nurse practitioner–led and 11,479 physician-led patient centered medical homes (PCMHs). They found that NP-led PCMHs were more likely to provide care to vulnerable populations in rural and other underserved areas. While NP-led PCMHs emphasized population health needs, physician-led PCMHs focused on practice improvements through enhanced access to care and informatics. As in this example, APRNs routinely use strategies that are not considered or fully incorporated by physicians. Ideally, attention should be directed at indicators that accurately measure all care providers' impacts as well as those that can serve as benchmarks for APRN practice alone.

Granting APRNs full practice authority can improve access, patient safety, and quality of care (Adams & Markowitz, 2018; Buerhaus, 2018; Buerhaus et al., 2018; Martsolf et al., 2015). Removing restrictive regulations that limit APRN scope of practice nationwide could therefore have a significant impact on a broader population scale. In addition, eliminating APRN scope of practice restrictions can result in annual Medicare cost savings estimated at $44.5 billion (Chattopadhyay & Zangaro, 2019).

Studies Comparing APRN to Physician and Other Provider Outcomes

Studies comparing APRNs with physicians have been reported internationally. A synthesis review of US APRN roles demonstrated that APRN care is equivalent to physician care and for some outcomes, such as patient satisfaction, APRN care was rated higher

TABLE 21.4

Examples of APRN-Sensitive Outcome Indicators Tested in Practice

Outcome Indicator	Study (Year)	Study Design	Focus of Indicator[a]	Findings
Activities of daily living	Counsell et al. (2007)	Randomized controlled trial	Population-generic	Significantly improved
	Krichbaum (2007)	Randomized controlled trial	Population-generic	Significantly improved over control group
Advance directives/ advance care planning completion	Splendore and Grant (2017)	Program evaluation	Population-specific	Increased completion of advanced care planning
	Walling et al. (2017)	Program evaluation	Population-specific	Increased documentation of advance care planning
Adverse events, unplanned incidents, including drug reactions	Simonson et al. (2007)	Retrospective comparison	Population-specific	Comparable to anesthesiologists
Amniotomy rates	Cheung et al. (2011)	Randomized controlled trial	Population-specific	Significant decreased rates compared with usual care
Anxiety, depression; mental health status; emotional state	McCorkle et al. (2007)	Secondary data analysis	Population-generic	Comparable to control group
Asthma control	Borgmeyer et al. (2008)	Observational	Population-specific	Significantly improved
Blood pressure	Partiprajak (2012)	Observational	Population-specific	Significantly decreased
Cardiac arrest rates after rapid response team call	Morse et al. (2006)	Observational	Population-generic	Significantly decreased
	Scherr et al. (2012)	Retrospective	Population-generic	Significantly decreased
Central line-associated bloodstream infections	Hsueh and Dorcy (2016)	Quality improvement pre- and post-data	Population-specific	Decreased with APRN Care Coordinator
Cesarean delivery	Cragin and Kennedy (2006)	Prospective descriptive cohort	Population-specific	Significantly lower than physician group
Cholesterol level	Paez and Allen (2006)	Randomized controlled trial	Population-generic	Significantly better than usual care group
Cost of care	Albers-Heitner et al. (2012)	Precomparison and postcomparison	Population-specific	Nurse practitioner (NP) care cost-effective for managing care for urinary incontinence
	Bethea et al. (2019)	Evaluation of trauma program	Population-specific	Significantly lower hospital costs for NP care
	Chattopadhyay and Zangaro (2019)	Compared Medicare cost of care to NP scope of practice restrictions	Population-generic	Estimate Medicare cost savings of $44.5 billion per year with removal of scope of practice restrictions
	Cowan et al. (2006)	Quasi-experimental comparison	Population-generic	Significantly improved compared with control

TABLE 21.4

Examples of APRN-Sensitive Outcome Indicators Tested in Practice—cont'd

Outcome Indicator	Study (Year)	Study Design	Focus of Indicator[a]	Findings
	Craswell et al. (2018)	NP-led heart failure medication titration program evaluation	Population-specific	Lower cost per patient and lower cost per visit compared with usual care
	Lutfiyya et al. (2017)	Cross-sectional analysis of Medicare claims data	Population-specific	Significantly lower costs per recipient with type 2 diabetes
	Moreton et al. (2020)	Palliative care service evaluation	Population-specific	Decreased cost of hospital care per patient
	Naylor et al. (2013)	Randomized controlled trial		Significantly less than control group
	Paez and Allen (2006)	Randomized controlled trial		Incremental costs offset by improved outcome
	Patel et al. (2021)	Retrospective cohort study	Population-generic	Statistically significant increase in cost per patient with significantly improved quality
Depression management	Hanrahan et al. (2011)	Randomized controlled trial	Population-specific	Significantly improved
Discharge disposition	Bethea et al. (2019)	Evaluation of trauma program	Population specific	Significantly higher percentage discharged to home for NP care cohort; significantly lower discharge to skilled nursing facilities for NP care cohort
Door-to-needle time for thrombolytic therapy for acute stroke patients	Sung et al. (2011)	Parallel comparison	Population-specific	Significantly better than physician control group
Eczema flare ups	Schuttelaar et al. (2011)	Randomized controlled trial	Population-specific	Significantly lower rates than physician comparison group
Emergency department use	Smith et al. (2016)	Case-control study	Population-specific	Decreased readmissions and fewer emergency department visits for patients who received postdischarge NP home visit
Episiotomy rates	Cheung et al. (2011)	Randomized controlled trial	Population-specific	Decreased rates with certified nurse-midwife care
Fall risk	Harrison (2017)	Before and after	Population specific	Decreased fall risk scores after NP education intervention
Functional status, ability	McCorkle et al. (2009)	Randomized controlled trial	Population-specific	Significantly improved
Hip fracture rate	Krichbaum (2007)	Care coordination program evaluation	Population-specific	Significantly decreased rate of fractures
Hip fractures with osteoporosis screening and treatment	Greene and Dell (2010)	Disease management program evaluation	Population-specific	Significantly decreased rate of fractures, increased rate of osteoporosis treatment

Continued

TABLE 21.4

Examples of APRN-Sensitive Outcome Indicators Tested in Practice—cont'd

Outcome Indicator	Study (Year)	Study Design	Focus of Indicator[a]	Findings
Hospice referrals	Walling et al. (2017)	Program evaluation	Population-specific	Significantly increased hospice referrals
Hospital-acquired conditions	Hu et al. (2018)	Evaluation	Population-generic	Outcomes better for APRN than resident physicians
Hospitalizations, including readmissions	Brandon et al. (2009)	Quasi-experimental comparison	Population-generic	Decreased readmissions, improved self-care behaviors
	Brandon et al. (2009)	Telehealth program evaluation	Population-specific	Decreased readmission rates, improved patient self-care behaviors
	Lowery et al. (2012)	Precomparison and postcomparison	Population-specific	Decreased readmissions for patients with heart failure
	Moreton et al. (2020)	Palliative care service evaluation	Population-specific	Decreased hospital admissions
Length of stay	Bethea et al. (2019)	Evaluation of trauma program	Population specific	Significantly lower length of stay for NP care
	Collins et al. (2014)	Precomparison and postcomparison	Population-specific	Decreased hospital length of stay for trauma patients cared for by NP
	Fanta et al. (2006)	Randomized controlled trial	Population-generic	Significantly shorter than for resident physicians
	Hsueh and Dorcy (2016)	Quality improvement pre- and post-data	Population-specific	Decreased average length of stay with APRN care coordinator
	Gershengorn et al. (2011)	Retrospective review	Population-generic	No difference in hospital mortality, length of stay (intensive care unit, hospital), and post–hospital discharge destination for NP care compared with physician care
	Patel et al. (2021)	Retrospective cohort study	Population-generic	Statistically significant increase in length of stay with significantly improved quality
	Rideout (2007)	Precomparison and postcomparison	Population generic	No difference in precomparison and postcomparison
Mortality	Costa et al. (2014)	Descriptive comparison	Population-generic	Comparable to physicians
	Jakobs and Bigbee (2016)	Compared health outcomes in rural counties with and without APRNs	Population-specific	Mortality (premature death rate) significantly lower in counties with APRNs
	Landsperger et al. (2015)	Descriptive comparison	Population-generic	Comparable to physicians
	Morse et al. (2006)	Observational	Population-generic	Significantly lower
	Patel et al. (2021)	Retrospective cohort study	Population-generic	Statistically significant decrease in hospital mortality
	Scherr et al. (2012)	Retrospective	Population-generic	Significantly decreased

TABLE 21.4

Examples of APRN-Sensitive Outcome Indicators Tested in Practice—cont'd

Outcome Indicator	Study (Year)	Study Design	Focus of Indicator[a]	Findings
Nurse satisfaction	Hu et al. (2018)	Survey	Population-generic	Higher satisfaction for APRN than resident physicians
	McMullen et al. (2001)	Program evaluation	Population-specific, organizational	Highly satisfied
	Rideout (2007)	Postcomparison	Population-specific	Highly satisfied postintervention
	Simonson et al. (2007)	Medical record review	Population-specific	Comparable to anesthesiologists
Patient, family satisfaction	Fanta et al. (2006)	Survey	Population-generic	Comparable to or significantly greater than residents
	Hu et al. (2018)	Survey	Population-generic	Higher satisfaction for APRN than resident physicians
	Sidani et al. (2005, 2006)	Cross-sectional comparison	Population-generic	Significantly greater than resident physicians
	Varughese et al. (2006)	Observational	Population-generic	Significantly improved
Physician satisfaction, perception of APRN performance	Rideout (2007)	Post implementation	Population-specific	Highly satisfied post implementation
Pulmonary function	Rideout (2007)	Precomparison and postcomparison	Population-specific	No difference in precomparison and postcomparison
Quality measure (QM) scores (nursing home)	Rantz et al. (2018)	Two-group comparison (nursing homes with and without APRNs)	Population-specific	APRN nursing home composite QM scores significantly better
Quality of life	Hamilton and Hawley (2006)	Retrospective review	Population-specific	Significant improvement over time
	Kutzleb and Reiner (2006)	Quasi-experimental comparison	Population-specific	Significantly better than control group
	McCorkle et al. (2009)	Randomized controlled trial	Population-specific	Significantly improved
Teen birth rate	Jakobs and Bigbee (2016)	Compared health outcomes in rural counties with and without APRNs	Population-specific	Significantly lower in counties with APRNs
Time to service delivery	Reigle et al. (2006)	Medical record review	Population-generic, organizational	Significantly less than physicians
Urinary tract infection	Elpern et al. (2009)	Retrospective	Population-generic	Significantly reduced
Vaginal delivery rates	Cheung et al. (2011)	Randomized controlled trial	Population-specific	Significantly reduced
Ventilator-associated pneumonia	Quenot et al. (2007)	Observational	Population-generic	Significantly decreased rates of pneumonia

Continued

TABLE 21.4

Examples of APRN-Sensitive Outcome Indicators Tested in Practice—cont'd

Outcome Indicator	Study (Year)	Study Design	Focus of Indicator[a]	Findings
Weight	Rideout (2007)	Precomparison and postcomparison	Population-generic	No difference in precomparison and postcomparison

Note: Some indicators that were used with specific populations in studies have been labeled as generic because they can be applied to multiple patient groups. The outcome measures listed here are not uniformly consistent with the measure properties of similar indicators endorsed by the National Quality Forum.

[a]Definition of terms for the focus of the indicator:

Population-generic—indicators that could be used with any patient population.

Population-specific—indicators that are relevant to specific populations only.

(Newhouse et al., 2011). Studies comparing NP care with that of physician residents have demonstrated comparable medical management skills and improved staff and family satisfaction (Gershengorn et al., 2011; Lakhan & Laird, 2009). Alexandrov et al. (2009, 2011) found that APRNs provided with postgraduate academic fellowship education and training in acute neurovascular care were able to diagnose acute ischemic stroke accurately through a combination of clinical localization and neuroimaging interpretation and make safe and effective tissue plasminogen activator (tPA) treatment decisions while also increasing the absolute number of tPA-treated patients with stroke at their facility.

In an analysis of 2012 Medicare claims, Lutfiyya et al. (2017) stratified patients with diabetes from healthiest to least healthy to compare outcomes for groups cared for by nurse practitioners to primary care physician (PCP) groups. Both overall and by stratification, patients in the NP group had significantly improved outcomes compared with PCPs for patient health outcomes, utilization of healthcare services, and healthcare costs. A systematic review on the management of patients with asthma found comparable clinical and financial outcomes when care was delivered by a nurse practitioner working independently or by a physician (Kuethe et al., 2013). When comparing primary care provided by advanced practice nurses to physician care, Laurant et al. (2018) found that APRN care resulted in higher satisfaction and quality of life, slightly fewer deaths, and better health outcomes for a broad range of patient conditions. Other studies have continued to demonstrate comparable outcomes of APRN and physician care (Costa et al., 2014; Gershengorn et al., 2011; Landsperger et al., 2015; Newhouse et al., 2011).

A number of studies comparing APRN care with physician care internationally have demonstrated similar results (Albers-Heitner et al., 2012; Hu et al., 2018; Scherr et al., 2012) with improved care in outcomes such as rates of vaginal deliveries and episiotomies (Cheung et al., 2011), eczema care (Schuttelaar et al., 2011), skilled procedures such as thoracostomy tube insertion (Bevis et al., 2008), and ophthalmic examination techniques in the ED (Lamirel et al., 2012). In an Australian study, Craswell et al. (2018) compared patients with heart failure who received care through nurse practitioner–led titration services to similar patients who received usual care. They found that the usual care group had a higher percentage of patients who failed to attend appointments and took longer to reach therapeutic levels for their prescribed medications, with some patients never reaching target dose. The total cost, cost per patient, and cost per visit were higher for usual care than for the NP services. In a study conducted in the Netherlands (Smits et al., 2020), experienced nurse practitioners replaced general practitioners for after-hour primary care home visits. The NP visits were significantly longer than those of physicians and the NPs referred significantly more patients to the hospital. NPs prescribed medications significantly less, the medications they prescribed were significantly more appropriate, and they adhered to the protocol significantly more often. There were no differences in the number of missed diagnoses or complications. Patient satisfaction was high for both groups and significantly higher for NPs on several items. A small study conducted in the United Kingdom (Machin,

2017) compared the clinical diagnosis and management decisions related to skin cancer between a nurse practitioner and a dermatologist. She found 97% diagnostic accuracy and 84% management accuracy, suggesting that independent practice may be safe.

Nurse Practitioner Outcomes

Other studies have examined the impact of care provided by NPs. A systematic review by Stanik-Hutt et al. (2013) summarized data from 37 studies based on 11 aggregated outcomes of NP care. In comparison to physician care or teams without NPs, outcomes for NPs were comparable or better for all 11 outcomes reviewed. A high level of evidence identified better serum lipid levels in patients managed by NPs in primary care practices and for patient outcomes related to satisfaction with care, health status, functional status, blood pressure control, blood glucose control, number of ED visits, hospitalizations, and mortality.

A parallel synthesis review by Newhouse et al. (2011) confirmed the positive outcomes from NP care in comparison to physician care. Other studies comparing care by NP-led teams to physician care have demonstrated no differences in care with respect to mortality rates, length of stay, or rehospitalization rates (Collins et al., 2014; Costa et al., 2014; Gershengorn et al., 2011; Landsperger et al., 2015). Patel et al. (2021) compared outcomes for hospitalized patients cared for by NPs to patients receiving usual care. They found lower hospital mortality and less frequent transfers to a higher level of care in the NP group. However, patients cared for by NPs had longer lengths of stay and higher cost per patient.

Studies have demonstrated improved disease management from NP care, including care for hypertension, cardiovascular disease, and diabetes (Newhouse et al., 2011) and specialty-based care such as Alzheimer disease management (Callahan et al., 2006), urology care (Albers-Heitner et al., 2012), cancer care (Cooper et al., 2009), and heart failure care (Case et al., 2010; Lowery et al., 2012).

Multiple studies related to NP care have demonstrated advantages to specific role components. Examples include NP-led rapid response teams (Barocas et al., 2014; Kapu, Wheeler, et al., 2014; Morse et al., 2006; Scherr et al., 2012; Sonday & Grecsek, 2010), NP-delivered post-discharge home visits in patients with medical conditions at high risk for readmission, (Smith et al., 2016), patients with clinical complexity (Coppa et al., 2018), patients after cardiac surgery (Sawatzky et al., 2013), NP-led renal teams (Lucatorto et al., 2016), NP-led titration centers for patients with heart failure (Craswell et al., 2018), NP-led community palliative care services (Moreton et al., 2020), a nursing home model of care (Lacny et al., 2016), and an outreach syncope clinic managed by an NP (Hamdan et al., 2018). In addition, research suggests benefits for specialty-based NP roles, including trauma care (Bethea et al., 2019; Collins et al., 2014), emergency care (Li et al., 2013), intensive care (White et al., 2017), inpatient medical services, geriatric inpatient care, cardiovascular care (Alexander-Banys, 2014; David et al., 2015; Horne & Estes, 2021), mental health (Alexander & Schnell, 2019), oncology and palliative care (Hsueh & Dorcy, 2016; Hutchinson et al., 2014; Kilpatrick et al., 2014; Spears, et al., 2017; Walling et al., 2017), and advance care planning (Splendore & Grant, 2017).

Clinical Nurse Specialist Outcomes

The impact of CNS care has been examined in several reviews, including a literature review on CNS competencies and outcome studies, highlighting the role of the CNS in specialty-based practice roles including chronic disease management, influence on the practice of nursing staff, and unit-level metrics such as pressure ulcer prevention, fall prevention, patient satisfaction, promotion of EBP, and staff turnover and satisfaction (Gordon et al., 2012). Salamanca-Balen et al. (2018) conducted a systematic review of international evidence. Based on a review of 79 papers, they found that CNS interventions may be effective in reducing hospitalizations, rehospitalizations, admissions, length of stay, and healthcare costs. There was mixed evidence regarding their cost-effectiveness of the interventions.

Several studies have explored outcomes related to CNS care and CNS productivity (Urden & Stacy, 2012). Fulton (2012) surveyed CNSs and found the most frequently monitored outcomes related to APRN nursing interventions (68% in the patient sphere, 87% in the EBP sphere, and 86% in the nurse and organizational spheres). The least monitored outcomes related to diagnosing (range 54%–57%) and cost and revenue (range 36%–55%). Other studies have focused on exploring outcomes related to specialty areas of care. Favorable outcomes have been seen for cancer patients managed by CNSs in outpatient settings (Dayhoff & Lyons, 2009). Studies related to CNS outcomes in acute care have demonstrated reductions in hospital length of stay and costs (Dayhoff & Lyons, 2009; Newhouse et al., 2011). A systematic review on the effectiveness and cost-effectiveness of CNSs in outpatient roles identified 11 randomized controlled trials with evidence of reduced resource use and costs of care favoring CNS care (Kilpatrick et al., 2014).

The outcomes of CNS care have also been investigated in international models of care. Begley and colleagues (2010) assessed the impact of the CNS and midwifery roles in Ireland. APRNs, including CNSs and nurse-midwives, were found to improve service delivery by leading the development of new clinical services; taking responsibility for guideline development, implementation, and evaluation; and positively influencing quality patient care through formal and informal education.

Certified Nurse-Midwife Outcomes

Studies of the outcomes of CNM care have demonstrated significant impact on vaginal delivery rates, decreased rates of episiotomies and amniotomies, less use of pain medication, and high satisfaction ratings (Arthur et al., 2009; Cheung et al., 2011; Johantgen et al., 2012; Malloy, 2010).

A study of CNM outcomes used an optimality index to compare midwifery and physician practices according to the extent of preexisting conditions at the time of treatment (Cragin & Kennedy, 2006). The optimality index contained a list of 40 care delivery processes and outcome measures pertaining to pregnancy, parturition, and neonatal and maternal postpartum conditions. Women cared for by physicians were 1.7 times as likely as those cared for by CNMs to have a cesarean section delivery. Women seen by physicians in this study had a significantly greater proportion of chronic illness and drug abuse, although these differences did not explain the higher rate of cesarean section for the group.

A Cochrane Database systematic review comparing midwife-led care with other models of care examined 15 clinical trials and found that midwife-led models of care resulted in primary outcomes of patients being less likely to experience regional analgesia, instrumental vaginal birth, and preterm birth less than 37 weeks; there were fewer fetal losses before and after 24 weeks, fewer neonatal deaths; and patients were more likely to have spontaneous vaginal births (Sandall et al., 2016). In terms of secondary outcomes, the midwife-led groups were less likely to have amniotomy, episiotomy, and fetal loss less than 24 weeks and during the neonatal period, and they were more likely to experience no intrapartum analgesia or anesthesia but had longer labor time and more likely to be attended by a known midwife. There were no statistically significant differences between groups for cesarean births or intact perineum. While data could not be pooled for statistical analysis, a narrative analysis indicated that most studies showed higher levels of maternal satisfaction with midwife-led care (Sandall et al., 2016).

Certified Registered Nurse Anesthetist Outcomes

In the United States, numerous studies suggest the provision of anesthesia by CRNAs to be cost-effective (Dulisse & Cromwell, 2010; French et al., 2016; Hogan et al., 2010; Kremer & Faut-Callahan, 2009; Lewin Group, 2016; Ohsfeldt et al., 2016). One study examined anesthesia services at four different hospitals: a large academic medical center, a large community hospital, a medium-sized community hospital, and a small community hospital (Cromwell & Snyder, 2000). Labor cost projections demonstrated that an all-CRNA care delivery model cost less than 50% of an all-anesthesiologist model. The cost savings for a mixed model composed of anesthesiologists and CRNAs in ratios of 1:1 to 1:4 ranged from 33% to 41% of the total costs for an all-anesthesiologist model.

Many studies have found care delivered by CRNAs to be equivalent to that delivered by anesthesiologists in terms of quality and safety across a variety of procedures and settings (Dulisse & Cromwell, 2010; Henrichs et al., 2019; Lewis et al., 2014; Pine et al., 2003; Simonson et al., 2007). However, Ohsfeldt et al. (2016) found that anesthesiologists had fewer unexpected dispositions (transfers to higher levels of care) for orthopedic ambulatory surgery patients compared with nurse anesthetists. A Cochrane systematic review of six CRNA studies demonstrated no difference in death rate when given anesthetic by either a nurse anesthetist or a licensed physician anesthetist (Lewis et al., 2014). Based on an analysis of 5.7 million commercial insurance claims, Negrusa et al. (2016) found no statistical differences in anesthesia-specific complications between CRNAs and anesthesiologists. Despite the demonstrated positive outcomes related to CNRA-provided anesthesia, multiple factors continue to influence anesthesia staffing models, including a misunderstanding of physician supervision, unfamiliarity with anesthesia payments, and resistance to a CRNA model by anesthesiologists and surgeons (Mills et al., 2020).

Studies Comparing APRN and Physician Productivity

One of the most difficult and contentious elements of APRN outcomes measurement is the assessment of APRN productivity, which is an organizational rather than a patient outcome. Productivity is an organizational indicator that measures provider efficiency rather than skill or capability. For example, Xue and Tuttle (2017) found that the estimated number of patients seen by an NP in a typical week is comparable to the number seen by a primary care physician; however, NPs had a significantly smaller patient panel. The authors concluded that NP clinical productivity can be improved. The issue with productivity is that reimbursement practices and the income generated by care providers are directly tied to productivity levels. Because APRNs have historically spent more time with patients, their overall productivity levels may result in changes in potential income for the organization or practice. Until reimbursement decisions are shifted to a care delivery outcomes approach, this will continue to be problematic for APRNs.

Relative Work Value of APRNs

Payment for services provided to Medicare patients is based on the resource-based relative value (RBRV) scale methodology, which incorporates an estimate of the amount of work, practice expense, and professional liability insurance associated with various procedures. The total relative value of each procedure is multiplied by a standard dollar conversion factor and adjusted for geographic differences in resource costs to determine the allowable service charge that providers can request for reimbursement of services (CMS, 2021b). CMS does not publish a separate fee schedule for APRNs, although NP data have been used to adjust the RBRVs for some payment codes (Sullivan-Marx, 2008). Demonstrating the quality and financial impact of APRN care is a priority area of focus but presents challenges in identifying the true impact of care on costs or through cost avoidance (Kapu, Kleinpell, et al., 2014).

Sullivan-Marx (2008) quantified NP time required for preservice, intraservice, and postservice. Complexity was measured by assessing mental effort, technical skill, physical effort, and the psychological stress associated with an iatrogenic event related to the Current Procedural Terminology (CPT) code. In all cases, NPs' estimated relative work values were comparable to those established for physician practice, suggesting that practice patterns were similar for the scenarios described (Sullivan-Marx, 2008). Because the CPT codes and descriptors were designed with physicians in mind, other APRN activities may not have been included in the estimation process. Until these are well defined and described by APRNs, the work of APRNs may not capture the actual relative value in the delivery of APRN care.

Research suggests that APRNs continue to spend considerable time on nonbillable but value added activities. In a survey of 509 NPs, Kippenbrock et al. (2018) found that nonbillable activities included reviewing laboratory reports, making phone calls to patients and family members, refilling prescriptions, reviewing image results, contacting consultants, responding to emails, and meeting with sales representatives. The amount of time spent on nonbillable activities ranged from 0 to 570 minutes per day and was influenced by workplace setting, number of support staff, and primary care provider role. Winter et al. (2021) examined nonbillable service activities that contribute to billable service provision, quality of care, and value of care. NPs and CNSs spent between 3.7 and 36.5 hours per month on these nonbillable activities. Most often, the activities were related to orders, chart review, and documentation.

Steuer and Kopan (2011) advocated tracking productivity and the work value of APRN care using productivity tools to capture outcomes. A workload analysis of a CNS role in a specialty lung cancer practice found that the role was primarily used to support processes and administrative components. Restructuring the role to implement standardized care based on national practice guidelines led to proactive case management that resulted in a decrease in admissions for nonacute healthcare problems (Baxter & Leary, 2011).

The number of international studies focusing on APRN outcomes has been increasing as APRN roles expand worldwide. Partiprajak (2012) followed 100 patients with type 2 diabetes in Thailand to assess the impact of an APRN-led support group. The results indicated that the APRN-led support group patients had lower systolic blood pressure, higher self-care abilities, and increased quality of life and satisfaction compared with a comparison group. Other international studies have demonstrated outcomes related to NP care (Ball et al., 2007), CNS care (Baxter & Leary, 2011; Begley et al., 2010; Oliver & Leary, 2010), and CNM care (Woods, 2007).

As noted, Table 21.4 provides a comprehensive summary of APRN outcome studies organized by outcome indicators. An impressive number of studies have examined specific outcomes. Most of the studies have demonstrated improved outcomes as a result of APRN care and/or comparable outcomes with other healthcare providers. As APRN roles continue to expand to different practice settings and to specialty-based practices, continued evaluation of the impact of APRN care is warranted to identify APRN contributions to care.

FUTURE DIRECTIONS FOR USING OUTCOMES IN APRN PRACTICE

The evidence suggests that the quality of care that APRNs deliver is comparable or superior to that of other care providers in the specialty. Various studies have explored the direct and indirect processes that APRNs use to manage patient care and the outcomes achieved. All have determined that APRN practice overlaps that of other care providers in some respects and differs in others. These distinctions, and their potential to confound comparisons with other care providers, contribute to the complexity inherent in measuring the effect of APRNs. Moreover, the limited research linking specific APRN processes to care delivery outcomes makes it difficult to determine which role components achieved the effect. Difficult or not, a clear distinction is needed if APRNs are ever to receive the recognition they deserve or the financial reimbursement they are due.

This review of APRN outcome studies suggests that the quality and quantity of research pertaining to APRN outcomes has improved over time, with initial studies focusing primarily on role description and acceptance issues and more recent studies addressing performance and outcomes. A variety of research designs are now being used to measure APRN impact, with an increasing number of investigators using prospective designs and including comparison groups. Although medical record reviews continue to provide much of the data for these comparison studies, methods to control for differences in patient populations and the use of more sophisticated data analysis techniques are providing more reliable, replicable, and generalizable information.

Despite these improvements, intensive work is needed in several areas. These include agreement on a consistent set of core outcomes, clear definitions of the specific role components within the APRN profession, the relationship between APRN care delivery and long-term clinical outcomes, research on the unique contributions made by APRNs, evaluation of the value-added impact of APRNs in collaborative practice, measurement related to the impact of the APRN role on social determinants of health, and research to investigate the role of APRNs in addressing health disparities, including studies that examine APRN interventions to dismantle institutional racism in health care. Each is briefly discussed below.

Additional work is needed to develop and implement a consistent set of core outcome indicators relevant and sensitive to differences in APRN practice. An important step in this direction is the work performed by the NQF to establish a list of endorsed measures, many of which are applicable to the work of APRNs (National Quality Forum, 2021). National APRN leadership groups should develop and test measures using the methods outlined by the NQF to guide their work; such a process would increase the number of measures in the domain of APRN practice and would ultimately facilitate a standardized approach to evaluating APRN effect and public reporting. Collaborations between APRNs and nurse researchers and the development of outcomes consortia will also facilitate this process. Bringing together experts in clinical practice and research design and measurement from multiple locations and specialties is the best approach for the development and subsequent testing of reliable and valid indicators of the effect of APRN-directed and APRN-delivered care. Networks of APRN groups and institutions in which APRNs practice should also play an active role in the collection of data to assist the development of APRN-sensitive measures. An understanding of the important role that the NQF plays in relation to endorsing measures recognized by the CMS is essential. Table 21.4 lists examples of the various APRN-sensitive outcome indicators that have been used in previous studies; however, the conformity of these measures with the NQF-endorsed measures for use by the CMS, third-party payers, and public reporting is inconsistent. This work must also consider the reporting burden that can result from requiring use of additional reporting metrics, an area of importance highlighted by the Institute for Healthcare Improvement in advocating for a reduction in data-gathering burden (Institute for Healthcare Improvement, 2017).

Second, the specific role components within the APRN role must be clearly defined. A systematic review identified 43 randomized controlled trials evaluating the cost-effectiveness of APRNs using criteria that meet current definitions of the roles. Incomplete reporting of study methods and lack of details about the APRN roles create challenges in evaluating the evidence of the cost-effectiveness of these roles (Donald et al., 2014).

Third, there is a need to determine how the increased patient and family satisfaction evident when interacting with APRN providers contributes to long-term care delivery outcomes. Because APRNs traditionally spend more time with patients and provide additional teaching and healthy behavior counseling, their impact may be most evident in the long-term prevention of diseases and adverse outcomes commonly associated with unhealthy behaviors. Studies thus far have followed patient outcomes for relatively short periods. Additional longitudinal studies are needed to determine the true long-term impact of these early outcomes on overall lifestyle, quality of life, and health.

A fourth future direction for APRN outcomes is to focus on the unique contributions that APRNs make in their roles. Many studies have focused on comparing APRNs with other providers, particularly attending physicians, physician residents, or physician assistants. Although these studies are useful, they do not address the unique contributions of APRN care, nor do they identify which outcome indicators are most sensitive to differences in APRN practices. The focus of outcomes assessment research needs to turn to the value of APRN care in patient and population outcomes, rather than comparison of care with other healthcare providers. Of course, when APRNs stretch the boundaries of their practice to incorporate new roles and responsibilities, comparisons to more traditional providers of these services are inevitable and important.

Fifth, evaluation of the value-added impact of APRNs in collaborative practice with physicians and other care providers is needed. Although the work of Newhouse and associates (2011) has highlighted that an impressive number of studies have been conducted that demonstrate outcomes of APRN care, additional research is needed as APRN roles continue to expand and as roles in novel practice areas develop. Because APRNs and physicians bring different perspectives about care and demonstrate distinct but complementary behaviors, studies are needed to determine how these combined practices reinforce and maximize the beneficial effects of one another. These studies may generate the data needed to determine the value-added benefits of combining APRN and physician practices. By accurately documenting outcomes when a collaborative APRN-physician approach is used, the profession can more effectively argue for altered reimbursement procedures and reveal the contributions of APRNs to the public.

Sixth, work is needed to examine the impact of the APRN role on social determinants of health. A body of literature has addressed how APRNs increase healthcare access and quality. However, APRNs function holistically and consider multiple factors. Research is needed to assess the interface between care delivered by APRNs and other social determinants of health, including economic stability, education access and quality, neighborhoods and environments, and the social and community context.

Last, additional research is needed to investigate the role of APRNs in addressing health disparities. As with social determinants of health, the role of APRNs in increasing healthcare access and quality has been examined. Additional factors that contribute to health disparities, including institutional racism in health care, must also be researched. The NASEM (2021) *Future of Nursing Report* provides valuable insights that can be used to structure research in the areas of social determinants of health and health disparities.

The literature highlights the difficulties evident in generating widespread interest in measuring care delivery outcomes. Many APRNs view the ongoing assessment of care delivery impact as an additional burden to an already full agenda. Because APRN outcome measurement activities begin immediately when an APRN is hired, graduate programs must prepare new APRNs to identify target outcomes, collect data, and manage and report findings. In addition to clinically focused outcomes content, several individuals and groups have recommended including content on healthcare financing, healthcare information systems, database query, and statistics for APRNs (AACN, 2021). Developing APRN-associated metrics for outcomes assessment is a strategy that holds promise for future work highlighting the impact of APRN care (Kapu & Kleinpell, 2013). Dashboards can then be used to outline the metrics, assign data definitions, and enable data transfer and display to assess trends over time. In well-conceived electronic health records (EHRs), downloadable data can self-populate APRN dashboards to promote ready viewing of APRN-led initiatives. For example, when promoting adherence to national quality guidelines such as VTE prophylaxis in hospitalized patients, tracking use of an EHR order set for eligible patients can enhance data capture and identify trends over time.

Several strategies can be used to develop APRN-associated outcomes metrics. These include identifying high-priority outcomes, outlining how these outcomes measure APRN core competencies, determining whether currently existing data sets can be used to abstract metrics, and evaluating whether informatics can be created to automatically collect the data (Kapu & Kleinpell, 2013). Ideally, APRNs should consider outcome assessment for regularly assigned duties and new projects.

CONCLUSION

Focusing on the outcomes of APRN care is an essential component in demonstrating the impact of the role. APRN care has been cited as being valuable but often invisible because APRNs traditionally have not focused on highlighting the impact of their care. This invisibility further undermines APRNs as viable and important providers of healthcare services. The current emphasis on health equity, quality of care, and care effectiveness mandates that APRNs demonstrate their impact on patient care, healthcare outcomes, and particularly disparity in outcomes related to social determinants of health and APRNs' ability to improve systems of care. The need for well-designed, longitudinal assessments of APRN impact has never been greater. Assessing the outcomes of APRN care has become a necessary rather than an optional endeavor. It is only through demonstrating the outcomes of APRN care for patients, providers, and healthcare systems that the value of this care can be defined.

In addition, focusing on APRN-sensitive outcome indicators is important for highlighting the unique contributions of APRNs. Addressing APRN-sensitive outcome indicators will require focused attention on the continued evolution of EHRs that support the identification and tracking of process and outcome data in line with APRN contributions. An important component in this process is national agreement on a core set of outcome indicators relevant to APRNs, the initiation of standards that support the collection of APRN-sensitive data, testing of these core measures, and ultimately measure endorsement by the NQF.

This chapter has presented a review of concepts related to APRN outcomes and several frameworks for measuring and monitoring APRN practice. Other approaches are also available; the APRN should begin the process by selecting one and refining it to meet individual and organizational needs. The best approach is to begin small and expand activities over time. Using a pragmatic model like structure, process, and outcome may help bring order and meaning to the process. Networking with other APRNs is useful for identifying beneficial outcomes and sharing personal experiences about what does and does not work when integrating outcomes measurement into busy practices. Disseminating outcome evaluations through presentations and publications will allow for replication.

Effective outcomes measurement requires APRNs to work collaboratively with others, plan and organize processes of care and assessment of quality in highly complex health services environments, and expose their individual practices to the scrutiny of others. Experience with organizational change behaviors and a willingness to seek information and assistance from others will help with these processes. In the end, the quality and value of care will improve, as will the community's recognition of the APRN's impact on outcomes of care.

KEY SUMMARY POINTS

- Performance indicators for APRN roles focus on two levels—the aggregate level, at which evidence addresses APRN role impact in one of the four APRN roles, and the individual level, with activities directed at the outcomes of a single APRN's practice.
- Studies evaluating care delivery processes of APRN practice often occur in combination with role definition research. The distinction between these process studies and role definition explorations is their attention to what APRNs do as part of their roles.
- Various studies have explored the direct and indirect processes that APRNs use to manage patient care and the outcomes achieved. These studies identify that APRN practice overlaps with that of other care providers in some respects and differs in others. These distinctions, and their potential to confound comparisons with other care providers, contribute to the complexity inherent in measuring the effect of APRNs.
- Effective outcomes measurement requires APRNs to work collaboratively with others, plan and organize processes of care and assessment of quality in highly complex health services environments, and expose their individual practices to the scrutiny of others.
- APRNs must respond to the urgent need to impact health disparities and demonstrate their impact to improve health equity.

REFERENCES

Adams, E. K., & Markowitz, S. (2018). Improving efficiency in the health care system: Removing anticompetitive barriers for advanced practice registered nurses and physician assistants. *Brookings*. https://www.brookings.edu/research/improving-efficiency-in-the-health-care-system-removing-anticompetitive-barriers-for-advanced-practice-registered-nurses-and-physician-assistants/

Agency for Healthcare Resarch and Quality (AHRQ). (n.d.). PSNet Patient Safety Network: Glossary. https://psnet.ahrq.gov/glossary?glossary%5B0%5D=term%3AB

Agency for Healthcare Research and Quality (AHRQ). (2020). AHRQ quality indicators. http://www.qualityindicators.ahrq.gov/

Albers-Heitner, C. P., Joore, M. A., Winkens, R. A., Lagro-Janssen, A. L. M., Severns, J. L., & Berghmans, L. C. (2012). Cost-effectiveness of involving nurse specialists for adult patients with urinary incontinence in primary care compared with care as usual: An economic evaluation alongside a pragmatic randomized controlled trial. *Neurology and Urodynamics, 31*, 526–534.

Alexander, D., & Schnell, M. (2019). Just what the nurse practitioner ordered: Independent prescriptive authority and population mental health. *Journal of Health Economics, 66*, 145–162.

Alexander-Banys, B. (2014). Acute care nurse practitioner managed home monitoring program for patients with complex congenital heart disease: A case study. *Journal of Pediatric Health Care, 28*, 97–100.

Alexandrov, A. W. (2011). Outcomes management. In H. R. Feldman, M. Jaffe-Ruiz, M. J. Greenberg, & T. D. Smith (Eds.), *Nursing leadership: A concise encyclopedia* (2nd ed., pp. 285–296). Springer.

Alexandrov, A. W., Baca, T., Albright, K. C., DiBiase, S., & Alexandrov, A. V. for the NET SMART Faculty and Fellows. (2011). Post-graduate academic neurovascular fellowship for advanced practice nurses and physician assistants significantly increases tPA treatment rates: Results from the first graduating class of the NET SMART program. [Abstract]. *Stroke: A Journal of Cerebral Circulation, 42*, e206.

Alexandrov, A. W., Brethour, M., Cudlip, F., Swatzell, V., Biby, S., Reiner, D., Kiernan, T., Handler, D., Tocco, S., & Yang, J. (2009). Post-graduate fellowship education and training for nurses: The NET SMART experience. *Critical Care Nursing Clinics of North America, 21*(4), 435–449.

Alexandrov, A. W., Brewer, T. L., & Brewer, B. B. (2019). The role of outcomes in evaluating practice change. In B. Melnyk, & E. Finout-Overholt (Eds.), *Evidence-based practice in nursing and health: A guide for translating research evidence into practice* (4th ed., pp. 293–312). Wolters Kluwer.

Amaral, A. F. S., Fereira, P. L., Cardoso, M. L., & Vidinha, T. (2014). Implementation of the nursing role effectiveness model. *International Journal of Caring Sciences, 7*(3), 757–770.

American Association of Colleges of Nursing. (2006). The essentials of doctoral education for advanced nursing practice. https://www.aacnnursing.org/Portals/42/Publications/DNPEssentials.pdf

American Association of Colleges of Nursing. (2021). The essentials: Core competencies for professional nursing education. https://www.aacnnursing.org/Portals/42/AcademicNursing/pdf/Essentials-2021.pdf

American Nurses Association. (2021). *Nursing: Scope and standards of practice* (4th ed.). Author.

Anetzberger, G. J., Stricklin, M. L., Gaunter, D., Banozic, R., & Laurie, R. (2006). VNA Housecalls of Greater Cleveland, Ohio: Development and pilot evaluation of a program for high-risk older adults offering primary medical care in the home. *Home Health Services Quarterly, 25*, 155–166.

Arthur, R., Marfell, J., & Ulrich, S. (2009). Outcomes measurement in nurse-midwifery practice. In R. M. Kleinpell (Ed.), *Outcome assessment in advanced practice nursing* (pp. 229–254). Springer.

Atkinson, S., Crutcher, T. D., & King, J. E. (2021). Improving efficiency within a trauma nurse practitioner team. *Journal of the American Association of Nurse Practitioners, 33*(3), 239–245.

Ball, S. T. E., Walton, K., & Hawes, S. (2007). Do emergency department physiotherapy practitioners, emergency nurse practitioners and doctors investigate, treat and refer patients with closed musculoskeletal injuries differently? *Emergency Medicine Journal, 24*, 185–188.

Barnum, T. J., Vaez, K., Cesarone, D., & Yingling, C. T. (2019). Your data looks good on a dashboard. *Online Journal of Nursing Informatics, 23*(3), 10–11.

Barocas, D. A., Kulahalli, C. S., Ehrenfeld, J. M., Kapu, A. N., Penson, D. F., You, C. C., Weavind, L., & Dmochowski, R. (2014). Benchmarking the use of a rapid response team by surgical services at a tertiary care hospital. *Journal of the American College of Surgeons, 218*(1), 66–72.

Baxter, J., & Leary, A. (2011). Productivity gains by specialist nurses. *Nursing Times, 107*, 15–17.

Begley, C., Murphy, K., Higgins, A., Elliot, N., Lalor, J., Sheerin, F., Coyne, I., Comiskey, C., Normand, C., Casey, C., Dowling, M., Devane, D., Cooney, A., Farrelly, F., Brennan, M., Meskell, P., & MacNeela, P. (2010). Evaluation of clinical nurse and midwife specialist and advanced nurse and midwife practitioner roles in Ireland (SCAPE): Final report. Dublin: National Council for the Professional Development of Nursing and Midwifery in Ireland.

Bethea, A., Samanta, D., White, T., Payne, N., & Hardway, J. (2019). Nurse practitioners' role in improving service for elderly trauma patients. *Journal of Trauma Nursing, 26*(4), 174–179.

Bevis, L. C., Berg-Copas, G. M., Thomas, B. W., Vasquez, D. G., Wetta-Hall, R., Brake, D., Lucas, E., Toumeh, K., & Harrison, P. (2008). Outcomes of tube thoracostomies performed by advanced practice providers vs. trauma surgeons. *American Journal of Critical Care, 17*(4), 357–363.

Bissonnette, J. M. (2011). Evaluation of an advanced practice nurse led inter-professional collaborative chronic care approach for kidney transplant patients: The TARGET study. http://www.ruor.uottawa.ca/en/handle/10393/19975

Borgmeyer, A., Gyr, P. M., Jamerson, P. A., & Henry, L. D. (2008). Evaluation of the role of the pediatric nurse practitioner in an inpatient asthma program. *Journal of Pediatric Health Care, 22*, 273–281.

Bradway, C., Trotta, R., Bixby, M. B., McPartland, E., Wollman, M. C., Kapustka, H., McCauley, K., & Naylor, Mary D. (2012). A qualitative analysis of an advanced practice nurse-directed transitional care model intervention. *The Gerontologist, 52*(3), 394–407.

Brandon, A. F., Schuessler, J. B., Ellison, K. J., & Lazenby, R. B. (2009). The effects of an advanced practice nurse led telephone intervention on outcomes of patients with heart failure. *Applied Nursing Research, 22*, e1–e7.

Brooks, P. B., & Fulton, M. E. (2019). Demonstrating advanced practice provider value: Implementing a new advanced practice provider billing algorithm. *Journal of American Academy of Physician Assistants, 32*(2), 1–10. doi:10.1097/01.JAA.0000550293.01522.01

Buchholz, S. W., & Purath, J. (2007). Physical activity and physical fitness counseling patterns of adult nurse practitioners. *Journal of the American Academy of Nurse Practitioners, 19*, 86–92.

Buerhaus, P. (September 2018). Nurse practitioners: A solution to America's primary care crisis. *American Enterprise Institute*. https://www.aei.org/research-products/report/nurse-practitioners-a-solution-to-americas-primary-care-crisis/

Buerhaus, P., Perloff, J., Clarke, S., O'Reilly-Jacob, M., Zolotusky, G., & DesRoches, C. M. (2018). Quality of primary care provided by Medicare beneficiaries by nurse practitioners and physicians. *Medical Care, 56*(6), 484–490. doi:10.1097/MLR.0000000000000908

Callahan, C. M., Boustani, M. A., Unverzagt, F. W., Austrom, M. G., Damush, T. M., Perkins, A. J., Fultz, B. A., Hui, S. L., Counsell, S. R., & Hendrie, H. C. (2006). Effectiveness of collaborative care for older adults with Alzheimer disease in primary care: A randomized controlled trial. *The Journal of the American Medical Association, 295*(18), 2148–2157.

Capezuti, E., Wagner, L. M., Brush, B. L., Boltz, M., Renz, S., & Talerico, K. A. (2007). Consequences of an intervention to reduce restrictive siderail use in nursing homes. *Journal of the American Geriatrics Society, 55*, 334–341.

Case, R., Haynes, D., Holaday, B., & Parker, V. G. (2010). Evidence-based nursing: The role of the advanced practice registered nurse in the management of heart failure patients in the outpatient setting. *Dimensions of Critical Care Nursing, 29*, 57–62.

Centers for Medicare & Medicaid Services. (2020). CMS hospital IQR program measures for FY 2023 payment update. https://qualitynet.cms.gov/inpatient/iqr/measures

Centers for Medicare & Medicaid Services. (2021a). Hospital value-based purchasing. https://www.cms.gov/Medicare/Quality-Initiatives-Patient-Assessment-Instruments/HospitalQualityInits/Hospital-Value-Based-Purchasing

Centers for Medicare and Medicaid Services. (2021b). Physician fee schedule. https://www.cms.gov/Medicare/Medicare-Fee-for-Service-Payment/PhysicianFeeSched

Chattopadhyay, S., & Zangaro, G. (2019). The economic cost and impacts of scope of practice restrictions on nurse practitioners. *Nursing Economic$, 37*(6), 273–283.

Cheng, C. (2012, August 20-22). In The impact of an APRN-led clinic on patients with psychosis. Paper presented at the 7th Annual International Nurse Practitioner/Advanced Practice Nursing Network Conference London.

Cheung, N. F., Mander, R., Wang, X., Fu, W., Zhou, H., & Zhang, L. (2011). Clinical outcomes of the first midwife-led normal birth unit in China: A retrospective cohort study. *Midwifery, 27*, 582–587.

Cibulka, N. J., Forney, S., Goodwin, K., Lazaroff, P., & Sarabia, R. (2011). Improving oral health in low-income pregnant women with a nurse practitioner-directed oral care program. *Journal of the American Academy of Nurse Practitioners, 23*, 249–257.

Coddington, J., Sands, L., Edwards, N., Kirkpatrick, J., & Chen, S. (2012). Quality of health care provided at a pediatric nurse-managed clinic. *Journal of the American Academy of Nurse Practitioners, 23*, 674–680.

Collins, N., Miller, R., Kapu, A., Martin, R., Morton, M., Forrester, M., Atkinson, S., Evans, B., & Wilkinson, L. (2014). Outcomes of adding acute care nurse practitioners to a Level I trauma service with the goal of decreased length of stay and improved physician and nursing satisfaction. *The Journal of Trauma and Acute Care Surgery, 76*(2), 353–357.

Cooper, J. M., Loeb, S., & Smith, C. A. (2009). The primary care nurse practitioner and cancer survivorship care. *Journal of the American Academy of Nurse Practitioners, 22*, 394–402.

Coppa, D., Winchester, S. B., & Roberts, M. B. (2018). Home-based nurse practitioners demonstrate reductions in rehospitalizations and emergency department visits in a clinically complex patient population through an academic-clinical partnership. *Journal of the American Association of Nurse Practitioners, 30*(6), 335–343.

Costa, D. K., Wallace, D. J., Barnato, A. E., & Kahn, J. M. (2014). Nurse practitioner/physician assistant staffing and critical care mortality. *Chest, 146*, 1566–1573.

Counsell, S. R., Callahan, C. M., Clark, D. O., Tu, W., Buttar, A. B., Stump, T. E., & Ricketts, G. D. (2007). Geriatric care management for low-income seniors: A randomized controlled trial. *The Journal of the American Medical Association, 298*(22), 2623–2633.

Cowan, M. J., Shapiro, M., Hays, R. D., Afifi, A., Vazirani, S., Ward, C. R., & Ettner, S. L. (2006). The effect of a multidisciplinary hospitalist/physician and advanced practice nurse collaboration on hospital costs. *Journal of Nursing Administration, 36*(2), 79–85.

Cragin, L., & Kennedy, H. P. (2006). Linking obstetric and midwifery practice with optimal outcomes. *Journal of Obstetric, Gynecologic, and Neonatal Nursing, 35*, 779–785.

Craswell, A., Dwyer, T., Rossi, D., Armstrong, C., & Akbar, D. (2018). Cost-effectiveness of nurse practitioner-led regional titration service for heart failure patients. *The Journal for Nurse Practitioners, 14*(2), 105–111.

Cromwell, J., & Snyder, K. (2000). Alternate cost-effective anesthesia care teams. *Nursing Economic$, 18*, 185–193.

David, D., Britting, L., & Dalton, J. (2015). Cardiac acute care nurse practitioner and 30-day readmission. *Journal of Cardiovascular Nursing, 30*, 248–255.

Dayhoff, N., & Lyons, B. (2009). Assessing outcomes of clinical nurse specialist practice. In R. M. Kleinpell (Ed.), *Outcome assessment in advanced practice nursing* (pp. 201–228). Springer.

Dickerson, S. S., Wu, Y. W. B., & Kennedy, M. C. (2006). A CNS-facilitated ICD support group: A clinical project evaluation. *Clinical Nurse Specialist, 20*, 146–153.

Donabedian, A. (1966). Evaluating the quality of medical care. *Milbank Quarterly, 44*, 166–206.

Donabedian, A. (1980). *Explorations in quality assessment and monitoring: The definition of quality and approaches to its assessment*. Ann Arbor, MI: Health Administration Press.

Donald, F., Kilpatrick, K., Reid, K., Carter, N., Martin-Misener, R., Bryant-Lukosius, D., Harbman, P., Kaasalainen, S., Marshall, D. A., Charbonneau-Smith, R., & Donald, E. E. (2014). A systematic review of the cost-effectiveness of nurse practitioners and clinical nurse specialists: What is the quality of the evidence? *Nursing Research and Practice*. Art. ID 896587. doi:10.1155/2014/896587

Doran, D. (2011). *Nursing outcomes: The state of the science* (2nd ed.). Jones & Bartlett.

Doran, D. I., Sidani, S., Keetings, M., & Doidge, D. (2002). An empirical testing of the nursing role effectiveness model. *Journal of Advanced Nursing, 38*(1), 29–39. doi:10.1046/j.1365-2648.2002.02143.x

Dulisse, B., & Cromwell, J. (2010). No harm found when nurse anesthetists work without supervision by physicians. *Health Affairs*, 29, 1469–1475.

Dwyer, T., Craswell, A., Rossi, D., & Holzberger, D. (2017). Evaluation of an aged care nurse practitioner service: Quality of care within a residential aged care facility hospital avoidance service. *BMC Health Services Research, 17*, 1–11. doi:10.1186/s12913-017-1977-x

Ellwood, P. M. (1988). Outcomes management: A technology of patient experience. *New England Journal of Medicine, 318*, 1549–1556.

Elpern, E. H., Killeen, K., Ketchem, A., Wiley, A., Patel, G., & Lateef, O. (2009). Reducing use of indwelling urinary catheters and associated urinary tract infections. *American Journal of Critical Care, 18*, 535–541.

Fanta, K., Cook, B., Falcone, R. A., Jr., Rickets, C., Schweer, L., Brown, R. L., & Garcia, V. F. (2006). Pediatric trauma nurse practitioners provide excellent care with superior patient satisfaction for injured children. *Journal of Pediatric Surgery, 41*(1), 277–281.

French, K. E., Guzman, A. B., Rubio, A. C., Frenzel, J. C., & Feeley, T. W. (2016). Value based care and bundled payments: Anesthesia care costs for outpatient oncology surgery using time-driven activity-based costing. *Healthcare, 4*(3), 173–180.

Fry, M. (2011). Literature review of the impact of nurse practitioners in critical care services. *Nursing in Critical Care, 16*, 58–66.

Fulton, J. S. (2012, August 20-22). In Validation of clinical nurse specialist core practice outcomes. Paper presented at the 7th Annual International Nurse Practitioner/Advanced Practice Nursing Network Conference, London, United Kingdom.

Fulton, J. S., Mayo, A., Walker, J., & Urden, L. D. (2019). Description of work processes used by clinical nurse specialists to improve patient outcomes. *Nursing Outlook, 67*(5), 511–522.

Gardner, G., Gardner, A., & O'Connell, J (2013). Using the Donabedian framework to examine the quality and safety of nursing service innovation. *Journal of Clinical Nursing, 23*, 145–155. doi:10.1111/jocn.12146

Garner, S., Lopatina, E., Rankin, J. A., & Marshall, D. A. (2017). Nurse-led care for patients with rheumatoid arthritis: A systematic review of the effect on quality of care. *Journal of Rheumatology, 44*(6), 557–565.

Gershengorn, H. B., Wunsch, H., Wahab, R., Leaf, D. E., Brodie, D., Li, G., & Factor, P. (2011). Impact of non-physician staffing on outcomes in a medical ICU. *Chest, 139*(6), 1347–1353.

Goncalves-Bradley, D., Khangura, J., Flodgren, G., Perera, R., Rowe, B. H., & Shepperd, S. (2018). Primary care professionals providing non-urgent care in hospital emergency departments.

Cochrane Database of Systematic Reviews, 11. https://doi.org/10.1002/14651858.CD002097.pub4

Goolsby, M. J. (2007). Antibiotic-prescribing habits of nurse practitioners treating adult patients: Antibiotic Use and Guidelines Survey adult. *Journal of the American Academy of Nurse Practitioners, 19*, 212–214.

Gordon, J. M., Lorilla, J. D., & Lehman, C. A. (2012). The role of the clinical nurse specialist in the future of health care in the United States. *Perioperative Nursing Clinics, 7*, 343–353.

Gracias, V. H., Sicoutris, C. P., Stawicki, S. P., Meredith, D. M., Horan, A. D., Gupta, R., Haut, E. R., Auerbach, S., Sonnad, S., Hanson, C. W., & Schwab, C. W. (2008). Critical care nurse practitioners improve compliance with clinical practice guidelines in "semiclosed" surgical intensive care unit. *Journal of Nursing Care Quality, 23*(4), 338–344.

Grant, J., Lines, L., Darbyshire, P., & Parry, Y. (2017). How do nurse practitioners work in primary health care settings? A scoping review. *International Journal of Nursing Studies, 75*, 51–57.

Greene, D., & Dell, R. M. (2010). Outcomes of an osteoporosis disease-management program managed by nurse practitioners. *Journal of the American Academy of Nurse Practitioners, 22*, 326–329.

Hamdan, M. H., Walsh, K. E., Brignole, M., & Key, J. (2018). Outreach syncope clinic managed by a nurse practitioner: Outcome and cost effectiveness. *Journal of Telemedicine & Telecare, 24*(8), 566–571.

Hamilton, R., & Hawley, S. (2006). Quality of life outcomes related to anemia management of patients with chronic renal failure. *Clinical Nurse Specialist, 20*, 139–143.

Hanrahan, N. P., Wu, E., Kelly, D., Aiken, L. H., & Blank, M. B. (2011). Randomized clinical trial of the effectiveness of a home-based advanced practice psychiatric nurse intervention: Outcomes for individuals with serious mental illness and HIV. *Nursing Research and Practice, 2011*, 840248.

Hardie, H., & Leary, A. (2010). Value to patients of a breast cancer clinical nurse specialist. *Nursing Standard, 24*, 42–48.

Harrison, B. E. (2017). Fall prevention program in the community: A nurse practitioner's contribution. *Journal for Nurse Practitioners, 13*(8), e395–e397.

Henrichs, B. M., Avidan, M. S., Murray, D. J., Boulet, J. R., Kras, J., Krause, B., & Evers, A. S. (2019). Performance of certified registered nurse anesthetists and anesthesiologists in a simulation-based skills assessment. *Anesthesia & Analgesia, 108*(1), 255–262.

Hogan, P., Seifert, R., Moore, C., & Simonson, B. (2010). Cost-effectiveness analysis of anesthesia providers. *Nursing Economic$, 28*, 159–169.

Holzemer, W. L. (1994). The impact of nursing care in Latin America and the Caribbean: A focus on outcomes. *Journal of Advanced Nursing, 20*, 5–12.

Horne, M. P., & Estes, K. R. (2021). Implementation of a new cardiology hospital service leveraging nurse practitioners to improve patient access and outcomes. *Journal of the American Association of Nurse Practitioners, 33*(3), 231–238.

Hsueh, M. T.-F. & Dorcy, K. S. (2016). Improving transitions of care with an advanced practice nurse: A pilot study. *Clinical Journal of Oncology Nursing, 20*(3), 240–243.

Hu, J.-Y., Tung, H.-H., Tsay, S.-L., & Lin, W.-C. (2018). An outcome analysis of nurse practitioner care in a community hospital in Taiwan. *Journal of the American Association of Nurse Practitioners, 30*(8), 464–471.

Hutchinson, M., East, L., Stasa, H., & Jackson, D. (2014). Deriving consensus on the characteristics of advanced practice nursing: Meta-summary of more than 2 decades of research. *Nursing Research, 63*(2), 116–128.

Institute for Healthcare Improvement. (2017). Outcome measures for spread. http://www.ihi.org/resources/Pages/Measures/OutcomeMeasuresforSpread.aspx (Accessed August 19, 2017).

Institute of Medicine (US). (2011). *The future of nursing: Leading change, advancing health*. National Academies Press.

Institute of Medicine Committee on Standards for Developing Trustworthy Clinical Practice Guidelines. (2011). *Clinical practice guidelines we can trust*. National Academies of Press.

Jakobs, L., & Bigbee, J. (2016). US frontier distribution of advanced practice registered nurses and population health. *Online Journal of Rural Nursing and Health Care, 16*(2), 196–218.

Jessee, B. T., & Rutledge, C. M. (2012). Effectiveness of nurse practitioner–coordinated team group visits for type 2 diabetes in medically underserved Appalachia. *Journal of the American Academy of Nurse Practitioners, 24*, 735–743.

Johantgen, M., Fountain, L., Zangaro, G., Newhouse, R., Stanik-Hutt, J., & White, K. (2012). Comparison of labor and delivery care provided by certified nurse midwives and physicians: A systematic review, 1990-2008. *Woman's Health Issues, 22*, e73–e81.

Johnson, R. L. (2016). Use of a handoff communication tool between certified registered nurse anesthetists, anesthesiologists, and post anesthesia care unit nurses: The University of Southern Mississippi Dissertation, ISBN 9781369349054.

The Joint Commission. (2021). National patient safety goals® Effective January 2021 for the hospital program. https://www.jointcommission.org/-/media/tjc/documents/standards/national-patient-safety-goals/2021/npsg_chapter_hap_jan2021.pdf

Kahn, S. A., Davis, S. A., Banes, C. T., Dennis, B. M., May, A. K., & Gunter, O. D. (2015). Impact of advanced practice providers (nurse practitioners and physician assistants) on surgical residents' critical care experience. *Journal of Surgical Research, 199*(1), 7–12. https://doi.org/10.1016/j.jss.2015.05.036

Kapu, A. N., & Kleinpell, R. (2013). Developing nurse practitioner associated metrics for outcomes assessment. *Journal of the American Association of Nurse Practitioners, 25*, 289–296.

Kapu, A. N., Kleinpell, R., & Pilon, B. (2014). Quality and financial impact of adding nurse practitioners to inpatient care teams. *Journal of Nursing Administration, 44*, 87–96.

Kapu, A. N., Wheeler, A. P., & Lee, B. (2014). Addition of acute care nurse practitioners to medical and surgical rapid response teams: A pilot project. *Critical Care Nurse, 34*, 51–59.

Kilpatrick, K., Kaasalainen, S., Donald, F., Reid, K., Carter, N., Bryant-Lukosius, D., Martin-Misener, R., Harbman, P., Marshall, D. A., Charbonneau-Smith, R., & DiCenso, A. (2014). The effectiveness and cost-effectiveness of clinical nurse specialists in outpatient roles: A systematic review. *Journal of Evaluation in Clinical Practice, 20*(6), 1106–1123.

Kippenbrock, T., Lo, W.-J., Emroy, J., Buron, B., Odell, E., & Reimers, J. (2018). Nurse practitioners' time on nonbillable activities. *Journal of the American Association of Nurse Practitioners, 30*(9), 48–490.

Kofler, S., Kobleder, A., Ott, S., & Senn, B. (2019). The effect of written information and counselling by an advanced practice nurse on resilience in women with vulvar neoplasia six months after surgical treatment and the influence of social support, recurrence, and age: A secondary analysis of a multicenter randomized controlled trial, WOMAN-PRO II. *Boston Medical Center Women's Health, 20*(1), 1–9.

Kremer, M. J., & Faut-Callahan, M. (2009). Outcome assessment in nurse anesthesia. In R. Kleinpell (Ed.), *Outcome assessment in advanced practice nursing* (pp. 255–276). Springer.

Krichbaum, K. (2007). GAPRN postacute care coordination improves hip fracture outcomes. *Western Journal of Nursing Research, 29*, 523–544.

Kuethe, M. C., Vaessen-Verberne, A. A. P. H., Elbers, R. G., & Van Aalderen, W. M. C. (2013). Nurse versus physician-led care for the management of asthma. *The Cochrane Database of Systematic Reviews*. Art. No.: CD009296. https://www.cochranelibrary.com/cdsr/doi/10.1002/14651858.CD009296.pub2/full

Kutzleb, J., & Reiner, D. (2006). The impact of nurse-directed patient education on quality of life and functional capacity in people with heart failure. *Journal of American Academy of Nurse Practitioners, 18*, 116–123.

Lacny, S., Zarrabi, M., Martin-Misener, R., Donald, F., Sketris, I., Murphy, A., DiCenso, A., & Marshall, D. A. (2016). Cost effectiveness of a nurse practitioner family physician model of care in a nursing home: Controlled before and after study. *Journal of Advanced Nursing, 72*(9), 2138–2152.

Lakhan, S. E., & Laird, C. (2009). Addressing the primary care physician shortage in an evolving medical workforce. *International Archives of Medicine, 2*, 14. https://intarchmed.biomedcentral.com/articles/10.1186/1755-7682-2-14

Lamirel, C., Bruce, B. B., Wright, D. W., Delaney, K. P., Newman, N. J., & Biousse, V. (2012). Quality of nonmydriatic digital fundus photography obtained by nurse practitioners in the emergency department: The FOTO-ED study. *Ophthalmology, 119*, 617–624.

Landsperger, J. S., Semler, M. W., Wang, L., Byrne, D. W., & Wheeler, A. P. (2015). Outcomes of nurse practitioner-delivered critical care: A prospective cohort study. *Chest, 149*, 1146–1154.

Laurant, M., van der Biezen, M., Watananirum, K., Kontopantelis, E., & van Vught, A. J. A. H. (2018). Nurses as substitutes for doctors by nurses in primary care. *The Cochrane Database of Systematic Reviews*. https://doi.org/10.1002/14651858.CD001271.pub3

Lewin Group. (2016). Update of cost effectiveness of anesthesia providers: Final report. American Association of Nurse Anesthetists.

Lewis, S. R., Nicholson, A., Smith, A. F., & Alderson, P. (2014). Physician anaesthetists versus non-physician providers of anaesthesia for surgical patients. *The Cochrane Database of Systematic Reviews*, (7), Art. No. CD010357.

Li, J., Westbrook, J., Callen, J., Georgiou, A., & Braithwaite, J. (2013). The impact of nurse practitioners on care delivery in the emergency department: A multiple perspectives qualitative study. *BMC Health Services Research, 13*, 1–8.

Lopatina, E., Donald, F., DiCenso, A., Martin-Misener, R., Kilpatrick, K., Bryant-Lukosius, D., Carter, N., Reid, K., & Marshall, D. A. (2017). Economic evaluation of nurse practitioner and clinical nurse specialist roles: A methodological review. *International Journal of Nursing Studies, 72*, 7–82. http://doi.org/10.1016/j.ijnurstu.2017.04.012

Lowery, J., Hopp, F., Subramanian, U., Wiitala, W., Welsh, D. E., Larkin, A., Stemmer, K., Zak, C., & Vaitkevicius, P. (2012). Evaluation of a nurse practitioner disease management model for chronic heart failure: A multi-site implementation study. *Congestive Heart Failure, 18*(1), 64–71.

Lucatorto, M. A., Watts, S. A., Kresevic, D., Burant, C., & Carney, K. J. (2016). Impacting the trajectory of chronic kidney disease with APRN-led renal teams. *Nursing Administration Quarterly, 40*(1), 76–86.

Lutfiyya, M. N., Tomai, L., Frogner, B., Cerra, F., Zismer, D., & Parente, S. (2017). Does primary care diabetes management provided to Medicare patients differ between primary care physicians and nurse practitioners? *Journal of Advanced Nursing, 73*(1), 240–252.

Lutgendorf, M. A., Spalding, C., Drake, E., Spence, D., Heaton, J. O., & Morocco, K. V. (2017). Multidisciplinary in situ simulation-based training as a postpartum hemorrhage quality improvement project. *Military Medicine, 182*(3/4), e1762–31766.

Machin, C. (2017). Can a nurse practitioner independently diagnose and manage skin cancer? *Dermatological Nursing, 16*(3), 10–15.

Malloy, M. H. (2010). Infant outcomes of certified nurse midwife–attended home births: United States: 2000-2004. *Journal of Perinatology, 30*, 622–627.

Martsolf, G. R., Auerbach, D. I., & Arifkhanova, A. (2015). The impact of full practice authority for nurse practitioners and other advanced practice registered nurses in Ohio. Rand Corporation.

McCorkle, R., Dowd, M. F., Ercolano, E., Schulman-Green, D., Williams, A. L., Siefert, M. L., Steiner, J., & Schwartz, P. (2009). Effects of a nursing intervention on quality of life outcomes in post-surgical women with gynecological cancer. *Psycho-Oncology, 18*(1), 62–70.

McCorkle, R., Dowd, M. F., Pickett, M., Siefert, M. L., & Robinson, J. P. (2007). Effects of advanced practice nursing on patient and spouse depressive symptoms, sexual function, and marital interaction after radical prostatectomy. *Urologic Nursing, 27*, 65–77.

McMullen, M., Alexander, M. K., Bourgeois, A., & Goodman, L. (2001). Evaluating a nurse practitioner service. *Dimensions of Critical Care Nursing, 20*, 30–34.

MeiLing, M. S. (2009). A proposed framework for evaluating the impact of advanced practice nursing roles in Singapore. *Singapore Nursing Journal, 36*(4), 31–34.

Mills, A., Sorensen, A., Gillen, E., Coomer, N. M., & Theis, E. (2020). Quality, costs, and policy: Factors influencing choice of anesthesia staffing models. *Journal of Healthcare Management, 65*(1), 45–60.

Moote, M., Krsek, C., Kleinpell, R., & Todd, B. (2011). Physician assistant and nurse practitioner utilization in academic medical centers. *American Journal of Medical Quality, 26*, 452–460.

Moreton, S. G., Saurman, E., Salkeld, G., Edwards, J., Hooper, D., Kneen, K., Rothwell, G., & Watson, J. (2020). Economic and clinical outcomes of the nurse practitioner-led Sydney Adventist Hospital community palliative care services. *Australian Health Review, 44*(5), 791–798.

Morse, K. J., Warshawsky, D., Moore, J. M., & Pecora, D. C. (2006). A new role for the ACNP: The rapid response team leader. *Critical Care Nursing Quarterly, 29*, 137–146.

National Academies of Sciences, Engineering, and Medicine. (2021). *The Future of nursing 2020-2030: Charting a path to achieve health equity*. The National Academies Press. doi:10.17226/25982

National Quality Forum. (2017). *Measuring performance: NQF-endorsed standards*. http://www.qualityforum.org/Measuring_Performance/Measuring_Performance.aspx

National Quality Forum. (2019). *Measure evaluation criteria and guidance for evaluating measures for endorsement*. https://www.qualityforum.org/Measuring_Performance/Endorsed_Performance_Measures_Maintenance.aspx

National Quality Forum. (2021). *Measuring performance*. https://www.qualityforum.org/Measuring_Performance/Measuring_Performance.aspx#:~:text=NQF%20has%20a%20portfolio%20of,to%20provide%20high%2Dquality%20care

Naylor, M. D., Bowles, K. H., McCauley, K. M., Maccoy, M. C., Maislin, G., Pauly, M. V., & Krakauer, R. (2013). High-value transitional care: Translation of research into practice. *Journal of Evaluation in Clinical Practice, 19*(5), 727–733.

Negrusa, B., Hogan, P. F., Warner, J. T., Schroeder, C. H., & Pang, B. (2016). Scope of practice laws and anesthesia complications: No measurable impact of certified registered nurse anesthetists expanded scope of practice on anesthesia-related complications. *Medical Care, 54*(1), 913–920.

Newhouse, R. P., Weiner, J. P., Stanik-Hutt, J., White, K. M., Johantgen, M., Bass, E. B., Zangaro, G., Wilson, R. F., Fountain, L., Steinwachs, D. M., Heindel, L., & Weiner, J. P. (2011). Advanced practice outcomes 1990-2008: A systematic review. *Nursing Economic$, 29*(5), 230–250.

O'Grady, E. (2008). Advanced practice registered nurses: The impact on patient safety and quality. In R. G. Hughes (Ed.), *Patient safety and quality: An evidence-based handbook for nurses*, (Ch. 43, pp. 601–620). Agency for Healthcare Research and Quality. https://archive.ahrq.gov/professionals/clinicians-providers/resources/nursing/resources/nurseshdbk/OGradyE_APRN.pdf

Ohsfeldt, R. L., Miller, T. R., Schneider, J. E., & Scheibling, C. M. (2016). Cost impact of unexpected disposition after orthopedic ambulatory surgery associated with category of anesthesia provider. *Journal of Clinical Anesthesia, 35*, 157–162.

Oliver, S., & Leary, A. (2010). Return on investment: Workload, complexity and value of the CNS. *British Journal of Nursing, 21*(32), 34–37.

Padula, W. V., Nagarajan, M., Davidson, P. M., & Pronovost, P. J. (2021). Investing in skilled specialists to grow hospital infrastructure for quality improvement. *Journal of Patient Safety, 17*(1), 51–55.

Paez, K. A., & Allen, J. K. (2006). Cost-effectiveness of nurse practitioner management of hypercholesterolemia following coronary revascularization. *Journal of the American Academy of Nurse Practitioners, 18*, 436–444.

Park, J., & Dowling, M. (2020). Do nurse practitioner-led medical homes differ from physician-led medical homes? *Nursing Outlook, 68*(5), 601–610.

Park, J., Han, X., & Pittman, P. (2020). Does expanded state scope of practice for nurse practitioners and physician assistants increase primary care utilization in community health centers? *Journal of the American Association of Nurse Practitioners, 32*(6), 447–460.

Partiprajak, S. (2012, August 20-22). Outcomes of advanced practice nurse–led type 2 diabetes support group. Paper presented at the 7th Annual International Nurse Practitioner/Advanced Practice Nursing Network Conference, London.

Patel, M. S., Hogshire, L. C., Noveck, H., Steinberg, M. B., Hoover, D. R., Rosenfeld, J., Arya, A., & Carson, J. L. (2021). A retrospective cohort study of the impact of nurse practitioners on hospitalized patient outcomes. *Nursing Reports, 11*(1), 28–35.

Patient-Centered Outcomes Research Institute. (2013). *2013 Annual Report*. https://www.pcori.org/assets/2014/06/PCORI-Annual-Report-2013.pdf

Patient-Centered Outcomes Research Institute. (2021). Glossary. https://www.pcori.org/glossary

Patient Protection and Affordable Care Act, 42 U.S.C. §18001 (2010).

Pearson, J. T. (2017). Implementation and evaluation of coronary heart disease outreach community education: Improvement in evidence based screening for nurse practitioner clinical office follow up: Dissertation, ISBN 9781369428988. Wilmington University (Delaware).

Pine, M., Holt, K. D., & Lou, Y. B. (2003). Surgical mortality and type of anesthesia provider. *AANA Journal, 71*(2), 109–116.

Prajankett, O., & Markaki, A. (2021). Integrating older people care and advanced practice nursing: An evidence-based review. *International Nursing Review, 68*(1), 67–77.

Quenot, J. P., Ladoire, S., Devoucoux, F., Doise, J. M., Cailliod, R., Cunin, N., Aubé, H., Blettery, B., & Charles, P. E. (2007). Effect of a nurse-implemented sedation protocol on the incidence of ventilator-associated pneumonia. *Critical Care Medicine, 35*(9), 2031–2036.

Rantz, M. J., Popejoy, L., Vogelsmeier, A., Galambos, C., Alexander, G., Flesner, M., Murray, C., Crecelius, C., Ge, B., & Petroski, G. (2018). Impact of advanced practice registered nurses on quality measures: The Missouri quality initiative experience. *Journal of the American Medical Directors Association, 19*(6), 541–550.

Reigle, J., Molnar, H. M., Howell, C., & Dumont, C. (2006). Evaluation of in-patient interventional cardiology. *Critical Care Nursing Clinics of North America, 18*(4), 523–529. https://doi.org/10.1016/j.ccell.2006.09.002

Reynolds, T. (2018). *Advanced practice nurse intervention and heart failure readmissions*: Dissertation, ISBN 978035572557. Walden University.

Rideout, K. (2007). Evaluation of a PNP care coordinator model for hospitalized children, adolescents, and young adults with cystic fibrosis. *Pediatric Nursing, 33*(29–34), 48.

Sackett, D. L., Rosenberg, W. M. C., Gray, J. A., Hayn, R. B., & Richardson, W. S. (1996). Evidence-based medicine: What it is and what it isn't. *British Medical Journal, 312*(7023), 71–72.

Salamanca-Balen, N., Symore, J., Cawell, G., Whynes, D., & Tod, A. (2018). The costs, resource use and cost-effectiveness of Clinical Nurse Specialist-led interventions for patients with palliative care needs: A systematic review of international evidence. *Palliative Medicine, 32*(2), 447–465.

Sandall, J., Soltani, H., Gates, S., Shennan, A., & Devane, D. (2016). Midwife-led versus other models of care for childbearing women. *The Cochrane Database of Systematic Reviews, 4*, Art. No.: CD004667. doi:10.1002/14651858.CD004667.pub5

Sawatzky, J.-A. V., Christie, S., & Singal, R. K. (2013). Exploring outcomes of a nurse practitioner-managed cardiac surgery follow-up intervention: A randomized trial. *Journal of Advanced Nursing, 69*(9), 2076–2087.

Scherr, K., Wilson, D. M., Wagner, J., & Haughian, M. (2012). Evaluating a new rapid response team: NP-led versus intensivist-led comparisons. *AACN Advanced Critical Care, 23*, 32–43.

Schuttelaar, M. L. A., Vermeulen, K. M., & Coenraads, P. J. (2011). Costs and cost-effectiveness analysis of treatment in children with eczema by nurse practitioner vs dermatologist: Results of a randomized, controlled trial and a review of international costs. *British Journal of Dermatology, 165*, 600 611.

Seabra, P. R. C., Amendoeira, J. J. P., & Sa, L. O. (2018). Testing nursing sensitive outcomes in out-patient drug addicts, with "nursing role effectiveness model." *Issues in Mental Health Nursing, 39*(3), 200–207. doi:10.1080/01612840.2017.1378783

Seale, C., Anderson, E., & Kinnersley, P. (2005). Comparison of GP and nurse practitioner consultations: An observational study. *British Journal of General Practice, 521*, 938–943.

Seale, C., Anderson, E., & Kinnersley, P. (2006). Treatment advice in primary care: A comparative study of nurse practitioners and general practitioners. *Journal of Advanced Nursing, 54*, 534–541.

Sidani, S., Doran, D., Porter, H., LeFort, S., O'Brien Pallas, L. L., Zahn, C., Laschinger, H., & Sarkissian, S. (2006). Processes of care: Comparison between nurse practitioners and physician residents in acute care. *Nursing Leadership, 19*(1), 69–85.

Sidani, S., Doran, D., Porter, H., LeFort, S., O'Brien-Pallas, L. L., Zahn, C., & Sarkissian, S. (2005). Outcomes of nurse practitioners in acute care: An exploration. *The Internet Journal of Advanced Nursing Practice, 8*(1). http://ispub.com/IJANP/8/1/12232

Sidani, S., & Irvine, D. (1999). A conceptual framework for evaluating the nurse practitioner role in acute care settings. *Journal of Advanced Nursing, 30*, 58–66.

Simonson, D. C., Ahern, M. M., & Hendryx, M. S. (2007). Anesthesia staffing and anesthetic complications during cesarean delivery: A retrospective analysis. *Nursing Research, 56*, 9–17.

Smith, J., Pan, D., & Novelli, M. (2016). A nurse practitioner–led intervention to reduce hospital readmissions. *The Journal for Nurse Practitioners, 12*(5), 311–316.

Smits, M., Peters, Y., Ranke, S., Plat, E., Laurant, M., & Giesen, P. (2020). Substitution of general practitioners by nurse practitioners in out-of-hours primary care home visits: A quasi-experimental study. *International Journal of Nursing Studies, 104*. https://pubmed.ncbi.nlm.nih.gov/32105972/

Sonday, C., & Grecsek, E. (2010). Rapid response teams: NPs lead the way. *Nurse Practitioner, 35*, 40–46.

Spears, J. A., Craft, M., & White, S. (2017). Outcomes of cancer survivorship care provided by advanced practice RNs compared to other models of care: A systematic review. *Oncology Nursing Forum, 44*(1), E34–E41.

Splendore, E., & Grant, C. (2017). A nurse practitioner-led community workshop: Increasing adult participation in advance care planning. *Journal of the American Association of Nurse Practitioners, 29*(9), 535–542.

Stanik-Hutt, J., Newhouse, R. P., White, K. M., Johantgen, M., Bass, E. B., Zangaro, G., Wilson, R., Fountain, L., Steinwachs, D. M., Heindel, L., & Weiner, J. P. (2013). The quality and effectiveness of care provided by nurse practitioners. *Journal for Nurse Practitioners, 9*(8), 492–500.

Steuer, J., & Kopan, K. (2011). Productivity tool serves as outcome measurement for NPs in acute care practice. *Nurse Practitioner, 36*, 6–7.

Stolee, P., Hillier, L. M., Esbaugh, J., Griffiths, N., & Borrie, M. J. (2006). Examining the nurse practitioner role in long-term care. *Journal of Gerontological Nursing, 32*, 28–36.

Sullivan-Marx, E. M. (2008). Lessons learned from advanced practice nursing payment. *Policy, Politics and Nursing Practice, 9*, 121–126.

Sung, S. F., Huang, Y. C., Ong, C. T., & Chen, Y. W. (2011). A parallel thrombolysis protocol with nurse practitioners as coordinators minimizing door-to-needle time for acute ischemic stroke. *Stroke Research and Treatment*, 2011–198518. 1–8.

Thamm, C., Teleni, L., Chan, R. J., Stone, L., & McCarthy, A. L. (2019). Nurse-led interventions for cancer patients in emergency department: Systematic review. *Collegian, 26*(2), 311–319.

Trentalange, M., Bielawski, M., Murphy, T. E., Lessard, K., Brandt, C., Bean-Maberry, B., Maisel, N. C., Wright, S. M., Allore, H., Skanderson, M., Reyes-Harvey, E., Gaetano, V., Haskell, S., & Bastian, L. A. (2016). Patient perception of enough time spent with provider is a mechanism for improving women veterans' experiences with VA outpatient health care. *Evaluation & the Health Professions, 39*(4), 460–474. doi:10.1177/0163278716629523

Urden, L., & Stacy, K. (2012, August 20-22). Clinical nurse specialist productivity and outcomes. Paper presented at the 7th Annual International Nurse Practitioner/Advanced Practice Nursing Network Conference, London.

US Department of Health and Human Services Administration for Children and Families. (2010). *Measuring outcomes*. https://www.acf.hhs.gov/sites/default/files/ocs/measuring_outcomes.pdf

Varughese, A. M., Byczkowski, T. L., Wittkugel, E. P., Kotagal, U., & Dean, K. (2006). Impact of a nurse practitioner–assisted preoperative assessment program on quality. *Pediatric Anesthesia, 16*, 723–733.

Wagner, L. M., Capezuti, E., Brush, B., Boltz, M., Renz, S., & Talerico, K. A. (2007). Description of an advanced practice nursing consultative model to reduce restrictive siderail use in nursing homes. *Research in Nursing & Health, 30*, 131–140.

Walling, A. M., D'Ambruoso, S. F., Malin, J. L., Huritz, S., Zisser, A., Coscarelli, A., Clarke, R., Hackbarth, A., Pietras, C., Watts, F., Ferrell, B., Skootsky, S., & Wenger, N. S. (2017). Effect and efficiency of an embedded palliative care nurse practitioner in an oncology clinic. *Journal of Oncology Practice, 13*(9), e792–e799.

White, T., Kokiousis, J., Ensminger, S., & Shirey, M. (2017). Supplementing intensivist staffing with nurse practitioners: Literature review. *AACN Advanced Critical Care, 28*(2), 111–123.

Winter, S., Chan., G. K., Kuriakose, C., Duderstadt, K., Spetz, J., Hsieh, D., Platon, C., & Chapman, S. A. (2021). Measurement of nonbillable service value activities by nurse practitioners, physician assistants, and clinical nurse specialists in ambulatory specialty care. *Journal of the American Association of Nurse Practitioners, 33*(3), 211–219.

Wong, I., Wright, E., Santomauro, D., How, R., Leary, C., & Harris, C. (2018). Implementing two nurse practitioner models of service at an Australian male prison: A quality assurance study. *Journal of Clinical Nursing, 27*(1-2), e287–e300.

Woods, L. (2007). Evaluating the clinical effectiveness of neonatal nurse practitioners: An exploratory study. *Journal of Clinical Nursing, 15*, 35–44.

Xue, Y., & Tuttle, J. (2017). Clinical productivity of primary care nurse practitioners in ambulatory settings. *Nursing Outlook, 65*(2), 162–171.

22 FUTURE TECHNOLOGIES INFLUENCING APRN PRACTICE

DEBORA SIMMONS ■ PAMELA SALYER

"Let us never consider ourselves as finished nurses. We must be learning all our lives."

~ Florence Nightingale

CHAPTER CONTENTS

ILLUSIONS OF TECHNOLOGY IN A PANDEMIC 711
MAKING SENSE OF COMPLEXITY IN HEALTH INFORMATION TECHNOLOGY 711
The Donabedian Model 711
James Reason Swiss Cheese Model 712
HUMAN-CENTERED DESIGN 713
TECHNOLOGY-ASSISTED COMMUNICATION 715
Written Communication Technologies 715
Verbal Communication Technologies 717
Nonverbal Communication Technologies 718
Visual Communication Technologies 719
Social Media as a Communication Tool 719
DIAGNOSTIC, THERAPEUTIC, AND PROCEDURAL DEVICES AND APPS 721
Diagnostic and Therapeutic Devices and Apps 721
Procedural Devices and Apps 724
SUPPORTIVE TECHNOLOGY 725
DATA, CLINICAL DECISION SUPPORT, AND ADVANCED ANALYTICS 727
Data 727
Clinical Decision Support 730
Advanced Analytics 731
CYBERSECURITY 732
Data Security and Privacy 732
States of Digital Data 732
Regulatory Compliance 733
Types of Cyberattack 734
Mobile Device Security 734
Blockchain 735
HIGH-TECH HOME CARE 735
FUTURE IMPLICATIONS OF TECHNOLOGY-ENABLED ADVANCED PRACTICE REGULATION AND GROWTH: A CALL TO PARTICIPATE 737
CONCLUSION 738
KEY SUMMARY POINTS 739

The purpose of this chapter is to inspire questions that will guide future advanced practice nurses (APRNs) to assess and critique technology applications and practices. There are two simple but profound overarching questions to ask after reading this chapter:

- What lessons can be applied to the evolution of advanced practice nursing enabled by technology?
- What are the skills needed to safely use future technology in the advanced practice of nursing in its many varied settings?

There is no doubt of the influence of technology on nursing practice today and its far-reaching impact on nursing practice in the future. Technology-enabled data fuel the ever-changing landscape of health care as evidence. At the core of the technology is data we use as evidence. Therefore, at its best, technology delivers data in forms easily assimilated into clinical knowledge and wisdom. However the data are created, captured, archived, or retrieved, the nature of data is foundational to understanding technology today and technology in our future. Understanding how we use data enables us to understand the technology we need and the intersections to advanced practice. It is essential to understand the implications of data acquisition and its functions and how the human mind uses technology.

Florence Nightingale's 200th birthday was celebrated in the notable year of 2020. Born on May 12, 1820, in Florence, Italy, Florence Nightingale came of age when medical care was locally understood and delivered. Descriptions of Florence Nightingale in Crimea are compelling, bringing severe conditions into sharp focus with many unknown dangers. Her reports from Crimea, where she became the Lady with the Lamp, relied heavily on her lifelong habit of documentation and categorizing (Halliday, 2019). In unlikely times, she created new understandings of health, nursing, and data. The data she used were manually collected, analyzed, and reported, which led to the modern concepts of nursing practice, epidemiology, and technology. Evergreen and timely, her methods of using documentation, data, and visualizations are easily reflected in today's technology-enabled care.

Medical documentation was not yet practiced during the Victorian era in England, and medical knowledge relied on the mercy of memory and a few books. However astute, Nightingale's early views could only be viewed as anecdotal, because there was no medical record, no systematic accounting of mortality and morbidity, and no data record of the events taking place. Nightingale knew she needed a breakthrough. The beliefs and inconsistent practices of the time did not serve the patients. She described her use of charts as meant "to affect through the eyes what we may fail to convey to the brains of the public through their word-proof ears" (Hammer, 2020, para. 18), which is poignant when we look at today's information systems; the goals are the same. The collection, aggregation, and visualization of the mortality and morbidity of the Crimean War soldiers was Nightingale's legacy, leading to an impact strong enough to effect change in healthcare practice and policy during the Victorian era. Nightingale originated a profoundly pivotal turning point for health care.

Florence Nightingale is widely known for her defining role in nursing's future and statistics. In Crimea, she also decisively pointed her revelations toward collected data. She used the power of data to insert her points into the rigid system of beliefs. Her Coxcomb diagrams were revolutionary at the time, graphically illustrating a complexity in easily understood terms. Nightingale was able to take data and turn it toward a shared understanding of the issues at hand. Her manipulation of information in the form of archived, analyzed, and disseminated data is a goal we still chase today.

To fully understand the current healthcare information technology or prepare for the future, we can still learn from Florence Nightingale's lessons of 200 years ago. We are moving through this century with increasingly sophisticated technology. Yet much like Nightingale, we struggle to use the right tools to find the data, transform data into information, and analyze the issues at hand. Today in health care, technology cannot easily aggregate patient data across the care continuum, leaving the patient as the sole repository for complex and sometimes confusing information. Reflecting on the current state, what we do as advanced practice nurses, and what we will do tomorrow, will not stray far from Nightingale's practice. We will use assessment, planning, intervention, and evaluation to create data to benefit patients.

We use technology-enabled data to share knowledge and make evidence-based decisions to inform and persuade, much as Nightingale did. Evidence-based data remain a large part of our power. Nightingale empowered nurses to observe, assess, gather data, analyze, and intervene (Reinking, 2020). These skills remain core to the success of APRNs today. The present models for advanced practice nursing evolved because data proved the critical role that nursing actions play in delivering care. APRNs must understand the technology as a source of data to represent and inform their practice.

While Nightingale's vision of nursing was undoubtedly close to our practice today, she did not foresee the technology that compels us to reexamine practice and safety. As APRNs hold a crucial role in both micro (patient to provider) and macro (clinical expert, administration) systems, APRNs use the same nursing process to analyze and address complex issues in patient care. The expansive role of the APRN takes this process to another level of patient and population health. Because of this comprehensive and holistic view, future technology design can only be enhanced with the full participation of advanced practice nurses. The APRN is positioned to advocate for safer and more usable technology solutions across the care continuum.

ILLUSIONS OF TECHNOLOGY IN A PANDEMIC

The spring of 2020 brought an event not seen for a century: a global pandemic. The pandemic was met with an arsenal of healthcare technology in the United States. However, the patina of technology began to tarnish in meeting the challenge. Severe impediments to receiving electronic data at health departments prevented reporting of hospital-level cases (Holmgren et al., 2020). Coronavirus disease 2019 (COVID-19) data were widely acknowledged as inconsistent, not reliable, and suspected as simply wrong. This problem with data led conversations down an increasingly argumentative winding path that did not serve the public and created derisive nonproductive conversations (Manski & Molinari, 2020). Painfully missing were integrated systems, interoperability, and public healthcare infrastructure. Outdated faxes and paper records remained where technology did not meet its promise, and the virus continued to spread (Tahir, 2020). Old problems persisted as vital information was not defined uniformly, not collected in real-time, and essentially siloed in hospitals, health departments, and other healthcare organizations that could not communicate with each other. As significant gaps and terse discourse about the virus increased, critical answers were irretrievable despite smartphones, artificial intelligence, and electronic medical records. The definitive agreement was that monitoring, transmission analysis, data aggregation, and trending in the pandemic were essentially nonexistent (Zhou et al., 2020).

The big question for today and the future is how we can be here after all of the money and effort to bring technology to health care. Trying to understand the technology while facing a dangerous viral adversary is not ideal. However, the pandemic has offered an opportunity to look at significant gaps in our present abilities, assess future needs, and give a chance for a redemptive future. Farzad Mostashari, past head of the Office of the National Coordinator (ONC) for Health Information Technology, has said that understanding technology is recognizing technology is not "auto magic"; implementation of technology does not instantly increase the quality of care (Porter, 2013, p. 388). It has been said that creating technology to preserve the same old way of doing things is not a path to efficiency but instead paving a well-worn inefficient cow path into technology cement. The pandemic has shown a bright light on the old way, perhaps opening an opportunity for APRNs in the future.

MAKING SENSE OF COMPLEXITY IN HEALTH INFORMATION TECHNOLOGY

For this chapter's discussions, we use two models to understand health information technology (HIT) systems. Multiple models help demystify complexity and technology. These models offer a foundational understanding and a starting point. While applying the models to technology may be new, the models' generalizability to the many different settings where APRNs practice is starkly apparent. Moreover, using a scientific and evidence-based approach, APRN core competencies, keeping the patient in the center, and applying systems knowledge are critical to any present or future technology. Assessing technology is within the skills of the APRN, whether considering an existing technology system or problem or the purchase of new technology by using the tools of nursing.

The Donabedian Model

Avedis Donabedian is often referred to as the father of healthcare quality and is responsible for one of the most widely used models for quality assessment (Donabedian, 1988). His contribution to the healthcare community was to simplify complex systems interactions by using his straightforward equation. His classic and simple model of structure (the environment) and process (the actions) equaling outcomes (the product of structure and process) can be applied easily to technology. While health care is immensely complex, his model has persisted through challenges over the decades and across patient care to organizational systems.

Although Donabedian did not live to see the technology-enabled healthcare environment or use the technology we do today, he predicted and described the perils of technology (Donabedian, 1988). He encouraged us to look at the quality of technology in its judicious and appropriate use and the extent it is used skillfully to improve the health of individuals and communities. Donabedian reminded us that technology assessment is a tool and is limited in how it assists the delivery of care (Donabedian, 1988). Using the Donabedian model to assess the interactions within the care process offers insight into the impact of technology as a tool for assisting patient care (Table 22.1).

James Reason Swiss Cheese Model

The James Reason Swiss cheese model (SCM) of system safety errors is applicable to high-risk industries such as nuclear energy, aviation, and health care (Perneger, 2005; Reason, 2000). Understanding health care from a systems approach, such as Reason's model, is essential to deconstruct and visualize the multilayered complexity of the healthcare system (Reason, 2016). Healthcare technology and information systems are a part of the massive network of care. Information may come from other hospitals with different electronic health records (EHRs), from a referring clinician through an EHR portal or a wearable data point on the patient. The data pass through servers and departments to the bedside silently, electronic records quietly archive vital data, and pharmacy systems dispense magnitudes of drugs without signals of distress. Most failures in these networks are silent and difficult to detect. The holes in the "Swiss cheese" technology systems are not readily apparent until the error reaches the patient. The SCM reminds us that there are layers of protection against errors in a system, including people, processes, and the environment in a dynamic state. Deconstructing the system into layers allows for a deeper look into causal factors and a hope for mitigating risk earlier in the trajectory before the error occurs.

James Reason's work with SCM was grounded in his understanding of the condition of fallibility. It is the combination of human fallibility and layers of defense that gives a sharper view of the role of technology in safety. Reason described accidents as having organizational characteristics of culture and layers that contribute to "catastrophic organisational accidents" (Reason, 2004, p. ii28), defying the layers of defense in place (Reason, 2004, 2016). The energy and transportation industries have relatively stable processes, whereas health care has a unique variation and randomness inherent in patients and conditions. Health care is highly technology-dependent, bound to human fallibility, and victim to the ambiguities and variation in human health. Accepting fallibility is key to understanding technology. If we learn from the past, other industries, and experiences, we begin to understand, acknowledge, and predict failures.

In 1999, the Institute of Medicine (IOM) Committee on Quality of Health Care in America released the report *To Err Is Human: Building a Safer Health System.* Based on 1984 data developed from reviews of medical records of patients treated in New York hospitals, the IOM estimated that up to 98,000 Americans die each year from medical errors (Hayward & Hofer, 2001; IOM, 1999; James, 2013; McDonald et al., 2000). The IOM report called for technology systems to address the medication errors that were a frequent cause of preventable harm, including EHRs, computerized order entry, and clinical decision support (CDS). Whether the technology has impacted the safety of patients in

TABLE 22.1

Examples of Care Processes Aligned With the Donabedian Model

Structure (Environment)	Process (How We Do It)	Outcome (Care Quality)
Admissions documentation in electronic health record (EHR)	Enter information into the EHR	Patient's correct information is readily accessible
Discharge documentation in EHR	Enter the discharge assessment while in the presence of the patient	Patient assessment at discharge is archived for later use
Home oxygen saturation monitoring	Place the sensor on the patient correctly	Oxygen saturation is correctly monitored

the United States is as controversial as the initial IOM report. Numerous attempts to quantify errors with technology implications have been made, but consensus remains elusive. Some experts believe that safety improvement has not been demonstrated (Chassin & Loeb, 2013; Singh & Sittig, 2015). Thus it is not surprising that HIT systems, therapeutic technology applications, and technology-based communication systems create a significant opportunity for error in a complex care environment (Perrow, 2011).

HUMAN-CENTERED DESIGN

The APRN must view technology within its full systems scope, complexity, and interconnected nature while not forgetting the human design needs of the user. Technology applications in health care involve software and hardware and the human social systems supporting the technology applications. The intentions of technology can be disrupted at any level of a system of care, whether that be training, the user, the interface design, the hardware support, or the organization's maintenance of the technology. In any role of the APRN, these organizational decisions about technology implementation and governance influence the quality of care providers can deliver and are relevant questions to ask whenever relying on technology. As evidence-based practitioners and systems thinkers, APRNs offer a unique view to assessing technology in health care.

Human-centered design includes an understanding and assessment of the interfaces between technology and humans and the processes in the technology and incorporates the cognitive aspects necessary for performance. The complexity of health care cannot be overstated. Staggers et al. (2018) researched health IT problems and found that vendors do not yet understand how to support nurses' work, critical thinking, and decision making. Workflow interruptions, delays, and prolonged searching activities have been identified in observational and anecdotal accounts, pointing toward the need for informed usability and human-centered technology design (Nolan et al., 2017). In a literature review, Carayon and Hoonakker (2019) reported significant problems in usability and human factors in design impacting patient safety and workplace quality. The difficulties span the entire scope of healthcare delivery.

Recommendations from standard settings agencies are consistent in prescribing human-centered design and formal usability testing (Lowry et al., 2015; Nolan et al., 2017). Researchers in human-centered design have suggested standardized testing requirements. Substantiated evidence supports that technology improvements would increase safety and satisfaction in using technology for providers and patients (ECRI Institute, 2019; Howe et al., 2018; Hunt et al., 1998; IOM, 2003, 2012; Staggers et al., 2018; Zhang & Walji, 2011). While significant federal funding has been spent to discover best practices, enforcement is still absent, and reporting technology-related errors is voluntary.

Organizations may lack expertise in current research in technology safety, informatics, data science, and human design factors. Data standards, data dictionaries, and regular data quality checks are necessary for data integrity in an organization's technology responsibilities (HealthIT.gov, 2018a). For some, there is never a consideration of the impact of technology on intertwined systems of care. It is easy to negate the influence of mitigatable factors in the face of unintended consequences and fall back to blaming singular causes, most likely the person involved (Reason, 2004). Exemplar 22.1 provides examples of common data entry errors and recommendations for how to avoid them.

There is a larger dynamic in technology systems, the change of systems over time. The changing of data in dynamic environments and in data streaming models and the large amounts of data moving through algorithms in health care should be anticipated and monitored. These changes are impactful to care delivery and an integral element to the ability of the practitioner to practice safely. It requires a strategic quality monitoring system to control the untoward drift of technology over time or detect untoward changes.

Human factors, workflow analysis, qualitative interviewing, Ishikawa diagrams, root cause analysis, and failure modes and effects analyses apply to systematic technology examinations and can be integrated into health care. Other industries with equal complexity to health care use tools for understanding problems and events that include a larger view of the system. Human factors tools have reliably informed complex systems and created safer technology in

EXEMPLAR 22.1
EXAMPLES OF DATA ENTRY ERRORS FROM THE JOINT COMMISSION'S SAFE USE OF HEALTH INFORMATION TECHNOLOGY, SENTINEL EVENT ALERT 54

The Joint Commission issued Sentinel Event Alert 54 (2015) to highlight the risk of incorrect data entry. Cited examples of data entry errors obtained from the Emergency Care Research Institute (ECRI) include (p. 1):

A chest x-ray was ordered for the wrong patient when the wrong patient room number was accidentally clicked. The orderer noticed the error right away and promptly discontinued the order but not in time for the x-ray technician to see that the order was withdrawn. The technician performed the test on the wrong patient.

A drug was ordered as an intramuscular injection when it was supposed to be administered intravenously. The physician did not choose the appropriate delivery route from the drop-down menu.

A nurse noted that a patient had a new order for acetaminophen. After speaking with the pharmacist, the nurse determined that the order was placed for the wrong patient. The pharmacist had two patient records open, was interrupted, and subsequently entered the order for the wrong patient.

Factors found in reported events include (p. 2):

1. Human–computer interface (33%) ergonomics and usability issues resulting in data-related errors
2. Workflow and communication (24%): issues relating to health IT support of communication and teamwork
3. Clinical content (23%): design or data issues relating to clinical content or decision support
4. Internal organizational policies, procedures, and culture (6%)
5. People (6%): training and failure to follow established processes
6. Hardware and software (6%) design issues and other hardware/software problems
7. External factors (1%): vendor and other external issues
8. System measurement and monitoring (1%)

Recommendations for safer use include developing proactive risk assessments and using the sociotechnical model to assess factors that may lead to adverse events (Sittig & Singh, 2010). Tools such as workflow modeling, failure modes and effects analysis, and the SAFER Guides can assist organizations in developing safer technology use.

From The Joint Commission (2015): https://www.jointcommission.org/-/media/tjc/documents/resources/patient-safety-topics/sentinel-event/sea_54_hit_4_26_16.pdf

other industries such as airlines and nuclear reactors. It is not unexpected that increases in healthcare technology will require applying the same quality monitoring, tools, and culture seen in other high-risk industries.

The *Safety Assurance Factors for EHR Resilience (SAFER) Guides* consist of nine self-assessment guides and recommended practices designed to help healthcare organizations assess and optimize the safety and safe use of EHRs (American Hospital Association, 2014) (Box 22.1).

Produced by The ONC in 2014 and updated in 2017, the *SAFER Guides* combine evidence-based guidelines with practical advice for using health information technology more safely (HealthIT.gov, 2018b). The guides were designed to assess an organization's conformance to recommended practices by completing a series of self-assessment checklists (HealthIT.gov, 2018b).

BOX 22.1
The SAFER Guides

Foundational Guides
- High Priority Practices
- Organizational Responsibilities

Infrastructure Guides
- Contingency Planning
- System Configuration
- System Interfaces

Clinical Process Guides
- Patient Identification
- Computerized Provider Order Entry With Decision Support
- Test Result Reporting and Follow-Up
- Clinician Communication

The SAFER Guides are available at www.healthit.gov/policy-researchers-implementers/safer

Technology is attractive in its promise; however, we are beginning to understand how it impacts health care and nursing practice. Whether the technology is a high-fidelity simulator, an electronic record, or a smartphone, APRNs have a reason to look at technology critically and systematically. Unfortunately, the direction of technology doesn't always include the largest group of healthcare providers in the United States: nurses (Brennan & Bakken, 2015). For this reason alone, nurses need to engage in technology assessment, implementation, and design. APRNs can become role models and lead those efforts, which begins with a basic understanding of health information technology in its varied forms, from technology-assisted communication to health-related devices and apps.

TECHNOLOGY-ASSISTED COMMUNICATION

Information and communication technologies in health care include all digital technologies that support the electronic capture, storage, processing, and exchange of information to promote health, prevent illness, treat disease, and manage chronic illness (Rouleau et al., 2017). These technologies enable patient-centered health care at a lower cost, a higher quality of care and information sharing, fewer medical errors, and increased efficiency and a new form of relationship between patients and their healthcare providers. As a result, APRNs are well positioned to leverage digital communication technologies in their practice to benefit themselves and their patients.

Technology increasingly supports the APRN core competencies of direct clinical practice, guidance and coaching, evidence-based practice, leadership, collaboration, and ethical practice. In each of these roles, APRNs frequently lead as communication director and care coordinator for patients and interprofessional teams in settings as diverse as critical care to home care. This demands a diverse technology skill set to ensure the delivery of optimal care (The Journal of MHealth, 2019).

Coordination of patient care and the quality of its delivery depend on accurate, timely, and detailed communication among all members of the patient's care team, including the patient. In today's healthcare era, technology plays an increasing role in communication in the form of written, verbal, nonverbal, and visual technologies that hold the potential to transform how APRNs communicate.

Written Communication Technologies

Thorough documentation demonstrates APRN knowledge and judgment skills and establishes professional accountability. It also serves as a legal document that verifies the APRN delivered care according to industry standards, state regulations, and an institution's policies.

Electronic records were developed to standardize documentation, improve accessibility, reduce errors, improve efficiency, improve privacy and security, and facilitate long-term storage and retrieval of medical records (Androus, 2020). With electronic records came several digital communication technologies that play an essential role in APRN documentation and written communication.

Electronic medical records (EMRs) are digital versions of the paper chart providers use for diagnosis and treatment. They are episodic and organized by specific medical encounters to facilitate medical record management and billing (Garrett & Seidman, 2011).

Electronic health records (EHRs), in contrast to EMRs, are longitudinal, holistic, and consider the body, mind, and spirit over time, across providers, and between institutions (Garrett & Seidman, 2011). The defining characteristic of an EHR is its design, allowing data collection and retrieval across multiple healthcare encounters, inpatient and outpatient, by numerous providers, prompting the adages womb to tomb and cradle to grave medical records.

Patient portals are secure websites that allow patients access to their personal health information anytime, anywhere there is an Internet connection (HealthIT.gov, 2017b). They are often integrated into a provider's EHR and share medication lists, test results, visit summaries, appointment reminders, and secure messaging with providers on the portal's network. In addition, some patient portals allow patients to schedule appointments, pay bills, and enter data through the portal to their EHR.

Personal health records (PHRs) are designed to be set up, accessed, and managed by patients (or their authorized representative), enabling them to maintain their health information in a safe, private, and secure digital environment. Like an EHR, the PHR contains health information such as diagnoses, medications, allergies, immunizations, family medical histories, and provider contact information. The PHR can accept data and information from various sources, including providers, home medical devices, and patients themselves (HealthIT.gov, 2019). A PHR can be a lifesaver in an emergency since it makes health information accessible to authorized users anytime via web-enabled devices such as smartphones and tablets. The key to a PHR is that it is maintained by the patient and is only as good as their ability to keep it up to date consistently.

Patient-generated health data (PGHD) is defined by the ONC as "health-related data created, recorded, or gathered by or from patients (or family members or other caregivers) to help address a health concern" (HealthIT.gov, 2018a, §2). To promote PGHD, the ONC included it in the 2015 Edition Health Information Technology Certification Rule. The rule states that to be an ONC-certified EHR, the EHR must provide at least one means for accepting patient health information directly and electronically from the patient in the most flexible way (HealthIT.gov, 2017a). For example, PGHD can be text, readings from medical devices, or anything that the patient or their authorized representative wants to include in their health record. Giving patients the ability to add their data to the health record has many benefits to APRNs, including insight into the patient's condition and activities between healthcare visits, monitoring or discovering opportunities for prevention and chronic care management, gathering information about medications and reactions, and obtaining valuable data for analysis to improve care and promote patient engagement.

Fax (short for facsimile) is the telephonic transmission of scanned printed material, usually to a telephone number associated with a printer or other output device. Although still prevalent in hospitals and clinics today, traditional fax machines pose significant security threats, especially when sending protected health information (PHI). In conventional fax, data are not encrypted. Fax output baskets are often unmonitored, and the fax can sit in the basket exposed to unintended view for extended periods. A fax with PHI can also be sent to the wrong number. Unauthorized document access and misdirected PHI are considered impermissible disclosures under the Health Insurance Portability and Accountability Act (HIPAA) privacy rules and should be treated as a privacy breach until proven otherwise (Serrano, 2020). Faxes can be sent securely by using a HIPAA-compliant solution. Online fax, cloud fax, and eFax products use the Internet and Internet protocols to securely send a HIPAA-compliant fax, mitigating the risk associated with the use of a standard fax machine or telephone connection (Total HIPAA, 2020).

Secure text messaging apps permit texting within a secure, encrypted network with access and audit controls that satisfy HIPAA requirements. This technology far exceeds the standard security offered by non-HIPAA-compliant solutions (e.g., personal phone). Secure texts are archived on a private cloud and logically separated from other data. Covered entities can apply role-based permissions and messaging policies and remotely retract or delete text messages if a device is lost or stolen, extract audit reports, and PIN-lock apps installed on mobile devices. The latest version of HIPAA-compliant messaging apps enables voice and video calls and remote group collaboration and facilitates sharing images and files with authorized users. When the app is integrated with an EHR, patient information can be securely sent directly from the app to the EHR. HIPAA-compliant texting is an efficient and safe way for APRNs to communicate with their teams and patients (HIPAA Journal, n.d.). Never text PHI over an unsecured network or with an unsecured device.

The growing amount of written data collected and stored in electronic records includes many unstructured free-text, structured and unstructured electronic data, and scanned paper-based records. The need to capture these data and transform them into a machine-readable format that can be used for patient care, research, and decision support has prompted the development of a range of purposeful technologies designed for text transformation. These include technologies for recognition of machine-printed text (OCR), hand-printed text (ICR), optical marks (OMR), and barcodes (OBR) (Box 22.2).

BOX 22.2

Text Recognition Technology

Optical character recognition (OCR) finds and extracts document-based, machine-printed data, without providing any intelligence (i.e., no context or meaning; Rowe, 2017).

Intelligent character recognition (ICR) is used to convert hand-printed characters to machine print, made possible by ICR's ability to identify variations in character shape. Advanced ICR software can recognize unstructured handprint and even cursive writing. ICR software also provides context, mimicking the human action of interpreting words by their overall context within the sentence. ICR does this by using dictionaries that contain possible field values consistent with the word's context within the script (Rowe, 2017).

Optical mark recognition (OMR) is used to collect data from "fill-in-the-bubble" types of forms, such as tests, surveys, ballots, evaluations, and other forms (Remark, n.d.).

Optical barcode readers (OBR) are devices that read and convert coded information in the form of printed images and text into digital data that can be edited, transmitted, and stored. The two most common images decoded by OBR are barcode and quick-response (QR) codes (Marder, 2017). Barcodes are used extensively in hospitals to manage supplies and inventory and in closed-loop medication processes.

Artificial intelligence (AI) and machine learning (ML) power are the most advanced data recognition and interpretation technologies used today. Primary data recognition results are combined, and alternate choices are considered to provide the best possible results (Rowe, 2017). AI provides pattern recognition and then uses ML and cognitive technology to identify and categorize unstructured data into classifications. ML can interpret unstructured data in any of its forms (e.g., text, images, video, quantitative data, anything that AI recognized). This pattern recognition and interpretation enable machines to mimic the human brain, identifying what we perceive in the real world (Schmelzer, 2020).

Verbal Communication Technologies

Verbal communication depends on words to deliver meaning and is an essential component of most interactions. It can be done face-to-face or remotely over various communication devices and is a vital part of nursing practice. Because health care is becoming increasingly specialized, care teams have grown larger, making interprofessional collaboration more important than ever (TigerConnect, 2019).

Hospitals typically employ four times more nurses than physicians, putting them at the forefront of team communication (TigerConnect, 2018). Indeed, APRNs are often the conduit between the patient and other caregivers, trying to convey and clarify what each has to say in terms that are understandable to all. Verbal communication has been aided by a variety of smart devices, many of which incorporate advanced technologies such as artificial intelligence (AI), machine learning (ML), and natural language processing (NLP) that can significantly benefit the APRN.

Artificial intelligence (AI) leverages computers and machines to mimic the decision-making and problem-solving capabilities of the human mind. It is a field that combines computer science and robust data sets to enable problem solving (IBM, 2020). AI is an umbrella term that includes multiple advanced technologies such as NLP for processing unstructured data and ML methods for processing structured data (Jiang et al., 2017). With the increasing availability of healthcare data and evolving big data analytics methods, the successful application of AI in health care has become a reality.

Machine learning (ML) is a form of AI based on the theory that systems can change actions and responses as they are exposed to more data; they can learn. ML is often categorized as supervised or unsupervised. Supervised ML involves software inferring functions from known inputs to known outputs. Unsupervised ML works with inputs only, independently transforming or finding patterns in the data without an expected or known output. ML is a method of teaching computers to adapt to changes in data (Paskin, 2018).

Natural language processing (NLP) is a field of AI that enables machines to read, understand, and derive meaning from unstructured human language. Unstructured data such as script, voice, graphics, and images do not fit neatly into the rows and columns of a traditional relational database. Yet these data represent most of the data available in the world. NLP and ML can understand the meaning and context of data in its varied forms and even detect figures of speech like irony or perform sentiment analysis (Yse, 2019).

Automated speech recognition (ASR) technology enables digital devices to listen and respond to human speech. Combining AI, ML, and NLP, ASR can now understand, interpret, and generate human speech to perform tasks such as transcription, translation, summarization, topic segmentation, and more, far exceeding traditional dictation (Sinhasane, 2020). ASR eases the burden of documentation, freeing up time to spend on face-to-face, personalized patient care. For example, an APRN could use ASR to update an EHR or complete a discharge summary by simply speaking, gaining back valuable time. Patients are also benefiting from voice recognition using smart ASR-enabled devices in their homes.

Virtual assistants (VA), also known as *digital assistants*, are advanced computer programs that simulate human conversation. In short, they allow humans to interact with machines. Using AI, ML, and NLP to learn as they go, they provide a personalized conversational experience. VAs collect and analyze data as the user interacts with the technology, allowing algorithms to create personalized data models that identify the user's behavior patterns and refine those patterns as more data about the user's preferences are added. By learning a user's history, preferences, and other characteristics and information, the VA can provide personalized recommendations, answer complex questions, make predictions, and even initiate conversations (Oracle, n.d.).

A less-advanced form of a VA is a chatbot. Chatbots are frequently used today in customer-facing interactions in written and verbal form; for example, the automated "drill down" questions you encounter when calling customer support or ordering something on the phone. It can understand your voice as a VA can, but its responses are rule-based or predetermined (Expert.ai, 2020). If an APRN wants to know the protocol for a specific intervention, a chatbot can assist. But if they want to know the protocol for a particular intervention for a patient of a certain age, body mass index, taking specific medications, and with specific comorbidities, then the advanced technology of a VA would be required.

VAs and chatbots are making their way into hospitals and homes and have many uses in health care. Patients can use chatbots in smart patient rooms to order meals and triage patient requests to the right person for the task. Patients can use a VA at home to remind them to take their medications, monitor compliance, and keep track of medication refills. The future for VAs for nurses and patients is bright, and its potential benefits should always be considered when APRNs are preparing a patient for discharge.

Smartphone and ***cellphone*** are terms that are often used interchangeably, but they are different devices. A cellphone is a digital device that can send and receive phone calls and text messages. A smartphone can do this and more (Fendelman, 2020). The smartphone can be considered a minicomputer, with functionality limited by its operating system, the software that runs its interface, the owner's phone, and the apps that the owner has chosen to run on the phone. Thousands of healthcare and other apps are available for APRNs and patients to enhance efficiency, safety, knowledge, overall health, and well-being. According to a 2019 survey by the Pew Research Center, 81% of Americans own a smartphone, making it a logical delivery mechanism for healthcare apps. As part of patient assessment and during discharge planning, the APRN should assess and document if the patient owns a smartphone and, if so, what model and year. That will inform the APRN about options the patient may have for useful mHealth (mobile health care) apps. As smartphones age, they may not be able to handle some new apps or be unable to accept updates for existing apps (Resnick, 2019). If the APRN follows data from a patient's app on a smartphone, characteristics such as the phone's age and operating system become essential parameters in care.

Nonverbal Communication Technologies

Nonverbal communication occurs when messages and meanings are sent or received without the use of words. Nonverbal communication is conveyed through facial expressions, body language, eye contact, hand gestures, touch, posture, and even appearance (Albuquerque Speech Language Hearing Center, 2016). It is estimated that 70% of all language is nonverbal (Orsini, 2018) and can be intentional or unintentional. It can also dramatically differ in meaning across cultures. For example, a hand gesture in one country may have a different meaning in another. Likewise, direct eye contact is another nonverbal cue that is acceptable in one culture and not another.

Nonverbal communication can present unique challenges for APRNs using telecommunication for care or consultation. Something as simple as your attire or the appearance of your setting during the telehealth encounter can send a message to the patient or colleague about how seriously you are taking the encounter. Orsini (2018) gave the following suggestions for how APRNs can continue to build a professional, trusting, and compassionate relationship with their patients during remote communication.

Give the patient your undivided attention. Maintain eye contact, limit notetaking, and be aware of your facial expression and body language.

Remember that the interaction is a conversation, not an interview. Don't interrupt, and hold follow-up questions until the patient has stopped speaking. Even though you are not in the same room, the patient should feel like they are the most important person to you at that moment.

Be a genuine person and relate to the patient on a personal level. Avoid the "all business" attitude by interjecting some casual talk at the beginning of the interaction.

Being aware of your patient's body language during a telehealth session is critical, as there may be disparities between what they say and what you observe. For example, the patient may say that they are fine but their facial expression or the way they move may say something else. Body language is only one source of information upon which to base a decision, but it is crucial. Reading a patient's body language can be as important as observing clinical symptoms during a telehealth session (Ali, 2018).

Developing telepresence skills, making two people in different locations feel like they are together, is essential for the modern APRN, as telehealth and telemedicine will remain in some form. Recording telehealth sessions and then reflectively reviewing them can be an effective way to assess, learn about, and improve your nonverbal and telepresence skills.

Visual Communication Technologies

Visualizing health data is a powerful way to communicate information quickly and effectively. Health data visualization methods can condense complex data into easy-to-understand presentation formats, including charts, graphs, tables, timelines, presentation slides, infographics, and dashboards. Pictorial representations of data offer many options, and the specific choice is usually based on the type of data and the intended audience (University of Illinois Chicago Online Health Informatics, 2020). Beginning with Florence Nightingale and her Coxcomb diagram, nurses have long turned to data to drive critical decisions and have used data visualization tools to communicate their message. As a result, using data visualization tools is becoming another essential technical skill for all APRN roles.

Visual communication techniques can aid APRNs in communicating with patients whose health literacy is low. The Health Resources and Services Administration (HRSA) defines health literacy as "the degree to which individuals can obtain, process, and understand basic health information needed to make appropriate health decisions" (HRSA, 2019, para. 1). There are many reasons for low health literacy, including low education skills, cultural barriers, limited English language proficiency (LEP), and words that healthcare providers use that patients simply do not understand (HRSA, 2019). Nurses who use visual aids like pictures, diagrams, 3D models, infographics, and international healthcare symbols can bridge gaps in understanding for all patient populations.

Social Media as a Communication Tool

Social media is any digital platform that connects and engages others for sharing information, thoughts, and ideas. When used responsibly, social media can be a very effective and efficient way for APRNs to collaborate with peers, coordinate care with a team, engage with and educate others, and meet people who can help them attain personal and professional goals (Leary & Charles, 2021). Nurses use social networking sites, blogs, online chat rooms, forums, and video sites to communicate with others in their personal and professional lives (The National Council of State Boards of Nursing [NCSBN], 2018).

While social media holds great promise for APRN communication, it can result in a breach of patient or institutional privacy, damage to reputation, and even involvement in litigation if not used responsibly. For that reason, many nursing organizations have written guidelines and best practices for nurses using social media (Leary & Charles, 2021).

The American Nurses Association (ANA) has created a set of principles for nurses that allows them to get the most out of using social media while protecting themselves, their patients, and their profession (ANA, n.d.) (Box 22.3). The ANA has also provided helpful social media tips for those new to social media or new to using social media as a nurse (ANA, n.d.) (Box 22.4).

Over 3.8 billion people worldwide use social media, making it a valuable communication medium for APRNs to amplify their voices, make connections, and educate the public (Leary & Charles, 2021). However, it can just as quickly ruin a reputation and cast a negative light on the nursing profession or the APRN. Therefore before you blog, tweet, or share information, take a moment to reflect on your intentions and possible consequences. Likewise, liking someone's unprofessional comments is just as serious as writing them yourself (International Nurse Regulator Collaborative, 2017).

According to the NCSBN (2018) in their brochure, *A Nurse's Guide to the Use of Social Media,* potential consequences of inappropriate use of social and electronic media may result in an investigation on the grounds of:

- unprofessional conduct
- unethical conduct
- moral turpitude (defined as conduct that is considered contrary to community standards of justice, honesty, or good morals)
- mismanagement of patient records
- revealing a privileged communication
- breach of confidentiality.

If allegations are found to be accurate, the nurse could face disciplinary action by their state board of nursing, including reprimand or sanction, assessment of a fine, or temporary or permanent loss of license. To assist nurses with self-checking before posting content on social media, the International Nurse Regulator Collaborative (2017) published the six Ps of Social Media Use (Box 22.5).

The explosion of technology-assisted communication in its various forms has added to the wealth of data available to APRNs for care delivery, research, and defining through documented evidence what and how they contribute to health care. Exemplar 22.2 provides a view into the everyday use of technology-enabled communication by APRNS. While technology and actionable data are essential to nursing's aims, they cannot be allowed to overtake the rich "story" of nursing care (Siegler, 2010). Nursing communication is most effective when data and the nurse's narrative are balanced and inform and support each other.

BOX 22.3

American Nurses Association Principles of Social Networking

Nurses must not transmit or place online individually identifiable patient information.

Nurses must observe ethically prescribed professional patient-nurse boundaries.

Nurses should understand that patients, colleagues, organizations, and employers may view postings.

Nurses should take advantage of privacy settings and seek to separate personal and professional information online.

Nurses should bring content that could harm a patient's privacy, right, or welfare to the attention of appropriate authorities.

Nurses should participate in developing organizational policies governing conduct. (https://www.nursingworld.org/social/)

BOX 22.4

American Nurses Association Social Media Tips

Remember that standards of professionalism are the same online as in any other circumstance.

Do not share or post information or photos gained through the nurse-patient relationship.

Maintain professional boundaries in the use of electronic media. Online contact with patients blurs this boundary.

Do not make disparaging remarks about patients, employers, or co-workers, even if they are not identified.

Do not take photos or videos of patients on personal devices, including cell phones.

Promptly report a breach of confidentiality or privacy. (https://www.nursingworld.org/social/)

BOX 22.5

International Nurse Regulator Collaborative 6 "P"s of Social Media

Professional—Act professionally at all times
Positive—Keep post positive
Patient/Person-free—Keep posts patient or person free
Protect yourself—Protect your professionalism, your reputation, and yourself
Privacy—Keep your personal and professional life separate; respect the privacy of others
Pause before you post—Consider implications; avoid posting in haste or anger

DIAGNOSTIC, THERAPEUTIC, AND PROCEDURAL DEVICES AND APPS

Diagnostic and Therapeutic Devices and Apps

mHealth, or mobile health care, using diagnostic, therapeutic, and procedural devices and apps is here to stay. In 2018, 75% of US consumers surveyed said that technology in some form is essential to managing their health. Consumers are increasingly willing to let intelligent devices and applications support some aspects of their care, and the use of self-service digital health tools is growing every year (Resnick, 2019).

While mHealth devices and apps are accepted and used by APRNs and patients, it can be challenging to identify what is safe to use and what is not. There are thousands of devices and apps available, and most are unregulated. Many do not live up to their claims and are short-lived. Ferretti et al. (2019) noted,

> *In most countries, medical device regulation applies only to a subset of high-risk health apps that have well-defined medical purposes. However, most health apps available on the market target a wide range of health-related issues, including diet and exercise, pregnancy, and mental health, while still being considered nonmedical devices. (p. e55)*

The United States is one such country, with only a subset of devices and apps regulated by the US Food and Drug Administration (FDA). While there are no clear guidelines for how an APRN or patient should decide

EXEMPLAR 22.2
TECHNOLOGY-ENABLING COMMUNICATION

APRN PRACTICE	ENABLING TECHNOLOGY
Morgan Gomez, MS, RN, ACNP-BC, starting her day in 2025	Voice recognition
7:00 am—After dropping the kids off at school, Morgan asks the Aly car app to connect to the patient care portal for the cancer center. As she drives to Meyerland Hospital, she hears her surgery and clinic schedules over a secure channel. The navigation system in her car notifies her of a traffic incident and plots a new course to the hospital.	Virtual assistant Secure portal Mobile app Global Positioning System Mobile security
7:45 am—Walking through the hospital doors, Morgan's phone communicates her location to the central scheduling office, where the building's visual 3D avatar tracks all employees, visitors, and patients at all times. The building's SMART system can locate and sequester any area in the hospital deemed a threat. This security layer allows the building to be secured for any danger (e.g., fire, weather, infection, or physical hazards). Theft of valuables, patient elopement, security threats, and other dangers have been reduced to near-zero levels.	Artificial intelligence Geofencing Real-time location system Artificial intelligence Machine learning Wireless radio frequency sensing devices
Morgan notices that the patients and families coming in are being screened for temperature, respiratory rate, skin moisture, and heart rate as they pass through the doorway. In addition, sensors scan for any cybersecurity issues, weapons, or other harmful devices. Anyone with irregularities is asked to have additional screening at the front door.	Decision support system Artificial intelligence Predictive analytics

about the safety and efficacy of a mHealth device or app, it is wise to follow hospital guidelines where possible. Devices that hospitals choose generally go through rigorous vetting by the purchasing department, usually in concert with an interprofessional product selection committee. When considering commercial consumer devices, always read product reviews and look for peer-reviewed studies. Other great resources are a nurse informaticist and the biomedical engineering and monitoring departments. For mHealth apps, look for opportunities to use those sponsored by your hospital or clinic. In addition, many facilities have a list of health apps that have been vetted by the IT department's security team and are compatible with the EHR.

mHealth medical devices and apps run the gamut from high-tech to basic and are a staple in the modern APRN's practice. Keeping up to date on the development of new technology and new uses for old technology is one of the responsibilities of the APRN. Some of the most promising mHealth technologies are presented here.

Virtual health care is an umbrella term that refers to the use of technology, including video, telephone, mobile apps, text messaging, and other communication platforms, to deliver health services to a patient outside of a health system (TigerConnect, n.d.b). The use of virtual health technologies exploded during the COVID-19 pandemic, as healthcare providers sought to remain in contact with their patients safely. As many as 20% of all medical visits in 2020 were by some form of virtual health. Such virtual care can fall into four models spanning the gamut of healthcare needs: virtual well-being, connected health, virtual health, and virtual medicine (Schrimpf et al., n.d.).

Virtual well-being is the use of digital technology to promote health and fitness and areas of prevention, remediation, and treatment of health conditions.

Connected health uses applications and devices to analyze and apply data to improve outcomes and ease communication between patients and providers.

Virtual health is the use of technologies to provide care. This can include direct clinical services such as remote patient monitoring and video consulting and nonclinical services such as professional training and collaboration among interprofessional teams.

Virtual medicine is the use of technology to provide person-to-person clinical health services via online person-to-person interfaces or over the phone.

Virtual health care is bidirectional, meaning provider to patient and patient to provider, and can be synchronous (happening in real-time) or asynchronous (data sharing and messaging; Schrimpf et al., n.d.). The benefits of virtual care are numerous for patients, providers, and health systems. Better access to care, better quality of care, convenience, managing chronic conditions, treating urgent symptoms, reducing cost, and promoting better self-care are just some of the benefits realized. The ability for APRNs to digitally connect with patients through voice, video, and text regardless of location can lead to healthier populations and better outcomes (TigerConnect, n.d.b). To be effective, the APRN must be diligent and self-aware and pay careful attention to build and retain the human component of the nurse–patient relationship in a digital world.

A ***universal image viewer*** is a single platform that can aggregate and support visualization of medical images in any format, both DICOM (digital communication standard) and non-DICOM, and imaging reports from any digital source. A universal viewer makes diverse images from diverse systems available anytime, anywhere, and to anyone authorized to view them. This eliminates the need to logon to separate digital radiology, cardiology, laboratory, ophthalmology, and wound care systems to access digital images (Tilmans, 2014). Advanced universal image viewers aggregate images in any format, from any connected departmental system, and make them available to authorized users via browsers or smartphones. Embedded tools allow caregivers to make precise measurements and annotate images as needed (GE Healthcare, n.d.). Many viewers can be integrated with an EHR for further efficiencies. Having all image-related data from all imaging systems in one place is a great time-saver for the APRN.

Point of care (POC) devices are used to obtain diagnostic results while with or near the patient. POC can be used to analyze blood, saliva, urine, stool, and skin cells. A sample is exposed to a medium intended to detect the presence of certain types of chemical markers or cells. The medium will react to the sample and show a visible result that indicates the presence or absence of the disease or condition that the test is performed to detect. Some common applications of POC device testing include blood glucose testing, cholesterol testing, electrolyte and enzyme analysis (present or absent), alcohol or drug testing, test for signs of infection, blood markers for cardiac conditions, fecal occult blood markers for colon cancer, and blood gas levels (Symbient, 2020).

There are many benefits to POC testing, such as portability, convenience, speed, and connectivity. Rapid test results can quickly help an APRN decide on a course of action or treatment, and the results from POC can be integrated with other healthcare applications and made available to others. Patients and caregivers can also use these devices in the home and transmit the results to authorized providers and health records.

Wearable technology ("wearables") is a category of electronic devices that can be worn as accessories, implanted in the body, embedded in clothing, and even tattooed on the skin. Wearables are hands-free devices with practical uses, powered by microprocessors, and are able to send and receive data over the Internet. This technology has been made possible by the growth in the Internet of Things (IoT), mobile networks, high-speed data transfer, and the miniaturization of microprocessors (Hayes, 2020).

Once seen as consumer gadgets, wearable technology today has blurred the lines between consumer gadget and medical device. Wearables allow APRNs and patients to partner as never before to monitor, analyze, and act upon parameters of health and well-being. APRNs can remotely monitor their patients' behaviors, such as activity, eating, and sleeping, and patients can be more active in their care by seeing the effects of their behaviors on their health in real time (Bove, 2019). There are wearable devices to monitor glucose, activity, vital signs, and sleep and to measure parameters of an electrocardiogram, electromyography, and electroencephalogram. Many of these devices can send their data to a patient's EHR portal or a PHR that can be shared with an APRN who is following their care. There are a growing number of intelligent devices equipped with predictive analytics capabilities, such as Intelligent Asthma Monitoring, which can forecast an oncoming asthma attack before the patient notices the oncoming symptoms. APRNs would be wise to stay abreast of developments in the health and wellness wearables market to recommend their use when opportunities present themselves.

Genetic and genomic research has shown a genetic component to diabetes, cancer, heart disease, and Alzheimer's disease, with new discoveries each year. The application of genetics and genomics has the potential to transform health care from one that focuses on curing disease to a preventive, diagnostic, genomic-based model that focuses on treating or preventing conditions that we know patients are likely to develop (Mohmmed et al., 2019). In its *State of the World's Nursing 2020* report, the World Health Organization (2020) stated, "Personalized medicine and genomics have the potential to better tailor patient care" (p. 73). The demands of this growing field have led to the creation of the *genetics nurse*, an RN, often with a master's degree or advanced practice nursing certification, who receives additional education and training in genetics. Genetics nurses care for patients who are affected by or at risk for diseases with a genetic component. They provide direct patient care, perform and analyze genetic risk assessments, educate patients and families on their risk for various genetic conditions, and counsel patients and families on how identified risks may impact their ongoing health and health management (International Society of Nurses in Genetics, n.d.).

A ***liquid biopsy*** is a blood test that looks for cancer cells from a tumor or pieces of DNA from tumor cells that circulate in the blood. This test can be used to find cancer at an early stage, plan for care, and determine how well treatments are working or if cancer has returned. Taking multiple samples over time can also illustrate what kind of molecular changes are taking place in a tumor (National Cancer Institute, n.d.). Liquid biopsies have many advantages over tissue biopsies. They are safer, quicker, and cheaper for patients and can be done repeatedly to track changes in the genetic profile of a tumor, a common occurrence when tumors develop resistance to treatment. A liquid biopsy can also be done when obtaining a tissue sample that is difficult or dangerous (Roberson, 2019). Liquid biopsies allow APRNs to target their therapy and counseling with patients and their families more precisely and open the door to precision medicine and nursing.

Global Pandemic Detection, using ML and AI, makes it possible to monitor known vectors of disease worldwide. An application called Bluedot scans over 100,000 media sources worldwide in over 65 languages daily to identify disease outbreaks in near real time. Bluedot was the first to publish an article predicting the worldwide spread of COVID-19. To predict the risk of disease becoming a pandemic, programs such as these can analyze the following threat vectors (Tsymbal, n.d.):

Global and regional climate conditions
Animal and insect populations
Flight and itinerary data worldwide
Health system capacity
Vaccine development

Procedural Devices and Apps

Dimensional (3D) printing is a process for making a physical object from a three-dimensional model by laying down many successive thin layers of materials specific to the intended application (3D Printing Industry, n.d.). 3D printing begins with computer-aided design (CAD) software used to design a three-dimensional model in precise terms. 3D printers require CAD software to provide the minute instructions needed to build a product, such as how much material is required and where it should be deposited (Monroe Engineering, 2020). Materials for 3D printing include plastics, metals, ceramics, paper, and biomaterials. Healthcare applications of 3D printing are extensive and growing, including orthopedic implants, personalized prosthetics, highly accurate 3D models to assist in presurgical planning, precision surgical instruments, dental implants, and a host of other uses (Additive Manufacturing, 2019). 3D printing holds great potential to meet the need for kinesthetic (hands-on) learning. With 3D printing, APRNs and APRN students can visualize anatomy and physiology concepts based on realistic or individualized structures rather than standard, static models. Rapid 3D prototypes can facilitate training for standard APRN procedures, simulating conditions, differences in tissues, and other anatomic differences without risk to a patient. Using 3D-enabled training could increase an APRN's or APRN student's confidence before performing a new procedure or entering a new clinical setting (Hatch & Shaw, 2019).

Robotics in health care has evolved alongside ML advancements, AI-enabled computer vision, data analytics, and other technologies. Robots come in many forms and can be used for many purposes in health care. A few examples are listed here (Alexander, 2020).

- **Robotic surgical assistants**, under the guidance of a surgeon, enable some minimally invasive operations to be performed with great precision through tiny incisions, resulting in less bleeding, faster healing, and a lower risk of infection.
- **Actuated and sensory prosthetics** have come a long way in the unification of humans and machines. For example, the Massachusetts Institute of Technology (MIT) has developed a gyroscopically actuated robotic limb that can track its position in three-dimensional space and adjust its joints up to 750 times per second. The robotic limb is covered in bionic skin and a neural implant system that interfaces with the nervous system to allow the user to receive tactile feedback and control the prosthesis at will just as they would their normal limb.
- **Orthoses (Exoskeletons)** help paralyzed people walk again and provide weak muscles the support they need to heal during rehabilitation following brain or spinal cord injury. Most exoskeletons work through a combination of preset movements and user input, but with advancements in neural interfaces, a directly mind-controlled exoskeleton may soon be available.
- **Capsule endoscopies** involve swallowing a pill-sized robot that travels through the digestive tract taking pictures and collecting data that is sent to a processor for diagnostic interpretation.
- **Targeted therapy microbots** deliver a drug or other therapy to a specific site within the body. Using near-microscopic mechanical particles, they can deliver radiation directly to a tumor.
- **Care assistant robots** are being used in hospitals to do many tasks such as taking vital signs, weighing patients, assisting patients with activities of daily living, retrieving equipment and supplies, delivering meal trays, and even helping patients in and out of beds and chairs.

Robotic process automation **(RPA)** is a technology that can create software robots, or "bots," that can mimic, learn, and execute rules-based business processes. RPA bots represent a digital workforce that can interact with an application or system just as a human worker would do. RPA bots can automate standard or repetitive business functions much faster and more accurately than humans. For example, bots can open and move files, parse email, make calculations, extract data, scrape web data, etc. (Automation Anywhere, n.d.). Bots can be used for good or harm. Several malicious bots can be threats to privacy and security and do great harm to people and businesses; thus most computer security software includes technologies to identify them.

The operational efficiencies and risk reductions that robots afford offer value in many areas of health care, including advanced practice nursing. As robotic technology evolves, it will function more autonomously, eventually performing specific tasks independently, freeing APRNs to provide the assessment, analysis, and care that only an APRN can provide (Intel, n.d.). Robots are here to assist the healthcare team, not replace it.

Vein visualization, also known as *vein illumination*, uses near-infrared (NIR) imaging technology to assist clinicians with finding the best vein for blood draws and IV starts. Using a handheld device, projected NIR light is absorbed by the blood and reflected by the surrounding tissue. Information is captured, processed, and digitally projected directly onto the skin surface, providing an image of the patient's blood pattern and allowing clinicians to see peripheral veins, bifurcations, and valves and assess the refill and flushing of veins in real-time (Emergency Medicine News, 2017).

Steth IO is a ***smartphone-based digital stethoscope*** with a stethoscope bell built directly into a smartphone's protective case, allowing the user to listen to and measure heart rates and lung sounds through an app while holding the phone to the patient's chest. APRNs can visualize the patient's heart and lung activity directly on the phone's screen while listening to the heart and breath sounds on any pair of headphones. Data can be recorded, organized by patient, annotated with notes, and exported or shared through the accompanying app. The device requires no Bluetooth pairing, batteries, or charging, as it draws power directly from the phone (Muoio, 2018).

SUPPORTIVE TECHNOLOGY

Companion robots have many applications that can benefit elderly, infirm, or mentally disabled people and those who suffer from chronic loneliness and lack of stimulation. These robots can do a range of functions from simply interacting with the patient and providing needed stimulus; helping with activities of daily living, such as reminding patients to take their medications; and sending monitoring data remotely to the healthcare team.

Smart bed technology can help APRNs track patient movement, weight, and vital signs. Data from the smart bed can provide regular updates and communications about a patient's activity, alerting the APRN to potential problems and saving them time that would have been spent on visually monitoring the patient and taking weights and vital signs. Advanced smart beds can remotely monitor in real time such things as safe side rail configuration for fall risk patients and Fowler-Philip angle for critical care patients. Real-time visibility can be monitored on any web-enabled device or a central console. Alerts can be directed to the APRN's smartphone if a patient's bed configuration is compromised (Tiger Connect, n.d.a).

Radiofrequency (RF)-based medical devices utilize wireless RF communication such as Bluetooth, Wi-Fi, and mobile/cellular phone to support healthcare delivery. Wireless technology can offer many benefits to patients and APRNs, including increased mobility, remote monitoring, programming of devices, and transferring data from a mobile device to another platform like a phone or another device. While wireless devices afford many benefits, they also carry risks. Without proper security, wireless devices can be breached, so keeping device security updated is paramount. They also share the airways with multiple other wireless devices that may interfere with a medical device causing data loss or disruption (US Food and Drug Administration, 2018b).

Radiofrequency identification (RFID) is a wireless system comprising two components: tags and readers. A reader is a device that emits radio waves and receives signals back from RFID tags. Tags use radio waves to communicate their identity and other information to nearby readers. RFID has multiple uses in health care, including asset tagging, equipment tracking, out-of-bed and fall detection, personnel tracking, and preventing the distribution of counterfeit drugs and medical devices. While there have been no reports of harm directly related to RFID, there is a potential hazard from electromagnetic interference to pacemakers, implantable cardioverter defibrillators, and other medical devices (US Food and Drug Administration,

2018a). The APRN should consider the impact on patients, warranting discussion about RFID safety when caring for patients with implantable devices.

A *real-time location system* (RTLS) uses tags and badges; wireless technology such as Wi-Fi, infrared, Bluetooth, and ultrasound; and readers to provide real-time tracking and management of assets, staff, and patients (CenTrak, n.d.). Users can typically log into the system to see location details as needed, reducing time spent looking for people and things. Some facilities are now tagging patients with RTLS-enabled wristbands that allow hospital workers to view their locations on an enterprise-wide digital map. While RTLS began in hospitals as a technology to track equipment and prevent theft and loss, use cases have grown to include staff and patient tracking in hospitals and outpatient clinics and managing operating room schedules, workflows, and availability and location of critical supplies. During the COVID-19 pandemic, some hospitals used RTLS for contact tracing of people and materials that came in contact with infected patients. RTLS collects a vast amount of data that can be analyzed to identify workflow and patient throughput, wait times, bottlenecks, and opportunities to improve the utilization of people and equipment (Lorenzi, 2020).

Geofencing is a location-based technology that uses the Global Positioning System (GPS), RFID, Wi-Fi, or cellular data to trigger an alert or action when a geo-enabled mobile device such as a smartphone enters or leaves the virtual boundary (geofence) set up around a geographic location (Croxton, 2021). Geofencing can be used in hospitals to identify when patients arrive for admission and push directions or instructions to their phones. Another application may notify a clinical trial manager when a subject enrolled in a clinical trial enters an emergency room. Recognition is triggered when a patient's cell phone crosses the geofence, announcing their arrival, location, and movement within the defined area.

Virtual reality (VR) is defined as "a medium composed of interactive computer simulations that sense the participant's position and replace or augment the feedback to one or more senses, giving the feeling of being immersed or being present in the simulation" (Craig, 2013, p. 22). The key to VR is that it is a complete immersion into an entirely synthetic world. APRN classrooms and simulation labs are increasingly using VR simulation training. Nurses find VR training effective and fun, leading them to spend more time practicing new skills (Lea, 2020). Patients also benefit from VR to simulate everything from going through the admission process to going into the operating room suite and being oriented virtually as part of preop teaching.

The National Academies of Sciences, Engineering, and Medicine (NASEM, 2021) states in *The Future of Nursing 2020–2030: Charting a Path to Achieve Health Equity*,

> *Simulation-based education is another useful tool for teaching nursing concepts and developing competencies and skills. It can range from very low-tech (e.g., using oranges to practice injections) to very high-tech (e.g., a virtual reality emergency room "game"), but all simulations share the ability to bridge the gap between education and practice by imparting skills in a low-risk environment. (p. 215)*

Augmented reality (AR) is an enhanced version of the real world that is achieved by introducing technology-enabled digital visual elements, sound, or other sensory stimuli (Hayes, 2020). You can still see the real world, but it is augmented with digital content that overlays it. An important aspect of AR is that you remain in the physical "real" world and there is no attempt to make you think otherwise. In AR, all of your senses work as normal (i.e., you can hear, smell, see, touch, and taste). The digital information is superimposed on, or added to, the physical world. AR has many uses in health care. For example, AR can be used to teach a patient crutch training before knee surgery. The stairs in the simulation are real, but the crutches that the patient is maneuvering are augmented reality.

Patients are more digitally savvy today, and they expect their APRN to use data they have collected on their smart and wearable devices. This requires that the APRN have a basic understanding of eHealth technology, as illustrated in Exemplars 22.3 and 22.4. In the American Association of Colleges of Nursing (AACN, 2021), *The Essentials: Core Competencies for Professional Nursing Education*, they state:

> *Informatics has increasingly been a focus in nursing education, correlating with the advancement in sophistication and reach of information technologies; the use of technology to support healthcare processes*

EXEMPLAR 22.3
TECHNOLOGY SUPPORTING APRN PRACTICE

APRN PRACTICE	SUPPORTING TECHNOLOGY
Kylie Bruno MS, RN, PCNS-BC, starts her day at home in her home office in Rhode Island, reviewing her population of patients with diabetes. Her telemedicine practice and her patients use various devices to communicate based on their preferences and abilities. Her teenage patient population loves the group chats and interactives. As they gain autonomy and understand diabetes, they have begun swapping stories and learning from each other. Recently the teen group built an online interactive game for newly diagnosed teen diabetics in an "app lab." Parents are guided by chatbots in off-hours and readily find answers from the virtual assistant. Food scanners on smartphones review food choices and make suggestions for diet control. This activity is logged and analyzed in an artificial intelligence (AI) model that predicts outcomes and alerts Kylie when a patient is starting a dangerous course. Finally, a centrally-located dietitian algorithm calculates values, makes adjustments, and aggregates recommendations. Based on data from the patient devices that monitor and control glucose levels, Kylie is presented with a list of patients who have blood glucoses out of control limits this morning. The first on the roster was already routed to the emergency department when the decision support system (DSS) with AI and machine learning (ML) detected an untoward trend in the patient's values. Because the AI considers each patient's unique characteristics, early detection before complications is the norm. Smartwatches, smartphones, and monitoring devices send data to a central data warehouse where data is normalized and analyzed in the aggregate and individually. Internal (patient values) and external (weather, seasonal, and social events) data are weighted against past trends. The AI sees into the immediate future to offer interventions before events occur.	Telehealth Smartphone Tablet Patient-generated health data Private social media site administered by Kylie's healthcare system Secure texting Virtual assistant Chatbots Algorithms Continuous glucose monitoring device Patient portal Decision support system Artificial intelligence Machine learning Smart secure devices Structured data Artificial intelligence Communication on a secure network Data cleaning before storage Data warehouse storage Rule-based DSS Analytics for trending

and clinical thinking; and the ability of informatics and technology to positively impact patient outcomes. Health information technology is required for person-centered service across the continuum and requires consistency in user input, proper process, and quality management. While different specialty roles in nursing may require varying depth and breadth of informatics competencies, basic informatics competencies are foundational to all nursing practice. Much work will be required to achieve full integration of core information and communication technologies competencies into nursing curricula. (p. 7)

Development and advances in healthcare technologies are rapid and ever-changing. Becoming and then staying competent will be a continuous learning process, a process that APRNs know well.

DATA, CLINICAL DECISION SUPPORT, AND ADVANCED ANALYTICS

Data

Many factors must be considered in planning and managing patient wellness and care. APRNs must remember the patient's history, diagnosis, allergies, vital signs, medications, treatments, comorbidities, and a myriad of other patient-specific details and consider these in the context of national best practices, institution-specific protocols, and, often, provider preferences. This challenge is exponentially compounded when caring for multiple patients and as patient acuity and level of care increase (Castillo & Kelemen, 2013).

The EHR is the core technology in the healthcare industry. It serves to collect, store, and make available patient data to support care planning and

EXEMPLAR 22.4
COMMUNICATION AND DEVICE TECHNOLOGY IN PATIENT CARE

CONGESTIVE HEART FAILURE CLINIC	SUPPORTING TECHNOLOGY
Meghan Asher, RN, ANP-BC, APNP, sees patients with congestive heart failure, locally and remotely. Often, they are young adults who have had COVID-19 in the pandemic of 2020. Meghan's clinic is in an acute care hospital in Houston where the team can see them quickly, but she also monitors patients seen in clinics many miles away, offers consults in other states, and communicates with her research lab in Galveston.	Telehealth technologies Wayfinding with radio frequency and Global Positioning System Remote monitoring Radio frequency Global Positioning System
Patients go to the welcome kiosk at any entrance and scan their cards. The kiosk gives detailed wayfinding information for their visit and instructions for how to get there. Screens along their path light with a green arrow as they pass or stop them to reroute them if they stray from the correct direction. Wait times are less than 5 minutes anywhere in the hospital, and throughput is at an all-time high.	Artificial intelligence geofencing Robotics Real-time location system Decision support system Radiofrequency identification UV light sterilization robot
The routing system alerts the unit when the assigned room is ready if the patient is to be admitted. An APRN checks the RTLS system to locate needed equipment and verifies the readiness of the room. A final UV light sterilization is done in the room by a robot. When the patient walks into the room, they hear a verbal welcome from the room's virtual assistant in their preferred language, known by the integrated DSS and the patient's EHR profile. They also see a welcome message on their digital foot wall that orients them to the unit as the APRN greets them.	Virtual assistant Artificial intelligence Point-of-care capnography Telehealth Technology-enabled patient-centered care
Meghan begins her day with an AI-supported report on her patients. AI has already triaged results, presenting the most acute issues first. The first patient's report suggests that he needs a follow-up echocardiogram and computed tomography (CT) scan. All are done in the exam room at the time of visit and before Meghan arrives. Blood draws are a thing of the past; the new system uses advanced capnography to collect and analyze blood tests in real-time at the bedside. A social worker and psychologist have already had home visits through telehealth. Her visit with the patient starts with all lab results and tests in front of her. This leaves the people-to-people interaction at the center of the visit. During the visit, the patient never leaves one room; the care team rotates around the patient. This model allows the team to support the patient's emotional needs, and often Meghan comes back to a room when the patient is distressed.	

decision making. Each day, APRNs successfully manage thousands of data points due to two embedded components of the EHR. First, the EHR supports the entry of patient data that are critical to all other embedded applications like pain scales, pressure ulcer risk scales, and others. Second, embedded within the EHR are other technologies such as clinical decision support systems (CDSSs) and interfaces connecting any number of different systems and clinical devices that push and pull their data into and out of the EHR (Nibbelink et al., 2018). These data can be structured or unstructured in form.

Structured data are predefined and formatted to a set structure before being placed into data storage (called schema-on-write). These data are formatted into precisely defined fields, such as dates, names, addresses, allergies, and formulary drug names, making the data easily available to manipulate and query (Talend, n.d.). This makes structured data readily available to APRNs for use in quality improvement or evidence-based practice (EBP) projects using standard data extraction tools like business software.

Unstructured data are stored in their native format and not processed until used (called schema-on-read).

These data come in many formats from many sources, including written text, chats, IoT sensors, device output, graphs, and waveforms. Because unstructured data are stored in their native format, they accumulate rapidly and require data science expertise and special tools for extraction and use in decision making (Talend, n.d.).

An example of common structured data is an EHR flowsheet, as data are either numeric or a known value selected from a pull-down list. An example of unstructured data is typed free-text notes. Structured and unstructured data are stored in progressively more sophisticated data stores called databases and data warehouses in massive volumes, ready to be analyzed by ever more sophisticated decision support and advanced analytic tools to provide insights never before possible (Box 22.6).

Essential to any form of analytics is the process of data mining, data cleaning, and having a complete and robust data dictionary.

Data mining is a process of extracting data from a large data set to determine patterns and relationships to enhance the decision-making process (Nibbelink et al., 2018).

Data cleaning, also called *data scrubbing*, is the process of fixing or removing incorrect, corrupted, duplicate, incomplete, or incorrectly formatted data within a data set. This process is essential when combining data from multiple sources since there are many opportunities for duplicate or mislabeled data. If data are incorrect, algorithms and outcomes will be unreliable (e.g., garbage in, garbage out; Tableau, n.d.). For example, a query regarding blood pressure will be affected if the person writing the query doesn't know that blood pressure is expressed as BP, bp, B/P, etc., in different systems. Unless the query is written to capture all expressions of blood pressure, the query results will not pick up all instances of the term. Data cleaning/scrubbing and a good data dictionary limit such errors. This is especially important when using data for individual patients and when making decisions for patient populations.

A **data dictionary** is a collection of the names, definitions, and attributes for data elements (i.e., the metadata about the database). The primary purpose of a data dictionary is to document and share data structures and other information with all persons involved with a database to ensure the same meaning, quality, and relevance for all data elements across teams (Derda, 2020). Without a data dictionary and rigorous adherence to keeping it current, the risk of creating duplicates and alternate versions of existing instances of terms is great, posing a significant risk to data quality. Data cleaning and having a current data dictionary help to ensure data quality, which is essential for advanced analytics and decision support.

BOX 22.6

Types of Data Storage

A **database** is an organized collection of data and is usually classified by the way it stores data. The two most common types of databases are relational databases, which store their data in tables, and object-oriented databases, which store their data in object classes and subclasses. Databases are usually set up to update and monitor real-time structured data, and usually have only the most recent data available (Tiao, 2020).

A **data warehouse** collects data from multiple sources, internal and external, and optimizes it for retrieval. Data are usually structured data from relational databases, but the warehouse can also accommodate some unstructured data. Primarily, a data warehouse is designed to integrate data from multiple sources, manage it, and analyze it at many levels.

An **enterprise data warehouse (EDW)** is a data warehouse that serves an entire enterprise, collecting data from all its key digital departmental systems (Tiao, 2020).

A **clinical data repository (CDR)** is a type of data warehouse that aggregates and stores patient-centric health data collected from multiple IT systems and organizes it for analytics and other uses (Gartner, n.d.). Because a data warehouse ingests data from multiple sources, it first cleans or scrubs all data before it enters the data warehouse, a laborious process in terms of process cycles and time but necessary to ensure that data are clean for analytic and other uses.

Tools for advanced analytics, such as AI, ML, and NLP, assist APRNs in their critical thinking, providing vast amounts of data in varied forms from disparate systems, offering insights into patient care and professional practice not otherwise available to them. AI, ML, and NLP used with APRN knowledge and judgment open the door to the generation of new knowledge, looking beyond the obvious and challenging traditional ways of thinking (Health Information and Management Systems Society, 2019).

Clinical Decision Support

Advanced analytics is a broad category of technologies, applications, and services designed to gather, store, analyze, and access data for decision making, whereas CDSSs are more purpose-built for supporting specific decisions (Olavsrud, 2020). APRNs commonly encounter CDSSs that depend on quality data in their day-to-day work with an EHR. The Centers for Medicare & Medicaid Services defines CDS as "HIT functionality that builds upon the foundation of an EHR to provide persons involved in care processes with general and person-specific information, intelligently filtered and organized, at appropriate times, to enhance health and health care" (Bresnick, 2017, para. 16). CDS may be deployed across various platforms, like cloud-based, server-based, or mobile, and is often integrated into the EHR to utilize existing data and streamline workflow. CDSSs are designed to sift through enormous amounts of digital data to alert providers to critical information, potential risk, and suggestions for care (Bresnick, 2017). CDS is not intended to replace clinician judgment but rather to provide a tool to APRNs in making timely, informed, and higher quality decisions.

Most CDS applications operate as a component of an EHR capable of obtaining computable biomedical knowledge and patient-specific data through data entry and data capture from connected digital devices. These data are then filtered through a reasoning or inference mechanism to combine knowledge and data to generate helpful information for clinicians at the point of care (Castillo & Kelemen, 2013).

CDSSs can be either active or passive. An active CDSS presents information to the clinician that is retrieved by comparing available patient information with programmed rules, protocols, and guidelines, utilizing a knowledge base, available patient information, and an inference engine. A knowledge database includes organizational protocols, guidelines, and rules developed using evidence-based research. Available patient data include data retrieved from physiologic monitors, test results, and data entered by clinicians. The inference engine compares the available patient information with the knowledge base to deliver pertinent information to the user. An active CDSS delivers an immediate presentation of alerts and suggestions; for example, medication interaction or dosage, allergies, critical lab values, and other reminders about patient care. A passive CDSS presents additional resources via links for the clinician to access further information (Castillo & Kelemen, 2013).

A CDSS encompasses a variety of tools to enhance decision making in the clinical workflow, including automated alerts and reminders to care providers and patients, clinical guidelines, condition-specific order sets, focused patient data reports and summaries, documentation templates, diagnostic support, and contextually relevant reference information, among other tools (Castillo & Kelemen, 2013). Simply stated, CDSSs are computer software tools that facilitate decision making by connecting specific patient data with evidence (Nibbelink et al., 2018).

CDSSs are often classified as knowledge-based or non-knowledge-based. In knowledge-based systems, rules are created in the form of IF–THEN statements, and the system retrieves data to evaluate against the rule to produce an action or output. Rules are created from literature-based, practice-based, or patient-directed evidence. Non-knowledge-based CDSSs still require a data source, but the decision leverages AI, ML, or statistical pattern recognition rather than being programmed to follow expert medical knowledge. Although growing in use, non-knowledge-based CDSS pose some challenges, such as problems with a care provider not understanding the AI logic used to generate recommendations, a situation known as a *black box* (Sutton et al., 2020).

Knowledge-based systems utilizing expert rules have a wealth of uses in patient care. Computerized provider order entry (CPOE) systems are now designed with drug safety safeguards for dosing, duplicate orders, allergy, and compatibility checking and recommend less-expensive drug alternatives at the point of order. The scope of functions provided by CDSSs is vast and includes alarm systems, diagnostics, medication and prescription management, and more (Sutton et al., 2020).

Non-knowledge-based CDSSs are garnering increased interest in enhanced imaging and precision radiology (radiomics). Images require extensive manual interpretation, leading providers to search for technologies to aid them in extracting, visualizing, and interpreting them. AI technologies are capable of providing insights into data beyond what humans can by using advanced pixel recognition and image classification algorithms (Sutton et al., 2020). These capabilities often exceed what a CDSS can provide, leading to the development of more advanced forms of analytics, which provide APRNs with an increased ability to aggregate and analyze data to discover trends, risks, and patterns to benchmark and improve safety, quality, and the cost of health care.

Advanced Analytics

With the evolution and pervasive use of healthcare technologies and devices, interoperability, and cross-platform connectivity, we are faced with an unprecedented amount of data in a wide array of formats. This offers the promise of large-scale analysis of disparate healthcare data from widely different sources to gain insights into correlations, patterns, trends, and patient care outcomes. Gone are the days of having automated queries look for keywords in computer-generated text. Now, these systems must glean data from textual and cursive writing; images, such as radiographs, pathology slides, and photographs; symbols, such as barcodes, QR codes, icons, and emojis; tracings, such as electrocardiographs and fetal monitoring strips; and sounds, such as voice recordings and the change in pitch of the reflected sound waves during a Doppler study (the Doppler effect).

Big data refers to data sets that are so large and complex that traditional data processing methods are inadequate (Paskin, 2018). Healthcare data include static data from patient records, diagnostic images, reports, and dynamic data from bedside monitors, biomedical devices, and remote patient monitoring. Most of these data are unstructured and go beyond the capabilities of traditional analytics tools to manage. Artificial intelligence and big data analytics techniques allow big data to be processed to obtain insights not otherwise possible with conventional methods (Mehta et al., 2019).

Three characteristics distinguish big data from traditional data used for decision making: the sheer volume, the velocity (speed) at which it moves, and its high variability in nature and structure, coming from so many sources in so many formats. Volume, velocity, and variability are known as the 3Vs of Big Data ("Healthcare Big Data and the Promise of Value-Based Care," 2018). These data require more than rules and data objects. They need advanced analytic technologies such as AI, ML, and NLP.

Precision health "refers to personalized health care based on a person's unique genetic, genomic, or omic composition within the context of lifestyle, social, economic, cultural and environmental influences to help individuals achieve wellbeing and optimal health" (Fu et al., 2020, p. 6). Precision health uses advanced analytics and big data sets that combine omics (i.e., genomic sequence, metabolite, protein, and microbiome data) with clinical information and health outcomes to optimize disease diagnosis, treatment, and prevention specific to each patient (Fu et al., 2020).

In an era of big data and precision medicine, advanced analytics techniques such as predictive analytics have been developed that exceed the abilities of a standard CDSS. Techniques in computer science, AI, ML, and NLP teach computers to mine EHR data in all of its forms to predict patient outcomes and risk for complications. Regardless of the type of technology used to extract data from any source, the Five Rights of Decision Support provide a best practices framework that can help APRNs decide between available options (Centers for Medicare & Medicaid Services, 2014). The decision support intervention, if beneficial, must provide:

The right information (evidence-based guidance, response to clinical need)
To the right people (entire care team – including the patient)
Through the right channels (e.g., EHR, mobile device, patient portal)
In the right intervention formats (e.g., order sets, flowsheets, dashboards, patient lists)
At the right points in the workflow (for decision making or action)

Recommendation 6 in The Future of Nursing 2020–2030: Charting a Path to Achieve Health Equity (NASEM, 2021) states, "All public and private health care systems should incorporate nursing expertise in designing, generating, analyzing and applying data to support initiatives focused on social determinants of health and health equity using diverse digital platforms, artificial intelligence, and other innovative technologies" (pp. 366–367). Big data, advances in data storage and analytics, and a more tech-savvy APRN bode well for APRN innovation, evidence, insights, and treatment methods for patient care and wellness. The opportunity to transform practice through insight into data has never been greater.

CYBERSECURITY

The National Institute of Standards and Technology (n.d.) defines *cybersecurity* as "prevention of damage to, protection of, and restoration of computers, electronic communications systems, electronic communication services, wire communication, and electronic communication, including information contained therein, to ensure its availability, integrity, authentication, confidentiality, and nonrepudiation" (para. 1). Health care was the most targeted sector for data breaches in 2020, with ransomware attacks responsible for almost 50% of all healthcare data breaches (US Department of Health and Human Services, 2021).

With the move to "work from home" caused by the COVID-19 pandemic in 2020, targeting of home environments and mobile devices increased, and these threats will continue for the foreseeable future (US Department of Health and Human Services, 2021). This has significant implications for APRNs and their digitally connected patients.

As the highest percentage of healthcare workers in the United States, nurses are well placed to take a lead role in cybersecurity, protecting their digital technology in all of its forms and educating patients to do the same. APRN practice of cybersecurity starts with an understanding of security and privacy, the states of digital data, regulatory compliance, types of cyberattacks, and best practices in cybersecurity.

Data Security and Privacy

Data security and privacy are differentiated by what data need to be protected, how, and from whom and who is responsible for the protection. At its most simple, security is about protecting data from malicious threats, while privacy is about using data responsibly (Phillips, 2020).

Data security focuses on preventing unauthorized data access via leaks or breaches, regardless of who the unauthorized person is. To prevent this, organizations use security tools and technologies like firewalls, network limitations, user authentication, encryption, and internal security practices (Phillips, 2020).

Privacy focuses on ensuring that the sensitive data an organization processes, stores, or transmits are collected compliantly and with the data owner's consent. This means that people are told upfront what data will be collected, for what purpose, how it will be used, and with whom it will be shared. Privacy is about using data responsibly and as the patient wishes (Phillips, 2020).

States of Digital Data

Understanding the characteristics and differences between data states helps APRNs handle sensitive data more securely and often dictates which regulation to apply. The three states of data are data at rest, data in motion, and data in use (Fitzgibbons, 2019).

- *Data at rest* describes data in computer storage that are not currently being accessed or transferred. These can be data stored in a file, hard drive, cloud backup, external drive, or company storage area network (SAN). Methods to protect data at rest include data encryption, strict data security protocols, multifactor authentication, hierarchical password protection, secure server rooms, and outside data protection services.
- *Data in motion* is data that are being transferred within or between computer systems. They may be data written to the computer's random-access memory (RAM), readily available for access and use. They can also be data moving between cloud storage and a local file storage point or moving between computer systems, files dragged from one folder to another, and even data transmitted in emails. The most common methods for protecting data in motion are encryption before they are transmitted or encrypting the tunnel through which the data are sent, such as HTTPS, virtual private network (VPN), and secure sockets layer (SSL).
- *Data in use* is data that are being accessed, updated, processed, or read by another system. Because data in use are directly accessible, this is the state at which data

are most vulnerable. Security measures for data in use include encryption, user authentication, strong identity management, and well-maintained permissions.

Regulatory Compliance

Regulatory compliance is the act of adhering to all international, federal, state, and local laws and regulations that apply to your business. As APRNs increasingly communicate with patients electronically, assuring the security and privacy of their and their patients' data, regardless of data state, becomes an essential part of APRN practice. When it comes to cybersecurity, APRNs must look to four predominant regulations that inform their practice: HIPAA, the Health Information Technology for Economic and Clinical Health Act of 2009 (HITECH), General Data Protection Regulation (GDPR), and California Consumer Privacy Act (CCPA).

HIPAA was created to improve health insurance portability, ensuring that employees retained coverage between jobs. It also made healthcare organizations accountable for health data and provided regulations to ensure health information remains private and secure (HIPAA Journal, 2018).

The HIPAA Privacy Rule, effective in December 2000, defines protected health information (PHI), how it can be used by covered entities, to whom it can be disclosed, and under what circumstances and gives patients the right to obtain a copy of their PHI held by a covered entity. The Privacy Rule also requires covered entities to implement appropriate safeguards to protect the privacy of patients (HIPAA Journal, 2018). Note that the Privacy Rule covers PHI in any form (e.g., electronic, paper, graphics, photos, recordings).

The HIPAA Security Rule became effective in February 2003 and is primarily concerned with establishing national standards for security to protect electronic protected health information (ePHI). The Security Rule requires covered entities to implement administrative, technical, and physical safeguards to ensure the confidentiality, integrity, and availability (CIA) of ePHI. It also requires covered entities to conduct risk assessments to identify threats to the ePHI or the CIA of data and mitigate those risks to a reasonable level (HIPAA Journal, 2018). Note that the Security Rule only covers ePHI in any of its states; that is, at rest, in motion, or use.

HITECH builds upon and expands the protections of HIPAA. HITECH added a Breach Notification Rule that requires covered entities to notify all individuals impacted by a data breach in less than 60 days, notify local media outlets if the breach affected more than 500 people, and report breaches to the Health and Human Services secretary. It also provided a new Enforcement Rule with additional penalties or fines for noncompliance and requirements for increased compliance auditing by Health and Human Service's Office of Civil Rights in conjunction with the US Department of Justice and broadened the definition of covered entity to include business associates (RSI Security, 2021).

The GDPR, effective May 2018, establishes privacy and security protections for the personal data of individuals in the European Economic Area (European Union [EU]) countries. The law covers any data gathered on an EU citizen *anywhere in the world.* The GDPR regulates the collection, use, disclosure, or other processing of personal data by controllers and processors. In US terms, a covered entity would equate to a controller, and a business associate would equate to a processor (Broccolo & Gottlieb, 2018).

Where HIPAA only protects an individual's 18 individual identifiers known as PHI, GDPR applies to all categories of health or other data that could directly or indirectly identify an EU resident. In addition, GDPR requires heightened protections for sensitive personal data, including data concerning health, genetic data, biometric data, and data revealing racial or ethnic origin (Broccolo & Gottlieb, 2018).

The extent of the impact of GDPR on US healthcare providers depends on the degree of their contact with patients who live in EU countries. APRNs should identify these patients to ensure compliance with GDPR requirements, as penalties for noncompliance can apply. EU patients may require additional consent forms to collect and process their information. EU patients also have certain access rights, breach notification, and they may even ask to be "forgotten," meaning have their data erased. APRNs should be forewarned that the law applies even after discharge as it covers data collected via remote access, cookies on websites, and data collected via remote monitoring after the patient returns home to their EU country (Broccolo & Gottlieb, 2018).

The CCPA went into effect on January 1, 2020. Like the GDPR and as written, the CCPA is the most restrictive consumer data protection regulation in the United States. It applies to the management of personal data of California residents around the world. CCPA guarantees California residents the right to know what personal information about them is being collected, from where, how it is used, and how it is shared. It also gives California residents the right to limit or stop collecting, using, sharing, or selling their personal information (Oranski, n.d.).

The CCPA contains an exemption for health information covered by federal and state data privacy laws, such as PHI covered by HIPAA. It also exempts covered entities governed by HIPAA to the extent that the entity handles its patient information in compliance with HIPAA. This exemption does not currently apply to business associates of the covered entity.

These healthcare exemptions are not as broad as they first appear; the devil is in the detail. Health information collected directly from patients or their representatives via an app is not considered PHI if it is not created by or on behalf of a healthcare plan or provider (e.g., device data, PGHD submitted voluntarily by the patient, etc.). Also, personal data collected outside the scope of PHI are not exempt from CCPA (e.g., information collected by the covered entity's website via cookies) and geolocation data collected by a website or app (e.g., geofencing, RTLS; O'Connor et al., 2020).

When in doubt about regulatory compliance, collaborate with nurse management or a business practices officer to determine the best course of action.

Types of Cyberattack

A cyberattack is an intentional act perpetrated by cybercriminals to steal data, fabricate information, or disable digital systems. Through such attacks, nefarious characters can gain illegal and unauthorized access to one or more computers or digital devices and use them to their benefit. Many cyberattacks exploit digital vulnerabilities, as illustrated in Box 22.7 (Upadhyay, 2021).

While cyberattacks involve various programmatic vectors like malicious code, most are triggered by human actions, like clicking on links or opening attachments in email, or falling for social engineering on a telephone call. The APRN's best defense against cyberattacks is knowledge, vigilance, and a healthy skepticism about suspicious emails, phone calls, and downloads from unknown sources.

BOX 22.7

Common Types of Cyberattacks

Phishing attacks involve an attacker trying to obtain personal information or data by disguising themselves as trustworthy entities. Phishing is mainly conducted via email and telephone.

Spear phishing attacks are a form of phishing attack that is targeted to a specific individual, again most often by email or telephone.

Malware attacks occur when an attacker deploys computer code to hack digital devices (e.g., computers, laptops, mobile devices) to gain unauthorized access. This may be in the form of a malicious Internet bot.

Man-in-the-Middle (MitM) attacks occur when an attacker intercepts data between two endpoints, thus gaining unauthorized access to data. MitM attacks are one of the risks of using unsecured networks such as public hot spots.

Ransomware is a form of malware that encrypts a victim's files and then holds restoration of function hostage until the victim pays a ransom. Phishing is a common method to deliver the ransomware, often as email attachments.

Mobile Device Security

Most APRNs use mobile communication devices like smartphones, tablets, and laptops in their personal and professional lives. While these devices increase efficiency, they also present serious vulnerabilities if not properly secured. Mobile communication devices, in general, are not as secure as computers and may not have the same protective technologies like firewalls, encryption, and antivirus software, making these devices very attractive to malicious actors. If you are not securing your mobile communication devices, you may be exposing your own, your organization's, and your patients' data to cyberattack. There are basic mobile security practices that every APRN should follow (Security Metrics, n.d.) (Box 22.8).

Mobile medical devices pose another risk to PHI and patient safety. The current IoT environment and the explosion of consumer medical devices and apps

BOX 22.8

Basic Mobile Security Practices

Accept all OS and app updates immediately. Mobile devices must be patched often to eliminate software or hardware vulnerabilities found after initial release.

Never connect to unsecured Wi-Fi (e.g., hotspots). Using unsecured websites and networks opens the door to man-in-the-middle attacks (interception) and exposure to malware.

Install firewall protection on your home network and ask your organization if they provide firewall software.

Use discretion when downloading apps. They may be infected with malware.

Make sure the devices you plug your mobile device into (e.g., your home computer, work laptop, etc.) are secure.

Implement a strong password/pin on your mobile device, never share it, and change it often.

Connect to your EHR via secured remote access (e.g., a virtual private network [VPN], through two-factor authentication).

Encrypt your data. If you must have sensitive data on your mobile device, make sure it's encrypted so that it remains secure even if malware steals it.

Use mobile vulnerability scanning, usually provided with security software to discover weaknesses.

Learn about your organization's mobile device policies. Employees should know about malware and take the right measures to avoid it.

Avoid suspicious email, text messages, and voicemail on your phone. Also avoid pop-ups and links in email.

can leave patients vulnerable to cyberattacks. Healthcare systems and providers encourage patients to use these devices to monitor health, promote wellness, and share these data via patient portals, PHRs, and PGHD. To do so safely, the device owner must apply security updates as soon as they are available, maintain strong password protection, and always operate on a secured network. The APRN can help with this by consistently reminding their patients who use connected medical devices to apply security best practices when using, storing, and transmitting data from their devices. If there are questions about best practices, a nurse informaticist or your IT department is a great interprofessional resource.

Blockchain

Blockchain is a system for recording data that makes it difficult to hack or change the system. It was created for cryptocurrency but holds promise for use in healthcare and other industries and is one of the technologies to watch in the healthcare security sector.

In simple terms, a blockchain consists of private digital information (the "block") stored in a public database (the "chain"). It is a form of distributed ledger technology consisting of a cluster of connected databases that record various transactions in such a way as to prevent the alternation of the transactions (Carroll, 2020). "Nurses can make a significant difference in the quality of patient care by harnessing the power of blockchain technology" (Carroll, 2020, p. 63). APRNs can utilize these immutable datastores to optimize patient data management and portability, manage professional nurse credentialing and education, expedite nursing research, and safeguard clinical trials, adding value to their practice (Carroll, 2020).

HIGH-TECH HOME CARE

Hospitals strive to discharge patients as soon as possible. Spurred by regulatory incentives to cut length-of-stay and costs, staffing shortages, the emphasis on patient-centered care, the baby boomers' desire for autonomy, the evolving view of patients as consumers, and the "age in place" movement, patients are going home "quicker and sicker," often still in need of care. Fortunately, the healthcare industry is steadily increasing its capacity to care for patients outside of the hospital. Thousands of healthcare apps, devices, and communication technologies are available to providers and patients, ranging from simple materials for use in first aid to complex devices to deliver advanced medical treatment and sustain life at home. In this era of high-tech home care, discharge planning requires that APRNs leverage their tried-and-true cognitive techniques in new ways to ensure the safe use of technology in the patient's home. Planning the discharge of a patient using medical technology at home starts with a patient technology readiness assessment.

A patient technology readiness assessment should begin as soon as the APRN knows that the patient will be discharged with orders to continue care with home care technology. It is essential to know what technology or device(s) the patient will be using, whether the patient has used this or similar technology before, and whether the patient will have help at home to assist with its use and maintenance. A readiness assessment will include this and a review of the personal characteristics that facilitate a patient's ability to operate the medical device or technology (Story, 2010) (Box 22.9).

Upon discharge, it is essential to remember that the effects of illness, medications, and stress can accentuate any preexisting limitations in the patient's physical, perceptual, or cognitive functions (Story, 2010). Their condition can negatively affect an otherwise tech-savvy user, so do not assume proficiency in this instance. Knowledge of the patient's characteristics, coupled with knowledge of the technology, can inform the APRN's plans for patient-specific education and preparation of discharge instructions specific to the patient's needs (e.g., literacy level, language, format).

The safe use of technology at home involves more than assessing whether the patient is willing or able to use it. A home environmental assessment is critical as the use of medical devices may be introduced into less than desirable or even dangerous conditions (Story, 2010) (Box 22.10). Therefore, before a medical device goes into a home with a patient, it is crucial to verify that the device is compatible with the patient's home. The FDA has developed a checklist with essential questions to ask when considering the use of home medical devices (US Food and Drug Administration, 2017).

Patients and families should have contingency plans for emergencies such as power outages and running out of supplies. There needs to be a written backup plan for each medical device, identifying a reliable source for medical supplies and a plan for proper storage and disposal of supplies. Patients should maintain device and supply inserts and instructions in an easily assessable location and read the material carefully before using new equipment.

Patients with implantable medical devices, such as cardiac pacemakers, cardioverter defibrillators, and

BOX 22.9

Personal Characteristics That Influence Ability to Operate a Medical Device

- Sensory capabilities (e.g., vision, hearing, tactile sensitivity)
- Cognitive abilities, including memory
- Physical size, strength, and stamina
- Physical dexterity, flexibility, and coordination
- Literacy, including language skills
- Mental and emotional state
- Level of education and training relative to their medical condition
- General health
- Knowledge of similar devices
- Knowledge of and experience with the actual device
- Ability to learn and adapt to a new device
- Willingness and motivation to use a new device

BOX 22.10

Environmental Issues for Home Use of Medical Devices

- Rooms that are physically crowded or cluttered, impeding maneuverability in the space
- Stairs or carpeting that can hinder device maneuverability or portability
- Low lighting level that makes it hard to see device controls and displays
- High noise level that makes it hard to hear device alarms and prompts
- Temperature that is too high or too low that can cause equipment to overheat or stall out
- Humidity that is too high, causing condensation, or too low, causing static electricity
- Cleanliness of the house may be an issue
- Distractions of a household busy with other people and activities
- Children, pets, vermin, or unauthorized users in the house can cause damage to patients, cause damage to devices, or change device settings
- Electromagnetic interference from other equipment in the home

cardiac resynchronization devices, may be subject to electromagnetic interference and require special instructions and precautions. Electromagnetic interference is a disruption of the operation of an electronic device by an electromagnetic field, usually in proximity to the device (Nunns, 2016). According to the FDA (2020), common electromagnetic emitters are RFID readers, electronic security systems (e.g., electronic article surveillance, metal detectors, airport security), near-field communications (NFC) systems (e.g., keyless access, E-wallets, credit cards, wearable devices), wireless power transfer (e.g., wireless chargers), and what the FDA calls "unique medical emitters," such as electrocautery, magnetic resonance imaging (MRI), diathermy equipment, and electrosurgical units. Device manufacturers are required to label devices that may present a risk of electromagnetic interference, so all medical and health devices used by a patient with an implantable device should have such a label.

Home device use by older patients brings challenges, especially if they struggle with impaired eyesight, hearing, mobility, or cognition. For this reason, devices with voice output are particularly beneficial to elderly patients (Box 22.11).

If the patient has a designated caregiver postdischarge, they should be involved in discharge planning and training from the beginning. Their knowledge about medical devices and equipment can be a lifesaver in an emergency. They can also be crucial to the use, maintenance, and acquisition of essential equipment and supplies.

BOX 22.11

Benefits to Elderly of Voice Output on Medical Devices

- Reinforce visual messages and provide redundant cuing
- Reduce misinterpreting visual messages; for example, words and icons
- Help infrequent users with prompts and feedback as they use the device
- Improve user confidence
- Provide vital support for the visually impaired who cannot perceive visual information on the device

Miniaturization of medical equipment previously limited to a hospital or clinic has opened many new opportunities in high-tech home care. The well-equipped home care APRN can now carry a wealth of advanced technology and digital tools in a typical "nurse bag." According to the medical futurist Bertalan Mesko (2020), the well-equipped practitioner will carry a digital stethoscope; a handheld electrocardiogram device; a digital blood pressure monitor, thermometer, and pulse oximeter; an ultraportable ultrasound machine; and a portable digital otoscope with built-in nano camera. The FDA recently approved the Viacom CheckMe Pro, a mobile device that measures electrocardiogram, blood oxygen level, temperature, blood pressure, heart rate, and steps all in one small device (Mesko, 2020). The devices and the many apps available to APRNs and patients are remarkable breakthroughs, but they are all dependent on the knowledge and skills of the APRN for best and safest use. The APRN must make the assessment, ask the questions, survey the environment, know the patient, and ultimately use traditional nurse logic and skill to determine the best course of action to take concerning what, when, and where to use technology. The APRN will analyze (critically think), apply (clinically reason), and act (clinically judge) when assessing and promoting the safe use of technology for the patient and home environment.

The future for high-tech home care is bright, and the potential for APRNs in this field is expanding. The disruption that digital health has brought about has radically changed how APRNs can consult with and care for patients in the home setting, resulting in an expansion of their scope of authority in this area. As of March 2020, APRNs can order home health services for Medicare patients, consistent with state law, including skilled medical care and respiratory, speech, and occupational therapies.

FUTURE IMPLICATIONS OF TECHNOLOGY-ENABLED ADVANCED PRACTICE REGULATION AND GROWTH: A CALL TO PARTICIPATE

Numerous reports have supported the pivotal role of advanced practice nurses in technology-enabled systems. The impact is no less than the transformation of the healthcare system (IOM, 2011). APRNs have repeatedly been called to practice to the full extent of their license and education, spend more time with patients, and improve the care environment (Bolton et al., 2008). It is imperative for the future of APRN practice that the linkage between data and outcomes be collected to support these findings. Further, data have the potential to create strong evidence that APRN practice should be unchained to fulfill its full potential for the public. Simplistically, but foundational to a future course, technology must capture the correct data to demonstrate the worth of the APRN.

Keeping our focus on technology use in advanced practice nursing will require a systems understanding of the relevant drivers of the data-driven future. While the patient is the center of advanced nursing practice, areas of focus for future monitoring and professional advocacy include:

Telehealth reimbursement models: Telehealth services have shown promise for increased reach for physical and mental health challenges (Nagel & Penner, 2016; Schlachta-Fairchild, 2001). Payers should fully reimburse for APRN visits. During the COVID-19 pandemic, many states relaxed or eliminated regulatory burdens in APRN practice to better serve the public. Advocacy groups are now pressing the case that the APRN should not suffer rollbacks to prepandemic restrictions once the crisis has waned (NCSBN, 2021).

Integrating telehealth and informatics into APRN curricula: Future APRNs must realize the full breadth of technology-enabled practice to keep current with healthcare changes and influence policy direction (Guenther et al., 2021). APRN students must gain skills in working with patients through telehealth. In addition, it is increasingly difficult to find practice settings for the APRN student. Telehealth offers an alternative to the traditional onsite preceptorship (Schweickert et al., 2018).

Standards and interoperability: ANA advisories have indicated that future electronic health records (EHRs) and other HIT solutions used to document, manage, and report nursing care in all phases and settings should promote the accurate capture and standardized representation of nursing knowledge, data collected by nurses in the context of patient care, and contributions to outcomes across the nursing process.

(ANA, 2014, para. 1)

Increasing the engagement of nurses and other front-line staff to work with developers and manufacturers in the design, development, purchase, implementation, and evaluation of medical and health devices and health information technology products is needed to progress technology in healthcare settings (IOM, 2012).

Education: Integrating skills, technology, and practice to inform the new generations of APRNs is vital for progress in the profession. Clearly stated guides are needed to make this transformative step (IOM, 2011).

Aligning data: There is an overwhelming need to understand healthcare practices and trends that influence policy decisions (Cipriano, 2011).

Creating clear regulatory guidance: Peer review, nomenclature, practice settings, education, continuing education, and prescriptive authority are among the areas impacted at the regulatory level (Pulcini et al., 2010). The statutory bodies must be competent in technology used in advanced practice nursing and understand the implication for technology failure on APRN practice.

CONCLUSION

Increasingly with technology, there is hope that the past ills of the US healthcare system will be eradicated, public health and healthcare disparities will be improved, and transparency into the healthcare delivery system will be achieved. These overarching goals will impact the advanced practice nurse in increasingly direct and indirect manners. If the full potential of advanced practice is realized, it will be because APRNs were fully involved in crafting the future. With scrutiny of the impact of technology and full participation by APRNs, the path forward for advanced practice nursing can be self-directed and aligned with a just and safe healthcare system.

KEY SUMMARY POINTS

- Florence Nightingale used data to transform health care and provide evidence for the power of nursing practice.
- Nursing skills include observation, assessment, gathering data, analyzing, and intervening. Nursing skills are readily applied to technology assessment now and in the future.
- Assessment of technology requirements is key to utilizing technology in practice.
- Understanding data, how it is acquired and manipulated, and consistent maintenance of the integrity of technology is a prerequisite for any technology application to patient care.
- Diagnostic and therapeutic medical devices and apps enhance nursing practice and education regardless of setting.
- It is essential for APRNs to participate in the assessment and acquisition of technology.

REFERENCES

3D Printing Industry. (n.d.). *The free beginner's guide*. 3D Printing Industry. Retrieved June 28, 2021, from https://3dprintingindustry.com/3d-printing-basics-free-beginners-guide/

Additive Manufacturing. (2019). *3D printing in healthcare: Where are we in 2021? (Updated)*. Additive Manufacturing. https://amfg.ai/2019/08/30/3d-printing-in-healthcare-where-are-we-in-2019/

Albuquerque Speech Language Hearing Center. (2016). *Three primary means of communication*. Albuquerque Speech Language Hearing Center Blog. https://aslhc.org/three-primary-forms-communication/

Alexander, D. (2020, November 3). *15 medical robots that are changing the world*. https://interestingengineering.com/15-medical-robots-that-are-changing-the-world

Ali, M. (2018). Communication skills 3: Non-verbal communication. *Nursing Times*. https://www.nursingtimes.net/clinical-archive/assessment-skills/communication-skills-3-non-verbal-communication-15-01-2018/

American Association of Colleges of Nursing (AACN). (2021). *The essentials: Core competencies for professional nursing education*. https://www.aacnnursing.org/Portals/42/AcademicNursing/pdf/Essentials-2021.pdf

American Hospital Association (AHA). (2014, January 16). *SAFER guides*. https://www.aha.org/guidesreports/2014-01-16-safer-guides

American Nurses Association (ANA). (n.d.). *ANA social media principles*. Retrieved June 7, 2021, from https://www.nursingworld.org/social/

American Nurses Association (ANA). (2014). *Standardization and interoperability of health information technology - ANA position statement*. June 11. https://www.nursingworld.org/practice-policy/nursing-excellence/official-position-statements/id/standardization-and-interoperability-of-health-information-technology/

Androus, A. B. (2020). What are some pros and cons of using electronic charting (EMR)? *Registered Nursing*. https://www.registerednursing.org/articles/pros-cons-using-electronic-charting/

Automation Anywhere. (n.d.). *What is RPA? Robotics process automation software*. Automation Anywhere. Retrieved June 2, 2021 from https://www.automationanywhere.com/rpa/robotic-process-automation

Bolton, L. B., Gassert, C. A., & Cipriano, P. F. (2008). Smart technology, enduring solutions. *Journal of Health Information Management, 22*(4), 26–30. http://medicalautomation.org/wp-content/uploads/2009/09/smart-technology-enduring-solutions-nursing-it-fall-2008.pdf

Bove, L. A. (2019). Increasing patient engagement through the use of wearable technology. *The Journal for Nurse Practitioners, 15*(8), 535–539.

Brennan, P. F., & Bakken, S. (2015). Nursing needs big data and big data needs nursing. *Journal of Nursing Scholarship, 47*(5), 477–484.

Bresnick, J. (2017, December 12). *Understanding the basics of clinical decision support systems*. HealthITAnalytics. https://healthitanalytics.com/features/understanding-the-basics-of-clinical-decision-support-systems

Broccolo, B. M., & Gottlieb, D. F. (2018). *Does GDPR regulate clinical care delivery by US health care providers?* February 26: The National Law Review. https://www.natlawreview.com/article/does-gdpr-regulate-clinical-care-delivery-us-health-care-providers

Carayon, P., & Hoonakker, P. (2019). Human factors and usability for health information technology: Old and new challenges. *International Medical Informatics Association (IMIA) Yearbook of Medical Informatics*, 71–77. 2019.

Carroll, W. (2020). How blockchain can improve nursing. *Nursing, 50*(8), 62–63. 2020.

Castillo, R. S., & Kelemen, A. (2013). Considerations for a successful clinical decision support system. *Computers, Informatics, Nursing: CIN, 31*(7), 319–326. quiz 327–328.

Centers for Medicare & Medicaid Services (CMS). (2014). *Clinical decision support tipsheet*. https://www.cms.gov/Regulations-and-Guidance/Legislation/EHRIncentivePrograms/Downloads/ClinicalDecisionSupport_Tipsheet-.pdf

CenTrak. (n.d.). *Real time location system (RTLS) for hospitals*. Retrieved May 30, 2021, from https://centrak.com/products/real-time-location-services/

Chassin, M. R., & Loeb, J. M. (2013). High-reliability health care: Getting there from here. *The Milbank Quarterly, 91*(3), 459–490.

Cipriano, P. F. (2011). The future of nursing and health IT: The quality elixir. *Nursing Economic$, 29*(5), 286–289.

Craig, A. B. (2013). *Understanding augmented reality: Concepts and applications*. Morgan Kaufmann.

Croxton, J. (2021). *What is geofencing and how does it work?* Propellant Media. https://propellant.media/what-is-geofencing/

Derda, M. (2020). *What is a data dictionary?* Trifacta Blog. https://www.trifacta.com/blog/data-dictionary/

Donabedian, A. (1988). The assessment of technology and quality: A comparative study of certainties and ambiguities. *International Journal of Technology Assessment in Health Care, 4*(4), 487–496.

ECRI Institute. (2019). *Top 10 health technology hazards for 2020.* http://www.smsendo.com/wp-content/uploads/2019/10/ECRI_Top_Ten_Health_Technology_Hazards_2020.pdf

Emergency Medicine News. (2017). Vein visualization aids providers. *Emergency Medicine News* (4B), 39.

Expert.ai. (2020). *Chatbot: What is a chatbot? Why are chatbots important?* Expert.Ai Blog. https://www.expert.ai/blog/chatbot/

Fendelman, A. (2020). *Cellphones vs. smartphones.* February 11: Lifewire. https://www.lifewire.com/cell-phones-vs-smartphones-577507

Ferretti, A., Ronchi, E., & Vayena, E. (2019). From principles to practice: Benchmarking government guidance on health apps. *The Lancet Digital Health, 1*(2), e55–e57.

Fitzgibbons, L. (2019). *States of Digital Data.* February: SearchDataManagement. https://searchdatamanagement.techtarget.com/reference/states-of-digital-data

Fu, M. R., Kurnat-Thoma, E., Starkweather, A., Henderson, W. A., Cashion, A. K., Williams, J. K., Katapodi, M. C., Reuter-Rice, K., Hickey, K. T., Barcelona de Mendoza, V., Calzone, K., Conley, Y. P., Anderson, C. M., Lyon, D. E., Weaver, M. T., Shiao, P. K., Constantino, R. E., Wung, S.-F., Hammer, M. J., & Coleman, B. (2020). Precision health: A nursing perspective. *International Journal of Nursing Sciences, 7*(1), 5–12.

Garrett, P., & Seidman, J. (2011). *EMR vs EHR – What is the difference?* Health IT Buzz Blog. https://www.healthit.gov/buzz-blog/electronic-health-and-medical-records/emr-vs-ehr-difference

Gartner. (n.d.). *Gartner Glossary.* https://www.gartner.com/en/information-technology/glossary/cdr-clinical-data-repository

GE Healthcare. (n.d.). *Centricity universal viewer zero footprint.* GE Healthcare. Retrieved June 14, 2021, from https://www.gehealthcare.com/products/healthcare-it/enterprise-imaging/centricity-universal-viewer-zero-footprint

Guenther, J., Branham, S., Calloway, S., Hilliard, W., Jimenez, R., & Merrill, E. (2021). Five steps to integrating telehealth into APRN curricula. *Telehealth, 17*(3), 322–325.

Halliday, S. (2019). *The lady with the stats: How Florence Nightingale's nursing by numbers is still influencing today's healthcare.* HistoryExtra. https://www.historyextra.com/period/victorian/project-nightingale-who-was-florence-influence-legacy-big-data/

Hammer, J. (2020, March). *The defiance of Florence Nightingale. Smithsonian Magazine.* Retrieved June 28, 2021, from https://www.smithsonianmag.com/history/the-worlds-most-famous-nurse-florence-nightingale-180974155/

Hatch, N., & Shaw, R. J. (2019). *3D printing: The future of nursing and clinical education.* MedTech Boston. https://medtechboston.medstro.com/blog/2019/01/18/3d-printing-the-future-of-nursing-and-clinical-education/

Hayes, A. (2020, May 11). *The ins and outs of wearable technology.* Investopedia. https://www.investopedia.com/terms/w/wearable-technology.asp

Hayward, R. A., & Hofer, T. P. (2001). Estimating hospital deaths due to medical errors preventability is in the eye of the reviewer. *Journal of the American Medical Association (JAMA), 286*(4), 415–420.

Health Information and Management Systems Society (HIMSS). (2019). *Artificial intelligence, critical thinking and the nursing process.* February 6. https://www.himss.org/resources/artificial-intelligence-critical-thinking-and-nursing-process

HealthIT.gov. (2017a). *What are the PGHD-related criteria in the health IT rules and programs?* December 21. https://www.healthit.gov/topic/otherhot-topics/what-are-pghd-related-criteria-health-it-rules-and-programs

HealthIT.gov. (2017b). *What is a patient portal?* September 29. https://www.healthit.gov/faq/what-patient-portal

HealthIT.gov. (2018a). *Patient-generated health data.* https://www.healthit.gov/topic/scientific-initiatives/patient-generated-health-data

HealthIT.gov. (2018b). *SAFER guides.* https://www.healthit.gov/topic/safety/safer-guides

HealthIT.gov. (2019). *What are the differences between electronic medical records, electronic health records, and personal health records?* May 2. https://www.healthit.gov/faq/what-are-differences-between-electronic-medical-records-electronic-health-records-and-personal

Health Resources & Services Administration (HRSA). (2019, August). *Health literacy.* Official Web Site of the US Health Resources & Services Administration. https://www.hrsa.gov/about/organization/bureaus/ohe/health-literacy/index.html

HIPAA Journal. (n.d.). Is text messaging HIPAA compliant? *HIPAA Journal.* Retrieved May 6, 2021 from https://www.hipaajournal.com/is-text-messaging-hipaa-compliant/

HIPAA Journal. (2018). When was HIPAA enacted? *HIPAA Journal.* https://www.hipaajournal.com/when-was-hipaa-enacted/

Holmgren, A. J., Apathy, N. C., & Adler-Milstein, J. (2020). Barriers to hospital electronic public health reporting and implications for the COVID-19 pandemic. *Journal of the American Medical Informatics Association, 27*(8), 1306–1309.

Howe, J. L., Adams, K. T., Hettinger, A. Z., & Ratwani, R. M. (2018). Electronic health record usability issues and potential contribution to patient harm. *Journal of the American Medical Association, 319*(12), 1276–1278.

Hunt, D. L., Haynes, R. B., Hanna, S. E., & Smith, K. (1998). Effects of computer-based clinical decision support systems on physician performance and patient outcomes: A systematic review. *Journal of the American Medical Association, 280*(15), 1339–1346.

IBM. (2020, June 3). *What is artificial intelligence (AI)?* IBM. https://www.ibm.com/cloud/learn/what-is-artificial-intelligence

Institute of Medicine. (1999). *To err is human: Building a safer health system.* National Academy Press.

Institute of Medicine. (2003). *Key capabilities of an electronic health record system: Letter report.* https://doi.org/10.17226/10781

Institute of Medicine (IOM). (2011). *The future of nursing: Leading change, advancing health.* National Academies Press. doi:10.17226/12956

Institute of Medicine. (2012). *Health IT and patient safety: Building safer systems for better care.* https://doi.org/10.17226/13269

Intel. (n.d.). *Robotics in healthcare to improve patient outcomes.* Intel. Retrieved June 2, 2021, from https://www.intel.com/content/www/us/en/healthcare-it/robotics-in-healthcare.html

International Nurse Regulator Collaborative. (2017). *Social media use: Common expectations for nurses.* https://inrc.com/112.htm

International Society of Nurses in Genetics. (n.d.). *What is a genetic nurse?* Retrieved June 1, 2021, from https://www.isong.org/page-1325153

James, J. T. (2013). A new, evidence-based estimate of patient harms associated with hospital care. *Journal of Patient Safety, 9*(3), 122–128.

Jiang, F., Jiang, Y., Zhi, H., Dong, Y., Li, H., Ma, S., Wang, Y., Dong, Q., Shen, H., & Wang, Y. (2017). Artificial intelligence in healthcare: Past, present, and future. *Stroke and Vascular Neurology, 2*(4), 230–243.

The Joint Commission. (2015). *Safe use of health information technology*. March 31 (pp. 54) Sentinel Event Alert. Retrieved May 30, 2021, from. https://www.jointcommission.org/-/media/tjc/documents/resources/patient-safety-topics/sentinel-event/sea_54_hit_4_26_16.pdf

Lea, M. (2020). *How VR simulation training is set to change nursing education*. May 20: HealthTech Magazine. https://healthtechmagazine.net/article/2020/05/how-virtual-training-set-change-nursing-education

Leary, M., & Charles, R. (2021, April 13). *Nurses on social media: A guide to your best practices*. American Nurse. https://www.myamericannurse.com/my-nurse-influencers-yes-and-nurses-on-social-media/

Lorenzi, N. (2020). RTLS applications grow with hospital data needs. *Health Facilities Management Magazine*. https://www.hfmmagazine.com/articles/4028-rtls-applications-grow-with-hospital-data-needs

Lowry, S. Z., Ramaiah, M., Taylor, S., Patterson, E. S., Prettymaan, S. S., Simmons, D., Brick, D., Latkany, P., & Gibbons, M. C. (2015, October 7). *NISTIR 7804-1 Technical evaluation, testing, and validation of the usability of electronic health records: empirically based use cases for validating safety enhanced usability and guidelines for standardization*. National Institute of Standards and Technology. doi:10.6028/NIST.IR.7804-1

Manski, C. F., & Molinari, F. (2020). Estimating the COVID 19 infection rate: Anatomy of an inference problem. *Journal of Econometrics, 220*(1), 181–192.

Marder, A. (2017). *Are barcodes or QR codes better for retailers?* Captera Blog. https://blog.capterra.com/are-barcodes-or-qr-codes-better-for-retailers/

McDonald, C. J., Weiner, M., & Hui, S. L. (2000). Deaths due to medical errors are exaggerated in Institute of Medicine Report. *Journal of the American Medical Association, 284*(1), 93–95.

Mehta, N., Pandit, A., & Shukla, S. (2019). Transforming healthcare with big data analytics and artificial intelligence: A systematic mapping study. *Journal of Biomedical Informatics, 100*(2019), Article 103311.

Mesko, B. (2020, March 5). *The 7 must-haves for the doctor of the 21st century*. The Medical Futurist. https://medicalfuturist.com/the-7-must-haves-for-the-doctor-of-the-21st-century

Mohmmed, R. G. A., Mohammed, H. M., El-sol, Hassane, & A., E.-S (2019). New technology in nursing education and practice. *International Organization of Scientific Research Journal of Nursing and Health Science (IOSR-JNHS), 6*(6), 29–38.

Monroe Engineering. (2020). *The role of computer-aided design (CAD) in 3D printing*. Monroe Engineering Blog. https://monroeengineering.com/blog/the-role-of-computer-aided-design-cad-in-3d-printing/

Muoio, D. (2018). *Steth IO launches digital stethoscope housed within smartphone case*. MobiHealthNews. https://www.mobihealthnews.com/content/steth-io-launches-digital-stethoscope-housed-within-smartphone-case

Nagel, D. A., & Penner, J. L. (2016). Conceptualizing telehealth in nursing practice: Advancing a conceptual model to fill a virtual gap. *Journal of Holistic Nursing, 34*(1), 91–104.

National Academies of Sciences, Engineering, and Medicine (NASEM). (2021). *The future of nursing 2020-2030: Charting a path to achieve health equity*. The National Academies Press. doi:10.17226/25982

National Cancer Institute. (n.d.). *Liquid biopsy*. NCI dictionaries. https://www.cancer.gov/publications/dictionaries/cancer-terms/def/liquid-biopsy

National Council of State Boards of Nursing (NCSBN). (2018). *A nurse's guide to the use of social media*. https://www.ncsbn.org/3739.htm

National Council of State Boards of Nursing (NCSBN). (2021). NCSBN's environmental scan COVID-19 and its impact on nursing and regulation. *Journal of Nursing Regulation, 11*(4), S1–S36. Supplement.

National Institute of Standards and Technology (NIST). (n.d.). Cybersecurity. In *NIST glossary*. Retrieved June 28, 2021, from https://csrc.nist.gov/glossary/term/cybersecurity

New England Journal of Medicine (NEJM) Catalyst. (2018, January 1). Healthcare big data and the promise of value-based care. https://catalyst.nejm.org/doi/full/10.1056/CAT.18.0290

Nibbelink, C. W., Young, J. R., Carrington, J. M., & Brewer, B. B. (2018). Informatics solutions for application of decision-making skills. *Critical Care Nursing Clinics of North America, 30*(2), 237–246.

Nolan, M. E., Siwani, R., Helmi, H., Pickering, B. W., Moreno-Franco, P., & Herasevich, V. (2017). Health IT usability focus section: Data use and navigation patterns among medical ICU clinicians during electronic chart review. *Applied Clinical Informatics, 8*(4), 1117–1126.

Nunns, J. (2016). *What is EMI?* Tech Monitor. https://techmonitor.ai/what-is/what-is-emi-4966134

O'Connor, M. C., Weiss, R. H., Erdmann, S. A., & Lockwood, B. A. (2020, January 28). *With CCPA in effect, what do health and life sciences entities need to know? And how does the new amendment affect you?* Lexology. https://www.lexology.com/library/detail.aspx?g=931a3a85-bf4d-470b-838a-c1b8c181f7ca

Olavsrud, T. (2020). *Decision support systems: Sifting data for better business decisions*. CIO. https://www.cio.com/article/3545813/decision-support-systems-sifting-data-for-better-business-decisions.html

Oracle. (n.d.). *What is a digital assistant?* Oracle. Retrieved May 13, 2021, from https://www.oracle.com/chatbots/what-is-a-digital-assistant/

Oranski, S. (n.d.). *The CCPA and healthcare: What you need to know*. CyberMDX Blog. https://blog.cybermdx.com/the-ccpa-and-healthcare-what-you-need-to-know

Orsini, A. (2018). *Techniques for bringing compassionate communication to telehealth interactions*. The Beryl Institute PX Blog. https://www.theberylinstitute.org/blogpost/947424/301876/Techniques-for-Bringing-Compassionate-Communication-to-Telehealth-Interactions

Paskin, S. (2018). *Machine learning, data science, artificial intelligence, deep learning, and statistics*. BMC Blogs. https://www.bmc.com/blogs/machine-learning-data-science-artificial-intelligence-deep-learning-and-statistics/

Perneger, T. V. (2005). The Swiss cheese model of safety incidents: Are there holes in the metaphor? *BMC Health Services Research, 5*, 1–7.

Perrow, C. (2011). *Normal accidents: Living with high risk technologies - updated edition*. Princeton University Press.

Phillips, D. (2020). *Data privacy vs. data security: What is the dore difference?* Tokenex Blog. https://www.tokenex.com/blog/data-privacy-vs-security

Porter, S. (2013). AAFP interview with Farzad Mostashari, MD, MS, National Coordinator for Health Information Technology. *The Annals of Family Medicine, 11*(4), 387–388.

Pulcini, J., Jelic, M., Gul, R., & Loke, A. Y. (2010). An international survey on advanced practice nursing education, practice, and regulation. *Journal of Nursing Scholarship, 42*(1), 31–39.

Reason, J. (2000). Human error: Models and management. *British Medical Journal, 320*(7237), 768–770.

Reason, J. (2004). Beyond the organizational accident: The need for "error wisdom" on the frontline. *BMJ Quality & Safety, 13*(suppl 2), ii28–ii33.

Reason, J. (2016). *Managing the risks of organizational accidents*. Routledge ISBN: 978-1-134-85535-3.

Reinking, C. (2020). Nurses transforming systems of care: The bicentennial of Florence Nightingale's legacy. *Nursing Management, 51*(5), 32–37.

Remark. (n.d.). *What is OMR (Optical Mark Recognition)?* Remark Software Blog. https://remarksoftware.com/omr-technology/what-is-omr-optical-mark-recognition/

Resnick, R. (2019, July 17). *What are the pros and cons of mHealth?* Cureatr Blog. https://blog.cureatr.com/pros-and-cons-mhealth

Roberson, M. R. (2019, April 18). *Liquid biopsies smooth way for personalized medicine*. Duke Cancer Institute. http://dukecancerinstitute.org/donors/your-gifts-at-work/liquid-biopsies-smooth-way-personalized-medicine

Rowe, R. (2017). *OCR, ICR recognition software 101*. Parascript Blog. https://www.parascript.com/blog/ocr-icr-recognition-software-101/

Rouleau, G., Gagnon, M.-P., Côté, J., Payne-Gagnon, J., Hudson, E., & Dubois, C.-A. (2017). Impact of information and communication technologies on nursing care: Results of an overview of systematic reviews. *Journal of Medical Internet Research, 19*(4), e122.

RSI Security. (2021). *Major components of the HITECH Act: What you should know*. RSI Security Blog. https://blog.rsisecurity.com/major-components-of-the-hitech-act-what-you-should-know/

Schlachta-Fairchild, L. (2001). Telehealth: A new venue for health care delivery. *Seminars in Oncology Nursing, 17*(1), 34–40.

Schmelzer, R. (2020, May 9). *Understanding the recognition pattern of AI*. Forbes. https://www.forbes.com/sites/cognitiveworld/2020/05/09/understanding-the-recognition-pattern-of-ai/

Schrimpf, P., Gourji, J., & Aneja, P. (n.d.). *Virtual care: From rarity to reality*. Prophet. Retrieved June 5, 2021, from https://www.prophet.com/download/virtual-care-from rarity-to-reality/

Schweickert, P., Rheuban, K. S., Cattell-Gordon, D., Rose, R. L., Wiles, L. L., Reed, K. E., Reid, K. B., Fowler, C. N., Haney, T., & Rutledge, C. (2018). The APN-PLACE telehealth education network: Legal and regulatory considerations. *Journal of Nursing Regulation, 9*(1), 47–51.

Security Metrics. (n.d.). *5 tips for HIPAA compliant mobile devices*. Security Metrics. Retrieved June 10, 2021, from https://www.securitymetrics.com/learn/hipaa-compliant-mobile-devices

Serrano, H. (2020, January 1). *How to handle a misdirected fax containing patient information*. HIPAAtrek. https://hipaatrek.com/misdirected-fax/

Siegler, E. (2010). The evolving medical record. *Annals of Internal Medicine, 153*(10), 671–677.

Singh, H., & Sittig, D. F. (2015). Advancing the science of measurement of diagnostic errors in healthcare: The Safer Dx framework. *BMJ Quality & Safety, 24*(2), 103–110.

Sinhasane, S. (2020, January 1). *Voice technology: Reinventing healthcare and exploring more possibilities*. Mobisoft Infotech. https://mobisoftinfotech.com/resources/blog/voice-technology-in-healthcare/

Sittig, D. F., & Singh, H. (2010). A new sociotechnical model for studying health information technology in complex adaptive healthcare systems. *Quality & Safety in Health Care, 19*(Suppl 3), i68–i74. Suppl 3.

Staggers, N., Elias, B. L., Makar, E., & Alexander, G. L. (2018). The imperative of solving nurses' usability problems with health information technology. *The Journal of Nursing Administration, 48*(4), 191–196.

Story, M. F. (2010). *Medical devices in home health care*. National Research Council 2010. In *The role of human factors in home health care: Workshop summary* (pp. 145–172). The National Academies Press. doi:10.17226/12927

Sutton, R. T., Pincock, D., Baumgart, D. C., Sadowski, D. C., Fedorak, R. N., & Kroeker, K. I. (2020). An overview of clinical decision support systems: Benefits, risks, and strategies for success. *NPJ Digital Medicine, 3*(1), 1–10.

Symbient. (2020, August 7). *Applications of point of care diagnostic devices*. SymbientProduct Development. https://www.symbientpd.com/applications-of-point-of-care-diagnostic-devices/

Tableau. (n.d.). Data cleaning: The benefits and steps to creating and using clean data. Tableau. Retrieved May 25, 2021, from https://www.tableau.com/learn/articles/what-is-data-cleaning

Tahir, D. (2020). *Coronavirus adds new stress to antiquated health record-keeping*. Politico. https://www.politico.com/news/2020/03/11/coronavirus-health-record-keeping-125841

Talend. (n.d.). *Structured vs. Unstructured data: A complete guide*. Talend. Retrieved May 23, 2021, from https://www.talend.com/resources/structured-vs-unstructured-data/

The Journal of MHealth. (2019). *Technology in Nursing Today*. Retrieved May 31, 2021, from. https://thejournalofmhealth.com/technology-in-nursing-today/

TigerConnect. (n.d.a). *Smart bed integration*.TigerConnect. Retrieved June 14, 2021, from https://tigerconnect.com/products/smart-bed-integration/

TigerConnect. (n.d.b). *What is virtual healthcare?* FAQs. TigerConnect. Retrieved June 7, 2021, from https://tigerconnect.com/about/faqs/what-is-virtual-healthcare/

TigerConnect. (2018). *6+ benefits of effective communication in nursing*. TigerConnect Blog. https://tigerconnect.com/blog/nine-ways-nurse-communication-improves-deliver-healthcare/

TigerConnect. (2019). *5 benefits of interprofessional collaboration in healthcare*. TigerConnect Blog. https://tigerconnect.com/blog/5-benefits-of-interprofessional-collaboration-in-healthcare/

Tilmans, T. (2014). The universal image viewer. *HealthManagement, 14(4).* https://healthmanagement.org/c/healthmanagement/issuearticle/the-universal-image-viewer

Total HIPAA. (2020, June 16). *HIPAA compliant efax provider recommendations.*Total HIPAA. https://www.totalhipaa.com/hipaa-compliant-efax-provider-recommendations/

Tsymbal, O. (n.d.). *Technology trends in healthcare in 2021: The rise of AI.* MobiDev Blog. Retrieved June 1, 2021, from https://mobidev.biz/blog/technology-trends-healthcare-digital-transformation

University of Illinois Chicago Online Health Informatics. (2020). *Tools and strategies for visualizing health data.* October 21: UIC Online Health Informatics. https://healthinformatics.uic.edu/blog/health-data-visualization/

Upadhyay, I. (2021). *20 types of cyber attacks to be aware of in 2021.* Jigsaw Academy Blog. Retrieved June 18, 2021, from https://www.jigsawacademy.com/blogs/cyber-security/types-of-cyber-attacks/

US Department of Health and Human Services (HHS). (2021). *A prescription for health sector cybersecurity.*https://www.hhs.gov/about/agencies/asa/ocio/hc3/index.html

US Food and Drug Administration (FDA). (2017). *Home healthcare medical devices: A checklist.* https://www.fda.gov/medical-devices/home-health-and-consumer-devices/brochure-home-healthcare-medical-devices-checklist

US Food and Drug Administration (FDA). (2018a). *Radio frequency identification (RFID).* https://www.fda.gov/radiation-emitting-products/electromagnetic-compatibility-emc/radio-frequency-identification-rfid

US Food and Drug Administration (FDA). (2018b). *Wireless medical devices.* https://www.fda.gov/medical-devices/digital-health-center-excellence/wireless-medical-devices

US Food and Drug Administration (FDA). (2020). Electromagnetic compatibility (EMC) of medical devices - draft guidance for industry and Food and Drug Administration staff. Retrieved from https://www.fda.gov/media/143716/download

World Health Organization. (2020). *State of the world's nursing 2020: Investing in education, jobs and leadership.* https://www.who.int/publications-detail-redirect/9789240003279

Yse, D. L. (2019). *Your guide to natural language processing (NLP).* Medium. https://towardsdatascience.com/your-guide-to-natural-language-processing-nlp-48ea2511f6e1

Zhang, J., & Walji, M. F. (2011). TURF: Toward a unified framework of EHR usability. *Journal of Biomedical Informatics, 44*(6), 1056–1067.

Zhou, C., Su, F., Pei, T., Zhang, A., Du, Y., Luo, B., Cao, Z., Wang, J., Yuan, W., Zhu, Y., Song, C., Chen, J., Xu, J., Li, F., Ma, T., Jiang, L., Yan, F., Yi, J., Hu, Y., … Xiao, H. (2020). COVID-19: Challenges to GIS with big data. *Geography and Sustainability, 1*(1), 77–87.

23 USING HEALTHCARE INFORMATION TECHNOLOGY TO EVALUATE AND IMPROVE PERFORMANCE AND PATIENT OUTCOMES

MARISA L. WILSON

"Better a diamond with a flaw than a pebble without."
~ Confucius

CHAPTER CONTENTS

INFORMATICS AND INFORMATION TECHNOLOGY SUPPORTING IMPROVED PERFORMANCE AND OUTCOMES 746
Coding Taxonomies and Classification Systems 747
REGULATORY REPORTING INITIATIVES THAT DRIVE PERFORMANCE IMPROVEMENT 751
Current Reporting Requirements 751
New Reporting Requirements of MACRA 755
RELEVANCE OF REGULATORY REPORTING TO ADVANCED PRACTICE NURSING OUTCOMES 761
The National Provider Identifier Number 762
FOUNDATIONAL COMPETENCIES IN MANAGING HEALTH INFORMATION TECHNOLOGY 762
Descriptive, Predictive, and Prescriptive Data Analytics 763
FOUNDATIONAL COMPETENCIES IN QUALITY IMPROVEMENT 768
Continuous Quality Improvement Frameworks 768
Organizational Structures and Cultures That Optimize Performance Improvement 769
STRATEGIES FOR DESIGNING QUALITY IMPROVEMENT AND OUTCOME EVALUATION PLANS FOR ADVANCED PRACTICE NURSING 770
Phases of Preparing a Plan for Outcome Evaluation 770
Define the Data Elements 774
Derive Meaning From Data and Act on Results 776
Clarify Purpose of the Advanced Practice Nurse's Role 778
CONCLUSION 779
KEY SUMMARY POINTS 780

This chapter will introduce the need for outcomes evaluation for advanced practice registered nurses (APRNs), the regulatory and reimbursement mandates pushing this forward, and the informatics and information technology tools and processes required for conducting this work. In this chapter, the terms *outcome evaluation* and *performance improvement* will be used interchangeably and may refer to three levels of outcome evaluation: (1) activities that evaluate individual APRN practice, such as peer review; (2) activities that evaluate the collective value of all APRNs to an organization or population, such as a research or demonstration project; or (3) outcomes in clinical populations served by all providers, including APRNs, in an organization or population. Depending on the nature of the outcome evaluation activity and metrics used to monitor performance, these activities may at times overlap *and* are not always mutually exclusive.

APRN contributions to patient or population outcomes, as an individual provider or as a member of a team, will become increasingly important in the transformation of care.

Early in 2021, two guiding documents emerged providing significant reconsideration of the expected foundational competencies of all nurses, including advanced practice nurses. The first is *The Essentials: Core Competencies for Professional Nursing Education* (American Association of Colleges of Nursing [AACN], 2021), and the second is *The Future of Nursing 2020–2030: Charting a Path to Achieve Health Equity* (National Academies of Science, Engineering, and Medicine [NASEM], 2021). The AACN outlined a new two-level model for academic nursing, entry to practice and advanced, with advanced inclusive of master's and doctor of nursing practice graduates (AACN, 2021). For each level, the AACN described reenvisioned essential competencies required to respond to practice partners' expressed needs and external healthcare and society demand (AACN, 2021). Ten domains are offered along with expected competencies and measurable subcompetencies for all graduates of nursing programs, entry and advanced (AACN, 2021). In addition to requiring advanced practice nurses to lead change with all forms of information technology available and in use in care settings, the AACN *Essentials* (2021), Domain 8, Informatics and Healthcare Technology, also directs that advanced practice nurses be competent to generate information and knowledge from the data gathered and stored within health information technology databases. The *Essentials* document also mandates that advanced practice nurses use standardized data to evaluate decision making and outcomes across all systems levels and that they have the knowledge and skill to use primary and secondary data to support and evaluate care (AACN, 2021). It provides a road map of demonstrable and measurable knowledge, skills, and attitudes that students must be able to attain in order to graduate.

In addition to the AACN *Essentials* and almost simultaneous to that document release, a select expert committee of the National Academy of Medicine released *The Future of Nursing 2020–2030: Charting a Path to Achieve Health Equity* (NASEM, 2021), which makes clear that the upcoming decade will test the competencies and expectations of nearly 4 million US nurses. The committee indicated that to advance health equity and improve the health outcomes of the nation, nursing capacity and expertise to address equity issues must be strengthened (NASEM, 2021). The authors state that barriers need to be lifted to expand the contributions of nurses and that payment models must be designed to reimburse team-based care that demonstrates a positive impact on social determinants of health and, ultimately, equity and outcomes. The authors offer several key recommendations that directly impact APRNs and their ability to manage data and information to guide program development and care. In addition to recommending expansion of the scope of practice for APRNs to increase access to care and decrease health inequities, the committee recommended (NASEM, 2021):

1. All organizations, including state and federal entities and employing organizations, should enable nurses to practice to the full extent of their education and training by removing barriers that prevent them from addressing social determinants of health.
2. All public and private healthcare systems should incorporate nursing expertise in designing, generating, analyzing, and applying data to support initiatives focused on social determinants of health and health equity using diverse digital platforms, artificial intelligence, and other innovative technologies.

Both of these recommendations address interventions of APRNs to positively impact the health outcomes of patients and populations; however, they require APRNs to be competent in data management and analysis and to act on the findings.

It is known that APRNs make positive impacts on the health outcomes of those they serve; however, to ensure full practice authority across the country, the impact must be quantified and demonstrated. In 1965 Dr. Loretta Ford and Dr. Henry Silver developed the first pediatric nurse practitioner program at the University of Colorado. Since that time, the role and professional practice of the APRN has been well described (Archibald & Fraser, 2013; Honeyfield, 2009; Sackett et al., 1974; Vleet & Paradise, 2015; Wang-Romjue, 2018). The impact of APRN professional practice, compared with similar care provided by physicians, has also been well described and has been demonstrated to be safe, of high quality, and cost effective (McCleery et al., 2014; Mundinger et al., 2000; Newhouse et al., 2011; Stanik-Hutt et al., 2013). However, studies with a purpose of comparison between providers individually or as a group have proven to have methodological challenges due to previous inconsistencies in automated data collection as a byproduct of care, lack of data specificity, and data storage. Other challenges have been the automated attribution, or misattribution, of interventions and outcomes to specific providers or groups of provider types. Despite these challenges and based on the available evidence, many state legislative bodies are following the recommendation of the National Academy of Medicine directing all nurses, including APRNs, to practice at the top of their license. According to the American Association of Nurse Practitioners, as of 2021, nurse practitioners in 28 states and the District of Columbia have full practice authority (American Academy of Nurse Practitioners, 2022). This is demonstrated as autonomous practice through the repeal of restrictive practice laws which serves to increase access to quality care for millions of citizens (NASEM, 2021; National Governor's Association, 2012). Thus APRNs have seen increasing independence, authority, and responsibility. However, there remains a need to continue to demonstrate comparable outcomes between and among providers. Kleinpell and Kapu (2017) highlighted the urgent need for APRNs to participate in and lead efforts to measure the impact of APRN practice as models of care continue to develop and expand and the external pressures to demonstrate the evidence remain unabated. Moreover, work that has been aimed at healthcare reform to improve quality and efficiency while containing escalating costs continues. Pressure to demonstrate impact of care using data collected and stored in electronic records remains a constant. The goal is to differentiate outcomes by provider type so that APRN full practice authority can be gained consistently across the country in an ever-changing healthcare system landscape.

Finally, this information is needed by the public to help raise awareness that APRNs can deliver quality care in cost-effective ways. This means that it is every APRN's responsibility to engage fully in evaluative activities, not only to fulfill regulatory and reimbursement mandates, but also to inform all stakeholders, including other APRNs, about the effectiveness of their practice.

INFORMATICS AND INFORMATION TECHNOLOGY SUPPORTING IMPROVED PERFORMANCE AND OUTCOMES

Since the 1960s, providers and facilities have slowly been implementing a variety of technologies to support care and provide data for outcomes measurement. Over the last decade, this movement toward technology has accelerated. As of 2017, electronic health records (EHRs), patient portals, bar code administration systems, point-of-care devices, wearable physiologic device monitors with integration, and system interoperability mechanisms are in use in over 96% of hospitals and over 75% of provider offices offering a foundation for safe, quality, and efficient care (US Department of Health and Human Services [DHHS], 2019). The APRN must be aware of and be able to manage the array of information systems and devices in use to collect patient data in order to evaluate fully the outcomes of care. These technologies are described in detail in Chapter 22. However, the APRN must consider that access to technology is not enough to provide the information needed to demonstrate or compare outcomes between and among providers and provider types. It is the ability of the APRN to use these technology tools to engage in informatics processes to collect data, generate information, form knowledge, and ultimately guide wisdom development (Nelson, 2020). This is a fundamental model of informatics.

The Health Information Technology for Economic and Clinical Health (HITECH) Act of 2009 was the impetus behind the wave of health information technology implementation, specifically EHRs, into healthcare settings over the last decade. The HITECH Act represented one of the largest federal investments ($29 billion) in health information technology (IT) demonstrating a broad and bipartisan commitment to realizing the potential of EHRs to transform care using data. The program widely became known as Meaningful Use (MU). To meet the requirements of MU, providers or facilities had to demonstrate:

1. the use of a certified EHR that met defined criteria,
2. the ability to exchange standardized health data and information,
3. technology to advance clinical processes, and
4. the ability to report quality measures.

The benefits of MU, upon implementation and deployment of EHRs, are to:

1. improve quality of patient care,
2. increase patient participation and engagement in their own care,
3. improve accuracy of diagnoses and outcomes through decision support and guideline use,
4. improve care coordination through data and information exchange,
5. increase efficiency and cost savings by reducing duplication, and
6. improve public and population health through data reporting, exchange, and analysis.

To benefit financially from the federal MU program, hospitals and providers had to demonstrate the ability to meet the mandates using certified technology, had to have adapted and adjusted processes to improve outcomes, and had to demonstrate adequate data collation and analysis to improve outcomes. Stage 1 of MU did result in increased adoption of health information technology, but the verdict on transformation of health care and the projected gains in cost savings and improved outcomes is still under consideration (Green, 2019). EHR technologies do play a vital role in advancing quality, safety, and efficiency; however, literature provides mixed impact on outcomes. Using a certified EHR and attesting to MU criteria are important drivers related to inpatient quality. A detailed review of inpatient hospitalization data, American Hospital Association data, and CMS Attestation data by Trout et al. (2021) indicated that healthcare leaders need to focus on improvement initiatives and advanced analytics to better leverage those EHRs in which they invested. To optimize the impact on quality and safety by the implementation of a certified EHR, multiple complex factors have to be considered. Workflow, cognitive processing, communication patterns, system sophistication and usage, and clinician buy-in all must be considered.

Coding Taxonomies and Classification Systems

In considering how the APRN can engage in evaluation of outcomes, they must consider the collection of standardized data for important concepts of interest such as diagnosis, treatment, and outcomes. Technology is built on databases with required reporting functions that use accurate, defined, and standardized terms to represent concepts of interest. These terms become the data. The data are the foundation of any solid database model from which quality measures and evaluation processes will come. In the most concrete description, concepts of interest must be clearly described and uniformly named by all providers who use the terms. Although providers still prefer to use free-text notes, concepts of interest should be coded and standardized across providers if the APRN is to use them in any evaluation process. Free-text notes can be harvested for information using natural language processing (NLP) techniques, but this is often a more difficult and time-consuming path to follow. In order to efficiently move from data to information to knowledge that can be acted on, data must be shared, compared, and standardized with taxonomies. Here are some of the most commonly used sets.

ICD-10, SNOMED CT, and LOINC

Data standards mandate how the concepts are aligned as data elements, which then allows comparisons and analysis of outcomes to occur. Good data are essential for the data–information–knowledge continuum, a foundational model of informatics. One cannot form information and knowledge without a solid foundation of accurate and comparable data. The APRN must be able to articulate the type of data they require to meet their information needs most effectively. In this regard, it is necessary for APRNs to understand how various coding taxonomies and terminology sets are used in health information management for documenting care and generating claims and how this information can be leveraged for purposes of outcome evaluation. For clarification, a *taxonomy* is a way to classify words or concepts into hierarchical groupings, while a *terminology* is a system of words that belong to something in common. For inpatient settings, this would include concepts within the *International Classification of Diseases* (ICD) version 10 or 11. ICD-10 codes are used for documentation and billing of diagnoses and procedures as well as documenting cause of mortality from death certificates. ICD codes are alphanumeric designations given to almost every diagnosis, description of symptoms, and cause of death attributed to humans. ICD codes are used worldwide. Browsing the ICD-10 website (World Health Organization, 2022), one can see a taxonomy organized under various diseases. Expanding any of the classes reveals conditions and diseases that all fall under the specific taxonomy or classification.

Concept standards also include the use of assessment and outcome terms housed within the Systematized Nomenclature of Medicine–Clinical Terms (SNOMED-CT) and the Logical Observation and Identifiers Names and Codes (LOINC), which are built into EHRs for seamless use. SNOMED-CT is a systematically organized collection of over 300,000 medical concepts that are essential for documenting clinical concepts such as problem lists and patient histories. LOINC is a clinical standardized terminology set important for laboratory test orders, results reporting, and other clinical observations. The HITECH Act mandated the use of these standards within certified EHRs so that reporting and interoperability (e.g., sharing of data between and across different EHRs, healthcare systems, and providers) can occur.

APRNs practicing in acute care hospitals must understand that for every claim there is a single principal ICD diagnosis code that indicates the primary reason for a patient's admission to the hospital. In addition, there may be multiple secondary ICD diagnosis codes that represent comorbid conditions that were present at the time of admission or conditions and complications that were acquired during the hospital stay. ICD procedure codes also have a designated principal procedure, which is typically the initial major procedure during the admission or care encounter. Many hospitals in the United States code as many as 25 to 50 secondary ICD-10 diagnoses and procedure codes in the medical claim for a hospital admission. In addition, the ICD diagnosis status flag of present on admission (POA) or not present on admission (NPOA) can be used to differentiate between hospital-acquired conditions and those acquired prior to hospitalization. This is useful when evaluating phenomenon such as hospital-acquired pneumonia, pressure ulcers, acute renal failure, and sepsis. The APRN should become familiar with the coding practices in their care settings, because not all countries or organizations have adopted the use of the POA and NPOA status flags.

APRNs practicing in the United States should also have a strong working knowledge of the Medicare Severity Diagnosis-Related Groups (MS-DRGs). The MS-DRG groupings categorize inpatient discharge diagnoses and adjust payments based on the weight of the DRGs. Each weight represents the average treatment patterns and resources used in the care of those patients (Centers for Medicare & Medicaid Services [CMS], 2022b). APRNs should understand how clinical documentation by the APRN and medical providers directly affects MS-DRG assignments and ultimately reimbursement. Many US healthcare organizations are actively implementing clinical documentation improvement (CDI) programs in their institutions for purposes of coaching and training medical providers and APRNs in improving their documentation skills for greater precision and accuracy in medical records coding and billing. Greater detail in the medical record can potentially lead to higher reimbursement and fewer denials and audits from payers, which are prevalent in the US healthcare payment system.

Finally, it may be useful for APRNs to understand other types of coding taxonomies and terminology sets that are available for purposes of quality reporting and research. Table 23.1 summarizes several common taxonomies used in inpatient and ambulatory settings. These taxonomies enable informaticians to take complex concepts and place them into databases for automated documentation, storage, and retrieval. As an example, the human brain can immediately form an image of acute abdominal pain as a complex, multifactorial concept, but a computer database cannot. This complex concept consists of three concepts: the concepts of acute (versus benign), abdominal (as a specified location), and pain (as a phenomenon of interest). Each of these concepts would be separate entities in a database. With this level of granularity, an APRN looking for all patients with acute abdominal pain could locate them in the database.

TABLE 23.1

Coding Taxonomies and Terminology Sets Commonly Used in Outcomes

Coding Taxonomy	Description	Website
ICD-10-CM	*International Classification of Diseases*, Tenth Revision, Clinical Modification Published by the World Health Organization and based upon the *International Classification of Diseases*, which houses unique alphanumeric codes to identify known diseases and other health problems. ICD 10 includes more than 68,000 diagnostic codes and reasons for visits	http://www.cdc.gov/nchs/icd/icd10cm.htm
ICD-10-PC	ICD-10 Procedure Codes Approximately 87,000 available codes, seven alphanumeric characters in length Used by most countries worldwide to classify procedures for inpatient hospital claims Coding set very specific, provides for precisely defined procedures and laterality	www.cms.gov/ICD10
CPT	Current Procedural Terminology Approximately 7800 available codes for reporting medical, surgical, and diagnostic services in outpatient and office settings, as well as acute care emergency settings, ambulatory surgery, and inpatient procedures done in some hospitals outside the United States CPT is a registered trademark of the American Medical Association and is considered a proprietary terminology set requiring licensure before using inside a health information technology application New codes are released each October	https://www.ama-assn.org/practice-management/cpt
HCPCS	Healthcare Common Procedure Coding System There are two types of HCPCS codes. Level 1 HCPCS codes are identical to CPT codes used for reporting services and procedures in outpatient and office settings to Medicare, Medicaid, and private health insurers. Level II HCPCS codes are used by medical suppliers other than physicians, such as ambulance services or durable medical equipment	https://www.cms.gov/Medicare/Coding/MedHCPCSGenInfo/index.html
SNOMED-CT	Systemized Nomenclature of Medicine–Clinical Terms Complex and highly hierarchical collection of over 1 million codes and medical terms that describe diseases, procedures, symptoms, findings, and more Developed by the College of American Pathologists and the National Health Service (Britain) Used extensively throughout the world, SNOMED-CT codes help organize content in the electronic health record and crosswalk to other terminologies such as ICD-10 and LOINC SDOH Z Codes	www.snomed.org https://www.cms.gov/files/document/zcodes-infographic.pdf
LOINC	Logical Observation Identifiers Names and Codes Universal standard containing 58,000 observation terms for identifying medical laboratory tests and clinical observations, as well as nursing diagnosis, nursing interventions, outcomes classification, and patient care data sets Originally developed in the United States in 1994; international adoption expanding rapidly	http://loinc.org
RxNorm	Standardized nomenclature for clinical drugs produced by the National Library of Medicine. This data set is updated monthly to stay abreast of the rapidly changing pharmaceutical industry. It contains links between national drug codes, which are used widely in EHRs and e-prescribing systems	https://www.nlm.nih.gov/research/umls/rxnorm/docs/index.html

Continued

TABLE 23.1

Coding Taxonomies and Terminology Sets Commonly Used in Outcomes—cont'd

Coding Taxonomy	Description	Website
MS-DRGs	Medicare Severity-Diagnosis Related Groups Each inpatient hospital stay in the United States is assigned one of over 750 MS-DRG codes, which are used for billing to Medicare and other payers. Codes are derived from ICD diagnoses and procedure codes. Many conditions are split into one, two, or three MS-DRGs based on whether any one of the secondary diagnoses has been categorized as a major complication or comorbidity (MCC), a complication or comorbidity (CC), or no CC and are weighted accordingly to reflect severity and reimbursement. Note that a separate MS-DRG code set for long-term care is used (MS-LTC-DRG). Additional coding sets apply to other areas of care (e.g., resource utilization groups [RUGs] apply to skilled nursing and rehabilitation stays)	https://www.cms.gov/Medicare/Medicare-Fee-for-Service-Payment/AcuteInpatientPPS/index.html?redirect=/AcuteInpatientPPS/FFD/list.asp

SNOMED Z Codes: Capturing Social Determinants of Health

In addition, with the increased focus on the impact of social determinants of health (SDOH) on outcomes and on health equity, it is important to note that SDOH factors have been codified within SNOMED as a set of Z codes. The *Future of Nursing 2020–2030* report places attention on all nurses, including APRNs, attending to the SDOH data among their patients and populations serving as a pathway to health equity (NASEM, 2021). This will require the APRN to collect SDOH data on their patients in order to develop a risk score so that the APRN can address the risk that is potentially driving poor health (CMS, 2021b). An infographic from CMS describes the Z codes, data collection tools, and best practice and process considerations (CMS, 2021c). The University of California San Francisco (2022) Social Interventions Research and Evaluation Network (SIREN) is an important source of SDOH data information. SIREN houses valid and reliable SDOH data collection tools along with exemplars of projects addressing SDOH. The Gravity Project is a collaboration of experts under SIREN who are working toward the complete and standardized collection of all SDOH concepts of interest (The Gravity Project, 2021). This website provides training videos, opportunities to participate in the process, and a listing of existing SDOH codes.

Data Types

Data that have alphanumeric identifiers such as ICD or SNOMED-CT codes and can be easily queried from a database are termed *discrete* or *structured data.* Data containing dictated sentences and phrases, such as radiology reports, operative summaries, or history and physical dictations, are termed *nondiscrete* or *unstructured.* Compiling and analyzing the unstructured data from free-text notes is more challenging. Unless the organization has technology with a sophisticated reporting system containing a tool for natural language processing (NLP) with a well-developed and tested rules engine, it is very difficult to mine information and knowledge from free-text notes. As an example, it would be difficult to differentiate between patients with active pneumonia and those without because the narrative may contain phrases such as "pneumonia ruled out" or "no signs of pneumonia." If the APRN was trying to review data on the outcomes of patients with active pneumonia, free-text mining may yield too many false-positives to be a reliable and valid screening tool. Manual extraction of these data is not typically feasible on an ongoing basis for the number of patients needed to measure outcomes effectively and accurately.

Although it is not necessary for the APRN to understand the nuances and precision behind coding processes, it is highly recommended that APRNs spend time interacting with a coder (also referred to as a health information management specialist) or an informatician to understand the timing and ways the various terminology sets are used. This is important to outcomes evaluation because some types of data are more useful than others, even though they represent similar concepts. For example, the phenomenon of pneumonia could be captured from a claim (using an ICD-10 diagnosis or Current Procedural Terminology [CPT]-4 code), laboratory culture and sensitivity report (using LOINC and RxNorm codes), problem list in the EHR (using SNOMED-CT codes), chest imaging report (using NLP), or a dictated history and physical report (requiring manual chart abstraction). Although each source of information in the EHR may be correct, the APRN may have to determine the best source of information to address the nature of the inquiry in the most timely, efficient, and accurate manner. Exemplar 23.1 illustrates the critical evaluation of the various data types that an APRN would explore when planning to deploy a new strategy to improve care, as well as the collaborative process with quality and informatics specialists that will benefit the APRN in the outcome evaluation efforts.

REGULATORY REPORTING INITIATIVES THAT DRIVE PERFORMANCE IMPROVEMENT

In the United States, legislative regulatory and reporting requirements are released by the CMS or DHHS and posted in the *Federal Registry* numerous times each year. Requirements were released in November 2016 that significantly impact the mandated reporting of performance and outcomes of providers, whether that provider is a physician or APRN.

Current Reporting Requirements

The United States is evolving from a pay-for-service and pay-for-reporting culture to one of pay-for-performance. In 2015 a significant change to provider reimbursement for services billed to the CMS was enacted to promote value. With the Medicare Access and CHIP Re-Authorization Act of 2015 (MACRA), CMS moved toward rewarding high-value, high-quality providers of care to Medicare patients with payment increases if performance standards are met; conversely payments are reduced if performance expectations are not met (Quality Payment Program, n.d.c). MACRA is a CMS initiative to improve quality of care through engagement of evidence-based practice to address a gap or quality issue, and by monitoring impact of the project on outcomes. MACRA requires qualified providers (inclusive of nurse practitioners [NPs], certified registered nurses anesthetists [CRNA], and clinical nurse specialists [CNSs]) to enroll in one of two Quality Payment Programs (QPPs). The QPPs are Merit-Based Incentive Payment Systems (MIPS) and the Alternative Payment Model (APM; CMS, 2021b)

The QPP started in January 2017 with the objectives to (1) improve beneficiary population health, (2) improve care received by Medicare beneficiaries, (3) lower costs to the Medicare program through improvement of care and health, and (4) educate, engage, and empower patients.

CMS is continually working to improve QPP clinician and practice participation through education, outreach, and support practices; expand the APM; provide accurate, timely, and actionable performance data and measures to clinicians, patients, and stakeholders; and continuously improve the QPP based on feedback (CMS, 2021b). This site does provide a Resource Library, access to webinars, and a CMS speaker list among other resources.

As part of this site, the reader will note the variety of performance measures. The reader should note that some measures cross multiple settings and multiple diagnoses. Measures such as central line–associated bloodstream infection (CLABSI) not only apply to multiple quality reporting programs in a single healthcare facility but they also apply to multiple care settings across the continuum, including acute care hospitals, cancer care hospitals, ambulatory surgery centers, and long-term care facilities. Therefore failure to address a quality gap with CLABSI or to comply with reporting requirements has the potential to affect reimbursement across an entire healthcare system. Additional measurement and reporting requirements for specialized services and healthcare systems also exist. Box 23.1 illustrates a set of measures that are required for healthcare systems reorganizing as accountable care organizations (ACOs). The CMS defines ACOs as groups of physicians, other providers, and hospitals who come together voluntarily to

EXEMPLAR 23.1

EVALUATING DATA TYPES WHEN USING HEALTH INFORMATION TECHNOLOGY TO IMPLEMENT PRACTICE CHANGE

An APRN working in a 400-bed acute care setting needs to identify all inpatients with an active diagnosis of pneumonia to ensure that all best practice interventions have been implemented in a timely and appropriate manner. Although the performance in these areas is retrospectively monitored and reported periodically by the quality management department, the APRN wishes to engage in the process concurrently to influence outcomes for this population. The APRN's intervention is to perform clinical rounds several times a day on this population to ensure optimal delivery of best practice standards. These standards include antibiotic timeliness, appropriateness of antibiotic selection in intensive care unit (ICU) and non-ICU patients, smoking cessation advice and counseling, and influenza and pneumococcal vaccinations. The APRN wants to leverage the hospital's information systems to create a real-time alert notification system to identify and track patients with pneumonia immediately on any nursing unit and then monitor performance trends to reflect the impact of interventions on this population.

The APRN recognizes that there are multiple taxonomies and methodologies that could be used to identify pneumonia patients in the organization and begins to inventory the pros and cons of each data type and source to create the best technology solution to obtain the required data. ICD-10 diagnosis codes are a typical taxonomy for identifying patients with pneumonia. Although these codes are readily available, reliable, and robust population identifiers in other types of outcome evaluation measures used in the organization, such as length of stay, mortality, and readmissions, this approach would not be optimal because ICD-10 codes are typically not assigned until after the patient is discharged and the medical record is coded for the claim. Using this type of data element is retrospective and therefore not useable to identify patients with pneumonia on a real-time basis.

The APRN next considers a more concurrent coding methodology, which is based on the active problem lists in the EHR. In collaboration with a health information management specialist, a list of problem types and their corresponding SNOMED-CT codes is established, which can be used to identify patients with an active diagnosis of pneumonia. The APRN has observed that many medical providers in the organization do not update the problem list in the electronic health record until the patient is being discharged, which makes a real-time query unreliable.

The final option that the APRN considers is the use of radiology and laboratory reports with the words containing *pneumonia* or other related terms. In discussing this option with a nursing informatics specialist at her organization, she learns that the EHR has been fully implemented to report laboratory results for all clinical areas in the hospital and that this includes microbiology results. Using the LOINC (Logical Observation Identifiers Names and Codes) coding terminology set, patients with pneumonia can be identified as soon as the laboratory result transaction is received in the EHR. In addition, she learns of a pilot project in the Quality Department in which cardiac catheterization reports are being processed by a natural language processing (NLP) engine to capture cardiac registry information. She asks about the potential to expand this pilot to include radiology reports to identify pneumonia patients. The Quality Department agrees to expand the project scope with the help of the APRN to begin formulating a list of phrases that will be used to identify a pneumonia diagnosis in a radiology report. The APRN collaborates with the medical director of radiology to create the final list of terms to be used in the pilot.

After 3 months of implementing the practice change, the APRN is able to demonstrate that performance in five best practice indicators for patients with pneumonia is almost 100% across the organization. She tracks the compliance rates in a statistical process control (SPC) chart, which demonstrates a statistically significant favorable change in the process. Furthermore, she is able to use the organization's value-based purchasing calculator to demonstrate a financial contribution to the hospital's Medicare reimbursement program of almost $68,000 simply by improving performance. The APRN plans to make a formal recommendation to expand similar APRN interventions to other key populations influenced by pay-for-performance initiatives, including cardiac, medical, orthopedics, and stroke. Thus the APRN is able to materially demonstrate the value-added benefit of APRN clinical interventions using financial and quality analytics.

give coordinated high-quality care to their Medicare patients to ensure that patients get the right care at the right time, while avoiding unnecessary duplication of services and preventing medical errors (CMS, 2021a). These measures focus on ambulatory populations and may overlap with several other reporting programs that exist simultaneously across an integrated health-care organization, such as the measures required by the Health Resources and Services Administration (HRSA) for federally qualified health centers (see

BOX 23.1

Shared Savings Program for Accountable Care Organizations Quality Measures

CONSUMER ASSESSMENT OF HEALTHCARE PROVIDERS AND SYSTEMS (CAHPS)

- Getting timely care, appointments, and information
- How well your doctors communicate
- Patients' rating of doctor
- Access to specialists
- Health promotion and education
- Shared decision making
- Health status/functional status

CARE COORDINATION AND PATIENT SAFETY

- Ambulatory-sensitive conditions admissions—chronic obstructive pulmonary disease and heart failure (Agency for Healthcare Research and Quality prevention quality indicator)
- Number of primary care providers (%) who successfully qualify for an electronic health record incentive program payment
- Medication reconciliation after discharge from an inpatient facility
- Screening for fall risk

PREVENTIVE HEALTH

- Influenza immunization
- Pneumococcal vaccination
- Adult weight screening and follow-up
- Tobacco use assessment and tobacco cessation intervention
- Depression screening
- Colorectal cancer screening
- Mammography screening
- Proportion of adults ≥18 years who had their blood pressure measured within the preceding 2 years

AT-RISK POPULATIONS

- Diabetes composite (all or nothing scoring)—non-use of tobacco, aspirin use
- Diabetes mellitus—HbA_{1c} poor control (>9%)
- Hypertension—blood pressure control
- Ischemic vascular disease—complete lipid profile and low-density lipoprotein control <100 mg/dL, use of aspirin or another antithrombotic
- Heart failure—beta blocker therapy for left ventricular systolic dysfunction
- Coronary artery disease composite (all or nothing scoring)—angiotensin-converting enzyme inhibitor or angiotensin receptor blocker therapy for patients with coronary artery disease and diabetes and/or left ventricular systolic dysfunction

Adapted from Health Resources and Services Administration Bureau of Primary Care (2020).

Box 23.2), or measures required by providers who care for patients within selected payer niches, such as the Medicaid Adult Quality Measures Program (Box 23.3).

In addition to payer-mandated reporting programs, healthcare organizations have specific reporting requirements for their accreditation bodies, including The Joint Commission (TJC), Healthcare Facilities Accreditation Program (HFAP), and Det Norske Veritas Healthcare (DNV). It is not unusual for many of the measures required for accreditation to overlap with those reported to the CMS, although accreditation measures typically reflect an all-payer population. What is important to note is that although many of these measures are similar across reporting programs, each program has specific requirements for data collection, data quality, and data submission, which must be strictly followed to ensure proper accreditation, achieve financial incentives, or avoid financial penalties.

Given this broad array of reporting mandates, APRNs should become familiar with the regulatory reporting requirements of their organization. The National Quality Forum (NQF) Community Tool to Align Measurement is a useful tool for the APRN to review. This tool will help the APRN become familiar with the measures required for a specific practice setting. This tool organizes NQF-endorsed clinical quality measures associated with major national and

BOX 23.2

Health Resources & Services Administration (HRSA) Uniform Data Set for Clinical Quality Measures and Related Healthy People 2020 Goals

- Early entry into prenatal care
- Childhood immunization status
- Cervical and breast cancer screening
- Weight assessment and counseling for nutrition and physical activity of children and adolescents
- Preventive care and screening: Body mass index (BMI) screening and follow-up
- Preventive care and screening: Tobacco use screening and cessation intervention
- Statin therapy for the prevention and treatment of cardiovascular disease
- Ischemic vascular disease: Use of aspirin or another antiplatelet
- Colorectal cancer screening
- Depression measures
- Human immunodeficiency virus (HIV) measures
- Dental sealant

Adapted from Health Resources and Services Administration Bureau of Primary Care (2020).

BOX 23.3

Medicaid Adult Quality Reporting Quality Measures

PREVENTION AND HEALTH PROMOTION

- Flu shots for adults ages 50 to 64 years (collected as part of HEDIS CAHPS supplemental survey)
- Adult body mass index assessment
- Breast cancer screening
- Cervical cancer screening
- Medical assistance with smoking and tobacco use cessation (collected as part of HEDIS CAHPS supplemental survey)
- Screening for clinical depression and follow-up plan
- Plan all-cause readmission
- Diabetes, short-term complications admission rate
- Chronic obstructive pulmonary disease admission rate
- Congestive heart failure admission rate
- Adult asthma admission rate
- Chlamydia screening in women ages 21 to 24 years

MANAGEMENT OF ACUTE CONDITIONS

- Follow-up after hospitalization for mental illness
- Elective delivery
- Antenatal steroids
- Heart failure admission rates
- Chronic obstructive pulmonary disease or asthma in older adults admission rate

BEHAVIORAL HEALTH AND SUBSTANCE ABUSE

- Initiation and engagement of alcohol and other drug dependence treatment
- Antidepressant medication management
- Follow-up after hospitalization for mental illness
- Diabetes screening for people with schizophrenia and bipolar disorder
- Adherence to antipsychotics for individuals with schizophrenia
- Use of opioids at high dosage

MANAGEMENT OF CHRONIC CONDITIONS

- Annual HIV/AIDS medical visit
- Controlling high blood pressure
- Comprehensive diabetes care: Low-density lipoprotein cholesterol screening, HbA_1c testing
- Antidepressant medication management
- Adherence to antipsychotics for individuals with schizophrenia
- Annual monitoring for patients on persistent medications

FAMILY EXPERIENCES OF CARE

- HCAHPS health plan survey v4.0—adult questionnaire with CAHPS health plan survey v4.0, H-NCQA supplemental

BOX 23.3

Medicaid Adult Quality Reporting Quality Measures—cont'd

CARE COORDINATION

- Care transition record transmitted to healthcare professional

AVAILABILITY

- Initiation and engagement of alcohol and other drug dependence treatment
- Prenatal and postpartum care—postpartum care rate

Adapted from Centers for Medicare & Medicaid Services. (2016). Adult health care quality measure. https://www.medicaid.gov/medicaid/quality-of-care/downloads/ffy-2016-adult-core-set-measurement-periods.pdf

state reporting initiatives for all practice settings into a single spreadsheet, which can then be sorted by various programs of interest. Hyperlinks are embedded in the spreadsheet so that it is easy to access the Quality Positioning System on the NQF website, on which measure definitions for each metric are maintained (NQF, 2022).

Traditionally, many reporting requirements required manual chart abstraction, along with an element of clinical judgment for accurate reporting on whether or not a particular standard of evidence-based best practice was met. Questions such as "Did the patient get smoking cessation advice prior to discharge?" are typically abstracted by a review of patient education documentation in the medical record. However, some questions, such as "Was the patient eligible for angiotensin-converting enzyme inhibitors at discharge?" may require a review and synthesis of multiple sources of information in the record, including the history and physical examination, cardiac imaging tests, or medical provider progress notes, before a determination can be made. These review activities can be time-consuming and may not always be reliable. APRNs may be engaged in many aspects of the data collection and analysis activities associated with chart-abstracted data. Today, through the MU provisions, EHRs need to demonstrate the ability for all providers including APRNs to electronically mine data and produce the needed reporting. However, even while the system can automate the reporting process, the data and results still need to be reviewed for accuracy of content and context, which requires human review. In addition, the quality reporting can only demonstrate outcomes. To produce true changes in outcomes, the APRN needs to engage in gap or need identification to determine what specific changes are needed in care. Once the gap or need is identified, the APRN has to seek evidence, weigh and grade literature, translate findings, accommodate local need, develop and implement interventions, and then evaluate outcomes through data analysis. The APRN needs to use quality improvement processes to truly address quality care, which requires the tools of data and technology along with informatics support. Table 23.2 provides resources for quality improvement activities that are needed to support the measures. For example, it is not enough just to report that smoking cessation advice was given to a proportion of patients based on EHR check box documentation. The APRN needs to use evidence to build a process to address smoking cessation successfully with patients, including options for intervention and referral, and then use the data to evaluate the success of the intervention outcome.

Moreover, additional regulatory reporting requirements are beginning to emerge in the areas of patient safety, an area in which APRNs can have significant impact. The Patient Safety and Quality Improvement Act of 2005 established a voluntary patient safety event reporting system and guidelines for the establishment of patient safety organizations (Agency for Healthcare Research and Quality [AHRQ], 2005). This act called for the standardization of data used for adverse event reporting based on the common formats established and maintained by AHRQ. Some of the risk events being reported include medication errors, patient falls, central line infections, and pressure ulcers.

New Reporting Requirements of MACRA

In April 2015, the Medicare Access and CHIP Reauthorization Act (MACRA) became law. MACRA then

TABLE 23.2

Quality Improvement and Outcome Assessment Website Resources

Resource and Information Available	Website
Agency for Healthcare Research and Quality (AHRQ) Supports evidence-based practice centers, outcomes and effectiveness trials, national quality measures clearinghouse	www.ahrq.gov
American Society for Quality (ASQ) Contains tools for cause analysis, evaluation and decision-making, data collection and analysis, idea creation, project planning, and implementation ASQ offers certification, training and ongoing education in quality improvement (QI) techniques	http://asq.org/learn-about-quality/quality-tools.html
Centers for Medicare and Medicaid Services Transforming Clinical Practice Initiative This initiative is designed to help clinicians achieve large-scale health transformation to improve quality of patient care and manage costs	https://innovation.cms.gov/initiatives/Transforming-Clinical-Practices/
Institute for Healthcare Improvement (IHI) Offers training and ongoing education in QI techniques Promotes healthcare innovation through fellowships, the IHI Open School, and networking	http://www.ihi.org/Pages/default.aspx
Mind Tools Excellent site for learning skills in change management, team-building, brainstorming, straw man concept, strategy tools, leadership skills, and project management	http://www.mindtools.com
National Association for Healthcare Quality Promotes continuous improvement of quality in health care by providing educational and development opportunities and national certification as a Certified Professional of Healthcare Quality	www.nahq.org
National Committee for Quality Assurance Develops the Health Effectiveness Data and Information Set (HEDIS) to measure quality of care delivered by US health plans Offers online training and seminars on a wide range of quality-related topics	www.ncqa.org
National Database of Nursing Quality Indicators Collects and evaluates unit-specific nurse-sensitive data from US hospitals	https://www.nursingquality.org
National Network of Public Health Institutes Dedicated to improving public health through innovation, QI and education Website includes QI tools and frameworks (e.g., aim statements, balanced scorecard templates, brainstorming, fishbone, cause and effect diagrams, force field analysis, Kaizen, Lean, story board, radar charts, tree diagrams, interrelationship diagrams, and others that may be useful in outcome evaluation)	https://nnphi.org/phln/
National Quality Forum (NQF), Community Tool to Align Measurement Excel spreadsheet inventory of NQF-endorsed measures for one or more of the national reporting programs, including the Aligning Forces for Quality Alliances in regions across the United States Also includes drill-down to the Quality Positioning System for quick access to measure definitions of NQF-endorsed measures These resources are in the public domain and do not require membership	http://www.qualityforum.org/AlignmentTool/

TABLE 23.2

Quality Improvement and Outcome Assessment Website Resources—cont'd

Resource and Information Available	Website
Public Health Foundation, QI Quick Guide Tutorial Online tutorial for review of the plan–do–check–act (PDCA) process, plus additional resources for population outcomes evaluation	http://www.phf.org/quickguide/LeftNavTwoPanel.aspx?Page=Introduction
The Joint Commission (TJC) Maintains measure definitions for hospital quality reporting programs Provides educational offerings for quality improvement and accreditation standards Expanding international presence	www.jointcommission.org

went into effect on January 1, 2017. In 2019 providers participating in the program who demonstrated positive performance measures under the domains of quality, costs, improvement activities, and the use of health information technology began receiving payment adjustments through Medicare. MACRA substantially changed how Medicare payments are made to all providers including NPs, CNSs, CRNAs, and physician assistants. As described earlier, MACRA mandates that Medicare payments be based on quality through the described QPP with two payment paths for designated providers: MIPS and APM (CMS, 2022a).

MACRA provides opportunities to use the data to compare outcomes across provider types if the data are aligned to a specific provider through an identifier. MACRA is broader than reimbursement as it ties payment and reward to outcomes and quality of care. MACRA consolidated three previous quality reporting programs: the Physician Quality Reporting System (PQRS), the Value-Based Payment Modifier, and Meaningful Use.

MACRA payment adjustments began January 1, 2019; however, data were retrospective to provider experiences from January 1, 2017.

Merit-Based Incentive Program System (MIPS)

MIPS is one of two payment models. MIPS-eligible providers do not have to participate in the MIPS program if they do not meet the volume threshold: if they have less than $90,000 in allowable charges, or less than or equal to 200 Medicare patients, or less than or equal to 200 charge line items. Based on the current proposed rule, MIPS attributes provider performance across four categories:

1. **Quality:** For 2021, quality constitutes 40% of the score. The provider chooses six measures to report on from a list of options that align with their patient population needs. CMS ensures these options accommodate differences among specialties and practices. One of the six quality measures must include a measure that tracks an outcome for a minimum of 90 days. Table 23.3 lists the categories of MIPS measures along with one example measure. For a complete listing of the over 200 measures across all specialties, go to https://qpp.cms.gov/mips/explore-measures?tab=qualityMeasures&py=2021. In addition, there are some core measures that cross all specialties such as care planning for patients over 65 years of age to document an advance care plan or surrogate decision maker in the medical record. Another example of a measure that crosses specialties is documentation of current medications in the medical record.
2. **Promoting Interoperability:** (EHR MU). For 2021, promoting interoperability is 25% of the total score. The provider will choose customizable measures reflecting daily technology use to manage and share patient information. CMS intends to emphasize interoperability and information exchange with the goal of having patient records available across all systems, allowing providers needed access. The Promoting Interoperability category also emphasizes patient access to their own record and improved patient engagement in their own care and health management. There are four objectives with multiple measures in this category: ePrescribing, Provider to Patient

TABLE 23.3

Quality Patient Program Measure Categories With Example Measures

Specialty Measure Set	Example Measure
Allergy/Immunology	Percentage of patients, aged 18 years and older, with a diagnosis of acute sinusitis who were prescribed an antibiotic within 10 days after onset of symptoms
Anesthesiology	Percentage of patients, regardless of age, who undergo surgical or therapeutic procedures under general or neuraxial anesthesia of 60 minutes duration or longer for whom at least one body temperature greater than or equal to 35.5°C (or 95.9°F) was recorded within the 30 minutes immediately before or the 15 minutes immediately after anesthesia end time
Cardiology	Percentage of patients aged 18 years and older with a diagnosis of coronary artery disease (CAD) seen within a 12-month period who were prescribed aspirin or clopidogrel
Dermatology	Percentage of patients, regardless of age, with a current diagnosis of melanoma or a history of melanoma whose information was entered, at least once within a 12-month period, into a recall system that includes: A target date for the next complete physical skin exam, AND A process to follow up with patients who either did not make an appointment within the specified time frame or who missed a scheduled appointment
Diagnostic Radiology	Percentage of final reports for computed tomography (CT) imaging studies of the thorax for patients aged 18 years and older with documented follow-up recommendations for incidentally detected pulmonary nodules (e.g., follow-up CT imaging studies needed or that no follow-up is needed) based at a minimum on nodule size AND patient risk factors
Electrophysiology/ Cardiac Specialist	Patients with physician-specific risk-standardized rates of procedural complications following the first-time implantation of an implantable cardio-defibrillator
Emergency Medicine	Percentage of children 3–18 years of age who were diagnosed with pharyngitis, ordered an antibiotic, and received a group A streptococcus (strep) test for the episode
Gastroenterology	The percentage of patients greater than 85 years of age who received a screening colonoscopy from January 1 to December 31
General Oncology	Proportion of female patients (aged 18 years and older) with breast cancer who are human epidermal growth factor receptor 2 (HER2)/neu negative who are not administered HER2-targeted therapies
General Practice/Family Medicine	Percentage of patients aged 2 years and older with a diagnosis of acute otitis externa (AOE) who were not prescribed systemic antimicrobial therapy
General Surgery	Percentage of patients aged 18 years and older who required an anastomotic leak intervention following gastric bypass or colectomy surgery
Hospitalists	Percentage of patients with sepsis due to methicillin-sensitive Staphylococcus aureus bacteremia who received beta-lactam antibiotic (e.g., nafcillin, oxacillin, or cefazolin) as definitive therapy
Internal Medicine	Percentage of patients, regardless of age, who are active injection drug users who received screening for hepatitis C virus infection within the 12-month reporting period
Interventional Radiology	Percentage of new patients whose biopsy results have been reviewed and communicated to the primary care/referring physician and patient by the performing physician
Mental/Behavioral Health	Percentage of individuals at least 18 years of age as of the beginning of the measurement period with schizophrenia or schizoaffective disorder who had at least two prescriptions filled for any antipsychotic medication and who had a proportion of days covered (PDC) of at least 0.8 for antipsychotic medications during the measurement period (12 consecutive months)
Neurology	Percentage of patients diagnosed with amyotrophic lateral sclerosis (ALS) who were offered assistance in planning for end-of-life issues (e.g., advance directives, invasive ventilation, hospice) at least once annually
Obstetrics/Gynecology	Percentage of women 50–74 years of age who had a mammogram to screen for breast cancer
Ophthalmology	Patients aged 18 years and older who had surgery for primary rhegmatogenous retinal detachment who did not require a return to the operating room within 90 days of surgery

TABLE 23.3

Quality Patient Program Measure Categories With Example Measures—cont'd

Specialty Measure Set	Example Measure
Orthopedic Surgery	Percentage of patients 18 years of age and older with primary total hip arthroplasty (THA) who completed baseline and follow-up patient-reported functional status assessments
Otolaryngology	Percentage of patients aged 2 years and older with a diagnosis of AOE who were prescribed topical preparations
Pathology	Percentage of esophageal biopsy reports that document the presence of Barrett's mucosa that also include a statement about dysplasia
Pediatrics	Percentage of children 2 years of age who had four diphtheria, tetanus, and acellular pertussis (DTaP); three polio (IPV); one measles, mumps, and rubella (MMR); three *Haemophilius influenza* type B (HiB); three hepatitis B (Hep B); one varicella zoster virus (chicken pox) (VZV); four pneumococcal conjugate (PCV); one hepatitis A (Hep A); two or three rotavirus (RV); and two influenza (flu) vaccines by their second birthday
Physical Medicine	Percentage of visits for patients aged 18 years and older with documentation of a current functional outcome assessment using a standardized functional outcome assessment tool on the date of the encounter AND documentation of a care plan based on identified functional outcome deficiencies on the date of the identified deficiencies
Plastic Surgery	Percentage of patients aged 18 years and older who had a surgical site infection (SSI)
Preventive Medicine	Percentage of patients 18–85 years of age who had a diagnosis of hypertension and whose blood pressure was adequately controlled (<140/90 mm Hg) during the measurement period
Radiation Oncology	Percentage of visits for patients, regardless of age, with a diagnosis of cancer currently receiving chemotherapy or radiation therapy who report having pain with a documented plan of care to address pain
Rheumatology	Percentage of patients aged 18 years and older with a diagnosis of rheumatoid arthritis (RA) who have an assessment and classification of disease prognosis at least once within 12 months
Thoracic Surgery	Percentage of patients who underwent a nonemergency surgery who had their personalized risks of postoperative complications assessed by their surgical team prior to surgery using a clinical data-based, patient-specific risk calculator and who received personal discussion of those risks with the surgeon
Urology	Percentage of new patients whose biopsy results have been reviewed and communicated to the primary care/referring physician and patient by the performing physician
Vascular Surgery	Percent of asymptomatic patients undergoing carotid endarterectomy who are discharged to home no later than postoperative day 2

For a complete and up-to-date list, see: Quality Payment Program. (n.d.a). Explore measures and activities. https://qpp.cms.gov/mips/explore measures?tab=qualityMeasures&py=2021

Exchange, Health Information Exchange, and Public Health and Clinical Data Exchange. This MIPS category is a reconfiguration of the original Meaningful Use measures. For a complete list of specific measures, see the Quality Payment Program, Promoting Interoperability Measures: Traditional MIPS Requirements at https://qpp.cms.gov/mips/promoting-interoperability

3. **Clinical Practice Improvement:** For 2021, the category Improvement Activities accounts for 15% of the final score. The provider must perform between one and four improvement activities depending on reporting requirements. There are multiple activities to choose from, including provide real-time access to patient medical records by providers, use telehealth services that expand practice, collect and use patient experience and satisfaction data, anticoagulant management improvement, glycemic management services, and engagement of community for health status improvement. Under each category, there are multiple activities from which to choose. MIPS participants attest to completing a combination of high-weighted and medium-weighted im-

provement activities for a minimum of 90 days (Quality Payment Program, n.d.b). Table 23.4 lists example activities under each of the nine categories. Improvement activities also include the use of health IT functions such as the capture of social, psychological, and behavioral data, as well as technology that can generate and exchange an electronic care plan to other providers to support these improvement activities.

4. **Cost/Resource Use:** For 2021, the category Cost Requirements accounts for 20% of the final score. However, for 2021, the cost performance category will be reweighted to 5% for MIPS entities that choose to report to traditional MIPS and report both quality and improvement activity data. A provider's score will be based on Medicare claims using episode-specific measures to account for differences among specialties. This category is based on the current Value-Based Payment Modifier program.

In the MIPS model, accountability and scoring of care outcomes are applied across an interprofessional team but team members are scored individually. In the future, provider quality and cost rankings will be publicly available through mechanisms such as Physician Compare. Everyone on the team needs to demonstrate high-quality care scores to achieve higher payment.

TABLE 23.4

Merit-Based Incentive Payment System (MIPS) Example Improvement Activities

Subcategory Name	Improvement Activity
Achieving Health Equity	Seeing new and follow-up Medicaid patients in a timely manner, including individuals dually eligible for Medicaid and Medicare
Behavioral and Mental Health	Depression screening and follow-up plan: Regular engagement of MIPS-eligible clinicians or groups in integrated prevention and treatment interventions, including depression screening and follow-up plan (refer to NQF #0418) for patients with co-occurring conditions of behavioral or mental health conditions
Beneficiary Engagement	Engage patients, family, and caregivers in developing a plan of care and prioritizing their goals for action, documented in the certified EHR technology
Care Coordination	Implementation of practices/processes for care transition that include documentation of how a MIPS-eligible clinician or group carried out a patient-centered action plan for first 30 days following a discharge (e.g., staff involved, phone calls conducted in support of transition, accompaniments, navigation actions, home visits, patient information access, etc.)
Emergency Response and Preparedness	Participation in disaster medical assistance teams or community emergency responder teams. Activities that simply involve registration are not sufficient. MIPS-eligible clinicians and MIPS-eligible clinician groups must be registered for a minimum of 6 months as a volunteer for disaster or emergency response
Expanded Practice Access	Collection of patient experience and satisfaction data on access to care and development of an improvement plan, such as outlining steps for improving communications with patients to help understanding of urgent access needs
Patient Safety and Practice Assessment	Administration of the AHRQ Survey of Patient Safety Culture and submission of data to the comparative database (refer to AHRQ Survey of Patient Safety Culture website http://www.ahrq.gov/professionals/quality-patient-safety/patientsafetyculture/index.html)
Population Management	Take steps to improve health status of communities, such as collaborating with key partners and stakeholders to implement evidenced-based practices to improve a specific chronic condition. Refer to the local quality improvement organization (QIO) for additional steps to take for improving health status of communities as there are many steps to select from for satisfying this activity. QIOs work under the direction of CMS to assist MIPS-eligible clinicians and groups with quality improvement and review quality concerns for the protection of beneficiaries and the Medicare Trust Fund.

Alternative Payment Model

Providers deciding to participate in an advanced APM through Medicare Part B will earn incentive payments for participating in an innovative payment model and for using certified EHR technology. Practitioners wanting to participate as an APM will take on more than nominal risk, as this means changing processes substantially. There are several types of programs that are categorized as APMs, among which are Accountable Care Communities; Comprehensive Joint Replacement Models; Emergency Triage, Treat, and Transport; Kidney Care Choices; End-Stage Renal Disease Treatment Choices; and Maternal Opioid Misuse Model programs (https://qpp.cms.gov/apms/mips-apms). MACRA was built on the foundation of the Affordable Care Act incentives that seek to transform care and delivery by rewarding the adoption of alternative payment models such as ACOs, bundled payment models, and patient-centered medical homes. In these models, providers accept the risk and reward for providing innovative, coordinated, high-quality, and efficient care. Most providers will participate in MACRA through the MIPS pathway; however, a group can participate through the APM. Providers participating in one or more of the APMs will be exempt from participating in MIPS. Table 23.5 provides a listing of APM categories and resources that describe specific services in detail.

It is clear how the mandated MACRA activities leading to better outcomes are aligned with the expected competencies of a doctor of nursing practice (DNP)-prepared APRN. Savas et al. (2019) described clearly how EHR quality indicator tracking can be implemented within a DNP process improvement project that meets both DNP and MACRA requirements.

RELEVANCE OF REGULATORY REPORTING TO ADVANCED PRACTICE NURSING OUTCOMES

The national quality, patient safety, and accreditation reporting requirements are relevant to APRN outcome evaluation for several reasons. First, they are of critical interest to the organizations that employ APRNs. Many healthcare organizations are carefully tracking key performance measures that affect their financial bottom line in scorecards or dashboards, which are then communicated to all stakeholders, from clinical units to the board room. In many organizations, financial incentives and annual bonuses for those in strategic and operational leadership roles, as well as other key clinical staff, are based on achieving designated performance thresholds. Organizations monitor their performance against competitive market segments using comparative benchmarking systems so that they can ensure their performance exceeds that of their peer groups. This is important not only to maintain their reputation within their community and market but also because CMS programs, specifically the current Value-Based Purchasing, Hospital Readmission Reduction Programs, and the MACRA program, basc financial incentives on the organization's ranking across thousands of US hospitals that are competing for incentive dollars in these programs.

TABLE 23.5

Alternative Payment Model (APMs) Resource Types

Comprehensive End-Stage Renal Disease (ESRD) Care Model	https://innovation.cms.gov/initiatives/comprehensive-esrd-care/
Comprehensive Primary Care Plus	https://innovation.cms.gov/initiatives/comprehensive-primary-care-plus
Next Generation Accountable Care Organization (ACO) Model	https://innovation.cms.gov/initiatives/Next-Generation-ACO-Model/
Shared Savings Program Track 2	https://www.cms.gov/Medicare/Medicare-Fee-for-Service-Payment/sharedsavingsprogram/index.html
Shared Savings Program Track 3	https://www.cms.gov/Medicare/Medicare-Fee-for-Service-Payment/sharedsavingsprogram/index.html
Oncology Care Model	https://innovation.cms.gov/initiatives/oncology-care/

The second and more compelling reason why national regulatory reporting initiatives are critical to APRN outcome evaluation is because so many of the clinical processes and outcomes reflected in these performance measures are directly sensitive to APRN intervention. Thus active participation in the data collection, data analysis, and resulting performance improvement initiatives provides a rich forum to make the value-added APRN contributions highly visible across the organization. In many organizations, key regulatory performance metrics are included in individual provider profiles and integrated into ongoing professional practice evaluation (OPPE) activities, thus rendering APRN value invisible. Although the APRN has a direct and immediate opportunity to influence outcomes for many of these measures, linking APRNs to the performance trend is often a challenge, particularly in an acute care hospital environment in which many providers contribute to the management of a single patient's care episode. For example, medical orders for a patient with heart failure who is eligible for angiotensin-converting enzyme inhibitors at discharge could be written by the patient's attending physician, cardiac specialist, or hospitalist or an acute care nurse practitioner who is accountable for overseeing the cardiac medical population.

The National Provider Identifier Number

Identifying the specific contributions of the APRN to outcomes of care, as a group or as an individual provider, is an essential element to ensuring that they can practice to the full extent of their license uniformly across the country. To accomplish this, there needs to be a data element that will identify the provider as an individual and as a type. Moreover, under MACRA, payment adjustments based on quality outcomes will be assigned at the level of the individual provider by use of the National Provider Identifier (NPI)/Tax Identification Number (TIN) combination. This means that all MIPS-eligible clinicians (physicians, NPs, physician assistants, CNSs, CRNAs) will be identified by the unique NPI and TIN combination. It will be imperative for information systems to capture the provider responsible for ordering individual medications or nonprocedural treatments. With MACRA, it will be essential for all providers to register for an NPI number so that all activity emanating from a singular provider across geography and time can be attributed to that provider and accounted for in a specific patient outcome. The NPI is a 10-digit numerical identifier for which the APRN should apply. Once assigned, an NPI should be permanent and remain with the provider regardless of job or location change. Having an NPI will allow comparisons of individual providers and provider groups and will allow for data to be rolled up into a team outcome. Providers can apply for an NPI number through CMS at https://nppes.cms.hhs.gov/NPPES/Welcome.do.

In addition, MACRA requires CMS to post a list of patient relationship categories. This will also allow for the evaluation of human resources used during care episodes, in addition to allowing attribution of patients to physicians or practitioners who have primary responsibility for the patient, who consider themselves to be the lead provider, who furnishes items and services to the patient on an ongoing basis or intermittent basis at the request of another provider. For a discussion of the categories and codes describing patient relationship to provider, go to https://www.cms.gov/Medicare/Quality-Initiatives-Patient-Assessment-Instruments/Value-Based-Programs/MACRA-MIPS-and-APMs/Patient-Relationship-Categories-and-Codes-Posting-FINAL.pdf.

Providing individual NPI and relationship codes allows for evaluation or comparison of outcomes and quality based on individual provider and/or specialties. This will provide opportunities to promote the value of the professional practice of APRNs using more efficient and accurate means.

FOUNDATIONAL COMPETENCIES IN MANAGING HEALTH INFORMATION TECHNOLOGY

At the heart of any performance measurement activity is the ability and competence to collect data and analyze results effectively so that one can reliably and accurately inform and educate stakeholders about an outcome or process. In health care, these outcomes typically consist of three types of information—clinical, financial, and administrative. Clinical data, such as a patient's medication list or laboratory results, are generally found in the EHR. In some cases, clinical data may be found in specialized registries, such as the registry of the Society of Thoracic Surgeons (STS), which collects data on open heart surgical outcomes and related cardiac diseases. Financial data, such as the cost of a given hospital stay or medication, are typically tied to a financial or billing system. Administrative data, such as a patient's age, gender, or address, are typically tied to a patient registration system (often referred to as an admission–discharge–transfer [ADT] system in acute care hospitals). The health information systems (HIS) that store these data types also include servers, cloud-based platforms, networks, clinical data warehouses, mobile applications, and point-of-care devices. Minimum informatics competencies are required before one may access the various health information technology (HIT) applications in an organization.

Although APRNs directly engage with these technologies at various levels, not all APRNs are able to independently manipulate the various HIS components to compile the data required to evaluate outcomes. More advanced skills from nurse informatics specialists or other expert report writers may be needed to capture necessary information, such as creating a customized report or merging files from multiple databases to assemble the required information. However, strong informatics competencies are needed by APRNs to design the evaluation strategy, validate the data, and interpret the findings effectively. For APRNs prepared at the DNP level, the expectation is that the APRN is able to apply new knowledge, manage individual and aggregate level information, and assess the efficacy of patient care technology appropriate to a specialized area of practice. DNP graduates are prepared to lead the design and select and use information systems technology to evaluate programs of care, outcomes of care, and care systems. The expectations for technology fluency are reflected in almost every advanced level nurse competency in the new *Essentials* (AACN, 2021). The DNP graduate needs to understand how to determine gaps in care or poor outcomes, find the literature, translate the evidence, and develop and implement a process to address the gap or problem. The DNP graduate uses the data to evaluate the new plan and to evaluate the impact of the information system, the informatics processes on the workflow and communications processes.

Although most healthcare organizations have quality management departments with the expertise to build an outcome evaluation plan and conduct the actual data collection and reporting tasks, the APRN should understand these concepts to participate in, and in some cases lead, performance measurement activities actively throughout the full data-information-knowledge continuum. Without these competencies and skill sets, APRNs may find that their level of participation is often limited to routine data collection tasks that do not require critical thinking or clinical judgment. APRNs should be validating the accuracy of the data, monitoring performance trends, and ensuring that best practices are implemented and fully adopted by the interprofessional team. Exemplar 23.2 also illustrates a scenario of appropriate APRN data collection activities associated with a professional peer review process for the purposes of outcome evaluation and performance improvement.

Descriptive, Predictive, and Prescriptive Data Analytics

Another component of outcomes evaluation in which APRNs need to become proficient involves understanding how data will ultimately be used to inform stakeholders about a phenomenon of interest. This may come in the form of performance metrics that describe historical trends for outcomes or processes that have happened in the past or tools that can be used in real time to alert providers to potential trends or events. Collectively, the activities of designing the measurement process, collecting and analyzing the data, and presenting the data back to stakeholders in a timely and effective manner are termed *data analytics.* As EHR data become more standardized and broadly adopted, the methods for performing data analytics will continue to evolve to automated capture and compilation of results, thus allowing data analytics to become more ingrained in every aspect of health care. Analytics in the healthcare industry can be organized into three main categories: descriptive, predictive, and prescriptive.

Descriptive Analytics

The term *descriptive analytics* essentially describes a retrospective trend or outcome. Typically, descriptive data are reported as percentages, rates, means, medians, ratios, or counts in which a value is assigned to inform

EXEMPLAR 23.2

PUTTING IT ALL TOGETHER: PLANNING AND MANAGING QUALITY REPORTING AT A NURSE-MANAGED CLINIC

Nancy Lawson (N.L.) is a nurse practitioner (NP) and clinical director of a nurse-managed health center (NMHC) in a large urban Midwestern city. Primary care services, including health promotion, preventive care, and chronic disease management, are provided to a diverse population consisting of college-aged students, children, adolescents, and an increasing number of adults with chronic diseases such as hypertension and diabetes. The center's population has a mix of commercial, Medicare, and Medicaid payers, with some patients having little to no insurance. This NMHC is staffed by a practice of six primary care NPs, one administrative assistant, and a part-time information systems analyst, whose position is shared by the NMHC's sponsoring healthcare system. Although owned and operated by a college of nursing, the NMHC is also partnered with a large healthcare system, which is participating in the Centers for Medicare & Medicaid Service (CMS) demonstration project as an accountable care organization (ACO). The NMHC is also committed to supporting nursing student placements at the undergraduate and graduate levels. As N.L. begins her annual review of the performance improvement plan, she creates a list of all quality and patient safety reporting requirements to which the NMHC must respond over the course of the next year. This year, the NMHC is planning to apply for status as a federally qualified health center (FQHC), which will expand their quality reporting requirements. N.L. discovers that many FQHC reporting requirements are now outlined in the new guidance found in the Uniform Data System 2020 reporting guidance manual (Health Resources and Services Administration Bureau of Primary Care, 2020). This guidance outlines the requirements for reporting. Here are some examples:

A. Uniform Data System Tables
   1. Patients by ZIP code
   2. Patients by age and sex assigned at birth
   3. Demographic characteristics
   4. Staffing and utilization
   5. Selected diagnoses
   6. Selected services rendered
   7. Quality of care measures
   8. Health outcomes and disparities
   9. Financial costs
   10. Patient service revenue

B. Health Center Health Information (HIT) Capabilities
   1. Does the health center currently have an electronic health record (EHR)?
   2. Is the EHR certified by the Office of the National Coordinator for Health Information Technology?
   3. Does your health center engage patients through health information technology?
   4. How do you collect the data for the Uniform Data Set clinical reporting?
   5. What standardized screener(s) for social risk factors did you use during the calendar year?

C. Workforce
   1. Does your health center provide health professional education/training that is hands-on, practical, or clinical?
   2. How does your health center conduct satisfaction surveys for general personnel working for the health center?

Knowing this information will also be useful to N.L. in her planning and prioritization for health information technology enhancements that need to be implemented at the NMHC to reduce the data collection burden on her team.

Next, N.L. considers her professional practice team and their areas of interest. She calls a meeting to bring the stakeholders together, including herself (information technology [IT]) analyst, and an informatician. N.L. then asks for input from the team to decide which quality measures they should select to meet their regulatory reporting requirements. She asks the stakeholders to consider the NMHC's population and mission, as well as the burden of data collection. The IT analyst contributes to this assessment by advising the team on whether their EHR and IT infrastructure are currently capable of capturing this information electronically or whether manual data collection methods would need to be incorporated to collect the necessary information. The IT analyst notes areas of future expansion and prioritizes these needs relative to quality reporting initiatives at the NMHC. This information will be shared in the upcoming meeting with the healthcare system's corporate HIT strategy team to build their integrated healthcare information system to support their work as an ACO.

Finally, N.L. asks the team to consider any other areas of interest that they would like to focus on over the course of the next year that are not already captured in the must measure list and that will inform them about the quality, effectiveness, efficacy, and efficiency of the group's practice. They suggest that the average waiting time to be seen by a clinic provider and the number of patients who are admitted to the emergency department (ED) or hospital within 72 hours after being seen at the NMHC would be valuable information in the year ahead. In collaboration with their IT analyst, they determine the best ways to capture waiting time to be seen and 72-hour admissions.

As the team completes their final assessment, they raise concerns that although the value of knowing the patient satisfaction and patient experience data is high, the data collection effort will be intensive and likely require the

EXEMPLAR 23.2

PUTTING IT ALL TOGETHER: PLANNING AND MANAGING QUALITY REPORTING AT A NURSE-MANAGED CLINIC—cont'd

assistance of additional staff or university students to collect and analyze this information. N.L. and the NPs in the practice suggest including the students from the college of nursing to partner with this project. N.L. schedules a meeting with the dean of academic affairs to discuss internship opportunities for nursing students. With enthusiasm from the dean that these would be good learning opportunities, these measures and the proposed data collection plan are added to the NMHC's performance improvement plan.

Finally, for each measure, the team identifies a target for their performance. Measures in which there are known national benchmarks associated with them, such as the Healthcare Effectiveness Data and Information Set (HEDIS) process measure for diabetes care, which measures the percentage of patients with diabetes receiving glycosylated hemoglobin (HbA_{1C}) tests in the reporting year or the outcome measure that reports the percentage of patients with diabetes with a controlled HbA_{1C} result, are set at higher percentiles of desired performance (e.g., 90%). Conversely, measures in which the benchmark for the phenomenon of interest are not established nationally, such as the number of patients admitted to the healthcare system's ED within 72 hours of a visit to the NMHC, may be set at lower thresholds of performance or have no specific target established until patterns in the performance data have been well established.

N.L. compiles the final list of measures to be reported, along with a data collection plan and schedule for periodic review and reporting to all stakeholders. She submits this performance improvement plan to the College of Nursing's Faculty Practice Plan group for feedback prior to submitting the plan to the sponsoring healthcare system's quality director for final review and approval. Over the course of the next year, the NMHC team monitors the results of their performance monthly. Measure rates and continuous variables are presented in a dashboard, using statistical process control (SPC) charts so that trends can be rapidly visualized. For each measure, a target is established so that all stakeholders reviewing the monthly dashboard can see briefly any performance trends that are falling below desired targets.

Midway through the year, the NMHC team observes that their performance in mammography screening is substantially below the national median as reported by HEDIS. The team decides to review their performance stratified by payer (commercial, Medicare, Medicaid, and self-pay or uninsured) to see whether any disparities might exist. No significant trends appear. However, when reviewing the inclusion and exclusion criteria for the measure, it is observed that the primary reason for failing to meet the criterion was that mammography results were not reported back to the NMHC. The team quickly realized that to understand their effectiveness in this referral metric fully, they had to correct an underlying system issue and secure mammography results back to the referring NP provider.

N.L. organized a small team of stakeholders, which included the administrator for the contracted imaging facility, medical director of the imaging facility, oversight physician for the NMHC, and IT systems analyst. During a 1-hour meeting, it was unanimously agreed by all parties that the NP provider ordering the mammogram required a copy of the results. It was further determined that the root cause for this omission was tied to the absence of the NP providers from the hospital information systems provider dictionary. The IT analyst was able to quickly add the six NPs to the required dictionary, enabling the admissions clerk at the imaging center to select the appropriate provider and route the results to them.

The next month, the performance trend for mammography referrals from the NMHC demonstrated a significant increase. Using the SPC software function to designate a phase change within a time-trended process, N.L. modified the SPC chart in the dashboard by inserting a phase line to distinguish between the pre- and postprocess improvement periods. In this manner, she will be able to document the impact of the PI initiative to have available for potential accreditation surveys and to detect any statistically significant changes in their new process moving forward that might indicate that they are not sustaining their improvements over time. N.L. makes a plan to reevaluate performance in mammography referrals monthly for the remainder of the year and at least once a quarter thereafter for the next 18 to 24 months, as long as the process appears to be stable.

the degree of positive or negative movement against a given target or norm. Another type of descriptive analytic would be time-trended comparison data, which could inform the audience about a hospital's overall and periodic fluctuations in performance, for example, a hospital's readmission rates compared with that of other hospitals. The limitation of descriptive analytic tools is that they do not illuminate the reasons behind a given pattern, suggest an improvement strategy, or help the audience understand the relative stability or predictability of the process that is currently producing outcomes to date.

One of the most effective methods for demonstrating that an intervention or process modification has resulted in meaningful change over time is statistical process control (SPC) analysis. SPC analysis examines variation within an individual process as well as the timing in which a change in process occurred. SPC uses control charts that visually display performance data against upper and lower control limits reflective of normal variation in a system. Fig. 23.1 provides an example of an SPC chart with an upper and lower limit. In contrast to comparative reports that display individual performance data compared with peer group performance, SPC charts display time-trended data only for individual performance data. No peer performance data are displayed in an SPC chart. Rather, the individual data are trended over time, with mathematically computed control limits that indicate the expected ranges for random variation within a given process. When data points within the time-trended process change in a manner indicative of a statistically significant change, a special cause signal is displayed in the SPC chart. Special cause signals can occur whenever a single data point exceeds the upper or lower control limits in the SPC charts. Additional trends in the data may also designate special cause signals, such as eight data points in a row above or below the center line or six points in a row increasing or decreasing in a single direction.

SPC charts have the added advantage of being able to distinguish results achieved during a pre-intervention process and the results achieved following a process change that occurs as a result of an innovation or practice change. This is done by inserting a phase change line between the two different processes and computing new control limits to monitor for statistical process capability moving forward. A detailed discussion of these data analysis techniques is beyond the scope of this chapter, although a basic knowledge of control charts is useful for most situations. The reader is referred to the classic reference on SPC chart theory (Wheeler, 1993) or an online reference for basic SPC chart theory and application such as that from the American Society for Quality (2021).

To understand why a hospital has fluctuations in their readmission performance data or why a hospital's performance differs from others, the inquiry must progress further. Additional descriptive analytics may be used to look at specific details within the population, such as readmissions by sex, age, provider, payer, disease severity, and other related criteria. This type of inquiry that drills down to explore more specific patterns in data sets is termed *data mining.* Typical tools that the APRN will use involve Excel spreadsheets or other types of statistical software tools. Data patterns may then be displayed in charts to describe the patterns in the data. Table 23.6 lists several tools and techniques that are commonly used when working with descriptive analytics.

Predictive Analytics

Predictive analytics are rapidly emerging in the science of performance improvement. In contrast to descriptive

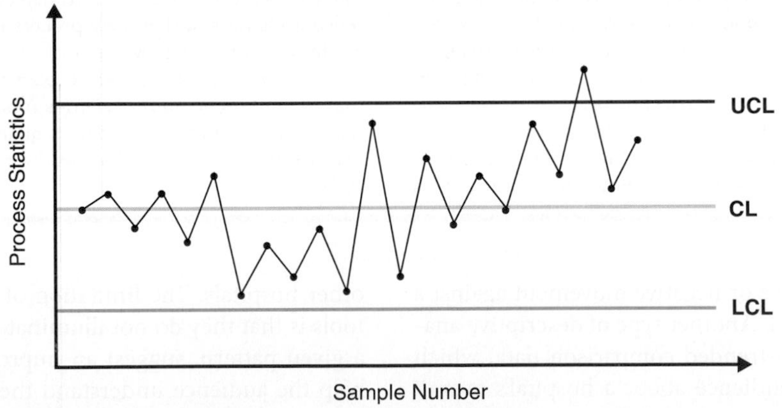

Fig. 23.1 ■ **Example statistical process control chart.** Source: Statistical Process Control. (2022). Control charts. http://www.processma.com/resource/spc.php

TABLE 23.6

Continuous Quality Improvement Tools and Techniques for Process Improvement

Tools and Techniques	Primary Function	Benefits
Flowchart	Displays the process	Facilitates understanding of the process Identifies stakeholders Clarifies potential gaps and system breakdowns
Run chart	Displays performance over time	Increases understanding of the problem Identifies changes over time
Control chart	Displays how predictable the process is over time	Identifies change in the process as a result of intentional or nonintentional changes in the process Identifies opportunities for improvement
Pie chart	Displays the percentage that each variable contributes to the whole	Identifies variables affecting process Increases understanding of the problem
Bar chart	Compares categories of data during a single point in time	Increases understanding of the problem Identifies differences in variables Compares performance with known standards
Pareto chart	Identifies the most frequent trend within a data set	Identifies principal variables impacting the process Identifies opportunities for improvement
Cause and effect	Displays multiple causes of a problem	Identifies root causes Identifies variables affecting the process Identifies opportunities for improvement Plans for change
Scatter diagram	Displays relationship between two variables	Increases understanding of the relationship between multiple variables
Brainstorming	Rapidly generates multiple ideas	Promotes stakeholder buy-in Increases understanding of the problem Identifies variables affecting the process
Multivoting	Consolidates ideas	Achieves consensus among stakeholders Prioritizes improvement strategies
Nominal group technique	Rapidly generates multiple ideas and prioritizes them	Identifies the problem Achieves consensus among stakeholders Prioritizes improvement strategies Plans for change
Root cause analysis	Identifies the cause of the problem	Increases understanding of the problem Identifies multicause variables affecting the process Identifies opportunities to improve Plans for change
Force field analysis	Identifies driving and restraining forces that impact proposed change	Identifies and lists variables affecting process Plans for change
Consensus	Generates agreement among stakeholders	Increases understanding of the problem Reduces resistance to change Plans for change

Adapted from *Fundamentals of Health Care Improvement: A Guide to Improving Your Patients Care* (3rd ed.), by G. S. Ogrinc, L. A. Headrick, A. J. Barton, M. A. Dolansky, & R. A. Miltner, 2018, Joint Commission Resources.

analytics, which only describe a process after it has happened, predictive analytics provide insight on what might happen in the future based on past patterns or other criteria so that the appropriate interventions may be applied to achieve desired outcomes. For example, a tool that would identify a patient's risk of readmission following discharge from a hospital would be considered a predictive analytic. CMS offers a free tool on the QualityNet web portal to predict the 30-day, all-cause readmission risk of individual patients hospitalized for pneumonia, heart failure, and acute myocardial infarction. This tool, developed by the Cooperative Cardiovascular Project initiative and under contract with CMS, uses sex, clinical history, physical examination findings, diagnostic and laboratory test results, and medications to compute an individual's overall risk of readmission (CMS, n.d.).

Currently, software engineers and clinical innovators are partnering to develop technology solutions that will assist in identifying individual patients at highest risk for readmissions, pressure ulcers, falls, and other hospital-acquired complications. Cerner Systems and Advocate Health Care have developed a predictive analytic for hospital readmissions based on 25 variables, including payer, race, prior hospitalization, emergency department use in the past 12 months, admission source, current use of insulin or warfarin, and 17 disease-related variables (Sikka et al., 2012). Most tools are not yet robust enough to have broad applicability to general populations; however, this area of performance improvement will likely accelerate particularly as Big Data techniques and visual analytics tools become more robust. Such development will allow measurement of more timely and proactive interventions to ensure that best practices are delivered at the right time for more high-risk patients. Kansagara and colleagues (2011) and Artetxe et al. (2018) both provided a systemic review of predictive analytics and risk predication models pertaining to hospital readmission.

Prescriptive Analytics

Finally, the term *prescriptive analytics* refers to tools that assist with modeling and longitudinal forecasting to inform users on how to respond to a given pattern in one's data. In prescriptive analytics, the evidence-based best practice is linked to the trend so that it indicates not only why there is a problem but what the most likely solutions would be to get a trend back on a desired course. Computer science and machine learning is rapidly accelerating scientific innovation which will change how evidence-based practice is deployed in the clinical environment. APRN participation in collaborative learning with medical and nursing informatics specialists, clinical researchers, HIT vendors, and scientists may lead to transformational technologies within the next 5 to 8 years.

FOUNDATIONAL COMPETENCIES IN QUALITY IMPROVEMENT

APRNs must be able to participate in and lead interprofessional teams effectively toward data-based conclusions and process improvements. Data analysis is a specific skill for evidence-based practice. APRNs are required to have the ability to manipulate and interpret raw data, query information within a database containing clinical or financial information, and use an information system to collect data and trend performance. If it is not possible for the APRN to directly query, the APRN must have the ability to work with an informatician or analyst to extract the correct data because the APRN has an appreciation for the content of the data needed and the context in which the data was collected. The purpose of this section is to elaborate on the specific skills that APRNs need to be knowledgeable participants and leaders in continuous quality improvement (CQI) efforts. APRN students need content on CQI knowledge and skills, and graduate APRNs should seek ongoing CQI knowledge through reading, continuing education, and participation in formal quality improvement (QI) training programs. A healthcare system's approach to CQI should be included in an APRN's orientation. If such programs are not in place, APRNs are strongly encouraged to include formal QI training in their performance and learning objectives within the first year of hire and to identify opportunities to initiate modest QI initiatives.

Continuous Quality Improvement Frameworks

There are numerous frameworks and related strategies for improving performance and evaluating outcomes in today's healthcare system. Some of these include the Institute for Healthcare Improvement's plan–do–study–act (PDSA) model, Six Sigma, and Lean Manufacturing techniques (Morgan & Brenig-Jones, 2012). APRNs can examine selected frameworks to understand the how-to mechanics of creating systems that are safe, effective, patient-centered, timely, efficient, and equitable. Generally, the employer will have selected a framework or philosophy that guides CQI efforts across an organization. Many of these methodologies have evolved from the work of Drs. W. Edwards Deming and Joseph M. Juran, both considered to be forefathers of modern-day statistical process control theory. Although a detailed review of the various CQI frameworks is not included here, APRNs are highly encouraged to contact the quality management department in their organization and request an orientation to the CQI framework used in their practice settings. The American Association of Family Physicians (2021) provides a review of the basic frameworks used in quality improvement.

Regardless of the type of QI approach an organization selects, the APRN should be competent in a variety of specific techniques, tools, and methodologies used to evaluate process performance and outcomes. Most approaches involve the use of different types of charts and analysis tools to examine findings and establish linkages. Some charts are easy to learn, such as flowcharts. Other charts, such as Pareto charts, SPC charts, scatter diagrams, and cause-and-effect diagrams, also termed *fishbone* or *Ishikawa diagrams,* require specific training and expertise in statistical software. APRNs may also need to become familiar with the software used in their agencies to conduct CQI analyses and reports.

APRNs prepared at a master's level should achieve beginning level competencies with these tools, including the ability to interpret the data in these reports and effectively participate in teams using CQI techniques. One exception is the CNS role, which has had expectations for leading QI efforts as part of system influence expectations embedded in their role; mastery is expected for any CNS, whether master's or DNP prepared. Other APRNs should achieve mastery of QI competencies at the DNP level, with full accountability for planning the CQI project, selecting and using appropriate tools and techniques, including the ability to enter data and run the reports, synthesize information from the reports, and coach others in deriving meaning from the information and making decisions. QI training should also include techniques for analyzing how people and processes work. Root cause analysis is one popular approach to identifying underlying causes of problems and process failures in a particular system. This approach may be particularly useful for examining adverse events and other patient safety issues.

Organizational Structures and Cultures That Optimize Performance Improvement

APRNs who practice in a hospital or an integrated delivery network may find that their span of influence crosses many units, departments, and points of service within the system. Thus it is important to consider carefully the reporting structures that will best support their roles. In many organizations, APRNs report to nurse or medical executives. Regardless of organizational placement, APRNs should seek to work within a reporting structure that supports whole-system thinking and places a high value on innovation and process improvement. Conversely, APRNs should avoid reporting structures that constrain their practices to one unit's or department's interests or seem to place a particular emphasis on task-oriented activities. Optimally, the organization and its administrators should recognize that the APRN is in a unique position to promote excellence in clinical practice and system performance. To achieve these outcomes, the APRN may at times require the formal and tacit authority that comes from others in an organization. This means that the APRN will work with and through leadership in order to achieve improved outcomes. Those who lead APRNs must be prepared to be responsible, if necessary, for changes perceived as coming from the APRN. Although APRNs will not need daily or even weekly supervision, they will need to be kept abreast of organizational issues that are likely to affect the practice and business environment. APRNs should have routine briefing sessions scheduled with their immediate supervisors to clarify goals and expected outcomes, identify any resource needs, discuss any barriers, and exchange information relating to pending contracts, changes in the product line, medical practice issues, or staff education needs.

Active membership on key medical and quality oversight committees and direct access to administrative decision makers are imperative. This access affords APRNs the opportunity to integrate clinical expertise with communication, negotiation, and leadership skills to promote effective and efficient clinical processes. For APRNs who contract independently, becoming familiar with the organizational structure and culture and becoming a trusted insider in the organization will be critical to successful contracting and service delivery.

STRATEGIES FOR DESIGNING QUALITY IMPROVEMENT AND OUTCOME EVALUATION PLANS FOR ADVANCED PRACTICE NURSING

As noted, much of healthcare practice in today's economic market is data driven, with APRNs assuming greater responsibility for collecting and using clinical, economic, and quality outcomes data. Interprofessional QI teams are increasingly charged with improving care delivery outcomes or redesigning workflow processes for greater effectiveness or efficiency. Because APRNs routinely monitor and maintain clinical care delivery systems, they are in an ideal position to plan QI initiatives by leading or actively participating in interprofessional QI teams. As clinical experts, APRNs influence practice patterns and develop meaningful standards, practice protocols, clinical guidelines, healthcare programs, and healthcare policies that promote teamwork, improve clinical outcomes, and reduce costs. Moreover, APRNs' pattern recognition skills facilitate the identification of system inefficiencies, barriers to continuity of care, and other ineffective ways of delivering healthcare services. These in turn become opportunities for APRNs to influence processes and outcomes positively at both the individual patient and system levels. With these opportunities comes the responsibility to be knowledgeable in outcome evaluation. In the remainder of this chapter, a stepwise approach is proposed to developing and implementing an outcome evaluation plan that demonstrates an APRN's value and contribution to the healthcare setting. Although the term *outcome evaluation* is used throughout this section, these steps can be applied to impact analysis, outcomes measurement, performance evaluation, process improvement, program evaluation, and clinical research.

Phases of Preparing a Plan for Outcome Evaluation

There are three phases in the organizing framework to develop an effective outcome evaluation plan—defining the core questions that need to be answered, determining the data required to answer the questions, and interpreting the data and acting on the results. Box 23.4 lists the phases and related steps in developing and conducting an outcomes evaluation. A description of each step follows.

Define the Core Questions

Whether the APRN is designing an outcome evaluation project to assess their own practice effectiveness or participating on an interprofessional team responsible for improving the care for a given clinical population, the first step is to clearly articulate and ask "What are the questions we should ask and why?" Clear questions will lay the foundation for an effective outcome evaluation and limit unintended project scope creep. In formulating clear core questions, it is helpful to define the target population, identify the relevant stakeholders, and articulate specific program goals and interventions to be evaluated. It is also useful to understand any key business drivers tied to the outcome evaluation or performance improvement initiative. Once these foundational aspects have been established, the APRN can progress to the mechanics of how the data for the project will be collected.

Define the Target Population for Evaluation

APRNs use a range of activities to manage heterogeneous clinical populations. When designing an outcome evaluation plan, it is necessary to focus on specific aspects of the practice with a particular patient group. This focus helps create a more manageable outcome evaluation plan and limits the impact of extraneous variables that could interfere with the interpretation of findings. Aspects of APRN activities used with the target population need to be identified and included in the design. Whenever possible, the target population should be comparable to other groups monitored through QI initiatives at the organizational or departmental level so that the vested interests of the organization's commitment to improving care and the APRN's activities are aligned. The decision to target subpopulations of patients may be based on a desire to

BOX 23.4

Summary of Outcome Evaluation Planning Process

PHASE I: DEFINE THE CORE QUESTIONS

I-1. Define the target population.
- Identify differences in patient characteristics within target population.
- Clarify relationships between APRN role behaviors and population needs and outcomes.
- Compare target group with other groups monitored through QI activities.
- Assess level of risk, complexity, and resource use of subpopulations within target group.

I-2. Identify the stakeholders.
- Facilitate participation by and input from key stakeholders.
- Isolate APRN interventions and actions from those of other care providers.
- Secure early buy-in from stakeholders.

I-3. Articulate program goals and interventions.
- Review literature for supportive evidence.
- Consider resources needed to implement and maintain the intervention.
- Formulate specific questions.
- Implement practice change or QI strategy.

PHASE II: DEFINE THE DATA ELEMENTS

II-1. Identify selection criteria for the population of interest.
- Clarify inclusion and exclusion criteria.
- Identify electronic data sources of information about the target population.

II-2. Establish performance and outcome indicators.
- Identify measures to determine evidence of APRN impact.
- Ensure alignment among program goals, proposed interventions, and outcome indicators.
- Consider the use of national databases for comparison and benchmarking purposes.

II-3. Identify and evaluate data elements, collection instruments, and procedures.
- Evaluate ease of collecting data and compare with need.
- Identify data resources available.
- Link use of intermediate outcome indicators to target goals and outcome achievement.
- Summarize the outcome evaluation plan.

PHASE III: DERIVE MEANING FROM DATA AND ACT ON RESULTS

III-1. Analyze data and interpret findings.
- Seek assistance from others, as needed.
- Select data analysis and reporting procedures.

III-2. Present and disseminate findings.
- Prepare reports according to audience and stakeholder needs and interests.
- Select software programs and other resources to support presentation approach.

III-3. Identify improvement opportunities.
- Work with stakeholders to identify most appropriate opportunity for improvement.
- Select most effective tools to facilitate performance improvement planning process.
- Conduct pilot studies to assess new program feasibility, cost, and resource needs.

III-4. Formulate a plan for ongoing monitoring and reevaluation.
- Summarize goals of performance improvement plan.
- Identify proposed interventions, responsible persons, and target dates for completion.
- Select indicators and measures based on goals and interventions identified.
- Provide educational programs to support intervention, as needed.

III-5. Clarify the purpose of the APRN's role.
- Review organization's mission, vision, and goals.
- Clarify role expectations.
- Confirm clinical and reporting accountability.

evaluate patients who are high risk, complex, or tend to use more services than others.

Other factors to consider when defining a target population include patient satisfaction and financial performance. For example, when a large pediatric medical group hires a pediatric nurse practitioner to provide routine physical examinations and vaccinations, parent satisfaction is likely to be an important component of the outcome evaluation plan. Patient factors such as insurance provider, age, ethnicity, or comorbid conditions also may be used to define the target population at risk for adverse outcomes. Finally, some populations are targeted because of the need for organizations to determine their level of compliance with national care delivery guidelines, best practice standards, or regulatory requirements, as illustrated in Exemplar 23.2. Frequently, APRNs are involved in the care of several populations of interest and, as such, must prioritize which populations warrant first review and evaluation. APRNs must be sensitive to the resource requirements of any outcome evaluation, working closely with information systems, QI, and medical records staff for the support required to conduct the review.

Identify the Stakeholders

APRNs must identify the structures and processes of care for which they share accountability. Although APRNs are rarely the only or primary stakeholder in the provision of care to the populations they serve, they often serve as the glue that holds the team together. As such, they often move the team, healthcare agency, and/or system toward a shared vision of desired outcome. Creating this vision is not an isolated APRN activity; APRNs must also facilitate the contributions, ideas, and creativity of professionals who participate in the care of the target population. Exemplar 23.3 demonstrates that small changes with multiple stakeholders using reminders within an EHR can make significant change. Stakeholders most commonly involved are physicians, physician assistants, other APRNs, registered nurses, pharmacists, administrators, and other members of the healthcare team. In some cases, APRNs will need to include stakeholders from outside their immediate practice settings. For example, a community-based APRN serving fragile older patients with chronic diseases may need to include stakeholders from managed care payers and insurers, primary care clinics, physicians' offices, skilled nursing facilities, home healthcare agencies, and hospitals. Although including all stakeholders in the development of an outcome evaluation plan may not be feasible or desirable, attention to the impact of primary stakeholders on care delivery outcomes will aid in the understanding and measurement of processes and outcomes interdependent with APRN practice.

Typically, APRNs are only one component of a greater whole, so they cannot receive full credit for the positive results. Therefore APRNs must articulate APRN-specific inputs and interventions that contribute to the team effect so that the value of the APRN to the organization can be documented and demonstrated. The need to carve out additional measures of role effectiveness results in a more complex outcomes plan, requiring multiple measurement methodologies, instruments, and analytic techniques. For example, part of an outcome evaluation plan may use quantitative methods to capture specific outcomes of treatment (e.g., average number of clinic visits per year, total costs, number of patients with diabetes who have a normal HbA_{1c} level within 2 months of diagnosis). Another part of the plan may use a qualitative approach, using verbal or written feedback from physician and dietitian colleagues about APRN effectiveness in facilitating the development of new patient care guidelines to manage patients with diabetes. Once the plan for an evaluation study has been shared with stakeholders, buy-in to any proposed change must be obtained to proceed. APRNs not only will be change recipients as a result of the outcome evaluation but also will serve as change implementers and change strategists for others and their organization. Involving stakeholders early in the process facilitates ongoing communication, reduces resistance to change, and promotes adoption of recommended changes.

Articulate Program Goals and Interventions

The easiest way to demonstrate positive outcomes of care is to do the right things, at the right times, for the right patients, in the right ways. The task of evaluation becomes an artful assembly of necessary data and information that reflect the outcomes and processes associated with the intervention. Determining which interventions to implement for a given population and

EXEMPLAR 23.3

SIMPLE CHANGES RESULT IN SUBSTANTIAL IMPROVEMENT

There is an identified need within an urban academic medical center to improve quality and outcomes around 30-day readmission for patients with heart failure. A literature review by the APRN indicates that it takes numerous transitions of care interventions to prevent the 30-day readmission of patients with heart failure after discharge. One key intervention is to ensure that the patients follow up with their primary care provider within 48 to 72 hours after discharge. The care team identified actions to increase use of this important intervention when it was discovered through data analytics that only 20% of patients with heart failure had appointments scheduled prior to discharge. All clinicians were educated on how important the follow-up appointment was to improving overall outcomes. Patients were educated by the discharging nurse. The unit care team made checking on the status of the follow-up appointment part of discharge planning processes. For some patients, case managers were assigned the task of contacting the primary care provider to establish the appointment. The information system was adapted to capture follow-up appointment information, making it clear to patient and providers whether this task was completed. A report was created listing all patients nearing discharge and the follow-up appointment information as a clinical decision support tool. This information on follow-up was collected within the electronic health record so that results could be monitored. The net result was an increase in the number of conversations about follow-up appointments, an increase in the number of appointments made (up to 90% compliance), and a decrease in the 30-day preventable readmission rate. In addition, patient satisfaction scores for the heart failure clinic improved.

which to include in an outcome evaluation plan may be based in part on the resources required to accomplish these interventions and maintain them in practice. To begin, APRNs should engage in a comprehensive literature review to examine all standards of care, regulatory requirements, national guidelines, and established or emerging evidence-based best practices relevant to their clinical population. The most current information may be found on websites that are relevant to the APRN's clinical specialty or through specialized fee-for-service vendor services that accumulate and organize best practice information and a meta-analysis of the literature for selected clinical topics, such as Zynx Health (www.zynxhealth.com).

Using information from literature and experience, APRNs can identify appropriate interventions for managing populations. For example, interventions may include attention to early detection and diagnostic modalities, timeliness of interventions, medication appropriateness, or patient education. The organization's needs and any political agendas should also be considered. APRNs should limit the number of evaluated interventions to keep the project scope manageable. A commitment to too many interventions or unrealistic data collection activities can overwhelm available resources and undermine or stall performance improvement and outcome evaluation initiatives.

Once the program goals and interventions have been defined, the APRN can begin to formulate specific questions of interest to stakeholders. Sketching out some basic questions serves as a useful exercise for establishing the outcome evaluation plan. The following are some sample questions:

- How cost effective is this program?
- How satisfied are patients with the services they received?
- How closely does the healthcare team adhere to best practice standards?
- How many patients experienced complications of care?
- What patient safety issues associated with this population should we examine?
- What can be done to reduce resource utilization and create efficiencies for this population?
- What do we need to do differently to become a center of excellence for this population?
- How has the APRN contributed to the training and development of other staff?
- What are the key business drivers behind the outcome evaluation project or performance improvement initiative?

Once the core questions have been formulated, the APRN can design the data collection methodology that will be used to answer key questions. Typically, this step occurs simultaneously with the actual implementation of a practice change or quality improvement strategy. Pre-intervention baseline performance measurement, whenever feasible, is important both to confirm that there is a gap that needs to be addressed and to assess any changes that occurred post-intervention.

Define the Data Elements

After APRNs clarify the program goals, identify the key interventions to evaluate in the outcome evaluation plan, and determine the core questions to be answered, they are ready to define the outcome indicators and data elements that they will use to measure the intervention's success. This phase in the outcome evaluation plan often poses the greatest challenge for APRNs, particularly for those who have had little or no exposure to QI principles and management information systems—both of which support outcome evaluation. There are three steps in this phase. First, APRNs decide how they will determine patients or encounters of care for inclusion in the outcome evaluation; second, they identify which indicators they will use to answer the project's core questions; and, third, they determine which data elements will be collected for each indicator chosen for the evaluation. As noted, APRNs with limited expertise in these areas should seek assistance from other healthcare professionals with experience in CQI principles, healthcare statistics, nursing informatics, program evaluation, and/or nursing research.

Identify Selection Criteria for the Population of Interest

Although this may seem like an obvious step, it is important to consider which patient characteristics will be included in the evaluation. Identifying electronic data sources that contain information about the target population is generally the most efficient way to begin. For example, APRNs who practice in a physician's office or clinic may be able to retrieve a list of all patients seen within a given time frame. This is possible because the APRN's provider number, which identifies their patients in the claims database and generates the bill for services rendered, can be used to define the population of interest. The APRN could further reduce this list to patients seen for a specific diagnosis or symptom through the use of ICD-10 codes, CPT-4 codes, or ambulatory payment classification (APC) codes. In behavioral health settings, *Diagnostic and Statistical Manual of Mental Disorders,* version 5 (DSM-V) codes are generally more useful. Additional coding taxonomies and terminology sets relevant to this level of query are listed and described in Table 23.1.

In contrast, CNSs who practice in acute care environments may have a more difficult time obtaining a list of patients whose care they managed or influenced because CNSs do not typically bill directly for services. In this scenario, the population may be identified by nonelectronic data sources, such as a log or referral list. If the CNS's influence extends to a general clinical population, specified MS-DRG or ICD-10 diagnostic or procedure codes can be used to obtain a patient list if the outcome evaluation design is retrospective. CRNAs and certified nurse-midwives (CNMs) who contract with the hospital for their services may be able to identify patients for whom they have provided care from the procedure provider that corresponds to the procedure code; however, they should confirm that they are listed as the procedure provider in the final claim, rather than the medical provider assigned to their practice. This information is generally available from hospital information systems and is rapidly being enhanced through the adoption of the EHR and meaningful use technologies (see earlier). As illustrated in Exemplar 23.1, APRNs should collaborate with health information management and nursing informatics specialists for this component of their analysis to ensure that the right inclusion variables have been identified to secure their population of interest.

Establish Performance and Outcome Indicators

Once the patient population has been defined, APRNs and their colleagues specify measures of performance that will be used to draw conclusions about how well the population was managed or the degree to which favorable outcomes were achieved. In general, descriptive measures are predominately classified into three types: (1) proportion measures (e.g., mortality rates, readmission rates, complication rates), (2) ratio measures (e.g., falls/1000 patient days, central line infections/1000 line days, restraint episodes per psychiatric patient days), and (3) continuous variable measures (e.g., median time to initial antibiotic, average length of stay). Some measures are direct counts of a particular phenomenon within a given time period, such as the number of allergic reactions in patients receiving antibiotics. Others are sums, such as total costs of care for a given population or total patient days. For rare events, such as ventilator-acquired pneumonia in hospitals that have implemented aggressive protocols to prevent this phenomenon from occurring, the days between undesirable events may be a more effective way to track and monitor outcomes, with longer time intervals being the more desirable trend, rather than fewer events.

The type of measure selected is less important than how well it answers the core questions of the study, although, ultimately, the type of measure will determine the approach required for data analysis and presentation to stakeholders. The best approach is to create a draft list of indicators and obtain feedback from stakeholders about how well the indicators address their core questions and concerns. Only after stakeholder buy-in is secured should the APRN formally establish the indicators for the evaluation plan. When informing the stakeholders of the outcome evaluation plan, the APRN should keep in mind that if data collection is concurrent and involves the clinical practice patterns of the clinical stakeholders, the potential exists to bias the results simply because the providers know that they are being observed and their performance is being monitored. This reaction, termed the *Hawthorne effect,* is troublesome for process measurement. The data collection period should continue for a sufficient period to ensure that the novelty of the intervention has worn off and the changes in behaviors are a true reflection of intervention effect and not the effect of providers being evaluated.

Alignment among program goals, interventions, and performance and outcome indicators is another important consideration when designing the outcome evaluation plan. This process ensures that the findings of the outcome evaluation can be traced back to APRN practice when appropriate. For example, if average length of stay is selected as one outcome indicator for a population of patients with acute myocardial infarction under the direction of a hospital-based CNS, this variable should be linked in theory and in practice to an intervention for which the CNS has or shares accountability (e.g., discharge planning or management of complications). Measures that reflect the subprocesses of other providers, such as time from first incision for patients undergoing angioplasty to the time the wire crosses the lesion in the coronary artery, may be of interest to invasive cardiologists and other stakeholders from the cardiac catheterization laboratory; however, they may have little to do with the APRN's direct practice role.

As noted earlier, APRNs are often lured into coordinating data collection for other providers as part of the performance monitoring process. APRNs may agree to perform these data coordination or data collection activities but must be careful not to become overburdened with tasks that diminish their own clinical effectiveness or assessment of intervention effect. If this happens, APRNs should examine other potential resources for data collection in the organization so they can continue to carry out their role and provide service to the institution. Staying focused on the interventions and specific program goals for which they are responsible will assist APRNs to formulate a meaningful and manageable outcome evaluation plan.

Identify and Evaluate Data Elements, Collection Instruments, and Procedures

To ensure an efficient data collection process, APRNs should evaluate the effort to collect each individual data element compared with the overall usefulness of the indicator. Data available only through specialized or resource-intensive instruments, such as phone surveys, home follow-up visits, or comprehensive chart reviews, are considered difficult to obtain and should be carefully considered before making a final decision to include them in the outcome evaluation plan. When data are obtained electronically, the specific source for each data element needs to be identified and understood. As noted earlier, running queries and reports from the EHR may or may not become an essential part of the APRN's role and, in most cases, expert resources are available in healthcare systems to assist APRNs in retrieving the information. However, in the era of the EHR, it is especially important that data obtained electronically be validated for accuracy before they can be reliably used. APRNs can collaborate with quality management and nursing informatics specialists to design a data validation strategy to ensure that data are complete, accurate, and sensitive to the issue of interest. This may involve the random review of records by expert clinicians and an inspection of an interface file by a technician in the IT department to ensure that all source systems are working as designed.

APRNs can avoid duplication of effort and data collection redundancy by becoming familiar with the many sources of data and information available in their respective organizations. This will require collaboration with interprofessional team members such as database administrators, report writers, data analysis experts, and administrators of the data warehouse. The APRN will be interacting with a variety of data storage systems. These may include registries, surgery scheduling systems, pharmacy or medication delivery systems, point-of-care laboratory devices, quality management systems, case management systems, risk management systems, infection control systems, and cost accounting systems. In some cases, information from one information system might be cross-checked against another system with a similar data set. If differences between two similar data sets are identified, they should be closely examined to understand why the differences are occurring. For example, the number of infections captured by a laboratory system might be different than those captured by an infection control practitioner using an infection control information system and still different from those captured in a medical record coding system. Common reasons for variance among similar HIT systems include variability in the start or end dates (or times) used to run the reports, a difference in the codes used to define the population of interest, or differences in how the data were captured in the source systems. In the case of medical records coding, variation is often the result of inconsistent documentation by medical and APRN providers. These types of variations should be understood during the design phase of the outcome evaluation plan so that the best data source can be selected to answer the core questions of the evaluation.

In some cases, questions about the effective management of clinical populations can be answered only through longitudinal studies. For example, for a population of patients with diabetes, clinical outcomes such as reduced hospitalization, improved functioning, reduced evidence of retinopathy, and reduced limb amputations may be sound and reasonable for research purposes, but they are typically too long range to be useful for performance improvement or outcome evaluation activities. The link between APRN practice and outcomes may be difficult to assess over long periods, making intermediate outcomes assessment more desirable for a short-term evaluation.

When collecting patient identifiable data, APRNs should be cognizant of the restrictions on their use. The Health Insurance Portability and Accountability Act of 1996 (govinfo, n.d.), commonly referred to as HIPAA, includes significant restrictions on the manner in which identifiable patient information may be used for research and QI activities. Typically, information used for quality improvement and outcome evaluations is less restrictive. In some circumstances, particularly if they are contracted in a fee-for-service arrangement with the healthcare agency, APRNs may be required to sign a business associate agreement with the healthcare provider to access or use patient data. For more information about HIPAA regulations and impact on evaluation activities, APRNs should refer to their organization's policies and procedures.

The APRN will have a full appreciation of the scope of the outcome evaluation project and resources required for successful completion only after all of the indicators within the plan are evaluated. Once the indicators and the individual data elements have been finalized and the sources of data secured, APRNs should summarize the outcome evaluation plan in a concise document that describes the plan and communicate it to all stakeholders.

Derive Meaning From Data and Act on Results

The final phase of the outcome evaluation process involves evaluation and dissemination of the findings and identification of opportunities for improvement. In these final steps, results are transformed into meaningful information that can be used to improve quality, cost, and patient satisfaction and to evaluate the contributions of the APRN. The final step involves formulating a plan to implement and reevaluate changes that occur as a result of the study.

Analyze Data and Interpret Findings

Typically, data analysis is the responsibility of the APRN, although the inclusion of other peer reviewers is useful, especially when the APRN has a vested interest in the outcomes. Including others helps eliminate any perceived bias during the final data analysis and reporting phases. In some cases, the APRN may wish to enlist the support and guidance of a statistician or a nurse researcher to ensure that the end product is methodologically sound and contains the information necessary to convince others.

Comparing pre-intervention with post-intervention performance data is one effective way to evaluate the degree of change resulting from APRN interventions. Pre-intervention performance data are commonly collected retrospectively and then compared with data collected during or after an APRN intervention. Retrospective data are generally available for measures constructed from electronic data sources. When electronic data are insufficient to provide adequate baseline information, APRNs may elect to collect more detailed data from noncomputerized medical records. Although this approach generally requires more effort, time, and planning, it may be warranted when specific processes of care are altered as part of the APRN's intervention. For example, a CRNA evaluating the frequency of intraoperative hypotensive episodes may have to manually review medical records, because this phenomenon may not be contained in common electronic source data. In some cases, baseline data collection must be conducted before the APRN intervention to ensure that appropriate baseline data are available for comparison. For example, a CNM who is implementing changes in clinic protocols to reduce waiting times for prenatal patients undergoing glucose tolerance testing may have to conduct a pre-intervention time and motion study to establish a baseline against which to compare post-intervention results.

Although baseline information is useful for evaluating outcomes, not everything measured by APRNs will have suitable baseline data for comparison. In these cases, performance can be evaluated against a known standard of care or benchmark, especially when an area of practice is supported by evidence-based practice. When no best practice standard of performance is known, APRNs may use comparative data provided by a national database if the measures used for comparison are the same as those contained within the national database.

Present and Disseminate Findings

Effective communication of data-based findings, conclusions, and recommendations for future practice is an essential component of the outcome evaluation process. How the findings are presented depends on the audience. Nonclinical audiences with a business focus, such as boards of directors or operations teams, will require briefings that summarize pertinent findings, draw conclusions, and provide reasonable options or recommendations for consideration. Clinical audiences generally require additional detail about how the evaluation was conducted and a more extensive discussion of the clinical and statistical strengths of the evidence. Clinical audiences are becoming more sophisticated in their understanding of data analysis techniques and their assessment of the applicability of evidence to practice.

The APRN may be responsible for packaging the project's findings to present to stakeholders. Assistance from the facility's media or publications department may be required, depending on the final forum for communicating findings. Findings are commonly presented in committee meetings and formal presentations, although the APRN should also consider posters, newsletters, APRN or clinical conference presentations, white papers, articles, bulk e-mail communications, or listserv communities as additional ways to disseminate information.

Identify Improvement Opportunities

Once the outcome evaluation findings have been interpreted, the APRN begins to work closely with stakeholders to evaluate the effectiveness of the practice change or QI strategy. This step may occur very quickly following a practice change or intervention, depending on the QI project. Many healthcare organizations are adopting a rapid cycle of learning, in which they perform smaller tests of change, evaluate the results, and then, if successful, expand to larger areas or populations. For example, an APRN intervention might be pilot-tested in one nursing unit before deploying the strategy across the hospital. If the intervention does not lead to the desired outcome in a timely manner, improvement opportunities are quickly identified and implemented and the results are reevaluated, with constant scrutiny on specific aspects of the care delivery processes, technology resources, or points in time that could be altered to achieve greater efficiency or effectiveness.

For example, an APRN working in an acute care hospital may identify opportunities to improve performance in teaching discharge instructions to patients with heart failure. For 1 week, a request report can be generated identifying patients who need heart failure instructions at discharge. The following week it is identified that during the weekends there is a gap in the use of the report because the APRN is not available. Rather than wait for a longer evaluation period to pass, an incremental improvement in the process is adopted whereby automated alerts are generated out of the HIT system to identify all patients with an active diagnosis of heart failure who are on the telemetry unit longer than 24 hours. Incremental improvement opportunities may be made over time until a larger and more sustainable strategy is identified and long-term adoption has been achieved. In this example, the most effective solution may ultimately be for the hospital to participate in the American Heart Association's Get With the Guidelines Program, a national demonstration of best practice performance for the treatment of acute myocardial infarction (http://www.heart.org/HEARTORG/). With this program, comprehensive Internet-based patient education materials are available to staff nurses and other clinicians, who can quickly customize the materials to meet the specific learning needs of individual patients. This solution may not have been part of the initial strategy at the onset of the project, but the APRN's stewardship of the process will assist team members to develop a shared vision of which intervention(s) to adopt and why. Bringing stakeholders together to review existing and ongoing processes of care and isolate any process failures or barriers that have contributed to suboptimal performance is essential in today's healthcare environment.

The process to identify opportunities for improvement is similar to any work redesign initiative. The APRN should identify champions and potential opponents of change. Change theory can serve as a useful foundation for APRNs responsible for preparing stakeholders and overcoming their resistance to new healthcare delivery practices. Issues such as difficulty with deploying the intervention should be addressed, as well as projected costs and the human and technology resources required to implement and sustain the plan. Consider how much time the APRN will be engaged in the project and how this may affect other areas of practice. A staged pilot test approach is useful for new or large-scale projects. As noted, these smaller scale versions can help identify potential implementation problems and determine whether the intervention can achieve the desired effect.

Formulate a Plan for Ongoing Monitoring and Reevaluation

Once an acceptable outcome has been achieved and sustained for a period of time, a final summary of the performance improvement initiative should be documented. This type of documentation is useful to a healthcare organization during an accreditation survey so that it can demonstrate that a culture of quality has been established and that it is actively engaged in improving care. In addition, this information is useful to demonstrate the APRN's value to their organization. Each goal should specify the primary interventions that were used to reach the goal, along with who was accountable for the actions required and the dates for completion. This reevaluation then becomes the basis for future outcome evaluation plans. Once performance in a particular area is stabilized, the APRN may elect to discontinue monitoring a given area of performance or periodically revisit performance through intermittent monitoring.

Clarify Purpose of the Advanced Practice Nurse's Role

A final step in the process may include a thoughtful review of the APRN's role and their effectiveness in achieving desired outcomes. An APRN's role may change as a direct result of performance improvement and outcome evaluation studies. Findings may indicate that APRN interventions are better suited to other points of care across the continuum of services than originally envisioned or may reveal that care may be delivered more efficiently by other providers. Conversely, findings may support the effectiveness and efficiency of the APRN intervention, which could lead to program growth and expansion to other populations or points of care. In all cases, outcome evaluation, APRN role definition, and scope of practice go hand in hand. If the purposes of their roles are unclear, APRNs may need to identify and discuss reasonable and appropriate expectations with administrators and collaborators. It is not possible to decide which outcomes to measure without clarity about the APRN's clinical populations and their accountability for the structures and processes of care. Finally, employers may not recognize the APRN's full range of services or potential benefit to the organization. In such situations, the APRN may need to take the lead in identifying specific processes and areas of focus within the setting and set appropriate goals and performance objectives to meet them.

Although the strategies discussed in this chapter to evaluate outcomes and improve performance are integral to the success of the APRN in any organization, it is important to remember that data are ultimately a tool that can be used to foster learning, improve quality, and assist APRNs in the nursing process to achieve their ultimate goal. Exemplar 23.3 reveals a unique and powerful perspective on QI and outcomes evaluation as it pertains to nursing practice.

CONCLUSION

This chapter illustrates the interconnectivity among policy, regulation, healthcare information technology, information management, outcomes measurement, systems thinking, and performance improvement with every aspect of APRN practice. Effective outcomes measurement and management require APRNs to master information technologies, work collaboratively with others, plan and organize processes of care and assessments of quality in highly complex health services environments, and effectively manage change within their sponsoring organizations. Because reimbursement decisions are increasingly driven by evidence of organizational and individual provider performance, APRNs who lack reliable and valid data to substantiate their impact will struggle for equitable reimbursement for their services, and possibly employment. For APRNs to be a visible and viable resource in today's healthcare delivery system, they must have visible and robust outcomes that demonstrate their value. APRNs in every practice setting must be willing and able to spearhead performance improvement initiatives in their institutions. Given the challenges of healthcare reform and the pioneering innovations of many healthcare systems across the United States and internationally, there are many opportunities to deploy APRNs to deliver primary, preventive, acute, and chronic care and episodic care services in a quality and cost-effective manner. It may be that APRNs who successfully steward safer care environments, improve clinical performance, and achieve greater efficiencies in caregiving processes will demonstrate their value more than they ever could have in the past, but they must be involved in the development of information systems to help carry this out. APRNs who develop robust and ongoing outcome evaluation plans place themselves in the strongest position to demonstrate their impact on outcomes of care delivery. In so doing, they also render advanced practice nursing visible to patients, other providers, administrators, payers, and communities. In addition, they ensure that patients continue to receive the best available, efficient, and cost effective care.

Given the many quality reporting initiatives that represent so many clinical specialty domains and care delivery settings, one must wonder why it has taken so long for the nursing profession to develop a quality data set that represents the best that advanced practice nursing has to offer to those to whom we are in service. Considering emerging HIT technologies, would it now be possible to develop a robust, reliable, and highly interoperable data set of clinical outcomes that are sensitive to APRN practice? Although these are important aspects of care, it seems long overdue to expand beyond the traditional measurement of outcomes, such as pressure ulcers, falls, and medication errors, and examine the difference that APRN practice brings to patient outcomes, the patient experience, and the entire care delivery system. Isn't it possible for APRNs to make a measurable difference in conditions such as childhood obesity, diabetes management, cardiac and pulmonary disease prevention, cancer treatment, and acute and episodic care? Isn't it possible for the APRN to address health disparities and poor outcomes by systematically collecting and scoring patient risk based on social determinants of health and then providing resources to patients to address their needs? The Social Interventions Research and Evaluation Network (SIREN) from the University of California San Francisco (2021) provides valid and reliable tools as well as study designs and outcomes.

Through advanced education and clinical expertise, APRNs are in a unique position to lead the way to this new level of thought leadership and clinical practice that is sorely needed in today's healthcare ecosystem.

KEY SUMMARY POINTS

- Information technology is a necessary tool for collection and storage of data used to measure outcomes and improvement.
- Informatics is the combination of computer science, information science, and nursing science that allows the development of information and knowledge from the data collected.
- It is mandatory for APRNs (and other providers) to be able to measure and report on care improvement and patient outcomes to benefit from a changing reimbursement structure that will pay for quality, and not quantity, of services performed.
- APRNs must be skillful leaders of quality improvement initiatives that optimize use of information technology and data that ensure quality care for patients and that meet mandatory reporting requirements.
- For APRNs to be able to practice at the top of their licenses uniformly across the nation, data collected in information systems must be robust enough to demonstrate equal or better outcomes compared with physician counterparts.

REFERENCES

Agency for Healthcare Research and Quality. (2005). Patient Safety and Quality Improvement Act of 2005. Retrieved from https://archive.ahrq.gov/news/newsroom/press-releases/2008/psoact.html

American Academy of Nurse Practitioners. (2022). State practice environment. Retrieved from https://www.aanp.org/advocacy/state/state-practice-environment

American Association of Colleges of Nursing (2021). The essentials: Core competencies for professional nursing practice. Retrieved from https://www.aacnnursing.org/Portals/42/AcademicNursing/pdf/Essentials-2021.pdf

American Association of Family Physicians. (2021). Basics of quality improvement. Retrieved from https://www.aafp.org/family-physician/practice-and-career/managing-your-practice/quality-improvement-basics.html

American Society for Quality. (2021). Control chart. Retrieved from: https://asq.org/quality-resources/control-chart

Archibald, M. M., & Fraser, K. (2013). The potential for nurse practitioners in health care reform. *Journal of Professional Nursing, 25*(5), 270–275. doi:10.1016/j.profnurs.2012.10.002

Artetxe, A., Beristain, A., & Grana, M. (2018). Predictive models for hospital readmission risk: A systematic review of method. *Computer Methods Programs Biomed, 164*, 49–64. doi:10.1016/j.cmpb.2018.06.006

Centers for Medicare & Medicaid Services [CMS]. (n.d.) Welcome to QualityNet. https://www.qualitynet.org

Centers for Medicare & Medicaid Services [CMS]. (2021a). Accountable care organizations (ACOs). https://www.cms.gov/Medicare/Medicare-Fee-for-Service-Payment/ACO

Centers for Medicare & Medicaid Services [CMS]. (2021b). Quality payment programs. Retrieved from https://qpp.cms.gov/about/qpp-overview

Centers for Medicare & Medicaid Services [CMS]. (2021c). Using SDOH Z codes can enhance your quality improvement initiatives. Retrieved from https://www.cms.gov/files/document/zcodes-infographic.pdf

Centers for Medicare & Medicaid Services [CMS]. (2022a). MACRA. Retrieved from https://www.cms.gov/Medicare/Quality-Initiatives-Patient-Assessment-Instruments/Value-Based-Programs/MACRA-MIPS-and-APMs/MACRA-MIPS-and-APMs.html

Centers for Medicare & Medicaid Services [CMS]. (2022b). MS-DRG classifications and software. Retrieved from https://www.cms.gov/Medicare/Medicare-Fee-for-Service-Payment/AcuteInpatientPPS/MS-DRG-Classifications-and-Software

govinfo. (n.d.). Public Law 104–191–Health Insurance Portability and Accountability Act of 1996. Retrieved from https://www.govinfo.gov/app/details/PLAW-104publ191

The Gravity Project. (2021). Educational and instructional materials. Retrieved from https://confluence.hl7.org/display/GRAV/Educational+and+Instructional+Materials

Green, J. (2019). *How EHR and meaningful use has transformed healthcare*. EHR in Practice. Retrieved from https://www.ehrinpractice.com/ehr-meaningful-use-transformed-healthcare.html

Health Resources and Services Administration [HRSA] Bureau of Primary Care. (2020). Uniform Data 2021 Health Center Data Reporting Tables. Retrieved from https://bphc.hrsa.gov/sites/default/files/bphc/data-reporting/2021-uds-manual.pdf

Honeyfield, M. E. (2009). Neonatal nurse practitioners: Past, present, and future. *Advances in Neonatal Care, 9*(3), 125–128.

Kansagara, D., Englander, H., Salanitro, A., Kagen, D., Theobald, C., Freeman, M., & Kripalani, S. (2011). Risk prediction models for hospital readmission: A systematic review. *Journal of the American Medical Association, 306*(15), 1688–1697.

Kleinpell, R., & Kapu, A. N. (2017). Quality measures for nurse practitioner practice evaluation. *Journal of the American Association of Nurse Practitioners, 29*, 446–451. doi:10.1002/2327-6924.12474

McCleery, E., Christensen, V., Peterson, K., Humphrey, L., & Helfand, M. (2014). Evidence brief: The quality of care provided by advance practice nurses. VA-ESP Project #09-199; US Department of Veteran Affairs. Retrieved from https://www.ncbi.nlm.nih.gov/books/NBK384613/

Morgan, J., & Brenig-Jones, M. (2012). *Lean six sigma for dummies*. West Sussex: John Wiley & Sons, Ltd.

Mundinger, M. O., Kane, R. L., Lentz, E. R., Totten, A. M., Tsai, W., Cleary, P. D., Friedewald, W. T., Siu, A. L., & Shelanski, M. L. (2000). Primary care outcomes in patients treated by nurses practitioners or physicians: A randomized trial. *Journal of the American Medical Association, 283*(1), 59–68.

National Academies of Science, Engineering and Medicine [NASEM]. (2021). *The future of nursing 2020-2030: Charting a path to achieve health equity*. The National Academies Press. doi:10.17226/25982

National Governors Association. (2012). Nurse practitioners have potential to improve access to primary care. Retrieved from https://www.nga.org/cms/home/news-room/news-releases/page_2012/col2-content/nurse-practitioners-have-potenti.html

National Quality Forum. (2022). Community tool to align measurement. Retrieved from http://www.qualityforum.org/AlignmentTool

Nelson, R. (2020). Informatics: The evolution of the Nelson data, information, knowledge, and wisdom model: Part 2. *The Online Journal of Issues in Nursing, 25*(3). doi:10.3912/OJIN.Vol-25No03InfoCol01

Newhouse, R., Stanik-Hutt, J., White, K. M., Johantgen, M., Bass, E. B., Zangaro, G., Wilson, R. F., Fountain, L., Steinwachs, D. M, Heindel, L., & Weiner, J. P. (2011). Advanced practice nurse outcomes 1990-2008: A systematic review. *Nurse Economics, 29*(5), 230–250. doi:10.1177/1077558719901216

Ogrinc, G. S., Headrick, L. A., Barton, A. J., Dolansky, M. A., & Miltner, R. A. (2018). *Fundamentals of health care improvement: A guide to improving your patients' care* (3rd ed.). Joint Commission Resources.

Quality Payment Program. (n.d.a.). Explore measures and activities. https://qpp.cms.gov/mips/explore-measures?tab=qualityMeasures&py=2021

Quality Payment Program. (n.d.b). Improvement activities performance categories: Traditional MIPS requirements. Retrieved from https://qpp.cms.gov/mips/improvement-activities

Quality Payment Program. (n.d.c). Latest updates. Retrieved from https://qpp.cms.gov/mips/explore-measures?tab=qualityMeasures&py=2021

Sackett, D. L., Spitzer, W. O., Gent, M., & Roberts, R. S. (1974). The Burlington randomized trial of the nurse practitioner: Health outcomes of patients. *Annals of Internal Medicine, 80*(2), 137–142.

Savas, A., Smith, E., & Hay, B. (2019). EHR quality indicator tracking: A process improvement pilot project to meet MACRA requirements. *The Nurse Practitioner, 44*(4), 30–39. doi:10.1097/01.NPR.0000554084.05450.0e. Retrieved from https://pubmed.ncbi.nlm.nih.gov/30889108/

Sikka, R., Gagen, M., Crayton, M., & Esposito, T. (2012). An administrative claims and electronic medical record derived risk prediction model for hospital readmissions. Presented at the Academy Health Annual Research Conference, Orlando, Florida, June 24, 2012.

Stanik-Hutt, J., Newhouse, R. P., White, K. M., Johantgen, M., Bass, E. B, Zangaro, G., Wilson, R., Fountain, L., Steinwachs, D. M., Heindel, L., & Weiner, JP. (2013). The quality and effectiveness of care provided by nurse practitioners. *The Journal for Nurse Practitioners, 9*(8), 492–500. doi:10.1016/j.nurpra.2013.07.004

Statistical Process Control. (2022). Control charts. http://www.processma.com/resource/spc.php

Trout, K. E., Chen, L-W., Wilson, F., Tak, H. J., & Palm, D. (2021). The impact of electronic health records and meaningful use on impatient quality. *Journal of Healthcare Quality, 44*(2), 15–23. doi:10.1097/JHQ.0000000000000314

University of California San Francisco. (2022). Social interventions research and evaluation network. Evidence and resource library. Retrieved from https://sirenetwork.ucsf.edu/tools/evidence-library

US Department of Health and Human Services (DHHS). (2019). Office of the National Coordinator for Health Information Technology. The Health IT Dashboard. Retrieved from https://dashboard.healthit.gov/quickstats/quickstats.php

Vleet, A.V., & Paradise, J. (2015). Tapping nurse practitioners to meet rising demand for primary care. Retrieved from http://kff.org/medicaid/issue-brief/tapping-nurse-practitioners-to-meet-rising-demand-for-primary-care/

Wang-Romjue, P. (2018). Meta-synthesis on nurse practitioner autonomy and roles in ambulatory care. *Nursing Forum, 53*(2), 148–155. Retrieved from https://onlinelibrary-wiley-com.ezproxy3.lhl.uab.edu/doi/pdfdirect/10.1111/nuf.12236

Wheeler, D. J. (1993). *Understanding variation: The key to managing chaos.* SPC Press.

World Health Organization. (2022). ICD-11 for mortality and morbidity statistics (Version: 02/2022). Retrieved from https://icd.who.int/browse11/l-m/en

INDEX

Pages followed by *b*, *t*, or *f* refer to boxes, tables, or figures, respectively.

A

AACN. *See* American Association of Colleges of Nursing
AACN Scope and Standards for Acute Care Nurse Practitioner Practice, 469, 472
AANA. *See* American Association of Nurse Anesthetists
AANA Nurse Anesthesia Scope of Practice Domains, 525*b*
AANA Standards for Nurse Anesthesia Practice, 524, 526*b*
AANP. *See* American Association of Nurse Practitioners
Abandonment of nursing identity, 307
Accelerators, additional dynamics and, 565
Accountability, 234*t*, 235
- collaboration and, 316

Accountable care organizations (ACOs), 321, 569, 751, 753
Accreditation. *See also* Credentialing requirements
- of advanced practice nurse, programs for, 654
- certified nurse-midwife (CNM), 492
- Consensus Model for APRN Regulation, 650

ACNM. *See* American College of Nurse-Midwives
ACNPs. *See* Acute care nurse practitioners
ACOs. *See* Accountable care organizations
Actions
- in APRN coaching process, 217
- and goal setting, 221*b*–222*b*, 235

Activities, APRN and, 179
Actuated and sensory prosthetics, 724
Acute and chronic care issues, ethical practice, 361
Acute care nurse practitioners (ACNPs), 25, 484, 680, 682*f*
- adult–gerontology, work activities arranged by criticality, 462*b*
- challenges, 483
- competencies of
  - collaboration, 468
  - diagnosing and managing disease, 461
  - direct clinical practice, 461
  - ethical practice, 468
  - evidence-based practice, 467
  - guidance and coaching, 466
  - health and preventing disease, promoting and protecting, 465
  - leadership, 467
- diagnoses, 463*t*
- emergence of, 458
- preparation of, 469
- procedures, 463*t*
- profiles, role and practice models, 475
  - advanced practice nurse and physician assistant roles, 478
- scope of practice, levels of influence
  - individual level, 475
  - institutional level, 473
  - national level (professional organizations), 472
  - service-related level, 474
  - state level (government), 473
- specialty services
  - bone marrow transplantation services, 481
  - critical care teams, 482
  - diagnostic and interventional services, 481
  - heart failure services, 482
  - orthopedic services, 482
  - rapid response teams, 482
  - supportive and palliative care, 482

Acute care pediatric nurse practitioner (AC-PNP), 464*b*–465*b*, 476*b*
Acute Care Pediatric Population-Focused Nurse Practitioner Competencies, 469
Adams, Dawn, 576*b*–577*b*
Adcock, Gale, 575*b*–576*b*
Admission-discharge-transfer (ADT), 763
Adult-gerontology acute care nurse practitioner (AG-ACNP) practice
- healthcare services, 477*b*
- hospitalist team, 480*b*
- role implementation, 471*b*
- work activities arranged by criticality, 462*b*

Adult NPs, 458–459
Advance care planning resources, 364*b*
Advanced analytics, 731
- cleaning, 729
- dictionary, 729
- mining, 729
- scrubbing, 729
- storage, types of, 729*b*
- structured, 728
- unstructured, 728–729
- warehouse, 729

"Advanced generalist", 81
Advanced nursing practice, advanced practice nursing *vs.*, 77
Advanced Nursing Practice: A National Framework, 46
Advanced physical assessment, 187
Advanced Practice, 23
Advanced Practice Committee, 668*b*
Advanced practice nurse (APN), 140, 554
- competencies, 84, 281, 498
  - central, 84, 84*f*
  - collaboration, 503
  - consultation, 504–505, 507
  - core, 85, 85*f*
  - direct clinical practice, 501
  - ethical practice, 505

Advanced practice nurse (APN) *(Continued)*
evidence-based practice, 502
guidance and coaching, 502
health professional education, evolution of, 281
leadership, 503
overview of, and certified nurse-midwife competencies, 498
conceptualizations of, 34, 37
conceptual models for, 37
Dunphy and Winland-Brown's Circle of Caring model for, 62, 63*f*
framework for, 33
implications for, 46
SickKids APRN Framework, 57
transitional care models for, 61
core values for, 75
definition of, 78, 137
advanced nursing practice *vs.*, 77
conceptual, 79
core, 78
implications of, 91
direct care practice of, 84
education, implications for, 84
environments
critical elements in managing, 89
implications for, 91
experienced, 668*b*
expert, 668*b*
features of, 138
funding and reimbursement arrangements, 152
future directions of, 65
global deployment, 138
global evolution of, 155*b*, 155
global health care context, 137
health policy of, 90
integrative approaches, identity, abandonment of, 301*b*
international development of, 137
introduction and integration of, 148, 148*t*
licensing and regulating, 77
models of
Calkin's, 50, 53*f*
Hamric's integrative, 48
new frontiers for future role development, 143
novice, 668*b*
operational definitions of, 87
organizational perspectives, 37
pan-approaches and collaboration, 148
policy issues, current, 566
Advanced practice nurse (APN) *(Continued)*
access, 569
cost, 568
quality, 569
primary criteria of, 80, 80*f*
certification as, 80*f*, 81
graduate education as, 80
practice focused on patient and family as, 82
profiles, role and practice models, 478
quality in, 91
recommendations of, 65
regulation and credentialing, 92
research on, 67
implication for, 92
role development, 147*b*
roles in
established, 87
scope of practice in, 86
specialization and, 76
systematic approaches to role planning, 153
timeline of, 11*b*
types of, 138
in United States, history of, 3
use and generation of evidence, 154
Advanced practice nurse and physician assistant roles, 478
ACNP practice models, 479
outcome studies, 479
physician hospitalists, ACNPs and, 479
Advanced practice providers (APPs), 468
Advanced practice registered nurse (APRN), 168–169, 170–171, 176*b*
access to health care, 617–618, 618*f*
acquisition of knowledge and skill, 99
additional compensation models, 644
advanced physical assessment, 187
adverse events and performance errors, 189
ambiguity in, role of, 98, 102
anticipatory planning for the first, 110–111
barriers of, 105, 125–126
billing for, 624
coding sets, 627
credentialing process, 625
inpatient billing, 633
Advanced practice registered nurse (APRN) *(Continued)*
medical decision making, 630
outpatient billing, 629
provider panels and contracts, 626
revenue cycle management, 635
building coalitions and, 581–582
building unity for, 581
characteristics of, 172
direct clinical care provided by, 172
classification schemas in, 170–171
clinical thinking, 182
coaching process, 233*f*, 233
action, 233
contemplation, 232
maintenance, 233
preparation, 232
readiness, of patient, 228
resistance, 228
skills, guidance and, 213
communicating findings on, 582*f*, 582
communication with patients, 179
competencies, 213
cross-mapping of, 427*t*–430*t*
conceptual models of, 67–68
APRN Consensus Model, 66
model for maximizing NP contributions to primary care, 60
model of exemplary midwifery practice, 57, 58*f*
and perceptions of team effectiveness, 59, 59*f*
SickKids APRN framework, 57
Consensus Model, 469
consensus model for regulation and implications, CNS, 406
cultural influences on partnerships, 180
direct care
vs. indirect care activities, 169, 170*b*
and information management, 203
provided by, 171*b*
directed program evaluations, 687*t*–689*t*
ethical reasoning, 186
in evidence-based practice, 192, 245
levels of, 245
quality improvement of, 250
research for, 252

Advanced practice registered nurse (APRN) *(Continued)*
facilitators, 124
frustration phase, 123
full practice authority in, 584
future technologies, 709
health and illness management, 194
health policy experiences for, 584*t*
impact of, 689, 690*t*–694*t*
implementation phase, 124
imposter phenomenon, 119
indirect care provided by, 171*b*
integrating telehealth and informatics into, 738
integration phase, 124
international experiences with, 98–99
interprofessional role conflict, 105, 106*b*
intraprofessional role conflict, 104
Joint Dialogue Group, 56
long-term collaboration for education and regulation of, 332*b*
marketing the role of, 590, 591*b*
activities, 595*t*
business and contractual arrangements, 611
characteristics of, 593
choosing between, 592
communication in, 600
core competencies, 596, 597*t*–598*t*
cover letters for, 601
employment contracts and, 611*b*, 611
entrepreneurial/freelancer, 592
independent contractor and, 611, 613*b*
innovative practices and, 593
interview process in, 603, 604*b*
malpractice insurance in, 612
professional networking in, 596
professional portfolio and, 601, 602*b*
professional recruiters in, 599
résumés and curricula vitae in, 602*b*, 602, 603*b*
success of, 593, 594*b*–595*b*
value of, 606*b*, 607
web-based resources in, 599, 600*t*
multisite practices of, 127*b*
novice, 183
nursing model/medical model, 175

Advanced practice registered nurse (APRN) *(Continued)*
orientation phase, 122
outcomes
future directions for, 698
integrative review of, 673
measures of, importance of, 678
physician and other provider *vs.*, 689
patient education, 176*b*, 188
perspectives on, 99
political competence in policy arena, 571
practice principles, 235, 235*t*
productivity, physicians *vs.*, 697
regulatory model, 66–67
reimbursement and payment for, 617
role acquisition
clinical knowledge development for, 111
developing supportive network for, 113
in graduate school, 98, 107
role rehearsal, 111
role concepts and development issues of, 98, 101
role conflict, 98, 104
role development of, 99
evaluation of, 127
role evolution, continued, 126
role implementation at work, 98, 114, 118
strategies to facilitate, 98, 110
role incongruity, 98, 102
role transitions, 107, 119
sensitive outcome indicators, 690*t*–694*t*
shared decision making, 179
skillful performance, 187
student role transition studies, 98, 108
surveillance, 197
technology supporting, 725, 727*b*
theory-based practice, 193
therapeutic partnerships with noncommunicative patients, 181
thinking errors, 184, 185*b*
time pressures, 184
transition from student to clinician, 101
Vision Paper, 37–38
workforce development, 586
Advance practice, definition of, 3
Adverse events, 189

Advocacy, 303
Affordable Care Act (ACA), 213–214
Agency for Healthcare Research and Quality (AHRQ), 257, 257*t*, 324, 662, 674–678, 679, 756*t*–757*t*
Agenda for Health Care Reform, 20
Agenda setting, 233*f*, 233, 564–565, 567*t*
AHRQ. *See* Agency for Healthcare Research and Quality
AI. *See* Appreciative inquiry; Artificial intelligence
Alternative ethical approaches, 347*b*
Ambiguity, role of, 102, 103*t*
American Academy of Nurse Practitioners Certification Program, 655
American Academy of Pediatrics, 270*t*
American Association of Colleges of Nursing (AACN), 13, 41, 280, 319, 571, 653, 745
American Association of Colleges of Nursing Essentials, 213
American Association of Colleges of Pharmacy, 319
American Association of Critical-Care Nurses, 17
and Oncology Nursing Society, 76
practice environments, 93
American Association of Nurse Anesthesiology (AANA), 519, 520
American Association of Nurse Anesthetists (AANA), 5, 43, 572, 653–654
American Association of Nurse-Midwives (AANM), 11
American Association of Nurse Practitioners (AANP), 26, 570–571
American Board of Nursing Specialties (ABNS), 41
American Cancer Society, 21
American College of Nurse-Midwives (ACNM), 45, 107, 490–491, 495*b*, 496, 653–654
Code of Ethics of, 45
philosophy of, 497*b*
American College of Obstetricians and Gynecologists (ACOG), 107, 495*b*
American Dental Education Association, 319

American Heart Association, Get With the Guidelines program, 778
American Journal of Nursing, 13
American Nurses Association (ANA), 5, 40
  for advanced practice nursing, 76
  Agenda for Health Care Reform, 15
  Congress of Nursing Practice, 17
  nursing practice defined by, 14
  Nursing's Social Policy Statement, 319
  Primary Health Care Nurse Practitioner Council, 25
  principles of social networking, 720*b*
  Scope and Standards of Practice, 41
  social media tips, 720*b*
  Social Policy Statement of, 17–18
American Nurses Credentialing Center (ANCC), 82, 272, 328, 655
American Society for Quality (ASQ), 756*t*–757*t*
American Society of Anesthesiologists (ASA), 572
Amicus curiae (friend of the court) briefs, 557
ANA. *See* American Nurses Association
ANCC. *See* American Nurses Credentialing Center
Anesthesia
  billing calculation, 545
  modifiers, 546
  nurse anesthesia organizations
    American Association of Nurse Anesthesiology, 546
    International Federation of Nurse Anesthetists (IFNA), 546
  practice models, 544
  time definitions, 545*b*
Anesthesia care modifiers, 546*b*
Anesthesia claim modifiers, 546
Anesthesiologist assistants (AAs), 531
Anticipatory guidance, 215
APN. *See* Advanced practice nurse; Advanced practice nurse (APN)
Appalachia, primary care in, 26
Appreciative inquiry (AI), 286
Apps, in health information technology, 721
APRN. *See* Advanced practice registered nurse
APRN Consensus Model, 35
APSM (Association for the Promotion and Standardization of Midwifery), 10
Artificial intelligence (AI)
  in verbal communication technologies, 717
  in written communication technologies, 717
ASA. *See* American Society of Anesthesiologists
ASR. *See* Automated speech recognition
Assessment
  advanced physical, 187
  of environmental factors, 334
  health, 187
  institutional, 310
  of outcome(s), 675*t*–677*t*
  of personal factors, 334
  quality, 263*f*
Association for the Promotion and Standardization of Midwifery (APSM), 10
Association of American Medical Colleges, 318
Association of Schools of Public Health, 328–329
Association of Women's Health, Obstetric, and Neonatal Nurses (AWHONN), 26
4 A's to Rise Above Moral Distress, The (AACCN), 169
Augmented reality (AR), 726
Authority
  perspective, 26
  prescriptive, 659
Automated speech recognition (ASR), 718
Awareness raising, 233*f*, 234
AWHONN (Association of Women's Health, Obstetric, and Neonatal Nurses), 26

B

Balanced Budget Act, 19
Bar chart, 767*t*
Bar code administration, 746
Barriers
  to collaboration, 316
  disciplinary, 330
  ethical practice, 371
    barriers internal to APRN, 371
    interprofessional barriers, 372
    organizational and environmental barriers, 373
    patient–provider barriers, 372
  organizational, 331
  regulatory, 331
Barry, Donna, 585*b*
Behavior-based question, for interview, 604*b*
Benchmark, 675*t*–677*t*
  performance, 675*t*–677*t*
Benchmarking, 653
Benner's model, 99
Benner's model of expert nursing practice, 49
Bethany Hospital, 15–16
Bhan v. NME Hospitals, Inc., et al. (1985), 7–8
Bias, 264
Big data, 731
Bipartisan support, 556*b*
Birth center setting, 509*b*–510*b*
Blockchain, 735
Bone marrow transplantation services, ACNPs, 481
Boundary awareness, 226
Boundary management, 298
Braden Scale for Pressure Sore Risk, 270–271
Brainstorming, 767*t*
Breckinridge, Mary, 9–10
Brew, Nancy, 560
Brown and Olshansky study, 119
Bryant-Lukosius education framework matrix, 65*f*
Buhler-Wilkerson, Karen, 19
Bullying, 306, 308
Bundled billing, 634
Bureau of Indian Affairs, 21
Bureau of Labor Statistics, 586
Business development
  reimbursement, 643
    additional APRN compensation models, 644
    business ownership, 644
    entrepreneurship, 643
Business ownership, 644

C

California Consumer Privacy Act (CCPA), 733
California Supreme Court, 5–6
Calkin, Joy, 23
Calkin's Model of Advanced Nursing Practice, 50, 53*f*
Callen, Maude, 11*b*
Campaign for Action, 92
Canadian Interprofessional Health Collaborative (CIHC), 32, 317
Canadian Nurses Association (CNA), 32
Capsule endoscopies, 724

CAQH. *See* Council for Affordable Quality Healthcare
Cardiopulmonary resuscitation (CPR), 464
Care assistant robots, 724
Care-based ethics, 347, 348
Care coordination, 421, 434
Care delivery impact, conceptual models of, 680
  by APRNs, 680
  nurse practitioner role effectiveness model, 680, 682*f*
  outcomes evaluation model, 680, 681*t*–682*t*
Care delivery process studies, 684
Care, quality of, 675*t*–677*t*
Case-control study, 261
Case study, 260
Casuistry approach, 347
  ethical practice, 347
Cause-and-effect diagrams, 767*t*, 769
CCNE. *See* Commission on Collegiate Nursing Education
CCPA. *See* California Consumer Privacy Act
CDR. *See* Clinical data repository
CEBM. *See* Centre for Evidence-Based Medicine
Cellphone, smartphone and, 718
Center for Preventive Medicine scale, 268
Centers for Disease Control and Prevention, 661
Centers for Medicare and Medicaid Services (CMS), 621, 674–678, 679, 747, 768
  Transforming Clinical Practice Initiative, 756*t*–757*t*
Central competency, in advanced practice nursing, 84, 84*f*
Central line-associated bloodstream infection (CLABSI), 751, 753
Centre for Evidence-Based Medicine (CEBM), 268
CER. *See* Comparative effectiveness research
Cerner Systems and Advocate Health Care, 768
Certification
  of advanced practice registered nurses
    continuing education requirements, 656
    mandatory requirements for, 656
    recertification, 655
  of clinical nurse specialist, 13
Certification *(Continued)*
  Consensus Model for, 650
  CRNAs, 520
  as primary criteria, of advanced practice nursing, 84*f*, 84
Certification and certification maintenance, 493
Certified nurse-midwife (CNM), 76
  certification and certification maintenance, 493
  definitions of, 490
  education and accreditation, 492
  historical perspective, 491
  outcomes, 696
  practice of, 506
  practice settings, 507
  professional issues, 508
  recognition of, 491
  reentry to practice, 493
  regulation, reimbursement and credentialing, 493
  scope of practice, 506
  summary of, 508
  in United States, 491
Certified professional midwife (CPM), 490, 491
Certified registered nurse anesthetist (CRNA)-PAC Mission, 572
Certified registered nurse anesthetists (CRNAs), 76, 572
  access to care, 543
  clinical competence, role development and measures of, 531
    collaboration, 538
    direct clinical practice, 531
    evidence-based practice (EBP), 535, 537*t*
    guidance and coaching, 534
    leadership, 536
    and opioid crisis, 534
    palliative care, 533
    specialty practice areas, 534
  continued professional competence, 521
  education and practice, brief history of, 520
  ethical practice, 541
  outcomes, 696
  pain management, role in, 535*b*
  practice, 521, 542, 547
  professional career, 538*b*
  professional journey, 532*b*
  profile of, 523
    education, 524
    institutional credentialing, 530
Certified registered nurse anesthetists (CRNAs) *(Continued)*
    practice doctorate, 530
    programs of study, 527
    scope and standards of practice, 524
  reimbursement, 544
    anesthesia practice models, 544
    anesthesiologist billing for medical direction *vs.* medical supervision, 544
  role differentiation, between CRNAs and anesthesiologists, 522
  strategies, opioid misuse, 536*b*
  workforce issues, 543
Chalmers-Frances v. Nelson (1936), 5–6
Chalmers-Frances, William, 5–6
Change-related contexts
  concepts related to, 286
    driving forces, 287
    opinion leadership, 287
    pace of change, 287
    restraining forces, 287
  culture of, 288*b*, 288
  institutional assessment of, 310
  leadership models of, 282
  pace of, 287
  readiness for, 310*b*
  transformational, 283*t*–284*t*
Children's Bureau, 10
Chloroform, instructions for administration of, 3*b*
Chronic illness
  burden of, 214
  management of, 202
Chronic noncommunicable diseases, s, 212
CIHC. *See* Canadian Interprofessional Health Collaborative
CINAHL. *See* Cumulative Index for Nursing and Allied Health Literature
Circle of Caring: Transformative, Collaborative Model (Dunphy and Winland-Brown), 62
Citizenship
  global, 302
  systems, 337
Civic engagement, 561, 564*t*
Civilian Health and Medical Program of the Uniformed Services (CHAMPUS), 12–13
CLABSI. *See* Central line-associated bloodstream infection

Classification systems, coding taxonomies and, 747, 752*b*
data types, 750
ICD-10, 747
LOINC, 747
SNOMED CT, 747
SNOMED Z codes, 750
Cleaning, data, 729
Clear communication, ethical practice, 345
CLIA. *See* Clinical Laboratory Improvement Amendments
Client advocacy, 506
Clinical data repository (CDR), 729
Clinical decision making, interpretation and use of evidence-based practice in, 247*b*
Clinical decision support systems (CDSSs), 730
knowledge-based, 730–731
non-knowledge-based, 731
Clinical Laboratory Improvement Amendments (CLIA), 663
Clinical mentoring, by preceptors, 111–113
Clinical nurse specialist (CNS), 13, 41, 76, 141, 478
APRN regulation and implications, consensus model for, 406
availability and standardization, of educational curricula, 409
care of complex and vulnerable patients, interventions in
collaboration and ethical practice, 387
direct care and evidence-based practice, 387
collaboration, 401
complex/multiple comorbidities, 392
continuous patient care, 392
declining demand for, 18
delegated authority, 405
direct clinical practice, 391
education and reimbursement for, 19
episodic patient care, 392
ethical practice, 401
evaluation of practice, 412
evidence-based practice (EBP), 396
future of nursing reports, 405
growth of, 12
guidance and coaching, 394
indirect practice, 393
individual clinical nurse specialist practices and prescriptive authority, variability in, 410
Clinical nurse specialist (CNS) *(Continued)*
interpretation and use of evidence in practice, 397
leadership, 398
marketplace forces and concerns, 402
National Certification for, 409
and nurse practitioners, 410
outcomes, 695
participation in collaborative research, 398
patient safety, 393
patients and families, 394
practice, competencies within spheres of impact, 387
reimbursement for, 408
role implementation, 412
transitional care CNSs, navigating patients across the care continuum, 403*b*–404*b*
unique situations, 392
Clinical practice/direct care
guidelines for, 258
leadership, 272
Clinical question, for interview, 604*b*
Clinical-related contexts
competence, 321
leadership, 284
Clinical transplant coordination, 76
CMS. *See* Centers for Medicare and Medicaid Services
CNA. *See* Canadian Nurses Association
CNS. *See* Clinical nurse specialist
Coaching. *See also* Guidance/coaching
definition of, 215, 216*t*
Cochrane Central Register of Controlled Trials, 256
Cochrane Collaboration, 256
Cochrane Database systematic review, in certified nurse-midwife outcomes, 696
Cochrane Nursing Care Field, 257
Cochrane Qualitative Research Methods Group, 257
Cochrane systematic review, in certified registered nurse anesthetist outcomes, 696–697
Code of Ethics of American College of Nurse-Midwives, 45
Coding sets, 627
CPT codes, 627
ICD-10 coding, 628
Coding taxonomies, 749*t*–750*t*
classification systems and, 747, 752*b*
Coding taxonomies *(Continued)*
data types, 750
ICD-10, 747
LOINC, 747
SNOMED CT, 747
SNOMED Z codes, 750
Cohort study, 260
Collaboration, 315
acute care nurse practitioners (ACNPs), 468
advanced practice nurse (APN), 503
barriers to, 316
communication, ineffective, 331
disciplinary, 330
organizational, 331
regulatory, 331
sociocultural, 331
team dysfunction, 331
benefits of, 324*t*
characteristics of, 320, 321*b*
accountability, 321
common purpose, 321
communication (effective), 321
competence (clinical), 321
competence (interpersonal), 321
humor, 322
mutual trust, 322
recognition, 322
trust and mutual respect, 322
clinical nurse specialist (CNS), 401
with clinicians, 325*b*
in contemporary health care, 329
core competencies, of advanced practice nursing, 78, 85*f*
definition of, 316
domains of, 318
elements of, 323*b*
evidence-based contexts and, 328
failure of, 326
faux, 317
in global arenas, 319
with groups, 319
impact (patients and clinicians), 324
imperatives for, 327
ethical, 327
institutional, 328
research, 329
implementing, 333
assessment of, 334
environmental factors, 334
personal factors, 334
incentives for, 329
with individuals, 318
interaction (mode of) with, 330

Collaboration *(Continued)*
comanagement, 318
consultation, 317
coordination, 317
faux collaboration, 317
information exchange, 317
one-sided compromise, 317
parallel communication, 316
parallel functioning, 317
referral, 318
supervision, 318
interprofessional, 320, 327*b*–328*b*
collaboration on costs, effects of, 326
evidence of, 324
impact on health outcomes, 325
research supporting, 325
opportunities for, 329
in organizational arenas, 319
with patients, 327*b*–328*b*
in policy arenas, 319
process, 332
conflict negotiation, 333
partnering, 333
recurring interactions, 332
resolution skills, 333
team building, 333
in quality improvement, 336*b*
strategies for, 334*b*, 334
individual, 334
organizational, 335
team, 335
with teams, 319
terms of, 319–320
types, 319
Comanagement, 318
Commission on Collegiate Nursing Education (CCNE), 41
Committee interviews, 604–605
Committee to Study Extended Roles for Nurses, 22–23
Common purpose, 321
Commonwealth Foundation, 22
Communication, 298
in advanced practice nurse, 600
device technology and, 728*b*
effective, 321
expert, 305
ineffective, 331
gaps, 104
modes of, 305
networking, 310
parallel, 316
with patients, 179
strategies for, 334*b*
technology-assisted, 715
Communication *(Continued)*
nonverbal communication technologies, 718
verbal communication technologies, 717
visual communication technologies, 719
written communication technologies, 715
technology-enabling, 721*b*
Communication
"Communicative power", 580–581
Community health centers, 443
Community, international
United States differs from, 557
Community Mental Health Centers Act of 1963, 15
Community Tool to Align Measurement, 753–755, 756*t*–757*t*
Companion robots, 725
Comparative effectiveness research (CER), 571, 675*t*–677*t*
Compassion, 226
Competencies
of advanced practice nursing, 41, 76
of advanced practice registered nurse, 653
central, 76
ethical practice, 354
ethical decision-making frameworks, 356
knowledge development, 355
skill acquisition, 355
clinical, 99, 321
collaboration and, 321
cultural, 301*b*
definition of, 85
development of
education and, 137–138, 146
foundational
in health information technology management, 762
in quality improvement, 768
global, 302*b*
interdisciplinary, 281
interpersonal, 321
leadership, 282, 283*t*–284*t*
characteristics of, 293
health care system, transformation of, 282
health professional education, evolution of, 281
of National Association of Clinical Nurse Specialists, 43*f*
Competencies *(Continued)*
of National Organization of Nurse Practitioner Faculties, 42
professional, 653, 654*f*
skill sets, leadership, 309
Competitive compensation packages, 645
Complacent phase, of role development, 127
Complementary therapies, 197
Complex/multiple comorbidities, patients with
clinical nurse specialist (CNS), 392
Complex situation management, 200, 201*b*–202*b*
Compromising, one-sided, 317
Computerized Provider Order Entry (CPOE), 730–731
Conceptualizations, of advance practice nursing, 42
for advanced practice nurses, 67
Donabedian structure/process/outcome model, 64
Dunphy and Winland-Brown's Circle of Caring model, 62
transitional care models, 61
Calkin's Model of Advanced Nursing Practice, 50, 53*f*
components of, 33
Fenton's and Brykczynski's expert practice domains of the CNS and NP, 49
Hamric's Integrative Model of, 48
imperatives of, 34
implications for, 61
international examples of, 57
nature of, 33
organizational perspectives of, 37
Advanced Practice Registered Nurse regulation, consensus model for, 37
American Association of Colleges of Nursing, 41
American Association of Nurse Anesthetists, 43
American College of Nurse-Midwives, 45
American Nurses Association, 40
international, 45
National Association of Clinical Nurse Specialists, 42
National Organization of Nurse Practitioner Faculties, 42
problems with, 50–52
purposes of, 54
recommendations and future directions of, 65

Conceptualizations, of advance practice nursing *(Continued)*
conceptualizations of, 65
consensus building, 66
for practice doctorate curricula, 67
research on advanced practice nurses, 67
role and perceptions of team effectiveness, 59
Shuler's Model of NP Practice, 56
Strong Memorial Hospital's model, 52, 54*f*
Texas Children's Hospital transformational Advanced Professional Practice (TAPP) APRN model, 55
Conceptual models, of care delivery impact, 680
by APRNs, 680
nurse practitioner role effectiveness model, 680, 682*f*
outcomes evaluation model, 679, 681*t*–682*t*
Conference calls, 294
Confidence interval (CI), 261–262
Conflict
negotiation in, 337
resolution of, 333*b*, 333
role, 103*t*, 129
Conflict Resolution Network, 298
Conflicts, ethical practice
addressing ethical conflict, 357
principle-based approach, 346
strategies used in resolving, 358*b*
Congress of Nursing Practice, 17
Consensus, 767*t*
building, 66
Consensus Conference, 37–38
Consensus Model for APRN Regulation, 32, 38*f*, 76, 457, 650
certification, 650
education, 650
implementation of, 650
licensure, 650
Consensus Work Group, 43
Consolidated Standards of Reporting Trials (CONSORT), 262–264
CONSORT. *See* Consolidated Standards of Reporting Trials
Consultation, 317
advanced practice nurse (APN), 504–505, 507
advanced practice nursing
implementing of, 498
core competencies of, 84, 85*f*
Contemplation, in APRN coaching process, 232
Contemporary health care, 329
Content expertise, APRN and, 577
Continued advanced practice nurse role evolution, 126, 127*b*
Continued competency assessments, 655
Continued professional certification assessment (CPCA), 521
Continued professional competence (CPC), 521
Continuing education, mandatory requirements of, 656
Continuous patient care, clinical nurse specialist (CNS), 392
Continuous quality improvement, 675*t*–677*t*, 768
Control chart, 767*t*
Controlled Substances Act, 25
Convenient care clinics, 447
Coordination, 317
Core competencies
of advanced practice nursing, 84
additional, 85
central competency as, 84
Core questions, 770
in interventions, 772
in program goals, 772
in stakeholders, 772, 773*b*
in target population, 770
Coronary care nursing specialist, 15–16
Coronary care unit (CCU), 15
Coronavirus disease 2019 (COVID-19), 711
Cost considerations, for current advanced practice nursing policy issues, 566
Cost-quality-access schema, 568*f*
Council for Affordable Quality Healthcare (CAQH), 626
Council on Certification of Nurse Anesthetists (CCNA), 520–521
Council on Recertification (COR) of Nurse Anesthetists, 520–521
Counseling, 216–217
Cover letters, 601*b*, 601
Covey, Stephen, 282–284
COVID-19 global pandemic, 586, 644
CPOE. *See* Computerized Provider Order Entry
CPT codes. *See* Current Procedural Terminology codes
Credentialing, certified nurse-midwife (CNM), 493
Credentialing process, 625
hospital, 625
insurance, 626
payment partnerships, 627*f*
Credentialing requirements, 649
of advanced practice nurse
issues affecting, 662
practice climate for, 667
scope of practice for, 661
visioning for, 667
of advanced practice registered nurse
accrediting bodies, 651*t*
competencies, professional, 653, 654*f*
Consensus Model for, 650
elements of, 656
future challenges facing, 669
institutional, 658
language associated with, 657
Master's and Doctoral education, 652
program oversight and accreditation, 654
regulatory model, 651*f*
role and population certification, 655
state licensure and recognition of, 657
in US health care system, 652
legal requirements for
collaborative practice arrangements, 662
elements of, 656
future challenges facing, 669
identifier numbers, 660
influencing, 667
institutional, 658
issues affecting, 662
language associated with, 657
malpractice, 664
negligence, 664
reimbursement, 663
risk management, 664
telehealth, 666
telepractice, 666
titling, 657
practice-related issues for
collaborative practice arrangements, 662
Consensus Model, 650
current, 667
identifier numbers, 660
malpractice, 664
negligence, 664
reimbursement, 663

Credentialing requirements (Continued)
risk management, 664
telehealth, 666
telepractice, 666
titling, 657
requirements for, 664b
for scope of practice
competencies, 653
education, benchmark of, 653
standards of practice and care, 662
Crile, George, 4
Criteria for Evaluation of Nurse Practitioner Programs, 469
Critical appraisal, 262
data extraction for, 267, 269f
evidence pyramid for, 260, 262t
of individual studies, 266–267
meta-analyses for, 264
for quantitative studies, 262t
systematic reviews and, 273
Critical Appraisal Guide for Quantitative Studies, 262–264, 262t
Critical care codes, 635
Critical care teams, ACNPs, 482
CRNA. *See* Certified registered nurse anesthetist
Crossing the Quality Chasm, 318
Cultivate unconditional positive regard, 219
Cultural contexts
of change, 301b, 301
cultural competence, 301b
Cumulative Index for Nursing and Allied Health Literature (CINAHL), 256
Current best evidence, 256
historical perspective of, 252
Current Procedural Terminology (CPT) codes, 624–625, 627, 628t, 697, 749t–750t
Curriculum vitae (CV), 602–603, 603b
CV. *See* Curriculum vitae
Cyberattacks, 734
types of, 734b, 734
Cybersecurity, 732
blockchain, 735
data security and privacy, 732
mobile device security, 734, 735b
regulatory compliance, 733
states of digital data, 732
type of cyberattacks and, 734b, 734

D

Dashboard, 675t–677t
Data at rest, 732
Database, 729
Database of Systematic Reviews, 256
Data entry errors, 714b
Data extraction, 267, 269f
Data in motion, 732
Data in use, 732–733
Data mining, 766
Data-related concepts
defining elements of, 774
deriving meaning from, 776
results of, 776
Data security and privacy, 732
Data types, 750
DEA (Drug Enforcement Administration) number, 25, 660
Death With Dignity Act (DWDA) requirements, 365b
Decision making, shared, 179
Decision support tools, 246
Deep knowledge, APRN and, 573
Definitions/fundamentals
for advanced practice nurse, 85, 137
advanced nursing practice *vs.*, 77
conceptual, 79
core, 78
implications of, 91
for advanced practice registered nurse, 658b
for coaching, 214
for collaboration, 316
for guidance, 214
for leadership, 280
empowerment, 301b, 306
innovation, 285
mentoring, 293
political activism, 296
Delegated authority, clinical nurse specialist (CNS), 405
Deming, W. Edwards, 769
Descriptive analytics, 763, 767t
Descriptive and interpretative phenomenology, 114t–118t
Descriptive qualitative focused ethnography, 114t–118t
Descriptive Qualitative Survey Questionnaire, 114t–118t
Design concept, 286
Destiny concept, 286
Det Norske Veritas Healthcare, 753
Developmental contexts. *See also* Historical perspectives
of leadership, 295

Developmental contexts. (Continued)
factors influencing, 302
skills of, 299
Developmental transitions, 221–223
Device technology and communication in patient care, 728b
Dewitt, Katherine, 13
Diabetes specialist nurses (DSNs), role development experiences of, 114t–118t
Diagnosis-related group, 18
Diagnostic and Statistical Manual of Mental Disorders 5th edition (DSM-V), 774
Diagnostic and therapeutic devices and apps, 721
in health information technology, 721
Diagnostic services, ACNPs, 481
Dictionary, data, 729
Diffusion of Innovation Theory, 268–270
Digital data states
data at rest, 732
data in motion, 732
data in use, 732–733
Digital stethoscope, smartphone-based, 725
Dignity, ten essential elements of, 343t
clinical situation, ethical comportment, 344b
Dilemma of guiding/leading from behind, 213
Dimensional (3D) printing, 724
Direct care/clinical practice, 79 *See also* Competencies
acute care nurse practitioners (ACNPs), 461
indirect care activities *vs.*, 169, 171b
information management and, 203
Direct clinical practice, 501
clinical nurse specialist (CNS), 391
and core competencies, clinical nurse specialist, 395b
Directed program evaluations, 686, 687t–689t
Direct entry midwife (DEM), 490–491
Disciplinary barriers, 330
Disciplinary split, 330
Discontinuous time, anesthesia, 545
Discovery concept, 286
Discrete or structured data, 750
Disease
diagnosing and managing, 461
management of, 675t–677t

Disruptive behavior, 331
Disruptive innovation, 41
Diversity, certified nurse-midwife, 511
DNAP. *See* Doctor of Nurse Anesthesia Practice
DNP. *See* Doctor of Nursing Practice
DNP Essentials, 41, 328–329
  APRNs and, 203
  task force, 199
Dock, Lavinia, 3
Doctoral education, 40
Doctoral programs in nurse anesthesia, 8
Doctorate of nursing practice (DNP), 32, 77, 128*b*, 244
  preparation, 471*b*
Doctor of Nurse Anesthesia Practice (DNAP), 8, 44–45
Doctor of Philosophy (PhD), programs, 244
Documentation in litigation process, 643
Domains
  clinical, 290
  collaboration, 318
  health policy contexts for, 292
  of National Organization of Nurse Practitioner Faculties, 40
  professional, 293–294
  systems, 300
Donabedian, Avedis, 711–712
Donabedian-guided model, 680
Donabedian model, 711, 712*t*
Donabedian structure/process/outcome model, 64
Dream concept, 286
Dreyfus model, 101
Driving forces, 305
Drug Enforcement Administration. *See* DEA (Drug Enforcement Administration) number
Dunphy and Winland-Brown's Circle of Caring: A Transformative, Collaborative Model, 62, 63*f*
Dysfunctional leadership styles, 306

E

Education
  certified nurse-midwife (CNM), 492
  and practice, CRNAs, 520
Educational-related contexts
  of advanced practice nurse
    benchmarks of, 653
    implications, 91
  Consensus Model for, 650
Educational-related contexts *(Continued)*
  continuing, mandatory requirements of, 656
  doctoral, 40
  evolution, leadership, 311
  graduate, 80, 80*f*
  health professional, 281
  for nurse-midwifery, 10
  patient, 213
    APRN and, 179
  postgraduate, 655
Educational Standards, 8
EDW. *See* Enterprise data warehouse
Effectiveness, definition of, 675*t*–677*t*
Efficiency, definition of, 675*t*–677*t*
EHRs. *See* Electronic health records
Electronic databases, 255*t*, 258
Electronic health records (EHRs), 712, 715, 746, 747, 762–763
Electronic medical records (EMRs), 715
Electronic Medical Record systems, 244
Electronic protected health information (ePHI), 733
Electronic technology, 89
Empathic stance, 223
Empathy, 226
Employer-based malpractice insurance, 612
Employment contracts, 611*b*, 611
Empowerment, 295
EMRs. *See* Electronic medical records
End time, anesthesia, 545
Enterprise data warehouse (EDW), 729
Entrepreneur, 591
Entrepreneurial leadership, 290–291
Entrepreneurship, 643
Environment, advanced practice nursing, 89
  implications for, 91
Environment-management convergence, assessment of, 334
ePHI. *See* Electronic protected health information
Episodic patient care, clinical nurse specialist (CNS), 392
ERIC, 259
Errors, clinical thinking, 184, 185*b*
Essential Evidence Plus, 257
Essentials, 745
Essentials: Core Competencies for Professional Nursing Education, The (AACN), 726–727
Essentials of Doctoral Education for Advanced Nursing Practice, The (AACN), 77, 78, 101, 280, 653, 674
Essentials of Master's Education in Nursing, The (AACN), 75
Ethical contexts. *See also* Ethical decision making
  collaboration, 334
Ethical decision making, 346
  barriers to. *See* Barriers
  sample APRN, 356*b*
Ethical dilemma, 342
Ethical practice, 505
  access to resources, 368
  acute care nurse practitioners (ACNPs), 468
  addressing ethical conflict, 357
    different approaches to, 357*b*
  APRN well-being, 373
  barriers, ethical practice and strategies, 371
    barriers internal to APRN, 371
    interprofessional barriers, 372
    organizational and environmental barriers, 373
    patient–provider barriers, 372
  casuistry approach, 347
  clear communication, 345
  clinical nurse specialist (CNS), 401
  clinical situation, demonstrating differing ethical approaches, 349*b*
  conflicts
    addressing ethical conflict, 357
    principle-based approach, 346
    strategies used in resolving, 358*b*
  conscientious objection, 365
    policies guiding, criteria to include in, 366*b*
  COVID-19 pandemic, 369
  creating ethical environments, 357
  cultural competence, Internet-based resources, 374*b*
  decision-making competency, 367*b*
  definitions and terms for APRNs, 342*b*
  end-of-life complexities
    advance directives, 362
    medical aid in dying (MAID), 363
    POLST, 363
    technological imperative, 362
  ethical competency, of APRNS, 354
    ethical decision-making frameworks, 356

Ethical practice *(Continued)*
knowledge development, 355
skill acquisition, 355
foundations of, 342
functional health patterns
context, 352
poster "Get to know me", 353*f*
relationships, 352
genomics, 369
goals of care model, prognosis, 350
gun violence, 370
interprofessional collaboration, 346
issues affecting APRN practice
acute and chronic care issues, 361
primary care issues, 361
landmark legal cases, end-of-life care, 363*b*
legal issues, 370
moral distress, 345
organizations with electronically available ethics resources, 375*b*–376*b*
ethics and legal search sites, 376
ethics policy statements or guidelines, 375
participation in research, 370
personal and professional values, 344
preventive ethics, 359
addressing staff moral distress through, 360*b*
professional codes and guidelines, 348
particulars, 352
professional boundaries, 350
values, beliefs and preferences, 352
societal issues, promoting social justice, 366
values and ethics competencies, 373*b*
Ethical reasoning, APRN and, 186
Evidence-based contexts, collaborations and, 318
Evidence-based medicine, 246
Evidence-based nursing, 246
Evidence-based practice (EBP), 243, 502
acute care nurse practitioners (ACNPs), 467
advantages of, 261
appraisal of systematic reviews and meta-analyses, 264
APRN and, 179, 244, 245
changes in, 273
clinical leadership support, 272
innovation feedback on, 273
organizational support, 271
stakeholder, 271
Evidence-based practice (EBP) *(Continued)*
clinical nurse specialist (CNS), 396
clinical practice guidelines, 192
competencies and core, of advanced practice nursing, 75
decision making in, 268
definition of, 675*t*–677*t*
evaluation of, for determination of standards of care, 249*b*
evidence pyramid, 260*f*, 260
extraction of evidence and, 259
feedback on, 273
future perspectives on, 273
historical perspective of, 252
in individual clinical decision making, interpretation and use of, 247*b*
literature for relevant studies, 254
clinical practice guidelines, 258
Cumulative Index for Nursing and Allied Health, 256
electronic database searching, 258
MEDLINE, 254
online evidence-based resources, 256
PubMed, 254
online resources for, 257, 257*t*
patient care policies for, 248*b*
principles of, 258
process for identifying, 245
steps of the, 253
pyramid illustrating, 260*f*
quality improvement, 250
research, 252
resources, 248
search/retrieval
allied health literature, 256
clinical practice guidelines, 258
cumulative index for nursing, 256
Evidence-informed policy, 583
development, resources and challenges in, 582, 583*b*
Evidence-informed Policy Network (EVIPNet), 583
Evidence to date, 683
literature assessment in, 683
care delivery process studies in, 684
role acceptance studies in, 684
role description studies in, 683
role perception studies in, 684
EVIPNet. *See* Evidence-informed Policy Network; Evidence-informed Policy Network (EVIPNet)
Evolution (education)
competencies, 281
interdisciplinary, 311
leadership, 311
Exemplary midwifery practice, model of, 57, 58*f*
Expert clinical performance, 182
Expert communication, 286
Expert, definition of, 84
Expert Practice Domains of the CNS and NP (Fenton's and Brykczynski's) model, 49, 51*f*
Extended reporting period/tail coverage, 641
Extracorporeal membrane oxygenation (ECMO), 464
Extraction, data, 267, 269*f*

F

Fagan, Cynthia M., 562
Failure-related issues
collaboration failure, 326–327
failure to mentor, 308
Family NPs, 458–459
Family nurse practitioner (FNP), 560*b*–561*b*, 664
qualitative study of, 110
Farm Security Administration (FSA), 20–21
Faulty thinking, 184
Faux collaboration, 317
Fax, 716
Federal funding, 14–15
Federal government
health professional shortage areas, designation of, 443*b*
Health resources and Services Administration, 441
Federalism, 559
Federally funded medical coverage, 621
Federal Medical Assistance Percentage (FMAP), 622–623
Feedback on evidence-based practice, 245
Fee-for-service reimbursement models, 153, 623, 636
Feeling, range of, 238
Fellowships, 121–122, 305
Feminist ethics, 347
Fenton's and Brykczynski's Expert Practice Domains of the CNS and NP model, 49
Financial reimbursement, 7
First nurse practitioners, primary care nurse practitioner (PCNP), 423

Fishbone diagrams, 769
Fixed mindset, 219–220
Flow chart, 767*t*
FNP. *See* Family nurse practitioner
Focused professional practice evaluation (FPPE), 480
Focus group method, 114*t*–118*t*
Followship, 311
Force field analysis, 767*t*
Force, *vs.* power, 579 *See also* Power
Ford, Loretta, 22*b*, 22
Forensic nursing, 76
Formal consultations. *See also* Consultation
Formal mentoring, 294
Foundational competencies
  in health information technology management, 762
  in quality improvement, 768
    continuous, 768
    performance improvement, 764*b*–765*b*, 769
4D cycle of leadership, 286
Frameworks/models
  change-related contexts, 285
    concepts related, 286
  federalism, 559
  incrementalism, 559
  innovation, 286
    concepts related to, 286
  Kingdon model, 564, 566*f*
  knowledge transfer, 565, 568*f*
  Longest model (policy formulation phase), 564, 565*f*
  modifications, 564
  National Association of Clinical Nurse Specialists, 43*f*
  transformation, 282
    of habits, 282, 284*b*
Framing current issues, 566
Frank, Louis, 4–5
Fraudulent billing practices, examples of, 640*b*
Freestanding birth center, 492, 498–500, 507–508
Freud, Sigmund, 14
From Novice to Expert, 49
Frontier Graduate School of Midwifery, 10
Frontier Nursing Service, 20, 20*f*
Frozen phase, of role development, 127
Frustration phase
  of role development, 119
  of role implementation, 121, 122*t*
FSA (Farm Security Administration), 26
Functional health patterns
  ethical practice
    context, 352
    poster "Get to know me", 353*f*
    relationships, 352
Fundamentals/definitions
  for advanced practice nurse, 85, 137
    advanced nursing practice *vs.*, 91–92
    conceptual, 79
    core, 84
    implications of, 91
  for advanced practice registered nurse, 658*b*
  for coaching, 214
  for collaboration, 316
  for guidance, 214
  for leadership, 284
    empowerment, 295, 301*b*
    innovation, 295
    mentoring, 293
    political activism, 296
Fundamentals, of midwifery care, 501
Funding and reimbursement arrangements, 152
Future directions
  for credentialing, 669
  of evidence-based practice, 273
  for regulations, 669
Future of Nursing 2020-2030: Charting a Path to Achieve Health Equity, The (NASEM), 726
Future of Nursing report (IOM), 280, 405, 520, 669, 673–674

G

Gallup Poll, 176, 581*t*
GDP. *See* Gross domestic product
GDPR. *See* General Data Protection Regulation
Geisinger Health System, 570
General anesthesia documentation requirements, 545*b*
General Data Protection Regulation (GDPR), 733
General physician competence, 441*b*
General question, for interview, 604
Genetic and genomic research, 723
Genetics nursing, 76
Genomics, ethical practice, 369
Geofencing, 726
Geographic practice cost index (GPCI), 636
Get With the Guidelines program, 778
Global arenas, 319
Global awareness, 302
Global citizenship, 302
Global competencies, 302*b*
Global deployment, APN and, 138
Global health care context, 137
Global pandemic detection, 723–724
Gloor, Dorothy Sandridge, 7*b*
Goals of care model, ethical practice, 350
Gordon's functional health pattern assessment categories, 352
GPCI. *See* geographic practice cost index
Grading of Recommendations Assessment, Development and Evaluation (GRADE) scales, 268
Graduate Nurse Education Demonstration project, 113
Graham, Edith, 3
"Granny midwives", 8
Gray literature, 246–248
Grey, Michael, 20–21
Gross domestic product (GDP), 568–569
Grounded theory, 114*t*–118*t*
Group leadership, 289
Growth mindset, 219
Guidance/coaching, 212
  acute care nurse practitioners (ACNPs), 466
  advanced practice nurse (APN), 502
  advanced practice nursing, core competencies of, 78, 85*f*
  anticipatory, 215
  building into practice, 238
  clinical nurse specialist (CNS), 394
  communication, 224
  conflicts, 227
  context of, 213
  counseling, 216–217
  definition of, 214
  mentoring, 216–217
  nonjudgmental (suspending judgment), 225
  nurse, 217
  patient education, 215
  patient engagement, 213
  patient readiness, 228, 229*b*
  process, four *A*s of, 233*f*, 233
  skills in, 213
    ask permission, 236
    courage to challenge, 236
    curiosity, 237
    getting to the feelings, 238
    support small changes, 237
  theories and research supporting APRN, 217

Guide for practice, use of evidence as, 174
Guidelines for the Economic Evaluation of Health Technologies: Canada, 673–674
Guide to Clinical Preventive Services, 199
Gun violence, ethical practice, 370

H

Hallmarks, of midwifery, 501
Hamric's Integrative Model, of advanced practice nursing, 48
Hartford CCU, 16
Harvard T.H. Chan School of Public Health (2015) website, 189
Harvey, Samuel, 5
Hatfield, Margaret, 4–5
Hawthorne effect, 775
HCPCS. *See* Healthcare Common Procedure Coding System
Health and preventing disease, promoting and protecting, 465
Health and illness management, diverse approaches and interventions for, 194
  clinical prevention, 198
  complementary therapies, 197
  individualized interventions, 197
  interpersonal interventions, 194, 195*b*–196*b*
  therapeutic interventions, 194
Health and illness transitions, 221–223
Health assessment, holism and, 173
Health care, 174
  access to cost-effective, quality, 24*b*
  changing face of, 128*b*
  contemporary, 329
  leadership and, transformation of, 289–290
Healthcare Common Procedure Coding System (HCPCS), 627, 749*t*–750*t*
Health care delivery settings, patient care problems and nurse practitioner management interventions, 470*t*
Healthcare Facilities Accreditation Program, 753
Health care information technology, 744
  management of, 762
  for performance improvement, 746
  for quality improvement
    foundational competencies in, 768
Health care information technology *(Continued)*
    outcome evaluation plans, 770
    strategies for designing, 770
  for regulatory reporting
    performance improvement, 751
    relevance of, 761
Health care safety net
  primary care nurse practitioner (PCNP)
    community health centers, 443
    nurse-led health centers, 444
    school-based health centers, 446
    veterans affairs, 446
Healthcare services, AG-ACNP, 477*b*
Health Information Portability and Accountability Act (HIPAA), 462
Health information technology
  complexity in
    Donabedian model, 711, 712*t*
    James Reason Swiss cheese model (SCM), 712
  cyberattacks, 734
  cybersecurity, 732
  data, clinical decision support and advanced analytics, 727
  data entry errors, 714*b*
  diagnostic and therapeutic devices and apps, 721
  future implications of, 737
  high-tech home care, 735
  human-centered design and, 713
  illusions of, in pandemic, 711
  influencing APRN practice, 709
  procedural devices and apps, 724
  supportive, 725
  technology-assisted communication, 715
  TJC's safe use of, 714*b*
Health Information Technology for Economic and Clinical Health (HITECH) Act, 733
Health Insurance Exchanges, 624
Health Insurance Portability and Accountability Act (HIPAA), 125–126, 625, 665–666, 716, 733, 776
Health Maintenance Organizations (HMOs), 624
Health policy contexts, 556
  for advanced practice nurses
    emerging, 584
    public health crisis, 586
  competencies for, individual skills, 573
Health policy contexts *(Continued)*
  frameworks for, 564
  historic core function of, 555
  Kingdon model, 564
  for leadership, 280, 281
    fellowships, 305
    internships, 305
    modes of communication, 305
    professional organizations, 305
  modern roles of, 555
  moving APRNs forward in, 582
  overview concepts of
    politics *vs.*, 556
    United States *vs.* international communities, 557
  political competence in policy arena, 571
Health policy knowledge, 574*b*
Health professional education, 281
Health professional shortage areas (HPSAs), 443
Health reform history on advanced practice registered nurses, 618
Health reform initiatives, 570
Health Resources and Services Administration (HRSA), 586, 751–753, 754*b*
Heart failure services, ACNPs, 482
Heath Information Technology for Economic and Clinical Health (HITECH) Act, 746–747
Henderson, Virginia, 7*b*
Henry Street Settlement (HSS) House, 19
High-deductible health plans, 624
High-tech home care, 735
  future for, 737
  medical devices
    benefits to elderly of voice output on, 737*b*
    environmental issues for home use of, 736*b*
    personal characteristics that influence ability to operate, 736*b*
HIPAA. *See* Health Insurance Portability and Accountability Act
Historical perspectives
  on certified nurse-midwife, 491
  on evidence-based practice, 246
  primary care nurse practitioner (PCNP), 423
  United States, history of, 5
HITECH Act. *See* Health Information Technology for Economic and Clinical Health Act

HMOs. *See* Health Maintenance Organizations
Hoarding (power), 307
Hodgins, Agatha, 4
Holism
description of, 173
and health assessment, 173
Holistic perspective, use of, 173, 174*b*
Home births, 495, 507
Horizontal violence, 104, 308
abandonment of nursing identity, 307
failure to mentor, 308
hoarding (power), 307
Hospital Compare, 571
Hospital credentialing, 625
Hospitalist team, AG-ACNP, 480*b*
House of Representatives, 561–564
HRSA. *See* Health Resources and Services Administration
Human resource policies and priorities, 149
Humor, 322
Hunt, Alice M., 5
Husband-and-wife nurse practitioner team, 560
Hypothetical question, for interview, 604

I

ICD. *See* International Classification of Diseases
ICF. *See* International Coach Federation
ICN. *See* International Council of Nurses
ICR. *See* Intelligent character recognition
ICUs. *See* Intensive care units
Idaho State Boards of Medicine and Nursing, 24
Identification processes
Medicaid provider numbers, 663
Medicare provider numbers, 663
national provider identifier number, 660
Identity, abandonment of, 307
IHI. *See* Institute for Healthcare Improvement
Illness, chronic, management of, 174
Illusions of technologies in pandemic, 711
Image, certified nurse-midwife, 508
"Immunization", 110–111
Impact measurement, 675*t*–677*t*
Implementation contexts
of clinical decision making, 244
of collaboration, 331–332
of Consensus Model, 650
leadership, 280
change implementation, 280
collaboration, 288
followship, 311
institutional assessment, 310
leadership portfolio, development of, 309
networking, 310
working with other leaders, 310
Implementation phase
of role development, 124
of role implementation, 124
Implicit Bias, 179
Imposter phenomenon, 119
Incentives, 329
Incident-to billing in reimbursement, 638, 639*b*, 639*t*
Incongruity, role, 102, 103*t*
Incrementalism, 559
Independent billing, 634
Independent midwifery practice, 494*b*
Indicators
of outcome(s), 675*t*–677*t*, 685
proxy, 675*t*–677*t*
Indirect care, 169 *See also* Direct care/clinical practice
Individual contexts, collaboration, strategies for successful, 334
Individual level, acute care nurse practitioners (ACNPs), 475
Individuals, collaboration with, 333
Individual studies
critical appraisal for, 262
quality assessment, 263*f*
Ineffective communication, 331
Influence levels, ACNPs
individual level, 475
institutional level, 473
national level (professional organizations), 472
service-related level, 474
state level (government), 473
Influence spheres
for advanced practice nurse
experienced, 668*b*
expert, 668*b*
novice, 668*b*
Informal mentoring, 294
Information exchange, 317
Information management, direct care and, 203
Information technology, health care, 744
management of, 762
for performance improvement, 746
for quality improvement
foundational competencies in, 768
outcome evaluation plans, 770
strategies for designing, 770
for regulatory reporting
performance improvement, 751
relevance of, 761
Innovation, 285
concepts related, 286
disruptive, 41
of leadership, 295
Inpatient billing, for reimbursement, 633
bundled billing, 634
critical care codes, 635
independent billing, 634
shared/split billing, 634
subsequent hospital visits, 635
Inpatient specialty service, AC-PNP practice, 476*b*
Inquiry (query) letters, 601
Institute for Healthcare Improvement (IHI), 281, 335–336, 756*t*–757*t*, 769
Institute of Medicine (IOM), 33, 92
Crossing the Quality Chasm, 319
Future of Nursing report, 280, 669
Institutional assessment, 310
Institutional credentialing, of advanced practice registered nurse, 658
Institutional issues, for collaboration, 328
Institutional level, acute care nurse practitioners (ACNPs), 473
Insufficiency, role, 103*t*
Insurance credentialing, 626
Insurance, malpractice, 612, 665
Integrated delivery network, 769
Integration of the AACN Essentials of Doctoral Education for Advanced Nursing Practice (2006) and the COA Standards for Accreditation of Nurse Anesthesia Educational Programs–Practice Doctorate (2019), 528*b*
Integration phase, of role implementation, 124
Integrative nurse coaching, midrange theory of, 217

Integrative therapies, 197–198
Intelligent character recognition (ICR), 717
Intensive care units (ICUs), 126
AC-PNP practice, 464*b*–465*b*
Interaction-related contexts, 330
comanagement, 318
consultation, 317
coordination, 317
faux collaboration, 317
information exchange, 317
one-sided compromise, 317
parallel communication, 316
parallel functioning, 317
recurring, 332
referral, 318
supervision, 318
International Classification of Diseases (ICD), 624–625, 748
ICD-10, 62, 628, 747, 748
Clinical Modification, 749*t*–750*t*
Procedure Coding System, 749*t*–750*t*
International Coach Federation (ICF), 223
International community, United States differs from, 557
International Confederation of Midwives (ICM, 2010), 139, 490
International Council of Nurses (ICN), 32, 302
International Federation of Nurse Anesthetists (IFNA), 139–140
International nurse regulator collaborative 6 "P"s of social media, 721*b*
International organizations and conceptualizations, of advanced practice nursing, 45
Internet-based search engines, 259
Internships, 305
Interpersonal competence, 321
Interpersonal Relations in Nursing: A Conceptual Frame of Reference for Psychodynamic Nursing (1952), 15
Interprofessional barriers, 372
Interprofessional contexts
collaboration, 321*b*, 326
driving forces of, 319
restraining forces of, 320
Interprofessional Education Collaborative (IPEC), 301, 316, 327*b*–328*b*
Expert Panel, 34, 106, 322–323
Interprofessional role conflict, 105, 106*b*
Interstate practice, 666*b*
Interventional services, ACNPs, 481
Interventions
APRN and, 197
effectiveness of, 675*t*–677*t*
Interview process, for APRNs, 603, 604*b*
committee or panel, 604–605
one-on-one, 604
preparation for, 606
questions and strategies, 604*b*, 605*b*
second, 605–606
tips for, 606*b*
videoconference, 604
Intrapreneurs, 290–291, 591
Intraprofessional role conflict, 104
IOM. *See* Institute of Medicine
Ishikawa diagrams, 769

J

James Reason Swiss cheese model (SCM), 712
Joanna Briggs Institute, 257
Johns Hopkins School of Nursing, 6–7
Johnson, Carene, 23
Joint Dialogue Group, 36
Joint Statement of Practice Relations Between Obstetricians and Gynecologists and Certified Nurse-Midwives/Certified Midwive, 495*b*
Josiah Macy Jr. Foundation, 281, 330, 669
Juran, Joseph M., 769

K

Kaiser Permanente, 570
Keane, Anne, 25
Key policy concepts, 559
APRNs, civic engagement, and money, 561, 564*t*
federalism, 559
incrementalism, 559
presidential politics, 561
Kingdon model, 564, 566*f*
Kitzman, Harriet, 23
Kleinpell-Nowell's surveys, 122

L

LACE (licensing, accreditation, certification, and education) issues, 39, 92, 650–651, 656*b*
Lakeside Hospital School of Anesthesia, 4
Landmark legal cases, end-of-life care, ethical practice, 363*b*
Language-related bias, 266
Latin America, APN roles and, 146
Leadership, 279 *See also* Competencies
in action, 300*b*
acute care nurse practitioners (ACNPs), 467
advanced practice nurse (APN), 503
of advance practice nurse
attributes of, 296
importance of, 280
skill development of, 286–287
attributes of, 296, 297*b*
and autonomy, CRNAs, 539*b*
change in, 287
clinical, 268, 287, 289
clinical nurse specialist (CNS), 398
competencies, 293, 293*t*, 302*b*, 309
concepts of, 295
core competencies, of advanced practice nursing, 92
definitions of, 282
development of, 302
clinical leadership issues, 305
dysfunctional styles, 306
horizontal violence, 306
professional obstacles, 306
system obstacles, 306
dysfunctional styles of, 306
entrepreneurial, 290–291
group, 289
health policy contexts for, 292, 302
fellowships, 305
internships, 305
modes of communication, 305
professional organizations, 305
health policy issues, 303
horizontal violence, for stopping, 306
implementation strategies, 310
collaboration, 309
fellowship, 305
institutional assessment, 310
leadership portfolio, development of, 309
networking, 310
working with other leaders, 310
models of, 285
for change, 310
for innovation, 286
opinion, 287
portfolio, 309
professional, 290, 305
roving, 284
situational, 284

Leadership *(Continued)*
skills development strategies, 286
acquiring competency, 303
factors influencing, 302
personal characteristics, 302
personal experiences, 302
systems, 290
transformational, 282, 283*t*–284*t*
Legal requirements, 649
for credentialing/regulation
certification, 655
collaborative practice arrangements, 662
Consensus Model, 650–651
elements of, 656
future challenges facing, 669
identifier numbers, 660
influencing, 668*b*
institutional, 658
issues affecting, 662
language associated with, 657
malpractice, 664
Master's and Doctoral education, 652
negligence, 664
practice-related issues, 667
reimbursement, 663
risk management, 664
telehealth, 666
telepractice, 666
titling, 657
scope of practice
competencies, 653
education, benchmark of, 653
standards of practice and care, 662
state licensure, 657
Drug Enforcement Administration number, 660
prescriptive authority, 659
visioning processes, 667
Legislation and Medical Specialization, 14
Legislative and regulatory policies, 150
Letterman General Hospital School of Anesthesia, 7
Levels-based compensation, 645
Liability/malpractice insurance, in reimbursement, 640, 642*f*
Library of Congress, 556
Licensed midwives (LMs), 490
Licensing, accreditation, certification, and educational issues. *See* LACE (licensing, accreditation, certification, and education) issues
Licensure, Consensus Model for, 650
LinkedIn profile, 599
Liquid biopsy, 723
Listening, 224, 225*f*
Literature
gray, 246–248
for relevant studies, 254
Lobenstine Midwifery School, 10
Logical Observation Identifiers Names and Codes (LOINC), 747, 748, 749*t*–750*t*
Longest model (policy formulation phase), 564, 565*f*
Los Angeles County Medical Association, 5
Low income, defined, 623

M

Machine learning (ML) power
in verbal communication technologies, 717
in written communication technologies, 717
Mackenzie, Elizabeth, 20
MACRA. *See* Medicare Access and CHIP Reauthorization Act
Magaw, Alice, 3
Magnet status, 272
Maintenance, in APRN coaching process, 233
Malpractice, negligence and, 664
Malpractice insurance, 612, 665
in reimbursement, 640
extended reporting period/tail coverage, 641
mitigating malpractice claims, 642
reimbursement pay parity, 643
steps to securing malpractice coverage, 641*t*
Managed care delivery systems, 623
comprehensive risk-based managed care, 623
limited benefit plans, 623
primary care case management, 623
Management environment convergence, assessment of, 334
Management process, of midwifery care, 501
Mandatory continuing education requirements, 656
Mandatory practice requirements, 656
Manhattan Midwifery School, 10
Marketing
for advanced practice nurse, 596
business and contractual arrangements, 611
Marketing *(Continued)*
communication in, 600
core competencies, 596, 597*t*–598*t*
cover letters for, 601*b*, 601
employment contracts and, 611*b*, 611
independent contractor and, 611, 613*b*
interview process in, 603, 604*b*
malpractice insurance in, 612
organizations, 599*t*
practice arrangements in, 612
professional issues in, 612
professional networking in, 596
professional portfolio and, 601, 602*b*
professional recruiters in, 599
résumés and curricula vitae in, 602*b*, 602, 603*b*
value of, 606*b*, 607
web-based resources in, 599, 600*t*
entrepreneurship/intrapreneurship in
characteristics of, 593
choosing between, 592
negotiation and renegotiation, 607, 608*b*, 609*b*–610*b*
overcoming invisibility in, 614
yourself as APRN, 590
Master's and Doctoral education
advanced practice registered nurse, 652
postgraduate education, 655
Maternity Center Association, 10
Mayo Clinic, 4*f*, 570
Mayo, William Worral, 5–6
McLean Hospital, 14
Meaningful Use (MU), 746, 747
Measurable clinical question, steps of evidence-based process, 253
Measurement
impact, 675*t*–677*t*
of outcome(s), 675*t*–677*t*
Medicaid, 559
provider numbers, 663
reimbursement, 623
dual eligibility for, 623
Medical decision making, 630
elements of, 631*t*–632*t*
modifiers, 633
time-based billing, 630, 633*t*
Medical direction, 541
Medical documentation, 710
Medical homes, 324

Medical malpractice policies, 613–614
Medical prognosis, 351*f*
Medical specialization, 14
Medicare, 559
  credentialing, 627
  Part B, 19
  provider numbers, 663
  reimbursement, 621, 622*t*
Medicare Access and CHIP Reauthorization Act (MACRA), 636, 751, 755
Medicare Payment Advisory Commission (MedPAC), 639
Medicare Severity Diagnosis-Related Groups (MS-DRGs), 748, 749*t*–750*t*
Medicare Shared Savings Program (MSSP), 570 571
MEDLINE, 254, 256
MedPAC. *See* Medicare Payment Advisory Commission
Meetings, conduct at, 578
Meltzer, Lawrence, 16*b*
Mentoring, 216–217, 293, 293*t*
  in community leadership, 304*b*
  failure-related issues, 308*b*, 308
  formal, 302
  informal, 310
  leadership, 293
Merit-based Incentive Payments System (MIPS), 636, 751, 757, 758*t*–759*t*, 760*t*
  clinical practice improvement, 759–760
  cost/resource use, 760
  promoting interoperability, 757–759
  quality, 757
Meta-analysis, 254, 267*t*
Metric, definition of, 675*t*–677*t*
mHealth apps, 721
Michigan Insane Hospital, 14
Middle Eastern countries, APN roles and, 145
Middle-Range Theories, 193*b*
Middle Range theory of integrative nurse coaching, 217
"Mid-level providers" (MLPs), 25, 93–94
Midwifery, 139
  care, components of, 499*t*–500*t*, 501
  core competencies, 501*b*
  internationally, 490, 497
  standards for practice, 499*t*–500*t*
  United States, 490
Mindfulness, 238
Mind Tools, 756*t*–757*t*
Mining, data, 729
MIPS. *See* Merit-Based Incentive Payments System
Mission of National Organization of Nurse Practitioner Faculties, 42
Missouri Supreme Court, 24
Misuse of power, 310
ML power. *See* Machine learning power
Mobile device security, 734, 735*b*
Model for APRN Regulation: Licensure, Accreditation, Certification and Education, 650
Models/frameworks
  change-related contexts, 295
    concepts related, 286
  federalism, 559
  incrementalism, 559
  innovation, 286
    concepts related, 286
  Kingdon model, 564, 566*f*
  knowledge transfer, 565, 568*f*
  Longest model (policy formulation phase), 564, 565*f*
  modifications, 564
  National Association of Clinical Nurse Specialists, 43*f*
  transformation, 282
    of habits, 282
Modifiers in reimbursement, 633
Moral distress, 345
  definition of, 186–187
Motivational interviewing (MI), 230, 231*b*–232*b*
MSSP. *See* Medicare Shared Savings Program (MSSP)
Multidisciplinary NP-coordinated team visits, effectiveness of, 686
Multisite roles, 126
Multivoting, 767*t*
Mutual trust, 321

N

NACNS. *See* National Association of Clinical Nurse Specialists
NACNS Strategies for Enacting the Institute of Medicine's (IOM's) The Future of Nursing Recommendations, 407*t*–408*t*
NAPNAP. *See* National Association of Pediatric Nurse Associates and Practitioners
NAQC. *See* Nursing Alliance for Quality of Care
Narrative analysis, 114*t*–118*t*
Narrative ethics, 347, 348
National Academy of Medicine, 746
National Advisory Commission on Health Manpower, 22
National Association for Healthcare Quality (NAHQ), 756*t*–757*t*
National Association of Clinical Nurse Specialists (NACNS), 19, 42, 281, 385, 386, 387, 409, 411, 653–654
  competencies of, 43*f*
  core competencies, 388*t*–389*t*
  Institute of Medicine's (IOM's) future of nursing recommendations, 407*t*–408*t*
  model of, 48
  in nurses and nursing practice sphere, 390*b*
    collaboration, 390
    evidence-based practice (EBP), 390
    guidance and coaching, 390
    leadership, 390
    patients and families, 394
  in organizations and systems sphere, 391*b*
National Association of Nurse Anesthetists (NANA), 520
National Association of Pediatric Nurse Associates and Practitioners (NAPNAP), 26, 459
National Board for Certification and Recertification of Nurse Anesthetists (NBCRNA), 520, 521
National Cancer Institute, 257
National Center for Biotechnology Information, 257
National Center for Nursing Research, 559–561
National Certification Examination (NCE), 521, 522*b*
National CNS Competency Task Force, 43
National Committee for Quality Assurance (NCQA), 756*t*–757*t*
National Council of State Boards of Nursing (NCSBN), 37–38, 584–585, 650
National Database of Nursing Quality Indicators, 756*t*–757*t*
National Guideline Clearinghouse (NGC), 258

National Institute for Health and Clinical Excellence (NICE), 257
National Institute for Health Research Health Technology Assessment Program, 257
National Institutes of Health (NIH), 329, 559–561
National level (professional organizations)
  acute care nurse practitioners (ACNPs), 472
National Mental Health Act, 14–15
National Network of Public Health Institutes, 756*t*–757*t*
National Nurse Practitioner Data Bank, 643
National Nurse Practitioner Sample Survey, 586
National Organization for Public Health Nursing (NOPHN), 17
National Organization of Nurse Practitioner Faculties (NONPF), 22, 42, 281, 427*t*–430*t*, 653–654
  competencies of, 42
  domains of, 42
  mission of, 42
National Patient Safety Goals of The Joint Commission, 679
National Provider Identifier (NPI), 660
  number, 624, 625, 762
National Quality Forum (NQF), 189, 674–678, 675*t*–677*t*, 679, 753–755
  Community Tool to Align Measurement, 753–755, 756*t*–757*t*
  Quality Positioning System, 755
National Sample Survey
  of Nurse Practitioners, 586
  of Registered Nurses, 8
Natural childbirth, 12
Natural language processing (NLP), 717–718, 747, 750
Neary, Elizabeth, 20
Negligence, malpractice and, 664
Negotiation, conflict, 333
Nelson, Dagmar, 5
Neonatal nurse practitioner (NNP), 26
Nested case-control design, 261
Networking, 123, 310
  professional, 596
Neurocognitive theory, 113–114
New England Hospital School of Nursing, 7
New York Medical College, 19
New York Medical Society, 19
New York State Medical Society, 4
New York Training School for Nurses, 19
NGC. *See* National Guideline Clearinghouse
NICE. *See* National Institute for Health and Clinical Excellence
Nightingale, Florence, 555, 710
Nightingale's environmental theory, 217
NIH. *See* National Institutes of Health
NLP. *See* Natural language processing
Nominal group technique, 767*t*
Nondiscrete or unstructured data, 750
NONPF. *See* National Organization of Nurse Practitioner Faculties
Nonpharmacologic techniques, 507
Nonverbal communication technologies, 718
North American Registry of Midwives (NARM), 490–491
"Not present on admission" (NPOA), 748
Novice-to-Expert Skill Acquisition Model, 99
NQF. *See* National Quality Forum
Nurse Anesthesia Educational Programs, 44–45
Nurse anesthesia practice, 532–533
Nurse anesthesia supervision opt-out states and territories, 540*b*
Nurse anesthetists, 3, 139, 533
  early challenges for, 3
  growth of, 12
  at Mayo Clinic, 4*f*
  reimbursement and education for, 12–13
  in 8th Evacuation Hospital, 7*b*
Nurse anesthetist traineeship (NAT), 529, 530
Nurse clinician, 14
Nurse coaching, 217
Nurse consultant, 143
Nurse in Washington Internship (NIWI), 305
Nurse-led clinic
  interprofessional, team-based education in, 445*b*
Nurse-led health centers, 444
Nurse-midwifery practice
  Alaska Native and American Indian people, intrastate practice for, 512*b*–513*b*
  in a birth center setting, 509*b*–510*b*
Nurse-midwives, 8, 139
  Callen, Maude, 11*b*
  education and organization for, 10
  frontier nursing service, 9
  "granny midwives", 8
  growth of, 12
  later education for, 14
  reimbursement for, 12
Nurse-patient interface, 83
Nurse Practice Acts, 24
Nurse practitioner (NP), 26, 85–86, 140, 145*b* *See also* Primary care nurse practitioner
  acute care, 25
  controversy for, 22
  education for, 26
  growth of, 12
  Henry Street Settlement and primary care in, 19
  intraprofessional conflict, 22
  neonatal, 25
  outcomes, 695
  pediatric, 21
  prescriptive privileges of, 24*b*
  primary care, 19
  resistance, organized medicine, 24
  role effectiveness model, 680, 682*f*
  role of, 16*b*
  scope of practice of, 24
  Shuler's model, 56
  support for, 22
  support from physicians, 23
Nurse Practitioner Core Competencies, 469
Nurse practitioners (NPs), 449*b*
Nurses' Association of the American College of Obstetricians and Gynecologists, 12
Nurse Training Act of 1964, 15*b*, 15
Nursing Alliance for Quality of Care (NAQC), 90–91, 569
Nursing competence, ten domains, 441*b*
Nursing discipline, advanced practice nursing in, 75
Nursing Model Act, 652–653
Nursing model/medical model, 175
Nursing Organizations Alliance, 305
Nursing parochialism, 579
Nursing practice
  coronary care unit, 15–16
  definition of, 15*b*

Nursing practice *(Continued)*
expanded role in, 16
extended role in, 22–23
identity, abandonment of, 311
specialist in, 17–18
Nursing Registration Bill, 19
Nursing research, 259
national center for, 559–561
Nursing: Scope and Standards of Practice (ANA), 41
Nursing's Social Policy Statement, 77, 324
Nursing surveillance, 172

O

OBR. *See* Optical barcode readers
Occurrence policies, in malpractice insurance, 612
OCR. *See* Optical character recognition
Office of Technology Assessment, 24
Office of the National Coordinator (ONC), 714
Ohio State Medical Board, 4
Oltz v. St. Peter's Community Hospital, 7–8
OMR. *See* Optical mark recognition
Oncology Nursing Society (ONS), 19, 254
One-on-one interview, 604
One sided compromise, 317
One-year longitudinal grounded theory, 114*t*–118*t*
Ongoing professional practice evaluation (OPPE), 480
Online evidence-based resources, 256
Online resources, 257*t*
ONS. *See* Oncology Nursing Society
Op-ed suggestions, 579*b*
Open and honest communication, shared decision-making and, 180
Open-ended question, for interview, 604
Opinion leadership, 287
Opportunities identification, 329
Optical barcode readers (OBR), 717
Optical character recognition (OCR), 717
Optical mark recognition (OMR), 717
Organizational and environmental barriers, 373
Organizational contexts
American Nurses Association, 40
barriers, 329
Organizational contexts *(Continued)*
collaboration strategies, 320
conceptualizations of advanced practice nursing roles, 45
Advanced Practice Registered Nurse, 37
American Association of Colleges of Nursing, 41
American Association of Nurse Anesthetists, 43
American College of Nurse-Midwives, 45
international, 45
evidence-based practice, 271
National Association of Clinical Nurse Specialists, 42
National Organization of Nurse Practitioner Faculties, 42
of nurse-midwifery, 13
performance improvement and, 764*b*–765*b*, 769
problems with, 291
Organized medicine
and evaluation, 17
resistance, 4
Orientation phase
of role development, 122
of role implementation, 122*t*, 125–126
Orthopedic services, ACNPs, 482
Orthoses (exoskeletons), 724
Outcomes
of advanced practice registered nurse (APRN) practice
future directions for, 698
integrative review of, 673
measures of, importance of, 678
assessment, 675*t*–677*t*
definition of, 675*t*–677*t*
indicators, 675*t*–677*t*, 685
management, 675*t*–677*t*, 686
measurement, 675*t*–677*t*
research, 675*t*–677*t*
Outcomes evaluation model, 680, 681*t*–682*t*
core questions, 770, 772
interventions, 772
program goals, 772
stakeholders, 772, 773*b*
data
deriving meaning from, 776
elements, 774
results of, 776
phases of, 770, 771*b*
target population for study, 770
Outpatient billing, 629
Overview concepts. *See also* Definitions/fundamentals
of health policy contexts
politics *vs.*, 556
United States *vs.* international communities, 557
Ovid, 254

P

PAC. *See* Political action committee
Page and Arena (1991), 123
Pan American Health Organization, 302
Pan-approaches and collaboration, 148
competency development and education, 151
human resource policies and priorities, 149
mentorship, 151
regulation, 150
Panel interviews, 604–605
Parallel communication, 316
Parallel functioning, 317
Pareto charts, 767*t*, 769
Partnerships
team building and, 333
therapeutic
with noncommunicative patients, 181, 182*b*
with patients, formation of, 176
Partnerships for Training initiative, 330
Patient care, device technology and communication in, 728*b*
Patient care technology, 89
Patient-centered outcomes research, 675*t*–677*t*
Patient-Centered Outcomes Research Institute (PCORI), 571
Patient-generated health data (PGHD), 716
Patient-Oriented Evidence that Matters (POEMs), 257
Patient portal, 715
Patient Protection and Affordable Care Act (PPACA), 32, 33, 37, 126, 127–129, 491, 492, 494, 559–561, 618–621
Patient–provider barriers, 372
Patient readiness, 228, 229*b*
Patient safety, clinical nurse specialist (CNS), 393

Patient safety organizations, 755
Patient-specific contexts
collaborations impact, 334
education, 217
APRN and, 188
noncommunicative, 181, 182*b*
Payment for advanced practice registered nurses (APRN) services, 617
PCORI. *See* Patient-Centered Outcomes Research Institute
PECOS. *See* Provider Enrollment Chain and Ownership System
Pediatric acute care nurse practitioner (AC-PNP) practice, 458
in inpatient specialty service, 476*b*
in intensive care unit, 464*b*–465*b*
Pediatric cardiac intensive care unit (PCICU), 464
Pediatric nurse practitioner (PNP), 22*b*
Peplau, Hildegarde E., 15
PEPPA framework, 107
Performance benchmark, 675*t*–677*t*
Performance errors, 189
Performance evaluation, 675*t*–677*t*
Performance improvement, 675*t*–677*t*, 685, 687*t*–689*t*
health care information technology for, 746
regulatory reporting and, 751
current reporting requirements, 751, 753*b*, 754*b*, 756*t*–757*t*
MACRA, 755, 758*t*–759*t*, 760*t*, 761*t*
research, 673
Persistence for Virginia NPS, 562*b*–563*b*
Personal contexts
personal factors, 334
professional and personal life balance, 298
Personal health records (PHRs), 715–716
Personal strengths and weaknesses questionnaire, 334*b*
PGHD. *See* Patient-generated health data
Pharmacology, 660
Phase 3 randomized controlled trials, 675*t*–677*t*
Phase 4 studies, 675*t*–677*t*
PHRs. *See* Personal health records
Physician assistants (PAs), 468, 478
ACNP practice models, 479
outcome studies, 479
Physician assistants (PAs) *(Continued)*
physician hospitalists, ACNPs and, 479
profiles, role and practice models, 478
Physician hospitalists, ACNPs, 479
Physician Orders for Life-Sustaining Treatment (POLST) approach, 363
Physician productivity, APRN and, 697
PICO model, 253*t*, 254
Pie chart, 767*t*
Pinneo, Rose, 16*b*
Plan-do-study-act (PDSA), 769
POEMs. *See* Patient-oriented evidence that matters
Point of care (POC) devices, 722–723, 746
Policy-related contexts
activators, 565
arena, APRN political competence in, 571
collaboration in, 332
evidence-based practice and, 247*b*
initiatives, in health reform, 570
value agenda, 570
for leadership, 292
fellowships, 305
internships, 305
modes of communication, 305
professional organizations, 305
models/frameworks
federalism, 559
knowledge transfer, 565, 568*f*
Longest model (policy formulation phase), 564, 565*f*
modifications, 565
modifications, 565
politics *vs.*, 556
process, 578
Political action committee (PAC), 561–564
Political activism, 296
Political antenna, 578
Political competence, 572, 580*f*
Politics, 556
Poor judgment, thinking errors and, 184
Population-based data, to inform practice, 198
Population focus, 92
Position Statement on the Practice Doctorate in Nursing, 77
Positive psychology, 219
Postgraduate education, 655
Postgraduate training, 121*b*
Postoperative pain management, anesthesia, 545
Power
force *vs.*, 579
misusing, 307
PPOs. *See* Preferred Provider Organizations
Practice Doctorate Nurse Practitioner Entry-Level Competencies, 469
Practice guidelines, 675*t*–677*t*
Practice redesign
primary care nurse practitioner (PCNP)
disruptive innovations, 447
team-based primary care, 447
Practice-related contexts (APN approaches)
for advanced practice nurse
family-focused, 80*f*, 82
patient-focused, 79
for credentialing requirements and contexts
collaborative practice arrangements, 662
Consensus Model, 650
current, 667
identifier numbers, 660
malpractice, 664
negligence, 664
reimbursement, 663
risk management, 664
telehealth, 666
telepractice, 666
titling, 657
guidelines, 662
Precision health, 731
Predictive analytics, 766
Preferred Provider Organizations (PPOs), 624
Preparation, in APRN coaching process, 226
Presbyterian Hospital, 15–16
Prescribers, requirements for, 660*b*
Prescriptive analytics, 768
Prescriptive authority, 659
Prescriptive privileges, 24*b*
Presence, 223
"Present on admission" (POA), 748
President Clinton, 25
Presidential politics, 561
Preston Retreat Hospital, 10
Preventive ethics, ethical practice, 359
Preventive services
in hospitals and home care, 200
in primary care, 199

Primary care, 88
Primary care nurse practitioner (PCNP), 458–459
ambulatory worksite settings, top clinical focus areas, 449*t*
burnout, COVID-19, 450
certification, 449*t*
collaboration, 438
coordinating transitional care services, care settings, 432
culturally sensitive and patient-centered care, 432
community health center, of New London, 433*b*–434*b*
current perspectives, 422
diagnosing and managing disease, 431
direct clinical practice, 426
ethical practice, 438
evidence-based practice, 437
and federal government, 441
guidance and coaching, 436
health promotion and disease prevention, 431
Health Resources and Services Administration (HRSA), 441
organization chart, 442*f*
historical perspective and the first nurse practitioners, 423
home care, 450
leadership, 437
learning, consulting, and working with specialists, new way of, 440*b*
models, in other nations and United States, 423*f*
postgraduate training, emergence of, 439
practice redesign in
disruptive innovations, 447
team-based primary care, 447
progress and change, 1970 to the present, 424
reflective practice, direct patient care, 436
safety net
community health centers, 443
nurse-led health centers, 444
school-based health centers, 446
veterans affairs, 446
shared competencies, 439
telecare, 434
virtual medical home collaborative practice, 435*b*
workforce and the context, PCNP practice, 448
Primary Health Care Nurse Practitioner Council, 25
Principle of beneficence, 342
Principle of formal justice, 342
Principle of nonmaleficence, 342
Principle of respect for autonomy, 342
Procedural devices and apps, 724
dimensional (3D) printing, 724
robotic process automation, 724–725
robotics, 724
smartphone-based digital stethoscope, 725
vein visualization, 725
Process
collaboration implementation, 330
conflict negotiation, 333
conflict resolution skills, 333
partnering, 333
recurring interactions, 332
team building, 333
identification
Medicaid provider numbers, 663
Medicare provider numbers, 663
national provider identifier number, 660
improvement of, 685, 687*t*–689*t*
indicator of, 675*t*–677*t*
measurement of, 675*t*–677*t*
"Process as outcome" studies, 685
Productivity-based compensation, 644
Professional codes and guidelines
ethical practice, 348
particulars, 352
professional boundaries, 350
values, beliefs and preferences, 352
Professional leadership, 290
Professional liability, certified nurse-midwife, 511
Professional networking, 596
Professional portfolio, 601, 602*b*
Professional recruiters, in advanced practice nurse, 599
Professional-related context
of certified nurse-midwife
diversity, 511
image, 508
professional liability, 511
quality and safety, 514
work life, 510
leadership of, 290
organizations for, 308
professional and personal life balance, 298
Professional responsibilities, of midwifery care, 501
Professional territoriality, 105
Programs
effectiveness of, 675*t*–677*t*
evaluation of, 675*t*–677*t*
Promotion-related contexts, collaboration, 310
Protected health information (PHI), 733
Provider Enrollment Chain and Ownership System (PECOS), 627
Proxy indicators, 675*t*–677*t*
Psychiatric nursing specialist, 14
PsycINFO, 259
Public comment, role of, 573*b*
Public discourse, contribute to, 578–579
Public health crisis, 586
Public Health Foundation, 756*t*–757*t*
Public law, 573
Public trust, take action to create, 580–581
PubMed, 254
PubMed Health, 256
Purpose-related contexts, common, 321

Q

QPPs. *See* Quality Payment Programs
Qualitative inquiry method, 114*t*–118*t*
Qualitative study
of critical care nurse, 110
of family nurse practitioner (FNP), 110
Quality and safety, certified nurse-midwife, 514
Quality improvement
collaboration in, 323*b*
competencies of
continuous, 768
foundational, 768
performance improvement, 764*b*–765*b*, 769
design strategies for, 770
evaluations
core questions, 770
data-related contexts, 774
phases of, 770, 771*b*
evidence-based practice and, 257*t*, 273
website resources for, 756*t*–757*t*
Quality of care, 675*t*–677*t*
Quality, of randomize and nonrandomized controlled trial, 265*t*

Quality Patient Program, 758*t*–759*t*
Quality Payment Programs (QPPs), 636, 638*f*, 751
Quality Positioning System, 755
Quantitative studies, 262*t*
Queen Bee syndrome, 306, 307
Questionnaire method, 114*t*–118*t*
Questions
- core, 770
- in interventions, 772
- in program goals, 772
- in stakeholders, 772, 773*b*
- in target population, 770

R

Radiofrequency, 725
Radiofrequency identification (RFID), 725–726
Random allocation, 252
Randomization, 252
Randomized controlled trial (RCT), 252
Rapid response teams, ACNPs, 482
Rationale-based clinical decision making, 246–248
RBRVS. *See* Resource-based relative value scale
Real-time location system (RTLS), 726
Recognition, 322
- of nurse-midwifery, 491

Recurring interactions, 332
Reentry to practice, CNM, 493
Referral, 318
Referral letters, 601
Reflection, 182–183
Reflection-in-action, 187
Reflective practice
- direct patient care, primary care nurse practitioner (PCNP), 436
- use of, 190

Regional anesthesia, 533
Registered Nurses Association of Ontario (RNAO), 258
Regulation, certified nurse-midwife (CNM), 493
Regulatory barriers, 332
Regulatory compliance, 733
Regulatory Model, 37–38
Regulatory requirements, 649
- credentialing
  - certification, 655
  - elements of, 656
  - future challenges facing, 669
  - influencing, 668*b*
  - institutional, 658

Regulatory requirements *(Continued)*
  - language associated with, 657
- elements, 656*b*, 656
- practice-related issues for
  - collaborative practice arrangements, 662
  - Consensus Model, 650
  - current, 667
  - identifier numbers, 660
  - language associated with, 657
  - malpractice, 664
  - negligence, 664
  - reimbursement, 663
  - risk management, 664
  - telehealth, 666
  - telepractice, 666
- for reporting
  - by advanced practice nurse, 761
  - performance improvement, 751
- state licensure, 657
  - Drug Enforcement Administration number, 660
  - prescriptive authority, 659
- visioning processes, 667

Reimbursement, 90–91, 663
- for APRN services, 617
- billing for APRN, 624
  - coding sets, 627
  - credentialing process, 625
  - inpatient billing, 633
  - medical decision making, 630
  - outpatient billing, 629
  - provider panels and contracts, 626
  - revenue cycle management, 635
- business development, 643
  - additional APRN compensation models, 644
  - business ownership, 644
  - entrepreneurship, 643
- certified nurse-midwife (CNM), 493
- for certified registered nurse anesthetist, 12
- for clinical nurse specialist (CNS), 408
- documentation of, 625*b*, 625
- future trends, 645
- health reform history of, 618, 619*t*–621*t*
- issues and challenges, 638
  - incident-to billing in, 638, 639*b*, 639*t*
  - liability/malpractice insurance, 640*b*, 640
- Medicaid, 623

Reimbursement *(Continued)*
  - dual eligibility for, 623
- Medicare, 621, 622*t*
  - dual eligibility for, 623
- models of, 621
  - federally funded medical coverage as, 621
  - fee-for-service model, 636
  - state-administered medical coverage as, 622
  - third-party payers, 624
  - value-based model, 636

Reimbursement pay parity, 643
Reiter, Frances, 14
Relationship building contexts, 298
Relative work value, of APRNs, 697
Relief, anesthesia, 545
Rescuing, 200
Research. *See also* Competencies
- collaboration imperatives for, 332
  - costs, 326
  - evidence-related contexts, 326
  - interprofessional, 320
- definition of, 258
- evidence-based practice (EBP) and, 246
- outcome(s), 675*t*–677*t*

Resolution, of conflict, 333*b*, 333
Resource-based relative value scale (RBRVS), 636, 637*f*, 697
Respect-related contexts, 337
- for cultural diversity, 301
- for gender diversity, 301

Restraining forces, 287
Résumés, 602*b*, 602
Retrieval/search
- allied health literature, 256
- clinical practice guidelines, 258
- electronic databases searching, 258
- online resources, 257

Retrospective interviews method, 114*t*–118*t*
Revenue cycle
- for health care, 633*f*
- management, 635

RFID. *See* Radiofrequency identification
Rich (2005), 120
Richards, Linda, 14
Richardson, Elliot, 22–23
Richmond, Therese, 25
Risk and severity adjustment, 675*t*–677*t*
Risk management, 664
Risk of Bias in Systematic Studies (ROBIS), 266–267
Risk taking, 297

Rites of passage, 111
RNAO. *See* Registered Nurses Association of Ontario
Robert Wood Johnson Foundation (RWJF), 330, 569
  Partnership for Training initiative, 334
ROBIS. *See* Risk of Bias in Systematic Studies
Robotic process automation, 724–725
Robotics, 724
Robotic surgical assistants, 724
Rogers, Carl, 225
Rogers, Martha, 22
Role acceptance studies, 684
Role acquisition
  clinical knowledge and development for APRN, 111, 112*t*
  developing a supportive network for, 113
  in graduate school, 107, 114*t*–118*t*
  purpose of, 128
  strategies to facilitate, 110
Role ambiguity, 110, 114*t*–118*t*
Role conflict, 103*t*, 104
  interprofessional, 105, 106*b*
  intraprofessional, 104
Role description studies, 683
Role evolution, advanced practice nurse, 126
Role implementation, 114
  strategies to facilitate, 110
Role incongruity, 102, 103*t*
Role insufficiency, 103*t*
Role of primary care nurse practitioner, 420
Role perception studies, 684
Role strain, concepts of, 103*t*, 107
Role stress, concepts of, 102, 103*t*
Role stressors, 103*t*
Role supplementation, 103*t*
Role transition, 103*t*, 108
Roosevelt, Franklin D., 20–21
Root cause analysis, 767*t*
Roving leadership, 284
Royal Statistical Society, 555
RTLS. *See* Real-time location system
Run chart, 767*t*
Rutgers University, 15
RxNorm, 749*t*–750*t*

S

Safe environment, 228
Safety Assurance Factors for EHR Resilience (SAFER) Guides, 714*b*, 714
Safriet, Barbara, 27, 661
Salaried compensation, 644
Scatter diagrams, 767*t*, 769
Schema-on-read. *See* Unstructured data
Schema-on-write. *See* Structured data
School-based health centers, 446
Schultz, Mark, 560
Scope of practice
  acute care nurse practitioners (ACNPs)
    individual level, 475
    institutional level, 473
    national level (professional organizations), 472
    service-related level, 474
    state level (government), 473
  for advanced practice nurse
    competencies, 653
    education, benchmark of, 653
    standards of practice and care, 662
  in advanced practice nursing, 86
  certified nurse-midwife (CNM), 506
  clinical nurse specialist (CNS), 405
Scottish Intercollegiate Guideline Network (SIGN), 268
Scrubbing, data, 729
SDOH. *See* Social determinants of health
Search/retrieval
  allied health literature, 254
  clinical practice guidelines, 258
  electronic databases searching, 258
  online resources, 257
Second interviews, 605–606
Secure text, 716
Self-awareness, APRN and, 573
Self-confidence, 297
Self-determination theory, 220*f*, 220
Self-efficacy theory, 102
Self-knowledge, as APRN, 227–228
  boundary awareness, 226
  empathic stance, 236
  feeling, range of, 238
  presence, 223
  somatic awareness, 238
Self-management education, 203
Self-management/emotional intelligence, 299
Self-reflection, 299
Sensitive outcome indicators, in advanced practice registered nurse (APRN) practice, 690*t*–694*t*
Serious reportable events (SRE), 569
Sermchief v. Gonzales (1983), 24
Servant leadership, 284, 285*b*
Shared Savings Program, 753*b*
Shared/split billing, 634
Shared vision, 286
SHARE Model, 607*b*, 607
Shuler's Model of NP Practice, 56, 175
SickKids APRN framework, 57
Sigma Theta Tau International, 302
SIGN. *See* Scottish Intercollegiate Guideline Network
SIREN. *See* Social Interventions Research and Evaluation Network
Situational leadership, 284
Skill acquisition, ethical practice, 355
Skillful performance, APRN and, 187
Skill sets/competencies, leadership, 309
  acquiring competency, 303
  factors influencing, 302
  personal characteristics, 302
  personal experiences, 302
Smart bed technology, 725
Smartphone and cellphone, 718
Smartphone-based digital stethoscope, 725
SNOMED Z codes, 750
Social determinants of health, 423
Social determinants of health (SDOH), 750
Social Interventions Research and Evaluation Network (SIREN), 750
Social media, International nurse regulator collaborative 6 "P"s of, 721*b*
Social media tips, ANA, 720*b*
Social networking, ANA principles of, 720*b*
Social Policy Statement, 17–18
Societal issues, promoting social justice, 366
Society for Opioid-Free Anesthesia (SOFA, 534
Society of Thoracic Surgeons, 763
Sociocultural issues, 331
Somatic awareness, 238
South Africa, APN roles and, 144–145
Specialization, definition of, 40, 76
"Specialties in Nursing", 13
Specialty services, ACNPs
  bone marrow transplantation services, 481
  critical care teams, 482

Specialty services, ACNPs *(Continued)*
diagnostic and interventional services, 481
heart failure services, 482
orthopedic services, 482
rapid response teams, 482
supportive and palliative care, 482
Spheres of influence
for advanced practice nurse
experienced, 668*b*
expert, 668*b*
novice, 668*b*
SRE. *See* Serious reportable events
Stage, in role development, 108–110
Stakeholder engagement, 271
Standards, definition of, 675*t*–677*t*
Standards for Nurse Anesthesia Practice, 44
Standards of practice and care
of advanced practice nurses, 662
evaluation of evidence-based practice to, 249*b*
midwifery, 499*t*–500*t*
Star complex, 306
Start time, anesthesia, 545
State-administered medical coverage, 622
State Children's Health Insurance Program, 559
State level (government), acute care nurse practitioners (ACNPs), 473
State licensure, 657
Drug Enforcement Administration number, 660
prescriptive authority and, 659
Statement on Clinical Nurse Specialist Practice and Education (NACNS), 42–43
State of the World's Nursing 2020 (WHO), 723
States of digital data. *See* Digital data states
Statistical process control (SPC) charts, 766, 766*f*
St. Mary's Hospital, 3
Storage, data, 729*b*
St. Paul's Medical Journal, 3–4
Strain, concepts of role, 102, 103*t*
Strategy-related contexts
of collaboration, 334–335
individual, 334
organizational, 329
team, 335
for electronic databases, 258
leadership competency, 293
outcome evaluation plan
Strategy-related contexts *(Continued)*
core questions, 770
date, 774
phases of, 770, 771*b*
for quality improvement, 770
Strength, building, 236
Strengthening Reporting of Observational Studies in Epidemiology (STROBE), 262–264
Strengthening skills in self-reflection, 191
Strength of Recommendation for Treatment taxonomy (SORT) scale, 268
Stress, concepts of role, 103*t*, 111
Stressors, role, 103*t*
Strong Memorial Hospital's model, of Advanced Practice Nursing, 52, 54*f*
Structural indicators, 675*t*–677*t*
Structured data, 728
Subsequent hospital visits, 635
Successful Political Action Committee, anatomy of, 572*b*
Sullivan, Harry Stack, 14
Supervision, 318
Supplemental security income (SSI) program, 623
Supplementation, role, 103*t*
Support interventions, 194
Supportive and palliative care, ACNPs, 482
Supportive technologies, 725, 727*b*
augmented reality, 726
companion robots, 725
geofencing, 726
radiofrequency, 725
radiofrequency identification, 725–726
real-time location system (RTLS), 726
smart bed technology, 725
virtual reality, 726
Surveillance, 197
Suspicion of fraud, 637*b*
Systematic approaches to role planning, 153
Systematic reviews, 261
Systematized Nomenclature of Medicine-Clinical Terms (SNOMED CT®), 747, 748, 749*t*–750*t*
Systems citizenship, 337
Systems leadership, 290
Systems thinking, 296

T

Tail coverage, of malpractice insurance, 612
Targeted therapy microbots, 724
Taunton Insane Hospital, 14
Taussig, Frederick, 6–7
Tax Equity and Financial Reform Act (TEFRA), 544, 545*b*
Taxonomy, 747–748
TCM. *See* Transitional care model
Team-based primary care, practice redesign in, 447
Team-related contexts
building, 333
collaboration with, 321
dysfunction, 331
Technology-assisted communication, 715
nonverbal communication technologies, 718
verbal communication technologies, 717
visual communication technologies, 719
written communication technologies, 715
Technology-enabling communication, 721*b*
Technology, health information
complexity in, 711
Donabedian model, 711, 712*t*
James Reason Swiss cheese model (SCM), 712
cyberattacks, 734
cybersecurity, 732
data, clinical decision support and advanced analytics, 727
data entry errors, 714*b*
diagnostic and therapeutic devices and apps, 721
future implications of, 737
high-tech home care, 735
human-centered design and, 713
illusions of, in pandemic, 711
influencing APRN practice, 709
procedural devices and apps, 724
supportive, 725, 727*b*
technology-assisted communication, 715
TJC's safe use of, 714*b*
Teec Nos Pas, 21
Telecare, 434
Telehealth, 666
Telehealth reimbursement models, 738
Telephone interviews, 114*t*–118*t*

Telepractice, 666
Terminology, 747–748
Tertiary nurse practitioner (TNP), 25
Tetralogy of Fallot, 6–7
Texas Children's Hospital
transformational Advanced Professional Practice (TAPP) APRN model, 55
Text recognition technology, 717*b*
The Essentials: Core Competencies for Professional Nursing Education, 427*t*–430*t*, 469, 745
The Future of Nursing 2020-2030: Charting a Path to Achieve Health Equity, 745
The Joint Commission (TJC), 296, 335–336, 659, 674–678, 679, 753, 756*t*–757*t*
safe use of health information technology, 714*b*
Theory-based practice, APRN and, 193
Therapeutic partnerships
with noncommunicative patients, 181, 182*b*
with patients, formation of, 176
8th Evacuation Hospital, 7*b*
Thinking errors, 184, 185*b*
Third-party payers, 624
types of, 624
Time-based billing, for reimbursement, 630, 633*t*
Time-related issues
bias, 265–266
clinical thinking and decision making, 186
leadership, 296
Title XIX of the Social Security Act, 622–623
Titling issues, 657
TJC. *See* The Joint Commission
TNP. *See* Tertiary nurse practitioner
To Err Is Human: Building a Safer Health System (IOM), 712–713
Total quality management, 675*t*–677*t*
Transformational change, 283*t*–284*t*
Transformational leadership, 283*t*–284*t*, 288
Transitional care, clinical nurse specialist (CNS), 403*b*–404*b*
Transitional care model (TCM), 61
Transition-related contexts, 216
developmental, 221–223
health and illness, 220
role, 114, 114*t*–118*t*
Transparency, concept of, 322
Transtheoretical model, 218

U

United States
American Association of Colleges of Nursing (AACN), 13
certified nurse-midwife (CNM), 491
clinical nurse specialists, 17*f*
declining demand for, 18
education and reimbursement for, 19
growth of, 12
coronary care nursing specialist, 15–16
Doctor of Nursing Practice (DNP), 8
healthcare reform history, 618, 619*t*–621*t*
history in, 2
international communities *vs.*, 557
nurse anesthetists, 3
early challenges for, 8
growth of, 12
at Mayo Clinic, 4*f*
reimbursement and education for, 12–13
in 8th Evacuation Hospital, 7*b*
nurse-midwifery profession, 491
nurse-midwives, 8
Callen, Maude, 11*b*
education and organization for, 19
frontier nursing service, 20
"granny midwives", 8
growth of, 12
later education for, 17
reimbursement for, 7
nurse practitioners, 19
acute care, 25
controversy for, 22
education for, 26
expanded scope of practice of, 20
growth of, 12
Henry Street Settlement and primary care, 19
neonatal, 25
pediatric, 21
prescriptive privileges of, 24*b*
role of, 16*b*
support for, 5
Universal image viewer, 722
Universal Provider Datasource, 626
University of Colorado, 22
University of Pennsylvania, 25
University of Rochester, 23
University of Virginia, 7*b*
Unstructured data, 728–729
U.S. Constitution, 559
US Health Resources and Services Administration (HRSA), 529
U.S. National Library of Medicine, 254–255
U.S. Preventive Services Task Force, 268, 270*t*, 335

V

Value-based model, 636
Value-based payments, 636
Value-based purchasing, 678
Value-related contexts, collaboration, 322
Vein illumination, 725
Vein visualization, 725
Verbal communication technologies, 717
artificial intelligence, 717
machine learning, 717
natural language processing, 717–718
smartphone and cellphone, 718
virtual assistants, 718
Veterans affairs, 446
Viacom CheckMe Pro, 737
Videoconference interviews, 604
Virginia's legislative journey to expand nurse practitioner (NP) autonomous practice licensure, 562
Virtual assistants (VA), 718
Virtual health, 722
Virtual health care, 722
Virtual medicine, 722
Virtual reality (VR), defined, 726
Virtual wellbeing, 722
Virtue-based ethics, 347
Visioning contexts for advanced practice nurse, 667
Vision Paper, 37–38
Visual communication technologies, 719
Vitae (curriculum), 602–603, 603*b*
VR. *See* Virtual reality

W

Wald, Lillian, 19
Walter Reed General Hospital, 7
Watson's model of caring, 219
Wearable technology, 723
Web-based resources, in APRN, 599, 600*t*

Well-functioning information systems, 204
Westchester Village Medical Group, 20
WHO. *See* World Health Organization
Wiley-Blackwell Publishers, 257
Williams, Dorothy, 21
Willingness, 291
Willow Ceremony, 111
Worcester Hospital for the Insane, 14
Work activities, AG-ACNP criticality, 462*b*
Workforce issues
data, of advanced practice nursing, 89
Work life certified nurse-midwife, 510
World Health Organization (WHO), 302
Written communication technologies, 715
electronic health records, 715
electronic medical records, 715
fax, 716
Written communication technologies *(Continued)*
patient-generated health data (PGHD), 716
patient portal, 715
personal health records (PHRs), 715–716
secure text, 716

Y

Yale Law School, 661
Yale Medical School, 5